2017 Annual
ICD-10-PCS

The Educational
Annotation of ICD-10-PCS

Procedure Index, Tables, and Appendices

CRAIG D. PUCKETT

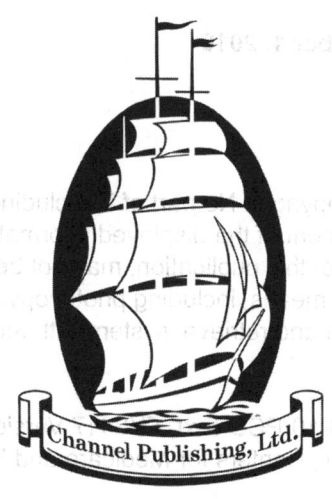

Channel Publishing, Ltd.

Complete Official ICD-10-PCS Text, FY2017 Version
Effective October 1, 2016
as standardized by
U.S. DEPARTMENT OF HEALTH AND HUMAN SERVICES
CENTERS FOR MEDICARE AND MEDICAID SERVICES

ISBN: 978-1-933053-81-3

DISCLAIMER

Every effort has been made to ensure the accuracy and reliability of the information contained in this publication. However, complete accuracy cannot be guaranteed. The editor and publisher will not be held responsible or liable for any errors.

Corrections Identification and Reporting

In an effort to provide our customers with the best code books possible, Channel Publishing has added a "Channel Errata Page" for each of its ICD-10 code books on its web site: www.channelpublishing.com. These Channel Errata Pages will be updated whenever an error is identified. Check the appropriate web page periodically for any changes to your Channel Publishing ICD-10 code book.

In addition, if at any time you identify a potential error, please copy the page and fax/mail/e-mail it to: Channel Publishing, Ltd., Attn: ICD-10 Book Production Department, 4750 Longley Lane, Suite 110, Reno, NV 89502. FAX (775) 825-5633. E-mail: info@channelpublishing.com

ICD-10-PCS, FY2017 Version, Effective October 1, 2016

This edition contains the Complete, Official ICD-10-PCS Text, FY2017 Version as standardized by the U.S. Department of Health and Human Services, Centers for Medicare and Medicaid Services.

Published by CHANNEL PUBLISHING, Ltd., Reno, Nevada

Produced by Craig Puckett, Editor; Susan Dely, Assistant Editor;
Jo Ann Jones, RHIA, CCS, Editorial Assistant; Charisse Puckett, Editorial Assistant;
Trey Puckett, Editorial Assistant

Printed in the United States of America

Additional sets may be ordered from Channel Publishing, Ltd., 4750 Longley Lane, Suite 110, Reno, Nevada 89502, 1-800-248-2882, www.channelpublishing.com

ISBN: 978-1-933053-81-3

Channel Publishing, Ltd.

Publishers of

"THE EDUCATIONAL ANNOTATION OF ICD-10-CM/PCS"

August 2016

Dear ICD-10 Colleague:

First, I would like to personally thank each and every Channel Publishing customer who has purchased and enjoyed our ICD-9-CM and ICD-10 coding products and services over these past 30 years.

Thank you for purchasing Channel Publishing's *2017 The Educational Annotation ICD-10-PCS* code book. I trust you will enjoy the new, innovative design, layout, and new, coder-helpful features that we have created for you. I would also like to thank everyone who shared their ICD-10 comments and suggestions over the years from our "Preparing for ICD-10" seminars sixteen years ago, to those of you who called or wrote in, and those who stopped by our booth at AHIMA. We listened and made note of those comments and suggestions to bring you what we believe is an excellent ICD-10-PCS code book, and at an incredibly low price.

In addition to this *2017 Educational Annotation of ICD-10-PCS* code book, I'd like to remind you about all our ICD-10 products and services. I strongly believe that the ICD-10 products and services we've developed will make this transition easier for you, both from a learning point of view and a budget point of view. Please visit our web site www.channelpublishing.com for details and sample content.

Once again, thank you for your purchase and I look forward to providing quality ICD-10 products and services to you in the years to come.

Sincerely,

Craig D. Puckett

Craig D. Puckett,
President, and Publisher

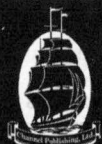
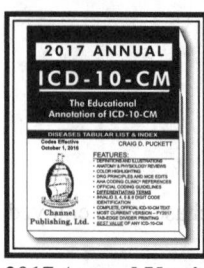
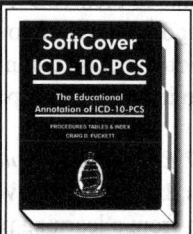
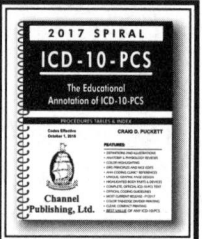
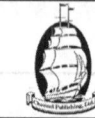
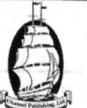

2016 FALL SALE ORDER FORM

Sale Prices Expire 12/31/16

1. CUSTOMER INFORMATION (Ship books to address below)

❑ Organization or ❑ Individual   ATTN: Name/Title/Dept.   Customer ID #   Order Date

Shipping Address (Street address required for FedEx delivery)   E-Mail Address

City   State   Zip   Telephone   Fax

2. ORDER INFORMATION

Product	See Web Site for Complete Product Descriptions and Sample Pages	Quantity	Regular Price	Fall Sale Price	Total(s)
				Exp. 12/31/16	
CODE BOOKS	**2017 ICD-10-CM, The Educational Annotation of ICD-10-CM**				
	Annual Version ICD-10-CM (Paperback) (ISBN: 9781933053-**76-9**)		$69⁹⁵ ea.	—	
	Spiral Version ICD-10-CM (Spiral coil) (ISBN: 9781933053-**77-6**)		$74⁹⁵ ea.	—	
	Spiral Version ICD-10-CM with Tabs (Spiral coil) (ISBN: 9781933053-**78-3**)		$89⁹⁵ ea.	—	
	SoftCover Version ICD-10-CM (Vinyl cover, updateable) (ISBN: 9781933053-**79-0**)		$79⁹⁵ ea.	—	
	2017 Update ICD-10-CM (Full text replacement) (ISBN: 9781933053-**80-6**)		$55⁹⁵ ea.	—	
	Tab Set for ICD-10-CM (SoftCover only, reusable) (ITEM: TABCM)		$17⁹⁵ ea.	—	
	2017 ICD-10-PCS, The Educational Annotation of ICD-10-PCS				
	Annual Version ICD-10-PCS (Paperback) (ISBN: 9781933053-**81-3**)		$59⁹⁵ ea.	—	
	Spiral Version ICD-10-PCS (Spiral coil) (ISBN: 9781933053-**82-0**)		$64⁹⁵ ea.	—	
	Spiral Version ICD-10-PCS with Tabs (Spiral coil) (ISBN: 9781933053-**83-7**)		$79⁹⁵ ea.	—	
	SoftCover Version ICD-10-PCS (Vinyl cover, updateable) (ISBN: 9781933053-**84-4**)		$69⁹⁵ ea.	—	
	2017 Update ICD-10-PCS (Full text replacement) (ISBN: 9781933053-**85-1**)		$48⁹⁵ ea.	—	
	Tab Set for ICD-10-PCS (SoftCover only, reusable) (ITEM: TABPCS)		$17⁹⁵ ea.	—	

(Professional Version – Includes: PowerPoint Slides, Instructor's Manual, DVD set, Workbook & Code Book)
(Individual Version – Includes: DVD set, Workbook & Code Book - CM-12 CEUs, PCS-20 CEUs)

Product		Quantity	Regular Price	Fall Sale Price	Total(s)
TRAINING	Professional Version – Learning ICD-10-CM (Step 1) (ITEM: SBCM-P)		$~~599⁹⁵~~ ea.	$559⁹⁵ ea.	
	Additional Learning ICD-10-CM Workbook & Book Packages (ITEM: ACM16W)		$65⁹⁵ ea.	—	
	Professional Version – Learning ICD-10-PCS (Step 1) (ITEM: SBPCS-P)		$~~699⁹⁵~~ ea.	$649⁹⁵ ea.	
	Additional Learning ICD-10-PCS Workbook & Book Packages (ITEM: APCS16W)		$55⁹⁵ ea.	—	
	Individual Version – Learning ICD-10-CM (Step 1) (12 CEUs) (ITEM: SBCM-I)		$~~299⁹⁵~~ ea.	$269⁹⁵ ea.	
	Individual Version – Learning ICD-10-PCS (Step 1) (20 CEUs) (ITEM: SBPCS-I)		$~~399⁹⁵~~ ea.	$359⁹⁵ ea.	
	2016 Mastering ICD-10-CM Exercise Book (Step 2) (ISBN: 9781933053-**88-2**)		$59⁹⁵ ea.	—	
	2016 Mastering ICD-10-PCS Exercise Book (Step 2) (ISBN: 9781933053-**89-9**)		$59⁹⁵ ea.	—	
	2016 Mastering ICD-10-CM Guidelines Exercise Book (Step 3) (ISBN: 9781933053-**90-5**)		$59⁹⁵ ea.	—	
	2016 Mastering ICD-10-PCS Guidelines Exercise Book (Step 3) (ISBN: 9781933053-**91-2**)		$59⁹⁵ ea.	—	
	The Last Word on ICD-10 (Step 4) (ISBN: 9781933053-**61-5**)		$69⁹⁵ ea.	—	
OTHER	2017 Clinotes for ICD-10-CM (ISBN: 9781933053-**87-5**)		$~~39⁹⁵~~ ea.	$29⁹⁵ ea.	
	2017 Expanded ICD-10-CM Table of Drugs & Chemicals (ISBN: 9781933053-**86-8**)		$~~39⁹⁵~~ ea.	$29⁹⁵ ea.	
	Acrylic Bookstand ❑ One-piece (ITEM: BSOP) ❑ Two-piece (ITEM: BSTP)		$34⁹⁵ ea.	—	
	CPT® 2017 Standard Edition (ISBN: 978162202-**398-1**)		$94⁹⁵ ea.	—	
	CPT® 2017 Professional Edition (ISBN: 978162202-**400-1**)		$119⁹⁵ ea.	—	

- OUTSIDE CONTINENTAL U.S.: Call for rates and shipping options. U.S. Dollars.
- EXPRESS SHIPPING: Call for delivery options and rates.

Fall Sale Prices Expire 12/31/16

Continental U.S. Shipping & Handling	
Less than $50	$7
$50-$99	$12
$100-$199	$19
$200-$299	$29
$300+	$39

Product Subtotal	
Shipping & Handling	
Nevada Res. Only Add Local Sales Tax	
Total Order Amount	

3. PAYMENT METHOD

❑ Purchase Order (Attach copy)   ❑ Check Enclosed
❑ Credit Card: MC, VISA, DISC, AMEX (Charged date order received)

_ _ _ _ _ _ _ _ _ _ _ _ _ _ _ _

_ _ _ / _ _ _   _ _ _ _

Exp. Date   Sec. Code   Authorized Cardholder Signature

Billing Address (Street number or PO Box and Zip Code) ❑ Same as shipping

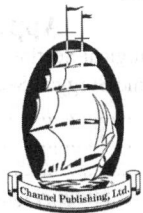

MAKE CHECKS PAYABLE AND MAIL TO:
Channel Publishing, Ltd.
4750 Longley Lane, Suite 110
Reno, NV 89502-5977
1-800-248-2882
(775) 825-0880
Fax (775) 825-5633
E-Mail: info@channelpublishing.com
Web Site: www.channelpublishing.com

THANK YOU FOR YOUR ORDER   FS99086-2

TABLE OF CONTENTS

Procedure Tabular – Medical and Surgical Section (Section 0)

Procedure Tabular – Medical/Surgical Related Sections

Procedure Tabular – Ancillary Sections

Appendices

INTRODUCTION TO ICD-10-PCS

THE INTERNATIONAL CLASSIFICATION OF DISEASES Tenth Revision Procedure Coding System (ICD-10-PCS) was created to accompany the World Health Organization's (WHO) ICD-10 diagnosis classification. The new procedure coding system was developed to replace ICD-9-CM procedure codes for reporting inpatient procedures.

Unlike the ICD-9-CM classification, ICD-10-PCS was designed to enable each code to have a standard structure and be very descriptive, and yet flexible enough to accommodate future needs.

This Introduction contains the following parts:
- What is ICD-10-PCS?
- ICD-10-PCS code structure
- ICD-10-PCS system organization
- ICD-10-PCS design
- ICD-10-PCS additional characteristics
- ICD-10-PCS applications

WHAT IS ICD-10-PCS?

ICD-10-PCS is a procedure coding system that will be used to collect data, determine payment, and support the electronic health record for all inpatient procedures performed in the United States.

History of ICD-10-PCS
The World Health Organization has maintained the International Classification of Diseases (ICD) for recording cause of death since 1893. It has updated the ICD periodically to reflect new discoveries in epidemiology and changes in medical understanding of disease.

The International Classification of Diseases Tenth Revision (ICD-10), published in 1992, is the latest revision of the ICD. The WHO authorized the National Center for Health Statistics (NCHS) to develop a clinical modification of ICD-10 for use in the United States. This version of ICD-10 is called ICD-10-CM. ICD-10-CM is intended to replace the previous U.S. clinical modification, ICD-9-CM, that has been in use since 1979. ICD-9-CM contains a procedure classification; ICD-10-CM does not.

The Centers for Medicare and Medicaid Services, the agency responsible for maintaining the inpatient procedure code set in the U.S., contracted with 3M Health Information Systems in 1993 to design and then develop a procedure classification system to replace Volume 3 of ICD-9-CM. ICD-10-PCS is the result. ICD-10-PCS was initially released in 1998. It has been updated annually since that time.

ICD-9-CM Volume 3 Compared with ICD-10-PCS
With ICD-10 implementation, the U.S. clinical modification of the ICD will not include a procedure classification based on the same principles of organization as the diagnosis classification. Instead, a separate procedure coding system has been developed to meet the rigorous and varied demands that are made of coded data in the healthcare industry. This represents a significant step toward building a health information infrastructure that functions optimally in the electronic age.

The following table highlights basic differences between ICD-9-CM Volume 3 and ICD-10-PCS.

ICD-9-CM Volume 3	ICD-10-PCS
Follows ICD structure (designed for diagnosis coding)	Designed/developed to meet healthcare needs for a procedure code system
Codes available as a fixed/finite set in list form	Codes constructed from flexible code components (values) using tables
Codes are numeric	Codes are alphanumeric
Codes are 3 through 4 digits long	All codes are seven characters long

ICD-10-PCS CODE STRUCTURE

Undergirding ICD-10-PCS is a logical, consistent structure that informs the system as a whole, down to the level of a single code. This means that the process of constructing codes in ICD-10-PCS is also logical and consistent: individual letters and numbers, called "values," are selected in sequence to occupy the seven spaces of the code, called "characters."

Characters
All codes in ICD-10-PCS are seven characters long. Each character in the seven-character code represents an aspect of the procedure, as shown in the following diagram of characters from the main section of ICD-10-PCS, called MEDICAL AND SURGICAL.

	Section	Body System	Root Operation	Body Part	Approach	Device	Qualifier
Characters of a PCS code	1	2	3	4	5	6	7

An ICD-10-PCS code is best understood as the result of a process rather than as an isolated, fixed quantity. The process consists of assigning values from among the valid choices for that part of the system, according to the rules governing the construction of codes.

Values
One of 34 possible values can be assigned to each character in a code: the numbers 0 through 9 and the alphabet (except I and O, because they are easily confused with the numbers 1 and 0). A finished code looks like the example below.

$$0\ 2\ 1\ 0\ 3\ D\ 4$$

This code is derived by choosing a specific value for each of the seven characters. Based on details about the procedure performed, values for each character specifying the section, body system, root operation, body part, approach, device, and qualifier are assigned.

Because the definition of each character is a function of its physical position in the code, the same value placed in a different position in the code means something different. The value 0 in the first character means something different than 0 in the second character, or 0 in the third character, and so on.

Code Structure: Medical and Surgical Section
The following character explanations define each character using the code 0 L B 5 0 Z Z, "Excision of right lower arm and wrist tendon, open approach" as an example. This example comes from the MEDICAL AND SURGICAL section of ICD-10-PCS.

Character 1: Section
The first character in the code determines the broad procedure category, or section, where the code is found. In this example, the section is MEDICAL AND SURGICAL.
0 is the value that represents MEDICAL AND SURGICAL in the 1ST character.

Character 2: Body System
The second character defines the body system—the general physiological system or anatomical region involved. Examples of body systems include LOWER ARTERIES, CENTRAL NERVOUS SYSTEM, and RESPIRATORY SYSTEM.
L is the value that represents the Body System, TENDONS in the 2ND character.

Character 3: Root Operation
The third character defines the root operation, or the objective of the procedure. Some examples of root operations are BYPASS, DRAINAGE, and REATTACHMENT. In the sample code below, the root operation is EXCISION.
B is the value that represents the Root Operation, EXCISION in the 3RD character.

Character 4: Body Part

The fourth character defines the body part, or specific anatomical site where the procedure was performed. The body system (second character) provides only a general indication of the procedure site. The body part and body system values together provide a precise description of the procedure site.

Examples of body parts are KIDNEY, TONSILS, and THYMUS. When the second character is L, the value 5 when used in the fourth character of the code represents the right lower arm and wrist tendon.
5 is the value that represents the Body Part, LOWER ARM AND WRIST, RIGHT in the 4TH character.

Character 5: Approach

The fifth character defines the approach, or the technique used to reach the procedure site. Seven different approach values are used in the MEDICAL AND SURGICAL section to define the approach. Examples of approaches include OPEN and PERCUTANEOUS ENDOSCOPIC.
0 is the value that represents the the Approach, OPEN in the 5TH character.

Character 6: Device

Depending on the procedure performed, there may or may not be a device left in place at the end of the procedure. The sixth character defines the device. Device values fall into four basic categories:
- Grafts and Prostheses
- Implants
- Simple or Mechanical Appliances
- Electronic Appliances

In this example, there is no device used in the procedure. The value Z is used to represent NO DEVICE, as shown below.
Z is the value that represents the Device, NO DEVICE in the 6TH character.

Character 7: Qualifier

The seventh character defines a qualifier for the code. A qualifier specifies an additional attribute of the procedure, if applicable.

Examples of qualifiers include DIAGNOSTIC and STEREOTACTIC. Qualifier choices vary depending on the previous values selected. In this example, there is no specific qualifier applicable to this procedure.
Z is the value that represents the Qualifier, NO QUALIFIER in the 7TH character.

0 L B 5 0 Z Z is the complete specification of the above procedure: "Excision of right lower arm and wrist tendon, open approach."

ICD-10-PCS SYSTEM ORGANIZATION

The ICD-10-PCS system is organized in three parts: the Tables, the Index, and the Definitions.

Tables (see example below)
The Tables are organized in a series, beginning with section 0, MEDICAL AND SURGICAL, and body system 0, CENTRAL NERVOUS SYSTEM, and proceeding in numerical order. Sections 0 through 9 are followed by sections B through D and F through H and X. The same convention is followed within each table for the second through the seventh characters—numeric values in order first, followed by alphabetical values in order.

The following examples use the MEDICAL AND SURGICAL section to describe the organization and format of the ICD-10-PCS Tables.

The MEDICAL AND SURGICAL section (first character 0) is organized by its 31 body system values. Each body system subdivision in the MEDICAL AND SURGICAL section contains tables that list the valid root operations for that body system. These are the root operation tables that form the the system. These tables provide the valid choices of values available to construct a code.

The root operation tables consist of four columns and a varying number of rows, as in the following example of the root operation EXCISION, in the TENDONS body system.

The values for characters 1 through 3 are provided at the top of each table. Four columns contain the applicable values for characters 4 through 7, given the values in characters 1 through 3.

A table may be separated into rows to specify the valid choices of values in characters 4 through 7. A code built using values from more than one row of a table is not a valid code.

For the complete list of ICD-10-PCS Official Coding Guidelines, please refer to the Official Coding Guidelines following this Introduction.

See Tables above for Table explanation.

EXCISION GROUP: Excision, Resection, Destruction, (Extraction), (Detachment)
Root Operations that take out some or all of a body part.

1ST – **0** Medical and Surgical (Section)	EXAMPLE: Ganglionectomy tendon sheath	CMS Ex: Liver biopsy
2ND – **L** Tendons (Body System)	**EXCISION:** Cutting out or off, without replacement, a portion of a body part.	
3RD – **B** EXCISION (Root Operation)	EXPLANATION: Qualifier "X Diagnostic" indicates biopsy …	

Body Part – 4TH		Approach – 5TH	Device – 6TH	Qualifier – 7TH
0 Head and Neck Tendon	F Abdomen Tendon, Right	0 Open	Z No device	X Diagnostic
1 Shoulder Tendon, Right	G Abdomen Tendon, Left	3 Percutaneous		Z No qualifier
2 Shoulder Tendon, Left	H Perineum Tendon	4 Percutaneous endoscopic		
3 Upper Arm Tendon, Right	J Hip Tendon, Right			
4 Upper Arm Tendon, Left	K Hip Tendon, Left			
5 Lower Arm and Wrist Tendon, Right	L Upper Leg Tendon, Right			
	M Upper Leg Tendon, Left			
6 Lower Arm and Wrist Tendon, Left	N Lower Leg Tendon, Right			
	P Lower Leg Tendon, Left			
7 Hand Tendon, Right	Q Knee Tendon, Right			
8 Hand Tendon, Left	R Knee Tendon, Left			
9 Trunk Tendon, Right	S Ankle Tendon, Right			
B Trunk Tendon, Left	T Ankle Tendon, Left			

Sections

ICD-10-PCS is composed of 17 sections, represented by the numbers 0 through 9 and the letters B through D, F through H, and X. The broad procedure categories contained in these sections range from surgical procedures to new technology.

The 17 sections are divided into three groups:
- Medical and Surgical Section
- Medical/Surgical Related Sections
- Ancillary Sections

Medical and Surgical Section

The first section, and the only section in the first group, MEDICAL AND SURGICAL, contains the great majority of procedures typically reported in an inpatient setting. As shown in the previous section discussing ICD-10-PCS code structure, all procedure codes in the MEDICAL AND SURGICAL section begin with the section value 0.

For a complete list of the Body Systems (Character 2) in the MEDICAL AND SURGICAL section, please see the Table of Contents located on page vi.

Medical/Surgical Related Sections

Sections 1 through 9 of ICD-10-PCS comprise the Medical and Surgical-related sections. These sections include obstetrical procedures, administration of substances, measurement and monitoring of body functions, and extracorporeal therapies, as listed below:

Section Value	Section Title
1	Obstetrics
2	Placement
3	Administration
4	Measurement and Monitoring
5	Extracorporeal Assistance and Performance
6	Extracorporeal Therapies
7	Osteopathic
8	Other Procedures
9	Chiropractic

In sections 1 and 2, all seven characters define the same aspects of the procedure as in the MEDICAL AND SURGICAL section.

Codes in sections 3 through 9 are structured for the most part like their counterparts in the MEDICAL AND SURGICAL section, with a few exceptions. For example, in sections 5 and 6, the fifth character is defined as duration instead of approach.

Additional differences include these uses of the sixth character:
- Section 3 defines the sixth character as substance.
- Sections 4 and 5 define the sixth character as function.
- Sections 7 through 9 define the sixth character as method.

Ancillary Sections

Sections B through D, F through H, and X comprise the ancillary sections of ICD-10-PCS. These seven sections include imaging procedures, nuclear medicine, and substance abuse treatment, as listed below:

Section Value	Section Title
B	Imaging
C	Nuclear Medicine
D	Radiation Therapy
F	Physical Rehabilitation and Diagnostic Audiology
G	Mental Health
H	Substance Abuse Treatment
X	New Technology

The definitions of some characters in the ancillary sections differs from that seen in previous sections. In the IMAGING section, the third character is defined as type, and the fifth and sixth characters define contrast and contrast/qualifier respectively.

Additional differences include:
- Section C defines the fifth character as radionuclide.
- Section D defines the fifth character as modality qualifier and the sixth character as isotope.
- Section F defines the fifth character as type qualifier and the sixth character as equipment.
- Sections G and H define the third character as a type qualifier.

Index

The ICD-10-PCS Index can be used to access the Tables. The Index mirrors the structure of the Tables, so it follows a consistent pattern of organization and use of hierarchies.

The Index is organized as an alphabetic lookup. Two types of main terms are listed in the Index:
- Based on the value of the third character (e.g., Root Operation, Root Type)
- Common procedure terms (e.g., Cholecystectomy)

Also included in the Index are the body parts identified in the Body Part Key and the devices identified in the Device Key.

Main Terms

For the MEDICAL AND SURGICAL and related sections, the root operation values are used as main terms in the Index. In other sections, the values representing the general type of procedure performed, such as nuclear medicine or imaging type, are listed as main terms.

For the MEDICAL AND SURGICAL and related sections, values such as EXCISION, BYPASS, and TRANSPLANTATION are included as main terms in the Index. The applicable body system entries are listed beneath the main term, and refer to a specific table. For the ancillary sections, values such as FLUOROSCOPY and POSITRON EMISSION TOMOGRAPHY are listed as main terms.

In the example below, the index entry "Bypass" refers to the MEDICAL AND SURGICAL section tables for all applicable body systems, including ANATOMICAL REGIONS and CENTRAL NERVOUS SYSTEM.

Bypass
  Cavity, Cranial 0W110J-
  Cerbral Ventricle 0016-

Common Procedure Terms

The second type of term listed in the Index uses procedure names, such as "appendectomy" or "fundoplication." These entries are listed as main terms, and refer to the possible valid Root Operations by using a "see" instruction, as shown in the following example.

Cholecystectomy
  – *see* Excision, Gallbladder 0FB4-
  – *see* Resection, Gallbladder 0FT4-

Definitions

The ICD-10-PCS Definitions contain the official definitions of ICD-10-PCS values in characters 3 through 7 of the seven-character code, and may also provide additional explanation or examples. The definitions are arranged in section order, and designate the section and the character within the section being defined.

The Medical and Surgical section body part value definitions refer from the body part value to corresponding anatomical terms. The Medical and Surgical section device definitions refer from the device value to corresponding device terms or manufacturer's names. The Substance value definitions in the Administration section refer from the substance value to a common substance name or manufacturer's substance name. These definitions are also sorted by common term and listed separately as the Body Part Key, Device Key, and Substance Key respectively.

The ICD-10-PCS Device Aggregation Table contains entries that correlate a specific ICD-10-PCS device value with a general device value to be used in tables containing only general device values.

Tabular Order File

The ICD-10-PCS Order file contains a unique "order number" for each valid code or table "header," a flag distinguishing valid codes from headers, and both long and short descriptions combined in a single file.

The code descriptions are generated using rules that produce standardized, complete, and easy-to-read code descriptions.

ICD-10-PCS DESIGN

ICD-10-PCS is fundamentally different from ICD-9-CM in its structure, organization, and capabilities. It was designed and developed to adhere to recommendations made by the National Committee on Vital and Health Statistics (NCVHS). It also incorporates input from a wide range of organizations, individual physicians, healthcare professionals, and researchers.

Several structural attributes were recommended for a new procedure coding system. These attributes include:
- Multiaxial structure
- Completeness
- Expandability

Multiaxial structure

The key attribute that provides the framework for all other structural attributes is multiaxial code structure. Multiaxial code structure makes it possible for the ICD-10-PCS to be complete, expandable, and to provide a high degree of flexibility and functionality.

As mentioned earlier, ICD-10-PCS codes are composed of seven characters. Each character represents a category of information that can be specified about the procedure performed. A character defines both the category of information and its physical position in the code.

A character's position can be understood as a semi-independent axis of classification that allows different specific values to be inserted into that space, and whose physical position remains stable. Within a defined code range, a character retains the general meaning that it confers on any value in that position. For example, the fifth character retains the general meaning "approach" in sections 0 through 4 and 7 through 9 of the system. Any specific value in the fifth character will define a specific approach, such as OPEN.

Each group of values for a character contains all of the valid choices in relation to the other characters of the code, giving the system completeness. In the fifth character, for example, each significantly distinct approach is assigned its own approach value and all applicable approach values are included to represent the possible versions of a procedure.

Each group of values for a character can be added to as needed, giving the system expandability. If a significantly distinct approach is used to perform procedures, a new approach value can be added to the system.

Each group of values is confined to its own character, giving ICD-10-PCS a stable, predictable readability across a wide range of codes. In sections 0 through 4 and 7 through 9 of the system, for example, the fifth character always represents the approach.

ICD-10-PCS' multiaxial structure houses its capacity for completeness, expandability, and flexibility, giving it a high degree of functionality for multiple uses.

Completeness

Completeness is considered a key structural attribute for a new procedure coding system. The specific recommendation for completeness includes these characteristics:
- A unique code is available for each significantly different procedure.
- Each code retains its unique definition. Codes are not reused.

In Volume 3 of ICD-9-CM, procedures performed on many different body parts using different approaches or devices may be assigned to the same procedure code. In ICD-10-PCS, a unique code can be constructed for every significantly different procedure.

Within each section, a character defines a consistent component of a code, and contains all applicable values for that character. The values define individual expressions (open, percutaneous) of the character's general meaning (approach) that are then used to construct unique procedure codes.

Because all approaches by which a procedure is performed are assigned a separate approach value in the system, every procedure which uses a different approach will have its own unique code. This is true of the other characters as well. The same procedure performed on a different body part has its own unique code, the same procedure performed using a different device has its own unique code, and so on.

Because ICD-10-PCS codes are constructed of individual values rather than lists of fixed codes and text descriptions, the unique, stable definition of a code in the system is retained. New values may be added to the system to represent a specific new approach or device or qualifier, but whole codes by design cannot be given new meanings and reused.

Expandability

Expandability was also recommended as a key structural attribute. The specific recommendation for expandability includes these characteristics:
- Accommodate new procedures and technologies
- Add new codes without disrupting the existing structure

ICD-10-PCS is designed to be easily updated as new codes are required for new procedures and new techniques. Changes to ICD-10-PCS can all be made within the existing structure, because whole codes are not added. Instead, one of two possible changes is made to the system:
- A new value for a character is added as needed to the system
- An existing value for a character is added to a table(s) in the system

ICD-10-PCS update: PICVA

An example of how the updating of ICD-10-PCS works can be seen in the coronary artery bypass procedure called Percutaneous in-situ coronary venous arterialization (PICVA). This procedure is no more invasive than a percutaneous coronary angioplasty, but achieves the benefits of a bypass procedure by placing a specialized stent into the diseased coronary artery, through its wall into the adjacent coronary vein, and diverting blood flow through the stent into the artery past the blockage.

ICD-10-PCS was updated in 2004 to include an appropriate range of codes for the PICVA procedure (16 possible codes). This was accomplished simply by adding another row to the relevant table (as shown in the example below) containing two approach values for the non-invasive approach, two device values for the possible types of stent, and a single qualifier defining the coronary vein as the source of the new blood flow, as in the example below.

The values for characters 1 through 3 at the top of each table are:
0: MEDICAL AND SURGICAL (Section)
2: HEART AND GREAT VESSELS (Body system)
1: BYPASS: Altering the route of passage of the contents of a tubular body part

Body Part Character 4	Approach Character 5	Device Character 6	Qualifier Character 7
0 Coronary Artery, One Artery 1 Coronary Artery, Two Arteries 2 Coronary Artery, Three Arteries 3 Coronary Artery, Four or More Arteries	3 Percutaneous 4 Percutaneous Endoscopic	4 Drug-eluting Intraluminal Device D Intraluminal Device	D Coronary Vein

Structural integrity

As shown in the previous example, ICD-10-PCS can be easily expanded without disrupting the structure of the system.

In the PICVA example, one new value—the qualifier value Coronary Vein—was added to the system to effect this change. All other values in the new row are existing values used to create unique, new codes.

This type of updating can be replicated anywhere in the system when a change is required. ICD-10-PCS allows unique new codes to be added to the system because values for the seven characters that make up a code can be combined as needed. The system can evolve as medical technology and clinical practice evolve, without disrupting the ICD-10-PCS structure.

ICD-10-PCS ADDITIONAL CHARACTERISTICS

ICD-10-PCS possesses several additional characteristics in response to government and industry recommendations. These characteristics are:
- Standardized terminology within the coding system
- Standardized level of specificity
- No diagnostic information
- No explicit "not otherwise specified" (NOS) code options
- Limited use of "not elsewhere classified" (NEC) code options

Standardized Terminology
Words commonly used in clinical vocabularies may have multiple meanings. This can cause confusion and result in inaccurate data. ICD-10-PCS is standardized and self-contained. Characters and values used in the system are defined in the system.

For example, the word "excision" is used to describe a wide variety of surgical procedures. In ICD-10-PCS, the word "excision" describes a single, precise surgical objective, defined as "Cutting out or off, without replacement, a portion of a body part."

No Eponyms or Common Procedure Names
The terminology used in ICD-10-PCS is standardized to provide precise and stable definitions of all procedures performed. This standardized terminology is used in all ICD-10-PCS code descriptions.

As a result, ICD-10-PCS code descriptions do not include eponyms or common procedure names. Two examples from ICD-9-CM are 22.61, "Excision of lesion of maxillary sinus with Caldwell-Luc approach," and 51.10, "Endoscopic retrograde cholangiopancreatography [ERCP]." In ICD-10-PCS, physicians' names are not included in a code description, nor are procedures identified by common terms or acronyms such as appendectomy or CABG. Instead, such procedures are coded to the root operation that accurately identifies the objective of the procedure.

The procedures described in the preceding paragraph by ICD-9-CM codes are coded in ICD-10-PCS according to the root operation that matches the objective of the procedure. Here the ICD-10-PCS equivalents would be EXCISION and INSPECTION respectively. By relying on the universal objectives defined in root operations rather than eponyms or specific procedure titles that change or become obsolete, ICD-10-PCS preserves the capacity to define past, present, and future procedures accurately using stable terminology in the form of characters and values.

No Combination Codes
With rare exceptions, ICD-10-PCS does not define multiple procedures with one code. This is to preserve standardized terminology and consistency across the system. Procedures that are typically performed together but are distinct procedures may be defined by a single "combination code" in ICD-9-CM. An example of a combination code in ICD-9-CM is 28.3, "Tonsillectomy with adenoidectomy."

A procedure that meets the reporting criteria for a separate procedure is coded separately in ICD-10-PCS. This allows the system to respond to changes in technology and medical practice with the maximum degree of stability and flexibility.

Standardized Level of Specificity
In ICD-9-CM, one code with its description and includes notes may encompass a vast number of procedure variations while another code defines a single specific procedure. ICD-10-PCS provides a standardized level of specificity for each code, so that each code represents a single procedure variation.

The ICD-9-CM code 39.31, "Suture of artery," does not specify the artery, whereas the code range 38.40 through 38.49, "Resection of artery with replacement," provides a fourth-digit subclassification for specifying the artery by anatomical region (thoracic, abdominal, etc.).

In ICD-10-PCS, the codes identifying all artery suture and artery replacement procedures possess the same degree of specificity. The ICD-9-CM examples above coded to their ICD-10-PCS equivalents would use the same artery body part values in all codes identifying the respective procedures.

In general, ICD-10-PCS code descriptions are much more specific than their ICD-9-CM counterparts, but sometimes an ICD-10-PCS code description is actually less specific. In most cases this is because the ICD-9-CM code contains diagnosis information. The standardized level of code specificity in ICD-10-PCS cannot always take account of these fluctuations in ICD-9-CM level of specificity. Instead, ICD-10-PCS provides a standardized level of specificity that can be predicted across the system.

Diagnosis Information Excluded
Another key feature of ICD-10-PCS is that information pertaining to a diagnosis is excluded from the code descriptions.

ICD-9-CM often contains information about the diagnosis in its procedure codes. Adding diagnosis information limits the flexibility and functionality of a procedure coding system. It has the effect of placing a code "off limits" because the diagnosis in the medical record does not match the diagnosis in the procedure code description. The code cannot be used even though the procedural part of the code description precisely matches the procedure performed.

Diagnosis information is not contained in any ICD-10-PCS code. The diagnosis codes, not the procedure codes, will specify the reason the procedure is performed.

NOS Code Options Restricted
ICD-9-CM often designates codes as "unspecified" or "not otherwise specified" codes. By contrast, the standardized level of specificity designed into ICD-10-PCS restricts the use of broadly applicable NOS or unspecified code options in the system. A minimal level of specificity is required to construct a valid code.

In ICD-10-PCS, each character defines information about the procedure and all seven characters must contain a specific value obtained from a single row of a table to build a valid code. Even values such as the sixth-character value Z, NO DEVICE and the seventh-character value Z, NO QUALIFIER, provide important information about the procedure performed.

Limited NEC Code Options
ICD-9-CM often designates codes as "not elsewhere classified" or "other specified" versions of a procedure throughout the code set. NEC options are also provided in ICD-10-PCS, but only for specific, limited use.

In the MEDICAL AND SURGICAL section, two significant "not elsewhere classified" options are the root operation value Q, REPAIR and the device value Y, OTHER DEVICE.

The root operation REPAIR is a true NEC value. It is used only when the procedure performed is not one of the other root operations in the MEDICAL AND SURGICAL section.

OTHER DEVICE, on the other hand, is intended to be used to temporarily define new devices that do not have a specific value assigned, until one can be added to the system. No categories of medical or surgical devices are permanently classified to OTHER DEVICE.

ICD-10-PCS APPLICATIONS

ICD-10-PCS code structure results in qualities that optimize the performance of the system in electronic applications, and maximize the usefulness of the coded healthcare data. These qualities include:

- Optimal search capability
- Consistent character definitions
- Consistent values wherever possible
- Code readability

Some have argued that, in the world of the electronic health record, the classification system as we know it is outmoded, that classification doesn't matter because a computer is able to find a code with equal ease whether the code has been generated at random or is part of a classification scheme. While this may be true from an IT perspective, assignment of randomly generated code numbers makes it impossible to aggregate data according to related ranges of codes. This is a critical capability for providers, payers, and researchers to make meaningful use of the data.

Optimal Search Capability

ICD-10-PCS is designed for maximum versatility in the ability to aggregate coded data. Values belonging to the same character as defined in a section or sections can be easily compared, since they occupy the same position in a code. This provides a high degree of flexibility and functionality for data mining.

For example, the body part value 6, STOMACH, retains its meaning for all codes in the MEDICAL AND SURGICAL section that define procedures performed on the stomach. Because the body part value is dependent for its meaning on the body system in which it is found, the body system value D, GASTROINTESTINAL, must also be included in the search.

A person wishing to examine data regarding all medical and surgical procedures performed on the stomach could do so simply by searching the following code range: 0D*6***

Consistent Characters and Values

In the previous example, the value 6 means STOMACH only when the body system value is D, GASTROINTESTINAL. In many other cases, values retain their meaning across a much broader range of codes. This provides consistency and readability.

For example, the value 0 in the fifth character defines the approach OPEN and the value 3 in the fifth character defines the approach PERCUTANEOUS across sections 0 through 4 and 7 through 9, where applicable. As a result, all open and percutaneous procedures represented by codes in sections 0-4 and 7-9 can be compared based on a single character—approach—by conducting a query on the following code ranges:
[0 through 4,7 through 9]***0** vs. [0 through 4,7 through 9]***3**

Searches can be progressively refined by adding specific values. For example, one could search on a body system value or range of body system values, plus a body part value or range of body part values, plus a root operation value or range of root operation values.

To refine the search above, one could add the body system value for GASTROINTESTINAL and the body part value for STOMACH to limit the search to open vs. percutaneous procedures performed on the stomach: 0D*60** vs. 0D*63**

To refine the search even further and limit the comparison to open and percutaneous biopsies of the stomach, one could add the third-character value for the root operation EXCISION and the seventh-character qualifier DIAGNOSTIC, as follows: 0DB60*X vs. 0DB63*X

Stability of characters and values across vast ranges of codes provides the maximum degree of functionality and flexibility for the collection and analysis of data. The search capabilities demonstrated above function equally well for all uses of healthcare data: investigating quality of care, resource utilization, risk management, conducting research, determining reimbursement, and many others.

Because the character definition is consistent, and only the individual values assigned to that character differ as needed, meaningful comparisons of data over time can be conducted across a virtually infinite range of procedures.

Code readability

ICD-10-PCS resembles a language in the sense that it is made up of semi-independent values combined by following the rules of the system, much the way a sentence is formed by combining words and following the rules of grammar and syntax. As with words in their context, the meaning of any single value is a combination of its position in the code and any preceding values on which it may be dependent.

For example, in the MEDICAL AND SURGICAL section, a body part value is always dependent for its meaning on the body system in which it is found. It cannot stand alone as a letter or a number and be meaningful. A fourth-character value of 6 by itself can mean 31 different things, but a fourth-character value of 6 in the context of a second-character value of D means one thing only—STOMACH.

On the other hand, a root operation value is not dependent on any character but the section for its meaning, and identifies a single consistent objective wherever the third character is defined as root operation. For example, the third-character value T identifies the root operation RESECTION in both the MEDICAL AND SURGICAL and OBSTETRICS sections.

The approach value also identifies a single consistent approach wherever the fifth character is defined as approach. The fifth-character value 3 identifies the approach PERCUTANEOUS in the MEDICAL AND SURGICAL section, the OBSTETRICS section, the ADMINISTRATION section, and others.

The sixth-character device value or seventh-character qualifier value identifies the same device or qualifier in the context of the body system where it is found. Although there may be consistencies across body systems or within whole sections, this is not true in all cases.

Values in their designated context have a precise meaning, like words in a language. As seen in the code example which began this chapter, 0LB50ZZ represents the text description of the specific procedure "Excision of right lower arm and wrist tendon, open approach." Since ICD-10-PCS values in context have a single, precise meaning, a complete, valid code can be read and understood without its accompanying text description, much like one would read a sentence.

Please see the Appendices following the Ancillary Sections for further detailed information on ICD-10-PCS and its components.

Channel Publishing 2017 ICD-10-PCS Additional *Enhanced* Features

Unique, Enhanced Table Design

The basic PCS tables have been significantly enhanced (graphic design) to help coders clearly and quickly identify the components of each PCS code table.

Inclusion of Example and Brief Explanation in PCS Table design

The addition of root operation examples and a brief explanation of the root operation (in addition to the root operation definition) helps coders understand each root operation without referring to a table in the appendices.

Unique, Graphic Page Design

The unique, graphic page design clearly identifies which PCS code tables are located on that page and helps coders stay focused on the particular root operation for that body system. In addition, code tables that are too extensive for one page have that continued information very clearly identified.

Highlighted First 3 Digits in Index

The first 3 digits of each code in the Alphabetic Index are in boldface type to help coders identify and search for the correct 3-digit PCS code table in the Tabular Table sections.

Highlighted Body Part & Device Terms

The body part and device terms in the index have blue screen bars placed over them to help coders more easily differentiate between standard index entries and the body part and device terms.

Body Part, Device & Device Aggregation Keys

The body part, device, and device aggregation keys (tables) are listed in separate appendices following the Tabular Table sections.

All 7 Characters Clearly Identified

All 7 characters of a PCS code are clearly identified in each PCS code table to help coders learn and properly select the appropriate character for each digit.

Tab-Edge Printing

Chapter-by-chapter, and section-by-section stair-stepped, tab-edge printing helps coders locate the correct section quickly.

Clear, Compact Type Face Printing

The use of clear, compact type face to allow coders to clearly and easily locate and read all text in the Alphabetic Index and Tabular Tables.

Clear, Compact Guidewords at the Top of Each Page

The use of clear, compact guidewords allow coders to clearly and easily locate the correct page in the Alphabetic Index and Tabular Tables.

Channel Publishing Additional 2017 *Enhanced* Features

Educational Annotations for Each Body System and Section

Anatomy and Physiology Reviews
Anatomy and physiology reviews that help coders understand the anatomical structures and physiology of the various systems.

Illustrations
Anatomical illustrations with call outs of body parts.

Definitions
Medical definitions of common procedures written by a coder for coders.

AHA Coding Clinic® Reference Notations
Identifies AHA Coding Clinic® articles and Q&As (with descriptive title) that have relevant information for certain codes or code categories.

Body Part Key Listings
Identifies the Body Part Key listings specific for that body system or section.

Device Key Listings
Identifies the Device Key listings specific for that body system or section.

Device Aggregation Table Listings
Identifies the Device Aggregation Table listings specific for that body system or section.

Coding Guidelines
Lists the Official Coding Guidelines specific for that body system or section.

PCS Reference Manual Exercises
Lists the exercises found in the PCS Reference Manual specific for that body system or section.

Tab-Edge Printing for Educational Annotations Pages
The Educational Annotations pages are identified by two digits in the screen bar: First digit – Section, Second digit – Body System.

Additional 2017 Features

Groups of Similar Root Operations
At the top of each table is a list of similar Root Operations that includes that table's Root Operation. The screened-out Root Operations are Root Operations that are not included in that Body System.

Body System Specific Root Operation Examples
Each table identifies the CMS general Root Operation example and a Channel Publishing created Body System Specific example.

Medicare Code Editor Edits
Identifies codes that are edit-reviewed for age and sex-related discrepancies and coverage conditions.

Blue Color Highlighting of Graphic Design and Selected Text
Color highlighting of Index:
- Highlighted Body Part Key terms – Screened Blue
- Highlighted Device Key terms – Screened Blue
- Tab-Edge Printing – Blue

Color highlighting of Tables:
- Tables – Blue
- Root Operation Definitions – Blue
- Medicare Code Editor Edits – Blue
- Tab-Edge Printing – Blue

INTRODUCTION TO AHA CODING CLINIC® REFERENCE NOTATIONS

BACKGROUND

AHA Coding Clinic® is a registered trademark of the American Hospital Association. AHA Coding Clinic® Reference Notations is not a product of the American Hospital Association, and Channel Publishing, Ltd. is not affiliated with or endorsed by the American Hospital Association. The American Hospital coding website can be accessed at www.ahacentraloffice.org.

The AHA Coding Clinic® for ICD-10-CM/PCS is published quarterly by the American Hospital Association. The *Coding Clinic* is the official publication for *ICD-10-CM/PCS* coding guidelines and advice as designated by the four cooperating parties. The cooperating parties listed below have final approval of the coding advice provided in the *Coding Clinic*: American Hospital Association, American Health Information Management Association, Centers for Medicare and Medicaid Services, National Center for Health Statistics.

The *Coding Clinic* provides specific information and guidelines that are helpful for determining proper coding, and is used by CMS in reviewing claims. The goal of the *Coding Clinic* is to provide coding advice, official coding decisions, and news. It promotes accuracy and consistency in the use of ICD-10-CM/PCS. It offers coding guidelines and advice based on adherence to the statistical classification scheme of ICD-10-CM/PCS and the definitions specified in the Uniform Hospital Discharge Data Set (UHDDS).

INTRODUCTION

Channel Publishing has developed the AHA Coding Clinic® Reference Notations to help coders access the official coding advice found throughout all issues of the *Coding Clinic*. This information has been referenced in three ways: 1) at the Educational Annotations portion of each Body System/Section, 2) at the identified Coding Guideline, and 3) a categorical index of articles (see below) that are too broad in scope to be assigned to 1) or 2). Any comments regarding these reference notations should be directed to: *Coding Clinic* Reference Notations, c/o Channel Publishing, Ltd., 4750 Longley Lane, Suite 110, Reno, Nevada 89502.

GUIDANCE IN USE

Coders are encouraged to reference all relevant information contained in the *Coding Clinic* to promote the most accurate coding possible for their organization. It is important to understand the basic criteria for assigning the *Coding Clinic* Reference Notations. The basic criteria consists of: Assignment to codes with direct or indirect information concerning the proper use of each particular code, assignment to a code category when the information is relevant to all codes in that category, and assignment to codes where a coder might commonly attempt to use a code in error.

MISCELLANEOUS AHA CODING CLINIC® REFERENCE NOTATIONS INDEX

MISCELLANEOUS AHA CODING CLINIC® REFERENCE NOTATIONS INDEX

NOTES

<u>**IMPORTANT NOTES REGARDING THESE PRINTED GUIDELINES**</u>

These guidelines are effective for the 2017 version (June 2016 posting) of ICD-10-PCS. A newer version may become available after this book has been printed. Coders should periodically check the Centers for Medicare and Medicaid Services (CMS) web site for the most current version. CMS Web Site: www.cms.gov

Any text printed in blue represents an addition, ~~deletion~~, or revision from the 2017 Official Guidelines.

Some Body System specific Guidelines have been reprinted on the Educational Annotations pages for those Body Systems. However, they are not a substitute for using the entire set of Official Coding Guidelines.

Channel Publishing, Ltd.

2017 ICD-10-PCS Official Guidelines for Coding and Reporting

The Centers for Medicare and Medicaid Services (CMS) and the National Center for Health Statistics (NCHS), two departments within the U.S. Federal Government's Department of Health and Human Services (DHHS) provide the following guidelines for coding and reporting using the International Classification of Diseases, 10th Revision, Procedure Coding System (ICD-10-PCS). These guidelines should be used as a companion document to the official version of the ICD-10-PCS as published on the CMS website. The ICD-10-PCS is a procedure classification published by the United States for classifying procedures performed in hospital inpatient healthcare settings.

These guidelines have been approved by the four organizations that make up the Cooperating Parties for the ICD-10-PCS: the American Hospital Association (AHA), the American Health Information Management Association (AHIMA), CMS, and NCHS.

These guidelines are a set of rules that have been developed to accompany and complement the official conventions and instructions provided within the ICD-10-PCS itself. The instructions and conventions of the classification take precedence over guidelines. These guidelines are based on the coding and sequencing instructions in the Tables, Index and Definitions of ICD-10-PCS, but provide additional instruction. Adherence to these guidelines when assigning ICD-10-PCS procedure codes is required under the Health Insurance Portability and Accountability Act (HIPAA). The procedure codes have been adopted under HIPAA for hospital inpatient healthcare settings. A joint effort between the healthcare provider and the coder is essential to achieve complete and accurate documentation, code assignment, and reporting of diagnoses and procedures. These guidelines have been developed to assist both the healthcare provider and the coder in identifying those procedures that are to be reported. The importance of consistent, complete documentation in the medical record cannot be overemphasized. Without such documentation accurate coding cannot be achieved.

Table of Contents

Conventions

A1
ICD-10-PCS codes are composed of seven characters. Each character is an axis of classification that specifies information about the procedure performed. Within a defined code range, a character specifies the same type of information in that axis of classification.
Example: The fifth axis of classification specifies the approach in sections 0 through 4 and 7 through 9 of the system.

A2
One of 34 possible values can be assigned to each axis of classification in the seven-character code: they are the numbers 0 through 9 and the alphabet (except I and O because they are easily confused with the numbers 1 and 0). The number of unique values used in an axis of classification differs as needed.
Example: Where the fifth axis of classification specifies the approach, seven different approach values are currently used to specify the approach.

A3
The valid values for an axis of classification can be added to as needed.
Example: If a significantly distinct type of device is used in a new procedure, a new device value can be added to the system.

A4
As with words in their context, the meaning of any single value is a combination of its axis of classification and any preceding values on which it may be dependent.
Example: The meaning of a body part value in the Medical and Surgical section is always dependent on the body system value. The body part value 0 in the Central Nervous body system specifies Brain and the body part value 0 in the Peripheral Nervous body system specifies Cervical Plexus.

A5
As the system is expanded to become increasingly detailed, over time more values will depend on preceding values for their meaning.
Example: In the Lower Joints body system, the device value 3 in the root operation Insertion specifies Infusion Device and the device value 3 in the root operation Replacement specifies Ceramic Synthetic Substitute.

A6

The purpose of the alphabetic index is to locate the appropriate table that contains all information necessary to construct a procedure code. The PCS Tables should always be consulted to find the most appropriate valid code.

A7

It is not required to consult the index first before proceeding to the tables to complete the code. A valid code may be chosen directly from the tables.

AHA Coding Clinic® Reference Notation(s) — Coding Guideline A7
Reconstruction, main index term ....AHA 14:2Q:p10

A8

All seven characters must be specified to be a valid code. If the documentation is incomplete for coding purposes, the physician should be queried for the necessary information.

A9

Within a PCS table, valid codes include all combinations of choices in characters 4 through 7 contained in the same row of the table. In the example below, 0JHT3VZ is a valid code, and 0JHW3VZ is *not* a valid code.

1ST- 0 Medical and Surgical	EXAMPLE: Placement pacemaker generator
2ND- J Subcutaneous Tissue and Fascia	INSERTION: Putting in a nonbiological appliance that monitors, assists, performs, or prevents a physiological function but does not physically take the place of a body part.
3RD- H INSERTION	EXPLANATION:None

4TH Body Part	5TH Approach	6TH Device	7TH Qualifier
S Subcutaneous Tissue and Fascia, Head and Neck V Subcutaneous Tissue and Fascia, Upper Extremity **W Subcutaneous Tissue and Fascia, Lower Extremity**	0 Open 3 Percutaneous	1 Radioactive Element 3 Infusion Device	Z No Qualifier
T Subcutaneous Tissue and Fascia, Trunk	0 Open 3 Percutaneous	1 Radioactive Element 3 Infusion Device **V Infusion Pump**	Z No Qualifier

A10

"And," when used in a code description, means "and/or."
Example: Lower Arm and Wrist Muscle means lower arm and/or wrist muscle.

A11

Many of the terms used to construct PCS codes are defined within the system. It is the coder's responsibility to determine what the documentation in the medical record equates to in the PCS definitions. The physician is not expected to use the terms used in PCS code descriptions, nor is the coder required to query the physician when the correlation between the documentation and the defined PCS terms is clear.
Example: When the physician documents "partial resection" the coder can independently correlate "partial resection" to the root operation Excision without querying the physician for clarification.

Medical and Surgical Section Guidelines (Section 0)

B2. Body System

General guidelines

B2.1a

The procedure codes in the general anatomical regions body systems ~~should only~~ can be used when the procedure is performed on an anatomical region rather than a specific body part (e.g., root operations Control and Detachment, Drainage of a body cavity) or on the rare occasion when no information is available to support assignment of a code to a specific body part.
Examples: Control of postoperative hemorrhage is coded to the root operation Control found in the general anatomical regions body systems.
Chest tube drainage of the pleural cavity is coded to the root operation Drainage found in the general anatomical regions body systems. Suture repair of the abdominal wall is coded to the root operation Repair in the General Anatomical Regions body system.

B2.1b

Where the general body part values "upper" and "lower" are provided as an option in the Upper Arteries, Lower Arteries, Upper Veins, Lower Veins, Muscles and Tendons body systems, "upper" and "lower" specifies body parts located above or below the diaphragm respectively.
Example: Vein body parts above the diaphragm are found in the Upper Veins body system; vein body parts below the diaphragm are found in the Lower Veins body system.

AHA Coding Clinic® Reference Notation(s) — Coding Guideline B2.1b
Upper or lower veins body system ....AHA 14:3Q:p25

B3. Root Operation

General guidelines

B3.1a

In order to determine the appropriate root operation, the full definition of the root operation as contained in the PCS Tables must be applied.

B3.1b

Components of a procedure specified in the root operation definition and explanation are not coded separately. Procedural steps necessary to reach the operative site and close the operative site, including anastomosis of a tubular body part, are also not coded separately.
Examples: Resection of a joint as part of a joint replacement procedure is included in the root operation definition of Replacement and is not coded separately.
Laparotomy performed to reach the site of an open liver biopsy is not coded separately.
In a resection of sigmoid colon with anastomosis of descending colon to rectum, the anastomosis is not coded separately.

AHA Coding Clinic® Reference Notation(s) — Coding Guideline B3.1b
Components in fusion procedures included in Fusion root operation ....AHA 14:3Q:p30
Coronary artery release prior to bypass ....AHA 13:2Q:p37
Debridement considered as procedure preparation ....AHA 14:3Q:p31
Decalcification of aorta in preparation for further surgery.....................AHA 16:2Q:p25
FloSeal on small bleeder during cholecystectomy ....AHA 13:3Q:p22
Injection of substances with vitrectomy ....AHA 15:2Q:p24

AHA Coding Clinic® Reference Notation(s) — Coding Guideline B3.1b - continued
Lysis of adhesions, integral or code separately.................................AHA 14:1Q:p3
Omental bleeding repair during cholecystectomy............................AHA 13:3Q:p23
Orthotopic liver transplant with end-to-side cavoplasty and choledochostomy AHA 14:3Q:p13
Repositioning of aorta inherent to release of esophageal vascular ring ....AHA 15:3Q:p15

Multiple procedures

B3.2

During the same operative episode, multiple procedures are coded if:

a. The same root operation is performed on different body parts as defined by distinct values of the body part character.

Examples: Diagnostic excision of liver and pancreas are coded separately.

Excision of lesion in the ascending colon and excision of lesion in the transverse colon are coded separately.

b. The same root operation is repeated in multiple body parts, and those body parts are separate and distinct body parts classified to a single ICD-10-PCS body part value.

AHA Coding Clinic® Reference Notation(s) — Coding Guideline B3.2b
Coil embolization of gastroduodenal artery, and chemoembolization
   of hepatic artery ....AHA 14:3Q:p26
Uterine fibroids, multiple ....AHA 14:4Q:p16

Examples: Excision of the sartorius muscle and excision of the gracilis muscle are both included in the upper leg muscle body part value, and multiple procedures are coded.

Extraction of multiple toenails are coded separately.

c. Multiple root operations with distinct objectives are performed on the same body part.

Example: Destruction of sigmoid lesion and bypass of sigmoid colon are coded separately.

AHA Coding Clinic® Reference Notation(s) — Coding Guideline B3.2c
Laminoplasty with two distinct objectives ....AHA 15:2Q:p20

d. The intended root operation is attempted using one approach, but is converted to a different approach.

Example: Laparoscopic cholecystectomy converted to an open cholecystectomy is coded as percutaneous endoscopic Inspection and open Resection.

AHA Coding Clinic® Reference Notation(s) — Coding Guideline B3.2d
Laparoscopic procedure converted to open ....AHA 15:1Q:p33

Discontinued procedures

B3.3

If the intended procedure is discontinued, code the procedure to the root operation performed. If a procedure is discontinued before any other root operation is performed, code the root operation Inspection of the body part or anatomical region inspected.

Example: A planned aortic valve replacement procedure is discontinued after the initial thoracotomy and before any incision is made in the heart muscle, when the patient becomes hemodynamically unstable. This procedure is coded as an open Inspection of the mediastinum.

AHA Coding Clinic® Reference Notation(s) — Coding Guideline B3.3
Discontinued coronary intervention ....AHA 15:3Q:p9
Discontinued procedure after angiogram ....AHA 15:3Q:p9

Biopsy procedures

B3.4a

Biopsy procedures are coded using the root operations Excision, Extraction, or Drainage and the qualifier Diagnostic.

Examples: Fine needle aspiration biopsy of fluid in the lung is coded to the root operation Drainage with the qualifier Diagnostic.

Biopsy of bone marrow is coded to the root operation Extraction with the qualifier Diagnostic.

Lymph node sampling for biospy is coded to the root operation Excision with the qualifier Diagnostic.

Biopsy followed by more definitive treatment

B3.4b

If a diagnostic Excision, Extraction, or Drainage procedure (biopsy) is followed by a more definitive procedure, such as Destruction, Excision or Resection at the same procedure site, both the biopsy and the more definitive treatment are coded.

Example: Biopsy of breast followed by partial mastectomy at the same procedure site, both the biopsy and the partial mastectomy procedure are coded.

Overlapping body layers

B3.5

If the root operations Excision, Repair or Inspection are performed on overlapping layers of the musculoskeletal system, the body part specifying the deepest layer is coded.

Example: Excisional debridement that includes skin and subcutaneous tissue and muscle is coded to the muscle body part.

AHA Coding Clinic® Reference Notation(s) — Coding Guideline B3.5
Deepest layer coded ....AHA 14:3Q:p14
Deepest layer coded - coccyx...AHA 15:3Q:p3-8
Obstetric perineal laceration repair ....AHA 16:1Q:p6-8

Bypass procedures

B3.6a

Bypass procedures are coded by identifying the body part bypassed "from" and the body part bypassed "to." The fourth character body part specifies the body part bypassed from, and the qualifier specifies the body part bypassed to.

Example: Bypass from stomach to jejunum, stomach is the body part and jejunum is the qualifier.

AHA Coding Clinic® Reference Notation(s) — Coding Guideline B3.6a
Creation of percutaneous cutaneoperitoneal fistula for peritoneal dialysis ......AHA 13:4Q:p126

B3.6b

~~Coronary arteries are classified by number of distinct sites treated, rather than number of coronary arteries or anatomic name of a coronary artery (e.g., left anterior descending).~~ Coronary artery bypass procedures are coded differently than other bypass procedures as described in the previous guideline. Rather than identifying the body part bypassed from, the body part identifies the number of coronary artery sites bypassed to, and the qualifier specifies the vessel bypassed from.

Example: Aortocoronary artery bypass of ~~one site on~~ the left anterior descending coronary artery and ~~one site on~~ the obtuse marginal coronary artery is classified in the body part axis of classification as two coronary ~~artery sites~~ arteries and the qualifier specifies the aorta as the body part bypassed from.

AHA Coding Clinic® Reference Notation(s) — Coding Guideline B3.6b
Distinct coronary lesion sites treated ....AHA 15:2Q:p3-5

B3.6c

If multiple coronary ~~artery sites~~ arteries are bypassed, a separate procedure is coded for each coronary artery ~~site~~ that uses a different device and/or qualifier.

Example: Aortocoronary artery bypass and internal mammary coronary artery bypass are coded separately.

Control vs. more definitive root operations

B3.7

The root operation Control is defined as, "Stopping, or attempting to stop, postprocedural or other acute bleeding." If an attempt to stop postprocedural or other acute bleeding is initially unsuccessful, and to stop the bleeding requires performing any of the definitive root operations Bypass, Detachment, Excision, Extraction, Reposition, Replacement, or Resection, then that root operation is coded instead of Control.

Example: Resection of spleen to stop ~~postprocedural~~ bleeding is coded to Resection instead of Control.

Excision vs. Resection

B3.8

PCS contains specific body parts for anatomical subdivisions of a body part, such as lobes of the lungs or liver and regions of the intestine. Resection of the specific body part is coded whenever all of the body part is cut out or off, rather than coding Excision of a less specific body part.

Example: Left upper lung lobectomy is coded to Resection of Upper Lung Lobe, Left rather than Excision of Lung, Left.

Excision for graft

B3.9

If an autograft is obtained from a different ~~body part~~ procedure site in order to complete the objective of the procedure, a separate procedure is coded.

Example: Coronary bypass with excision of saphenous vein graft, excision of saphenous vein is coded separately.

AHA Coding Clinic® Reference Notation(s) — Coding Guideline B3.9
Harvesting of fat graft from abdomen ....AHA 14:3Q:p22

Fusion procedures of the spine

B3.10a

The body part coded for a spinal vertebral joint(s) rendered immobile by a spinal fusion procedure is classified by the level of the spine (e.g. thoracic). There are distinct body part values for a single vertebral joint and for multiple vertebral joints at each spinal level.

Example: Body part values specify Lumbar Vertebral Joint, Lumbar Vertebral Joints, 2 or More and Lumbosacral Vertebral Joint.

AHA Coding Clinic® Reference Notation(s) — Coding Guideline B3.10a
Fusion, level of spine ....AHA 13:1Q:p29
Fusion of multiple vertebral joints..AHA 13:1Q:p21

B3.10b

If multiple vertebral joints are fused, a separate procedure is coded for each vertebral joint that uses a different device and/or qualifier.

Example: Fusion of lumbar vertebral joint, posterior approach, anterior column and fusion of lumbar vertebral joint, posterior approach, posterior column are coded separately.

B3.10c

Combinations of devices and materials are often used on a vertebral joint to render the joint immobile. When combinations of devices are used on the same vertebral joint, the device value coded for the procedure is as follows:

- If an interbody fusion device is used to render the joint immobile (alone or containing other material like bone graft), the procedure is coded with the device value Interbody Fusion Device
- If bone graft is the *only* device used to render the joint immobile, the procedure is coded with the device value Nonautologous Tissue Substitute or Autologous Tissue Substitute
- If a mixture of autologous and nonautologous bone graft (with or without biological or synthetic extenders or binders) is used to render the joint immobile, code the procedure with the device value Autologous Tissue Substitute

Examples: Fusion of a vertebral joint using a cage style interbody fusion device containing morsellized bone graft is coded to the device Interbody Fusion Device.

Fusion of a vertebral joint using a bone dowel interbody fusion device made of cadaver bone and packed with a mixture of local morsellized bone and demineralized bone matrix is coded to the device Interbody Fusion Device.

© 2016 Channel Publishing, Ltd.

B3.10c – *Examples: — continued*

Fusion of a vertebral joint using both autologous bone graft and bone bank bone graft is coded to the device Autologous Tissue Substitute.

<u>AHA Coding Clinic® Reference Notation(s) — Coding Guideline B3.10c</u>
Interbody fusion device...AHA 13:1Q:p29
Bone graft with mixture of autologous and nonautologous bone ....AHA 13:3Q:p25
Fusion of multiple vertebral joints...AHA 13:1Q:p21

Inspection procedures

B3.11a

Inspection of a body part(s) performed in order to achieve the objective of a procedure is not coded separately.

Example: Fiberoptic bronchoscopy performed for irrigation of bronchus, only the irrigation procedure is coded.

B3.11b

If multiple tubular body parts are inspected, the most distal body part (the body part furthest from the starting point of the inspection) is coded. If multiple non-tubular body parts in a region are inspected, the body part that specifies the entire area inspected is coded.

Examples: Cystoureteroscopy with inspection of bladder and ureters is coded to the ureter body part value. Exploratory laparotomy with general inspection of abdominal contents is coded to the peritoneal cavity body part value.

B3.11c

When both an Inspection procedure and another procedure are performed on the same body part during the same episode, if the Inspection procedure is performed using a different approach than the other procedure, the Inspection procedure is coded separately.

Example: Endoscopic Inspection of the duodenum is coded separately when open Excision of the duodenum is performed during the same procedural episode.

Occlusion vs. Restriction for vessel embolization procedures

B3.12

If the objective of an embolization procedure is to completely close a vessel, the root operation Occlusion is coded. If the objective of an embolization procedure is to narrow the lumen of a vessel, the root operation Restriction is coded.

Examples: Tumor embolization is coded to the root operation Occlusion, because the objective of the procedure is to cut off the blood supply to the vessel. Embolization of a cerebral aneurysm is coded to the root operation Restriction, because the objective of the procedure is not to close off the vessel entirely, but to narrow the lumen of the vessel at the site of the aneurysm where it is abnormally wide.

Release procedures

B3.13

In the root operation Release, the body part value coded is the body part being freed and not the tissue being manipulated or cut to free the body part.

Example: Lysis of intestinal adhesions is coded to the specific intestine body part value.

<u>AHA Coding Clinic® Reference Notation(s) — Coding Guideline B3.13</u>
Lysis of adhesions, integral or code separately.......................AHA 14:1Q:p3

Release vs. Division

B3.14

If the sole objective of the procedure is freeing a body part without cutting the body part, the root operation is Release. If the sole objective of the procedure is separating or transecting a body part, the root operation is Division.

Examples: Freeing a nerve root from surrounding scar tissue to relieve pain is coded to the root operation Release.
Severing a nerve root to relieve pain is coded to the root operation Division.

Reposition for fracture treatment

B3.15

Reduction of a displaced fracture is coded to the root operation Reposition and the application of a cast or splint in conjunction with the Reposition procedure is not coded separately. Treatment of a nondisplaced fracture is coded to the procedure performed.

Examples: Casting of a nondisplaced fracture is coded to the root operation Immobilization in the Placement section.
Putting a pin in a nondisplaced fracture is coded to the root operation Insertion.

Transplantation vs. Administration

B3.16

Putting in a mature and functioning living body part taken from another individual or animal is coded to the root operation Transplantation. Putting in autologous or nonautologous cells is coded to the Administration section.

Example: Putting in autologous or nonautologous bone marrow, pancreatic islet cells or stem cells is coded to the Administration section.

B4. Body Part

General guidelines

B4.1a

If a procedure is performed on a portion of a body part that does not have a separate body part value, code the body part value corresponding to the whole body part.

Example: A procedure performed on the alveolar process of the mandible is coded to the mandible body part.

B4.1b

If the prefix "peri" is combined with a body part to identify the site of the procedure, and the site of the procedure is not further specified, then the procedure is coded to the body part named. This guideline applies only when a more specific body part value is not available.

Examples: A procedure site identified as perirenal is coded to the kidney body part when the site of the procedure is not further specified.

A procedure site described in the documentation as peri-urethral, and the documentation also indicates that it is the vulvar tissue and not the urethral tissue that is the site of the procedure, then the procedure is coded to the vulva body part.

AHA Coding Clinic® Reference Notation(s) — Coding Guideline B4.1b

Catheter ablation of peripulmonary veins to target the conduction pathway
of left atrium ....AHA 14:4Q:p47
Periurethral obstetric laceration repair ....AHA 14:4Q:p18

Branches of body parts

B4.2

Where a specific branch of a body part does not have its own body part value in PCS, the body part is typically coded to the closest proximal branch that has a specific body part value. In the cardiovascular body systems, if a general body part is available in the correct root operation table, and coding to a proximal branch would require assigning a code in a different body system, the procedure is coded using the general body part value.

Examples: A procedure performed on the mandibular branch of the trigeminal nerve is coded to the trigeminal nerve body part value.

Occlusion of the bronchial artery is coded to the body part value Upper Artery in the body system Upper Arteries, and not to the body part value Thoracic Aorta, Descending in the body system Heart and Great Vessels.

Bilateral body part values

B4.3

Bilateral body part values are available for a limited number of body parts. If the identical procedure is performed on contralateral body parts, and a bilateral body part value exists for that body part, a single procedure is coded using the bilateral body part value. If no bilateral body part value exists, each procedure is coded separately using the appropriate body part value.

Examples: The identical procedure performed on both fallopian tubes is coded once using the body part value Fallopian Tubes, Bilateral.

The identical procedure performed on both knee joints is coded twice using the body part values Knee Joint, Right and Knee Joint, Left.

AHA Coding Clinic® Reference Notation(s) — Coding Guideline B4.3

Repair of midline diaphragm (paraesophageal) hernia ....AHA 14:3Q:p28
Removal of bilateral nonviable TRAM flap..AHA 16:2Q:p27

Coronary arteries

B4.4

The coronary arteries are classified as a single body part that is further specified by number of ~~sites~~ arteries treated. ~~and not by name or number of arteries.~~ One procedure code specifying multiple arteries is used when the same procedure is performed, including the same device and qualifier values. ~~Separate body part values are used to specify the number of sites treated when the same procedure is performed on multiple sites in the coronary arteries.~~

Examples: Angioplasty of two distinct ~~sites in the left anterior descending coronary artery~~ coronary arteries with placement of two stents is coded as Dilation of Coronary Arteries, Two ~~Sites~~ Arteries, with Two Intraluminal Devices.

Angioplasty of two distinct ~~sites in the left anterior descending coronary artery~~ coronary arteries, one with stent placed and one without, is coded separately as Dilation of Coronary Artery, One ~~Site~~ Artery with Intraluminal Device, and Dilation of Coronary Artery, One ~~Site~~ Artery with no device.

Tendons, ligaments, bursae and fascia near a joint

B4.5

Procedures performed on tendons, ligaments, bursae and fascia supporting a joint are coded to the body part in the respective body system that is the focus of the procedure. Procedures performed on joint structures themselves are coded to the body part in the joint body systems.

Examples: Repair of the anterior cruciate ligament of the knee is coded to the knee bursa and ligament body part in the bursae and ligaments body system.

Knee arthroscopy with shaving of articular cartilage is coded to the knee joint body part in the Lower Joints body system.

Skin, subcutaneous tissue and fascia overlying a joint

B4.6

If a procedure is performed on the skin, subcutaneous tissue or fascia overlying a joint, the procedure is coded to the following body part:
- Shoulder is coded to Upper Arm
- Elbow is coded to Lower Arm
- Wrist is coded to Lower Arm
- Hip is coded to Upper Leg
- Knee is coded to Lower Leg
- Ankle is coded to Foot

Fingers and toes

B4.7

If a body system does not contain a separate body part value for fingers, procedures performed on the fingers are coded to the body part value for the hand. If a body system does not contain a separate body part value for toes, procedures performed on the toes are coded to the body part value for the foot.

Example: Excision of finger muscle is coded to one of the hand muscle body part values in the Muscles body system.

Upper and lower intestinal tract

B4.8

In the Gastrointestinal body system, the general body part values Upper Intestinal Tract and Lower Intestinal Tract are provided as an option for the root operations Change, Inspection, Removal and Revision. Upper Intestinal Tract includes the portion of the gastrointestinal tract from the esophagus down to and including the duodenum, and Lower Intestinal Tract includes the portion of the gastrointestinal tract from the jejunum down to and including the rectum and anus.

Example: In the root operation Change table, change of a device in the jejunum is coded using the body part Lower Intestinal Tract.

B5. Approach

Open approach with percutaneous endoscopic assistance

B5.2

Procedures performed using the open approach with percutaneous endoscopic assistance are coded to the approach Open.

Example: Laparoscopic-assisted sigmoidectomy is coded to the approach Open.

External approach

B5.3a

Procedures performed within an orifice on structures that are visible without the aid of any instrumentation are coded to the approach External.

Example: Resection of tonsils is coded to the approach External.

B5.3b

Procedures performed indirectly by the application of external force through the intervening body layers are coded to the approach External.

Example: Closed reduction of fracture is coded to the approach External.

Percutaneous procedure via device

B5.4

Procedures performed percutaneously via a device placed for the procedure are coded to the approach Percutaneous.

Example: Fragmentation of kidney stone performed via percutaneous nephrostomy is coded to the approach Percutaneous.

B6. Device

General guidelines

B6.1a

A device is coded only if a device remains after the procedure is completed. If no device remains, the device value No Device is coded.

B6.1b

Materials such as sutures, ligatures, radiological markers and temporary post-operative wound drains are considered integral to the performance of a procedure and are not coded as devices.

AHA Coding Clinic® Reference Notation(s) — Coding Guideline B6.1b
Bronchoscopic placement of fiducial marker...AHA 14:1Q:p20
Fluoroscopic guided fiducial marker placement ....AHA 14:1Q:p20

B6.1c

Procedures performed on a device only and not on a body part are specified in the root operations Change, Irrigation, Removal and Revision, and are coded to the procedure performed.

Example: Irrigation of percutaneous nephrostomy tube is coded to the root operation Irrigation of indwelling device in the Administration section.

AHA Coding Clinic® Reference Notation(s) — Coding Guideline B6.1c
Replacement of arterial conduit is not coded as Removal of device ....AHA 14:3Q:p30

Drainage device

B6.2

A separate procedure to put in a drainage device is coded to the root operation Drainage with the device value Drainage Device.

Obstetric Section Guidelines (Section 1)

C. Obstetrics Section

Products of conception

C1

Procedures performed on the products of conception are coded to the Obstetrics section. Procedures performed on the pregnant female other than the products of conception are coded to the appropriate root operation in the Medical and Surgical section.

Example: Amniocentesis is coded to the products of conception body part in the Obstetrics section. Repair of obstetric urethral laceration is coded to the urethra body part in the Medical and Surgical section.

Procedures following delivery or abortion

C2

Procedures performed following a delivery or abortion for curettage of the endometrium or evacuation of retained products of conception are all coded in the Obstetrics section, to the root operation Extraction and the body part Products of Conception, Retained. Diagnostic or therapeutic dilation and curettage performed during times other than the postpartum or post-abortion period are all coded in the Medical and Surgical section, to the root operation Extraction and the body part Endometrium.

New Technology Section Guidelines (Section X)

D. New Technology Section

General guidelines

D1

Section X codes are standalone codes. They are not supplemental codes. Section X codes fully represent the specific procedure described in the code title, and do not require any additional codes from other sections of ICD-10-PCS. When section X contains a code title which describes a specific new technology procedure, only that X code is reported for the procedure. There is no need to report a broader, non-specific code in another section of ICD-10-PCS.

Example: XW04321 Introduction of Ceftazidime-Avibactam Anti-infective into Central Vein, Percutaneous Approach, New Technology Group 1, can be coded to indicate that Ceftazidime-Avibactam Anti-infective was administered via a central vein. A separate code from table 3E0 in the Administration section of ICD-10-PCS is not coded in addition to this code.

Selection of Principal Procedure

Selection of Principal Procedure

The following instructions should be applied in the selection of principal procedure and clarification on the importance of the relation to the principal diagnosis when more than one procedure is performed:

1. Procedure performed for definitive treatment of both principal diagnosis and secondary diagnosis.
   a. Sequence procedure performed for definitive treatment most related to principal diagnosis as principal procedure.
2. Procedure performed for definitive treatment and diagnostic procedures performed for both principal and secondary diagnosis.
   a. Sequence procedure performed for definitive treatment most related to principal diagnosis as principal procedure.
3. A diagnostic procedure was performed for the principal diagnosis and a procedure is performed for definitive treatment of a secondary diagnosis.
   a. Sequence diagnostic procedure as principal procedure, since the procedure most related to the principal diagnosis takes precedence.
4. No procedures performed that are related to principal diagnosis; procedures performed for definitive treatment and diagnostic procedures were performed for secondary diagnosis.
   a. Sequence procedure performed for definitive treatment of secondary diagnosis as principal procedure, since there are no procedures (definitive or nondefinitive treatment) related to principal diagnosis.

<u>AHA Coding Clinic® Reference Notation(s) — Coding Guideline Selection of Principal Procedure</u>
Sequencing of mechanical ventilation with other procedures ....AHA 14:4Q:p11

© 2016 Channel Publishing, Ltd.

A

3f (Aortic) Bioprosthesis valve
  use Zooplastic Tissue in Heart and Great Vessels
Abdominal aortic plexus
  use Nerve, Abdominal Sympathetic
Abdominal esophagus
  use Esophagus, Lower
Abdominohysterectomy
  see Resection, Cervix **0UTC**-
  see Resection, Uterus **0UT9**-
Abdominoplasty
  see Alteration, Abdominal Wall **0W0F**-
  see Repair, Abdominal Wall **0WQF**-
  see Supplement, Abdominal Wall **0WUF**-
Abductor hallucis muscle
  use Muscle, Foot, Left
  use Muscle, Foot, Right
AbioCor® Total Replacement Heart
  use Synthetic Substitute
Ablation *see* Destruction
Abortion
  Products of Conception **10A0**-
    Abortifacient **10A07ZX**
    Laminaria **10A07ZW**
    Vacuum **10A07Z6**
Abrasion *see* Extraction
Absolute Pro Vascular (OTW) Self-Expanding Stent System
  use Intraluminal Device
Accessory cephalic vein
  use Vein, Cephalic, Left
  use Vein, Cephalic, Right
Accessory obturator nerve
  use Nerve, Lumbar Plexus
Accessory phrenic nerve
  use Nerve, Phrenic
Accessory spleen
  use Spleen
Acculink (RX) Carotid Stent System
  use Intraluminal Device
Acellular Hydrated Dermis
  use Nonautologous Tissue Substitute
Acetabular cup
  use Liner in Lower Joints
Acetabulectomy
  see Excision, Lower Bones **0QB**-
  see Resection, Lower Bones **0QT**-
Acetabulofemoral joint
  use Joint, Hip, Left
  use Joint, Hip, Right
Acetabuloplasty
  see Repair, Lower Bones **0QQ**-
  see Replacement, Lower Bones **0QR**-
  see Supplement, Lower Bones **0QU**-
Achilles tendon
  use Tendon, Lower Leg, Left
  use Tendon, Lower Leg, Right
Achillorrhaphy *see* Repair, Tendons **0LQ**-
Achillotenotomy, achillotomy
  see Division, Tendons **0L8**-
  see Drainage, Tendons **0L9**-
Acromioclavicular ligament
  use Bursa and Ligament, Shoulder, Left
  use Bursa and Ligament, Shoulder, Right
Acromion (process)
  use Scapula, Left
  use Scapula, Right
Acromionectomy
  see Excision, Upper Joints **0RB**-
  see Resection, Upper Joints **0RT**-
Acromioplasty
  see Repair, Upper Joints **0RQ**-
  see Replacement, Upper Joints **0RR**-
  see Supplement, Upper Joints **0RU**-

Activa PC neurostimulator
  use Stimulator Generator, Multiple Array in **0JH**-
Activa RC neurostimulator
  use Stimulator Generator, Multiple Array Rechargeable in **0JH**-
Activa SC neurostimulator
  use Stimulator Generator, Single Array in **0JH**-
Activities of Daily Living Assessment F02-
Activities of Daily Living Treatment F08-
ACUITY™ Steerable Lead
  use Cardiac Lead, Defibrillator in **02H**-
  use Cardiac Lead, Pacemaker in **02H**-
Acupuncture
  Breast
    Anesthesia **8E0H300**
    No Qualifier **8E0H30Z**
  Integumentary System
    Anesthesia **8E0H300**
    No Qualifier **8E0H30Z**
Adductor brevis muscle
  use Muscle, Upper Leg, Left
  use Muscle, Upper Leg, Right
Adductor hallucis muscle
  use Muscle, Foot, Left
  use Muscle, Foot, Right
Adductor longus muscle
  use Muscle, Upper Leg, Left
  use Muscle, Upper Leg, Right
Adductor magnus muscle
  use Muscle, Upper Leg, Left
  use Muscle, Upper Leg, Right
Adenohypophysis
  use Gland, Pituitary
Adenoidectomy
  see Excision, Adenoids **0CBQ**-
  see Resection, Adenoids **0CTQ**-
Adenoidotomy *see* Drainage, Adenoids **0C9Q**-
Adhesiolysis *see* Release
Administration
  Blood products *see* Transfusion
  Other substance *see* Introduction of substance in or on
Adrenalectomy
  see Excision, Endocrine System **0GB**-
  see Resection, Endocrine System **0GT**-
Adrenalorrhaphy *see* Repair, Endocrine System **0GQ**-
Adrenalotomy *see* Drainage, Endocrine System **0G9**-
Advancement
  see Reposition
  see Transfer
Advisa (MRI)
  use Pacemaker, Dual Chamber in **0JH**-
AFX® Endovascular AAA System
  use Intraluminal Device
AIGISRx Antibacterial Envelope
  use Anti-Infective Envelope
Alar ligament of axis
  use Bursa and Ligament, Head and Neck
Alimentation *see* Introduction of substance in or on
Alteration
  Abdominal Wall **0W0F**-
  Ankle Region
    Left **0Y0L**-
    Right **0Y0K**-
  Arm
    Lower
      Left **0X0F**-
      Right **0X0D**-
    Upper
      Left **0X09**-
      Right **0X08**-
  Axilla
    Left **0X05**-
    Right **0X04**-

Alteration — *continued*
  Back
    Lower **0W0L**-
    Upper **0W0K**-
  Breast
    Bilateral **0H0V**-
    Left **0H0U**-
    Right **0H0T**-
  Buttock
    Left **0Y01**-
    Right **0Y00**-
  Chest Wall **0W08**-
  Ear
    Bilateral **0902**-
    Left **0901**-
    Right **0900**-
  Elbow Region
    Left **0X0C**-
    Right **0X0B**-
  Extremity
    Lower
      Left **0Y0B**-
      Right **0Y09**-
    Upper
      Left **0X07**-
      Right **0X06**-
  Eyelid
    Lower
      Left **080R**-
      Right **080Q**-
    Upper
      Left **080P**-
      Right **080N**-
  Face **0W02**-
  Head **0W00**-
  Jaw
    Lower **0W05**-
    Upper **0W04**-
  Knee Region
    Left **0Y0G**-
    Right **0Y0F**-
  Leg
    Lower
      Left **0Y0J**-
      Right **0Y0H**-
    Upper
      Left **0Y0D**-
      Right **0Y0C**-
  Lip
    Lower **0C01X**-
    Upper **0C00X**-
  Neck **0W06**-
  Nose **090K**-
  Perineum
    Female **0W0N**-
    Male **0W0M**-
  Shoulder Region
    Left **0X03**-
    Right **0X02**-
  Subcutaneous Tissue and Fascia
    Abdomen **0J08**-
    Back **0J07**-
    Buttock **0J09**-
    Chest **0J06**-
    Face **0J01**-
    Lower Arm
      Left **0J0H**-
      Right **0J0G**-
    Lower Leg
      Left **0J0P**-
      Right **0J0N**-
    Neck
      Anterior **0J04**-
      Posterior **0J05**-
    Upper Arm
      Left **0J0F**-
      Right **0J0D**-
    Upper Leg
      Left **0J0M**-
      Right **0J0L**-
  Wrist Region
    Left **0X0H**-
    Right **0X0G**-

Alveolar process of mandible
  use Mandible, Left
  use Mandible, Right
Alveolar process of maxilla
  use Maxilla, Left
  use Maxilla, Right
Alveolectomy
  see Excision, Head and Facial Bones **0NB**-
  see Resection, Head and Facial Bones **0NT**-
Alveoloplasty
  see Repair, Head and Facial Bones **0NQ**-
  see Replacement, Head and Facial Bones **0NR**-
  see Supplement, Head and Facial Bones **0NU**-
Alveolotomy
  see Division, Head and Facial Bones **0N8**-
  see Drainage, Head and Facial Bones **0N9**-
Ambulatory cardiac monitoring 4A12X45
Amniocentesis *see* Drainage, Products of Conception **1090**-
Amnioinfusion *see* Introduction of substance in or on, Products of Conception **3E0E**-
Amnioscopy 10J08ZZ
Amniotomy *see* Drainage, Products of Conception **1090**-
AMPLATZER® Muscular VSD Occluder
  use Synthetic Substitute
Amputation *see* Detachment
AMS 800® Urinary Control System
  use Artificial Sphincter in Urinary System
Anal orifice
  use Anus
Analog radiography *see* Plain Radiography
Analog radiology *see* Plain Radiography
Anastomosis *see* Bypass
Anatomical snuffbox
  use Muscle, Lower Arm and Wrist, Left
  use Muscle, Lower Arm and Wrist, Right
Andexanet Alfa, Factor Xa Inhibitor Reversal Agent XW0-
AneuRx® AAA Advantage®
  use Intraluminal Device
Angiectomy
  see Excision, Heart and Great Vessels **02B**-
  see Excision, Lower Arteries **04B**-
  see Excision, Lower Veins **06B**-
  see Excision, Upper Arteries **03B**-
  see Excision, Upper Veins **05B**-
Angiocardiography
  Combined right and left heart *see* Fluoroscopy, Heart, Right and Left **B216**-
  Left Heart *see* Fluoroscopy, Heart, Left **B215**-
  Right Heart *see* Fluoroscopy, Heart, Right **B214**-
  SPY system intravascular fluorescence *see* Monitoring, Physiological Systems **4A1**-
Angiography
  see Plain Radiography, Heart **B20**-
  see Fluoroscopy, Heart **B21**-

Angioplasty
see Dilation, Heart and Great Vessels **027-**
see Dilation, Lower Arteries **047-**
see Dilation, Upper Arteries **037-**
see Repair, Heart and Great Vessels **02Q-**
see Repair, Lower Arteries **04Q-**
see Repair, Upper Arteries **03Q-**
see Replacement, Heart and Great Vessels **02R-**
see Replacement, Lower Arteries **04R-**
see Replacement, Upper Arteries **03R-**
see Supplement, Heart and Great Vessels **02U-**
see Supplement, Lower Arteries **04U-**
see Supplement, Upper Arteries **03U-**
Angiorrhaphy
see Repair, Heart and Great Vessels **02Q-**
see Repair, Lower Arteries **04Q-**
see Repair, Upper Arteries **03Q-**
Angioscopy
02JY4ZZ
03JY4ZZ
04JY4ZZ
Angiotripsy
see Occlusion, Lower Arteries **04L-**
see Occlusion, Upper Arteries **03L-**
Angular artery
use Artery, Face
Angular vein
use Vein, Face, Left
use Vein, Face, Right
Annular ligament
use Bursa and Ligament, Elbow, Left
use Bursa and Ligament, Elbow, Right
Annuloplasty
see Repair, Heart and Great Vessels **02Q-**
see Supplement, Heart and Great Vessels **02U-**
Annuloplasty ring
use Synthetic Substitute
Anoplasty
see Repair, Anus **0DQQ-**
see Supplement, Anus **0DUQ-**
Anorectal junction
use Rectum
Anoscopy 0DJD8ZZ
Ansa cervicalis
use Nerve, Cervical Plexus
Antabuse therapy HZ93ZZZ
Antebrachial fascia
use Subcutaneous Tissue and Fascia, Lower Arm, Left
use Subcutaneous Tissue and Fascia, Lower Arm, Right
Anterior (pectoral) lymph node
use Lymphatic, Axillary, Left
use Lymphatic, Axillary, Right
Anterior cerebral artery
use Artery, Intracranial
Anterior cerebral vein
use Vein, Intracranial
Anterior choroidal artery
use Artery, Intracranial
Anterior circumflex humeral artery
use Artery, Axillary, Left
use Artery, Axillary, Right
Anterior communicating artery
use Artery, Intracranial
Anterior cruciate ligament (ACL)
use Bursa and Ligament, Knee, Left
use Bursa and Ligament, Knee, Right
Anterior crural nerve
use Nerve, Femoral

Anterior facial vein
use Vein, Face, Left
use Vein, Face, Right
Anterior intercostal artery
use Artery, Internal Mammary, Left
use Artery, Internal Mammary, Right
Anterior interosseous nerve
use Nerve, Median
Anterior lateral malleolar artery
use Artery, Anterior Tibial, Left
use Artery, Anterior Tibial, Right
Anterior lingual gland
use Gland, Minor Salivary
Anterior medial malleolar artery
use Artery, Anterior Tibial, Left
use Artery, Anterior Tibial, Right
Anterior spinal artery
use Artery, Vertebral, Left
use Artery, Vertebral, Right
Anterior tibial recurrent artery
use Artery, Anterior Tibial, Left
use Artery, Anterior Tibial, Right
Anterior ulnar recurrent artery
use Artery, Ulnar, Left
use Artery, Ulnar, Right
Anterior vagal trunk
use Nerve, Vagus
Anterior vertebral muscle
use Muscle, Neck, Left
use Muscle, Neck, Right
Antihelix
use Ear, External, Bilateral
use Ear, External, Left
use Ear, External, Right
Antimicrobial envelope
use Anti-Infective Envelope
Antitragus
use Ear, External, Bilateral
use Ear, External, Left
use Ear, External, Right
Antrostomy see Drainage, Ear, Nose, Sinus **099-**
Antrotomy see Drainage, Ear, Nose, Sinus **099-**
Antrum of Highmore
use Sinus, Maxillary, Left
use Sinus, Maxillary, Right
Aortic annulus
use Valve, Aortic
Aortic arch
use Thoracic Aorta, Ascending/Arch
Aortic intercostal artery
use Upper Artery
Aortography
see Fluoroscopy, Lower Arteries **B41-**
see Fluoroscopy, Upper Arteries **B31-**
see Plain Radiography, Lower Arteries **B40-**
see Plain Radiography, Upper Arteries **B30-**
Aortoplasty
see Repair, Aorta, Abdominal **04Q0-**
see Repair, Aorta, Thoracic, Ascending/Arch **02QX-**
see Repair, Aorta, Thoracic, Descending **02QW-**
see Replacement, Aorta, Abdominal **04R0-**
see Replacement, Aorta, Thoracic, Ascending/Arch **02RX-**
see Replacement, Aorta, Thoracic, Descending **02RW-**
see Supplement, Aorta, Abdominal **04U0-**
see Supplement, Aorta, Thoracic, Ascending/Arch **02UX-**
see Supplement, Aorta, Thoracic, Descending **02UW-**

Apical (subclavicular) lymph node
use Lymphatic, Axillary, Left
use Lymphatic, Axillary, Right
Apneustic center
use Pons
Appendectomy
see Excision, Appendix **0DBJ-**
see Resection, Appendix **0DTJ-**
Appendicolysis see Release, Appendix **0DNJ-**
Appendicotomy see Drainage, Appendix **0D9J-**
Application see Introduction of substance in or on
Aquapheresis 6A550Z3
Aqueduct of Sylvius
use Cerebral Ventricle
Aqueous humour
use Anterior Chamber, Left
use Anterior Chamber, Right
Arachnoid mater, intracranial
use Cerebral Meninges
Arachnoid mater, spinal
use Spinal Meninges
Arcuate artery
use Artery, Foot, Left
use Artery, Foot, Right
Areola
use Nipple, Left
use Nipple, Right
AROM (artificial rupture of membranes) 10907ZC
Arterial canal (duct)
use Artery, Pulmonary, Left
Arterial pulse tracing see Measurement, Arterial **4A03-**
Arteriectomy see Excision, Heart and Great Vessels **02B-**
see Excision, Lower Arteries **04B-**
see Excision, Upper Arteries **03B-**
Arteriography
see Fluoroscopy, Heart **B21-**
see Fluoroscopy, Lower Arteries **B41-**
see Fluoroscopy, Upper Arteries **B31-**
see Plain Radiography, Heart **B20-**
see Plain Radiography, Lower Arteries **B40-**
see Plain Radiography, Upper Arteries **B30-**
Arterioplasty
see Repair, Heart and Great Vessels **02Q-**
see Repair, Lower Arteries **04Q-**
see Repair, Upper Arteries **03Q-**
see Replacement, Heart and Great Vessels **02R-**
see Replacement, Lower Arteries **04R-**
see Replacement, Upper Arteries **03R-**
see Supplement, Heart and Great Vessels **02U-**
see Supplement, Lower Arteries **04U-**
see Supplement, Upper Arteries **03U-**
Arteriorrhaphy
see Repair, Heart and Great Vessels **02Q-**
see Repair, Lower Arteries **04Q-**
see Repair, Upper Arteries **03Q-**
Arterioscopy
see Inspection, Artery, Lower **04JY-**
see Inspection, Artery, Upper **03JY-**
see Inspection, Great Vessel **02JY-**
Arthrectomy
see Excision, Lower Joints **0SB-**
see Excision, Upper Joints **0RB-**
see Resection, Lower Joints **0ST-**
see Resection, Upper Joints **0RT-**
Arthrocentesis
see Drainage, Lower Joints **0S9-**
see Drainage, Upper Joints **0R9-**

Arthrodesis
see Fusion, Lower Joints **0SG-**
see Fusion, Upper Joints **0RG-**
Arthrography
see Plain Radiography, Non-Axial Lower Bones **BQ0-**
see Plain Radiography, Non-Axial Upper Bones **BP0-**
see Plain Radiography, Skull and Facial Bones **BN0-**
Arthrolysis
see Release, Lower Joints **0SN-**
see Release, Upper Joints **0RN-**
Arthropexy
see Repair, Lower Joints **0SQ-**
see Repair, Upper Joints **0RQ-**
see Reposition, Lower Joints **0SS-**
see Reposition, Upper Joints **0RS-**
Arthroplasty
see Repair, Lower Joints **0SQ-**
see Repair, Upper Joints **0RQ-**
see Replacement, Lower Joints **0SR-**
see Replacement, Upper Joints **0RR-**
see Supplement, Lower Joints **0SU-**
see Supplement, Upper Joints **0RU-**
Arthroscopy
see Inspection, Lower Joints **0SJ-**
see Inspection, Upper Joints **0RJ-**
Arthrotomy
see Drainage, Lower Joints **0S9-**
see Drainage, Upper Joints **0R9-**
Artificial anal sphincter (AAS)
use Artificial Sphincter in Gastrointestinal System
Artificial bowel sphincter (neosphincter)
use Artificial Sphincter in Gastrointestinal System
Artificial Sphincter
Insertion of device in
Anus **0DHQ-**
Bladder **0THB-**
Bladder Neck **0THC-**
Urethra **0THD-**
Removal of device from
Anus **0DPQ-**
Bladder **0TPB-**
Urethra **0TPD-**
Revision of device in
Anus **0DWQ-**
Bladder **0TWB-**
Urethra **0TWD-**
Artificial urinary sphincter (AUS)
use Artificial Sphincter in Urinary System
Aryepiglottic fold
use Larynx
Arytenoid cartilage
use Larynx
Arytenoid muscle
use Muscle, Neck, Left
use Muscle, Neck, Right
Arytenoidectomy see Excision, Larynx **0CBS-**
Arytenoidopexy
see Repair, Larynx **0CQS-**
Ascenda Intrathecal Catheter
use Infusion Device
Ascending aorta
use Thoracic Aorta, Ascending/Arch
Ascending palatine artery
use Artery, Face
Ascending pharyngeal artery
use Artery, External Carotid, Left
use Artery, External Carotid, Right
Aspiration, fine needle
Fluid or gas see Drainage
Tissue see Excision

Assessment
　Activities of daily living *see* Activities of Daily Living Assessment, Rehabilitation **F02**-
　Hearing *see* Hearing Assessment, Diagnostic Audiology **F13**-
　Hearing aid *see* Hearing Aid Assessment, Diagnostic Audiology **F14**-
　Intravascular perfusion, using indocyanine green (ICG) dye *see* Monitoring, Physiological Systems **4A1**-
　Motor function *see* Motor Function Assessment, Rehabilitation **F01**-
　Nerve function *see* Motor Function Assessment, Rehabilitation **F01**-
　Speech *see* Speech Assessment, Rehabilitation **F00**-
　Vestibular *see* Vestibular Assessment, Diagnostic Audiology **F15**-
　Vocational *see* Activities of Daily Living Treatment, Rehabilitation **F08**-
Assistance
　Cardiac
　　Continuous
　　　Balloon Pump **5A0**2210
　　　Impeller Pump **5A0**221D
　　　Other Pump **5A0**2216
　　　Pulsatile Compression **5A0**2215
　　Intermittent
　　　Balloon Pump **5A0**2110
　　　Impeller Pump **5A0**211D
　　　Other Pump **5A0**2116
　　　Pulsatile Compression **5A0**2115
　Circulatory
　　Continuous
　　　Hyperbaric **5A0**5221
　　　Supersaturated **5A0**522C
　　Intermittent
　　　Hyperbaric **5A0**5121
　　　Supersaturated **5A0**512C
　Respiratory
　　24-96 Consecutive Hours
　　　Continuous Negative Airway Pressure **5A0**9459
　　　Continuous Positive Airway Pressure **5A0**9457
　　　Intermittent Negative Airway Pressure **5A0**945B
　　　Intermittent Positive Airway Pressure **5A0**9458
　　　No Qualifier **5A0**945Z
　　Greater than 96 Consecutive Hours
　　　Continuous Negative Airway Pressure **5A0**9559
　　　Continuous Positive Airway Pressure **5A0**9557
　　　Intermittent Negative Airway Pressure **5A0**955B
　　　Intermittent Positive Airway Pressure **5A0**9558
　　　No Qualifier **5A0**955Z
　　Less than 24 Consecutive Hours
　　　Continuous Negative Airway Pressure **5A0**9359
　　　Continuous Positive Airway Pressure **5A0**9357
　　　Intermittent Negative Airway Pressure **5A0**935B
　　　Intermittent Positive Airway Pressure **5A0**9358
　　　No Qualifier **5A0**935Z
Assurant (Cobalt) stent
　use Intraluminal Device
Atherectomy
　see Extirpation, Heart and Great Vessels **02C**-
　see Extirpation, Lower Arteries **04C**-
　see Extirpation, Upper Arteries **03C**-

Atlantoaxial joint
　use Joint, Cervical Vertebral
Atmospheric Control 6A0Z-
Atrioseptoplasty
　see Repair, Heart and Great Vessels **02Q**-
　see Replacement, Heart and Great Vessels **02R**-
　see Supplement, Heart and Great Vessels **02U**-
Atrioventricular node
　use Conduction Mechanism
Atrium dextrum cordis
　use Atrium, Right
Atrium pulmonale
　use Atrium, Left
Attain Ability® lead
　use Cardiac Lead, Defibrillator in **02H**-
　use Cardiac Lead, Pacemaker in **02H**-
Attain StarFix® (OTW) lead
　use Cardiac Lead, Defibrillator in **02H**-
　use Cardiac Lead, Pacemaker in **02H**-
Audiology, diagnostic
　see Hearing Aid Assessment, Diagnostic Audiology **F14**-
　see Hearing Assessment, Diagnostic Audiology **F13**-
　see Vestibular Assessment, Diagnostic Audiology **F15**-
Audiometry *see* Hearing Assessment, Diagnostic Audiology **F13**-
Auditory tube
　use Eustachian Tube, Left
　use Eustachian Tube, Right
Auerbach's (myenteric) plexus
　use Nerve, Abdominal Sympathetic
Auricle
　use Ear, External, Bilateral
　use Ear, External, Left
　use Ear, External, Right
Auricularis muscle
　use Muscle, Head
Autograft
　use Autologous Tissue Substitute
Autologous artery graft
　use Autologous Arterial Tissue in Heart and Great Vessels
　use Autologous Arterial Tissue in Lower Arteries
　use Autologous Arterial Tissue in Lower Veins
　use Autologous Arterial Tissue in Upper Arteries
　use Autologous Arterial Tissue in Upper Veins
Autologous vein graft
　use Autologous Venous Tissue in Heart and Great Vessels
　use Autologous Venous Tissue in Lower Arteries
　use Autologous Venous Tissue in Lower Veins
　use Autologous Venous Tissue in Upper Arteries
　use Autologous Venous Tissue in Upper Veins
Autotransfusion *see* Transfusion
Autotransplant
　Adrenal tissue *see* Reposition, Endocrine System **0GS**-
　Kidney *see* Reposition, Urinary System **0TS**-
　Pancreatic tissue *see* Reposition, Pancreas **0FS**G-
　Parathyroid tissue *see* Reposition, Endocrine System **0GS**-
　Thyroid tissue *see* Reposition, Endocrine System **0GS**-
　Tooth *see* Reattachment, Mouth and Throat **0CM**-

Avulsion *see* Extraction
Axial Lumbar Interbody Fusion System
　use Interbody Fusion Device in Lower Joints
AxiaLIF® System
　use Interbody Fusion Device in Lower Joints
Axillary fascia
　use Subcutaneous Tissue and Fascia, Upper Arm, Left
　use Subcutaneous Tissue and Fascia, Upper Arm, Right
Axillary nerve
　use Nerve, Brachial Plexus

B

BAK/C® Interbody Cervical Fusion System
　use Interbody Fusion Device in Upper Joints
BAL (bronchial alveolar lavage), diagnostic
　see Drainage, Respiratory System **0B9**-
Balanoplasty
　see Repair, Penis **0VQ**S-
　see Supplement, Penis **0VU**S-
Balloon Pump
　Continuous, Output **5A0**2210
　Intermittent, Output **5A0**2110
Bandage, Elastic *see* Compression
Banding
　see Occlusion
　see Restriction
Bard® Composix® (E/X) (LP) mesh
　use Synthetic Substitute
Bard® Composix® Kugel® patch
　use Synthetic Substitute
Bard® Dulex™ mesh
　use Synthetic Substitute
Bard® Ventralex™ hernia patch
　use Synthetic Substitute
Barium swallow *see* Fluoroscopy, Gastrointestinal System **BD1**-
Baroreflex Activation Therapy® (BAT®)
　use Stimulator Generator in Subcutaneous Tissue and Fascia
　use Stimulator Lead in Upper Arteries
Bartholin's (greater vestibular) gland
　use Gland, Vestibular
Basal (internal) cerebral vein
　use Vein, Intracranial
Basal metabolic rate (BMR) *see* Measurement, Physiological Systems **4A0**Z-
Basal nuclei
　use Basal Ganglia
Base of tongue
　use Pharnyx
Basilar artery
　use Artery, Intracranial
Basis pontis
　use Pons
Beam Radiation
　Abdomen **DW0**3-
　　Intraoperative **DW0**33Z0
　Adrenal Gland **DG0**2-
　　Intraoperative **DG0**23Z0
　Bile Ducts **DF0**2-
　　Intraoperative **DF0**23Z0
　Bladder **DT0**2-
　　Intraoperative **DT0**23Z0
　Bone
　　Intraoperative **DP0**C3Z0
　　Other **DP0**C-
　Bone Marrow **D70**0-
　　Intraoperative **D70**03Z0
　Brain **D00**0-
　　Intraoperative **D00**03Z0
　Brain Stem **D00**1-
　　Intraoperative **D00**13Z0
　Breast
　　Left **DM0**0-
　　　Intraoperative **DM0**03Z0
　　Right **DM0**1-
　　　Intraoperative **DM0**13Z0
　Bronchus **DB0**1-
　　Intraoperative **DB0**13Z0
　Cervix **DU0**1-
　　Intraoperative **DU0**13Z0
　Chest **DW0**2-
　　Intraoperative **DW0**23Z0
　Chest Wall **DB0**7-
　　Intraoperative **DB0**73Z0

Beam Radiation — *continued*
Colon **DD05**-
  Intraoperative **DD05**3Z0
Diaphragm **DB08**-
  Intraoperative **DB08**3Z0
Duodenum **DD02**-
  Intraoperative **DD02**3Z0
Ear **D900**-
  Intraoperative **D900**3Z0
Esophagus **DD00**-
  Intraoperative **DD00**3Z0
Eye **D800**-
  Intraoperative **D800**3Z0
Femur **DP09**-
  Intraoperative **DP09**3Z0
Fibula **DP0B**-
  Intraoperative **DP0B**3Z0
Gallbladder **DF01**-
  Intraoperative **DF01**3Z0
Gland
  Adrenal **DG02**-
    Intraoperative **DG02**3Z0
  Parathyroid **DG04**-
    Intraoperative **DG04**3Z0
  Pituitary **DG00**-
    Intraoperative **DG00**3Z0
  Thyroid **DG05**-
    Intraoperative **DG05**3Z0
Glands
  Intraoperative **D906**3Z0
  Salivary **D906**-
Head and Neck **DW01**-
  Intraoperative **DW01**3Z0
Hemibody **DW04**-
  Intraoperative **DW04**3Z0
Humerus **DP06**-
  Intraoperative **DP06**3Z0
Hypopharynx **D903**-
  Intraoperative **D903**3Z0
Ileum **DD04**-
  Intraoperative **DD04**3Z0
Jejunum **DD03**-
  Intraoperative **DD03**3Z0
Kidney **DT00**-
  Intraoperative **DT00**3Z0
Larynx **D90B**-
  Intraoperative **D90B**3Z0
Liver **DF00**-
  Intraoperative **DF00**3Z0
Lung **DB02**-
  Intraoperative **DB02**3Z0
Lymphatics
  Abdomen **D706**-
    Intraoperative **D706**3Z0
  Axillary **D704**-
    Intraoperative **D704**3Z0
  Inguinal **D708**-
    Intraoperative **D708**3Z0
  Neck **D703**-
    Intraoperative **D703**3Z0
  Pelvis **D707**-
    Intraoperative **D707**3Z0
  Thorax **D705**-
    Intraoperative **D705**3Z0
Mandible **DP03**-
  Intraoperative **DP03**3Z0
Maxilla **DP02**-
  Intraoperative **DP02**3Z0
Mediastinum **DB06**-
  Intraoperative **DB06**3Z0
Mouth **D904**-
  Intraoperative **D904**3Z0
Nasopharynx **D90D**-
  Intraoperative **D90D**3Z0
Neck and Head **DW01**-
  Intraoperative **DW01**3Z0
Nerve
  Intraoperative **D007**3Z0
  Peripheral **D007**-
Nose **D901**-
  Intraoperative **D901**3Z0
Oropharynx **D90F**-
  Intraoperative **D90F**3Z0

Beam Radiation — *continued*
Ovary **DU00**-
  Intraoperative **DU00**3Z0
Palate
  Hard **D908**-
    Intraoperative **D908**3Z0
  Soft **D909**-
    Intraoperative **D909**3Z0
Pancreas **DF03**-
  Intraoperative **DF03**3Z0
Parathyroid Gland **DG04**-
  Intraoperative **DG04**3Z0
Pelvic Bones **DP08**-
  Intraoperative **DP08**3Z0
Pelvic Region **DW06**-
  Intraoperative **DW06**3Z0
Pineal Body **DG01**-
  Intraoperative **DG01**3Z0
Pituitary Gland **DG00**-
  Intraoperative **DG00**3Z0
Pleura **DB05**-
  Intraoperative **DB05**3Z0
Prostate **DV00**-
  Intraoperative **DV00**3Z0
Radius **DP07**-
  Intraoperative **DP07**3Z0
Rectum **DD07**-
  Intraoperative **DD07**3Z0
Rib **DP05**-
  Intraoperative **DP05**3Z0
Sinuses **D907**-
  Intraoperative **D907**3Z0
Skin
  Abdomen **DH08**-
    Intraoperative **DH08**3Z0
  Arm **DH04**-
    Intraoperative **DH04**3Z0
  Back **DH07**-
    Intraoperative **DH07**3Z0
  Buttock **DH09**-
    Intraoperative **DH09**3Z0
  Chest **DH06**-
    Intraoperative **DH06**3Z0
  Face **DH02**-
    Intraoperative **DH02**3Z0
  Leg **DH0B**-
    Intraoperative **DH0B**3Z0
  Neck **DH03**-
    Intraoperative **DH03**3Z0
Skull **DP00**-
  Intraoperative **DP00**3Z0
Spinal Cord **D006**-
  Intraoperative **D006**3Z0
Spleen **D702**-
  Intraoperative **D702**3Z0
Sternum **DP04**-
  Intraoperative **DP04**3Z0
Stomach **DD01**-
  Intraoperative **DD01**3Z0
Testis **DV01**-
  Intraoperative **DV01**3Z0
Thymus **D701**-
  Intraoperative **D701**3Z0
Thyroid Gland **DG05**-
  Intraoperative **DG05**3Z0
Tibia **DP0B**-
  Intraoperative **DP0B**3Z0
Tongue **D905**-
  Intraoperative **D905**3Z0
Trachea **DB00**-
  Intraoperative **DB00**3Z0
Ulna **DP07**-
  Intraoperative **DP07**3Z0
Ureter **DT01**-
  Intraoperative **DT01**3Z0
Urethra **DT03**-
  Intraoperative **DT03**3Z0
Uterus **DU02**-
  Intraoperative **DU02**3Z0
Whole Body **DW05**-
  Intraoperative **DW05**3Z0

Bedside swallow **F00**ZJWZ
Berlin Heart Ventricular Assist Device
  use Implantable Heart Assist System in Heart and Great Vessels
Biceps brachii muscle
  use Muscle, Upper Arm, Left
  use Muscle, Upper Arm, Right
Biceps femoris muscle
  use Muscle, Upper Leg, Left
  use Muscle, Upper Leg, Right
Bicipital aponeurosis
  use Subcutaneous Tissue and Fascia, Lower Arm, Left
  use Subcutaneous Tissue and Fascia, Lower Arm, Right
Bicuspid valve
  use Valve, Mitral
Bililite therapy *see* Ultraviolet Light Therapy, Skin **6A80**-
Bioactive embolization coil(s)
  use Intraluminal Device, Bioactive in Upper Arteries
Biofeedback **GZC9**ZZZ
Biopsy
  see Drainage with qualifier Diagnostic
  see Excision with qualifier Diagnostic
  Bone Marrow *see* Extraction with qualifier Diagnostic
BiPAP *see* Assistance, Respiratory **5A09**-
Bisection *see* Division
Biventricular external heart assist system
  use External Heart Assist System in Heart and Great Vessels
Blepharectomy
  see Excision, Eye **08B**-
  see Resection, Eye **08T**-
Blepharoplasty
  see Repair, Eye **08Q**-
  see Replacement, Eye **08R**-
  see Reposition, Eye **08S**-
  see Supplement, Eye **08U**-
Blepharorrhaphy *see* Repair, Eye **08Q**-
Blepharotomy *see* Drainage, Eye **089**-
Blinatumomab antineoplastic immunothrerapy XW0-
Block, Nerve, anesthetic injection 3E0T3CZ
Blood glucose monitoring system
  use Monitoring Device
Blood pressure *see* Measurement, Arterial **4A03**-
BMR (basal metabolic rate) *see* Measurement, Physiological Systems **4A0Z**-
Body of femur
  use Femoral Shaft, Left
  use Femoral Shaft, Right
Body of fibula
  use Fibula, Left
  use Fibula, Right
Bone anchored hearing device
  use Hearing Device, Bone Conduction in **09H**-
  use Hearing Device in Head and Facial Bones
Bone bank bone graft
  use Nonautologous Tissue Substitute
Bone growth stimulator
  Insertion of device in
    Bone
      Facial **0NHW**-
      Lower **0QHY**-
      Nasal **0NHB**-
      Upper **0PHY**-
      Skull **0NH0**-

Bone growth stimulator — *continued*
  Removal of device from
    Bone
      Facial **0NPW**-
      Lower **0QPY**-
      Nasal **0NPB**-
      Upper **0PPY**-
      Skull **0NP0**-
  Revision of device in
    Bone
      Facial **0NWW**-
      Lower **0QWY**-
      Nasal **0NWB**-
      Upper **0PWY**-
      Skull **0NW0**-
Bone marrow transplant *see* Transfusion, Circulatory **302**-
Bone morphogenetic protein 2 (BMP 2)
  use Recombinant Bone Morphogenetic Protein
Bone screw (interlocking) (lag) (pedicle) (recessed)
  use Internal Fixation Device in Head and Facial Bones
  use Internal Fixation Device in Lower Bones
  use Internal Fixation Device in Upper Bones
Bony labyrinth
  use Ear, Inner, Left
  use Ear, Inner, Right
Bony orbit
  use Orbit, Left
  use Orbit, Right
Bony vestibule
  use Ear, Inner, Left
  use Ear, Inner, Right
Botallo's duct
  use Artery, Pulmonary, Left
Bovine pericardial valve
  use Zooplastic Tissue in Heart and Great Vessels
Bovine pericardium graft
  use Zooplastic Tissue in Heart and Great Vessels
BP (blood pressure) *see* Measurement, Arterial **4A03**-
Brachial (lateral) lymph node
  use Lymphatic, Axillary, Left
  use Lymphatic, Axillary, Right
Brachialis muscle
  use Muscle, Upper Arm, Left
  use Muscle, Upper Arm, Right
Brachiocephalic artery
  use Artery, Innominate
Brachiocephalic trunk
  use Artery, Innominate
Brachiocephalic vein
  use Vein, Innominate, Left
  use Vein, Innominate, Right
Brachioradialis muscle
  use Muscle, Lower Arm and Wrist, Left
  use Muscle, Lower Arm and Wrist, Right
Brachytherapy
  Abdomen **DW13**-
  Adrenal Gland **DG12**-
  Bile Ducts **DF12**-
  Bladder **DT12**-
  Bone Marrow **D710**-
  Brain **D010**-
  Brain Stem **D011**-
  Breast
    Left **DM10**-
    Right **DM11**-
  Bronchus **DB11**-
  Cervix **DU11**-
  Chest **DW12**-

PROCEDURE INDEX

Brachytherapy — *continued*
Chest Wall **DB17**-
Colon **DD15**-
Diaphragm **DB18**-
Duodenum **DD12**-
Ear **D910**-
Esophagus **DD10**-
Eye **D810**-
Gallbladder **DF11**-
Gland
  Adrenal **DG12**-
  Parathyroid **DG14**-
  Pituitary **DG10**-
  Thyroid **DG15**-
Glands, Salivary **D916**-
Head and Neck **DW11**-
Hypopharynx **D913**-
Ileum **DD14**-
Jejunum **DD13**-
Kidney **DT10**-
Larynx **D91B**-
Liver **DF10**-
Lung **DB12**-
Lymphatics
  Abdomen **D716**-
  Axillary **D714**-
  Inguinal **D718**-
  Neck **D713**-
  Pelvis **D717**-
  Thorax **D715**-
Mediastinum **DB16**-
Mouth **D914**-
Nasopharynx **D91D**-
Neck and Head **DW11**-
Nerve, Peripheral **D017**-
Nose **D911**-
Oropharynx **D91F**-
Ovary **DU10**-
Palate
  Hard **D918**-
  Soft **D919**-
Pancreas **DF13**-
Parathyroid Gland **DG14**-
Pelvic Region **DW16**-
Pineal Body **DG11**-
Pituitary Gland **DG10**-
Pleura **DB15**-
Prostate **DV10**-
Rectum **DD17**-
Sinuses **D917**-
Spinal Cord **D016**-
Spleen **D712**-
Stomach **DD11**-
Testis **DV11**-
Thymus **D711**-
Thyroid Gland **DG15**-
Tongue **D915**-
Trachea **DB10**-
Ureter **DT11**-
Urethra **DT13**-
Uterus **DU12**-

Brachytherapy seeds
use Radioactive Element
Broad ligament
use Uterine Supporting Structure
Bronchial artery
use Upper Artery
Bronchography
see Fluoroscopy, Respiratory System
  BB1-
see Plain Radiography, Respiratory
  System **BB0**-
Bronchoplasty
see Repair, Respiratory System **0BQ**-
see Supplement, Respiratory System
  0BU-
Bronchorrhaphy *see* Repair,
  Respiratory System **0BQ**-
Bronchoscopy 0BJ08ZZ
Bronchotomy *see* Drainage,
  Respiratory System **0B9**-

Bronchus intermedius
use Main Bronchus, Right
BRYAN® Cervical Disc System
use Synthetic Substitute
Buccal gland
use Buccal Mucosa
Buccinator lymph node
use Lymphatic, Head
Buccinator muscle
use Muscle, Facial
Buckling, scleral with implant *see*
  Supplement, Eye **08U**-
Bulbospongiosus muscle
use Muscle, Perineum
Bulbourethral (Cowper's) gland
use Urethra
Bundle of His
use Conduction Mechanism
Bundle of Kent
use Conduction Mechanism
Bunionectomy *see* Excision, Lower
  Bones **0QB**-
Bursectomy
see Excision, Bursae and Ligaments
  0MB-
see Resection, Bursae and Ligaments
  0MT-
Bursocentesis *see* Drainage, Bursae
  and Ligaments **0M9**-
Bursography
see Plain Radiography, Non-Axial
  Lower Bones **BQ0**-
see Plain Radiography, Non-Axial
  Upper Bones **BP0**-
Bursotomy
see Division, Bursae and Ligaments
  0M8-
see Drainage, Bursae and Ligaments
  0M9-
BVS 5000 Ventricular Assist Device
use External Heart Assist System in
  Heart and Great Vessels
Bypass
Anterior Chamber
  Left **08133**-
  Right **08123**-
Aorta
  Abdominal **0410**-
  Thoracic
    Ascending/Arch **021X**-
    Descending **021W**-
Artery
  Axillary
    Left **03160**-
    Right **03150**-
  Brachial
    Left **03180**-
    Right **03170**-
  Common Carotid
    Left **031J0**-
    Right **031H0**-
  Common Iliac
    Left **041D**-
    Right **041C**-
  Coronary
    Four or More Arteries **0213**-
    One Artery **0210**-
    Three Arteries **0212**-
    Two Arteries **0211**-
  External Carotid
    Left **031N0**-
    Right **031M0**-
  External Iliac
    Left **041J**-
    Right **041H**-
  Femoral
    Left **041L**-
    Right **041K**-
  Innominate **03120**-
  Internal Carotid
    Left **031L0**-
    Right **031K0**-

Bypass — *continued*
Artery — *continued*
  Internal Iliac
    Left **041F**-
    Right **041E**-
  Intracranial **031G0**-
  Popliteal
    Left **041N**-
    Right **041M**-
  Pulmonary
    Left **021R**-
    Right **021Q**-
  Pulmonary Trunk **021P**-
  Radial
    Left **031C0**-
    Right **031B0**-
  Splenic **0414**-
  Subclavian
    Left **03140**-
    Right **03130**-
  Temporal
    Left **031T0**-
    Right **031S0**-
  Ulnar
    Left **031A0**-
    Right **03190**-
Atrium
  Left **0217**-
  Right **0216**-
Bladder **0T1B**-
Cavity, Cranial **0W110J**-
Cecum **0D1H**-
Cerebral Ventricle **0016**-
Colon
  Ascending **0D1K**-
  Descending **0D1M**-
  Sigmoid **0D1N**-
  Transverse **0D1L**-
Duct
  Common Bile **0F19**-
  Cystic **0F18**-
  Hepatic
    Left **0F16**-
    Right **0F15**-
  Lacrimal
    Left **081Y**-
    Right **081X**-
  Pancreatic **0F1D**-
    Accessory **0F1F**-
Duodenum **0D19**-
Ear
  Left **091E0**-
  Right **091D0**-
Esophagus **0D15**-
  Lower **0D13**-
  Middle **0D12**-
  Upper **0D11**-
Fallopian Tube
  Left **0U16**-
  Right **0U15**-
Gallbladder **0F14**-
Ileum **0D1B**-
Jejunum **0D1A**-
Kidney Pelvis
  Left **0T14**-
  Right **0T13**-
Pancreas **0F1G**-
Pelvic Cavity **0W1J**-
Peritoneal Cavity **0W1G**-
Pleural Cavity
  Left **0W1B**-
  Right **0W19**-
Spinal Canal **001U**-
Stomach **0D16**-
Trachea **0B11**-
Ureter
  Left **0T17**-
  Right **0T16**-
Ureters, Bilateral **0T18**-
Vas Deferens
  Bilateral **0V1Q**-
  Left **0V1P**-
  Right **0V1N**-

Bypass — *continued*
Vein
  Axillary
    Left **0518**-
    Right **0517**-
  Azygos **0510**-
  Basilic
    Left **051C**-
    Right **051B**-
  Brachial
    Left **051A**-
    Right **0519**-
  Cephalic
    Left **051F**-
    Right **051D**-
  Colic **0617**-
  Common Iliac
    Left **061D**-
    Right **061C**-
  Esophageal **0613**-
  External Iliac
    Left **061G**-
    Right **061F**-
  External Jugular
    Left **051Q**-
    Right **051P**-
  Face
    Left **051V**-
    Right **051T**-
  Femoral
    Left **061N**-
    Right **061M**-
  Foot
    Left **061V**-
    Right **061T**-
  Gastric **0612**-
  Greater Saphenous
    Left **061Q**-
    Right **061P**-
  Hand
    Left **051H**-
    Right **051G**-
  Hemiazygos **0511**-
  Hepatic **0614**-
  Hypogastric
    Left **061J**-
    Right **061H**-
  Inferior Mesenteric **0616**-
  Innominate
    Left **0514**-
    Right **0513**-
  Internal Jugular
    Left **051N**-
    Right **051M**-
  Intracranial **051L**-
  Lesser Saphenous
    Left **061S**-
    Right **061R**-
  Portal **0618**-
  Renal
    Left **061B**-
    Right **0619**-
  Splenic **0611**-
  Subclavian
    Left **0516**-
    Right **0515**-
  Superior Mesenteric **0615**-
  Vertebral
    Left **051S**-
    Right **051R**-
Vena Cava
  Inferior **0610**-
  Superior **021V**-
Ventricle
  Left **021L**-
  Right **021K**-
Bypass, cardiopulmonary 5A1221Z

© 2016 Channel Publishing, Ltd.

PROCEDURE INDEX

C

Caesarean section *see* Extraction, Products of Conception **10D0-**

Calcaneocuboid joint
use Joint, Tarsal, Left
use Joint, Tarsal, Right

Calcaneocuboid ligament
use Bursa and Ligament, Foot, Left
use Bursa and Ligament, Foot, Right

Calcaneofibular ligament
use Bursa and Ligament, Ankle, Left
use Bursa and Ligament, Ankle, Right

Calcaneus
use Tarsal, Left
use Tarsal, Right

Cannulation
see Bypass
see Dilation
see Drainage
see Irrigation

Canthorrhaphy *see* Repair, Eye **08Q-**

Canthotomy *see* Release, Eye **08N-**

Capitate bone
use Carpal, Left
use Carpal, Right

Capsulectomy, lens *see* Excision, Eye **08B-**

Capsulorrhaphy, joint
see Repair, Lower Joints **0SQ-**
see Repair, Upper Joints **0RQ-**

Cardia
use Esophagogastric Junction

Cardiac contractility modulation lead
use Cardiac Lead in Heart and Great Vessels

Cardiac event recorder
use Monitoring Device

Cardiac Lead
Defibrillator
Atrium
Left **02H7-**
Right **02H6-**
Pericardium **02HN-**
Vein, Coronary **02H4-**
Ventricle
Left **02HL-**
Right **02HK-**
Insertion of device in
Atrium
Left **02H7-**
Right **02H6-**
Pericardium **02HN-**
Vein, Coronary **02H4-**
Ventricle
Left **02HL-**
Right **02HK-**
Pacemaker
Atrium
Left **02H7-**
Right **02H6-**
Pericardium **02HN-**
Vein, Coronary **02H4-**
Ventricle
Left **02HL-**
Right **02HK-**
Removal of device from, Heart **02PA-**
Revision of device in, Heart **02WA-**

Cardiac plexus
use Nerve, Thoracic Sympathetic

Cardiac Resynchronization Defibrillator Pulse Generator
Abdomen **0JH8-**
Chest **0JH6-**

Cardiac Resynchronization Pacemaker Pulse Generator
Abdomen **0JH8-**
Chest **0JH6-**

Cardiac resynchronization therapy (CRT) lead
use Cardiac Lead, Defibrillator in **02H-**
use Cardiac Lead, Pacemaker in **02H-**

Cardiac Rhythm Related Device
Insertion of device in
Abdomen **0JH8-**
Chest **0JH6-**
Removal of device from, Subcutaneous Tissue and Fascia, Trunk **0JPT-**
Revision of device in, Subcutaneous Tissue and Fascia, Trunk **0JWT-**

Cardiocentesis *see* Drainage, Pericardial Cavity **0W9D-**

Cardioesophageal junction
use Esophagogastric Junction

Cardiolysis *see* Release, Heart and Great Vessels **02N-**

CardioMEMS® pressure sensor
use Monitoring Device, Pressure Sensor in **02H-**

Cardiomyotomy *see* Division, Esophagogastric Junction **0D84-**

Cardioplegia *see* Introduction of substance in or on, Heart **3E08-**

Cardiorrhaphy *see* Repair, Heart and Great Vessels **02Q-**

Cardioversion 5A2204Z

Caregiver Training F0FZ-

Caroticotympanic artery
use Artery, Internal Carotid, Left
use Artery, Internal Carotid, Right

Carotid (artery) sinus (baroreceptor) lead
use Stimulator Lead in Upper Arteries

Carotid glomus
use Carotid Bodies, Bilateral
use Carotid Body, Left
use Carotid Body, Right

Carotid sinus
use Artery, Internal Carotid, Left
use Artery, Internal Carotid, Right

Carotid sinus nerve
use Nerve, Glossopharyngeal

Carotid WALLSTENT® Monorail® Endoprosthesis
use Intraluminal Device

Carpectomy
see Excision, Upper Bones **0PB-**
see Resection, Upper Bones **0PT-**

Carpometacarpal (CMC) joint
use Joint, Metacarpocarpal, Left
use Joint, Metacarpocarpal, Right

Carpometacarpal ligament
use Bursa and Ligament, Hand, Left
use Bursa and Ligament, Hand, Right

Casting *see* Immobilization

CAT scan *see* Computerized Tomography (CT Scan)

Catheterization
see Dilation
see Drainage
see Insertion of device in
see Irrigation
Heart *see* Measurement, Cardiac **4A02-**
Umbilical vein, for infusion **06H033T**

Cauda equina
use Spinal Cord, Lumbar

Cauterization
see Destruction
see Repair

Cavernous plexus
use Nerve, Head and Neck Sympathetic

Cecectomy
see Excision, Cecum **0DBH-**
see Resection, Cecum **0DTH-**

Cecocolostomy
see Bypass, Gastrointestinal System **0D1-**
see Drainage, Gastrointestinal System **0D9-**

Cecopexy
see Repair, Cecum **0DQH-**
see Reposition, Cecum **0DSH-**

Cecoplication *see* Restriction, Cecum **0DVH-**

Cecorrhaphy *see* Repair, Cecum **0DQH-**

Cecostomy
see Bypass, Cecum **0D1H-**
see Drainage, Cecum **0D9H-**

Cecotomy *see* Drainage, Cecum **0D9H-**

Ceftazidime-avibactam anti-infective XW0-

Celiac (solar) plexus
use Nerve, Abdominal Sympathetic

Celiac ganglion
use Nerve, Abdominal Sympathetic

Celiac lymph node
use Lymphatic, Aortic

Celiac trunk
use Artery, Celiac

Central axillary lymph node
use Lymphatic, Axillary, Left
use Lymphatic, Axillary, Right

Central venous pressure *see* Measurement, Venous **4A04-**

Centrimag® Blood Pump
use External Heart Assist System in Heart and Great Vessels

Cephalogram BN00ZZZ

Ceramic on ceramic bearing surface
use Synthetic Substitute, Ceramic in **0SR-**

Cerclage *see* Restriction

Cerebral aqueduct (Sylvius)
use Cerebral Ventricle

Cerebral embolic filtration, dual filter X2A5312

Cerebrum
use Brain

Cervical esophagus
use Esophagus, Upper

Cervical facet joint
use Joint, Cervical Vertebral
use Joint, Cervical Vertebral, 2 or more

Cervical ganglion
use Nerve, Head and Neck Sympathetic

Cervical interspinous ligament
use Bursa and Ligament, Head and Neck

Cervical intertransverse ligament
use Bursa and Ligament, Head and Neck

Cervical ligamentum flavum
use Bursa and Ligament, Head and Neck

Cervical lymph node
use Lymphatic, Neck, Left
use Lymphatic, Neck, Right

Cervicectomy
see Excision, Cervix **0UBC-**
see Resection, Cervix **0UTC-**

Cervicothoracic facet joint
use Joint, Cervicothoracic Vertebral

Cesarean section *see* Extraction, Products of Conception **10D0-**

Change device in
Abdominal Wall **0W2FX-**
Back
Lower **0W2LX-**
Upper **0W2KX-**
Bladder **0T2BX-**
Bone
Facial **0N2WX-**
Lower **0Q2YX-**
Nasal **0N2BX-**
Upper **0P2YX-**
Bone Marrow **072TX-**
Brain **0020X-**
Breast
Left **0H2UX-**
Right **0H2TX-**
Bursa and Ligament
Lower **0M2YX-**
Upper **0M2XX-**
Cavity, Cranial **0W21X-**
Chest Wall **0W28X-**
Cisterna Chyli **072LX-**
Diaphragm **0B2TX-**
Duct
Hepatobiliary **0F2BX-**
Pancreatic **0F2DX-**
Ear
Left **092JX-**
Right **092HX-**
Epididymis and Spermatic Cord **0V2MX-**
Extremity
Lower
Left **0Y2BX-**
Right **0Y29X-**
Upper
Left **0X27X-**
Right **0X26X-**
Eye
Left **0821X-**
Right **0820X-**
Face **0W22X-**
Fallopian Tube **0U28X-**
Gallbladder **0F24X-**
Gland
Adrenal **0G25X-**
Endocrine **0G2SX-**
Pituitary **0G20X-**
Salivary **0C2AX-**
Head **0W20X-**
Intestinal Tract
Lower **0D2DXUZ**
Upper **0D20XUZ**
Jaw
Lower **0W25X-**
Upper **0W24X-**
Joint
Lower **0S2YX-**
Upper **0R2YX-**
Kidney **0T25X-**
Larynx **0C2SX-**
Liver **0F20X-**
Lung
Left **0B2LX-**
Right **0B2KX-**
Lymphatic **072NX-**
Thoracic Duct **072KX-**
Mediastinum **0W2CX-**
Mesentery **0D2VX-**
Mouth and Throat **0C2YX-**
Muscle
Lower **0K2YX-**
Upper **0K2XX-**
Neck **0W26X-**
Nerve
Cranial **002EX-**
Peripheral **012YX-**
Nose **092KX-**
Omentum **0D2UX-**
Ovary **0U23X-**

Change device in — *continued*
Pancreas **0F2**GX-
Parathyroid Gland **0G2**RX-
Pelvic Cavity **0W2**JX-
Penis **0V2**SX-
Pericardial Cavity **0W2**DX-
Perineum
   Female **0W2**NX-
   Male **0W2**MX-
Peritoneal Cavity **0W2**GX-
Peritoneum **0D2**WX-
Pineal Body **0G2**1X-
Pleura **0B2**QX-
Pleural Cavity
   Left **0W2**BX-
   Right **0W2**9X-
Products of Conception **1020**7-
Prostate and Seminal Vesicles **0V2**4X-
Retroperitoneum **0W2**HX-
Scrotum and Tunica Vaginalis **0V2**8X-
Sinus **092**YX-
Skin **0H2**PX-
Skull **0N2**0X-
Spinal Canal **002**UX-
Spleen **072**PX-
Subcutaneous Tissue and Fascia
   Head and Neck **0J2**SX-
   Lower Extremity **0J2**WX-
   Trunk **0J2**TX-
   Upper Extremity **0J2**VX-
Tendon
   Lower **0L2**YX-
   Upper **0L2**XX-
Testis **0V2**DX-
Thymus **072**MX-
Thyroid Gland **0G2**KX-
Trachea **0B2**1-
Tracheobronchial Tree **0B2**0X-
Ureter **0T2**9X-
Urethra **0T2**DX-
Uterus and Cervix **0U2**DXHZ
Vagina and Cul-de-sac **0U2**HXGZ
Vas Deferens **0V2**RX-
Vulva **0U2**MX-
Change device in or on
Abdominal Wall **2W0**3X-
Anorectal **2Y0**3X5Z
Arm
   Lower
      Left **2W0**DX-
      Right **2W0**CX-
   Upper
      Left **2W0**BX-
      Right **2W0**AX-
Back **2W0**5X-
Chest Wall **2W0**4X-
Ear **2Y0**2X5Z
Extremity
   Lower
      Left **2W0**MX-
      Right **2W0**LX-
   Upper
      Left **2W0**9X-
      Right **2W0**8X-
Face **2W0**1X-
Finger
   Left **2W0**KX-
   Right **2W0**JX-
Foot
   Left **2W0**TX-
   Right **2W0**SX-
Genital Tract, Female **2Y0**4X5Z
Hand
   Left **2W0**FX-
   Right **2W0**EX-
Head **2W0**0X-
Inguinal Region
   Left **2W0**7X-
   Right **2W0**6X-

Change device in or on — *continued*
Leg
   Lower
      Left **2W0**RX-
      Right **2W0**QX-
   Upper
      Left **2W0**PX-
      Right **2W0**NX-
Mouth and Pharynx **2Y0**0X5Z
Nasal **2Y0**1X5Z
Neck **2W0**2X-
Thumb
   Left **2W0**HX-
   Right **2W0**GX-
Toe
   Left **2W0**VX-
   Right **2W0**UX-
Urethra **2Y0**5X5Z
Chemoembolization *see* Introduction of substance in or on
Chemosurgery, Skin **3E0**0XTZ
Chemothalamectomy *see* Destruction, Thalamus **0059**-
Chemotherapy, Infusion for cancer *see* Introduction of substance in or on
Chest x-ray *see* Plain Radiography, Chest **BW0**3-
Chiropractic Manipulation
Abdomen **9WB**9X-
Cervical **9WB**1X-
Extremities
   Lower **9WB**6X-
   Upper **9WB**7X-
Head **9WB**0X-
Lumbar **9WB**3X-
Pelvis **9WB**5X-
Rib Cage **9WB**8X-
Sacrum **9WB**4X-
Thoracic **9WB**2X-
Choana
use Nasopharynx
Cholangiogram
see Fluoroscopy, Hepatobiliary System and Pancreas **BF1**-
see Plain Radiography, Hepatobiliary System and Pancreas **BF0**-
Cholecystectomy
see Excision, Gallbladder **0FB**4-
see Resection, Gallbladder **0FT**4-
Cholecystojejunostomy
see Bypass, Hepatobiliary System and Pancreas **0F1**-
see Drainage, Hepatobiliary System and Pancreas **0F9**-
Cholecystopexy
see Repair, Gallbladder **0FQ**4-
see Reposition, Gallbladder **0FS**4-
Cholecystoscopy **0FJ**44ZZ
Cholecystostomy
see Drainage, Gallbladder **0F9**4-
see Bypass, Gallbladder **0F1**4-
Cholecystotomy *see* Drainage, Gallbladder **0F9**4-
Choledochectomy
see Excision, Hepatobiliary System and Pancreas **0FB**-
see Resection, Hepatobiliary System and Pancreas **0FT**-
Choledocholithotomy *see* Extirpation, Duct, Common Bile **0FC**9-
Choledochoplasty
see Repair, Hepatobiliary System and Pancreas **0FQ**-
see Replacement, Hepatobiliary System and Pancreas **0FR**-
see Supplement, Hepatobiliary System and Pancreas **0FU**-

Choledochoscopy **0FJ**B8ZZ
Choledochotomy *see* Drainage, Hepatobiliary System and Pancreas **0F9**-
Cholelithotomy *see* Extirpation, Hepatobiliary System and Pancreas **0FC**-
Chondrectomy
see Excision, Lower Joints **0SB**-
see Excision, Upper Joints **0RB**-
Knee *see* Excision, Lower Joints **0SB**-
Semilunar cartilage *see* Excision, Lower Joints **0SB**-
Chondroglossus muscle
use Muscle, Tongue, Palate, Pharynx
Chorda tympani
use Nerve, Facial
Chordotomy *see* Division, Central Nervous System **008**-
Choroid plexus
use Cerebral Ventricle
Choroidectomy
see Excision, Eye **08B**-
see Resection, Eye **08T**-
Ciliary body
use Eye, Left
use Eye, Right
Ciliary ganglion
use Nerve, Head and Neck Sympathetic
Circle of Willis
use Artery, Intracranial
Circumcision **0VT**TXZZ
Circumflex iliac artery
use Artery, Femoral, Left
use Artery, Femoral, Right
Clamp and rod internal fixation system (CRIF)
use Internal Fixation Device in Lower Bones
use Internal Fixation Device in Upper Bones
Clamping *see* Occlusion
Claustrum
use Basal Ganglia
Claviculectomy
see Excision, Upper Bones **0PB**-
see Resection, Upper Bones **0PT**-
Claviculotomy
see Division, Upper Bones **0P8**-
see Drainage, Upper Bones **0P9**-
Clipping, aneurysm *see* Restriction using Extraluminal Device
Clitorectomy, clitoridectomy
see Excision, Clitoris **0UBJ**-
see Resection, Clitoris **0UTJ**-
Clolar
use Clofarabine
Closure
see Occlusion
see Repair
Clysis *see* Introduction of substance in or on
Coagulation *see* Destruction
CoAxia NeuroFlo catheter
use Intraluminal Device
Cobalt/chromium head and polyethylene socket
use Synthetic Substitute, Metal on Polyethylene in **0SR**-
Cobalt/chromium head and socket
use Synthetic Substitute, Metal in **0SR**-
Coccygeal body
use Coccygeal Glomus
Coccygeus muscle
use Muscle, Trunk, Left
use Muscle, Trunk, Right

Cochlea
use Ear, Inner, Left
use Ear, Inner, Right
Cochlear implant (CI), multiple channel (electrode)
use Hearing Device, Multiple Channel Cochlear Prosthesis in **09H**-
Cochlear implant (CI), single channel (electrode)
use Hearing Device, Single Channel Cochlear Prosthesis in **09H**-
Cochlear Implant Treatment **F0B**Z0
Cochlear nerve
use Nerve, Acoustic
COGNIS® CRT-D
use Cardiac Resynchronization Defibrillator Pulse Generator in **0JH**-
Colectomy
see Excision, Gastrointestinal System **0DB**-
see Resection, Gastrointestinal System **0DT**-
Collapse *see* Occlusion
Collection from
Breast, Breast Milk **8E0**HX62
Indwelling Device
   Circulatory System
      Blood **8C0**2X6K
      Other Fluid **8C0**2X6L
   Nervous System
      Cerebrospinal Fluid **8C0**1X6J
      Other Fluid **8C0**1X6L
Integumentary System, Breast Milk **8E0**HX62
Reproductive System, Male, Sperm **8E0**VX63
Colocentesis *see* Drainage, Gastrointestinal System **0D9**-
Colofixation
see Repair, Gastrointestinal System **0DQ**-
see Reposition, Gastrointestinal System **0DS**-
Cololysis *see* Release, Gastrointestinal System **0DN**-
Colonic Z-Stent®
use Intraluminal Device
Colonoscopy **0DJ**D8ZZ
Colopexy
see Repair, Gastrointestinal System **0DQ**-
see Reposition, Gastrointestinal System **0DS**-
Coloplication *see* Restriction, Gastrointestinal System **0DV**-
Coloproctectomy
see Excision, Gastrointestinal System **0DB**-
see Resection, Gastrointestinal System **0DT**-
Coloproctostomy
see Bypass, Gastrointestinal System **0D1**-
see Drainage, Gastrointestinal System **0D9**-
Colopuncture *see* Drainage, Gastrointestinal System **0D9**-
Colorrhaphy *see* Repair, Gastrointestinal System **0DQ**-
Colostomy
see Bypass, Gastrointestinal System **0D1**-
see Drainage, Gastrointestinal System **0D9**-
Colpectomy
see Excision, Vagina **0UB**G-
see Resection, Vagina **0UT**G-
Colpocentesis *see* Drainage, Vagina **0U9**G-

PROCEDURE INDEX

Colpopexy
  see Repair, Vagina **0UQ**G-
  see Reposition, Vagina **0US**G-
Colpoplasty
  see Repair, Vagina **0UQ**G-
  see Supplement, Vagina **0UU**G-
Colporrhaphy *see* Repair, Vagina
  0UQG-
Colposcopy 0UJH8ZZ
Columella
  use Nose
Common digital vein
  use Vein, Foot, Left
  use Vein, Foot, Right
Common facial vein
  use Vein, Face, Left
  use Vein, Face, Right
Common fibular nerve
  use Nerve, Peroneal
Common hepatic artery
  use Artery, Hepatic
Common iliac (subaortic) lymph node
  use Lymphatic, Pelvis
Common interosseous artery
  use Artery, Ulnar, Left
  use Artery, Ulnar, Right
Common peroneal nerve
  use Nerve, Peroneal
Complete (SE) stent
  use Intraluminal Device
Compression
  see Restriction
  Abdominal Wall **2W1**3X-
  Arm
    Lower
      Left **2W1**DX-
      Right **2W1**CX-
    Upper
      Left **2W1**BX-
      Right **2W1**AX-
  Back **2W1**5X-
  Chest Wall **2W1**4X-
  Extremity
    Lower
      Left **2W1**MX-
      Right **2W1**LX-
    Upper
      Left **2W1**9X-
      Right **2W1**8X-
  Face **2W1**1X-
  Finger
    Left **2W1**KX-
    Right **2W1**JX-
  Foot
    Left **2W1**TX-
    Right **2W1**SX-
  Hand
    Left **2W1**FX-
    Right **2W1**EX-
  Head **2W1**0X-
  Inguinal Region
    Left **2W1**7X-
    Right **2W1**6X-
  Leg
    Lower
      Left **2W1**RX-
      Right **2W1**QX-
    Upper
      Left **2W1**PX-
      Right **2W1**NX-
  Neck **2W1**2X-
  Thumb
    Left **2W1**HX-
    Right **2W1**GX-
  Toe
    Left **2W1**VX-
    Right **2W1**UX-

Computer Assisted Procedure
  Extremity
    Lower
      No Qualifier **8E0**YXBZ
      With Computerized Tomography **8E0**YXBG
      With Fluoroscopy **8E0**YXBF
      With Magnetic Resonance Imaging **8E0**YXBH
    Upper
      No Qualifier **8E0**XXBZ
      With Computerized Tomography **8E0**XXBG
      With Fluoroscopy **8E0**XXBF
      With Magnetic Resonance Imaging **8E0**XXBH
  Head and Neck Region
    No Qualifier **8E0**9XBZ
    With Computerized Tomography **8E0**9XBG
    With Fluoroscopy **8E0**9XBF
    With Magnetic Resonance Imaging **8E0**9XBH
  Trunk Region
    No Qualifier **8E0**WXBZ
    With Computerized Tomography **8E0**WXBG
    With Fluoroscopy **8E0**WXBF
    With Magnetic Resonance Imaging **8E0**WXBH

Computerized Tomography (CT Scan)
  Abdomen **BW2**0-
  Chest and Pelvis **BW2**5-
  Abdomen and Chest **BW2**4-
  Abdomen and Pelvis **BW2**1-
  Airway, Trachea **BB2**F-
  Ankle
    Left **BQ2**H-
    Right **BQ2**G-
  Aorta
    Abdominal **B42**0-
      Intravascular Optical Coherence **B42**0Z2Z
    Thoracic **B32**0-
      Intravascular Optical Coherence **B32**0Z2Z
  Arm
    Left **BP2**F-
    Right **BP2**E-
  Artery
    Celiac **B42**1-
      Intravascular Optical Coherence **B42**1Z2Z
    Common Carotid
      Bilateral **B32**5-
      Intravascular Optical Coherence **B32**5Z2Z
    Coronary
      Bypass Graft
        Multiple **B22**3-
          Intravascular Optical Coherence **B22**3Z2Z
      Multiple **B22**1-
        Intravascular Optical Coherence **B22**1Z2Z
    Internal Carotid
      Bilateral **B32**8-
      Intravascular Optical Coherence **B32**8Z2Z
    Intracranial **B32**R-
      Intravascular Optical Coherence **B32**RZ2Z
    Lower Extremity
      Bilateral **B42**H-
        Intravascular Optical Coherence **B42**HZ2Z
      Left **B42**G-
        Intravascular Optical Coherence **B42**GZ2Z
      Right **B42**F-
        Intravascular Optical Coherence **B42**FZ2Z

Computerized Tomography (CT Scan) — *continued*
  Artery — *continued*
    Pelvic **B42**C-
      Intravascular Optical Coherence **B42**CZ2Z
    Pulmonary
      Left **B32**T-
        Intravascular Optical Coherence **B32**TZ2Z
      Right **B32**S-
        Intravascular Optical Coherence **B32**SZ2Z
    Renal
      Bilateral **B42**8-
        Intravascular Optical Coherence **B42**8Z2Z
      Transplant **B42**M-
        Intravascular Optical Coherence **B42**MZ2Z
    Superior Mesenteric **B42**4-
      Intravascular Optical Coherence **B42**4Z2Z
    Vertebral
      Bilateral **B32**G-
        Intravascular Optical Coherence **B32**GZ2Z
  Bladder **BT2**0-
  Bone
    Facial **BN2**5-
    Temporal **BN2**F-
  Brain **B02**0-
  Calcaneus
    Left **BQ2**K-
    Right **BQ2**J-
  Cerebral Ventricle **B02**8-
  Chest, Abdomen and Pelvis **BW2**5-
  Chest and Abdomen **BW2**4-
  Cisterna **B02**7-
  Clavicle
    Left **BP2**5-
    Right **BP2**4-
  Coccyx **BR2**F-
  Colon **BD2**4-
  Ear **B92**0-
  Elbow
    Left **BP2**H-
    Right **BP2**G-
  Extremity
    Lower
      Left **BQ2**S-
      Right **BQ2**R-
    Upper
      Bilateral **BP2**V-
      Left **BP2**U-
      Right **BP2**T-
  Eye
    Bilateral **B82**7-
    Left **B82**6-
    Right **B82**5-
  Femur
    Left **BQ2**4-
    Right **BQ2**3-
  Fibula
    Left **BQ2**C-
    Right **BQ2**B-
  Finger
    Left **BP2**S-
    Right **BP2**R-
  Foot
    Left **BQ2**M-
    Right **BQ2**L-
  Forearm
    Left **BP2**K-
    Right **BP2**J-
  Gland
    Adrenal, Bilateral **BG2**2-
    Parathyroid **BG2**3-
    Parotid, Bilateral **B92**6-
    Salivary, Bilateral **B92**D-
    Submandibular, Bilateral **B92**9-
    Thyroid **BG2**4-

Computerized Tomography (CT Scan) — *continued*
  Hand
    Left **BP2**P-
    Right **BP2**N-
  Hands and Wrists, Bilateral **BP2**Q-
  Head **BW2**8-
  Head and Neck **BW2**9-
  Heart
    Intravascular Optical Coherence **B22**6Z2Z
    Right and Left **B22**6-
  Hepatobiliary System, All **BF2**C-
  Hip
    Left **BQ2**1-
    Right **BQ2**0-
  Humerus
    Left **BP2**B-
    Right **BP2**A-
  Intracranial Sinus **B52**2-
    Intravascular Optical Coherence **B52**2Z2Z
  Joint
    Acromioclavicular, Bilateral **BP2**3-
    Finger
      Left **BP2**DZZZ
      Right **BP2**CZZZ
    Foot
      Left **BQ2**Y-
      Right **BQ2**X-
    Hand
      Left **BP2**DZZZ
      Right **BP2**CZZZ
    Sacroiliac **BR2**D-
    Sternoclavicular
      Bilateral **BP2**2-
      Left **BP2**1-
      Right **BP2**0-
    Temporomandibular, Bilateral **BN2**9-
    Toe
      Left **BQ2**Y-
      Right **BQ2**X-
  Kidney
    Bilateral **BT2**3-
    Left **BT2**2-
    Right **BT2**1-
    Transplant **BT2**9-
  Knee
    Left **BQ2**8-
    Right **BQ2**7-
  Larynx **B92**J-
  Leg
    Left **BQ2**F-
    Right **BQ2**D-
  Liver **BF2**5-
  Liver and Spleen **BF2**6-
  Lung, Bilateral **BB2**4-
  Mandible **BN2**6-
  Nasopharynx **B92**F-
  Neck **BW2**F-
  Neck and Head **BW2**9-
  Orbit, Bilateral **BN2**3-
  Oropharynx **B92**F-
  Pancreas **BF2**7-
  Patella
    Left **BQ2**W-
    Right **BQ2**V-
  Pelvic Region **BW2**G-
  Pelvis **BR2**C-
    Chest and Abdomen **BW2**5-
  Pelvis and Abdomen **BW2**1-
  Pituitary Gland **B02**9-
  Prostate **BV2**3-
  Ribs
    Left **BP2**Y-
    Right **BP2**X-
  Sacrum **BR2**F-
  Scapula
    Left **BP2**7-
    Right **BP2**6-

Computerized Tomography (CT Scan) — *continued*
Sella Turcica **B02**9-
Shoulder
  Left **BP29**-
  Right **BP28**-
Sinus
  Intracranial **B522**-
    Intravascular Optical Coherence **B522**Z2Z
  Paranasal **B922**-
Skull **BN20**-
Spinal Cord **B02**B-
Spine
  Cervical **BR20**-
  Lumbar **BR29**-
  Thoracic **BR27**-
Spleen and Liver **BF26**-
Thorax **BP2**W-
Tibia
  Left **BQ2**C-
  Right **BQ2**B-
Toe
  Left **BQ2**Q-
  Right **BQ2**P-
Trachea **BB2**F-
Tracheobronchial Tree
  Bilateral **BB29**-
  Left **BB28**-
  Right **BB27**-
Vein
  Pelvic (Iliac)
    Left **B52**G-
      Intravascular Optical Coherence **B52**GZ2Z
    Right **B52**F-
      Intravascular Optical Coherence **B52**FZ2Z
  Pelvic (Iliac) Bilateral **B52**H-
    Intravascular Optical Coherence **B52**HZ2Z
  Portal **B52**T-
    Intravascular Optical Coherence **B52**TZ2Z
  Pulmonary
    Bilateral **B52**S-
      Intravascular Optical Coherence **B52**SZ2Z
    Left **B52**R-
      Intravascular Optical Coherence **B52**RZ2Z
    Right **B52**Q-
      Intravascular Optical Coherence **B52**QZ2Z
  Renal
    Bilateral **B52**L-
      Intravascular Optical Coherence **B52**LZ2Z
    Left **B52**K-
      Intravascular Optical Coherence **B52**KZ2Z
    Right **B52**J-
      Intravascular Optical Coherence **B52**JZ2Z
  Spanchnic **B52**T-
    Intravascular Optical Coherence **B52**TZ2Z
  Vena Cava
    Inferior **B529**-
      Intravascular Optical Coherence **B529**Z2Z
    Superior **B528**-
      Intravascular Optical Coherence **B528**Z2Z
Ventricle, Cerebral **B028**-
Wrist
  Left **BP2**M-
  Right **BP2**L-

Concerto II CRT-D
use Cardiac Resynchronization Defibrillator Pulse Generator **0JH**-
Condylectomy
see Excision, Head and Facial Bones **0NB**-
see Excision, Lower Bones **0QB**-
see Excision, Upper Bones **0PB**-
Condyloid process
use Mandible, Left
use Mandible, Right
Condylotomy
see Division, Head and Facial Bones **0N8**-
see Division, Lower Bones **0Q8**-
see Division, Upper Bones **0P8**-
see Drainage, Head and Facial Bones **0N9**-
see Drainage, Lower Bones **0Q9**-
see Drainage, Upper Bones **0P9**-
Condylysis
see Release, Head and Facial Bones **0NN**-
see Release, Lower Bones **0QN**-
see Release, Upper Bones **0PN**-
Conization, cervix *see* Excision, Cervix **0UB**C-
Conjunctivoplasty
see Repair, Eye **08Q**-
see Replacement, Eye **08R**-
CONSERVE® PLUS Total Resurfacing Hip System
use Resurfacing Device in Lower Joints
Construction
Auricle, ear *see* Replacement, Ear, Nose, Sinus **09R**-
Ileal conduit *see* Bypass, Urinary System **0T1**-
Consulta CRT-D
use Cardiac Resynchronization Defibrillator Pulse Generator in **0JH**-
Consulta CRT-P
use Cardiac Resynchronization Pacemaker Pulse Generator in **0JH**-
Contact Radiation
Abdomen **DWY37ZZ**
Adrenal Gland **DGY27ZZ**
Bile Ducts **DFY27ZZ**
Bladder **DTY27ZZ**
Bone, Other **DPYC7ZZ**
Brain **D0Y07ZZ**
Brain Stem **D0Y17ZZ**
Breast
  Left **DMY07ZZ**
  Right **DMY17ZZ**
Bronchus **DBY17ZZ**
Cervix **DUY17ZZ**
Chest **DWY27ZZ**
Chest Wall **DBY77ZZ**
Colon **DDY57ZZ**
Diaphragm **DBY87ZZ**
Duodenum **DDY27ZZ**
Ear **D9Y07ZZ**
Esophagus **DDY07ZZ**
Eye **D8Y07ZZ**
Femur **DPY97ZZ**
Fibula **DPYB7ZZ**
Gallbladder **DFY17ZZ**
Gland
  Adrenal **DGY27ZZ**
  Parathyroid **DGY47ZZ**
  Pituitary **DGY07ZZ**
  Thyroid **DGY57ZZ**
Glands, Salivary **D9Y67ZZ**
Head and Neck **DWY17ZZ**
Hemibody **DWY47ZZ**
Humerus **DPY67ZZ**
Hypopharynx **D9Y37ZZ**

Contact Radiation — *continued*
Ileum **DDY47ZZ**
Jejunum **DDY37ZZ**
Kidney **DTY07ZZ**
Larynx **D9YB7ZZ**
Liver **DFY07ZZ**
Lung **DBY27ZZ**
Mandible **DPY37ZZ**
Maxilla **DPY27ZZ**
Mediastinum **DBY67ZZ**
Mouth **D9Y47ZZ**
Nasopharynx **D9YD7ZZ**
Neck and Head **DWY17ZZ**
Nerve, Peripheral **D0Y77ZZ**
Nose **D9Y17ZZ**
Oropharynx **D9YF7ZZ**
Ovary **DUY07ZZ**
Palate
  Hard **D9Y87ZZ**
  Soft **D9Y97ZZ**
Pancreas **DFY37ZZ**
Parathyroid Gland **DGY47ZZ**
Pelvic Bones **DPY87ZZ**
Pelvic Region **DWY67ZZ**
Pineal Body **DGY17ZZ**
Pituitary Gland **DGY07ZZ**
Pleura **DBY57ZZ**
Prostate **DVY07ZZ**
Radius **DPY77ZZ**
Rectum **DDY77ZZ**
Rib **DPY57ZZ**
Sinuses **D9Y77ZZ**
Skin
  Abdomen **DHY87ZZ**
  Arm **DHY47ZZ**
  Back **DHY77ZZ**
  Buttock **DHY97ZZ**
  Chest **DHY67ZZ**
  Face **DHY27ZZ**
  Leg **DHYB7ZZ**
  Neck **DHY37ZZ**
Skull **DPY07ZZ**
Spinal Cord **D0Y67ZZ**
Sternum **DPY47ZZ**
Stomach **DDY17ZZ**
Testis **DVY17ZZ**
Thyroid Gland **DGY57ZZ**
Tibia **DPYB7ZZ**
Tongue **D9Y57ZZ**
Trachea **DBY07ZZ**
Ulna **DPY77ZZ**
Ureter **DTY17ZZ**
Urethra **DTY37ZZ**
Uterus **DUY27ZZ**
Whole Body **DWY57ZZ**
CONTAK RENEWAL® 3 RF (HE) CRT-D
use Cardiac Resynchronization Defibrillator Pulse Generator in **0JH**-
Contegra Pulmonary Valved Conduit
use Zooplastic Tissue in Heart and Great Vessels
Continuous Glucose Monitoring (CGM) device
use Monitoring Device
Continuous Negative Airway Pressure
24-96 Consecutive Hours, Ventilation **5A09459**
Greater than 96 Consecutive Hours, Ventilation **5A09559**
Less than 24 Consecutive Hours, Ventilation **5A09359**
Continuous Positive Airway Pressure
24-96 Consecutive Hours, Ventilation **5A09457**
Greater than 96 Consecutive Hours, Ventilation **5A09557**
Less than 24 Consecutive Hours, Ventilation **5A09357**

Contraceptive Device
Change device in, Uterus and Cervix **0U2DXHZ**
Insertion of device in
  Cervix **0UHC**-
  Subcutaneous Tissue and Fascia
    Abdomen **0JH8**-
    Chest **0JH6**-
    Lower Arm
      Left **0JHH**-
      Right **0JHG**-
    Lower Leg
      Left **0JHP**-
      Right **0JHN**-
    Upper Arm
      Left **0JHF**-
      Right **0JHD**-
    Upper Leg
      Left **0JHM**-
      Right **0JHL**-
  Uterus **0UH9**-
Removal of device from
  Subcutaneous Tissue and Fascia
    Lower Extremity **0JPW**-
    Trunk **0JPT**-
    Upper Extremity **0JPV**-
  Uterus and Cervix **0UPD**-
Revision of device in
  Subcutaneous Tissue and Fascia
    Lower Extremity **0JWW**-
    Trunk **0JWT**-
    Upper Extremity **0JWV**-
  Uterus and Cervix **0UWD**-
Contractility Modulation Device
Abdomen **0JH8**-
Chest **0JH6**-
Control bleeding in
Abdominal Wall **0W3F**-
Ankle Region
  Left **0Y3L**-
  Right **0Y3K**-
Arm
  Lower
    Left **0X3F**-
    Right **0X3D**-
  Upper
    Left **0X39**-
    Right **0X38**-
Axilla
  Left **0X35**-
  Right **0X34**-
Back
  Lower **0W3L**-
  Upper **0W3K**-
Buttock
  Left **0Y31**-
  Right **0Y30**-
Cavity, Cranial **0W31**-
Chest Wall **0W38**-
Elbow Region
  Left **0X3C**-
  Right **0X3B**-
Extremity
  Lower
    Left **0Y3B**-
    Right **0Y39**-
  Upper
    Left **0X37**-
    Right **0X36**-
Face **0W32**-
Femoral Region
  Left **0Y38**-
  Right **0Y37**-
Foot
  Left **0Y3N**-
  Right **0Y3M**-
Gastrointestinal Tract **0W3P**-
Genitourinary Tract **0W3R**-

Control bleeding in — *continued*
Hand
  Left **0X3K-**
  Right **0X3J-**
Head **0W30-**
Inguinal Region
  Left **0Y36-**
  Right **0Y35-**
Jaw
  Lower **0W35-**
  Upper **0W34-**
Knee Region
  Left **0Y3G-**
  Right **0Y3F-**
Leg
  Lower
    Left **0Y3J-**
    Right **0Y3H-**
  Upper
    Left **0Y3D-**
    Right **0Y3C-**
Mediastinum **0W3C-**
Neck **0W36-**
Oral Cavity and Throat **0W33-**
Pelvic Cavity **0W3J-**
Pericardial Cavity **0W3D-**
Perineum
  Female **0W3N-**
  Male **0W3M-**
Peritoneal Cavity **0W3G-**
Pleural Cavity
  Left **0W3B-**
  Right **0W39-**
Respiratory Tract **0W3Q-**
Retroperitoneum **0W3H-**
Shoulder Region
  Left **0X33-**
  Right **0X32-**
Wrist Region
  Left **0X3H-**
  Right **0X3G-**
Conus arteriosus
use Ventricle, Right
Conus medullaris
use Spinal Cord, Lumbar
Conversion
Cardiac rhythm **5A2204Z**
Gastrostomy to jejunostomy feeding device *see* Insertion of device in, Jejunum **0DHA-**
Cook Biodesign® Fistula Plug(s)
use Nonautologous Tissue Substitute
Cook Biodesign® Hernia Graft(s)
use Nonautologous Tissue Substitute
Cook Biodesign® Layered Graft(s)
use Nonautologous Tissue Substitute
Cook Zenapro™ Layered Graft(s)
use Nonautologous Tissue Substitute
Cook Zenith AAA Endovascular Graft
use Intraluminal Device
use Intraluminal Device, Branched or Fenestrated, One or Two Arteries in **04V-**
use Intraluminal Device, Branched or Fenestrated, Three or More Arteries in **04V-**
Coracoacromial ligament
use Bursa and Ligament, Shoulder, Left
use Bursa and Ligament, Shoulder, Right
Coracobrachialis muscle
use Muscle, Upper Arm, Left
use Muscle, Upper Arm, Right
Coracoclavicular ligament
use Bursa and Ligament, Shoulder, Left
use Bursa and Ligament, Shoulder, Right

Coracohumeral ligament
use Bursa and Ligament, Shoulder, Left
use Bursa and Ligament, Shoulder, Right
Coracoid process
use Scapula, Left
use Scapula, Right
Cordotomy *see* Division, Central Nervous System **008-**
Core needle biopsy *see* Excision with qualifier Diagnostic
CoreValve transcatheter aortic valve
use Zooplastic Tissue in Heart and Great Vessels
Cormet Hip Resurfacing System
use Resurfacing Device in Lower Joints
Corniculate cartilage
use Larynx
CoRoent® XL
use Interbody Fusion Device in Lower Joints
Coronary arteriography
see Fluoroscopy, Heart **B21-**
see Plain Radiography, Heart **B20-**
Corox OTW (Bipolar) Lead
use Cardiac Lead, Defibrillator in **02H-**
use Cardiac Lead, Pacemaker in **02H-**
Corpus callosum
use Brain
Corpus cavernosum
use Penis
Corpus spongiosum
use Penis
Corpus striatum
use Basal Ganglia
Corrugator supercilii muscle
use Muscle, Facial
Cortical strip neurostimulator lead
use Neurostimulator Lead in Central Nervous System
Costatectomy
see Excision, Upper Bones **0PB-**
see Resection, Upper Bones **0PT-**
Costectomy
see Excision, Upper Bones **0PB-**
see Resection, Upper Bones **0PT-**
Costocervical trunk
use Artery, Subclavian, Left
use Artery, Subclavian, Right
Costochondrectomy
see Excision, Upper Bones **0PB-**
see Resection, Upper Bones **0PT-**
Costoclavicular ligament
use Bursa and Ligament, Shoulder, Left
use Bursa and Ligament, Shoulder, Right
Costosternoplasty
see Repair, Upper Bones **0PQ-**
see Replacement, Upper Bones **0PR-**
see Supplement, Upper Bones **0PU-**
Costotomy
see Division, Upper Bones **0P8-**
see Drainage, Upper Bones **0P9-**
Costotransverse joint
use Joint, Thoracic Vertebral
Costotransverse ligament
use Bursa and Ligament, Thorax, Left
use Bursa and Ligament, Thorax, Right
Costovertebral joint
use Joint, Thoracic Vertebral

Costoxiphoid ligament
use Bursa and Ligament, Thorax, Left
use Bursa and Ligament, Thorax, Right
Counseling
Family, for substance abuse, Other Family Counseling **HZ63ZZZ**
Group
  12-Step **HZ43ZZZ**
  Behavioral **HZ41ZZZ**
  Cognitive **HZ40ZZZ**
  Cognitive-Behavioral **HZ42ZZZ**
  Confrontational **HZ48ZZZ**
  Continuing Care **HZ49ZZZ**
  Infectious Disease
    Post-Test **HZ4CZZZ**
    Pre-Test **HZ4CZZZ**
  Interpersonal **HZ44ZZZ**
  Motivational Enhancement **HZ47ZZZ**
  Psychoeducation **HZ46ZZZ**
  Spiritual **HZ4BZZZ**
  Vocational **HZ45ZZZ**
Individual
  12-Step **HZ33ZZZ**
  Behavioral **HZ31ZZZ**
  Cognitive **HZ30ZZZ**
  Cognitive-Behavioral **HZ32ZZZ**
  Confrontational **HZ38ZZZ**
  Continuing Care **HZ39ZZZ**
  Infectious Disease
    Post-Test **HZ3CZZZ**
    Pre-Test **HZ3CZZZ**
  Interpersonal **HZ34ZZZ**
  Motivational Enhancement **HZ37ZZZ**
  Psychoeducation **HZ36ZZZ**
  Spiritual **HZ3BZZZ**
  Vocational **HZ35ZZZ**
Mental Health Services
  Educational **GZ60ZZZ**
  Other Counseling **GZ63ZZZ**
  Vocational **GZ61ZZZ**
Countershock, cardiac 5A2204Z
Cowper's (bulbourethral) gland
use Urethra
CPAP (continuous positive airway pressure)
see Assistance, Respiratory **5A09-**
Craniectomy
see Excision, Head and Facial Bones **0NB-**
see Resection, Head and Facial Bones **0NT-**
Cranioplasty
see Repair, Head and Facial Bones **0NQ-**
see Replacement, Head and Facial Bones **0NR-**
see Supplement, Head and Facial Bones **0NU-**
Craniotomy
see Division, Head and Facial Bones **0N8-**
see Drainage, Central Nervous System **009-**
see Drainage, Head and Facial Bones **0N9-**
Creation
Perineum
  Female **0W4N0-**
  Male **0W4M0-**
Valve
  Aortic **024F0-**
  Mitral **024G0-**
  Tricuspid **024J0-**
Cremaster muscle
use Muscle, Perineum

Cribriform plate
use Bone, Ethmoid, Left
use Bone, Ethmoid, Right
Cricoid cartilage
use Trachea
Cricoidectomy *see* Excision, Larynx **0CB**S-
Cricothyroid artery
use Artery, Thyroid, Left
use Artery, Thyroid, Right
Cricothyroid muscle
use Muscle, Neck, Left
use Muscle, Neck, Right
Crisis Intervention GZ2ZZZZ
Crural fascia
use Subcutaneous Tissue and Fascia, Upper Leg, Left
use Subcutaneous Tissue and Fascia, Upper Leg, Right
Crushing, nerve
Cranial *see* Destruction, Central Nervous System **005-**
Peripheral *see* Destruction, Peripheral Nervous System **015-**
Cryoablation *see* Destruction
Cryotherapy *see* Destruction
Cryptorchidectomy
see Excision, Male Reproductive System **0VB-**
see Resection, Male Reproductive System **0VT-**
Cryptorchiectomy
see Excision, Male Reproductive System **0VB-**
see Resection, Male Reproductive System **0VT-**
Cryptotomy
see Division, Gastrointestinal System **0D8-**
see Drainage, Gastrointestinal System **0D9-**
CT scan *see* Computerized Tomography (CT Scan)
CT sialogram *see* Computerized Tomography (CT Scan), Ear, Nose, Mouth and Throat **B92-**
Cubital lymph node
use Lymphatic, Upper Extremity, Left
use Lymphatic, Upper Extremity, Right
Cubital nerve
use Nerve, Ulnar
Cuboid bone
use Tarsal, Left
use Tarsal, Right
Cuboideonavicular joint
use Joint, Tarsal, Left
use Joint, Tarsal, Right
Culdocentesis *see* Drainage, Cul-de-sac **0U9F-**
Culdoplasty
see Repair, Cul-de-sac **0UQF-**
see Supplement, Cul-de-sac **0UUF-**
Culdoscopy 0UJH8ZZ
Culdotomy *see* Drainage, Cul-de-sac **0U9F-**
Culmen
use Cerebellum
Cultured epidermal cell autograft
use Autologous Tissue Substitute
Cuneiform cartilage
use Larynx
Cuneonavicular joint
use Joint, Tarsal, Left
use Joint, Tarsal, Right
Cuneonavicular ligament
use Bursa and Ligament, Foot, Left
use Bursa and Ligament, Foot, Right

Curettage
see Excision
see Extraction
Cutaneous (transverse) cervical nerve
use Nerve, Cervical Plexus
CVP (central venous pressure) see Measurement, Venous **4A04**-
Cyclodiathermy see Destruction, Eye **085**-
Cyclophotocoagulation see Destruction, Eye **085**-
CYPHER® Stent
use Intraluminal Device, Drug-eluting in Heart and Great Vessels
Cystectomy
see Excision, Bladder **0TBB**-
see Resection, Bladder **0TTB**-
Cystocele repair see Repair, Subcutaneous Tissue and Fascia, Pelvic Region **0JQC**-
Cystography
see Fluoroscopy, Urinary System **BT1**-
see Plain Radiography, Urinary System **BT0**-
Cystolithotomy see Extirpation, Bladder **0TCB**-
Cystopexy
see Repair, Bladder **0TQB**-
see Reposition, Bladder **0TSB**-
Cystoplasty
see Repair, Bladder **0TQB**-
see Replacement, Bladder **0TRB**-
see Supplement, Bladder **0TUB**-
Cystorrhaphy see Repair, Bladder **0TQB**-
Cystoscopy 0TJB8ZZ
Cystostomy see Bypass, Bladder **0T1B**-
Cystostomy tube
use Drainage Device
Cystotomy see Drainage, Bladder **0T9B**-
Cystourethrography
see Fluoroscopy, Urinary System **BT1**-
see Plain Radiography, Urinary System **BT0**-
Cystourethroplasty
see Repair, Urinary System **0TQ**-
see Replacement, Urinary System **0TR**-
see Supplement, Urinary System **0TU**-

D

DBS lead
use Neurostimulator Lead in Central Nervous System
DeBakey Left Ventricular Assist Device
use Implantable Heart Assist System in Heart and Great Vessels
Debridement
Excisional see Excision
Non-excisional see Extraction
Decompression, Circulatory 6A15-
Decortication, lung see Extraction, Respiratory System **0BD**-
Deep brain neurostimulator lead
use Neurostimulator Lead in Central Nervous System
Deep cervical fascia
use Subcutaneous Tissue and Fascia, Neck, Anterior
Deep cervical vein
use Vein, Vertebral, Left
use Vein, Vertebral, Right
Deep circumflex iliac artery
use Artery, External Iliac, Left
use Artery, External Iliac, Right
Deep facial vein
use Vein, Face, Left
use Vein, Face, Right
Deep femoral (profunda femoris) vein
use Vein, Femoral, Left
use Vein, Femoral, Right
Deep femoral artery
use Artery, Femoral, Left
use Artery, Femoral, Right
Deep Inferior Epigastric Artery Perforator Flap
Bilateral **0HRV077**
Left **0HRU077**
Right **0HRT077**
Deep palmar arch
use Artery, Hand, Left
use Artery, Hand, Right
Deep transverse perineal muscle
use Muscle, Perineum
Deferential artery
use Artery, Internal Iliac, Left
use Artery, Internal Iliac, Right
Defibrillator Generator
Abdomen **0JH8**-
Chest **0JH6**-
Defibrotide sodium anticoagulant XW0-
Defitelio
use Defibrotide sodium anticoagulant
Delivery
Cesarean see Extraction, Products of Conception **10D0**-
Forceps see Extraction, Products of Conception **10D0**-
Manually assisted **10E0XZZ**
Products of Conception **10E0XZZ**
Vacuum assisted see Extraction, Products of Conception **10D0**-
Delta frame external fixator
use External Fixation Device, Hybrid in **0PH**-
use External Fixation Device, Hybrid in **0PS**-
use External Fixation Device, Hybrid in **0QH**-
use External Fixation Device, Hybrid in **0QS**-

Delta III Reverse shoulder prosthesis
use Synthetic Substitute, Reverse Ball and Socket in **0RR**-
Deltoid fascia
use Subcutaneous Tissue and Fascia, Upper Arm, Left
use Subcutaneous Tissue and Fascia, Upper Arm, Right
Deltoid ligament
use Bursa and Ligament, Ankle, Left
use Bursa and Ligament, Ankle, Right
Deltoid muscle
use Muscle, Shoulder, Left
use Muscle, Shoulder, Right
Deltopectoral (infraclavicular) lymph node
use Lymphatic, Upper Extremity, Left
use Lymphatic, Upper Extremity, Right
Denervation
Cranial nerve see Destruction, Central Nervous System **005**-
Peripheral nerve see Destruction, Peripheral Nervous System **015**-
Densitometry
Plain Radiography
Femur
Left **BQ04ZZ1**
Right **BQ03ZZ1**
Hip
Left **BQ01ZZ1**
Right **BQ00ZZ1**
Spine
Cervical **BR00ZZ1**
Lumbar **BR09ZZ1**
Thoracic **BR07ZZ1**
Whole **BR0GZZ1**
Ultrasonography
Elbow
Left **BP4HZZ1**
Right **BP4GZZ1**
Hand
Left **BP4PZZ1**
Right **BP4NZZ1**
Shoulder
Left **BP49ZZ1**
Right **BP48ZZ1**
Wrist
Left **BP4MZZ1**
Right **BP4LZZ1**
Denticulate (dentate) ligament
use Spinal Meninges
Depressor anguli oris muscle
use Muscle, Facial
Depressor labii inferioris muscle
use Muscle, Facial
Depressor septi nasi muscle
use Muscle, Facial
Depressor supercilii muscle
use Muscle, Facial
Dermabrasion see Extraction, Skin and Breast **0HD**-
Dermis
use Skin
Descending genicular artery
use Artery, Femoral, Left
use Artery, Femoral, Right
Destruction
Acetabulum
Left **0Q55**-
Right **0Q54**-
Adenoids **0C5Q**-
Ampulla of Vater **0F5C**-
Anal Sphincter **0D5R**-
Anterior Chamber
Left **08533ZZ**
Right **08523ZZ**
Anus **0D5Q**-

Destruction — continued
Aorta
Abdominal **0450**-
Thoracic
Ascending/Arch **025X**-
Descending **025W**-
Aortic Body **0G5D**-
Appendix **0D5J**-
Artery
Anterior Tibial
Left **045Q**-
Right **045P**-
Axillary
Left **0356**-
Right **0355**-
Brachial
Left **0358**-
Right **0357**-
Celiac **045I**-
Colic
Left **0457**-
Middle **0458**-
Right **0456**-
Common Carotid
Left **035J**-
Right **035H**-
Common Iliac
Left **045D**-
Right **045C**-
External Carotid
Left **035N**-
Right **035M**-
External Iliac
Left **045J**-
Right **045H**-
Face **035R**-
Femoral
Left **045L**-
Right **045K**-
Foot
Left **045W**-
Right **045V**-
Gastric **0452**-
Hand
Left **035F**-
Right **035D**-
Hepatic **0453**-
Inferior Mesenteric **045B**-
Innominate **0352**-
Internal Carotid
Left **035L**-
Right **035K**-
Internal Iliac
Left **045F**-
Right **045E**-
Internal Mammary
Left **0351**-
Right **0350**-
Intracranial **035G**-
Lower **045Y**-
Peroneal
Left **045U**-
Right **045T**-
Popliteal
Left **045N**-
Right **045M**-
Posterior Tibial
Left **045S**-
Right **045R**-
Pulmonary
Left **025R**-
Right **025Q**-
Pulmonary Trunk **025P**-
Radial
Left **035C**-
Right **035B**-
Renal
Left **045A**-
Right **0459**-
Splenic **0454**-
Subclavian
Left **0354**-
Right **0353**-

PROCEDURE INDEX

Destruction — *continued*
Artery — *continued*
    Superior Mesenteric **0455**-
   Temporal
    Left **035**T-
    Right **035**S-
   Thyroid
    Left **035**V-
    Right **035**U-
   Ulnar
    Left **035**A-
    Right **0359**-
   Upper **035**Y-
   Vertebral
    Left **035**Q-
    Right **035**P-
Atrium
   Left **0257**-
   Right **0256**-
Auditory Ossicle
   Left **095**A0ZZ
   Right **0959**0ZZ
Basal Ganglia **0058**-
Bladder **0T5**B-
Bladder Neck **0T5**C-
Bone
   Ethmoid
    Left **0N5**G-
    Right **0N5**F-
   Frontal
    Left **0N52**-
    Right **0N51**-
   Hyoid **0N5**X-
   Lacrimal
    Left **0N5**J-
    Right **0N5**H-
   Nasal **0N5**B-
   Occipital
    Left **0N58**-
    Right **0N57**-
   Palatine
    Left **0N5**L-
    Right **0N5**K-
   Parietal
    Left **0N54**-
    Right **0N53**-
   Pelvic
    Left **0Q53**-
    Right **0Q52**-
   Sphenoid
    Left **0N5**D-
    Right **0N5**C-
   Temporal
    Left **0N56**-
    Right **0N55**-
   Zygomatic
    Left **0N5**N-
    Right **0N5**M-
Brain **0050**-
Breast
   Bilateral **0H5**V-
   Left **0H5**U-
   Right **0H5**T-
Bronchus
   Lingula **0B59**-
   Lower Lobe
    Left **0B5**B-
    Right **0B56**-
   Main
    Left **0B57**-
    Right **0B53**-
   Middle Lobe, Right **0B55**-
   Upper Lobe
    Left **0B58**-
    Right **0B54**-
Buccal Mucosa **0C54**-

Destruction — *continued*
Bursa and Ligament
   Abdomen
    Left **0M5**J-
    Right **0M5**H-
   Ankle
    Left **0M5**R-
    Right **0M5**Q-
   Elbow
    Left **0M54**-
    Right **0M53**-
   Foot
    Left **0M5**T-
    Right **0M5**S-
   Hand
    Left **0M58**-
    Right **0M57**-
   Head and Neck **0M50**-
   Hip
    Left **0M5**M-
    Right **0M5**L-
   Knee
    Left **0M5**P-
    Right **0M5**N-
   Lower Extremity
    Left **0M5**W-
    Right **0M5**V-
   Perineum **0M5**K-
   Shoulder
    Left **0M52**-
    Right **0M51**-
   Thorax
    Left **0M5**G-
    Right **0M5**F-
   Trunk
    Left **0M5**D-
    Right **0M5**C-
   Upper Extremity
    Left **0M5**B-
    Right **0M59**-
   Wrist
    Left **0M56**-
    Right **0M55**-
Carina **0B52**-
Carotid Bodies, Bilateral **0G58**-
Carotid Body
   Left **0G56**-
   Right **0G57**-
Carpal
   Left **0P5**N-
   Right **0P5**M-
Cecum **0D5**H-
Cerebellum **005**C-
Cerebral Hemisphere **0057**-
Cerebral Meninges **0051**-
Cerebral Ventricle **0056**-
Cervix **0U5**C-
Chordae Tendineae **0259**-
Choroid
   Left **085**B-
   Right **085**A-
Cisterna Chyli **075**L-
Clavicle
   Left **0P5**B-
   Right **0P59**-
Clitoris **0U5**J-
Coccygeal Glomus **0G5**B-
Coccyx **0Q5**S-
Colon
   Ascending **0D5**K-
   Descending **0D5**M-
   Sigmoid **0D5**N-
   Transverse **0D5**L-
Conduction Mechanism **0258**-
Conjunctiva
   Left **085**TXZZ
   Right **085**SXZZ

Destruction — *continued*
Cord
   Bilateral **0V5**H-
   Left **0V5**G-
   Right **0V5**F-
Cornea
   Left **0859**XZZ
   Right **0858**XZZ
Cul-de-sac **0U5**F-
Diaphragm
   Left **0B5**S-
   Right **0B5**R-
Disc
   Cervical Vertebral **0R53**-
   Cervicothoracic Vertebral **0R55**-
   Lumbar Vertebral **0S52**-
   Lumbosacral **0S54**-
   Thoracic Vertebral **0R59**-
   Thoracolumbar Vertebral **0R5**B-
Duct
   Common Bile **0F59**-
   Cystic **0F58**-
   Hepatic
    Left **0F56**-
    Right **0F55**-
   Lacrimal
    Left **085**Y-
    Right **085**X-
   Pancreatic **0F5**D-
    Accessory **0F5**F-
   Parotid
    Left **0C5**C-
    Right **0C5**B-
Duodenum **0D59**-
Dura Mater **0052**-
Ear
   External
    Left **0951**-
    Right **0950**-
   External Auditory Canal
    Left **0954**-
    Right **0953**-
   Inner
    Left **095**E0ZZ
    Right **095**D0ZZ
   Middle
    Left **0956**0ZZ
    Right **0955**0ZZ
Endometrium **0U5**B-
Epididymis
   Bilateral **0V5**L-
   Left **0V5**K-
   Right **0V5**J-
Epiglottis **0C5**R-
Esophagogastric Junction **0D54**-
Esophagus **0D55**-
   Lower **0D53**-
   Middle **0D52**-
   Upper **0D51**-
Eustachian Tube
   Left **095**G-
   Right **095**F-
Eye
   Left **0851**XZZ
   Right **0850**XZZ
Eyelid
   Lower
    Left **085**R-
    Right **085**Q-
   Upper
    Left **085**P-
    Right **085**N-
Fallopian Tube
   Left **0U56**-
   Right **0U55**-
Fallopian Tubes, Bilateral **0U57**-
Femoral Shaft
   Left **0Q59**-
   Right **0Q58**-

Destruction — *continued*
Femur
   Lower
    Left **0Q5**C-
    Right **0Q5**B-
   Upper
    Left **0Q57**-
    Right **0Q56**-
Fibula
   Left **0Q5**K-
   Right **0Q5**J-
Finger Nail **0H5**QXZZ
Gallbladder **0F54**-
Gingiva
   Lower **0C56**-
   Upper **0C55**-
Gland
   Adrenal
    Bilateral **0G54**-
    Left **0G52**-
    Right **0G53**-
   Lacrimal
    Left **085**W-
    Right **085**V-
   Minor Salivary **0C5**J-
   Parotid
    Left **0C59**-
    Right **0C58**-
   Pituitary **0G50**-
   Sublingual
    Left **0C5**F-
    Right **0C5**D-
   Submaxillary
    Left **0C5**H-
    Right **0C5**G-
   Vestibular **0U5**L-
Glenoid Cavity
   Left **0P58**-
   Right **0P57**-
Glomus Jugulare **0G5**C-
Humeral Head
   Left **0P5**D-
   Right **0P5**C-
Humeral Shaft
   Left **0P5**G-
   Right **0P5**F-
Hymen **0U5**K-
Hypothalamus **005**A-
Ileocecal Valve **0D5**C-
Ileum **0D5**B-
Intestine
   Large **0D5**E-
    Left **0D5**G-
    Right **0D5**F-
   Small **0D58**-
Iris
   Left **085**D3ZZ
   Right **085**C3ZZ
Jejunum **0D5**A-
Joint
   Acromioclavicular
    Left **0R5**H-
    Right **0R5**G-
   Ankle
    Left **0S5**G-
    Right **0S5**F-
   Carpal
    Left **0R5**R-
    Right **0R5**Q-
   Cervical Vertebral **0R51**-
   Cervicothoracic Vertebral **0R54**-
   Coccygeal **0S56**-
   Elbow
    Left **0R5**M-
    Right **0R5**L-
   Finger Phalangeal
    Left **0R5**X-
    Right **0R5**W-

Destruction — *continued*
Joint — *continued*
  Hip
    Left 0S5B-
    Right 0S59-
  Knee
    Left 0S5D-
    Right 0S5C-
  Lumbar Vertebral 0S50-
  Lumbosacral 0S53-
  Metacarpocarpal
    Left 0R5T-
    Right 0R5S-
  Metacarpophalangeal
    Left 0R5V-
    Right 0R5U-
  Metatarsal-Phalangeal
    Left 0S5N-
    Right 0S5M-
  Metatarsal-Tarsal
    Left 0S5L-
    Right 0S5K-
  Occipital-cervical 0R50-
  Sacrococcygeal 0S55-
  Sacroiliac
    Left 0S58-
    Right 0S57-
  Shoulder
    Left 0R5K-
    Right 0R5J-
  Sternoclavicular
    Left 0R5F-
    Right 0R5E-
  Tarsal
    Left 0S5J-
    Right 0S5H-
  Temporomandibular
    Left 0R5D-
    Right 0R5C-
  Thoracic Vertebral 0R56-
  Thoracolumbar Vertebral 0R5A-
  Toe Phalangeal
    Left 0S5Q-
    Right 0S5P-
  Wrist
    Left 0R5P-
    Right 0R5N-
Kidney
  Left 0T51-
  Right 0T50-
Kidney Pelvis
  Left 0T54-
  Right 0T53-
Larynx 0C5S-
Lens
  Left 085K3ZZ
  Right 085J3ZZ
Lip
  Lower 0C51-
  Upper 0C50-
Liver 0F50-
  Left Lobe 0F52-
  Right Lobe 0F51-
Lung
  Bilateral 0B5M-
  Left 0B5L-
  Lower Lobe
    Left 0B5J-
    Right 0B5F-
  Middle Lobe, Right 0B5D-
  Right 0B5K-
  Upper Lobe
    Left 0B5G-
    Right 0B5C-
Lung Lingula 0B5H-

Destruction — *continued*
Lymphatic
  Aortic 075D-
  Axillary
    Left 0756-
    Right 0755-
  Head 0750-
  Inguinal
    Left 075J-
    Right 075H-
  Internal Mammary
    Left 0759-
    Right 0758-
  Lower Extremity
    Left 075G-
    Right 075F-
  Mesenteric 075B-
  Neck
    Left 0752-
    Right 0751-
  Pelvis 075C-
  Thoracic Duct 075K-
  Thorax 0757-
  Upper Extremity
    Left 0754-
    Right 0753-
Mandible
  Left 0N5V-
  Right 0N5T-
Maxilla
  Left 0N5S-
  Right 0N5R-
Medulla Oblongata 005D-
Mesentery 0D5V-
Metacarpal
  Left 0P5Q-
  Right 0P5P-
Metatarsal
  Left 0Q5P-
  Right 0Q5N-
Muscle
  Abdomen
    Left 0K5L-
    Right 0K5K-
  Extraocular
    Left 085M-
    Right 085L-
  Facial 0K51-
  Foot
    Left 0K5W-
    Right 0K5V-
  Hand
    Left 0K5D-
    Right 0K5C-
  Head 0K50-
  Hip
    Left 0K5P-
    Right 0K5N-
  Lower Arm and Wrist
    Left 0K5B-
    Right 0K59-
  Lower Leg
    Left 0K5T-
    Right 0K5S-
  Neck
    Left 0K53-
    Right 0K52-
  Papillary 025D-
  Perineum 0K5M-
  Shoulder
    Left 0K56-
    Right 0K55-
  Thorax
    Left 0K5J-
    Right 0K5H-
  Tongue, Palate, Pharynx 0K54-
  Trunk
    Left 0K5G-
    Right 0K5F-

Destruction — *continued*
Muscle — *continued*
  Upper Arm
    Left 0K58-
    Right 0K57-
  Upper Leg
    Left 0K5R-
    Right 0K5Q-
Nasopharynx 095N-
Nerve
  Abdominal Sympathetic 015M-
  Abducens 005L-
  Accessory 005R-
  Acoustic 005N-
  Brachial Plexus 0153-
  Cervical 0151-
  Cervical Plexus 0150-
  Facial 005M-
  Femoral 015D-
  Glossopharyngeal 005P-
  Head and Neck Sympathetic 015K-
  Hypoglossal 005S-
  Lumbar 015B-
  Lumbar Plexus 0159-
  Lumbar Sympathetic 015N-
  Lumbosacral Plexus 015A-
  Median 0155-
  Oculomotor 005H-
  Olfactory 005F-
  Optic 005G-
  Peroneal 015H-
  Phrenic 0152-
  Pudendal 015C-
  Radial 0156-
  Sacral 015R-
  Sacral Plexus 015Q-
  Sacral Sympathetic 015P-
  Sciatic 015F-
  Thoracic 0158-
  Thoracic Sympathetic 015L-
  Tibial 015G-
  Trigeminal 005K-
  Trochlear 005J-
  Ulnar 0154-
  Vagus 005Q-
Nipple
  Left 0H5X-
  Right 0H5W-
Nose 095K-
Omentum
  Greater 0D5S-
  Lesser 0D5T-
Orbit
  Left 0N5Q-
  Right 0N5P-
Ovary
  Bilateral 0U52-
  Left 0U51-
  Right 0U50-
Palate
  Hard 0C52-
  Soft 0C53-
Pancreas 0F5G-
Para-aortic Body 0G59-
Paraganglion Extremity 0G5F-
Parathyroid Gland 0G5R-
  Inferior
    Left 0G5P-
    Right 0G5N-
  Multiple 0G5Q-
  Superior
    Left 0G5M-
    Right 0G5L-
Patella
  Left 0Q5F-
  Right 0Q5D-
Penis 0V5S-
Pericardium 025N-
Peritoneum 0D5W-

Destruction — *continued*
Phalanx
  Finger
    Left 0P5V-
    Right 0P5T-
  Thumb
    Left 0P5S-
    Right 0P5R-
  Toe
    Left 0Q5R-
    Right 0Q5Q-
Pharynx 0C5M-
Pineal Body 0G51-
Pleura
  Left 0B5P-
  Right 0B5N-
Pons 005B-
Prepuce 0V5T-
Prostate 0V50-
Radius
  Left 0P5J-
  Right 0P5H-
Rectum 0D5P-
Retina
  Left 085F3ZZ
  Right 085E3ZZ
Retinal Vessel
  Left 085H3ZZ
  Right 085G3ZZ
Rib
  Left 0P52-
  Right 0P51-
Sacrum 0Q51-
Scapula
  Left 0P56-
  Right 0P55-
Sclera
  Left 0857XZZ
  Right 0856XZZ
Scrotum 0V55-
Septum
  Atrial 0255-
  Nasal 095M-
  Ventricular 025M-
Sinus
  Accessory 095P-
  Ethmoid
    Left 095V-
    Right 095U-
  Frontal
    Left 095T-
    Right 095S-
  Mastoid
    Left 095C-
    Right 095B-
  Maxillary
    Left 095R-
    Right 095Q-
  Sphenoid
    Left 095X-
    Right 095W-
Skin
  Abdomen 0H57XZ-
  Back 0H56XZ-
  Buttock 0H58XZ-
  Chest 0H55XZ-
  Ear
    Left 0H53XZ-
    Right 0H52XZ-
  Face 0H51XZ-
  Foot
    Left 0H5NXZ-
    Right 0H5MXZ-
  Genitalia 0H5AXZ-
  Hand
    Left 0H5GXZ-
    Right 0H5FXZ-
  Lower Arm
    Left 0H5EXZ-
    Right 0H5DXZ-

PROCEDURE INDEX

Destruction — *continued*
Skin — *continued*
  Lower Leg
    Left **0H5**LXZ-
    Right **0H5**KXZ-
  Neck **0H54**XZ-
  Perineum **0H59**XZ-
  Scalp **0H50**XZ-
  Upper Arm
    Left **0H5**CXZ-
    Right **0H5**BXZ-
  Upper Leg
    Left **0H5**JXZ-
    Right **0H5**HXZ-
Skull **0N50**-
Spinal Cord
  Cervical **005**W-
  Lumbar **005**Y-
  Thoracic **005**X-
Spinal Meninges **005**T-
Spleen **075**P-
Sternum **0P50**-
Stomach **0D56**-
  Pylorus **0D57**-
Subcutaneous Tissue and Fascia
  Abdomen **0J58**-
  Back **0J57**-
  Buttock **0J59**-
  Chest **0J56**-
  Face **0J51**-
  Foot
    Left **0J5**R-
    Right **0J5**Q-
  Hand
    Left **0J5**K-
    Right **0J5**J-
  Lower Arm
    Left **0J5**H-
    Right **0J5**G-
  Lower Leg
    Left **0J5**P-
    Right **0J5**N-
  Neck
    Anterior **0J54**-
    Posterior **0J55**-
  Pelvic Region **0J5**C-
  Perineum **0J5**B-
  Scalp **0J50**-
  Upper Arm
    Left **0J5**F-
    Right **0J5**D-
  Upper Leg
    Left **0J5**M-
    Right **0J5**L-
Tarsal
  Left **0Q5**M-
  Right **0Q5**L-
Tendon
  Abdomen
    Left **0L5**G-
    Right **0L5**F-
  Ankle
    Left **0L5**T-
    Right **0L5**S-
  Foot
    Left **0L5**W-
    Right **0L5**V-
  Hand
    Left **0L58**-
    Right **0L57**-
  Head and Neck **0L50**-
  Hip
    Left **0L5**K-
    Right **0L5**J-
  Knee
    Left **0L5**R-
    Right **0L5**Q-
  Lower Arm and Wrist
    Left **0L56**-
    Right **0L55**-

Destruction — *continued*
Tendon — *continued*
  Lower Leg
    Left **0L5**P-
    Right **0L5**N-
  Perineum **0L5**H-
  Shoulder
    Left **0L52**-
    Right **0L51**-
  Thorax
    Left **0L5**D-
    Right **0L5**C-
  Trunk
    Left **0L5**B-
    Right **0L59**-
  Upper Arm
    Left **0L54**-
    Right **0L53**-
  Upper Leg
    Left **0L5**M-
    Right **0L5**L-
Testis
  Bilateral **0V5**C-
  Left **0V5**B-
  Right **0V59**-
Thalamus **0059**-
Thymus **075**M-
Thyroid Gland **0G5**K-
  Left Lobe **0G5**G-
  Right Lobe **0G5**H-
Tibia
  Left **0Q5**H-
  Right **0Q5**G-
Toe Nail **0H5**RXZZ
Tongue **0C57**-
Tonsils **0C5**P-
Tooth
  Lower **0C5**X-
  Upper **0C5**W-
Trachea **0B51**-
Tunica Vaginalis
  Left **0V57**-
  Right **0V56**-
Turbinate, Nasal **095**L-
Tympanic Membrane
  Left **0958**-
  Right **0957**-
Ulna
  Left **0P5**L-
  Right **0P5**K-
Ureter
  Left **0T57**-
  Right **0T56**-
Urethra **0T5**D-
Uterine Supporting Structure **0U54**-
Uterus **0U59**-
Uvula **0C5**N-
Vagina **0U5**G-
Valve
  Aortic **025**F-
  Mitral **025**G-
  Pulmonary **025**H-
  Tricuspid **025**J-
Vas Deferens
  Bilateral **0V5**Q-
  Left **0V5**P-
  Right **0V5**N-
Vein
  Axillary
    Left **0558**-
    Right **0557**-
  Azygos **0550**-
  Basilic
    Left **055**C-
    Right **055**B-
  Brachial
    Left **055**A-
    Right **0559**-

Destruction — *continued*
Vein — *continued*
  Cephalic
    Left **055**F-
    Right **055**D-
  Colic **0657**-
  Common Iliac
    Left **065**D-
    Right **065**C-
  Coronary **0254**-
  Esophageal **0653**-
  External Iliac
    Left **065**G-
    Right **065**F-
  External Jugular
    Left **055**Q-
    Right **055**P-
  Face
    Left **055**V-
    Right **055**T-
  Femoral
    Left **065**N-
    Right **065**M-
  Foot
    Left **065**V-
    Right **065**T-
  Gastric **0652**-
  Greater Saphenous
    Left **065**Q-
    Right **065**P-
  Hand
    Left **055**H-
    Right **055**G-
  Hemiazygos **0551**-
  Hepatic **0654**-
  Hypogastric
    Left **065**J-
    Right **065**H-
  Inferior Mesenteric **0656**-
  Innominate
    Left **0554**-
    Right **0553**-
  Internal Jugular
    Left **055**N-
    Right **055**M-
  Intracranial **055**L-
  Lesser Saphenous
    Left **065**S-
    Right **065**R-
  Lower **065**Y-
  Portal **0658**-
  Pulmonary
    Left **025**T-
    Right **025**S-
  Renal
    Left **065**B-
    Right **0659**-
  Splenic **0651**-
  Subclavian
    Left **0556**-
    Right **0555**-
  Superior Mesenteric **0655**-
  Upper **055**Y-
  Vertebral
    Left **055**S-
    Right **055**R-
Vena Cava
  Inferior **0650**-
  Superior **025**V-
Ventricle
  Left **025**L-
  Right **025**K-
Vertebra
  Cervical **0P53**-
  Lumbar **0Q50**-
  Thoracic **0P54**-
Vesicle
  Bilateral **0V53**-
  Left **0V52**-
  Right **0V51**-

Destruction — *continued*
Vitreous
  Left **08553**ZZ
  Right **08543**ZZ
Vocal Cord
  Left **0C5**V-
  Right **0C5**T-
Vulva **0U5**M-
Detachment
Arm
  Lower
    Left **0X6**F0Z-
    Right **0X6**D0Z-
  Upper
    Left **0X69**0Z-
    Right **0X68**0Z-
Elbow Region
  Left **0X6**C0ZZ
  Right **0X6**B0ZZ
Femoral Region
  Left **0Y68**0ZZ
  Right **0Y67**0ZZ
Finger
  Index
    Left **0X6**P0Z-
    Right **0X6**N0Z-
  Little
    Left **0X6**W0Z-
    Right **0X6**V0Z-
  Middle
    Left **0X6**R0Z-
    Right **0X6**Q0Z-
  Ring
    Left **0X6**T0Z-
    Right **0X6**S0Z-
Foot
  Left **0Y6**N0Z-
  Right **0Y6**M0Z-
Forequarter
  Left **0X6**10ZZ
  Right **0X6**00ZZ
Hand
  Left **0X6**K0Z-
  Right **0X6**J0Z-
Hindquarter
  Bilateral **0Y6**40ZZ
  Left **0Y6**30ZZ
  Right **0Y6**20ZZ
Knee Region
  Left **0Y6**G0ZZ
  Right **0Y6**F0ZZ
Leg
  Lower
    Left **0Y6**J0Z-
    Right **0Y6**H0Z-
  Upper
    Left **0Y6**D0Z-
    Right **0Y6**C0Z-
Shoulder Region
  Left **0X6**30ZZ
  Right **0X6**20ZZ
Thumb
  Left **0X6**M0Z-
  Right **0X6**L0Z-
Toe
  1st
    Left **0Y6**Q0Z-
    Right **0Y6**P0Z-
  2nd
    Left **0Y6**S0Z-
    Right **0Y6**R0Z-
  3rd
    Left **0Y6**U0Z-
    Right **0Y6**T0Z-
  4th
    Left **0Y6**W0Z-
    Right **0Y6**V0Z-
  5th
    Left **0Y6**Y0Z-
    Right **0Y6**X0Z-

Determination, Mental status
GZ14ZZZ
Detorsion
see Release
see Reposition
Detoxification Services, for
substance abuse HZ2ZZZZ
Device Fitting F0DZ-
Diagnostic Audiology *see*
Audiology, Diagnostic
Diagnostic imaging *see* Imaging,
Diagnostic
Diagnostic radiology *see* Imaging,
Diagnostic
Dialysis
Hemodialysis 5A1D00Z
Peritoneal 3E1M39Z
Diaphragma sellae
use Dura Mater
Diaphragmatic pacemaker
generator
use Stimulator Generator in
Subcutaneous Tissue and Fascia
Diaphragmatic Pacemaker Lead
Insertion of device in
Left 0BHS-
Right 0BHR-
Removal of device from, Diaphragm
0BPT-
Revision of device in, Diaphragm
0BWT-
Digital radiography, plain *see* Plain
Radiography
Dilation
Ampulla of Vater 0F7C-
Anus 0D7Q-
Aorta
Abdominal 0470-
Thoracic
Ascending/Arch 027X-
Descending 027W-
Artery
Anterior Tibial
Left 047Q-
Right 047P-
Axillary
Left 0376-
Right 0375-
Brachial
Left 0378-
Right 0377-
Celiac 0471-
Colic
Left 0477-
Middle 0478-
Right 0476-
Common Carotid
Left 037J-
Right 037H-
Common Iliac
Left 047D-
Right 047C-
Coronary
Four or More Arteries 0273-
One Artery 0270-
Three Arteries 0272-
Two Arteries 0271-
External Carotid
Left 037N-
Right 037M-
External Iliac
Left 047J-
Right 047H-
Face 037R-
Femoral
Left 047L-
Right 047K-
Foot
Left 047W-
Right 047V-
Gastric 0472-

Dilation — *continued*
Artery — *continued*
Hand
Left 037F-
Right 037D-
Hepatic 0473-
Inferior Mesenteric 047B-
Innominate 0372-
Internal Carotid
Left 037L-
Right 037K-
Internal Iliac
Left 047F-
Right 047E-
Internal Mammary
Left 0371-
Right 0370-
Intracranial 037G-
Lower 047Y-
Peroneal
Left 047U-
Right 047T-
Popliteal
Left 047N-
Right 047M-
Posterior Tibial
Left 047S-
Right 047R-
Pulmonary
Left 027R-
Right 027Q-
Pulmonary Trunk 027P-
Radial
Left 037C-
Right 037B-
Renal
Left 047A-
Right 0479-
Splenic 0474-
Subclavian
Left 0374-
Right 0373-
Superior Mesenteric 0475-
Temporal
Left 037T-
Right 037S-
Thyroid
Left 037V-
Right 037U-
Ulnar
Left 037A-
Right 0379-
Upper 037Y-
Vertebral
Left 037Q-
Right 037P-
Bladder 0T7B-
Bladder Neck 0T7C-
Bronchus
Lingula 0B79-
Lower Lobe
Left 0B7B-
Right 0B76-
Main
Left 0B77-
Right 0B73-
Middle Lobe, Right 0B75-
Upper Lobe
Left 0B78-
Right 0B74-
Carina 0B72-
Cecum 0D7H-
Cervix 0U7C-
Colon
Ascending 0D7K-
Descending 0D7M-
Sigmoid 0D7N-
Transverse 0D7L-

Dilation — *continued*
Duct
Common Bile 0F79-
Cystic 0F78-
Hepatic
Left 0F76-
Right 0F75-
Lacrimal
Left 087Y-
Right 087X-
Pancreatic 0F7D-
Accessory 0F7F-
Parotid
Left 0C7C-
Right 0C7B-
Duodenum 0D79-
Esophagogastric Junction 0D74-
Esophagus 0D75-
Lower 0D73-
Middle 0D72-
Upper 0D71-
Eustachian Tube
Left 097G-
Right 097F-
Fallopian Tube
Left 0U76-
Right 0U75-
Fallopian Tubes, Bilateral 0U77-
Hymen 0U7K-
Ileocecal Valve 0D7C-
Ileum 0D7B-
Intestine
Large 0D7E-
Left 0D7G-
Right 0D7F-
Small 0D78-
Jejunum 0D7A-
Kidney Pelvis
Left 0T74-
Right 0T73-
Larynx 0C7S-
Pharynx 0C7M-
Rectum 0D7P-
Stomach 0D76-
Pylorus 0D77-
Trachea 0B71-
Ureter
Left 0T77-
Right 0T76-
Ureters, Bilateral 0T78-
Urethra 0T7D-
Uterus 0U79-
Vagina 0U7G-
Valve
Aortic 027F-
Mitral 027G-
Pulmonary 027H-
Tricuspid 027J-
Vas Deferens
Bilateral 0V7Q-
Left 0V7P-
Right 0V7N-
Vein
Axillary
Left 0578-
Right 0577-
Azygos 0570-
Basilic
Left 057C-
Right 057B-
Brachial
Left 057A-
Right 0579-
Cephalic
Left 057F-
Right 057D-
Colic 0677-
Common Iliac
Left 067D-
Right 067C-

Dilation — *continued*
Vein — *continued*
Esophageal 0673-
External Iliac
Left 067G-
Right 067F-
External Jugular
Left 057Q-
Right 057P-
Face
Left 057V-
Right 057T-
Femoral
Left 067N-
Right 067M-
Foot
Left 067V-
Right 067T-
Gastric 0672-
Greater Saphenous
Left 067Q-
Right 067P-
Hand
Left 057H-
Right 057G-
Hemiazygos 0571-
Hepatic 0674-
Hypogastric
Left 067J-
Right 067H-
Inferior Mesenteric 0676-
Innominate
Left 0574-
Right 0573-
Internal Jugular
Left 057N-
Right 057M-
Intracranial 057L-
Lesser Saphenous
Left 067S-
Right 067R-
Lower 067Y-
Portal 0678-
Pulmonary
Left 027T-
Right 027S-
Renal
Left 067B-
Right 0679-
Splenic 0671-
Subclavian
Left 0576-
Right 0575-
Superior Mesenteric 0675-
Upper 057Y-
Vertebral
Left 057S-
Right 057R-
Vena Cava
Inferior 0670-
Superior 027V-
Ventricle, Right 027K-
Direct Lateral Interbody Fusion
(DLIF) device
use Interbody Fusion Device in Lower
Joints
Disarticulation *see* Detachment
Discectomy, diskectomy
see Excision, Lower Joints 0SB-
see Excision, Upper Joints 0RB-
see Resection, Lower Joints 0ST-
see Resection, Upper Joints 0RT-
Discography
see Fluoroscopy, Axial Skeleton,
Except Skull and Facial Bones
BR1-
see Plain Radiography, Axial
Skeleton, Except Skull and Facial
Bones BR0-

PROCEDURE INDEX

Distal humerus
  use Humeral Shaft, Left
  use Humeral Shaft, Right
Distal humerus, involving joint
  use Joint, Elbow, Left
  use Joint, Elbow, Right
Distal radioulnar joint
  use Joint, Wrist, Left
  use Joint, Wrist, Right
Diversion *see* Bypass
Diverticulectomy *see* Excision,
  Gastrointestinal System 0DB-
Division
  Acetabulum
    Left 0Q85-
    Right 0Q84-
  Anal Sphincter 0D8R-
  Basal Ganglia 0088-
  Bladder Neck 0T8C-
  Bone
    Ethmoid
      Left 0N8G-
      Right 0N8F-
    Frontal
      Left 0N82-
      Right 0N81-
    Hyoid 0N8X-
    Lacrimal
      Left 0N8J-
      Right 0N8H-
    Nasal 0N8B-
    Occipital
      Left 0N88-
      Right 0N87-
    Palatine
      Left 0N8L-
      Right 0N8K-
    Parietal
      Left 0N84-
      Right 0N83-
    Pelvic
      Left 0Q83-
      Right 0Q82-
    Sphenoid
      Left 0N8D-
      Right 0N8C-
    Temporal
      Left 0N86-
      Right 0N85-
    Zygomatic
      Left 0N8N-
      Right 0N8M-
  Brain 0080-
  Bursa and Ligament
    Abdomen
      Left 0M8J-
      Right 0M8H-
    Ankle
      Left 0M8R-
      Right 0M8Q-
    Elbow
      Left 0M84-
      Right 0M83-
    Foot
      Left 0M8T-
      Right 0M8S-
    Hand
      Left 0M88-
      Right 0M87-
    Head and Neck 0M80-
    Hip
      Left 0M8M-
      Right 0M8L-
    Knee
      Left 0M8P-
      Right 0M8N-
    Lower Extremity
      Left 0M8W-
      Right 0M8V-
    Perineum 0M8K-
    Shoulder
      Left 0M82-
      Right 0M81-

Division — *continued*
  Bursa and Ligament — *continued*
    Thorax
      Left 0M8G-
      Right 0M8F-
    Trunk
      Left 0M8D-
      Right 0M8C-
    Upper Extremity
      Left 0M8B-
      Right 0M89-
    Wrist
      Left 0M86-
      Right 0M85-
  Carpal
    Left 0P8N-
    Right 0P8M-
  Cerebral Hemisphere 0087-
  Chordae Tendineae 0289-
  Clavicle
    Left 0P8B-
    Right 0P89-
  Coccyx 0Q8S-
  Conduction Mechanism 0288-
  Esophagogastric Junction 0D84-
  Femoral Shaft
    Left 0Q89-
    Right 0Q88-
  Femur
    Lower
      Left 0Q8C-
      Right 0Q8B-
    Upper
      Left 0Q87-
      Right 0Q86-
  Fibula
    Left 0Q8K-
    Right 0Q8J-
  Gland, Pituitary 0G80-
  Glenoid Cavity
    Left 0P88-
    Right 0P87-
  Humeral Head
    Left 0P8D-
    Right 0P8C-
  Humeral Shaft
    Left 0P8G-
    Right 0P8F-
  Hymen 0U8K-
  Kidneys, Bilateral 0T82-
  Mandible
    Left 0N8V-
    Right 0N8T-
  Maxilla
    Left 0N8S-
    Right 0N8R-
  Metacarpal
    Left 0P8Q-
    Right 0P8P-
  Metatarsal
    Left 0Q8P-
    Right 0Q8N-
  Muscle
    Abdomen
      Left 0K8L-
      Right 0K8K-
    Facial 0K81-
    Foot
      Left 0K8W-
      Right 0K8V-
    Hand
      Left 0K8D-
      Right 0K8C-
    Head 0K80-
    Hip
      Left 0K8P-
      Right 0K8N-
    Lower Arm and Wrist
      Left 0K8B-
      Right 0K89-

Division — *continued*
  Muscle — *continued*
    Lower Leg
      Left 0K8T-
      Right 0K8S-
    Neck
      Left 0K83-
      Right 0K82-
    Papillary 028D-
    Perineum 0K8M-
    Shoulder
      Left 0K86-
      Right 0K85-
    Thorax
      Left 0K8J-
      Right 0K8H-
    Tongue, Palate, Pharynx 0K84-
    Trunk
      Left 0K8G-
      Right 0K8F-
    Upper Arm
      Left 0K88-
      Right 0K87-
    Upper Leg
      Left 0K8R-
      Right 0K8Q-
  Nerve
    Abdominal Sympathetic 018M-
    Abducens 008L-
    Accessory 008R-
    Acoustic 008N-
    Brachial Plexus 0183-
    Cervical 0181-
    Cervical Plexus 0180-
    Facial 008M-
    Femoral 018D-
    Glossopharyngeal 008P-
    Head and Neck Sympathetic 018K-
    Hypoglossal 008S-
    Lumbar 018B-
    Lumbar Plexus 0189-
    Lumbar Sympathetic 018N-
    Lumbosacral Plexus 018A-
    Median 0185-
    Oculomotor 008H-
    Olfactory 008F-
    Optic 008G-
    Peroneal 018H-
    Phrenic 0182-
    Pudendal 018C-
    Radial 0186-
    Sacral 018R-
    Sacral Plexus 018Q-
    Sacral Sympathetic 018P-
    Sciatic 018F-
    Thoracic 0188-
    Thoracic Sympathetic 018L-
    Tibial 018G-
    Trigeminal 008K-
    Trochlear 008J-
    Ulnar 0184-
    Vagus 008Q-
  Orbit
    Left 0N8Q-
    Right 0N8P-
  Ovary
    Bilateral 0U82-
    Left 0U81-
    Right 0U80-
  Pancreas 0F8G-
  Patella
    Left 0Q8F-
    Right 0Q8D-
  Perineum, Female 0W8NXZZ
  Phalanx
    Finger
      Left 0P8V-
      Right 0P8T-
    Thumb
      Left 0P8S-
      Right 0P8R-

Division — *continued*
  Phalanx — *continued*
    Toe
      Left 0Q8R-
      Right 0Q8Q-
  Radius
    Left 0P8J-
    Right 0P8H-
  Rib
    Left 0P82-
    Right 0P81-
  Sacrum 0Q81-
  Scapula
    Left 0P86-
    Right 0P85-
  Skin
    Abdomen 0H87XZZ
    Back 0H86XZZ
    Buttock 0H88XZZ
    Chest 0H85XZZ
    Ear
      Left 0H83XZZ
      Right 0H82XZZ
    Face 0H81XZZ
    Foot
      Left 0H8NXZZ
      Right 0H8MXZZ
    Genitalia 0H8AXZZ
    Hand
      Left 0H8GXZZ
      Right 0H8FXZZ
    Lower Arm
      Left 0H8EXZZ
      Right 0H8DXZZ
    Lower Leg
      Left 0H8LXZZ
      Right 0H8KXZZ
    Neck 0H84XZZ
    Perineum 0H89XZZ
    Scalp 0H80XZZ
    Upper Arm
      Left 0H8CXZZ
      Right 0H8BXZZ
    Upper Leg
      Left 0H8JXZZ
      Right 0H8HXZZ
  Skull 0N80-
  Spinal Cord
    Cervical 008W-
    Lumbar 008Y-
    Thoracic 008X-
  Sternum 0P80-
  Stomach, Pylorus 0D87-
  Subcutaneous Tissue and Fascia
    Abdomen 0J88-
    Back 0J87-
    Buttock 0J89-
    Chest 0J86-
    Face 0J81-
    Foot
      Left 0J8R-
      Right 0J8Q-
    Hand
      Left 0J8K-
      Right 0J8J-
    Head and Neck 0J8S-
    Lower Arm
      Left 0J8H-
      Right 0J8G-
    Lower Extremity 0J8W-
    Lower Leg
      Left 0J8P-
      Right 0J8N-
    Neck
      Anterior 0J84-
      Posterior 0J85-
    Pelvic Region 0J8C-
    Perineum 0J8B-
    Scalp 0J80-

PROCEDURE INDEX

Division — *continued*
Subcutaneous Tissue and Fascia — *continued*
  Trunk 0J8T-
  Upper Arm
    Left 0J8F-
    Right 0J8D-
  Upper Extremity 0J8V-
  Upper Leg
    Left 0J8M-
    Right 0J8L-
Tarsal
  Left 0Q8M-
  Right 0Q8L-
Tendon
  Abdomen
    Left 0L8G-
    Right 0L8F-
  Ankle
    Left 0L8T-
    Right 0L8S-
  Foot
    Left 0L8W-
    Right 0L8V-
  Hand
    Left 0L88-
    Right 0L87-
  Head and Neck 0L80-
  Hip
    Left 0L8K-
    Right 0L8J-
  Knee
    Left 0L8R-
    Right 0L8Q-
  Lower Arm and Wrist
    Left 0L86-
    Right 0L85-
  Lower Leg
    Left 0L8P-
    Right 0L8N-
  Perineum 0L8H-
  Shoulder
    Left 0L82-
    Right 0L81-
  Thorax
    Left 0L8D-
    Right 0L8C-
  Trunk
    Left 0L8B-
    Right 0L89-
  Upper Arm
    Left 0L84-
    Right 0L83-
  Upper Leg
    Left 0L8M-
    Right 0L8L-
Thyroid Gland Isthmus 0G8J-
Tibia
  Left 0Q8H-
  Right 0Q8G-
Turbinate, Nasal 098L-
Ulna
  Left 0P8L-
  Right 0P8K-
Uterine Supporting Structure 0U84-
Vertebra
  Cervical 0P83-
  Lumbar 0Q80-
  Thoracic 0P84-
Doppler study *see* Ultrasonography
Dorsal digital nerve
  use Nerve, Radial
Dorsal metacarpal vein
  use Vein, Hand, Left
  use Vein, Hand, Right
Dorsal metatarsal artery
  use Artery, Foot, Left
  use Artery, Foot, Right

Dorsal metatarsal vein
  use Vein, Foot, Left
  use Vein, Foot, Right
Dorsal scapular artery
  use Artery, Subclavian, Left
  use Artery, Subclavian, Right
Dorsal scapular nerve
  use Nerve, Brachial Plexus
Dorsal venous arch
  use Vein, Foot, Left
  use Vein, Foot, Right
Dorsalis pedis artery
  use Artery, Anterior Tibial, Left
  use Artery, Anterior Tibial, Right
Drainage
Abdominal Wall 0W9F-
Acetabulum
  Left 0Q95-
  Right 0Q94-
Adenoids 0C9Q-
Ampulla of Vater 0F9C-
Anal Sphincter 0D9R-
Ankle Region
  Left 0Y9L-
  Right 0Y9K-
Anterior Chamber
  Left 0893-
  Right 0892-
Anus 0D9Q-
Aorta, Abdominal 0490-
Aortic Body 0G9D-
Appendix 0D9J-
Arm
  Lower
    Left 0X9F-
    Right 0X9D-
  Upper
    Left 0X99-
    Right 0X98-
Artery
  Anterior Tibial
    Left 049Q-
    Right 049P-
  Axillary
    Left 0396-
    Right 0395-
  Brachial
    Left 0398-
    Right 0397-
  Celiac 0491-
  Colic
    Left 0497-
    Middle 0498-
    Right 0496-
  Common Carotid
    Left 039J-
    Right 039H-
  Common Iliac
    Left 049D-
    Right 049C-
  External Carotid
    Left 039N-
    Right 039M-
  External Iliac
    Left 049J-
    Right 049H-
  Face 039R-
  Femoral
    Left 049L-
    Right 049K-
  Foot
    Left 049W-
    Right 049V-
  Gastric 0492-
  Hand
    Left 039F-
    Right 039D-
  Hepatic 0493-
  Inferior Mesenteric 049B-

Drainage — *continued*
Artery — *continued*
  Innominate 0392-
  Internal Carotid
    Left 039L-
    Right 039K-
  Internal Iliac
    Left 049F-
    Right 049E-
  Internal Mammary
    Left 0391-
    Right 0390-
  Intracranial 039G-
  Lower 049Y-
  Peroneal
    Left 049U-
    Right 049T-
  Popliteal
    Left 049N-
    Right 049M-
  Posterior Tibial
    Left 049S-
    Right 049R-
  Radial
    Left 039C-
    Right 039B-
  Renal
    Left 049A-
    Right 0499-
  Splenic 0494-
  Subclavian
    Left 0394-
    Right 0393-
  Superior Mesenteric 0495-
  Temporal
    Left 039T-
    Right 039S-
  Thyroid
    Left 039V-
    Right 039U-
  Ulnar
    Left 039A-
    Right 0399-
  Upper 039Y-
  Vertebral
    Left 039Q-
    Right 039P-
Auditory Ossicle
  Left 099A-
  Right 0999-
Axilla
  Left 0X95-
  Right 0X94-
Back
  Lower 0W9L-
  Upper 0W9K-
Basal Ganglia 0098-
Bladder 0T9B-
Bladder Neck 0T9C-
Bone
  Ethmoid
    Left 0N9G-
    Right 0N9F-
  Frontal
    Left 0N92-
    Right 0N91-
  Hyoid 0N9X-
  Lacrimal
    Left 0N9J-
    Right 0N9H-
  Nasal 0N9B-
  Occipital
    Left 0N98-
    Right 0N97-
  Palatine
    Left 0N9L-
    Right 0N9K-
  Parietal
    Left 0N94-
    Right 0N93-

Drainage — *continued*
Bone — *continued*
  Pelvic
    Left 0Q93-
    Right 0Q92-
  Sphenoid
    Left 0N9D-
    Right 0N9C-
  Temporal
    Left 0N96-
    Right 0N95-
  Zygomatic
    Left 0N9N-
    Right 0N9M-
Bone Marrow 079T-
Brain 0090-
Breast
  Bilateral 0H9V-
  Left 0H9U-
  Right 0H9T-
Bronchus
  Lingula 0B99-
  Lower Lobe
    Left 0B9B-
    Right 0B96-
  Main
    Left 0B97-
    Right 0B93-
  Middle Lobe, Right 0B95-
  Upper Lobe
    Left 0B98-
    Right 0B94-
Buccal Mucosa 0C94-
Bursa and Ligament
  Abdomen
    Left 0M9J-
    Right 0M9H-
  Ankle
    Left 0M9R-
    Right 0M9Q-
  Elbow
    Left 0M94-
    Right 0M93-
  Foot
    Left 0M9T-
    Right 0M9S-
  Hand
    Left 0M98-
    Right 0M97-
  Head and Neck 0M90-
  Hip
    Left 0M9M-
    Right 0M9L-
  Knee
    Left 0M9P-
    Right 0M9N-
  Lower Extremity
    Left 0M9W-
    Right 0M9V-
  Perineum 0M9K-
  Shoulder
    Left 0M92-
    Right 0M91-
  Thorax
    Left 0M9G-
    Right 0M9F-
  Trunk
    Left 0M9D-
    Right 0M9C-
  Upper Extremity
    Left 0M9B-
    Right 0M99-
  Wrist
    Left 0M96-
    Right 0M95-
Buttock
  Left 0Y91-
  Right 0Y90-
Carina 0B92-
Carotid Bodies, Bilateral 0G98-

Drainage — *continued*
  Carotid Body
    Left 0G96-
    Right 0G97-
  Carpal
    Left 0P9N-
    Right 0P9M-
  Cavity, Cranial 0W91-
  Cecum 0D9H-
  Cerebellum 009C-
  Cerebral Hemisphere 0097-
  Cerebral Meninges 0091-
  Cerebral Ventricle 0096-
  Cervix 0U9C-
  Chest Wall 0W98-
  Choroid
    Left 089B-
    Right 089A-
  Cisterna Chyli 079L-
  Clavicle
    Left 0P9B-
    Right 0P99-
  Clitoris 0U9J-
  Coccygeal Glomus 0G9B-
  Coccyx 0Q9S-
  Colon
    Ascending 0D9K-
    Descending 0D9M-
    Sigmoid 0D9N-
    Transverse 0D9L-
  Conjunctiva
    Left 089T-
    Right 089S-
  Cord
    Bilateral 0V9H-
    Left 0V9G-
    Right 0V9F-
  Cornea
    Left 0899-
    Right 0898-
  Cul-de-sac 0U9F-
  Diaphragm
    Left 0B9S-
    Right 0B9R-
  Disc
    Cervical Vertebral 0R93-
    Cervicothoracic Vertebral 0R95-
    Lumbar Vertebral 0S92-
    Lumbosacral 0S94-
    Thoracic Vertebral 0R99-
    Thoracolumbar Vertebral 0R9B-
  Duct
    Common Bile 0F99-
    Cystic 0F98-
    Hepatic
      Left 0F96-
      Right 0F95-
    Lacrimal
      Left 089Y-
      Right 089X-
    Pancreatic 0F9D-
      Accessory 0F9F-
    Parotid
      Left 0C9C-
      Right 0C9B-
  Duodenum 0D99-
  Dura Mater 0092-
  Ear
    External
      Left 0991-
      Right 0990-
    External Auditory Canal
      Left 0994-
      Right 0993-
    Inner
      Left 099E-
      Right 099D-
    Middle
      Left 0996-
      Right 0995-

Drainage — *continued*
  Elbow Region
    Left 0X9C-
    Right 0X9B-
  Epididymis
    Bilateral 0V9L-
    Left 0V9K-
    Right 0V9J-
  Epidural Space 0093-
  Epiglottis 0C9R-
  Esophagogastric Junction 0D94-
  Esophagus 0D95-
    Lower 0D93-
    Middle 0D92-
    Upper 0D91-
  Eustachian Tube
    Left 099G-
    Right 099F-
  Extremity
    Lower
      Left 0Y9B-
      Right 0Y99-
    Upper
      Left 0X97-
      Right 0X96-
  Eye
    Left 0891-
    Right 0890-
  Eyelid
    Lower
      Left 089R-
      Right 089Q-
    Upper
      Left 089P-
      Right 089N-
  Face 0W92-
  Fallopian Tube
    Left 0U96-
    Right 0U95-
  Fallopian Tubes, Bilateral 0U97-
  Femoral Region
    Left 0Y98-
    Right 0Y97-
  Femoral Shaft
    Left 0Q99-
    Right 0Q98-
  Femur
    Lower
      Left 0Q9C-
      Right 0Q9B-
    Upper
      Left 0Q97-
      Right 0Q96-
  Fibula
    Left 0Q9K-
    Right 0Q9J-
  Finger Nail 0H9Q-
  Foot
    Left 0Y9N-
    Right 0Y9M-
  Gallbladder 0F94-
  Gingiva
    Lower 0C96-
    Upper 0C95-
  Gland
    Adrenal
      Bilateral 0G94-
      Left 0G92-
      Right 0G93-
    Lacrimal
      Left 089W-
      Right 089V-
    Minor Salivary 0C9J-
    Parotid
      Left 0C99-
      Right 0C98-
    Pituitary 0G90-
    Sublingual
      Left 0C9F-
      Right 0C9D-

Drainage — *continued*
  Gland — *continued*
    Submaxillary
      Left 0C9H-
      Right 0C9G-
    Vestibular 0U9L-
  Glenoid Cavity
    Left 0P98-
    Right 0P97-
  Glomus Jugulare 0G9C-
  Hand
    Left 0X9K-
    Right 0X9J-
  Head 0W90-
  Humeral Head
    Left 0P9D-
    Right 0P9C-
  Humeral Shaft
    Left 0P9G-
    Right 0P9F-
  Hymen 0U9K-
  Hypothalamus 009A-
  Ileocecal Valve 0D9C-
  Ileum 0D9B-
  Inguinal Region
    Left 0Y96-
    Right 0Y95-
  Intestine
    Large 0D9E-
      Left 0D9G-
      Right 0D9F-
    Small 0D98-
  Iris
    Left 089D-
    Right 089C-
  Jaw
    Lower 0W95-
    Upper 0W94-
  Jejunum 0D9A-
  Joint
    Acromioclavicular
      Left 0R9H-
      Right 0R9G-
    Ankle
      Left 0S9G-
      Right 0S9F-
    Carpal
      Left 0R9R-
      Right 0R9Q-
    Cervical Vertebral 0R91-
    Cervicothoracic Vertebral 0R94-
    Coccygeal 0S96-
    Elbow
      Left 0R9M-
      Right 0R9L-
    Finger Phalangeal
      Left 0R9X-
      Right 0R9W-
    Hip
      Left 0S9B-
      Right 0S99-
    Knee
      Left 0S9D-
      Right 0S9C-
    Lumbar Vertebral 0S90-
    Lumbosacral 0S93-
    Metacarpocarpal
      Left 0R9T-
      Right 0R9S-
    Metacarpophalangeal
      Left 0R9V-
      Right 0R9U-
    Metatarsal-Phalangeal
      Left 0S9N-
      Right 0S9M-
    Metatarsal-Tarsal
      Left 0S9L-
      Right 0S9K-
    Occipital-cervical 0R90-
    Sacrococcygeal 0S95-

Drainage — *continued*
  Joint — *continued*
    Sacroiliac
      Left 0S98-
      Right 0S97-
    Shoulder
      Left 0R9K-
      Right 0R9J-
    Sternoclavicular
      Left 0R9F-
      Right 0R9E-
    Tarsal
      Left 0S9J-
      Right 0S9H-
    Temporomandibular
      Left 0R9D-
      Right 0R9C-
    Thoracic Vertebral 0R96-
    Thoracolumbar Vertebral 0R9A-
    Toe Phalangeal
      Left 0S9Q-
      Right 0S9P-
    Wrist
      Left 0R9P-
      Right 0R9N-
  Kidney
    Left 0T91-
    Right 0T90-
  Kidney Pelvis
    Left 0T94-
    Right 0T93-
  Knee Region
    Left 0Y9G-
    Right 0Y9F-
  Larynx 0C9S-
  Leg
    Lower
      Left 0Y9J-
      Right 0Y9H-
    Upper
      Left 0Y9D-
      Right 0Y9C-
  Lens
    Left 089K-
    Right 089J-
  Lip
    Lower 0C91-
    Upper 0C90-
  Liver 0F90-
    Left Lobe 0F92-
    Right Lobe 0F91-
  Lung
    Bilateral 0B9M-
    Left 0B9L-
    Lower Lobe
      Left 0B9J-
      Right 0B9F-
    Middle Lobe, Right 0B9D-
    Right 0B9K-
    Upper Lobe
      Left 0B9G-
      Right 0B9C-
  Lung Lingula 0B9H-
  Lymphatic
    Aortic 079D-
    Axillary
      Left 0796-
      Right 0795-
    Head 0790-
    Inguinal
      Left 079J-
      Right 079H-
    Internal Mammary
      Left 0799-
      Right 0798-
    Lower Extremity
      Left 079G-
      Right 079F-
    Mesenteric 079B-

Drainage — continued
Lymphatic — continued
Neck
  Left **0792**-
  Right **0791**-
Pelvis **079C**-
Thoracic Duct **079K**-
Thorax **0797**-
Upper Extremity
  Left **0794**-
  Right **0793**-
Mandible
  Left **0N9V**-
  Right **0N9T**-
Maxilla
  Left **0N9S**-
  Right **0N9R**-
Mediastinum **0W9C**-
Medulla Oblongata **009D**-
Mesentery **0D9V**-
Metacarpal
  Left **0P9Q**-
  Right **0P9P**-
Metatarsal
  Left **0Q9P**-
  Right **0Q9N**-
Muscle
Abdomen
  Left **0K9L**-
  Right **0K9K**-
Extraocular
  Left **089M**-
  Right **089L**-
Facial **0K91**-
Foot
  Left **0K9W**-
  Right **0K9V**-
Hand
  Left **0K9D**-
  Right **0K9C**-
Head **0K90**-
Hip
  Left **0K9P**-
  Right **0K9N**-
Lower Arm and Wrist
  Left **0K9B**-
  Right **0K99**-
Lower Leg
  Left **0K9T**-
  Right **0K9S**-
Neck
  Left **0K93**-
  Right **0K92**-
Perineum **0K9M**-
Shoulder
  Left **0K96**-
  Right **0K95**-
Thorax
  Left **0K9J**-
  Right **0K9H**-
Tongue, Palate, Pharynx **0K94**-
Trunk
  Left **0K9G**-
  Right **0K9F**-
Upper Arm
  Left **0K98**-
  Right **0K97**-
Upper Leg
  Left **0K9R**-
  Right **0K9Q**-
Nasopharynx **099N**-
Neck **0W96**-
Nerve
Abdominal Sympathetic **019M**-
Abducens **009L**-
Accessory **009R**-
Acoustic **009N**-
Brachial Plexus **0193**-
Cervical **0191**-
Cervical Plexus **0190**-

Drainage — continued
Nerve — continued
Facial **009M**-
Femoral **019D**-
Glossopharyngeal **009P**-
Head and Neck Sympathetic **019K**-
Hypoglossal **009S**-
Lumbar **019B**-
Lumbar Plexus **0199**-
Lumbar Sympathetic **019N**-
Lumbosacral Plexus **019A**-
Median **0195**-
Oculomotor **009H**-
Olfactory **009F**-
Optic **009G**-
Peroneal **019H**-
Phrenic **0192**-
Pudendal **019C**-
Radial **0196**-
Sacral **019R**-
Sacral Plexus **019Q**-
Sacral Sympathetic **019P**-
Sciatic **019F**-
Thoracic **0198**-
Thoracic Sympathetic **019L**-
Tibial **019G**-
Trigeminal **009K**-
Trochlear **009J**-
Ulnar **0194**-
Vagus **009Q**-
Nipple
  Left **0H9X**-
  Right **0H9W**-
Nose **099K**-
Omentum
  Greater **0D9S**-
  Lesser **0D9T**-
Oral Cavity and Throat **0W93**-
Orbit
  Left **0N9Q**-
  Right **0N9P**-
Ovary
  Bilateral **0U92**-
  Left **0U91**-
  Right **0U90**-
Palate
  Hard **0C92**-
  Soft **0C93**-
Pancreas **0F9G**-
Para-aortic Body **0G99**-
Paraganglion Extremity **0G9F**-
Parathyroid Gland **0G9R**-
Inferior
  Left **0G9P**-
  Right **0G9N**-
Multiple **0G9Q**-
Superior
  Left **0G9M**-
  Right **0G9L**-
Patella
  Left **0Q9F**-
  Right **0Q9D**-
Pelvic Cavity **0W9J**-
Penis **0V9S**-
Pericardial Cavity **0W9D**-
Perineum
  Female **0W9N**-
  Male **0W9M**-
Peritoneal Cavity **0W9G**-
Peritoneum **0D9W**-
Phalanx
Finger
  Left **0P9V**-
  Right **0P9T**-
Thumb
  Left **0P9S**-
  Right **0P9R**-
Toe
  Left **0Q9R**-
  Right **0Q9Q**-

Drainage — continued
Pharynx **0C9M**-
Pineal Body **0G91**-
Pleura
  Left **0B9P**-
  Right **0B9N**-
Pleural Cavity
  Left **0W9B**-
  Right **0W99**-
Pons **009B**-
Prepuce **0V9T**-
Products of Conception
Amniotic Fluid
  Diagnostic **1090**-
  Therapeutic **1090**-
Fetal Blood **1090**-
Fetal Cerebrospinal Fluid **1090**-
Fetal Fluid, Other **1090**-
Fluid, Other **1090**-
Prostate **0V90**-
Radius
  Left **0P9J**-
  Right **0P9H**-
Rectum **0D9P**-
Retina
  Left **089F**-
  Right **089E**-
Retinal Vessel
  Left **089H**-
  Right **089G**-
Retroperitoneum **0W9H**-
Rib
  Left **0P92**-
  Right **0P91**-
Sacrum **0Q91**-
Scapula
  Left **0P96**-
  Right **0P95**-
Sclera
  Left **0897**-
  Right **0896**-
Scrotum **0V95**-
Septum, Nasal **099M**-
Shoulder Region
  Left **0X93**-
  Right **0X92**-
Sinus
Accessory **099P**-
Ethmoid
  Left **099V**-
  Right **099U**-
Frontal
  Left **099T**-
  Right **099S**-
Mastoid
  Left **099C**-
  Right **099B**-
Maxillary
  Left **099R**-
  Right **099Q**-
Sphenoid
  Left **099X**-
  Right **099W**-
Skin
Abdomen **0H97**-
Back **0H96**-
Buttock **0H98**-
Chest **0H95**-
Ear
  Left **0H93**-
  Right **0H92**-
Face **0H91**-
Foot
  Left **0H9N**-
  Right **0H9M**-
Genitalia **0H9A**-
Hand
  Left **0H9G**-
  Right **0H9F**-

Drainage — continued
Skin — continued
Lower Arm
  Left **0H9E**-
  Right **0H9D**-
Lower Leg
  Left **0H9L**-
  Right **0H9K**-
Neck **0H94**-
Perineum **0H99**-
Scalp **0H90**-
Upper Arm
  Left **0H9C**-
  Right **0H9B**-
Upper Leg
  Left **0H9J**-
  Right **0H9H**-
Skull **0N90**-
Spinal Canal **009U**-
Spinal Cord
Cervical **009W**-
Lumbar **009Y**-
Thoracic **009X**-
Spinal Meninges **009T**-
Spleen **079P**-
Sternum **0P90**-
Stomach **0D96**-
Pylorus **0D97**-
Subarachnoid Space **0095**-
Subcutaneous Tissue and Fascia
Abdomen **0J98**-
Back **0J97**-
Buttock **0J99**-
Chest **0J96**-
Face **0J91**-
Foot
  Left **0J9R**-
  Right **0J9Q**-
Hand
  Left **0J9K**-
  Right **0J9J**-
Lower Arm
  Left **0J9H**-
  Right **0J9G**-
Lower Leg
  Left **0J9P**-
  Right **0J9N**-
Neck
  Anterior **0J94**-
  Posterior **0J95**-
Pelvic Region **0J9C**-
Perineum **0J9B**-
Scalp **0J90**-
Upper Arm
  Left **0J9F**-
  Right **0J9D**-
Upper Leg
  Left **0J9M**-
  Right **0J9L**-
Subdural Space **0094**-
Tarsal
  Left **0Q9M**-
  Right **0Q9L**-
Tendon
Abdomen
  Left **0L9G**-
  Right **0L9F**-
Ankle
  Left **0L9T**-
  Right **0L9S**-
Foot
  Left **0L9W**-
  Right **0L9V**-
Hand
  Left **0L98**-
  Right **0L97**-
Head and Neck **0L90**-
Hip
  Left **0L9K**-
  Right **0L9J**-

Drainage — *continued*
Tendon — *continued*
Knee
Left **0L9R**-
Right **0L9Q**-
Lower Arm and Wrist
Left **0L96**-
Right **0L95**-
Lower Leg
Left **0L9P**-
Right **0L9N**-
Perineum **0L9H**-
Shoulder
Left **0L92**-
Right **0L91**-
Thorax
Left **0L9D**-
Right **0L9C**-
Trunk
Left **0L9B**-
Right **0L99**-
Upper Arm
Left **0L94**-
Right **0L93**-
Upper Leg
Left **0L9M**-
Right **0L9L**-
Testis
Bilateral **0V9C**-
Left **0V9B**-
Right **0V99**-
Thalamus **0099**-
Thymus **079M**-
Thyroid Gland **0G9K**-
Left Lobe **0G9G**-
Right Lobe **0G9H**-
Tibia
Left **0Q9H**-
Right **0Q9G**-
Toe Nail **0H9R**-
Tongue **0C97**-
Tonsils **0C9P**-
Tooth
Lower **0C9X**-
Upper **0C9W**-
Trachea **0B91**-
Tunica Vaginalis
Left **0V97**-
Right **0V96**-
Turbinate, Nasal **099L**-
Tympanic Membrane
Left **0998**-
Right **0997**-
Ulna
Left **0P9L**-
Right **0P9K**-
Ureter
Left **0T97**-
Right **0T96**-
Ureters, Bilateral **0T98**-
Urethra **0T9D**-
Uterine Supporting Structure **0U94**-
Uterus **0U99**-
Uvula **0C9N**-
Vagina **0U9G**-
Vas Deferens
Bilateral **0V9Q**-
Left **0V9P**-
Right **0V9N**-
Vein
Axillary
Left **0598**-
Right **0597**-
Azygos **0590**-
Basilic
Left **059C**-
Right **059B**-
Brachial
Left **059A**-
Right **0599**-

Drainage — *continued*
Vein — *continued*
Cephalic
Left **059F**-
Right **059D**-
Colic **0697**-
Common Iliac
Left **069D**-
Right **069C**-
Esophageal **0693**-
External Iliac
Left **069G**-
Right **069F**-
External Jugular
Left **059Q**-
Right **059P**-
Face
Left **059V**-
Right **059T**-
Femoral
Left **069N**-
Right **069M**-
Foot
Left **069V**-
Right **069T**-
Gastric **0692**-
Greater Saphenous
Left **069Q**-
Right **069P**-
Hand
Left **059H**-
Right **059G**-
Hemiazygos **0591**-
Hepatic **0694**-
Hypogastric
Left **069J**-
Right **069H**-
Inferior Mesenteric **0696**-
Innominate
Left **0594**-
Right **0593**-
Internal Jugular
Left **059N**-
Right **059M**-
Intracranial **059L**-
Lesser Saphenous
Left **069S**-
Right **069R**-
Lower **069Y**-
Portal **0698**-
Renal
Left **069B**-
Right **0699**-
Splenic **0691**-
Subclavian
Left **0596**-
Right **0595**-
Superior Mesenteric **0695**-
Upper **059Y**-
Vertebral
Left **059S**-
Right **059R**-
Vena Cava, Inferior **0690**-
Vertebra
Cervical **0P93**-
Lumbar **0Q90**-
Thoracic **0P94**-
Vesicle
Bilateral **0V93**-
Left **0V92**-
Right **0V91**-
Vitreous
Left **0895**-
Right **0894**-
Vocal Cord
Left **0C9V**-
Right **0C9T**-
Vulva **0U9M**-
Wrist Region
Left **0X9H**-
Right **0X9G**-

Dressing
Abdominal Wall **2W23X4Z**
Arm
Lower
Left **2W2DX4Z**
Right **2W2CX4Z**
Upper
Left **2W2BX4Z**
Right **2W2AX4Z**
Back **2W25X4Z**
Chest Wall **2W24X4Z**
Extremity
Lower
Left **2W2MX4Z**
Right **2W2LX4Z**
Upper
Left **2W29X4Z**
Right **2W28X4Z**
Face **2W21X4Z**
Finger
Left **2W2KX4Z**
Right **2W2JX4Z**
Foot
Left **2W2TX4Z**
Right **2W2SX4Z**
Hand
Left **2W2FX4Z**
Right **2W2EX4Z**
Head **2W20X4Z**
Inguinal Region
Left **2W27X4Z**
Right **2W26X4Z**
Leg
Lower
Left **2W2RX4Z**
Right **2W2QX4Z**
Upper
Left **2W2PX4Z**
Right **2W2NX4Z**
Neck **2W22X4Z**
Thumb
Left **2W2HX4Z**
Right **2W2GX4Z**
Toe
Left **2W2VX4Z**
Right **2W2UX4Z**

Driver stent (RX) (OTW)
use Intraluminal Device
Drotrecogin alfa *see* Introduction of Recombinant Human-activated Protein C
Duct of Santorini
use Duct, Pancreatic, Accessory
Duct of Wirsung
use Duct, Pancreatic
Ductogram, mammary *see* Plain Radiography, Skin, Subcutaneous Tissue and Breast **BH0**-
Ductography, mammary *see* Plain Radiography, Skin, Subcutaneous Tissue and Breast **BH0**-
Ductus deferens
use Vas Deferens
use Vas Deferens, Bilateral
use Vas Deferens, Left
use Vas Deferens, Right
Duodenal ampulla
use Ampulla of Vater
Duodenectomy
see Excision, Duodenum **0DB9**-
see Resection, Duodenum **0DT9**-
Duodenocholedochotomy *see* Drainage, Gallbladder **0F94**-
Duodenocystostomy
see Bypass, Gallbladder **0F14**-
see Drainage, Gallbladder **0F94**-
Duodenoenterostomy
see Bypass, Gastrointestinal System **0D1**-
see Drainage, Gastrointestinal System **0D9**-

Duodenojejunal flexure
use Jejunum
Duodenolysis *see* Release, Duodenum **0DN9**-
Duodenorrhaphy *see* Repair, Duodenum **0DQ9**-
Duodenostomy
see Bypass, Duodenum **0D19**-
see Drainage, Duodenum **0D99**-
Duodenotomy *see* Drainage, Duodenum **0D99**-
Dura mater, intracranial
use Dura Mater
Dura mater, spinal
use Spinal Meninges
DuraHeart Left Ventricular Assist System
use Implantable Heart Assist System in Heart and Great Vessels
Dural venous sinus
use Vein, Intracranial
Durata® Defibrillation Lead
use Cardiac Lead, Defibrillator in **02H**-
Dynesys® Dynamic Stabilization System
use Spinal Stabilization Device, Pedicle-Based in **0RH**-
use Spinal Stabilization Device, Pedicle-Based in **0SH**-

E

E-Lum1nexx™ (Biliary) (Vascular) Stent
use Intraluminal Device
Earlobe
use Ear, External, Bilateral
use Ear, External, Left
use Ear, External, Right
Echocardiogram *see* Ultrasonography, Heart **B24-**
Echography *see* Ultrasonography
ECMO *see* Performance, Circulatory **5A15-**
EDWARDS INTUITY Elite valve system
use Zooplastic Tissue, Rapid Deployment Technique in New Technology
EEG (electroencephalogram) *see* Measurement, Central Nervous **4A00-**
EGD (esophagogastroduoden- oscopy) 0DJ08ZZ
Eighth cranial nerve
use Nerve, Acoustic
Ejaculatory duct
use Vas Deferens
use Vas Deferens, Bilateral
use Vas Deferens, Left
use Vas Deferens, Right
EKG (electrocardiogram) *see* Measurement, Cardiac **4A02-**
Electrical bone growth stimulator (EBGS)
use Bone Growth Stimulator in Head and Facial Bones
use Bone Growth Stimulator in Lower Bones
use Bone Growth Stimulator in Upper Bones
Electrical muscle stimulation (EMS) lead
use Stimulator Lead in Muscles
Electrocautery
Destruction *see* Destruction
Repair *see* Repair
Electroconvulsive Therapy
Bilateral-Multiple Seizure **GZB3ZZZ**
Bilateral-Single Seizure **GZB2ZZZ**
Electroconvulsive Therapy, Other **GZB4ZZZ**
Unilateral-Multiple Seizure **GZB1ZZZ**
Unilateral-Single Seizure **GZB0ZZZ**
Electroencephalogram (EEG) *see* Measurement, Central Nervous **4A00-**
Electromagnetic Therapy
Central Nervous **6A22-**
Urinary **6A21-**
Electronic muscle stimulator lead
use Stimulator Lead in Muscles
Electrophysiologic stimulation (EPS) *see* Measurement, Cardiac **4A02-**
Electroshock therapy *see* Electroconvulsive Therapy
Elevation, bone fragments, skull *see* Reposition, Head and Facial Bones **0NS-**
Eleventh cranial nerve
use Nerve, Accessory

E-Luminexx™ (Biliary) (Vascular) Stent
use Intraluminal Device
Embolectomy *see* Extirpation
Embolization
see Occlusion
see Restriction
Embolization coil(s)
use Intraluminal Device
EMG (electromyogram) *see* Measurement, Musculoskeletal **4A0F-**
Encephalon
use Brain
Endarterectomy
see Extirpation, Lower Arteries **04C-**
see Extirpation, Upper Arteries **03C-**
Endeavor® (III) (IV) (Sprint) Zotarolimus-eluting Coronary Stent System
use Intraluminal Device, Drug-eluting in Heart and Great Vessels
Endologix AFX® Endovascular AAA System
use Intraluminal Device
EndoSure® sensor
use Monitoring Device, Pressure Sensor in **02H-**
ENDOTAK RELIANCE® (G) Defibrillation Lead
use Cardiac Lead, Defibrillator in **02H-**
Endotracheal tube (cuffed) (double-lumen)
use Intraluminal Device, Endotracheal Airway in Respiratory System
Endurant® II AAA stent graft system
use Intraluminal Device
Endurant® Endovascular Stent Graft
use Intraluminal Device
Enlargement
see Dilation
see Repair
EnRhythm
use Pacemaker, Dual Chamber **0JH-**
Enterorrhaphy *see* Repair, Gastrointestinal System **0DQ-**
Enterra gastric neurostimulator
use Stimulator Generator, Multiple Array in **0JH-**
Enucleation
Eyeball *see* Resection, Eye **08T-**
Eyeball with prosthetic implant *see* Replacement, Eye **08R-**
Ependyma
use Cerebral Ventricle
Epicel® cultured epidermal autograft
use Autologous Tissue Substitute
Epic™ Stented Tissue Valve (aortic)
use Zooplastic Tissue in Heart and Great Vessels
Epidermis
use Skin
Epididymectomy
see Excision, Male Reproductive System **0VB-**
see Resection, Male Reproductive System **0VT-**
Epididymoplasty
see Repair, Male Reproductive System **0VQ-**
see Supplement, Male Reproductive System **0VU-**

Epididymorrhaphy *see* Repair, Male Reproductive System **0VQ-**
Epididymotomy *see* Drainage, Male Reproductive System **0V9-**
Epidural space, intracranial
use Epidural Space
Epidural space, spinal
use Spinal Canal
Epiphysiodesis
see Fusion, Lower Joints **0SG-**
see Fusion, Upper Joints **0RG-**
Epiploic foramen
use Peritoneum
Epiretinal Visual Prosthesis
Left **08H105Z**
Right **08H005Z**
Episiorrhaphy *see* Repair, Perineum, Female **0WQN-**
Episiotomy *see* Division, Perineum, Female **0W8N-**
Epithalamus
use Thalamus
Epitrochlear lymph node
use Lymphatic, Upper Extremity, Left
use Lymphatic, Upper Extremity, Right
EPS (electrophysiologic stimulation) *see* Measurement, Cardiac **4A02-**
Eptifibatide, infusion *see* Introduction of Platelet Inhibitor
ERCP (endoscopic retrograde cholangiopancreatography) *see* Fluoroscopy, Hepatobiliary System and Pancreas **BF1-**
Erector spinae muscle
use Muscle, Trunk, Left
use Muscle, Trunk, Right
Esophageal artery
use Upper Artery
Esophageal obturator airway (EOA)
use Intraluminal Device, Airway in Gastrointestinal System
Esophageal plexus
use Nerve, Thoracic Sympathetic
Esophagectomy
see Excision, Gastrointestinal System **0DB-**
see Resection, Gastrointestinal System **0DT-**
Esophagocoloplasty
see Repair, Gastrointestinal System **0DQ-**
see Supplement, Gastrointestinal System **0DU-**
Esophagoenterostomy
see Bypass, Gastrointestinal System **0D1-**
see Drainage, Gastrointestinal System **0D9-**
Esophagoesophagostomy
see Bypass, Gastrointestinal System **0D1-**
see Drainage, Gastrointestinal System **0D9-**
Esophagogastrectomy
see Excision, Gastrointestinal System **0DB-**
see Resection, Gastrointestinal System **0DT-**
Esophagogastroduodenoscopy (EGD) 0DJ08ZZ
Esophagogastroplasty
see Repair, Gastrointestinal System **0DQ-**
see Supplement, Gastrointestinal System **0DU-**

Esophagogastroscopy 0DJ68ZZ
Esophagogastrostomy
see Bypass, Gastrointestinal System **0D1-**
see Drainage, Gastrointestinal System **0D9-**
Esophagojejunoplasty *see* Supplement, Gastrointestinal System **0DU-**
Esophagojejunostomy
see Bypass, Gastrointestinal System **0D1-**
see Drainage, Gastrointestinal System **0D9-**
Esophagomyotomy *see* Division, Esophagogastric Junction **0D84-**
Esophagoplasty
see Repair, Gastrointestinal System **0DQ-**
see Replacement, Esophagus **0DR5-**
see Supplement, Gastrointestinal System **0DU-**
Esophagoplication *see* Restriction, Gastrointestinal System **0DV-**
Esophagorrhaphy *see* Repair, Gastrointestinal System **0DQ-**
Esophagoscopy 0DJ08ZZ
Esophagotomy *see* Drainage, Gastrointestinal System **0D9-**
Esteem® implantable hearing system
use Hearing Device in Ear, Nose, Sinus
ESWL (extracorporeal shock wave lithotripsy) *see* Fragmentation
Ethmoidal air cell
use Sinus, Ethmoid, Left
use Sinus, Ethmoid, Right
Ethmoidectomy
see Excision, Ear, Nose, Sinus **09B-**
see Excision, Head and Facial Bones **0NB-**
see Resection, Ear, Nose, Sinus **09T-**
see Resection, Head and Facial Bones **0NT-**
Ethmoidotomy *see* Drainage, Ear, Nose, Sinus **099-**
Evacuation
Hematoma *see* Extirpation
Other Fluid *see* Drainage
Evera (XT) (S) (DR/VR)
use Defibrillator Generator in **0JH-**
Everolimus-eluting coronary stent
use Intraluminal Device, Drug-eluting in Heart and Great Vessels
Evisceration
Eyeball *see* Resection, Eye **08T-**
Eyeball with prosthetic implant *see* Replacement, Eye **08R-**
Ex-PRESS™ mini glaucoma shunt
use Synthetic Substitute
Examination *see* Inspection
Exchange *see* Change device in

Excision
Abdominal Wall 0WBF-
Acetabulum
  Left 0QB5-
  Right 0QB4-
Adenoids 0CBQ-
Ampulla of Vater 0FBC-
Anal Sphincter 0DBR-
Ankle Region
  Left 0YBL-
  Right 0YBK-
Anus 0DBQ-
Aorta
  Abdominal 04B0-
  Thoracic
    Ascending/Arch 02BX-
    Descending 02BW-
Aortic Body 0GBD-
Appendix 0DBJ-
Arm
  Lower
    Left 0XBF-
    Right 0XBD-
  Upper
    Left 0XB9-
    Right 0XB8-
Artery
  Anterior Tibial
    Left 04BQ-
    Right 04BP-
  Axillary
    Left 03B6-
    Right 03B5-
  Brachial
    Left 03B8-
    Right 03B7-
  Celiac 04B1-
  Colic
    Left 04B7-
    Middle 04B8-
    Right 04B6-
  Common Carotid
    Left 03BJ-
    Right 03BH
  Common Iliac
    Left 04BD-
    Right 04BC-
  External Carotid
    Left 03BN-
    Right 03BM-
  External Iliac
    Left 04BJ-
    Right 04BH-
  Face 03BR-
  Femoral
    Left 04BL-
    Right 04BK-
  Foot
    Left 04BW-
    Right 04BV-
  Gastric 04B2-
  Hand
    Left 03BF-
    Right 03BD-
  Hepatic 04B3-
  Inferior Mesenteric 04BB-
  Innominate 03B2-
  Internal Carotid
    Left 03BL-
    Right 03BK-
  Internal Iliac
    Left 04BF-
    Right 04BE-
  Internal Mammary
    Left 03B1-
    Right 03B0-
  Intracranial 03BG-
  Lower 04BY-
  Peroneal
    Left 04BU-
    Right 04BT-
  Popliteal
    Left 04BN-
    Right 04BM-

Excision — continued
Artery — continued
  Posterior Tibial
    Left 04BS-
    Right 04BR-
  Pulmonary
    Left 02BR-
    Right 02BQ-
  Pulmonary Trunk 02BP-
  Radial
    Left 03BC-
    Right 03BB-
  Renal
    Left 04BA-
    Right 04B9-
  Splenic 04B4-
  Subclavian
    Left 03B4-
    Right 03B3-
  Superior Mesenteric 04B5-
  Temporal
    Left 03BT-
    Right 03BS-
  Thyroid
    Left 03BV-
    Right 03BU-
  Ulnar
    Left 03BA-
    Right 03B9-
  Upper 03BY-
  Vertebral
    Left 03BQ-
    Right 03BP-
Atrium
  Left 02B7-
  Right 02B6-
Auditory Ossicle
  Left 09BA0Z-
  Right 09B90Z-
Axilla
  Left 0XB5-
  Right 0XB4-
Back
  Lower 0WBL-
  Upper 0WBK-
Basal Ganglia 00B8-
Bladder 0TBB-
Bladder Neck 0TBC-
Bone
  Ethmoid
    Left 0NBG-
    Right 0NBF-
  Frontal
    Left 0NB2-
    Right 0NB1-
  Hyoid 0NBX-
  Lacrimal
    Left 0NBJ-
    Right 0NBH-
  Nasal 0NBB-
  Occipital
    Left 0NB8-
    Right 0NB7-
  Palatine
    Left 0NBL-
    Right 0NBK-
  Parietal
    Left 0NB4-
    Right 0NB3-
  Pelvic
    Left 0QB3-
    Right 0QB2-
  Sphenoid
    Left 0NBD-
    Right 0NBC-
  Temporal
    Left 0NB6-
    Right 0NB5-
  Zygomatic
    Left 0NBN-
    Right 0NBM-

Excision — continued
Brain 00B0-
Breast
  Bilateral 0HBV-
  Left 0HBU-
  Right 0HBT-
  Supernumerary 0HBY-
Bronchus
  Lingula 0BB9-
  Lower Lobe
    Left 0BBB-
    Right 0BB6-
  Main
    Left 0BB7-
    Right 0BB3-
  Middle Lobe, Right 0BB5-
  Upper Lobe
    Left 0BB8-
    Right 0BB4-
Buccal Mucosa 0CB4-
Bursa and Ligament
  Abdomen
    Left 0MBJ-
    Right 0MBH-
  Ankle
    Left 0MBR-
    Right 0MBQ-
  Elbow
    Left 0MB4-
    Right 0MB3-
  Foot
    Left 0MBT-
    Right 0MBS-
  Hand
    Left 0MB8-
    Right 0MB7-
  Head and Neck 0MB0-
  Hip
    Left 0MBM-
    Right 0MBL-
  Knee
    Left 0MBP-
    Right 0MBN-
  Lower Extremity
    Left 0MBW-
    Right 0MBV-
  Perineum 0MBK-
  Shoulder
    Left 0MB2-
    Right 0MB1-
  Thorax
    Left 0MBG-
    Right 0MBF-
  Trunk
    Left 0MBD-
    Right 0MBC-
  Upper Extremity
    Left 0MBB-
    Right 0MB9-
  Wrist
    Left 0MB6-
    Right 0MB5-
Buttock
  Left 0YB1-
  Right 0YB0-
Carina 0BB2-
Carotid Bodies, Bilateral 0GB8-
Carotid Body
  Left 0GB6-
  Right 0GB7-
Carpal
  Left 0PBN-
  Right 0PBM-
Cecum 0DBH-
Cerebellum 00BC-
Cerebral Hemisphere 00B7-
Cerebral Meninges 00B1-
Cerebral Ventricle 00B6-
Cervix 0UBC-

Excision — continued
Chest Wall 0WB8-
Chordae Tendineae 02B9-
Choroid
  Left 08BB-
  Right 08BA-
Cisterna Chyli 07BL-
Clavicle
  Left 0PBB-
  Right 0PB9-
Clitoris 0UBJ-
Coccygeal Glomus 0GBB-
Coccyx 0QBS-
Colon
  Ascending 0DBK-
  Descending 0DBM-
  Sigmoid 0DBN-
  Transverse 0DBL-
Conduction Mechanism 02B8-
Conjunctiva
  Left 08BTXZ-
  Right 08BSXZ-
Cord
  Bilateral 0VBH-
  Left 0VBG-
  Right 0VBF-
Cornea
  Left 08B9XZ-
  Right 08B8XZ-
Cul-de-sac 0UBF-
Diaphragm
  Left 0BBS-
  Right 0BBR-
Disc
  Cervical Vertebral 0RB3-
  Cervicothoracic Vertebral 0RB5-
  Lumbar Vertebral 0SB2-
  Lumbosacral 0SB4-
  Thoracic Vertebral 0RB9-
  Thoracolumbar Vertebral 0RBB-
Duct
  Common Bile 0FB9-
  Cystic 0FB8-
  Hepatic
    Left 0FB6-
    Right 0FB5-
  Lacrimal
    Left 08BY-
    Right 08BX-
  Pancreatic 0FBD-
    Accessory 0FBF-
  Parotid
    Left 0CBC-
    Right 0CBB-
Duodenum 0DB9-
Dura Mater 00B2-
Ear
  External
    Left 09B1-
    Right 09B0-
  External Auditory Canal
    Left 09B4-
    Right 09B3-
  Inner
    Left 09BE0Z-
    Right 09BD0Z-
  Middle
    Left 09B60Z-
    Right 09B50Z-
Elbow Region
  Left 0XBC-
  Right 0XBB-
Epididymis
  Bilateral 0VBL-
  Left 0VBK-
  Right 0VBJ-
Epiglottis 0CBR-

Excision — *continued*
Esophagogastric Junction **0DB**4 -
Esophagus **0DB**5-
  Lower **0DB**3-
  Middle **0DB**2-
  Upper **0DB**1-
Eustachian Tube
  Left **09B**G-
  Right **09B**F-
Extremity
  Lower
    Left **0YB**B-
    Right **0YB**9-
  Upper
    Left **0XB**7-
    Right **0XB**6-
Eye
  Left **08B**1-
  Right **08B**0-
Eyelid
  Lower
    Left **08B**R-
    Right **08B**Q-
  Upper
    Left **08B**P-
    Right **08B**N-
Face **0WB**2-
Fallopian Tube
  Left **0UB**6-
  Right **0UB**5-
Fallopian Tubes, Bilateral **0UB**7-
Femoral Region
  Left **0YB**8-
  Right **0YB**7-
Femoral Shaft
  Left **0QB**9-
  Right **0QB**8-
Femur
  Lower
    Left **0QB**C-
    Right **0QB**B-
  Upper
    Left **0QB**7-
    Right **0QB**6-
Fibula
  Left **0QB**K-
  Right **0QB**J-
Finger Nail **0HB**QXZ-
Foot
  Left **0YB**N-
  Right **0YB**M-
Gallbladder **0FB**4-
Gingiva
  Lower **0CB**6-
  Upper **0CB**5-
Gland
  Adrenal
    Bilateral **0GB**4-
    Left **0GB**2-
    Right **0GB**3-
  Lacrimal
    Left **08B**W-
    Right **08B**V-
  Minor Salivary **0CB**J-
  Parotid
    Left **0CB**9-
    Right **0CB**8-
  Pituitary **0GB**0-
  Sublingual
    Left **0CB**F-
    Right **0CB**D-
  Submaxillary
    Left **0CB**H-
    Right **0CB**G-
  Vestibular **0UB**L-
Glenoid Cavity
  Left **0PB**8-
  Right **0PB**7-
Glomus Jugulare **0GB**C-

Excision — *continued*
Hand
  Left **0XB**K-
  Right **0XB**J-
Head **0WB**0-
Humeral Head
  Left **0PB**D-
  Right **0PB**C-
Humeral Shaft
  Left **0PB**G-
  Right **0PB**F-
Hymen **0UB**K-
Hypothalamus **00B**A-
Ileocecal Valve **0DB**C-
Ileum **0DB**B-
Inguinal Region
  Left **0YB**6-
  Right **0YB**5-
Intestine
  Large **0DB**E-
    Left **0DB**G-
    Right **0DB**F-
  Small **0DB**8-
Iris
  Left **08B**D3Z-
  Right **08B**C3Z-
Jaw
  Lower **0WB**5-
  Upper **0WB**4-
Jejunum **0DB**A-
Joint
  Acromioclavicular
    Left **0RB**H-
    Right **0RB**G-
  Ankle
    Left **0SB**G-
    Right **0SB**F-
  Carpal
    Left **0RB**R-
    Right **0RB**Q-
  Cervical Vertebral **0RB**1-
  Cervicothoracic Vertebral **0RB**4-
  Coccygeal **0SB**6-
  Elbow
    Left **0RB**M-
    Right **0RB**L-
  Finger Phalangeal
    Left **0RB**X-
    Right **0RB**W-
  Hip
    Left **0SB**B-
    Right **0SB**9-
  Knee
    Left **0SB**D-
    Right **0SB**C-
  Lumbar Vertebral **0SB**0-
  Lumbosacral **0SB**3-
  Metacarpocarpal
    Left **0RB**T-
    Right **0RB**S-
  Metacarpophalangeal
    Left **0RB**V-
    Right **0RB**U-
  Metatarsal-Phalangeal
    Left **0SB**N-
    Right **0SB**M-
  Metatarsal-Tarsal
    Left **0SB**L-
    Right **0SB**K-
  Occipital-cervical **0RB**0-
  Sacrococcygeal **0SB**5-
  Sacroiliac
    Left **0SB**8-
    Right **0SB**7-
  Shoulder
    Left **0RB**K-
    Right **0RB**J-
  Sternoclavicular
    Left **0RB**F-
    Right **0RB**E-

Excision — *continued*
Joint — *continued*
  Tarsal
    Left **0SB**J-
    Right **0SB**H-
  Temporomandibular
    Left **0RB**D-
    Right **0RB**C-
  Thoracic Vertebral **0RB**6-
  Thoracolumbar Vertebral **0RB**A-
  Toe Phalangeal
    Left **0SB**Q-
    Right **0SB**P-
  Wrist
    Left **0RB**P-
    Right **0RB**N-
Kidney
  Left **0TB**1-
  Right **0TB**0-
Kidney Pelvis
  Left **0TB**4-
  Right **0TB**3-
Knee Region
  Left **0YB**G-
  Right **0YB**F-
Larynx **0CB**S-
Leg
  Lower
    Left **0YB**J-
    Right **0YB**H-
  Upper
    Left **0YB**D-
    Right **0YB**C-
Lens
  Left **08B**K3Z-
  Right **08B**J3Z-
Lip
  Lower **0CB**1-
  Upper **0CB**0-
Liver **0FB**0-
  Left Lobe **0FB**2-
  Right Lobe **0FB**1-
Lung
  Bilateral **0BB**M-
  Left **0BB**L-
  Lower Lobe
    Left **0BB**J-
    Right **0BB**F-
  Middle Lobe, Right **0BB**D-
  Right **0BB**K-
  Upper Lobe
    Left **0BB**G-
    Right **0BB**C-
Lung Lingula **0BB**H-
Lymphatic
  Aortic **07B**D-
  Axillary
    Left **07B**6-
    Right **07B**5-
  Head **07B**0-
  Inguinal
    Left **07B**J-
    Right **07B**H-
  Internal Mammary
    Left **07B**9-
    Right **07B**8-
  Lower Extremity
    Left **07B**G-
    Right **07B**F-
  Mesenteric **07B**B-
  Neck
    Left **07B**2-
    Right **07B**1-
  Pelvis **07B**C-
  Thoracic Duct **07B**K-
  Thorax **07B**7-
  Upper Extremity
    Left **07B**4-
    Right **07B**3-

Excision — *continued*
Mandible
  Left **0NB**V-
  Right **0NB**T-
Maxilla
  Left **0NB**S-
  Right **0NB**R-
Mediastinum **0WB**C-
Medulla Oblongata **00B**D-
Mesentery **0DB**V-
Metacarpal
  Left **0PB**Q-
  Right **0PB**P-
Metatarsal
  Left **0QB**P-
  Right **0QB**N-
Muscle
  Abdomen
    Left **0KB**L-
    Right **0KB**K-
  Extraocular
    Left **08B**M-
    Right **08B**L-
  Facial **0KB**1-
  Foot
    Left **0KB**W-
    Right **0KB**V-
  Hand
    Left **0KB**D-
    Right **0KB**C-
  Head **0KB**0-
  Hip
    Left **0KB**P-
    Right **0KB**N-
  Lower Arm and Wrist
    Left **0KB**B-
    Right **0KB**9-
  Lower Leg
    Left **0KB**T-
    Right **0KB**S-
  Neck
    Left **0KB**3-
    Right **0KB**2-
  Papillary **02B**D-
  Perineum **0KB**M-
  Shoulder
    Left **0KB**6-
    Right **0KB**5-
  Thorax
    Left **0KB**J-
    Right **0KB**H-
  Tongue, Palate, Pharynx **0KB**4-
  Trunk
    Left **0KB**G-
    Right **0KB**F-
  Upper Arm
    Left **0KB**8-
    Right **0KB**7-
  Upper Leg
    Left **0KB**R-
    Right **0KB**Q-
Nasopharynx **09B**N-
Neck **0WB**6-
Nerve
  Abdominal Sympathetic **01B**M-
  Abducens **00B**L-
  Accessory **00B**R-
  Acoustic **00B**N-
  Brachial Plexus **01B**3-
  Cervical **01B**1-
  Cervical Plexus **01B**0-
  Facial **00B**M-
  Femoral **01B**D-
  Glossopharyngeal **00B**P-
  Head and Neck Sympathetic **01B**K-
  Hypoglossal **00B**S-
  Lumbar **01B**B-
  Lumbar Plexus **01B**9-
  Lumbar Sympathetic **01B**N-
  Lumbosacral Plexus **01B**A-
  Median **01B**5-

PROCEDURE INDEX

PROCEDURE INDEX

Excision — *continued*
  Nerve — *continued*
    Oculomotor **00BH**-
    Olfactory **00BF**-
    Optic **00BG**-
    Peroneal **01BH**-
    Phrenic **01B2**-
    Pudendal **01BC**-
    Radial **01B6**-
    Sacral **01BR**-
    Sacral Plexus **01BQ**-
    Sacral Sympathetic **01BP**-
    Sciatic **01BF**-
    Thoracic **01B8**-
    Thoracic Sympathetic **01BL**-
    Tibial **01BG**-
    Trigeminal **00BK**-
    Trochlear **00BJ**-
    Ulnar **01B4**-
    Vagus **00BQ**-
  Nipple
    Left **0HBX**-
    Right **0HBW**-
  Nose **09BK**-
  Omentum
    Greater **0DBS**-
    Lesser **0DBT**-
  Orbit
    Left **0NBQ**-
    Right **0NBP**-
  Ovary
    Bilateral **0UB2**-
    Left **0UB1**-
    Right **0UB0**-
  Palate
    Hard **0CB2**-
    Soft **0CB3**-
  Pancreas **0FBG**-
  Para-aortic Body **0GB9**-
  Paraganglion Extremity **0GBF**-
  Parathyroid Gland **0GBR**-
    Inferior
      Left **0GBP**-
      Right **0GBN**-
    Multiple **0GBQ**-
    Superior
      Left **0GBM**-
      Right **0GBL**-
  Patella
    Left **0QBF**-
    Right **0QBD**-
  Penis **0VBS**-
  Pericardium **02BN**-
  Perineum
    Female **0WBN**-
    Male **0WBM**-
  Peritoneum **0DBW**-
  Phalanx
    Finger
      Left **0PBV**-
      Right **0PBT**-
    Thumb
      Left **0PBS**-
      Right **0PBR**-
    Toe
      Left **0QBR**-
      Right **0QBQ**-
  Pharynx **0CBM**-
  Pineal Body **0GB1**-
  Pleura
    Left **0BBP**-
    Right **0BBN**-
  Pons **00BB**-
  Prepuce **0VBT**-
  Prostate **0VB0**-
  Radius
    Left **0PBJ**-
    Right **0PBH**-
  Rectum **0DBP**-

Excision — *continued*
  Retina
    Left **08BF3Z**-
    Right **08BE3Z**-
  Retroperitoneum **0WBH**-
  Rib
    Left **0PB2**-
    Right **0PB1**-
  Sacrum **0QB1**-
  Scapula
    Left **0PB6**-
    Right **0PB5**-
  Sclera
    Left **08B7XZ**-
    Right **08B6XZ**-
  Scrotum **0VB5**-
  Septum
    Atrial **02B5**-
    Nasal **09BM**-
    Ventricular **02BM**-
  Shoulder Region
    Left **0XB3**-
    Right **0XB2**-
  Sinus
    Accessory **09BP**-
    Ethmoid
      Left **09BV**-
      Right **09BU**-
    Frontal
      Left **09BT**-
      Right **09BS**-
    Mastoid
      Left **09BC**-
      Right **09BB**-
    Maxillary
      Left **09BR**-
      Right **09BQ**-
    Sphenoid
      Left **09BX**-
      Right **09BW**-
  Skin
    Abdomen **0HB7XZ**-
    Back **0HB6XZ**-
    Buttock **0HB8XZ**-
    Chest **0HB5XZ**-
    Ear
      Left **0HB3XZ**-
      Right **0HB2XZ**-
    Face **0HB1XZ**-
    Foot
      Left **0HBNXZ**-
      Right **0HBMXZ**-
    Genitalia **0HBAXZ**-
    Hand
      Left **0HBGXZ**-
      Right **0HBFXZ**-
    Lower Arm
      Left **0HBEXZ**-
      Right **0HBDXZ**-
    Lower Leg
      Left **0HBLXZ**-
      Right **0HBKXZ**-
    Neck **0HB4XZ**-
    Perineum **0HB9XZ**-
    Scalp **0HB0XZ**-
    Upper Arm
      Left **0HBCXZ**-
      Right **0HBBXZ**-
    Upper Leg
      Left **0HBJXZ**-
      Right **0HBHXZ**-
  Skull **0NB0**-
  Spinal Cord
    Cervical **00BW**-
    Lumbar **00BY**-
    Thoracic **00BX**-
  Spinal Meninges **00BT**-
  Spleen **07BP**-
  Sternum **0PB0**-
  Stomach **0DB6**-
    Pylorus **0DB7**-

Excision — *continued*
  Subcutaneous Tissue and Fascia
    Abdomen **0JB8**-
    Back **0JB7**-
    Buttock **0JB9**-
    Chest **0JB6**-
    Face **0JB1**-
    Foot
      Left **0JBR**-
      Right **0JBQ**-
    Hand
      Left **0JBK**-
      Right **0JBJ**-
    Lower Arm
      Left **0JBH**-
      Right **0JBG**-
    Lower Leg
      Left **0JBP**-
      Right **0JBN**-
    Neck
      Anterior **0JB4**-
      Posterior **0JB5**-
    Pelvic Region **0JBC**-
    Perineum **0JBB**-
    Scalp **0JB0**-
    Upper Arm
      Left **0JBF**-
      Right **0JBD**-
    Upper Leg
      Left **0JBM**-
      Right **0JBL**-
  Tarsal
    Left **0QBM**-
    Right **0QBL**-
  Tendon
    Abdomen
      Left **0LBG**-
      Right **0LBF**-
    Ankle
      Left **0LBT**-
      Right **0LBS**-
    Foot
      Left **0LBW**-
      Right **0LBV**-
    Hand
      Left **0LB8**-
      Right **0LB7**-
    Head and Neck **0LB0**-
    Hip
      Left **0LBK**-
      Right **0LBJ**-
    Knee
      Left **0LBR**-
      Right **0LBQ**-
    Lower Arm and Wrist
      Left **0LB6**-
      Right **0LB5**-
    Lower Leg
      Left **0LBP**-
      Right **0LBN**-
    Perineum **0LBH**-
    Shoulder
      Left **0LB2**-
      Right **0LB1**-
    Thorax
      Left **0LBD**-
      Right **0LBC**-
    Trunk
      Left **0LBB**-
      Right **0LB9**-
    Upper Arm
      Left **0LB4**-
      Right **0LB3**-
    Upper Leg
      Left **0LBM**-
      Right **0LBL**-
  Testis
    Bilateral **0VBC**-
    Left **0VBB**-
    Right **0VB9**-

Excision — *continued*
  Thalamus **00B9**-
  Thymus **07BM**-
  Thyroid Gland
    Left Lobe **0GBG**-
    Right Lobe **0GBH**-
  Tibia
    Left **0QBH**-
    Right **0QBG**-
  Toe Nail **0HBRXZ** -
  Tongue **0CB7**-
  Tonsils **0CBP**-
  Tooth
    Lower **0CBX**-
    Upper **0CBW**-
  Trachea **0BB1**-
  Tunica Vaginalis
    Left **0VB7**-
    Right **0VB6**-
  Turbinate, Nasal **09BL**-
  Tympanic Membrane
    Left **09B8**-
    Right **09B7**-
  Ulna
    Left **0PBL**-
    Right **0PBK**-
  Ureter
    Left **0TB7**-
    Right **0TB6**-
  Urethra **0TBD**-
  Uterine Supporting Structure **0UB4**-
  Uterus **0UB9**-
  Uvula **0CBN**-
  Vagina **0UBG**-
  Valve
    Aortic **02BF**-
    Mitral **02BG**-
    Pulmonary **02BH**-
    Tricuspid **02BJ**-
  Vas Deferens
    Bilateral **0VBQ**-
    Left **0VBP**-
    Right **0VBN**-
  Vein
    Axillary
      Left **05B8**-
      Right **05B7**-
    Azygos **05B0**-
    Basilic
      Left **05BC**-
      Right **05BB**-
    Brachial
      Left **05BA**-
      Right **05B9**-
    Cephalic
      Left **05BF**-
      Right **05BD**-
    Colic **06B7**-
    Common Iliac
      Left **06BD**-
      Right **06BC**-
    Coronary **02B4**-
    Esophageal **06B3**-
    External Iliac
      Left **06BG**-
      Right **06BF**-
    External Jugular
      Left **05BQ**-
      Right **05BP**-
    Face
      Left **05BV**-
      Right **05BT**-
    Femoral
      Left **06BN**-
      Right **06BM**-
    Foot
      Left **06BV**-
      Right **06BT**-

Excision — *continued*
Vein — *continued*
Gastric **06B2**-
Greater Saphenous
Left **06BQ**-
Right **06BP**-
Hand
Left **05BH**-
Right **05BG**-
Hemiazygos **05B1**-
Hepatic **06B4**-
Hypogastric
Left **06BJ**-
Right **06BH**-
Inferior Mesenteric **06B6**-
Innominate
Left **05B4**-
Right **05B3**-
Internal Jugular
Left **05BN**-
Right **05BM**-
Intracranial **05BL**-
Lesser Saphenous
Left **06BS**-
Right **06BR**-
Lower **06BY**-
Portal **06B8**-
Pulmonary
Left **02BT** -
Right **02BS**-
Renal
Left **06BB**-
Right **06B9**-
Splenic **06B1**-
Subclavian
Left **05B6**-
Right **05B5**-
Superior Mesenteric **06B5**-
Upper **05BY**-
Vertebral
Left **05BS**-
Right **05BR**-
Vena Cava
Inferior **06B0**-
Superior **02BV**-
Ventricle
Left **02BL**-
Right **02BK**-
Vertebra
Cervical **0PB3**-
Lumbar **0QB0**-
Thoracic **0PB4**-
Vesicle
Bilateral **0VB3**-
Left **0VB2**-
Right **0VB1**-
Vitreous
Left **08B53Z**-
Right **08B43Z**-
Vocal Cord
Left **0CBV**-
Right **0CBT**-
Vulva **0UBM**-
Wrist Region
Left **0XBH**-
Right **0XBG**-

EXCLUDER® AAA Endoprosthesis
use Intraluminal Device
use Intraluminal Device, Branched or Fenestrated, One or Two Arteries in **04V**-
use Intraluminal Device, Branched or Fenestrated, Three or More in Arteries **04V**-
EXCLUDER® IBE Endoprosthesis
use Intraluminal Device, Branched or Fenestrated, One or Two Arteries in **04V**-
Exclusion, Left atrial appendage (LAA) *see* Occlusion, Atrium, Left **02L7**-
Exercise, rehabilitation *see* Motor Treatment, Rehabilitation **F07**-
Exploration *see* Inspection
Express® (LD) Premounted Stent System
use Intraluminal Device
Express® Biliary SD Monorail® Premounted Stent System
use Intraluminal Device
Ex-PRESS™ mini glaucoma shunt
use Synthetic Substitute
Express® SD Renal Monorail® Premounted Stent System
use Intraluminal Device
Extensor carpi radialis muscle
use Muscle, Lower Arm and Wrist, Left
use Muscle, Lower Arm and Wrist, Right
Extensor carpi ulnaris muscle
use Muscle, Lower Arm and Wrist, Left
use Muscle, Lower Arm and Wrist, Right
Extensor digitorum brevis muscle
use Muscle, Foot, Left
use Muscle, Foot, Right
Extensor digitorum longus muscle
use Muscle, Lower Leg, Left
use Muscle, Lower Leg, Right
Extensor hallucis brevis muscle
use Muscle, Foot, Left
use Muscle, Foot, Right
Extensor hallucis longus muscle
use Muscle, Lower Leg, Left
use Muscle, Lower Leg, Right
External anal sphincter
use Anal Sphincter
External auditory meatus
use Ear, External Auditory Canal, Left
use Ear, External Auditory Canal, Right
External fixator
use External Fixation Device in Head and Facial Bones
use External Fixation Device in Lower Bones
use External Fixation Device in Lower Joints
use External Fixation Device in Upper Bones
use External Fixation Device in Upper Joints
External maxillary artery
use Artery, Face
External naris
use Nose
External oblique aponeurosis
use Subcutaneous Tissue and Fascia, Trunk
External oblique muscle
use Muscle, Abdomen, Left
use Muscle, Abdomen, Right

External popliteal nerve
use Nerve, Peroneal
External pudendal artery
use Artery, Femoral, Left
use Artery, Femoral, Right
External pudendal vein
use Vein, Greater Saphenous, Left
use Vein, Greater Saphenous, Right
External urethral sphincter
use Urethra
Extirpation
Acetabulum
Left **0QC5**-
Right **0QC4**-
Adenoids **0CCQ**-
Ampulla of Vater **0FCC**-
Anal Sphincter **0DCR**-
Anterior Chamber
Left **08C3**-
Right **08C2**-
Anus **0DCQ**-
Aorta
Abdominal **04C0**-
Thoracic
Ascending/Arch **02CX**-
Descending **02CW**-
Aortic Body **0GCD**-
Appendix **0DCJ**-
Artery
Anterior Tibial
Left **04CQ**-
Right **04CP**-
Axillary
Left **03C6**-
Right **03C5**-
Brachial
Left **03C8**-
Right **03C7**-
Celiac **04C1**-
Colic
Left **04C7**-
Middle **04C8**-
Right **04C6**-
Common Carotid
Left **03CJ**-
Right **03CH**-
Common Iliac
Left **04CD**-
Right **04CC**-
Coronary
Four or More Arteries **02C3**-
One Artery **02C0**-
Three Arteries **02C2**-
Two Arteries **02C1**-
External Carotid
Left **03CN**-
Right **03CM**-
External Iliac
Left **04CJ**-
Right **04CH**-
Face **03CR**-
Femoral
Left **04CL**-
Right **04CK**-
Foot
Left **04CW**-
Right **04CV**-
Gastric **04C2**-
Hand
Left **03CF**-
Right **03CD**-
Hepatic **04C3**-
Inferior Mesenteric **04CB**-
Innominate **03C2**-
Internal Carotid
Left **03CL**-
Right **03CK**-
Internal Iliac
Left **04CF**-
Right **04CE**-
Internal Mammary
Left **03C1**-
Right **03C0**-

Extirpation — *continued*
Artery — *continued*
Intracranial **03CG**-
Lower **04CY**-
Peroneal
Left **04CU**-
Right **04CT**-
Popliteal
Left **04CN**-
Right **04CM**-
Posterior Tibial
Left **04CS**-
Right **04CR**-
Pulmonary
Left **02CR**-
Right **02CQ**-
Pulmonary Trunk **02CP**-
Radial
Left **03CC**-
Right **03CB**-
Renal
Left **04CA**-
Right **04C9**-
Splenic **04C4**-
Subclavian
Left **03C4**-
Right **03C3**-
Superior Mesenteric **04C5**-
Temporal
Left **03CT**-
Right **03CS**-
Thyroid
Left **03CV**-
Right **03CU**-
Ulnar
Left **03CA**-
Right **03C9**-
Upper **03CY**-
Vertebral
Left **03CQ**-
Right **03CP**-
Atrium
Left **02C7**-
Right **02C6**-
Auditory Ossicle
Left **09CA0ZZ**-
Right **09C90ZZ**-
Basal Ganglia **00C8**-
Bladder **0TCB**-
Bladder Neck **0TCC**-
Bone
Ethmoid
Left **0NCG**-
Right **0NCF**-
Frontal
Left **0NC2**-
Right **0NC1**-
Hyoid **0NCX**-
Lacrimal
Left **0NCJ**-
Right **0NCH**-
Nasal **0NCB**-
Occipital
Left **0NC8**-
Right **0NC7**-
Palatine
Left **0NCL**-
Right **0NCK**-
Parietal
Left **0NC4**-
Right **0NC3**-
Pelvic
Left **0QC3**-
Right **0QC2**-
Sphenoid
Left **0NCD**-
Right **0NCC**-
Temporal
Left **0NC6**-
Right **0NC5**-
Zygomatic
Left **0NCN**-
Right **0NCM**-

Extirpation — *continued*
Brain 00C0-
Breast
 Bilateral 0HCV-
 Left 0HCU-
 Right 0HCT-
Bronchus
 Lingula 0BC9-
 Lower Lobe
  Left 0BCB-
  Right 0BC6-
 Main
  Left 0BC7-
  Right 0BC3-
 Middle Lobe, Right 0BC5-
 Upper Lobe
  Left 0BC8-
  Right 0BC4-
Buccal Mucosa 0CC4-
Bursa and Ligament
 Abdomen
  Left 0MCJ-
  Right 0MCH-
 Ankle
  Left 0MCR-
  Right 0MCQ-
 Elbow
  Left 0MC4-
  Right 0MC3-
 Foot
  Left 0MCT-
  Right 0MCS-
 Hand
  Left 0MC8-
  Right 0MC7-
 Head and Neck 0MC0-
 Hip
  Left 0MCM-
  Right 0MCL-
 Knee
  Left 0MCP-
  Right 0MCN-
 Lower Extremity
  Left 0MCW-
  Right 0MCV-
 Perineum 0MCK-
 Shoulder
  Left 0MC2-
  Right 0MC1-
 Thorax
  Left 0MCG-
  Right 0MCF-
 Trunk
  Left 0MCD-
  Right 0MCC-
 Upper Extremity
  Left 0MCB-
  Right 0MC9-
 Wrist
  Left 0MC6-
  Right 0MC5-
Carina 0BC2-
Carotid Bodies, Bilateral 0GC8-
Carotid Body
 Left 0GC6-
 Right 0GC7-
Carpal
 Left 0PCN-
 Right 0PCM-
Cavity, Cranial 0WC1-
Cecum 0DCH-
Cerebellum 00CC-
Cerebral Hemisphere 00C7-
Cerebral Meninges 00C1-
Cerebral Ventricle 00C6-
Cervix 0UCC-
Chordae Tendineae 02C9-
Choroid
 Left 08CB-
 Right 08CA-

Extirpation — *continued*
Cisterna Chyli 07CL-
Clavicle
 Left 0PCB-
 Right 0PC9-
Clitoris 0UCJ-
Coccygeal Glomus 0GCB-
Coccyx 0QCS-
Colon
 Ascending 0DCK-
 Descending 0DCM-
 Sigmoid 0DCN-
 Transverse 0DCL-
Conduction Mechanism 02C8-
Conjunctiva
 Left 08CTXZZ
 Right 08CSXZZ
Cord
 Bilateral 0VCH-
 Left 0VCG-
 Right 0VCF-
Cornea
 Left 08C9XZZ
 Right 08C8XZZ
Cul-de-sac 0UCF-
Diaphragm
 Left 0BCS-
 Right 0BCR-
Disc
 Cervical Vertebral 0RC3-
 Cervicothoracic Vertebral 0RC5-
 Lumbar Vertebral 0SC2-
 Lumbosacral 0SC4-
 Thoracic Vertebral 0RC9-
 Thoracolumbar Vertebral 0RCB-
Duct
 Common Bile 0FC9-
 Cystic 0FC8-
 Hepatic
  Left 0FC6-
  Right 0FC5-
 Lacrimal
  Left 08CY-
  Right 08CX-
 Pancreatic 0FCD-
  Accessory 0FCF-
 Parotid
  Left 0CCC-
  Right 0CCB-
Duodenum 0DC9-
Dura Mater 00C2-
Ear
 External
  Left 09C1-
  Right 09C0-
 External Auditory Canal
  Left 09C4-
  Right 09C3-
 Inner
  Left 09CE0ZZ
  Right 09CD0ZZ
 Middle
  Left 09C60ZZ
  Right 09C50ZZ
Endometrium 0UCB-
Epididymis
 Bilateral 0VCL-
 Left 0VCK-
 Right 0VCJ-
Epidural Space 00C3-
Epiglottis 0CCR-
Esophagogastric Junction 0DC4-
Esophagus 0DC5-
 Lower 0DC3-
 Middle 0DC2-
 Upper 0DC1-

Extirpation — *continued*
Eustachian Tube
 Left 09CG-
 Right 09CF-
Eye
 Left 08C1XZZ
 Right 08C0XZZ
Eyelid
 Lower
  Left 08CR-
  Right 08CQ-
 Upper
  Left 08CP-
  Right 08CN-
Fallopian Tube
 Left 0UC6-
 Right 0UC5-
Fallopian Tubes, Bilateral 0UC7-
Femoral Shaft
 Left 0QC9-
 Right 0QC8-
Femur
 Lower
  Left 0QCC-
  Right 0QCB-
 Upper
  Left 0QC7-
  Right 0QC6-
Fibula
 Left 0QCK-
 Right 0QCJ-
Finger Nail 0HCQXZZ
Gallbladder 0FC4-
Gastrointestinal Tract 0WCP-
Genitourinary Tract 0WCR-
Gingiva
 Lower 0CC6-
 Upper 0CC5-
Gland
 Adrenal
  Bilateral 0GC4-
  Left 0GC2-
  Right 0GC3-
 Lacrimal
  Left 08CW-
  Right 08CV-
 Minor Salivary 0CCJ-
 Parotid
  Left 0CC9-
  Right 0CC8-
 Pituitary 0GC0-
 Sublingual
  Left 0CCF-
  Right 0CCD-
 Submaxillary
  Left 0CCH-
  Right 0CCG-
 Vestibular 0UCL-
Glenoid Cavity
 Left 0PC8-
 Right 0PC7-
Glomus Jugulare 0GCC-
Humeral Head
 Left 0PCD-
 Right 0PCC-
Humeral Shaft
 Left 0PCG-
 Right 0PCF-
Hymen 0UCK-
Hypothalamus 00CA-
Ileocecal Valve 0DCC-
Ileum 0DCB-
Intestine
 Large 0DCE-
  Left 0DCG-
  Right 0DCF-
 Small 0DC8-

Extirpation — *continued*
Iris
 Left 08CD-
 Right 08CC-
Jejunum 0DCA-
Joint
 Acromioclavicular
  Left 0RCH-
  Right 0RCG-
 Ankle
  Left 0SCG-
  Right 0SCF-
 Carpal
  Left 0RCR-
  Right 0RCQ-
 Cervical Vertebral 0RC1-
 Cervicothoracic Vertebral 0RC4-
 Coccygeal 0SC6-
 Elbow
  Left 0RCM-
  Right 0RCL-
 Finger Phalangeal
  Left 0RCX-
  Right 0RCW-
 Hip
  Left 0SCB-
  Right 0SC9-
 Knee
  Left 0SCD-
  Right 0SCC-
 Lumbar Vertebral 0SC0-
 Lumbosacral 0SC3-
 Metacarpocarpal
  Left 0RCT-
  Right 0RCS-
 Metacarpophalangeal
  Left 0RCV-
  Right 0RCU-
 Metatarsal-Phalangeal
  Left 0SCN-
  Right 0SCM-
 Metatarsal-Tarsal
  Left 0SCL-
  Right 0SCK-
 Occipital-cervical 0RC0-
 Sacrococcygeal 0SC5-
 Sacroiliac
  Left 0SC8-
  Right 0SC7-
 Shoulder
  Left 0RCK-
  Right 0RCJ-
 Sternoclavicular
  Left 0RCF-
  Right 0RCE-
 Tarsal
  Left 0SCJ-
  Right 0SCH-
 Temporomandibular
  Left 0RCD-
  Right 0RCC-
 Thoracic Vertebral 0RC6-
 Thoracolumbar Vertebral 0RCA-
 Toe Phalangeal
  Left 0SCQ-
  Right 0SCP-
 Wrist
  Left 0RCP-
  Right 0RCN-
Kidney
 Left 0TC1-
 Right 0TC0-
Kidney Pelvis
 Left 0TC4-
 Right 0TC3-

Extirpation — *continued*
  Larynx **0CCS**-
  Lens
    Left **08CK**-
    Right **08CJ**-
  Lip
    Lower **0CC**1-
    Upper **0CC**0-
  Liver **0FC**0-
    Left Lobe **0FC**2-
    Right Lobe **0FC**1-
  Lung
    Bilateral **0BC**M-
    Left **0BC**L-
    Lower Lobe
      Left **0BC**J-
      Right **0BC**F-
    Middle Lobe, Right **0BC**D-
    Right **0BC**K-
    Upper Lobe
      Left **0BC**G-
      Right **0BC**C-
  Lung Lingula **0BC**H-
  Lymphatic
    Aortic **07C**D-
    Axillary
      Left **07C**6-
      Right **07C**5-
    Head **07C**0-
    Inguinal
      Left **07C**J-
      Right **07C**H-
    Internal Mammary
      Left **07C**9-
      Right **07C**8-
    Lower Extremity
      Left **07C**G-
      Right **07C**F-
    Mesenteric **07C**B-
    Neck
      Left **07C**2-
      Right **07C**1-
    Pelvis **07C**C-
    Thoracic Duct **07C**K-
    Thorax **07C**7-
    Upper Extremity
      Left **07C**4-
      Right **07C**3-
  Mandible
    Left **0NC**V-
    Right **0NC**T-
  Maxilla
    Left **0NC**S-
    Right **0NC**R-
  Mediastinum **0WC**C-
  Medulla Oblongata **00C**D-
  Mesentery **0DC**V-
  Metacarpal
    Left **0PC**Q-
    Right **0PC**P-
  Metatarsal
    Left **0QC**P-
    Right **0QC**N-
  Muscle
    Abdomen
      Left **0KC**L-
      Right **0KC**K-
    Extraocular
      Left **08C**M-
      Right **08C**L-
    Facial **0KC**1-
    Foot
      Left **0KC**W-
      Right **0KC**V-
    Hand
      Left **0KC**D-
      Right **0KC**C-
    Head **0KC**0-
    Hip
      Left **0KC**P-
      Right **0KC**N-

Extirpation — *continued*
  Muscle — *continued*
    Lower Arm and Wrist
      Left **0KC**B-
      Right **0KC**9-
    Lower Leg
      Left **0KC**T-
      Right **0KC**S-
    Neck
      Left **0KC**3-
      Right **0KC**2-
    Papillary **02C**D-
    Perineum **0KC**M-
    Shoulder
      Left **0KC**6-
      Right **0KC**5-
    Thorax
      Left **0KC**J-
      Right **0KC**H-
    Tongue, Palate, Pharynx **0KC**4-
    Trunk
      Left **0KC**G-
      Right **0KC**F-
    Upper Arm
      Left **0KC**8-
      Right **0KC**7-
    Upper Leg
      Left **0KC**R-
      Right **0KC**Q-
  Nasopharynx **09C**N-
  Nerve
    Abdominal Sympathetic **01C**M-
    Abducens **00C**L-
    Accessory **00C**R-
    Acoustic **00C**N-
    Brachial Plexus **01C**3-
    Cervical **01C**1-
    Cervical Plexus **01C**0-
    Facial **00C**M-
    Femoral **01C**D-
    Glossopharyngeal **00C**P-
    Head and Neck Sympathetic **01C**K-
    Hypoglossal **00C**S-
    Lumbar **01C**B-
    Lumbar Plexus **01C**9-
    Lumbar Sympathetic **01C**N-
    Lumbosacral Plexus **01C**A-
    Median **01C**5-
    Oculomotor **00C**H-
    Olfactory **00C**F-
    Optic **00C**G-
    Peroneal **01C**H-
    Phrenic **01C**2-
    Pudendal **01C**C-
    Radial **01C**6-
    Sacral **01C**R-
    Sacral Plexus **01C**Q-
    Sacral Sympathetic **01C**P-
    Sciatic **01C**F-
    Thoracic **01C**8-
    Thoracic Sympathetic **01C**L-
    Tibial **01C**G-
    Trigeminal **00C**K-
    Trochlear **00C**J-
    Ulnar **01C**4-
    Vagus **00C**Q-
  Nipple
    Left **0HC**X-
    Right **0HC**W-
  Nose **09C**K-
  Omentum
    Greater **0DC**S-
    Lesser **0DC**T-
  Oral Cavity and Throat **0WC**3-
  Orbit
    Left **0NC**Q-
    Right **0NC**P-
  Orbital Atherectomy Technology **X2C**-

Extirpation — *continued*
  Ovary
    Bilateral **0UC**2-
    Left **0UC**1-
    Right **0UC**0-
  Palate
    Hard **0CC**2-
    Soft **0CC**3-
  Pancreas **0FC**G-
  Para-aortic Body **0GC**9-
  Paraganglion Extremity **0GC**F-
  Parathyroid Gland **0GC**R-
    Inferior
      Left **0GC**P-
      Right **0GC**N-
    Multiple **0GC**Q-
    Superior
      Left **0GC**M-
      Right **0GC**L-
  Patella
    Left **0QC**F-
    Right **0QC**D-
  Pelvic Cavity **0WC**J-
  Penis **0VC**S-
  Pericardial Cavity **0WC**D-
  Pericardium **02C**N-
  Peritoneal Cavity **0WC**G-
  Peritoneum **0DC**W-
  Phalanx
    Finger
      Left **0PC**V-
      Right **0PC**T-
    Thumb
      Left **0PC**S-
      Right **0PC**R-
    Toe
      Left **0QC**R-
      Right **0QC**Q-
  Pharynx **0CC**M-
  Pineal Body **0GC**1-
  Pleura
    Left **0BC**P-
    Right **0BC**N-
  Pleural Cavity
    Left **0WC**B-
    Right **0WC**9-
  Pons **00C**B-
  Prepuce **0VC**T-
  Prostate **0VC**0-
  Radius
    Left **0PC**J-
    Right **0PC**H-
  Rectum **0DC**P-
  Respiratory Tract **0WC**Q-
  Retina
    Left **08C**F-
    Right **08C**E-
  Retinal Vessel
    Left **08C**H-
    Right **08C**G-
  Rib
    Left **0PC**2-
    Right **0PC**1-
  Sacrum **0QC**1-
  Scapula
    Left **0PC**6-
    Right **0PC**5-
  Sclera
    Left **08C**7XZZ
    Right **08C**6XZZ
  Scrotum **0VC**5-
  Septum
    Atrial **02C**5-
    Nasal **09C**M-
    Ventricular **02C**M-

Extirpation — *continued*
  Sinus
    Accessory **09C**P-
    Ethmoid
      Left **09C**V-
      Right **09C**U-
    Frontal
      Left **09C**T-
      Right **09C**S-
    Mastoid
      Left **09C**C-
      Right **09C**B-
    Maxillary
      Left **09C**R-
      Right **09C**Q-
    Sphenoid
      Left **09C**X-
      Right **09C**W-
  Skin
    Abdomen **0HC**7XZZ
    Back **0HC**6XZZ
    Buttock **0HC**8XZZ
    Chest **0HC**5XZZ
    Ear
      Left **0HC**3XZZ
      Right **0HC**2XZZ
    Face **0HC**1XZZ
    Foot
      Left **0HC**NXZZ
      Right **0HC**MXZZ
    Genitalia **0HC**AXZZ
    Hand
      Left **0HC**GXZZ
      Right **0HC**FXZZ
    Lower Arm
      Left **0HC**EXZZ
      Right **0HC**DXZZ
    Lower Leg
      Left **0HC**LXZZ
      Right **0HC**KXZZ
    Neck **0HC**4XZZ
    Perineum **0HC**9XZZ
    Scalp **0HC**0XZZ
    Upper Arm
      Left **0HC**CXZZ
      Right **0HC**BXZZ
    Upper Leg
      Left **0HC**JXZZ
      Right **0HC**HXZZ
  Spinal Cord
    Cervical **00C**W-
    Lumbar **00C**Y-
    Thoracic **00C**X-
  Spinal Meninges **00C**T-
  Spleen **07C**P-
  Sternum **0PC**0-
  Stomach **0DC**6-
    Pylorus **0DC**7-
  Subarachnoid Space **00C**5-
  Subcutaneous Tissue and Fascia
    Abdomen **0JC**8-
    Back **0JC**7-
    Buttock **0JC**9-
    Chest **0JC**6-
    Face **0JC**1-
    Foot
      Left **0JC**R-
      Right **0JC**Q-
    Hand
      Left **0JC**K-
      Right **0JC**J-
    Lower Arm
      Left **0JC**H-
      Right **0JC**G-
    Lower Leg
      Left **0JC**P-
      Right **0JC**N-

PROCEDURE INDEX

PROCEDURE INDEX

Extirpation — *continued*
  Subcutaneous Tissue and Fascia — *continued*
    Neck
      Anterior **0JC**4-
      Posterior **0JC**5-
    Pelvic Region **0JC**C-
    Perineum **0JC**B-
    Scalp **0JC**0-
    Upper Arm
      Left **0JC**F-
      Right **0JC**D-
    Upper Leg
      Left **0JC**M-
      Right **0JC**L-
  Subdural Space **00C**4-
  Tarsal
    Left **0QC**M-
    Right **0QC**L-
  Tendon
    Abdomen
      Left **0LC**G-
      Right **0LC**F-
    Ankle
      Left **0LC**T-
      Right **0LC**S-
    Foot
      Left **0LC**W-
      Right **0LC**V-
    Hand
      Left **0LC**8-
      Right **0LC**7-
    Head and Neck **0LC**0-
    Hip
      Left **0LC**K-
      Right **0LC**J-
    Knee
      Left **0LC**R-
      Right **0LC**Q-
    Lower Arm and Wrist
      Left **0LC**6-
      Right **0LC**5-
    Lower Leg
      Left **0LC**P-
      Right **0LC**N-
    Perineum **0LC**H-
    Shoulder
      Left **0LC**2-
      Right **0LC**1-
    Thorax
      Left **0LC**D-
      Right **0LC**C-
    Trunk
      Left **0LC**B-
      Right **0LC**9-
    Upper Arm
      Left **0LC**4-
      Right **0LC**3-
    Upper Leg
      Left **0LC**M-
      Right **0LC**L-
  Testis
    Bilateral **0VC**C-
    Left **0VC**B-
    Right **0VC**9-
  Thalamus **00C**9-
  Thymus **07C**M-
  Thyroid Gland **0GC**K-
    Left Lobe **0GC**G-
    Right Lobe **0GC**H-
  Tibia
    Left **0QC**H-
    Right **0QC**G-
  Toe Nail **0HC**RXZZ
  Tongue **0CC**7-
  Tonsils **0CC**P-
  Tooth
    Lower **0CC**X-
    Upper **0CC**W-

Extirpation — *continued*
  Trachea **0BC**1-
  Tunica Vaginalis
    Left **0VC**7-
    Right **0VC**6-
  Turbinate, Nasal **09C**L-
  Tympanic Membrane
    Left **09C**8-
    Right **09C**7-
  Ulna
    Left **0PC**L-
    Right **0PC**K-
  Ureter
    Left **0TC**7-
    Right **0TC**6-
  Urethra **0TC**D-
  Uterine Supporting Structure **0UC**4-
  Uterus **0UC**9-
  Uvula **0CC**N-
  Vagina **0UC**G-
  Valve
    Aortic **02C**F-
    Mitral **02C**G-
    Pulmonary **02C**H-
    Tricuspid **02C**J-
  Vas Deferens
    Bilateral **0VC**Q-
    Left **0VC**P-
    Right **0VC**N-
  Vein
    Axillary
      Left **05C**8-
      Right **05C**7-
    Azygos **05C**0-
    Basilic
      Left **05C**C-
      Right **05C**B-
    Brachial
      Left **05C**A-
      Right **05C**9-
    Cephalic
      Left **05C**F-
      Right **05C**D-
    Colic **06C**7-
    Common Iliac
      Left **06C**D-
      Right **06C**C-
    Coronary **02C**4-
    Esophageal **06C**3-
    External Iliac
      Left **06C**G-
      Right **06C**F-
    External Jugular
      Left **05C**Q-
      Right **05C**P-
    Face
      Left **05C**V-
      Right **05C**T-
    Femoral
      Left **06C**N-
      Right **06C**M-
    Foot
      Left **06C**V-
      Right **06C**T-
    Gastric **06C**2-
    Greater Saphenous
      Left **06C**Q-
      Right **06C**P-
    Hand
      Left **05C**H-
      Right **05C**G-
    Hemiazygos **05C**1-
    Hepatic **06C**4-
    Hypogastric
      Left **06C**J-
      Right **06C**H-
    Inferior Mesenteric **06C**6-
    Innominate
      Left **05C**4-
      Right **05C**3-

Extirpation — *continued*
  Vein — *continued*
    Internal Jugular
      Left **05C**N-
      Right **05C**M-
    Intracranial **05C**L-
    Lesser Saphenous
      Left **06C**S-
      Right **06C**R-
    Lower **06C**Y-
    Portal **06C**8-
    Pulmonary
      Left **02C**T-
      Right **02C**S-
    Renal
      Left **06C**B-
      Right **06C**9-
    Splenic **06C**1-
    Subclavian
      Left **05C**6-
      Right **05C**5-
    Superior Mesenteric **06C**5-
    Upper **05C**Y-
    Vertebral
      Left **05C**S-
      Right **05C**R-
    Vena Cava
      Inferior **06C**0-
      Superior **02C**V-
  Ventricle
    Left **02C**L-
    Right **02C**K-
  Vertebra
    Cervical **0PC**3-
    Lumbar **0QC**0-
    Thoracic **0PC**4-
  Vesicle
    Bilateral **0VC**3-
    Left **0VC**2-
    Right **0VC**1-
  Vitreous
    Left **08C**5-
    Right **08C**4-
  Vocal Cord
    Left **0CC**V-
    Right **0CC**T-
  Vulva **0UC**M-
Extracorporeal shock wave lithotripsy *see* Fragmentation
Extracranial-intracranial bypass (EC-IC) *see* Bypass, Upper Arteries **031**-
Extraction
  Auditory Ossicle
    Left **09D**A0ZZ
    Right **09D**90ZZ
  Bone Marrow
    Iliac **07D**R-
    Sternum **07D**Q-
    Vertebral **07D**S-
  Bursa and Ligament
    Abdomen
      Left **0MD**J-
      Right **0MD**H-
    Ankle
      Left **0MD**R-
      Right **0MD**Q-
    Elbow
      Left **0MD**4-
      Right **0MD**3-
    Foot
      Left **0MD**T-
      Right **0MD**S-
    Hand
      Left **0MD**8-
      Right **0MD**7-
    Head and Neck **0MD**0-
    Hip
      Left **0MD**M-
      Right **0MD**L-

Extraction — *continued*
  Bursa and Ligament — *continued*
    Knee
      Left **0MD**P-
      Right **0MD**N-
    Lower Extremity
      Left **0MD**W-
      Right **0MD**V-
    Perineum **0MD**K-
    Shoulder
      Left **0MD**2-
      Right **0MD**1-
    Thorax
      Left **0MD**G-
      Right **0MD**F-
    Trunk
      Left **0MD**D-
      Right **0MD**C-
    Upper Extremity
      Left **0MD**B-
      Right **0MD**9-
    Wrist
      Left **0MD**6-
      Right **0MD**5-
  Cerebral Meninges **00D**1-
  Cornea
    Left **08D**9XZ
    Right **08D**8XZ
  Dura Mater **00D**2-
  Endometrium **0UD**B-
  Finger Nail **0HD**QXZZ
  Hair **0HD**SXZZ
  Kidney
    Left **0TD**1-
    Right **0TD**0-
  Lens
    Left **08D**K3ZZ
    Right **08D**J3ZZ
  Nerve
    Abdominal Sympathetic **01D**M-
    Abducens **00D**L-
    Accessory **00D**R-
    Acoustic **00D**N-
    Brachial Plexus **01D**3-
    Cervical **01D**1-
    Cervical Plexus **01D**0-
    Facial **00D**M-
    Femoral **01D**D-
    Glossopharyngeal **00D**P-
    Head and Neck Sympathetic **01D**K-
    Hypoglossal **00D**S-
    Lumbar **01D**B-
    Lumbar Plexus **01D**9-
    Lumbar Sympathetic **01D**N-
    Lumbosacral Plexus **01D**A-
    Median **01D**5-
    Oculomotor **00D**H-
    Olfactory **00D**F-
    Optic **00D**G-
    Peroneal **01D**H-
    Phrenic **01D**2-
    Pudendal **01D**C-
    Radial **01D**6-
    Sacral **01D**R-
    Sacral Plexus **01D**Q-
    Sacral Sympathetic **01D**P-
    Sciatic **01D**F-
    Thoracic **01D**8-
    Thoracic Sympathetic **01D**L-
    Tibial **01D**G-
    Trigeminal **00D**K-
    Trochlear **00D**J-
    Ulnar **01D**4-
    Vagus **00D**Q-
  Ova **0UD**N-
  Pleura
    Left **0BD**P-
    Right **0BD**N-

Extraction — *continued*
  Products of Conception
    Classical **10D**00Z0
    Ectopic **10D**2-
    Extraperitoneal **10D**00Z2
    High Forceps **10D**07Z5
    Internal Version **10D**07Z7
    Low Cervical **10D**00Z1
    Low Forceps **10D**07Z3
    Mid Forceps **10D**07Z4
    Other **10D**07Z8
    Retained **10D**1-
    Vacuum **10D**07Z6
  Septum, Nasal **09DM**-
  Sinus
    Accessory **09D**P-
    Ethmoid
      Left **09D**V-
      Right **09D**U-
    Frontal
      Left **09D**T-
      Right **09D**S-
    Mastoid
      Left **09D**C-
      Right **09D**B-
    Maxillary
      Left **09D**R-
      Right **09D**Q-
    Sphenoid
      Left **09D**X-
      Right **09D**W-
  Skin
    Abdomen **0HD**7XZZ
    Back **0HD**6XZZ
    Buttock **0HD**8XZZ
    Chest **0HD**5XZZ
    Ear
      Left **0HD**3XZZ
      Right **0HD**2XZZ
    Face **0HD**1XZZ
    Foot
      Left **0HD**NXZZ
      Right **0HD**MXZZ
    Genitalia **0HD**AXZZ
    Hand
      Left **0HD**GXZZ
      Right **0HD**FXZZ
    Lower Arm
      Left **0HD**EXZZ
      Right **0HD**DXZZ
    Lower Leg
      Left **0HD**LXZZ
      Right **0HD**KXZZ
    Neck **0HD**4XZZ
    Perineum **0HD**9XZZ
    Scalp **0HD**0XZZ
    Upper Arm
      Left **0HD**CXZZ
      Right **0HD**BXZZ
    Upper Leg
      Left **0HD**JXZZ
      Right **0HD**HXZZ
  Spinal Meninges **00D**T-
  Subcutaneous Tissue and Fascia
    Abdomen **0JD**8-
    Back **0JD**7-
    Buttock **0JD**9-
    Chest **0JD**6-
    Face **0JD**1-
    Foot
      Left **0JD**R-
      Right **0JD**Q-
    Hand
      Left **0JD**K-
      Right **0JD**J-
    Lower Arm
      Left **0JD**H-
      Right **0JD**G-
    Lower Leg
      Left **0JD**P-
      Right **0JD**N-

Extraction — *continued*
  Subcutaneous Tissue and Fascia — *continued*
    Neck
      Anterior **0JD**4-
      Posterior **0JD**5-
    Pelvic Region **0JD**C-
    Perineum **0JD**B-
    Scalp **0JD**0-
    Upper Arm
      Left **0JD**F-
      Right **0JD**D-
    Upper Leg
      Left **0JD**M-
      Right **0JD**L-
  Toe Nail **0HD**RXZZ
  Tooth
    Lower **0CD**XXZ-
    Upper **0CD**WXZ-
  Turbinate, Nasal **09D**L-
  Tympanic Membrane
    Left **09D**8-
    Right **09D**7-
  Vein
    Basilic
      Left **05D**C-
      Right **05D**B-
    Brachial
      Left **05D**A-
      Right **05D**9-
    Cephalic
      Left **05D**F-
      Right **05D**D-
    Femoral
      Left **06D**N-
      Right **06D**M-
    Foot
      Left **06D**V-
      Right **06D**T-
    Greater Saphenous
      Left **06D**Q-
      Right **06D**P-
    Hand
      Left **05D**H-
      Right **05D**G-
    Lesser Saphenous
      Left **06D**S-
      Right **06D**R-
    Lower **06D**Y-
    Upper **05D**Y-
  Vocal Cord
    Left **0CD**V-
    Right **0CD**T-

Extradural space, intracranial
  use Epidural Space
Extradural space, spinal
  use Spinal Canal
EXtreme Lateral Interbody Fusion (XLIF) device
  use Interbody Fusion Device in Lower Joints

F

Face lift *see* Alteration, Face 0W02-
Facet replacement spinal stabilization device
  use Spinal Stabilization Device, Facet Replacement in **0RH**-
  use Spinal Stabilization Device, Facet Replacement in **0SH**-
Facial artery
  use Artery, Face
Factor Xa Inhibitor Reversal Agent, Andexanet Alfa
  use Andexanet Alfa, Factor Xa Inhibitor Reversal Agent
False vocal cord
  use Larynx
Falx cerebri
  use Dura Mater
Fascia lata
  use Subcutaneous Tissue and Fascia, Upper Leg, Left
  use Subcutaneous Tissue and Fascia, Upper Leg, Right
Fasciaplasty, fascioplasty
  see Repair, Subcutaneous Tissue and Fascia **0JQ**-
  see Replacement, Subcutaneous Tissue and Fascia **0JR**-
Fasciectomy *see* Excision, Subcutaneous Tissue and Fascia **0JB**-
Fasciorrhaphy *see* Repair, Subcutaneous Tissue and Fascia **0JQ**-
Fasciotomy
  see Division, Subcutaneous Tissue and Fascia **0J8**-
  see Drainage, Subcutaneous Tissue and Fascia **0J9**-
  see Release
Feeding Device
  Change device in
    Lower **0D2**DXUZ
    Upper **0D2**0XUZ
  Insertion of device in
    Duodenum **0DH**9-
    Esophagus **0DH**5-
    Ileum **0DH**B-
    Intestine, Small **0DH**8-
    Jejunum **0DH**A-
    Stomach **0DH**6-
  Removal of device from
    Esophagus **0DP**5-
    Intestinal Tract
      Lower **0DP**D-
      Upper **0DP**0-
    Stomach **0DP**6-
  Revision of device in
    Intestinal Tract
      Lower **0DW**D-
      Upper **0DW**0-
    Stomach **0DW**6-
Femoral head
  use Femur, Upper, Left
  use Femur, Upper, Right
Femoral lymph node
  use Lymphatic, Lower Extremity, Left
  use Lymphatic, Lower Extremity, Right
Femoropatellar joint
  use Joint, Knee, Left
  use Joint, Knee, Right
  use Joint, Knee, Left, Femoral Surface
  use Joint, Knee, Right, Femoral Surface
Femorotibial joint
  use Joint, Knee, Left
  use Joint, Knee, Right
  use Joint, Knee, Left, Tibial Surface
  use Joint, Knee, Right, Tibial Surface

Fibular artery
  use Artery, Peroneal, Left
  use Artery, Peroneal, Right
Fibularis brevis muscle
  use Muscle, Lower Leg, Left
  use Muscle, Lower Leg, Right
Fibularis longus muscle
  use Muscle, Lower Leg, Left
  use Muscle, Lower Leg, Right
Fifth cranial nerve
  use Nerve, Trigeminal
Filum terminale
  use Spinal Meninges
Fimbriectomy
  see Excision, Female Reproductive System **0UB**-
  see Resection, Female Reproductive System **0UT**-
Fine needle aspiration
  Fluid or gas *see* Drainage
  Tissue *see* Excision
First cranial nerve
  use Nerve, Olfactory
First intercostal nerve
  use Brachial Plexus
Fistulization
  see Bypass
  see Drainage
  see Repair
Fitting
  Arch bars, for fracture reduction *see* Reposition, Mouth and Throat **0CS**-
  Arch bars, for immobilization *see* Immobilization, Face **2W31**-
  Artificial limb *see* Device Fitting, Rehabilitation **F0D**-
  Hearing aid *see* Device Fitting, Rehabilitation **F0D**-
  Ocular prosthesis **F0D**Z8UZ
  Prosthesis, limb *see* Device Fitting, Rehabilitation **F0D**-
  Prosthesis, ocular **F0D**Z8UZ
Fixation, bone
  External, with fracture reduction *see* Reposition
  External, without fracture reduction *see* Insertion
  Internal, with fracture reduction *see* Reposition
  Internal, without fracture reduction *see* Insertion
FLAIR® Endovascular Stent Graft
  use Intraluminal Device
Flexible Composite Mesh
  use Synthetic Substitute
Flexor carpi radialis muscle
  use Muscle, Lower Arm and Wrist, Left
  use Muscle, Lower Arm and Wrist, Right
Flexor carpi ulnaris muscle
  use Muscle, Lower Arm and Wrist, Left
  use Muscle, Lower Arm and Wrist, Right
Flexor digitorum brevis muscle
  use Muscle, Foot, Left
  use Muscle, Foot, Right
Flexor digitorum longus muscle
  use Muscle, Lower Leg, Left
  use Muscle, Lower Leg, Right
Flexor hallucis brevis muscle
  use Muscle, Foot, Left
  use Muscle, Foot, Right
Flexor hallucis longus muscle
  use Muscle, Lower Leg, Left
  use Muscle, Lower Leg, Right
Flexor pollicis longus muscle
  use Muscle, Lower Arm and Wrist, Left
  use Muscle, Lower Arm and Wrist, Right

Fluoroscopy
Abdomen and Pelvis **BW11**-
Airway, Upper **BB1**DZZZ
Ankle
  Left **BQ1**H-
  Right **BQ1**G-
Aorta
  Abdominal **B410**-
    Laser, Intraoperative **B410**-
  Thoracic **B310**-
    Laser, Intraoperative **B310**-
  Thoraco-Abdominal **B31**P-
    Laser, Intraoperative **B31**P-
Aorta and Bilateral Lower Extremity
  Arteries **B41**D-
  Laser, Intraoperative **B41**D-
Arm
  Left **BP1**FZZZ
  Right **BP1**EZZZ
Artery
  Brachiocephalic-Subclavian
    Laser, Intraoperative **B311**-
    Right **B311**-
  Bronchial **B31**L-
    Laser, Intraoperative **B31**L-
  Bypass Graft, Other **B21**F-
  Cervico-Cerebral Arch **B31**Q-
    Laser, Intraoperative **B31**Q-
  Common Carotid
    Bilateral **B315**-
      Laser, Intraoperative **B315**-
    Left **B314**-
      Laser, Intraoperative **B314**-
    Right **B313**-
      Laser, Intraoperative **B313**-
  Coronary
    Bypass Graft
      Multiple **B213**-
        Laser, Intraoperative **B213**-
      Single **B212**-
        Laser, Intraoperative **B212**-
    Multiple **B211**-
      Laser, Intraoperative **B211**-
    Single **B210**-
      Laser, Intraoperative **B210**-
  External Carotid
    Bilateral **B31**C-
      Laser, Intraoperative **B31**C-
    Left **B31**B-
      Laser, Intraoperative **B31**B-
    Right **B319**-
      Laser, Intraoperative **B319**-
  Hepatic **B412**-
    Laser, Intraoperative **B412**-
  Inferior Mesenteric **B415**-
    Laser, Intraoperative **B415**-
  Intercostal **B31**L-
    Laser, Intraoperative **B31**L-
  Internal Carotid
    Bilateral **B318**-
      Laser, Intraoperative **B318**-
    Left **B317**-
      Laser, Intraoperative **B317**-
    Right **B316**-
      Laser, Intraoperative **B316**-
  Internal Mammary Bypass Graft
    Left **B218**-
    Right **B217**-
  Intra-Abdominal
    Other **B41**B-
    Laser, Intraoperative **B41**B-
  Intracranial **B31**R-
    Laser, Intraoperative **B31**R-
  Lower
    Other **B41**J-
    Laser, Intraoperative **B41**J-

Fluoroscopy — continued
Artery — continued
  Lower Extremity
    Bilateral and Aorta **B41**D-
      Laser, Intraoperative **B41**D-
    Left **B41**G-
      Laser, Intraoperative **B41**G-
    Right **B41**F-
      Laser, Intraoperative **B41**F-
  Lumbar **B419**-
    Laser, Intraoperative **B419**-
  Pelvic **B41**C-
    Laser, Intraoperative **B41**C -
  Pulmonary
    Left **B31**T-
      Laser, Intraoperative **B31**T-
    Right **B31**S-
      Laser, Intraoperative **B31**S-
  Renal
    Bilateral **B418**-
      Laser, Intraoperative **B418**-
    Left **B417**-
      Laser, Intraoperative **B417**-
    Right **B416**-
      Laser, Intraoperative **B416**-
  Spinal **B31**M-
    Laser, Intraoperative **B31**M-
  Splenic **B413**-
    Laser, Intraoperative **B413**-
  Subclavian
    Left **B312**-
      Laser, Intraoperative **B312**-
  Superior Mesenteric **B414**-
    Laser, Intraoperative **B414**-
  Upper
    Laser, Intraoperative **B31**N-
    Other **B31**N-
  Upper Extremity
    Bilateral **B31**K-
      Laser, Intraoperative **B31**K-
    Left **B31**J-
      Laser, Intraoperative **B31**J-
    Right **B31**H-
      Laser, Intraoperative **B31**H-
  Vertebral
    Bilateral **B31**G-
      Laser, Intraoperative **B31**G-
    Left **B31**F-
      Laser, Intraoperative **B31**F-
    Right **B31**D-
      Laser, Intraoperative **B31**D-
Bile Duct **BF10**-
  Pancreatic Duct and Gallbladder
    BF14-
Bile Duct and Gallbladder **BF13**-
Biliary Duct **BF11**-
Bladder **BT10**-
  Kidney and Ureter **BT14**-
    Left **BT1**F-
    Right **BT1**D-
Bladder and Urethra **BT1**B-
Bowel, Small **BD1**-
Calcaneus
  Left **BQ1**KZZZ
  Right **BQ1**JZZZ
Clavicle
  Left **BP15**ZZZ
  Right **BP14**ZZZ
Coccyx **BR1**F-
Colon **BD14**-
Corpora Cavernosa **BV10**-
Dialysis Fistula **B51**W-
Dialysis Shunt **B51**W-
Diaphragm **BB16**ZZZ-
Disc
  Cervical **BR11**-
  Lumbar **BR13**-
  Thoracic **BR12**-
  Duodenum **BD19**-

Fluoroscopy — continued
Elbow
  Left **BP1**H-
  Right **BP1**G-
Epiglottis **B91**G-
Esophagus **BD11**-
Extremity
  Lower **BW1**C-
  Upper **BW1**J-
Facet Joint
  Cervical **BR14**-
  Lumbar **BR16**-
  Thoracic **BR15**-
Fallopian Tube
  Bilateral **BU12**-
  Left **BU11**-
  Right **BU10**-
Fallopian Tube and Uterus **BU18**-
Femur
  Left **BQ14**ZZZ
  Right **BQ13**ZZZ
Finger
  Left **BP1**SZZZ
  Right **BP1**RZZZ
Foot
  Left **BQ1**MZZZ
  Right **BQ1**LZZZ
Forearm
  Left **BP1**KZZZ
  Right **BP1**JZZZ
Gallbladder **BF12**-
  Bile Duct and Pancreatic Duct **BF14**-
Gallbladder and Bile Duct **BF13**-
Gastrointestinal, Upper **BD1**-
Hand
  Left **BP1**PZZZ
  Right **BP1**NZZZ
Head and Neck **BW19**-
Heart
  Left **B215**-
  Right **B214**-
  Right and Left **B216**-
Hip
  Left **BQ11**-
  Right **BQ10**-
Humerus
  Left **BP1**BZZZ
  Right **BP1**AZZZ
Ileal Diversion Loop **BT1**C-
Ileal Loop, Ureters and Kidney **BT1**G-
Intracranial Sinus **B512**-
Joint
  Acromioclavicular, Bilateral
    BP13ZZZ
  Finger
    Left **BP1**D-
    Right **BP1**C-
  Foot
    Left **BQ1**Y-
    Right **BQ1**X-
  Hand
    Left **BP1**D-
    Right **BP1**C-
  Lumbosacral **BR1**B-
  Sacroiliac **BR1**D-
  Sternoclavicular
    Bilateral **BP12**ZZZ
    Left **BP11**ZZZ
    Right **BP10**ZZZ
  Temporomandibular
    Bilateral **BN19**-
    Left **BN18**-
    Right **BN17**-
  Thoracolumbar **BR18**-
  Toe
    Left **BQ1**Y-
    Right **BQ1**X-

Fluoroscopy — continued
Kidney
  Bilateral **BT13**-
  Ileal Loop and Ureter **BT1**G-
  Left **BT12**-
  Right **BT11**-
  Ureter and Bladder **BT14**-
    Left **BT1**F-
    Right **BT1**D-
Knee
  Left **BQ18**-
  Right **BQ17**-
Larynx **B91**J-
Leg
  Left **BQ1**FZZZ
  Right **BQ1**DZZZ
Lung
  Bilateral **BB14**ZZZ
  Left **BB13**ZZZ
  Right **BB12**ZZZ
Mediastinum **BB1**CZZZ
Mouth **BD1**B-
Neck and Head **BW19**-
Oropharynx **BD1**B-
Pancreatic Duct **BF1**-
  Gallbladder and Bile Buct **BF14**-
Patella
  Left **BQ1**WZZZ
  Right **BQ1**VZZZ
Pelvis **BR1**C-
Pelvis and Abdomen **BW11**-
Pharynix **B91**G-
Ribs
  Left **BP1**YZZZ
  Right **BP1**XZZZ
Sacrum **BR1**F-
Scapula
  Left **BP17**ZZZ
  Right **BP16**ZZZ
Shoulder
  Left **BP19**-
  Right **BP18**-
Sinus, Intracranial **B512**-
Spinal Cord **B01**B-
Spine
  Cervical **BR10**-
  Lumbar **BR19**-
  Thoracic **BR17**-
  Whole **BR1**G-
Sternum **BR1**H-
Stomach **BD12**-
Toe
  Left **BQ1**QZZZ
  Right **BQ1**PZZZ
Tracheobronchial Tree
  Bilateral **BB19**YZZ
  Left **BB18**YZZ
  Right **BB17**YZZ
Ureter
  Ileal Loop and Kidney **BT1**G-
  Kidney and Bladder **BT14**-
    Left **BT1**F-
    Right **BT1**D-
  Left **BT17**-
  Right **BT16**-
Urethra **BT15**-
Urethra and Bladder **BT1**B-
Uterus **BU16**-
Uterus and Fallopian Tube **BU18**-
Vagina **BU19**-
Vasa Vasorum **BV18**-

Fluoroscopy — *continued*
Vein
Cerebellar **B511**-
Cerebral **B511**-
Epidural **B510**-
Jugular
Bilateral **B515**-
Left **B514**-
Right **B513**-
Lower Extremity
Bilateral **B51**D-
Left **B51**C-
Right **B51**B-
Other **B51**V-
Pelvic (Iliac)
Left **B51**G-
Right **B51**F-
Pelvic (Iliac) Bilateral **B51**H-
Portal **B51**T-
Pulmonary
Bilateral **B51**S-
Left **B51**R-
Right **B51**Q-
Renal
Bilateral **B51**L-
Left **B51**K-
Right **B51**J-
Spanchnic **B51**T-
Subclavian
Left **B51**7-
Right **B51**6-
Upper Extremity
Bilateral **B51**P-
Left **B51**N-
Right **B51**M-
Vena Cava
Inferior **B51**9-
Superior **B51**8-
Wrist
Left **BP1**M-
Right **BP1**L-
Fluoroscopy, laser intraoperative
see Fluoroscopy, Heart **B21**-
see Fluoroscopy, Lower Arteries **B41**-
see Fluoroscopy, Upper Arteries **B31**-
Flushing *see* Irrigation
Foley catheter
use Drainage Device
Foramen magnum
use Bone, Occipital, Left
use Bone, Occipital, Right
Foramen of Monro (intraventricular)
use Cerebral Ventricle
Foreskin
use Prepuce
Formula™ Balloon-Expandable Renal Stent System
use Intraluminal Device
Fossa of Rosenmuller
use Nasopharynx
Fourth cranial nerve
use Nerve, Trochlear
Fourth ventricle
use Cerebral Ventricle
Fovea
use Retina, Left
use Retina, Right

Fragmentation
Ampulla of Vater **0FF**C-
Anus **0DF**Q-
Appendix **0DF**J-
Bladder **0TF**B-
Bladder Neck **0TF**C-
Bronchus
Lingula **0BF**9-
Lower Lobe
Left **0BF**B-
Right **0BF**6-
Main
Left **0BF**7-
Right **0BF**3-
Middle Lobe, Right **0BF**5-
Upper Lobe
Left **0BF**8-
Right **0BF**4-
Carina **0BF**2-
Cavity, Cranial **0WF**1-
Cecum **0DF**H-
Cerebral Ventricle **00F**6-
Colon
Ascending **0DF**K-
Descending **0DF**M-
Sigmoid **0DF**N-
Transverse **0DF**L-
Duct
Common Bile **0FF**9-
Cystic **0FF**8-
Hepatic
Left **0FF**6-
Right **0FF**5-
Pancreatic **0FF**D-
Accessory **0FF**F-
Parotid
Left **0CF**C-
Right **0CF**B-
Duodenum **0DF**9-
Epidural Space **00F**3-
Esophagus **0DF**5-
Fallopian Tube
Left **0UF**6-
Right **0UF**5-
Fallopian Tubes, Bilateral **0UF**7-
Gallbladder **0FF**4-
Gastrointestinal Tract **0WF**P-
Genitourinary Tract **0WF**R-
Ileum **0DF**B-
Intestine
Large **0DF**E-
Left **0DF**G-
Right **0DF**F-
Small **0DF**8-
Jejunum **0DF**A-
Kidney Pelvis
Left **0TF**4-
Right **0TF**3-
Mediastinum **0WF**C-
Oral Cavity and Throat **0WF**3-
Pelvic Cavity **0WF**J-
Pericardial Cavity **0WF**D-
Pericardium **02F**N-
Peritoneal Cavity **0WF**G-
Pleural Cavity
Left **0WF**B-
Right **0WF**9-
Rectum **0DF**P-
Respiratory Tract **0WF**Q-
Spinal Canal **00F**U-
Stomach **0DF**6-
Subarachnoid Space **00F**5-
Subdural Space **00F**4-
Trachea **0BF**1-
Ureter
Left **0TF**7-
Right **0TF**6-
Urethra **0TF**D-
Uterus **0UF**9-
Vitreous
Left **08F**5-
Right **08F**4-

Freestyle (Stentless) Aortic Root Bioprosthesis
use Zooplastic Tissue in Heart and Great Vessels
Frenectomy
see Excision, Mouth and Throat **0CB**-
see Resection, Mouth and Throat **0CT**-
Frenoplasty, frenuloplasty
see Repair, Mouth and Throat **0CQ**-
see Replacement, Mouth and Throat **0CR**-
see Supplement, Mouth and Throat **0CU**-
Frenotomy
see Drainage, Mouth and Throat **0C9**-
see Release, Mouth and Throat **0CN**-
Frenulotomy
see Drainage, Mouth and Throat **0C9**-
see Release, Mouth and Throat **0CN**-
Frenulum labii inferioris
use Lip, Lower
Frenulum labii superioris
use Lip, Upper
Frenulum linguae
use Tongue
Frenulumectomy
see Excision, Mouth and Throat **0CB**-
see Resection, Mouth and Throat **0CT**-
Frontal lobe
use Cerebral Hemisphere
Frontal vein
use Vein, Face, Left
use Vein, Face, Right
Fulguration *see* Destruction
Fundoplication, gastroesophageal *see* Restriction, Esophagogastric Junction **0DV**4-
Fundus uteri
use Uterus
Fusion
Acromioclavicular
Left **0RG**H-
Right **0RG**G-
Ankle
Left **0SG**G-
Right **0SG**F-
Carpal
Left **0RG**R-
Right **0RG**Q-
Cervical Vertebral **0RG**1-
2 or more **0RG**2-
Interbody Fusion Device, Nanotextured Surface **XRG**2092
Interbody Fusion Device, Nanotextured Surface **XRG**1092
Cervicothoracic Vertebral **0RG**4-
Interbody Fusion Device, Nanotextured Surface **XRG**4092
Coccygeal **0SG**6-
Elbow
Left **0RG**M-
Right **0RG**L-
Finger Phalangeal
Left **0RG**X-
Right **0RG**W-
Hip
Left **0SG**B-
Right **0SG**9-
Knee
Left **0SG**D-
Right **0SG**C-

Fusion — *continued*
Lumbar Vertebral **0SG**0-
2 or more **0SG**1-
Interbody Fusion Device, Nanotextured Surface **XRG**C092
Interbody Fusion Device, Nanotextured Surface **XRG**B092
Lumbosacral **0SG**3-
Interbody Fusion Device, Nanotextured Surface **XRG**D092
Metacarpocarpal
Left **0RG**T-
Right **0RG**S-
Metacarpophalangeal
Left **0RG**V-
Right **0RG**U-
Metatarsal-Phalangeal
Left **0SG**N-
Right **0SG**M-
Metatarsal-Tarsal
Left **0SG**L-
Right **0SG**K-
Occipital-cervical **0RG**0-
Interbody Fusion Device, Nanotextured Surface **XRG**0092
Sacrococcygeal **0SG**5-
Sacroiliac
Left **0SG**8-
Right **0SG**7-
Shoulder
Left **0RG**K-
Right **0RG**J-
Sternoclavicular
Left **0RG**F-
Right **0RG**E-
Tarsal
Left **0SG**J-
Right **0SG**H-
Temporomandibular
Left **0RG**D-
Right **0RG**C-
Thoracic Vertebral **0RG**6-
2 to 7 **0RG**7-
Interbody Fusion Device, Nanotextured Surface **XRG**7092
8 or more **0RG**8-
Interbody Fusion Device, Nanotextured Surface **XRG**8092
Interbody Fusion Device, Nanotextured Surface **XRG**6092
Thoracolumbar Vertebral **0RG**A-
Interbody Fusion Device, Nanotextured Surface **XRG**A092
Toe Phalangeal
Left **0SG**Q-
Right **0SG**P-
Wrist
Left **0RG**P-
Right **0RG**N-
Fusion screw (compression) (lag) (locking)
use Internal Fixation Device in Lower Joints
use Internal Fixation Device in Upper Joints

PROCEDURE INDEX

G

Gait training *see* Motor Treatment, Rehabilitation **F07-**
Galea aponeurotica
  use Subcutaneous Tissue and Fascia, Scalp
Ganglion impar (ganglion of Walther)
  use Nerve, Sacral Sympathetic
Ganglionectomy
  Destruction of lesion *see* Destruction
  Excision of lesion *see* Excision
Gasserian ganglion
  use Nerve, Trigeminal
Gastrectomy
  Partial *see* Excision, Stomach **0DB6-**
  Total *see* Resection, Stomach **0DT6-**
  Vertical (sleeve) *see* Excision, Stomach **0DB6-**
Gastric electrical stimulation (GES) lead
  use Stimulator Lead in Gastrointestinal System
Gastric lymph node
  use Lymphatic, Aortic
Gastric pacemaker lead
  use Stimulator Lead in Gastrointestinal System
Gastric plexus
  use Nerve, Abdominal Sympathetic
Gastrocnemius muscle
  use Muscle, Lower Leg, Left
  use Muscle, Lower Leg, Right
Gastrocolic ligament
  use Omentum, Greater
Gastrocolic omentum
  use Omentum, Greater
Gastrocolostomy
  see Bypass, Gastrointestinal System **0D1-**
  see Drainage, Gastrointestinal System **0D9-**
Gastroduodenal artery
  use Artery, Hepatic
Gastroduodenectomy
  see Excision, Gastrointestinal System **0DB-**
  see Resection, Gastrointestinal System **0DT-**
Gastroduodenoscopy 0DJ08ZZ
Gastroenteroplasty
  see Repair, Gastrointestinal System **0DQ-**
  see Supplement, Gastrointestinal System **0DU-**
Gastroenterostomy
  see Bypass, Gastrointestinal System **0D1-**
  see Drainage, Gastrointestinal System **0D9-**
Gastroesophageal (GE) junction
  use Esophagogastric Junction
Gastrogastrostomy
  see Bypass, Stomach **0D16-**
  see Drainage, Stomach **0D96-**
Gastrohepatic omentum
  use Omentum, Lesser
Gastrojejunostomy
  see Bypass, Stomach **0D16-**
  see Drainage, Stomach **0D96-**
Gastrolysis *see* Release, Stomach **0DN6-**
Gastropexy
  see Repair, Stomach **0DQ6-**
  see Reposition, Stomach **0DS6-**
Gastrophrenic ligament
  use Omentum, Greater

Gastroplasty
  see Repair, Stomach **0DQ6-**
  see Supplement, Stomach **0DU6-**
Gastroplication *see* Restriction, Stomach **0DV6-**
Gastropylorectomy *see* Excision, Gastrointestinal System **0DB-**
Gastrorrhaphy *see* Repair, Stomach **0DQ6-**
Gastroscopy 0DJ68ZZ
Gastrosplenic ligament
  use Omentum, Greater
Gastrostomy
  see Bypass, Stomach **0D16-**
  see Drainage, Stomach **0D96-**
Gastrotomy *see* Drainage, Stomach **0D96-**
Gemellus muscle
  use Muscle, Hip, Left
  use Muscle, Hip, Right
Geniculate ganglion
  use Nerve, Facial
Geniculate nucleus
  use Thalamus
Genioglossus muscle
  use Muscle, Tongue, Palate, Pharynx
Genioplasty *see* Alteration, Jaw, Lower **0W05-**
Genitofemoral nerve
  use Nerve, Lumbar Plexus
Gingivectomy *see* Excision, Mouth and Throat **0CB-**
Gingivoplasty
  see Repair, Mouth and Throat **0CQ-**
  see Replacement, Mouth and Throat **0CR-**
  see Supplement, Mouth and Throat **0CU-**
Glans penis
  use Prepuce
Glenohumeral joint
  use Joint, Shoulder, Left
  use Joint, Shoulder, Right
Glenohumeral ligament
  use Bursa and Ligament, Shoulder, Left
  use Bursa and Ligament, Shoulder, Right
Glenoid fossa (of scapula)
  use Glenoid Cavity, Left
  use Glenoid Cavity, Right
Glenoid ligament (labrum)
  use Shoulder Joint, Left
  use Shoulder Joint, Right
Globus pallidus
  use Basal Ganglia
Glomectomy
  see Excision, Endocrine System **0GB-**
  see Resection, Endocrine System **0GT-**
Glossectomy
  see Excision, Tongue **0CB7-**
  see Resection, Tongue **0CT7-**
Glossoepiglottic fold
  use Epiglottis
Glossopexy
  see Repair, Tongue **0CQ7-**
  see Reposition, Tongue **0CS7-**
Glossoplasty
  see Repair, Tongue **0CQ7-**
  see Replacement, Tongue **0CR7-**
  see Supplement, Tongue **0CU7-**
Glossorrhaphy *see* Repair, Tongue **0CQ7-**
Glossotomy *see* Drainage, Tongue **0C97-**
Glottis
  use Larynx

Gluteal Artery Perforator Flap
  Bilateral **0HRV079**
  Left **0HRU079**
  Right **0HRT079**
Gluteal lymph node
  use Lymphatic, Pelvis
Gluteal vein
  use Vein, Hypogastric, Left
  use Vein, Hypogastric, Right
Gluteus maximus muscle
  use Muscle, Hip, Left
  use Muscle, Hip, Right
Gluteus medius muscle
  use Muscle, Hip, Left
  use Muscle, Hip, Right
Gluteus minimus muscle
  use Muscle, Hip, Left
  use Muscle, Hip, Right
GORE® DUALMESH®
  use Synthetic Substitute
GORE® EXCLUDER® AAA Endoprosthesis
  use Intraluminal Device
  use Intraluminal Device, Branched or Fenestrated, One or Two Arteries in **04V-**
  use Intraluminal Device, Branched or Fenestrated, Three or More Arteries in **04V-**
GORE® EXCLUDER® IBE Endoprosthesis
  use Intraluminal Device, Branched or Fenestrated, One or Two Arteries in **04V-**
GORE® TAG® Thoracic Endoprosthesis
  use Intraluminal Device
Gracilis muscle
  use Muscle, Upper Leg, Left
  use Muscle, Upper Leg, Right
Graft
  see Replacement
  see Supplement
Great auricular nerve
  use Cervical Plexus
Great cerebral vein
  use Vein, Intracranial
Great saphenous vein
  use Vein, Greater Saphenous, Left
  use Vein, Greater Saphenous, Right
Greater alar cartilage
  use Nose
Greater occipital nerve
  use Nerve, Cervical
Greater splanchnic nerve
  use Nerve, Thoracic Sympathetic
Greater superficial petrosal nerve
  use Nerve, Facial
Greater trochanter
  use Femur, Upper, Left
  use Femur, Upper, Right
Greater tuberosity
  use Humeral Head, Left
  use Humeral Head, Right
Greater vestibular (Bartholin's) gland
  use Gland, Vestibular
Greater wing
  use Bone, Sphenoid, Left
  use Bone, Sphenoid, Right
Guedel airway
  use Intraluminal Device, Airway in Mouth and Throat
Guidance, catheter placement
  EKG *see* Measurement, Physiological Systems **4A0-**
  Fluoroscopy *see* Fluoroscopy, Veins **B51-**
  Ultrasound *see* Ultrasonography, Veins **B54-**

PROCEDURE INDEX

H

Hallux
  use Toe, 1st, Left
  use Toe, 1st, Right
Hamate bone
  use Carpal, Left
  use Carpal, Right
Hancock Bioprosthesis (aortic) (mitral) valve
  use Zooplastic Tissue in Heart and Great Vessels
Hancock Bioprosthetic Valved Conduit
  use Zooplastic Tissue in Heart and Great Vessels
Harvesting, stem cells *see* Pheresis, Circulatory **6A55**-
Head of fibula
  use Fibula, Left
  use Fibula, Right
Hearing Aid Assessment F14Z-
Hearing Assessment F13Z-
Hearing Device
  Bone Conduction
    Left **09HE**-
    Right **09HD**-
  Insertion of device in
    Left **0NH6**-
    Right **0NH5**-
  Multiple Channel Cochlear Prosthesis
    Left **09HE**-
    Right **09HD**-
  Removal of device from, Skull **0NP0**-
  Revision of device in, Skull **0NW0**-
  Single Channel Cochlear Prosthesis
    Left **09HE**-
    Right **09HD**-
Hearing Treatment F09Z-
Heart Assist System
  External
    Insertion of device in, Heart **02HA**-
    Removal of device from, Heart **02PA**-
    Revision of device in, Heart **02WA**-
  Implantable
    Insertion of device in, Heart **02HA**-
    Removal of device from, Heart **02PA**-
    Revision of device in, Heart **02WA**-
HeartMate II® Left Ventricular Assist Device (LVAD)
  use Implantable Heart Assist System in Heart and Great Vessels
HeartMate XVE® Left Ventricular Assist Device (LVAD)
  use Implantable Heart Assist System in Heart and Great Vessels
HeartMate® implantable heart assist system *see* Insertion of device in, Heart **02HA**-
Helix
  use Ear, External, Bilateral
  use Ear, External, Left
  use Ear, External, Right
Hematopoietic cell transplant (HCT) *see* Transfusion, Circulatory **302**-
Hemicolectomy *see* Resection, Gastrointestinal System **0DT**-
Hemicystectomy *see* Excision, Urinary System **0TB**-
Hemigastrectomy *see* Excision, Gastrointestinal System **0DB**-
Hemiglossectomy *see* Excision, Mouth and Throat **0CB**-
Hemilaminectomy
  see Excision, Lower Bones **0QB**-
  see Excision, Upper Bones **0PB**-

Hemilaminotomy
  see Drainage, Lower Bones **0Q9**-
  see Drainage, Upper Bones **0P9**-
  see Excision, Lower Bones **0QB**-
  see Excision, Upper Bones **0PB**-
  see Release, Central Nervous System **00N**-
  see Release, Lower Bones **0QN**-
  see Release, Peripheral Nervous System **01N**-
  see Release, Upper Bones **0PN**-
Hemilaryngectomy *see* Excision, Larynx **0CB**S-
Hemimandibulectomy *see* Excision, Head and Facial Bones **0NB**-
Hemimaxillectomy *see* Excision, Head and Facial Bones **0NB**-
Hemipylorectomy *see* Excision, Gastrointestinal System **0DB**-
Hemispherectomy
  see Excision, Central Nervous System **00B**-
  see Resection, Central Nervous System **00T**-
Hemithyroidectomy
  see Excision, Endocrine System **0GB**-
  see Resection, Endocrine System **0GT**-
Hemodialysis 5A1D00Z
Hepatectomy
  see Excision, Hepatobiliary System and Pancreas **0FB**-
  see Resection, Hepatobiliary System and Pancreas **0FT**-
Hepatic artery proper
  use Artery, Hepatic
Hepatic flexure
  use Colon, Ascending
Hepatic lymph node
  use Lymphatic, Aortic
Hepatic plexus
  use Nerve, Abdominal Sympathetic
Hepatic portal vein
  use Vein, Portal
Hepaticoduodenostomy
  see Bypass, Hepatobiliary System and Pancreas **0F1**-
  see Drainage, Hepatobiliary System and Pancreas **0F9**-
Hepaticotomy *see* Drainage, Hepatobiliary System and Pancreas **0F9**-
Hepatocholedochostomy *see* Drainage, Duct, Common Bile **0F9**9-
Hepatogastric ligament
  use Omentum, Lesser
Hepatopancreatic ampulla
  use Ampulla of Vater
Hepatopexy
  see Repair, Hepatobiliary System and Pancreas **0FQ**-
  see Reposition, Hepatobiliary System and Pancreas **0FS**-
Hepatorrhaphy *see* Repair, Hepatobiliary System and Pancreas **0FQ**-
Hepatotomy *see* Drainage, Hepatobiliary System and Pancreas **0F9**-
Herculink (RX) Elite Renal Stent System
  use Intraluminal Device

Herniorrhaphy
  see Repair, Anatomical Regions, General **0WQ**-
  see Repair, Anatomical Regions, Lower Extremities **0YQ**-
  With synthetic substitute
    see Supplement, Anatomical Regions, General **0WU**-
    see Supplement, Anatomical Regions, Lower Extremities **0YU**-
Hip (joint) liner
  use Liner in Lower Joints
Holter monitoring 4A12X45
Holter valve ventricular shunt
  use Synthetic Substitute
Humeroradial joint
  use Joint, Elbow, Left
  use Joint, Elbow, Right
Humeroulnar joint
  use Joint, Elbow, Left
  use Joint, Elbow, Right
Humerus, distal
  use Humeral Shaft, Left
  use Humeral Shaft, Right
Hydrocelectomy *see* Excision, Male Reproductive System **0VB**-
Hydrotherapy
  Assisted exercise in pool *see* Motor Treatment, Rehabilitation **F07**-
  Whirlpool *see* Activities of Daily Living Treatment, Rehabilitation **F08**-
Hymenectomy
  see Excision, Hymen **0UB**K-
  see Resection, Hymen **0UT**K-
Hymenoplasty
  see Repair, Hymen **0UQ**K-
  see Supplement, Hymen **0UU**K-
Hymenorrhaphy *see* Repair, Hymen **0UQ**K-
Hymenotomy
  see Division, Hymen **0U8**K-
  see Drainage, Hymen **0U9**K-
Hyoglossus muscle
  use Muscle, Tongue, Palate, Pharynx
Hyoid artery
  use Artery, Thyroid, Left
  use Artery, Thyroid, Right
Hyperalimentation *see* Introduction of substance in or on
Hyperbaric oxygenation
  Decompression sickness treatment *see* Decompression, Circulatory **6A15**-
  Wound treatment *see* Assistance, Circulatory **5A05**-
Hyperthermia
  Radiation Therapy
    Abdomen **DWY38ZZ**
    Adrenal Gland **DGY28ZZ**
    Bile Ducts **DFY28ZZ**
    Bladder **DTY28ZZ**
    Bone, Other **DPYC8ZZ**
    Bone Marrow **D7Y08ZZ**
    Brain **D0Y08ZZ**
    Brain Stem **D0Y18ZZ**
    Breast
      Left **DMY08ZZ**
      Right **DMY18ZZ**
    Bronchus **DBY18ZZ**
    Cervix **DUY18ZZ**
    Chest **DWY28ZZ**
    Chest Wall **DBY78ZZ**
    Colon **DDY58ZZ**
    Diaphragm **DBY88ZZ**
    Duodenum **DDY28ZZ**
    Ear **D9Y08ZZ**
    Esophagus **DDY08ZZ**
    Eye **D8Y08ZZ**

Hyperthermia — *continued*
  Radiation Therapy — *continued*
    Femur **DPY98ZZ**
    Fibula **DPYB8ZZ**
    Gallbladder **DFY18ZZ**
    Gland
      Adrenal **DGY28ZZ**
      Parathyroid **DGY48ZZ**
      Pituitary **DGY08ZZ**
      Thyroid **DGY58ZZ**
    Glands, Salivary **D9Y68ZZ**
    Head and Neck **DWY18ZZ**
    Hemibody **DWY48ZZ**
    Humerus **DPY68ZZ**
    Hypopharynx **D9Y38ZZ**
    Ileum **DDY48ZZ**
    Jejunum **DDY38ZZ**
    Kidney **DTY08ZZ**
    Larynx **D9YB8ZZ**
    Liver **DFY08ZZ**
    Lung **DBY28ZZ**
    Lymphatics
      Abdomen **D7Y68ZZ**
      Axillary **D7Y48ZZ**
      Inguinal **D7Y88ZZ**
      Neck **D7Y38ZZ**
      Pelvis **D7Y78ZZ**
      Thorax **D7Y58ZZ**
    Mandible **DPY38ZZ**
    Maxilla **DPY28ZZ**
    Mediastinum **DBY68ZZ**
    Mouth **D9Y48ZZ**
    Nasopharynx **D9YD8ZZ**
    Neck and Head **DWY18ZZ**
    Nerve, Peripheral **D0Y78ZZ**
    Nose **D9Y18ZZ**
    Oropharynx **D9YF8ZZ**
    Ovary **DUY08ZZ**
    Palate
      Hard **D9Y88ZZ**
      Soft **D9Y98ZZ**
    Pancreas **DFY38ZZ**
    Parathyroid Gland **DGY48ZZ**
    Pelvic Bones **DPY88ZZ**
    Pelvic Region **DWY68ZZ**
    Pineal Body **DGY18ZZ**
    Pituitary Gland **DGY08ZZ**
    Pleura **DBY58ZZ**
    Prostate **DVY08ZZ**
    Radius **DPY78ZZ**
    Rectum **DDY78ZZ**
    Rib **DPY58ZZ**
    Sinuses **D9Y78ZZ**
    Skin
      Abdomen **DHY88ZZ**
      Arm **DHY48ZZ**
      Back **DHY78ZZ**
      Buttock **DHY98ZZ**
      Chest **DHY68ZZ**
      Face **DHY28ZZ**
      Leg **DHYB8ZZ**
      Neck **DHY38ZZ**
    Skull **DPY08ZZ**
    Spinal Cord **D0Y68ZZ**
    Spleen **D7Y28ZZ**
    Sternum **DPY48ZZ**
    Stomach **DDY18ZZ**
    Testis **DVY18ZZ**
    Thymus **D7Y18ZZ**
    Thyroid Gland **DGY58ZZ**
    Tibia **DPYB8ZZ**
    Tongue **D9Y58ZZ**
    Trachea **DBY08ZZ**
    Ulna **DPY78ZZ**
    Ureter **DTY18ZZ**
    Urethra **DTY38ZZ**
    Uterus **DUY28ZZ**
    Whole Body **DWY58ZZ**
  Whole Body **6A3Z**-

PROCEDURE INDEX

Hypnosis GZFZZZZ
Hypogastric artery
  use Artery, Internal Iliac, Left
  use Artery, Internal Iliac, Right
Hypopharynx
  use Pharynx
Hypophysectomy
  see Excision, Gland, Pituitary **0GB**0-
  see Resection, Gland, Pituitary **0GT**0-
Hypophysis
  use Gland, Pituitary
Hypothalamotomy *see* Destruction, Thalamus **0059**-
Hypothenar muscle
  use Muscle, Hand, Left
  use Muscle, Hand, Right
Hypothermia, Whole Body 6A4Z-
Hysterectomy
  Supracervical
    see Resection, Uterus **0UT**9-
  Total
    see Resection, Cervix **0UT**C-
    see Resection, Uterus **0UT**9-
Hysterolysis *see* Release, Uterus **0UN**9-
Hysteropexy
  see Repair, Uterus **0UQ**9-
  see Reposition, Uterus **0US**9-
Hysteroplasty *see* Repair, Uterus **0UQ**9-
Hysterorrhaphy *see* Repair, Uterus **0UQ**9-
Hysteroscopy 0UJD8ZZ
Hysterotomy *see* Drainage, Uterus **0U9**9-
Hysterotrachelectomy
  see Resection, Cervix **0UT**C-
  see Resection, Uterus **0UT**9-
Hysterotracheloplasty *see* Repair, Uterus **0UQ**9-
Hysterotrachelorrhaphy *see* Repair, Uterus **0UQ**9-

I

IABP (Intra-aortic balloon pump)
  see Assistance, Cardiac **5A02**-
IAEMT (Intraoperative anesthetic effect monitoring and titration) *see* Monitoring, Central Nervous **4A10**-
Idarucizumab, Dabigatran reversal agent XW0-
Ileal artery
  use Artery, Superior Mesenteric
Ileectomy
  see Excision, Ileum **0DB**B-
  see Resection, Ileum **0DT**B-
Ileocolic artery
  use Artery, Superior Mesenteric
Ileocolic vein
  use Vein, Colic
Ileopexy
  see Repair, Ileum **0DQ**B-
  see Reposition, Ileum **0DS**B-
Ileorrhaphy *see* Repair, Ileum **0DQ**B-
Ileoscopy 0DJD8ZZ
Ileostomy
  see Bypass, Ileum **0D1**B-
  see Drainage, Ileum **0D9**B-
Ileotomy *see* Drainage, Ileum **0D9**B-
Ileoureterostomy *see* Bypass, Urinary System **0T1**-
Iliac crest
  use Bone, Pelvic, Left
  use Bone, Pelvic, Right
Iliac fascia
  use Subcutaneous Tissue and Fascia, Upper Leg, Left
  use Subcutaneous Tissue and Fascia, Upper Leg, Right
Iliac lymph node
  use Lymphatic, Pelvis
Iliacus muscle
  use Muscle, Hip, Left
  use Muscle, Hip, Right
Iliofemoral ligament
  use Bursa and Ligament, Hip, Left
  use Bursa and Ligament, Hip, Right
Iliohypogastric nerve
  use Nerve, Lumbar Plexus
Ilioinguinal nerve
  use Nerve, Lumbar Plexus
Iliolumbar artery
  use Artery, Internal Iliac, Left
  use Artery, Internal Iliac, Right
Iliolumbar ligament
  use Bursa and Ligament, Trunk, Left
  use Bursa and Ligament, Trunk, Right
Iliotibial tract (band)
  use Subcutaneous Tissue and Fascia, Upper Leg, Left
  use Subcutaneous Tissue and Fascia, Upper Leg, Right
Ilium
  use Bone, Pelvic, Left
  use Bone, Pelvic, Right
Ilizarov external fixator
  use External Fixation Device, Ring in **0PH**-
  use External Fixation Device, Ring in **0PS**-
  use External Fixation Device, Ring in **0QH**-
  use External Fixation Device, Ring in **0QS**-
Ilizarov-Vecklich device
  use External Fixation Device, Limb Lengthening in **0PH**-
  use External Fixation Device, Limb Lengthening in **0QH**-

Imaging, diagnostic
  see Computerized Tomography (CT Scan)
  see Fluoroscopy
  see Magnetic Resonance Imaging (MRI)
  see Plain Radiography
  see Ultrasonography
Immobilization
  Abdominal Wall 2W33X-
  Arm
    Lower
      Left 2W3DX-
      Right 2W3CX-
    Upper
      Left 2W3BX-
      Right 2W3AX-
  Back 2W35X-
  Chest Wall 2W34X-
  Extremity
    Lower
      Left 2W3MX-
      Right 2W3LX-
    Upper
      Left 2W39X-
      Right 2W38X-
  Face 2W31X-
  Finger
    Left 2W3KX-
    Right 2W3JX-
  Foot
    Left 2W3TX-
    Right 2W3SX-
  Hand
    Left 2W3FX-
    Right 2W3EX-
  Head 2W30X-
  Inguinal Region
    Left 2W37X-
    Right 2W36X-
  Leg
    Lower
      Left 2W3RX-
      Right 2W3QX-
    Upper
      Left 2W3PX-
      Right 2W3NX-
  Neck 2W32X-
  Thumb
    Left 2W3HX-
    Right 2W3GX-
  Toe
    Left 2W3VX-
    Right 2W3UX-
Immunization *see* Introduction of Serum, Toxoid, and Vaccine
Immunotherapy *see* Introduction of Immunotherapeutic Substance
Immunotherapy, antineoplastic
  Interferon *see* Introduction of Low-dose Interleukin-2
  Interleukin-2, high-dose *see* Introduction of High-dose Interleukin-2
  Interleukin-2, low-dose *see* Introduction of Low-dose Interleukin-2
  Monoclonal antibody *see* Introduction of Monoclonal Antibody
  Proleukin, high-dose *see* Introduction of High-dose Interleukin-2
  Proleukin, low-dose *see* Introduction of Low-dose Interleukin-2

Impeller Pump
  Continuous, Output 5A0221D
  Intermittent, Output 5A0211D
Implantable cardioverter-defibrillator (ICD)
  use Defibrillator Generator in **0JH**-
Implantable drug infusion pump (anti-spasmodic) (chemotherapy) (pain)
  use Infusion Device, Pump in Subcutaneous Tissue and Fascia
Implantable gastric pacemaker generator
  use Stimulator Generator in Subcutaneous Tissue and Fascia
Implantable glucose monitoring device
  use Monitoring Device
Implantable hemodynamic monitor (IHM)
  use Monitoring Device, Hemodynamic in **0JH**-
Implantable hemodynamic monitoring system (IHMS)
  use Monitoring Device, Hemodynamic in **0JH**-
Implantable Miniature Telescope™ (IMT)
  use Synthetic Substitute, Intraocular Telescope in **08R**-
Implantation
  see Insertion
  see Replacement
Implanted (venous) (access) port
  use Vascular Access Device, Reservoir in Subcutaneous Tissue and Fascia
IMV (intermittent mandatory ventilation) *see* Assistance, Respiratory **5A09**-
In Vitro Fertilization 8E0ZXY1
Incision, abscess *see* Drainage
Incudectomy
  see Excision, Ear, Nose, Sinus **09B**-
  see Resection, Ear, Nose, Sinus **09T**-
Incudopexy
  see Repair, Ear, Nose, Sinus **09Q**-
  see Reposition, Ear, Nose, Sinus **09S**-
Incus
  use Auditory Ossicle, Left
  use Auditory Ossicle, Right
Induction of labor
  Artificial rupture of membranes *see* Drainage, Pregnancy **109**-
  Oxytocin *see* Introduction of Hormone
InDura, intrathecal catheter (1P) (spinal)
  use Infusion Device
Inferior cardiac nerve
  use Nerve, Thoracic Sympathetic
Inferior cerebellar vein
  use Vein, Intracranial
Inferior cerebral vein
  use Vein, Intracranial
Inferior epigastric artery
  use Artery, External Iliac, Left
  use Artery, External Iliac, Right
Inferior epigastric lymph node
  use Lymphatic, Pelvis
Inferior genicular artery
  use Artery, Popliteal, Left
  use Artery, Popliteal, Right
Inferior gluteal artery
  use Artery, Internal Iliac, Left
  use Artery, Internal Iliac, Right
Inferior gluteal nerve
  use Nerve, Sacral Plexus

Inferior hypogastric plexus
  use Nerve, Abdominal Sympathetic
Inferior labial artery
  use Artery, Face
Inferior longitudinal muscle
  use Muscle, Tongue, Palate, Pharynx
Inferior mesenteric ganglion
  use Nerve, Abdominal Sympathetic
Inferior mesenteric lymph node
  use Lymphatic, Mesenteric
Inferior mesenteric plexus
  use Nerve, Abdominal Sympathetic
Inferior oblique muscle
  use Muscle, Extraocular, Left
  use Muscle, Extraocular, Right
Inferior pancreaticoduodenal artery
  use Artery, Superior Mesenteric
Inferior phrenic artery
  use Aorta, Abdominal
Inferior rectus muscle
  use Muscle, Extraocular, Left
  use Muscle, Extraocular, Right
Inferior suprarenal artery
  use Artery, Renal, Left
  use Artery, Renal, Right
Inferior tarsal plate
  use Eyelid, Lower, Left
  use Eyelid, Lower, Right
Inferior thyroid vein
  use Vein, Innominate, Left
  use Vein, Innominate, Right
Inferior tibiofibular joint
  use Joint, Ankle, Left
  use Joint, Ankle, Right
Inferior turbinate
  use Turbinate, Nasal
Inferior ulnar collateral artery
  use Artery, Brachial, Left
  use Artery, Brachial, Right
Inferior vesical artery
  use Artery, Internal Iliac, Left
  use Artery, Internal Iliac, Right
Infraauricular lymph node
  use Lymphatic, Head
Infraclavicular (deltopectoral) lymph node
  use Lymphatic, Upper Extremity, Left
  use Lymphatic, Upper Extremity, Right
Infrahyoid muscle
  use Muscle, Neck, Left
  use Muscle, Neck, Right
Infraparotid lymph node
  use Lymphatic, Head
Infraspinatus fascia
  use Subcutaneous Tissue and Fascia, Upper Arm, Left
  use Subcutaneous Tissue and Fascia, Upper Arm, Right
Infraspinatus muscle
  use Muscle, Shoulder, Left
  use Muscle, Shoulder, Right
Infundibulopelvic ligament
  use Uterine Supporting Structure

Infusion see Introduction of substance in or on
Infusion Device, Pump
  Insertion of device in
    Abdomen 0JH8-
    Back 0JH7-
    Chest 0JH6-
    Lower Arm
      Left 0JHH-
      Right 0JHG-
    Lower Leg
      Left 0JHP-
      Right 0JHN-
    Trunk 0JHT-
    Upper Arm
      Left 0JHF-
      Right 0JHD-
    Upper Leg
      Left 0JHM-
      Right 0JHL-
  Removal of device from
    Lower Extremity 0JPW-
    Trunk 0JPT-
    Upper Extremity 0JPV-
  Revision of device in
    Lower Extremity 0JWW-
    Trunk 0JWT-
    Upper Extremity 0JWV-
Infusion, glucarpidase
    Central vein 3E043GQ
    Peripheral vein 3E033GQ
Inguinal canal
  use Inguinal Region, Bilateral
  use Inguinal Region, Left
  use Inguinal Region, Right
Inguinal triangle
  use Inguinal Region, Bilateral
  use Inguinal Region, Left
  use Inguinal Region, Right
Injection see Introduction of substance in or on
Injection reservoir, port
  use Vascular Access Device, Reservoir in Subcutaneous Tissue and Fascia
Injection reservoir, pump
  use Infusion Device, Pump in Subcutaneous Tissue and Fascia
Insemination, artificial 3E0P7LZ
Insertion
  Antimicrobial envelope see Introduction of Anti-infective
  Aqueous drainage shunt
    see Bypass, Eye 081-
    see Drainage, Eye 089-
  Products of Conception 10H0-
  Spinal Stabilization Device
    see Insertion of device in, Lower Joints 0SH-
    see Insertion of device in, Upper Joints 0RH-
Insertion of device in
  Abdominal Wall 0WHF-
  Acetabulum
    Left 0QH5-
    Right 0QH4-
  Anal Sphincter 0DHR-
  Ankle Region
    Left 0YHL-
    Right 0YHK-
  Anus 0DHQ-
  Aorta
    Abdominal 04H0-
    Thoracic
      Ascending/Arch 02HX-
      Descending 02HW-
  Arm
    Lower
      Left 0XHF-
      Right 0XHD-
    Upper
      Left 0XH9-
      Right 0XH8-

Insertion of device in — continued
  Artery
    Anterior Tibial
      Left 04HQ-
      Right 04HP-
    Axillary
      Left 03H6-
      Right 03H5-
    Brachial
      Left 03H8-
      Right 03H7-
    Celiac 04H1-
    Colic
      Left 04H7-
      Middle 04H8-
      Right 04H6-
    Common Carotid
      Left 03HJ-
      Right 03HH-
    Common Iliac
      Left 04HD-
      Right 04HC-
    External Carotid
      Left 03HN-
      Right 03HM-
    External Iliac
      Left 04HJ-
      Right 04HH-
    Face 03HR-
    Femoral
      Left 04HL-
      Right 04HK-
    Foot
      Left 04HW-
      Right 04HV-
    Gastric 04H2-
    Hand
      Left 03HF-
      Right 03HD-
    Hepatic 04H3-
    Inferior Mesenteric 04HB-
    Innominate 03H2-
    Internal Carotid
      Left 03HL-
      Right 03HK-
    Internal Iliac
      Left 04HF-
      Right 04HE-
    Internal Mammary
      Left 03H1-
      Right 03H0-
    Intracranial 03HG-
    Lower 04HY-
    Peroneal
      Left 04HU-
      Right 04HT-
    Popliteal
      Left 04HN-
      Right 04HM-
    Posterior Tibial
      Left 04HS-
      Right 04HR-
    Pulmonary
      Left 02HR-
      Right 02HQ-
    Pulmonary Trunk 02HP-
    Radial
      Left 03HC-
      Right 03HB-
    Renal
      Left 04HA-
      Right 04H9-
    Splenic 04H4-
    Subclavian
      Left 03H4-
      Right 03H3-
    Superior Mesenteric 04H5-
    Temporal
      Left 03HT-
      Right 03HS-
    Thyroid
      Left 03HV-
      Right 03HU-

Insertion of device in — continued
  Artery — continued
    Ulnar
      Left 03HA-
      Right 03H9-
    Upper 03HY-
    Vertebral
      Left 03HQ-
      Right 03HP-
  Atrium
    Left 02H7-
    Right 02H6-
  Axilla
    Left 0XH5-
    Right 0XH4-
  Back
    Lower 0WHL-
    Upper 0WHK-
  Bladder 0THB-
  Bladder Neck 0THC-
  Bone
    Ethmoid
      Left 0NHG-
      Right 0NHF-
    Facial 0NHW-
    Frontal
      Left 0NH2-
      Right 0NH1-
    Hyoid 0NHX-
    Lacrimal
      Left 0NHJ-
      Right 0NHH-
    Lower 0QHY-
    Nasal 0NHB-
    Occipital
      Left 0NH8-
      Right 0NH7-
    Palatine
      Left 0NHL-
      Right 0NHK-
    Parietal
      Left 0NH4-
      Right 0NH3-
    Pelvic
      Left 0QH3-
      Right 0QH2-
    Sphenoid
      Left 0NHD-
      Right 0NHC-
    Temporal
      Left 0NH6-
      Right 0NH5-
    Upper 0PHY-
    Zygomatic
      Left 0NHN-
      Right 0NHM-
  Brain 00H0-
  Breast
    Bilateral 0HHV-
    Left 0HHU-
    Right 0HHT-
  Bronchus
    Lingula 0BH9-
    Lower Lobe
      Left 0BHB-
      Right 0BH6-
    Main
      Left 0BH7-
      Right 0BH3-
    Middle Lobe, Right 0BH5-
    Upper Lobe
      Left 0BH8-
      Right 0BH4-
  Buttock
    Left 0YH1-
    Right 0YH0-
  Carpal
    Left 0PHN-
    Right 0PHM-
  Cavity, Cranial 0WH1-
  Cerebral Ventricle 00H6-
  Cervix 0UHC-

PROCEDURE INDEX

Insertion of device in — *continued*
Chest Wall 0WH8-
Cisterna Chyli 07HL-
Clavicle
  Left 0PHB-
  Right 0PH9-
Coccyx 0QHS-
Cul-de-sac 0UHF-
Diaphragm
  Left 0BHS-
  Right 0BHR-
Disc
  Cervical Vertebral 0RH3-
  Cervicothoracic Vertebral 0RH5-
  Lumbar Vertebral 0SH2-
  Lumbosacral 0SH4-
  Thoracic Vertebral 0RH9-
  Thoracolumbar Vertebral 0RHB-
Duct
  Hepatobiliary 0FHB-
  Pancreatic 0FHD-
Duodenum 0DH9-
Ear
  Left 09HE-
  Right 09HD-
Elbow Region
  Left 0XHC-
  Right 0XHB-
Epididymis and Spermatic Cord 0VHM-
Esophagus 0DH5-
Extremity
  Lower
    Left 0YHB-
    Right 0YH9-
  Upper
    Left 0XH7-
    Right 0XH6-
Eye
  Left 08H1-
  Right 08H0-
Face 0WH2-
Fallopian Tube 0UH8-
Femoral Region
  Left 0YH8-
  Right 0YH7-
Femoral Shaft
  Left 0QH9-
  Right 0QH8-
Femur
  Lower
    Left 0QHC-
    Right 0QHB-
  Upper
    Left 0QH7-
    Right 0QH6-
Fibula
  Left 0QHK-
  Right 0QHJ-
Foot
  Left 0YHN-
  Right 0YHM-
Gallbladder 0FH4-
Gastrointestinal Tract 0WHP-
Genitourinary Tract 0WHR-
Gland, Endocrine 0GHS-
Glenoid Cavity
  Left 0PH8-
  Right 0PH7-
Hand
  Left 0XHK-
  Right 0XHJ-
Head 0WH0-
Heart 02HA-
Humeral Head
  Left 0PHD-
  Right 0PHC-
Humeral Shaft
  Left 0PHG-
  Right 0PHF-

Insertion of device in — *continued*
Ileum 0DHB-
Inguinal Region
  Left 0YH6-
  Right 0YH5-
Intestine
  Large 0DHE-
  Small 0DH8-
Jaw
  Lower 0WH5-
  Upper 0WH4-
Jejunum 0DHA-
Joint
  Acromioclavicular
    Left 0RHH-
    Right 0RHG-
  Ankle
    Left 0SHG-
    Right 0SHF-
  Carpal
    Left 0RHR-
    Right 0RHQ-
  Cervical Vertebral 0RH1-
  Cervicothoracic Vertebral 0RH4-
  Coccygeal 0SH6-
  Elbow
    Left 0RHM-
    Right 0RHL-
  Finger Phalangeal
    Left 0RHX-
    Right 0RHW-
  Hip
    Left 0SHB-
    Right 0SH9-
  Knee
    Left 0SHD-
    Right 0SHC-
  Lumbar Vertebral 0SH0-
  Lumbosacral 0SH3-
  Metacarpocarpal
    Left 0RHT-
    Right 0RHS-
  Metacarpophalangeal
    Left 0RHV-
    Right 0RHU-
  Metatarsal-Phalangeal
    Left 0SHN-
    Right 0SHM-
  Metatarsal-Tarsal
    Left 0SHL-
    Right 0SHK-
  Occipital-cervical 0RH0-
  Sacrococcygeal 0SH5-
  Sacroiliac
    Left 0SH8-
    Right 0SH7-
  Shoulder
    Left 0RHK-
    Right 0RHJ-
  Sternoclavicular
    Left 0RHF-
    Right 0RHE-
  Tarsal
    Left 0SHJ-
    Right 0SHH-
  Temporomandibular
    Left 0RHD-
    Right 0RHC-
  Thoracic Vertebral 0RH6-
  Thoracolumbar Vertebral 0RHA-
  Toe Phalangeal
    Left 0SHQ-
    Right 0SHP-
  Wrist
    Left 0RHP-
    Right 0RHN-

Insertion of device in — *continued*
Kidney 0TH5-
Knee Region
  Left 0YHG-
  Right 0YHF-
Leg
  Lower
    Left 0YHJ-
    Right 0YHH-
  Upper
    Left 0YHD-
    Right 0YHC-
Liver 0FH0-
  Left Lobe 0FH2-
  Right Lobe 0FH1-
Lung
  Left 0BHL-
  Right 0BHK-
Lymphatic 07HN-
  Thoracic Duct 07HK-
Mandible
  Left 0NHV-
  Right 0NHT
Maxilla
  Left 0NHS-
  Right 0NHR-
Mediastinum 0WHC-
Metacarpal
  Left 0PHQ-
  Right 0PHP-
Metatarsal
  Left 0QHP-
  Right 0QHN-
Mouth and Throat 0CHY-
Muscle
  Lower 0KHY-
  Upper 0KHX-
Nasopharynx 09HN-
Neck 0WH6-
Nerve
  Cranial 00HE-
  Peripheral 01HY-
Nipple
  Left 0HHX-
  Right 0HHW-
Oral Cavity and Throat 0WH3-
Orbit
  Left 0NHQ-
  Right 0NHP-
Ovary 0UH3-
Pancreas 0FHG-
Patella
  Left 0QHF-
  Right 0QHD-
Pelvic Cavity 0WHJ-
Penis 0VHS-
Pericardial Cavity 0WHD-
Pericardium 02HN-
Perineum
  Female 0WHN-
  Male 0WHM-
Peritoneal Cavity 0WHG-
Phalanx
  Finger
    Left 0PHV-
    Right 0PHT-
  Thumb
    Left 0PHS-
    Right 0PHR-
  Toe
    Left 0QHR-
    Right 0QHQ-
Pleural Cavity
  Left 0WHB-
  Right 0WH9-
Prostate 0VH0-
Prostate and Seminal Vesicles 0VH4-

Insertion of device in — *continued*
Radius
  Left 0PHJ-
  Right 0PHH-
Rectum 0DHP-
Respiratory Tract 0WHQ-
Retroperitoneum 0WHH-
Rib
  Left 0PH2-
  Right 0PH1-
Sacrum 0QH1-
Scapula
  Left 0PH6-
  Right 0PH5-
Scrotum and Tunica Vaginalis 0VH8-
Shoulder Region
  Left 0XH3-
  Right 0XH2-
Skull 0NH0-
Spinal Canal 00HU-
Spinal Cord 00HV-
Spleen 07HP-
Sternum 0PH0-
Stomach 0DH6-
Subcutaneous Tissue and Fascia
  Abdomen 0JH8-
  Back 0JH7-
  Buttock 0JH9-
  Chest 0JH6-
  Face 0JH1-
  Foot
    Left 0JHR-
    Right 0JHQ-
  Hand
    Left 0JHK-
    Right 0JHJ-
  Head and Neck 0JHS-
  Lower Arm
    Left 0JHH-
    Right 0JHG-
  Lower Extremity 0JHW-
  Lower Leg
    Left 0JHP-
    Right 0JHN-
  Neck
    Anterior 0JH4-
    Posterior 0JH5-
  Pelvic Region 0JHC-
  Perineum 0JHB-
  Scalp 0JH0-
  Trunk 0JHT-
  Upper Arm
    Left 0JHF-
    Right 0JHD-
  Upper Extremity 0JHV-
  Upper Leg
    Left 0JHM-
    Right 0JHL-
Tarsal
  Left 0QHM-
  Right 0QHL-
Testis 0VHD-
Thymus 07HM-
Tibia
  Left 0QHH-
  Right 0QHG-
Tongue 0CH7-
Trachea 0BH1-
Tracheobronchial Tree 0BH0-
Ulna
  Left 0PHL-
  Right 0PHK-
Ureter 0TH9-
Urethra 0THD-
Uterus 0UH9-
Uterus and Cervix 0UHD-
Vagina 0UHG-
Vagina and Cul-de-sac 0UHH-
Vas Deferens 0VHR-

Insertion of device in — *continued*
Vein
　Axillary
　　Left **05H8-**
　　Right **05H7-**
　Azygos **05H0-**
　Basilic
　　Left **05HC-**
　　Right **05HB-**
　Brachial
　　Left **05HA-**
　　Right **05H9-**
　Cephalic
　　Left **05HF-**
　　Right **05HD-**
　Colic **06H7-**
　Common Iliac
　　Left **06HD-**
　　Right **06HC-**
　Coronary **02H4-**
　Esophageal **06H3-**
　External Iliac
　　Left **06HG-**
　　Right **06HF-**
　External Jugular
　　Left **05HQ-**
　　Right **05HP-**
　Face
　　Left **05HV-**
　　Right **05HT-**
　Femoral
　　Left **06HN-**
　　Right **06HM-**
　Foot
　　Left **06HV-**
　　Right **06HT-**
　Gastric **06H2-**
　Greater Saphenous
　　Left **06HQ-**
　　Right **06HP-**
　Hand
　　Left **05HH-**
　　Right **05HG-**
　Hemiazygos **05H1-**
　Hepatic **06H4-**
　Hypogastric
　　Left **06HJ-**
　　Right **06HH-**
　Inferior Mesenteric **06H6-**
　Innominate
　　Left **05H4-**
　　Right **05H3-**
　Internal Jugular
　　Left **05HN-**
　　Right **05HM-**
　Intracranial **05HL-**
　Lesser Saphenous
　　Left **06HS-**
　　Right **06HR-**
　Lower **06HY-**
　Portal **06H8-**
　Pulmonary
　　Left **02HT-**
　　Right **02HS-**
　Renal
　　Left **06HB-**
　　Right **06H9-**
　Splenic **06H1-**
　Subclavian
　　Left **05H6-**
　　Right **05H5-**
　Superior Mesenteric **06H5-**
　Upper **05HY-**
　Vertebral
　　Left **05HS-**
　　Right **05HR-**
Vena Cava
　Inferior **06H0-**
　Superior **02HV-**

Insertion of device in — *continued*
Ventricle
　Left **02HL-**
　Right **02HK-**
Vertebra
　Cervical **0PH3-**
　Lumbar **0QH0-**
　Thoracic **0PH4-**
Wrist Region
　Left **0XHH-**
　Right **0XHG-**

Inspection
Abdominal Wall **0WJF-**
Ankle Region
　Left **0YJL-**
　Right **0YJK-**
Arm
　Lower
　　Left **0XJF-**
　　Right **0XJD-**
　Upper
　　Left **0XJ9-**
　　Right **0XJ8-**
Artery
　Lower **04JY-**
　Upper **03JY-**
Axilla
　Left **0XJ5-**
　Right **0XJ4-**
Back
　Lower **0WJL-**
　Upper **0WJK-**
Bladder **0TJB-**
Bone
　Facial **0NJW-**
　Lower **0QJY-**
　Nasal **0NJB-**
　Upper **0PJY-**
Bone Marrow **07JT-**
Brain **00J0-**
Breast
　Left **0HJU-**
　Right **0HJT-**
Bursa and Ligament
　Lower **0MJY-**
　Upper **0MJX-**
Buttock
　Left **0YJ1-**
　Right **0YJ0-**
Cavity, Cranial **0WJ1-**
Chest Wall **0WJ8-**
Cisterna Chyli **07JL-**
Diaphragm **0BJT-**
Disc
　Cervical Vertebral **0RJ3-**
　Cervicothoracic Vertebral **0RJ5-**
　Lumbar Vertebral **0SJ2-**
　Lumbosacral **0SJ4-**
　Thoracic Vertebral **0RJ9-**
　Thoracolumbar Vertebral **0RJB-**
Duct
　Hepatobiliary **0FJB-**
　Pancreatic **0FJD-**
Ear
　Inner
　　Left **09JE-**
　　Right **09JD-**
　Left **09JJ-**
　Right **09JH-**
Elbow Region
　Left **0XJC-**
　Right **0XJB-**
Epididymis and Spermatic Cord
　0VJM-
Extremity
　Lower
　　Left **0YJB-**
　　Right **0YJ9-**
　Upper
　　Left **0XJ7-**
　　Right **0XJ6-**

Inspection — *continued*
Eye
　Left **08J1XZZ**
　Right **08J0XZZ**
Face **0WJ2-**
Fallopian Tube **0UJ8-**
Femoral Region
　Bilateral **0YJE-**
　Left **0YJ8-**
　Right **0YJ7-**
Finger Nail **0HJQXZZ**
Foot
　Left **0YJN-**
　Right **0YJM-**
Gallbladder **0FJ4-**
Gastrointestinal Tract **0WJP**
Genitourinary Tract **0WJR**
Gland
　Adrenal **0GJ5-**
　Endocrine **0GJS-**
　Pituitary **0GJ0-**
　Salivary **0CJA-**
Great Vessel **02JY-**
Hand
　Left **0XJK-**
　Right **0XJJ-**
Head **0WJ0-**
Heart **02JA-**
Inguinal Region
　Bilateral **0YJA-**
　Left **0YJ6-**
　Right **0YJ5-**
Intestinal Tract
　Lower **0DJD-**
　Upper **0DJ0-**
Jaw
　Lower **0WJ5-**
　Upper **0WJ4-**
Joint
　Acromioclavicular
　　Left **0RJH-**
　　Right **0RJG-**
　Ankle
　　Left **0SJG-**
　　Right **0SJF-**
　Carpal
　　Left **0RJR-**
　　Right **0RJQ-**
　Cervical Vertebral **0RJ1-**
　Cervicothoracic Vertebral **0RJ4-**
　Coccygeal **0SJ6-**
　Elbow
　　Left **0RJM-**
　　Right **0RJL-**
　Finger Phalangeal
　　Left **0RJX-**
　　Right **0RJW-**
　Hip
　　Left **0SJB-**
　　Right **0SJ9-**
　Knee
　　Left **0SJD-**
　　Right **0SJC-**
　Lumbar Vertebral **0SJ0-**
　Lumbosacral **0SJ3-**
　Metacarpocarpal
　　Left **0RJT-**
　　Right **0RJS-**
　Metacarpophalangeal
　　Left **0RJV-**
　　Right **0RJU-**
　Metatarsal-Phalangeal
　　Left **0SJN-**
　　Right **0SJM-**
　Metatarsal-Tarsal
　　Left **0SJL-**
　　Right **0SJK-**
　Occipital-cervical **0RJ0-**

Inspection — *continued*
Joint — *continued*
　Sacrococcygeal **0SJ5-**
　Sacroiliac
　　Left **0SJ8-**
　　Right **0SJ7-**
　Shoulder
　　Left **0RJK-**
　　Right **0RJJ-**
　Sternoclavicular
　　Left **0RJF-**
　　Right **0RJE-**
　Tarsal
　　Left **0SJJ-**
　　Right **0SJH-**
　Temporomandibular
　　Left **0RJD-**
　　Right **0RJC-**
　Thoracic Vertebral **0RJ6-**
　Thoracolumbar Vertebral **0RJA-**
　Toe Phalangeal
　　Left **0SJQ-**
　　Right **0SJP-**
　Wrist
　　Left **0RJP-**
　　Right **0RJN-**
Kidney **0TJ5-**
Knee Region
　Left **0YJG-**
　Right **0YJF-**
Larynx **0CJS-**
Leg
　Lower
　　Left **0YJJ-**
　　Right **0YJH-**
　Upper
　　Left **0YJD-**
　　Right **0YJC-**
Lens
　Left **08JKXZZ**
　Right **08JJXZZ**
Liver **0FJ0-**
Lung
　Left **0BJL-**
　Right **0BJK-**
Lymphatic **07JN-**
　Thoracic Duct **07JK-**
Mediastinum **0WJC-**
Mesentery **0DJV-**
Mouth and Throat **0CJY-**
Muscle
　Extraocular
　　Left **08JM-**
　　Right **08JL-**
　Lower **0KJY-**
　Upper **0KJX-**
Neck **0WJ6-**
Nerve
　Cranial **00JE-**
　Peripheral **01JY-**
Nose **09JK-**
Omentum **0DJU-**
Oral Cavity and Throat **0WJ3-**
Ovary **0UJ3-**
Pancreas **0FJG-**
Parathyroid Gland **0GJR-**
Pelvic Cavity **0WJJ-**
Penis **0VJS-**
Pericardial Cavity **0WJD-**
Perineum
　Female **0WJN-**
　Male **0WJM-**
Peritoneal Cavity **0WJG-**
Peritoneum **0DJW-**
Pineal Body **0GJ1-**
Pleura **0BJQ-**
Pleural Cavity
　Left **0WJB-**
　Right **0WJ9-**
Products of Conception **10J0-**
　Ectopic **10J2-**
　Retained **10J1-**
Prostate and Seminal Vesicles **0VJ4-**

P R O C E D U R E   I N D E X

Inspection — *continued*
Respiratory Tract **0WJQ**-
Retroperitoneum **0WJH**-
Scrotum and Tunica Vaginalis **0VJ8**-
Shoulder Region
  Left **0XJ3**-
  Right **0XJ2**-
Sinus **09JY**-
Skin **0HJPXZZ**
Skull **0NJ0**-
Spinal Canal **00JU**-
Spinal Cord **00JV**-
Spleen **07JP**-
Stomach **0DJ6**-
Subcutaneous Tissue and Fascia
  Head and Neck **0JJS**-
  Lower Extremity **0JJW**-
  Trunk **0JJT**-
  Upper Extremity **0JJV**-
Tendon
  Lower **0LJY**-
  Upper **0LJX**-
Testis **0VJD**-
Thymus **07JM**-
Thyroid Gland **0GJK**-
Toe Nail **0HJRXZZ**
Trachea **0BJ1**-
Tracheobronchial Tree **0BJ0**-
Tympanic Membrane
  Left **09J8**-
  Right **09J7**-
Ureter **0TJ9**-
Urethra **0TJD**-
Uterus and Cervix **0UJD**-
Vagina and Cul-de-sac **0UJH**-
Vas Deferens **0VJR**-
Vein
  Lower **06JY**-
  Upper **05JY**-
Vulva **0UJM**-
Wrist Region
  Left **0XJH**-
  Right **0XJG**-
Instillation *see* Introduction of
  substance in or on
Insufflation *see* Introduction of
  substance in or on
Interatrial septum
  use Septum, Atrial
Interbody fusion device,
  nanotextured surface
Cervical Vertebral **XRG1092**
  2 or more **XRG2092**
Cervicothoracic Vertebral **XRG4092**
Lumbar Vertebral **XRGB092**
  2 or more **XRGC092**
Lumbosacral **XRGD092**
Occipital-cervical **XRG0092**
Thoracic Vertebral **XRG6092**
  2 to 7 **XRG7092**
  8 or more **XRG8092**
Thoracolumbar Vertebral **XRGA092**
Interbody fusion (spine) cage
  use Interbody Fusion Device in Lower
    Joints
  use Interbody Fusion Device in Upper
    Joints
Intercarpal joint
  use Joint, Carpal, Left
  use Joint, Carpal, Right
Intercarpal ligament
  use Bursa and Ligament, Hand, Left
  use Bursa and Ligament, Hand, Right
Interclavicular ligament
  use Bursa and Ligament, Shoulder,
    Left
  use Bursa and Ligament, Shoulder,
    Right

Intercostal lymph node
  use Lymphatic, Thorax
Intercostal muscle
  use Muscle, Thorax, Left
  use Muscle, Thorax, Right
Intercostal nerve
  use Nerve, Thoracic
Intercostobrachial nerve
  use Nerve, Thoracic
Intercuneiform joint
  use Joint, Tarsal, Left
  use Joint, Tarsal, Right
Intercuneiform ligament
  use Bursa and Ligament, Foot, Left
  use Bursa and Ligament, Foot, Right
Intermediate bronchus
  use Main Bronchus, Right
Intermediate cuneiform bone
  use Tarsal, Left
  use Tarsal, Right
Intermittent mandatory
  ventilation *see* Assistance,
  Respiratory **5A09**-
Intermittent Negative Airway
  Pressure
24-96 Consecutive Hours, Ventilation
  5A0945B
Greater than 96 Consecutive Hours,
  Ventilation **5A0955B**
Less than 24 Consecutive Hours,
  Ventilation **5A0935B**
Intermittent Positive Airway
  Pressure
24-96 Consecutive Hours, Ventilation
  5A09458
Greater than 96 Consecutive Hours,
  Ventilation **5A09558**
Less than 24 Consecutive Hours,
  Ventilation **5A09358**
Intermittent positive pressure
  breathing *see* Assistance,
  Respiratory **5A09**-
Internal (basal) cerebral vein
  use Vein, Intracranial
Internal anal sphincter
  use Anal Sphincter
Internal carotid artery,
  intracranial portion
  use Intracranial Artery
Internal carotid plexus
  use Nerve, Head and Neck
    Sympathetic
Internal iliac vein
  use Vein, Hypogastric, Left
  use Vein, Hypogastric, Right
Internal maxillary artery
  use Artery, External Carotid, Left
  use Artery, External Carotid, Right
Internal naris
  use Nose
Internal oblique muscle
  use Muscle, Abdomen, Left
  use Muscle, Abdomen, Right
Internal pudendal artery
  use Artery, Internal Iliac, Left
  use Artery, Internal Iliac, Right
Internal pudendal vein
  use Vein, Hypogastric, Left
  use Vein, Hypogastric, Right
Internal thoracic artery
  use Artery, Internal Mammary, Left
  use Artery, Internal Mammary, Right
  use Artery, Subclavian, Left
  use Artery, Subclavian, Right
Internal urethral sphincter
  use Urethra

Interphalangeal (IP) joint
  use Joint, Finger Phalangeal, Left
  use Joint, Finger Phalangeal, Right
  use Joint, Toe Phalangeal, Left
  use Joint, Toe Phalangeal, Right
Interphalangeal ligament
  use Bursa and Ligament, Foot, Left
  use Bursa and Ligament, Foot, Right
  use Bursa and Ligament, Hand, Left
  use Bursa and Ligament, Hand, Right
Interrogation, cardiac rhythm
  related device
Interrogation only *see* Measurement,
  Cardiac **4B02**-
With cardiac function testing *see*
  Measurement, Cardiac **4A02**-
Interruption *see* Occlusion
Interspinalis muscle
  use Muscle, Trunk, Left
  use Muscle, Trunk, Right
Interspinous ligament
  use Bursa and Ligament, Head and
    Neck
  use Bursa and Ligament, Trunk, Left
  use Bursa and Ligament, Trunk, Right
Interspinous process spinal
  stabilization device
  use Spinal Stabilization Device,
    Interspinous Process in **0RH**-
  use Spinal Stabilization Device,
    Interspinous Process in **0SH**-
InterStim® Therapy lead
  use Neurostimulator Lead in
    Peripheral Nervous System
InterStim® Therapy
  neurostimulator
  use Stimulator Generator, Single
    Array in **0JH**-
Intertransversarius muscle
  use Muscle, Trunk, Left
  use Muscle, Trunk, Right
Intertransverse ligament
  use Bursa and Ligament, Trunk, Left
  use Bursa and Ligament, Trunk, Right
Interventricular foramen (Monro)
  use Cerebral Ventricle
Interventricular septum
  use Septum, Ventricular
Intestinal lymphatic trunk
  use Cisterna Chyli
Intraluminal Device
Airway
  Esophagus **0DH5**-
  Mouth and Throat **0CHY**-
  Nasopharynx **09HN**-
Bioactive
  Occlusion
    Common Carotid
      Left **03LJ**-
      Right **03LH**-
    External Carotid
      Left **03LN**-
      Right **03LM**-
    Internal Carotid
      Left **03LL**-
      Right **03LK**-
    Intracranial **03LG**-
    Vertebral
      Left **03LQ**-
      Right **03LP**-
Restriction
  Common Carotid
    Left **03VJ**-
    Right **03VH**-
  External Carotid
    Left **03VN**-
    Right **03VM**-
  Internal Carotid
    Left **03VL**-
    Right **03VK**-
  Intracranial **03VG**-
  Vertebral
    Left **03VQ**-
    Right **03VP**-

Intraluminal Device — *continued*
Endobronchial Valve
  Lingula **0BH9**-
  Lower Lobe
    Left **0BHB**-
    Right **0BH6**-
  Main
    Left **0BH7**-
    Right **0BH3**-
  Middle Lobe, Right **0BH5**-
  Upper Lobe
    Left **0BH8**-
    Right **0BH4**-
Endotracheal Airway
  Change device in, Trachea
    0B21XEZ
  Insertion of device in, Trachea
    0BH1-
Pessary
  Change device in, Vagina and
    Cul-de-sac **0U2HXGZ**
  Insertion of device in
    Cul-de-sac **0UHF**-
    Vagina **0UHG**-
Intramedullary (IM) rod (nail)
  use Internal Fixation Device,
    Intramedullary in Lower Bones
  use Internal Fixation Device,
    Intramedullary in Upper Bones
Intramedullary skeletal kinetic
  distractor (ISKD)
  use Internal Fixation Device,
    Intramedullary in Lower Bones
  use Internal Fixation Device,
    Intramedullary in Upper Bones
Intraocular Telescope
Left **08RK30Z**
Right **08RJ30Z**
Intraoperative knee replacement
  sensor XR2-
Intraoperative Radiation Therapy
  (IORT)
Anus **DDY8CZZ**
Bile Ducts **DFY2CZZ**
Bladder **DTY2CZZ**
Cervix **DUY1CZZ**
Colon **DDY5CZZ**
Duodenum **DDY2CZZ**
Gallbladder **DFY1CZZ**
Ileum **DDY4CZZ**
Jejunum **DDY3CZZ**
Kidney **DTY0CZZ**
Larynx **D9YBCZZ**
Liver **DFY0CZZ**
Mouth **D9Y4CZZ**
Nasopharynx **D9YDCZZ**
Ovary **DUY0CZZ**
Pancreas **DFY3CZZ**
Pharynx **D9YCCZZ**
Prostate **DVY0CZZ**
Rectum **DDY7CZZ**
Stomach **DDY1CZZ**
Ureter **DTY1CZZ**
Urethra **DTY3CZZ**
Uterus **DUY2CZZ**
Intrauterine device (IUD)
  use Contraceptive Device in Female
    Reproductive System
Intravascular fluorescence
  angiography (IFA) *see*
  Monitoring, Physiological Systems
  4A1-

Introduction of substance in or on

Artery
  Central **3E06-**
    Analgesics **3E06-**
    Anesthetic, Intracirculatory **3E06-**
    Antiarrhythmic **3E06-**
    Anti-infective **3E06-**
    Anti-inflammatory **3E06-**
    Antineoplastic **3E06-**
    Destructive Agent **3E06-**
    Diagnostic Substance, Other **3E06-**
    Electrolytic Substance **3E06-**
    Hormone **3E06-**
    Hypnotics **3E06-**
    Immunotherapeutic **3E06-**
    Nutritional Substance **3E06-**
    Platelet Inhibitor **3E06-**
    Radioactive Substance **3E06-**
    Sedatives **3E06-**
    Serum **3E06-**
    Thrombolytic **3E06-**
    Toxoid **3E06-**
    Vaccine **3E06-**
    Vasopressor **3E06-**
    Water Balance Substance **3E06-**
  Coronary **3E07-**
    Diagnostic Substance, Other **3E07-**
    Platelet Inhibitor **3E07-**
    Thrombolytic **3E07-**
  Peripheral **3E05-**
    Analgesics **3E05-**
    Anesthetic, Intracirculatory **3E05-**
    Antiarrhythmic **3E05-**
    Anti-infective **3E05-**
    Anti-inflammatory **3E05-**
    Antineoplastic **3E05-**
    Destructive Agent **3E05-**
    Diagnostic Substance, Other **3E05-**
    Electrolytic Substance **3E05-**
    Hormone **3E05-**
    Hypnotics **3E05-**
    Immunotherapeutic **3E05-**
    Nutritional Substance **3E05-**
    Platelet Inhibitor **3E05-**
    Radioactive Substance **3E05-**
    Sedatives **3E05-**
    Serum **3E05-**
    Thrombolytic **3E05-**
    Toxoid **3E05-**
    Vaccine **3E05-**
    Vasopressor **3E05-**
    Water Balance Substance **3E05-**
Biliary Tract **3E0J-**
  Analgesics **3E0J-**
  Anesthetic, Local **3E0J-**
  Anti-infective **3E0J**
  Anti-inflammatory **3E0J**
  Antineoplastic **3E0J-**
  Destructive Agent **3E0J-**
  Diagnostic Substance, Other **3E0J-**
  Electrolytic Substance **3E0J-**
  Gas **3E0J-**
  Hypnotics **3E0J-**
  Islet Cells, Pancreatic **3E0J-**
  Nutritional Substance **3E0J-**
  Radioactive Substance **3E0J-**
  Sedatives **3E0J-**
  Water Balance Substance **3E0J-**

Introduction of substance in or on — *continued*

Bone **3E0V-**
  Analgesics **3E0V3NZ**
  Anesthetic, Local **3E0V3BZ**
  Anti-infective **3E0V32-**
  Anti-inflammatory **3E0V33Z**
  Antineoplastic **3E0V30-**
  Destructive Agent **3E0V3TZ**
  Diagnostic Substance, Other **3E0V3KZ**
  Electrolytic Substance **3E0V37Z**
  Hypnotics **3E0V3NZ**
  Nutritional Substance **3E0V36Z**
  Radioactive Substance **3E0V3HZ**
  Sedatives **3E0V3NZ**
  Water Balance Substance **3E0V37Z**
Bone Marrow **3E0A3GC**
  Antineoplastic **3E0A30-**
Brain **3E0Q-**
  Analgesics **3E0Q-**
  Anesthetic, Local **3E0Q-**
  Anti-infective **3E0Q-**
  Anti-inflammatory **3E0Q-**
  Antineoplastic **3E0Q-**
  Destructive Agent **3E0Q-**
  Diagnostic Substance, Other **3E0Q-**
  Electrolytic Substance **3E0Q-**
  Gas **3E0Q-**
  Hypnotics **3E0Q-**
  Nutritional Substance **3E0Q-**
  Radioactive Substance **3E0Q-**
  Sedatives **3E0Q-**
  Stem Cells
    Embryonic **3E0Q-**
    Somatic **3E0Q-**
  Water Balance Substance **3E0Q-**
Cranial Cavity **3E0Q-**
  Analgesics **3E0Q-**
  Anesthetic, Local **3E0Q-**
  Anti-infective **3E0Q-**
  Anti-inflammatory **3E0Q-**
  Antineoplastic **3E0Q-**
  Destructive Agent **3E0Q-**
  Diagnostic Substance, Other **3E0Q-**
  Electrolytic Substance **3E0Q-**
  Gas **3E0Q-**
  Hypnotics **3E0Q-**
  Nutritional Substance **3E0Q-**
  Radioactive Substance **3E0Q-**
  Sedatives **3E0Q-**
  Stem Cells
    Embryonic **3E0Q-**
    Somatic **3E0Q-**
  Water Balance Substance **3E0Q-**
Ear **3E0B**
  Analgesics **3E0B-**
  Anesthetic, Local **3E0B-**
  Anti-infective **3E0B-**
  Anti-inflammatory **3E0B-**
  Antineoplastic **3E0B-**
  Destructive Agent **3E0B-**
  Diagnostic Substance, Other **3E0B-**
  Hypnotics **3E0B-**
  Radioactive Substance **3E0B-**
  Sedatives **3E0B-**
Epidural Space **3E0S3GC**
  Analgesics **3E0S3NZ**
  Anesthetic
    Local **3E0S3BZ**
    Regional **3E0S3CZ**
  Anti-infective **3E0S32-**
  Anti-inflammatory **3E0S33Z**
  Antineoplastic **3E0S30-**
  Destructive Agent **3E0S3TZ**
  Diagnostic Substance, Other **3E0S3KZ**
  Electrolytic Substance **3E0S37Z**
  Gas **3E0S-**
  Hypnotics **3E0S3NZ**
  Nutritional Substance **3E0S36Z**
  Radioactive Substance **3E0S3HZ**
  Sedatives **3E0S3NZ**
  Water Balance Substance **3E0S37Z**

Introduction of substance in or on — *continued*

Eye **3E0C-**
  Analgesics **3E0C-**
  Anesthetic, Local **3E0C-**
  Anti-infective **3E0C-**
  Anti-inflammatory **3E0C-**
  Antineoplastic **3E0C-**
  Destructive Agent **3E0C-**
  Diagnostic Substance, Other **3E0C-**
  Gas **3E0C-**
  Hypnotics **3E0C-**
  Pigment **3E0C-**
  Radioactive Substance **3E0C-**
  Sedatives **3E0C-**
Gastrointestinal Tract
  Lower **3E0H-**
    Analgesics **3E0H-**
    Anesthetic, Local **3E0H-**
    Anti-infective **3E0H-**
    Anti-inflammatory **3E0H-**
    Antineoplastic **3E0H-**
    Destructive Agent **3E0H-**
    Diagnostic Substance, Other **3E0H-**
    Electrolytic Substance **3E0H-**
    Gas **3E0H-**
    Hypnotics **3E0H-**
    Nutritional Substance **3E0H-**
    Radioactive Substance **3E0H-**
    Sedatives **3E0H-**
    Water Balance Substance **3E0H-**
  Upper **3E0G-**
    Analgesics **3E0G-**
    Anesthetic, Local **3E0G-**
    Anti-infective **3E0G-**
    Anti-inflammatory **3E0G-**
    Antineoplastic **3E0G-**
    Destructive Agent **3E0G-**
    Diagnostic Substance, Other **3E0G-**
    Electrolytic Substance **3E0G-**
    Gas **3E0G-**
    Hypnotics **3E0G-**
    Nutritional Substance **3E0G-**
    Radioactive Substance **3E0G-**
    Sedatives **3E0G-**
    Water Balance Substance **3E0G-**
Genitourinary Tract **3E0K-**
  Analgesics **3E0K-**
  Anesthetic, Local **3E0K-**
  Anti-infective **3E0K-**
  Anti-inflammatory **3E0K-**
  Antineoplastic **3E0K-**
  Destructive Agent **3E0K-**
  Diagnostic Substance, Other **3E0K-**
  Electrolytic Substance **3E0K-**
  Gas **3E0K-**
  Hypnotics **3E0K-**
  Nutritional Substance **3E0K-**
  Radioactive Substance **3E0K-**
  Sedatives **3E0K-**
  Water Balance Substance **3E0K-**
Heart **3E08-**
  Diagnostic Substance, Other **3E08-**
  Platelet Inhibitor **3E08-**
  Thrombolytic **3E08-**
Joint **3E0U-**
  Analgesics **3E0U3NZ**
  Anesthetic, Local **3E0U3BZ**
  Anti-infective **3E0U-**
  Anti-inflammatory **3E0U33Z**
  Antineoplastic **3E0U30-**
  Destructive Agent **3E0U3TZ**
  Diagnostic Substance, Other **3E0U3KZ**
  Electrolytic Substance **3E0U37Z**
  Gas **3E0U3SF**
  Hypnotics **3E0U3NZ**
  Nutritional Substance **3E0U36Z**
  Radioactive Substance **3E0U3HZ**
  Sedatives **3E0U3NZ**
  Water Balance Substance **3E0U37Z**

Introduction of substance in or on — *continued*

Lymphatic **3E0W3GC**
  Analgesics **3E0W3NZ**
  Anesthetic, Local **3E0W3BZ**
  Anti-infective **3E0W32-**
  Anti-inflammatory **3E0W33Z**
  Antineoplastic **3E0W30-**
  Destructive Agent **3E0W3TZ**
  Diagnostic Substance, Other **3E0W3KZ**
  Electrolytic Substance **3E0W37Z**
  Hypnotics **3E0W3NZ**
  Nutritional Substance **3E0W36Z**
  Radioactive Substance **3E0W3HZ**
  Sedatives **3E0W3NZ**
  Water Balance Substance **3E0W37Z**
Mouth **3E0D-**
  Analgesics **3E0D-**
  Anesthetic, Local **3E0D-**
  Antiarrhythmic **3E0D-**
  Anti-infective **3E0D-**
  Anti-inflammatory **3E0D-**
  Antineoplastic **3E0D-**
  Destructive Agent **3E0D-**
  Diagnostic Substance, Other **3E0D-**
  Electrolytic Substance **3E0D-**
  Hypnotics **3E0D-**
  Nutritional Substance **3E0D-**
  Radioactive Substance **3E0D-**
  Sedatives **3E0D-**
  Serum **3E0D-**
  Toxoid **3E0D-**
  Vaccine **3E0D-**
  Water Balance Substance **3E0D-**
Mucous Membrane **3E00XGC**
  Analgesics **3E00XNZ**
  Anesthetic, Local **3E00XBZ**
  Anti-infective **3E00X2-**
  Anti-inflammatory **3E00X3Z**
  Antineoplastic **3E00X0-**
  Destructive Agent **3E00XTZ**
  Diagnostic Substance, Other **3E00XKZ**
  Hypnotics **3E00XNZ**
  Pigment **3E00XMZ**
  Sedatives **3E00XNZ**
  Serum **3E00X4Z**
  Toxoid **3E00X4Z**
  Vaccine **3E00X4Z**
Muscle **3E023GC**
  Analgesics **3E023NZ**
  Anesthetic, Local **3E023BZ**
  Anti-infective **3E0232-**
  Anti-inflammatory **3E0233Z**
  Antineoplastic **3E0230-**
  Destructive Agent **3E023TZ**
  Diagnostic Substance, Other **3E023KZ**
  Electrolytic Substance **3E0237Z**
  Hypnotics **3E023NZ**
  Nutritional Substance **3E0236Z**
  Radioactive Substance **3E023HZ**
  Sedatives **3E023NZ**
  Serum **3E0234Z**
  Toxoid **3E0234Z**
  Vaccine **3E0234Z**
  Water Balance Substance **3E0237Z**

Introduction of substance in or on — continued
Nerve
  Cranial 3E0X3GC
    Anesthetic
      Local 3E0X3BZ
      Regional 3E0X3CZ
    Anti-inflammatory 3E0X33Z
    Destructive Agent 3E0X3TZ
  Peripheral 3E0T3GC
    Anesthetic
      Local 3E0T3BZ
      Regional 3E0T3CZ
    Anti-inflammatory 3E0T33Z
    Destructive Agent 3E0T3TZ
  Plexus 3E0T3GC
    Anesthetic
      Local 3E0T3BZ
      Regional 3E0T3CZ
    Anti-inflammatory 3E0T33Z
    Destructive Agent 3E0T3TZ
Nose 3E09-
  Analgesics 3E09-
  Anesthetic, Local 3E09-
  Anti-infective 3E09-
  Anti-inflammatory 3E09-
  Antineoplastic 3E09-
  Destructive Agent 3E09-
  Diagnostic Substance, Other 3E09-
  Hypnotics 3E09-
  Radioactive Substance 3E09-
  Sedatives 3E09-
  Serum 3E09-
  Toxoid 3E09-
  Vaccine 3E09-
Pancreatic Tract 3E0J-
  Analgesics 3E0J-
  Anesthetic, Local 3E0J-
  Anti-infective 3E0J-
  Anti-inflammatory 3E0J-
  Antineoplastic 3E0J-
  Destructive Agent 3E0J-
  Diagnostic Substance, Other 3E0J-
  Electrolytic Substance 3E0J-
  Gas 3E0J-
  Hypnotics 3E0J-
  Islet Cells, Pancreatic 3E0J-
  Nutritional Substance 3E0J-
  Radioactive Substance 3E0J-
  Sedatives 3E0J-
  Water Balance Substance 3E0J-
Pericardial Cavity 3E0Y3GC
  Analgesics 3E0Y3NZ
  Anesthetic, Local 3E0Y3BZ
  Anti-infective 3E0Y32-
  Anti-inflammatory 3E0Y33Z
  Antineoplastic 3E0Y-
  Destructive Agent 3E0Y3TZ
  Diagnostic Substance, Other 3E0Y3KZ
  Electrolytic Substance 3E0Y37Z
  Gas 3E0Y-
  Hypnotics 3E0Y3NZ
  Nutritional Substance 3E0Y36Z
  Radioactive Substance 3E0Y3HZ
  Sedatives 3E0Y3NZ
  Water Balance Substance 3E0Y37Z
Peritoneal Cavity 3E0M3GC
  Adhesion Barrier 3E0M05Z
  Analgesics 3E0M3NZ
  Anesthetic, Local 3E0M3BZ
  Anti-infective 3E0M32-
  Anti-inflammatory 3E0M33Z
  Antineoplastic 3E0M-
  Destructive Agent 3E0M3TZ
  Diagnostic Substance, Other 3E0M3KZ
  Electrolytic Substance 3E0M37Z
  Gas 3E0M-
  Hypnotics 3E0M3NZ
  Nutritional Substance 3E0M36Z
  Radioactive Substance 3E0M3HZ
  Sedatives 3E0M3NZ
  Water Balance Substance 3E0M37Z

Introduction of substance in or on — continued
Pharynx 3E0D-
  Analgesics 3E0D-
  Anesthetic, Local 3E0D-
  Antiarrhythmic 3E0D-
  Anti-infective 3E0D-
  Anti-inflammatory 3E0D-
  Antineoplastic 3E0D-
  Destructive Agent 3E0D-
  Diagnostic Substance, Other 3E0D-
  Electrolytic Substance 3E0D-
  Hypnotics 3E0D-
  Nutritional Substance 3E0D-
  Radioactive Substance 3E0D-
  Sedatives 3E0D-
  Serum 3E0D-
  Toxoid 3E0D-
  Vaccine 3E0D-
  Water Balance Substance 3E0D-
Pleural Cavity 3E0L3GC
  Adhesion Barrier 3E0L05Z
  Analgesics 3E0L3NZ
  Anesthetic, Local 3E0L3BZ
  Anti-infective 3E0L32-
  Anti-inflammatory 3E0L33Z
  Antineoplastic 3E0L-
  Destructive Agent 3E0L3TZ
  Diagnostic Substance, Other 3E0L3KZ
  Electrolytic Substance 3E0L37Z
  Gas 3E0L-
  Hypnotics 3E0L3NZ
  Nutritional Substance 3E0L36Z
  Radioactive Substance 3E0L3HZ
  Sedatives 3E0L3NZ
  Water Balance Substance 3E0L37Z
Products of Conception 3E0E-
  Analgesics 3E0E-
  Anesthetic, Local 3E0E-
  Anti-infective 3E0E-
  Anti-inflammatory 3E0E-
  Antineoplastic 3E0E-
  Destructive Agent 3E0E-
  Diagnostic Substance, Other 3E0E-
  Electrolytic Substance 3E0E-
  Gas 3E0E-
  Hypnotics 3E0E-
  Nutritional Substance 3E0E-
  Radioactive Substance 3E0E-
  Sedatives 3E0E-
  Water Balance Substance 3E0E-
Reproductive
  Female 3E0P-
    Adhesion Barrier 3E0P05Z
    Analgesics 3E0P-
    Anesthetic, Local 3E0P-
    Anti-infective 3E0P-
    Anti-inflammatory 3E0P-
    Antineoplastic 3E0P-
    Destructive Agent 3E0P-
    Diagnostic Substance, Other 3E0P-
    Electrolytic Substance 3E0P-
    Gas 3E0P-
    Hypnotics 3E0P-
    Nutritional Substance 3E0P-
    Ovum, Fertilized 3E0P-
    Radioactive Substance 3E0P-
    Sedatives 3E0P-
    Sperm 3E0P-
    Water Balance Substance 3E0P-

Introduction of substance in or on — continued
Reproductive — continued
  Male 3E0N-
    Analgesics 3E0N-
    Anesthetic, Local 3E0N-
    Anti-infective 3E0N-
    Anti-inflammatory 3E0N-
    Antineoplastic 3E0N-
    Destructive Agent 3E0N-
    Diagnostic Substance, Other 3E0N-
    Electrolytic Substance 3E0N-
    Gas 3E0N-
    Hypnotics 3E0N-
    Nutritional Substance 3E0N-
    Radioactive Substance 3E0N-
    Sedatives 3E0N-
    Water Balance Substance 3E0N-
Respiratory Tract 3E0F-
  Analgesics 3E0F-
  Anesthetic
    Inhalation 3E0F-
    Local 3E0F-
  Anti-infective 3E0F-
  Anti-inflammatory 3E0F-
  Antineoplastic 3E0F-
  Destructive Agent 3E0F-
  Diagnostic Substance, Other 3E0F-
  Electrolytic Substance 3E0F-
  Gas 3E0F-
  Hypnotics 3E0F-
  Nutritional Substance 3E0F-
  Radioactive Substance 3E0F-
  Sedatives 3E0F-
  Water Balance Substance 3E0F-
Skin 3E00XGC
  Analgesics 3E00XNZ
  Anesthetic, Local 3E00XBZ
  Anti-infective 3E00X2-
  Anti-inflammatory 3E00X3Z
  Antineoplastic 3E00X0-
  Destructive Agent 3E00XTZ
  Diagnostic Substance, Other 3E00XKZ
  Hypnotics 3E00XNZ
  Pigment 3E00XMZ
  Sedatives 3E00XNZ
  Serum 3E00X4Z
  Toxoid 3E00X4Z
  Vaccine 3E00X4Z
Spinal Canal 3E0R3GC
  Analgesics 3E0R3NZ
  Anesthetic
    Local 3E0R3BZ
    Regional 3E0R3CZ
  Anti-infective 3E0R32-
  Anti-inflammatory 3E0R33Z
  Antineoplastic 3E0R30-
  Destructive Agent 3E0R3TZ
  Diagnostic Substance, Other 3E0R3KZ
  Electrolytic Substance 3E0R37Z
  Gas 3E0R-
  Hypnotics 3E0R3NZ
  Nutritional Substance 3E0R36Z
  Radioactive Substance 3E0R3HZ
  Sedatives 3E0R3NZ
  Stem Cells
    Embryonic 3E0R-
    Somatic 3E0R-
  Water Balance Substance 3E0R37Z

Introduction of substance in or on — continued
Subcutaneous Tissue 3E013GC
  Analgesics 3E013NZ
  Anesthetic, Local 3E013BZ
  Anti-infective 3E01-
  Anti-inflammatory 3E0133Z
  Antineoplastic 3E0130-
  Destructive Agent 3E013TZ
  Diagnostic Substance, Other 3E013KZ
  Electrolytic Substance 3E0137Z
  Hormone 3E013V-
  Hypnotics 3E013NZ
  Nutritional Substance 3E0136Z
  Radioactive Substance 3E013HZ
  Sedatives 3E013NZ
  Serum 3E0134Z
  Toxoid 3E0134Z
  Vaccine 3E0134Z
  Water Balance Substance 3E0137Z
Vein
  Central 3E04-
    Analgesics 3E04-
    Anesthetic, Intracirculatory 3E04-
    Antiarrhythmic 3E04-
    Anti-infective 3E04-
    Anti-inflammatory 3E04-
    Antineoplastic 3E04-
    Destructive Agent 3E04-
    Diagnostic Substance, Other 3E04-
    Electrolytic Substance 3E04-
    Hormone 3E04-
    Hypnotics 3E04-
    Immunotherapeutic 3E04-
    Nutritional Substance 3E04-
    Platelet Inhibitor 3E04-
    Radioactive Substance 3E04-
    Sedatives 3E04-
    Serum 3E04-
    Thrombolytic 3E04-
    Toxoid 3E04-
    Vaccine 3E04-
    Vasopressor 3E04-
    Water Balance Substance 3E04-
  Peripheral 3E03-
    Analgesics 3E03-
    Anesthetic, Intracirculatory 3E03-
    Antiarrhythmic 3E03-
    Anti-infective 3E03-
    Anti-inflammatory 3E03-
    Antineoplastic 3E03-
    Destructive Agent 3E03-
    Diagnostic Substance, Other 3E03-
    Electrolytic Substance 3E03-
    Hormone 3E03-
    Hypnotics 3E03-
    Immunotherapeutic 3E03-
    Islet Cells, Pancreatic 3E03-
    Nutritional Substance 3E03-
    Platelet Inhibitor 3E03-
    Radioactive Substance 3E03-
    Sedatives 3E03-
    Serum 3E03-
    Thrombolytic 3E03-
    Toxoid 3E03-
    Vaccine 3E03-
    Vasopressor 3E03-
    Water Balance Substance 3E03-

Intubation
Airway
see Insertion of device in, Esophagus **0DH**5-
see Insertion of device in, Mouth and Throat **0CH**Y-
see Insertion of device in, Trachea **0BH**1-
Drainage device see Drainage
Feeding Device see Insertion of device in, Gastrointestinal System **0DH**-
INTUITY Elite valve system, EDWARDS
use Zooplastic Tissue, Rapid Deployment Technique in New Technology
IPPB (intermittent positive pressure breathing) see Assistance, Respiratory **5A09**-
Iridectomy
see Excision, Eye **08B**-
see Resection, Eye **08T**-
Iridoplasty
see Repair, Eye **08Q**-
see Replacement, Eye **08R**-
see Supplement, Eye **08U**-
Iridotomy see Drainage, Eye **089**-
Irrigation
Biliary Tract, Irrigating Substance **3E1**J-
Brain, Irrigating Substance **3E1Q38Z**
Cranial Cavity, Irrigating Substance **3E1Q38Z**
Ear, Irrigating Substance **3E1**B-
Epidural Space, Irrigating Substance **3E1S38Z**
Eye, Irrigating Substance **3E1**C-
Gastrointestinal Tract
Lower, Irrigating Substance **3E1**H-
Upper, Irrigating Substance **3E1**G-
Genitourinary Tract, Irrigating Substance **3E1**K-
Irrigating Substance **3C1ZX8Z**
Joint, Irrigating Substance **3E1U38Z**
Mucous Membrane, Irrigating Substance **3E10**-
Nose, Irrigating Substance **3E19**-
Pancreatic Tract, Irrigating Substance **3E1**J-
Pericardial Cavity, Irrigating Substance **3E1Y38Z**
Peritoneal Cavity
Dialysate **3E1M39Z**
Irrigating Substance **3E1M38Z**
Pleural Cavity, Irrigating Substance **3E1L38Z**
Reproductive
Female, Irrigating Substance **3E1**P-
Male, Irrigating Substance **3E1**N-
Respiratory Tract, Irrigating Substance **3E1**F-
Skin, Irrigating Substance **3E10**-
Spinal Canal, Irrigating Substance **3E1R38Z**
Isavuconazole anti-infective XW0-
Ischiatic nerve
use Nerve, Sciatic
Ischiocavernosus muscle
use Muscle, Perineum
Ischiofemoral ligament
use Bursa and Ligament, Hip, Left
use Bursa and Ligament, Hip, Right
Ischium
use Bone, Pelvic, Left
use Bone, Pelvic, Right
Isolation 8E0ZXY6
Isotope Administration, Whole Body DWY5G-
Itrel (3) (4) neurostimulator
use Stimulator Generator, Single Array in **0JH**-

J

Jejunal artery
use Artery, Superior Mesenteric
Jejunectomy
see Excision, Jejunum **0DBA**-
see Resection, Jejunum **0DTA**-
Jejunocolostomy
see Bypass, Gastrointestinal System **0D1**-
see Drainage, Gastrointestinal System **0D9**-
Jejunopexy
see Repair, Jejunum **0DQA**-
see Reposition, Jejunum **0DSA**-
Jejunostomy
see Bypass, Jejunum **0D1A**-
see Drainage, Jejunum **0D9A**-
Jejunotomy see Drainage, Jejunum **0D9A**-
Joint fixation plate
use Internal Fixation Device in Lower Joints
use Internal Fixation Device in Upper Joints
Joint liner (insert)
use Liner in Lower Joints
Joint spacer (antibiotic)
use Spacer in Lower Joints
use Spacer in Upper Joints
Jugular body
use Glomus Jugulare
Jugular lymph node
use Lymphatic, Neck, Left
use Lymphatic, Neck, Right

K

Kappa
use Pacemaker, Dual Chamber in **0JH**-
Kcentra
use 4-Factor Prothrombin Complex Concentrate
Keratectomy, kerectomy
see Excision, Eye **08B**-
see Resection, Eye **08T**-
Keratocentesis see Drainage, Eye **089**-
Keratoplasty
see Repair, Eye **08Q**-
see Replacement, Eye **08R**-
see Supplement, Eye **08U**-
Keratotomy
see Drainage, Eye **089**-
see Repair, Eye **08Q**-
Kirschner wire (K-wire)
use Internal Fixation Device in Head and Facial Bones
use Internal Fixation Device in Lower Bones
use Internal Fixation Device in Lower Joints
use Internal Fixation Device in Upper Bones
use Internal Fixation Device in Upper Joints
Knee (implant) insert
use Liner in Lower Joints
KUB x-ray see Plain Radiography, Kidney, Ureter and Bladder **BT04**-
Kuntscher nail
use Internal Fixation Device, Intramedullary in Lower Bones
use Internal Fixation Device, Intramedullary in Upper Bones

L

Labia majora
use Vulva
Labia minora
use Vulva
Labial gland
use Lip, Lower
use Lip, Upper
Labiectomy
see Excision, Female Reproductive System **0UB**-
see Resection, Female Reproductive System **0UT**-
Lacrimal canaliculus
use Duct, Lacrimal, Left
use Duct, Lacrimal, Right
Lacrimal punctum
use Duct, Lacrimal, Left
use Duct, Lacrimal, Right
Lacrimal sac
use Duct, Lacrimal, Left
use Duct, Lacrimal, Right
Laminectomy
see Excision, Lower Bones **0QB**-
see Excision, Upper Bones **0PB**-
see Release, Central Nervous System **00N**-
see Release, Peripheral Nervous System **01N**-
Laminotomy
see Drainage, Lower Bones **0Q9**-
see Drainage, Upper Bones **0P9**-
see Excision, Lower Bones **0QB**-
see Excision, Upper Bones **0PB**-
see Release, Central Nervous System **00N**-
see Release, Lower Bones **0QN**-
see Release, Peripheral Nervous System **01N**-
see Release, Upper Bones **0PN**-
LAP-BAND® adjustable gastric banding system
use Extraluminal Device
Laparoscopy see Inspection
Laparotomy
Drainage see Drainage, Peritoneal Cavity **0W9G**-
Exploratory see Inspection, Peritoneal Cavity **0WJG**-
Laryngectomy
see Excision, Larynx **0CBS**-
see Resection, Larynx **0CTS**-
Laryngocentesis see Drainage, Larynx **0C9S**-
Laryngogram see Fluoroscopy, Larynx **B91J**-
Laryngopexy see Repair, Larynx **0CQS**-
Laryngopharynx
use Pharynx
Laryngoplasty
see Repair, Larynx **0CQS**-
see Replacement, Larynx **0CRS**-
see Supplement, Larynx **0CUS**-
Laryngorrhaphy see Repair, Larynx **0CQS**-
Laryngoscopy 0CJS8ZZ
Laryngotomy see Drainage, Larynx **0C9S**-

PROCEDURE INDEX

PROCEDURE INDEX

Laser Interstitial Thermal Therapy
Adrenal Gland **DGY**2KZZ
Anus **DDY**8KZZ
Bile Ducts **DFY**2KZZ
Brain **D0Y**0KZZ
Brain Stem **D0Y**1KZZ
Breast
   Left **DMY**0KZZ
   Right **DMY**1KZZ
Bronchus **DBY**1KZZ
Chest Wall **DBY**7KZZ
Colon **DDY**5KZZ
Diaphragm **DBY**8KZZ
Duodenum **DDY**2KZZ
Esophagus **DDY**0KZZ
Gallbladder **DFY**1KZZ
Gland
   Adrenal **DGY**2KZZ
   Parathyroid **DGY**4KZZ
   Pituitary **DGY**0KZZ
   Thyroid **DGY**5KZZ
Ileum **DDY**4KZZ
Jejunum **DDY**3KZZ
Liver **DFY**0KZZ
Lung **DBY**2KZZ
Mediastinum **DBY**6KZZ
Nerve, Peripheral **D0Y**7KZZ
Pancreas **DFY**3KZZ
Parathyroid Gland **DGY**4KZZ
Pineal Body **DGY**1KZZ
Pituitary Gland **DGY**0KZZ
Pleura **DBY**5KZZ
Prostate **DVY**0KZZ
Rectum **DDY**7KZZ
Spinal Cord **D0Y**6KZZ
Stomach **DDY**1KZZ
Thyroid Gland **DGY**5KZZ
Trachea **DBY**0KZZ
Lateral (brachial) lymph node
use Lymphatic, Axillary, Left
use Lymphatic, Axillary, Right
Lateral canthus
use Eyelid, Upper, Left
use Eyelid, Upper, Right
Lateral collateral ligament (LCL)
use Bursa and Ligament, Knee, Left
use Bursa and Ligament, Knee, Right
Lateral condyle of femur
use Femur, Lower, Left
use Femur, Lower, Right
Lateral condyle of tibia
use Tibia, Left
use Tibia, Right
Lateral cuneiform bone
use Tarsal, Left
use Tarsal, Right
Lateral epicondyle of femur
use Femur, Lower, Left
use Femur, Lower, Right
Lateral epicondyle of humerus
use Humeral Shaft, Left
use Humeral Shaft, Right
Lateral femoral cutaneous nerve
use Nerve, Lumbar Plexus
Lateral malleolus
use Fibula, Left
use Fibula, Right
Lateral meniscus
use Joint, Knee, Left
use Joint, Knee, Right
Lateral nasal cartilage
use Nose
Lateral plantar artery
use Artery, Foot, Left
use Artery, Foot, Right
Lateral plantar nerve
use Nerve, Tibial
Lateral rectus muscle
use Muscle, Extraocular, Left
use Muscle, Extraocular, Right
Lateral sacral artery
use Artery, Internal Iliac, Left
use Artery, Internal Iliac, Right

Lateral sacral vein
use Vein, Hypogastric, Left
use Vein, Hypogastric, Right
Lateral sural cutaneous nerve
use Nerve, Peroneal
Lateral tarsal artery
use Artery, Foot, Left
use Artery, Foot, Right
Lateral temporomandibular ligament
use Bursa and Ligament, Head and Neck
Lateral thoracic artery
use Artery, Axillary, Left
use Artery, Axillary, Right
Latissimus dorsi muscle
use Muscle, Trunk, Left
use Muscle, Trunk, Right
Latissimus Dorsi Myocutaneous Flap
Bilateral **0HR**V075
Left **0HR**U075
Right **0HR**T075
Lavage
see Irrigation
Bronchial alveolar, diagnostic *see* Drainage, Respiratory System **0B9**-
Least splanchnic nerve
use Nerve, Thoracic Sympathetic
Left ascending lumbar vein
use Vein, Hemiazygos
Left atrioventricular valve
use Valve, Mitral
Left auricular appendix
use Atrium, Left
Left colic vein
use Vein, Colic
Left coronary sulcus
use Heart, Left
Left gastric artery
use Artery, Gastric
Left gastroepiploic artery
use Artery, Splenic
Left gastroepiploic vein
use Vein, Splenic
Left inferior phrenic vein
use Vein, Renal, Left
Left inferior pulmonary vein
use Vein, Pulmonary, Left
Left jugular trunk
use Lymphatic, Thoracic Duct
Left lateral ventricle
use Cerebral Ventricle
Left ovarian vein
use Vein, Renal, Left
Left second lumbar vein
use Vein, Renal, Left
Left subclavian trunk
use Lymphatic, Thoracic Duct
Left subcostal vein
use Vein, Hemiazygos
Left superior pulmonary vein
use Vein, Pulmonary, Left
Left suprarenal vein
use Vein, Renal, Left
Left testicular vein
use Vein, Renal, Left
Lengthening
Bone, with device *see* Insertion of Limb Lengthening Device
Muscle, by incision *see* Division, Muscles **0K8**-
Tendon, by incision *see* Division, Tendons **0L8**-
Leptomeninges, intracranial
use Cerebral Meninges
Leptomeninges, spinal
use Spinal Meninges

Lesser alar cartilage
use Nose
Lesser occipital nerve
use Nerve, Cervical Plexus
Lesser splanchnic nerve
use Nerve, Thoracic Sympathetic
Lesser trochanter
use Femur, Upper, Left
use Femur, Upper, Right
Lesser tuberosity
use Humeral Head, Left
use Humeral Head, Right
Lesser wing
use Bone, Sphenoid, Left
use Bone, Sphenoid, Right
Leukopheresis, therapeutic *see* Pheresis, Circulatory **6A5**5-
Levator anguli oris muscle
use Muscle, Facial
Levator ani muscle
use Perineum Muscle
Levator labii superioris alaeque nasi muscle
use Muscle, Facial
Levator labii superioris muscle
use Muscle, Facial
Levator palpebrae superioris muscle
use Eyelid, Upper, Left
use Eyelid, Upper, Right
Levator scapulae muscle
use Muscle, Neck, Left
use Muscle, Neck, Right
Levator veli palatini muscle
use Muscle, Tongue, Palate, Pharynx
Levatores costarum muscle
use Muscle, Thorax, Left
use Muscle, Thorax, Right
LifeStent® (Flexstar) (XL) Vascular Stent System
use Intraluminal Device
Ligament of head of fibula
use Bursa and Ligament, Knee, Left
use Bursa and Ligament, Knee, Right
Ligament of the lateral malleolus
use Bursa and Ligament, Ankle, Left
use Bursa and Ligament, Ankle, Right
Ligamentum flavum
use Bursa and Ligament, Trunk, Left
use Bursa and Ligament, Trunk, Right
Ligation *see* Occlusion
Ligation, hemorrhoid *see* Occlusion, Lower Veins, Hemorrhoidal Plexus
Light Therapy GZJZZZZ
Liner
Removal of device from
  Hip
    Left **0SP**B09Z
    Right **0SP**909Z
  Knee
    Left **0SP**D09Z
    Right **0SP**C09Z
Revision of device in
  Hip
    Left **0SW**B09Z
    Right **0SW**909Z
  Knee
    Left **0SW**D09Z
    Right **0SW**C09Z
Supplement
  Hip
    Left **0SU**B09Z
      Acetabular Surface **0SU**E09Z
      Femoral Surface **0SU**S09Z
    Right **0SU**909Z
      Acetabular Surface **0SU**A09Z
      Femoral Surface **0SU**R09Z
  Knee
    Left **0SU**D09-
      Femoral Surface **0SU**U09Z
      Tibial Surface **0SU**W09Z
    Right **0SU**C09-
      Femoral Surface **0SU**T09Z
      Tibial Surface **0SU**V09Z

Lingual artery
use Artery, External Carotid, Left
use Artery, External Carotid, Right
Lingual tonsil
use Tongue
Lingulectomy, lung
see Excision, Lung Lingula **0BB**H-
see Resection, Lung Lingula **0BT**H-
Lithotripsy
see Fragmentation
With removal of fragments *see* Extirpation
LITT (laser interstitial thermal therapy)
see Laser Interstitial Thermal Therapy
LIVIAN™ CRT-D
use Cardiac Resynchronization Defibrillator Pulse Generator in **0JH**-
Lobectomy
see Excision, Central Nervous System **00B**-
see Excision, Endocrine System **0GB**-
see Excision, Hepatobiliary System and Pancreas **0FB**-
see Excision, Respiratory System **0BB**-
see Resection, Endocrine System **0GT**-
see Resection, Hepatobiliary System and Pancreas **0FT**-
see Resection, Respiratory System **0BT**-
Lobotomy *see* Division, Brain **008**0-
Localization
see Imaging
see Map
Locus ceruleus
use Pons
Long thoracic nerve
use Nerve, Brachial Plexus
Loop ileostomy *see* Bypass, Ileum **0D1**B-
Loop recorder, implantable
use Monitoring Device
Lower GI series *see* Fluoroscopy, Colon **BD1**4-
Lumbar artery
use Aorta, Abdominal
Lumbar facet joint
use Joint, Lumbar Vertebral
Lumbar ganglion
use Nerve, Lumbar Sympathetic
Lumbar lymph node
use Lymphatic, Aortic
Lumbar lymphatic trunk
use Cisterna Chyli
Lumbar splanchnic nerve
use Nerve, Lumbar Sympathetic
Lumbosacral facet joint
use Joint, Lumbosacral
Lumbosacral trunk
use Nerve, Lumbar
Lumpectomy *see* Excision
Lunate bone
use Carpal, Left
use Carpal, Right
Lunotriquetral ligament
use Bursa and Ligament, Hand, Left
use Bursa and Ligament, Hand, Right
Lymphadenectomy
see Excision, Lymphatic and Hemic Systems **07B**-
see Resection, Lymphatic and Hemic Systems **07T**-
Lymphadenotomy *see* Drainage, Lymphatic and Hemic Systems **079**-
Lymphangiectomy
see Excision, Lymphatic and Hemic Systems **07B**-
see Resection, Lymphatic and Hemic Systems **07T**-

Lymphangiogram *see* Plain Radiography, Lymphatic System **B70**-
Lymphangioplasty
  see Repair, Lymphatic and Hemic Systems **07Q**-
  see Supplement, Lymphatic and Hemic Systems **07U**-
Lymphangiorrhaphy *see* Repair, Lymphatic and Hemic Systems **07Q**-
Lymphangiotomy *see* Drainage, Lymphatic and Hemic Systems **079**-
Lysis *see* Release

M

Macula
  use Retina, Left
  use Retina, Right
MAGEC® Spinal Bracing and Distraction System
  use Magnetically Controlled Growth Rod(s) in New Technology
Magnet extraction, ocular foreign body *see* Extirpation, Eye **08C**-
Magnetically controlled growth rod(s)
  Cervical **XNS3**-
  Lumbar **XNS0**-
  Thoracic **XNS4**-
Magnetic Resonance Imaging (MRI)
  Abdomen **BW30**-
  Ankle
    Left **BQ3H**-
    Right **BQ3G**-
  Aorta
    Abdominal **B430**-
    Thoracic **B330**-
  Arm
    Left **BP3F**-
    Right **BP3E**-
  Artery
    Celiac **B431**-
    Cervico-Cerebral Arch **B33Q**-
    Common Carotid, Bilateral **B335**-
    Coronary
      Bypass Graft, Multiple **B233**-
      Multiple **B231**-
    Internal Carotid, Bilateral **B338**-
    Intracranial **B33R**-
    Lower Extremity
      Bilateral **B43H**-
      Left **B43G**-
      Right **B43F**-
    Pelvic **B43C**-
    Renal, Bilateral **B438**-
    Spinal **B33M**-
    Superior Mesenteric **B434**-
    Upper Extremity
      Bilateral **B33K**-
      Left **B33J**-
      Right **B33H**-
    Vertebral, Bilateral **B33G**-
  Bladder **BT30**-
  Brachial Plexus **BW3P**-
  Brain **B030**-
  Breast
    Bilateral **BH32**-
    Left **BH31**-
    Right **BH30**-
  Calcaneus
    Left **BQ3K**-
    Right **BQ3J**-
  Chest **BW33Y**-
  Coccyx **BR3F**-
  Connective Tissue
    Lower Extremity **BL31**-
    Upper Extremity **BL30**-
  Corpora Cavernosa **BV30**-
  Disc
    Cervical **BR31**-
    Lumbar **BR33**-
    Thoracic **BR32**-
  Ear **B930**-
  Elbow
    Left **BP3H**-
    Right **BP3G**-
  Eye
    Bilateral **B837**-
    Left **B836**-
    Right **B835**-

Magnetic Resonance Imaging (MRI) — *continued*
  Femur
    Left **BQ34**-
    Right **BQ33**-
  Fetal Abdomen **BY33**-
  Fetal Extremity **BY35**-
  Fetal Head **BY30**-
  Fetal Heart **BY31**-
  Fetal Spine **BY34**-
  Fetal Thorax **BY32**-
  Fetus, Whole **BY36**-
  Foot
    Left **BQ3M**-
    Right **BQ3L**-
  Forearm
    Left **BP3K**-
    Right **BP3J**-
  Gland
    Adrenal, Bilateral **BG32**-
    Parathyroid **BG33**-
    Parotid, Bilateral **B936**-
    Salivary, Bilateral **B93D**-
    Submandibular, Bilateral **B939**-
    Thyroid **BG34**-
  Head **BW38**-
  Heart, Right and Left **B236**-
  Hip
    Left **BQ31**-
    Right **BQ30**-
  Intracranial Sinus **B532**-
  Joint
    Finger
      Left **BP3D**-
      Right **BP3C**-
    Hand
      Left **BP3D**-
      Right **BP3C**-
    Temporomandibular, Bilateral **BN39**-
  Kidney
    Bilateral **BT33**-
    Left **BT32**-
    Right **BT31**-
    Transplant **BT39**-
  Knee
    Left **BQ38**-
    Right **BQ37**-
  Larynx **B93J**-
  Leg
    Left **BQ3F**-
    Right **BQ3D**-
  Liver **BF35**-
  Liver and Spleen **BF36**-
  Lung Apices **BB3G**-
  Nasopharynx **B93F**-
  Neck **BW3F**-
  Nerve
    Acoustic **B03C**-
    Brachial Plexus **BW3P**-
  Oropharynx **B93F**-
  Ovary
    Bilateral **BU35**-
    Left **BU34**-
    Right **BU33**-
  Ovary and Uterus **BU3C**-
  Pancreas **BF37**-
  Patella
    Left **BQ3W**-
    Right **BQ3V**-
  Pelvic Region **BW3G**-
  Pelvis **BR3C**-
  Pituitary Gland **B039**-
  Plexus, Brachial **BW3P**-
  Prostate **BV33**-
  Retroperitoneum **BW3H**-
  Sacrum **BR3F**-
  Scrotum **BV34**-
  Sella Turcica **B039**-

Magnetic Resonance Imaging (MRI) — *continued*
  Shoulder
    Left **BP39**-
    Right **BP38**-
  Sinus
    Intracranial **B532**-
    Paranasal **B932**-
  Spinal Cord **B03B**-
  Spine
    Cervical **BR30**-
    Lumbar **BR39**-
    Thoracic **BR37**-
  Spleen and Liver **BF36**-
  Subcutaneous Tissue
    Abdomen **BH3H**-
    Extremity
      Lower **BH3J**-
      Upper **BH3F**-
    Head **BH3D**-
    Neck **BH3D**-
    Pelvis **BH3H**-
    Thorax **BH3G**-
  Tendon
    Lower Extremity **BL33**-
    Upper Extremity **BL32**-
  Testicle
    Bilateral **BV37**-
    Left **BV36**-
    Right **BV35**-
  Toe
    Left **BQ3Q**-
    Right **BQ3P**-
  Uterus **BU36**-
    Pregnant **BU3B**-
  Uterus and Ovary **BU3C**-
  Vagina **BU39**-
  Vein
    Cerebellar **B531**-
    Cerebral **B531**-
    Jugular, Bilateral **B535**-
    Lower Extremity
      Bilateral **B53D**-
      Left **B53C**-
      Right **B53B**-
    Other **B53V**-
    Pelvic (Iliac) Bilateral **B53H**-
    Portal **B53T**-
    Pulmonary, Bilateral **B53S**-
    Renal, Bilateral **B53L**-
    Spanchnic **B53T**-
    Upper Extremity
      Bilateral **B53P**-
      Left **B53N**-
      Right **B53M**-
  Vena Cava
    Inferior **B539**-
    Superior **B538**-
  Wrist
    Left **BP3M**-
    Right **BP3L**-
Malleotomy *see* Drainage, Ear, Nose, Sinus **099**-
Malleus
  use Auditory Ossicle, Left
  use Auditory Ossicle, Right
Mammaplasty, mammoplasty
  see Alteration, Skin and Breast **0H0**-
  see Repair, Skin and Breast **0HQ**-
  see Replacement, Skin and Breast **0HR**-
  see Supplement, Skin and Breast **0HU**-
Mammary duct
  use Breast, Bilateral
  use Breast, Left
  use Breast, Right
Mammary gland
  use Breast, Bilateral
  use Breast, Left
  use Breast, Right

PROCEDURE INDEX

Mammectomy
see Excision, Skin and Breast **0HB**-
see Resection, Skin and Breast **0HT**-

Mammillary body
use Hypothalamus

Mammography *see* Plain Radiography, Skin, Subcutaneous Tissue and Breast **BH0**-

Mammotomy *see* Drainage, Skin and Breast **0H9**-

Mandibular nerve
use Nerve, Trigeminal

Mandibular notch
use Mandible, Left
use Mandible, Right

Mandibulectomy
see Excision, Head and Facial Bones **0NB**-
see Resection, Head and Facial Bones **0NT**-

Manipulation
Adhesions *see* Release
Chiropractic *see* Chiropractic Manipulation

Manubrium
use Sternum

Map
Basal Ganglia **00K8**-
Brain **00K0**-
Cerebellum **00KC**-
Cerebral Hemisphere **00K7**-
Conduction Mechanism **02K8**-
Hypothalamus **00KA**-
Medulla Oblongata **00KD**-
Pons **00KB**-
Thalamus **00K9**-

Mapping
Doppler ultrasound *see* Ultrasonography
Electrocardiogram only *see* Measurement, Cardiac **4A02**-

Mark IV Breathing Pacemaker System
use Stimulator Generator in Subcutaneous Tissue and Fascia

Marsupialization
see Drainage
see Excision

Massage, cardiac
External **5A12012**
Open **02QA0ZZ**

Masseter muscle
use Muscle, Head

Masseteric fascia
use Subcutaneous Tissue and Fascia, Face

Mastectomy
see Excision, Skin and Breast **0HB**-
see Resection, Skin and Breast **0HT**-

Mastoid (postauricular) lymph node
use Lymphatic, Neck, Left
use Lymphatic, Neck, Right

Mastoid air cells
use Sinus, Mastoid, Left
use Sinus, Mastoid, Right

Mastoid process
use Bone, Temporal, Left
use Bone, Temporal, Right

Mastoidectomy
see Excision, Ear, Nose, Sinus **09B**-
see Resection, Ear, Nose, Sinus **09T**-

Mastoidotomy *see* Drainage, Ear, Nose, Sinus **099**-

Mastopexy
see Reposition, Skin and Breast **0HS**-
see Repair, Skin and Breast **0HQ**-

Mastorrhaphy *see* Repair, Skin and Breast **0HQ**-

Mastotomy *see* Drainage, Skin and Breast **0H9**-

Maxillary artery
use Artery, External Carotid, Left
use Artery, External Carotid, Right

Maxillary nerve
use Nerve, Trigeminal

Maximo II DR (VR)
use Defibrillator, Generator in **0JH**-

Maximo II DR CRT-D
use Cardiac Resynchronization Defibrillator Pulse Generator in **0JH**-

Measurement
Arterial
Flow
Coronary **4A03**-
Peripheral **4A03**-
Pulmonary **4A03**-
Pressure
Coronary **4A03**-
Peripheral **4A03**-
Pulmonary **4A03**-
Thoracic, Other **4A03**-
Pulse
Coronary **4A03**-
Peripheral **4A03**-
Pulmonary **4A03**-
Saturation, Peripheral **4A03**-
Sound, Peripheral **4A03**-
Biliary
Flow **4A0C**-
Pressure **4A0C**-
Cardiac
Action Currents **4A02**-
Defibrillator **4B02XTZ**
Electrical Activity **4A02**-
Guidance **4A02X4A**
No Qualifier **4A02X4Z**
Output **4A02**-
Pacemaker **4B02XSZ**
Rate **4A02**-
Rhythm **4A02**-
Sampling and Pressure
Bilateral **4A02**-
Left Heart **4A02**-
Right Heart **4A02**-
Sound **4A02**-
Total Activity, Stress **4A02XM4**
Central Nervous
Conductivity **4A00**-
Electrical Activity **4A00**-
Pressure **4A000BZ**
Intracranial **4A00**-
Saturation, Intracranial **4A00**-
Stimulator **4B00XVZ**
Temperature, Intracranial **4A00**-
Circulatory, Volume **4A05XLZ**
Gastrointestinal
Motility **4A0B**-
Pressure **4A0B**-
Secretion **4A0B**-
Lymphatic
Flow **4A06**-
Pressure **4A06**-
Metabolism **4A0Z**-
Musculoskeletal
Contractility **4A0F**-
Stimulator **4B0FXVZ**
Olfactory, Acuity **4A08X0Z**
Peripheral Nervous
Conductivity
Motor **4A01**-
Sensory **4A01**-
Electrical Activity **4A01**-
Stimulator **4B01XVZ**

Measurement — *continued*
Products of Conception
Cardiac
Electrical Activity **4A0H**-
Rate **4A0H**-
Rhythm **4A0H**-
Sound **4A0H**-
Nervous
Conductivity **4A0J**-
Electrical Activity **4A0J**-
Pressure **4A0J**-
Respiratory
Capacity **4A09**-
Flow **4A09**-
Pacemaker **4B09XSZ**
Rate **4A09**-
Resistance **4A09**-
Total Activity **4A09**-
Volume **4A09**-
Sleep **4A0ZXQZ**
Temperature **4A0Z**-
Urinary
Contractility **4A0D73Z**
Flow **4A0D75Z**
Pressure **4A0D7BZ**
Resistance **4A0D7DZ**
Volume **4A0D7LZ**
Venous
Flow
Central **4A04**-
Peripheral **4A04**-
Portal **4A04**-
Pulmonary **4A04**-
Pressure
Central **4A04**-
Peripheral **4A04**-
Portal **4A04**-
Pulmonary **4A04**-
Pulse
Central **4A04**-
Peripheral **4A04**-
Portal **4A04**-
Pulmonary **4A04**-
Saturation, Peripheral **4A04**-
Visual
Acuity **4A07X0Z**
Mobility **4A07X7Z**
Pressure **4A07XBZ**

Meatoplasty, urethra *see* Repair, Urethra **0TQD**-

Meatotomy *see* Drainage, Urinary System **0T9**-

Mechanical ventilation *see* Performance, Respiratory **5A19**-

Medial canthus
use Eyelid, Lower, Left
use Eyelid, Lower, Right

Medial collateral ligament (MCL)
use Bursa and Ligament, Knee, Left
use Bursa and Ligament, Knee, Right

Medial condyle of femur
use Femur, Lower, Left
use Femur, Lower, Right

Medial condyle of tibia
use Tibia, Left
use Tibia, Right

Medial cuneiform bone
use Tarsal, Left
use Tarsal, Right

Medial epicondyle of femur
use Femur, Lower, Left
use Femur, Lower, Right

Medial epicondyle of humerus
use Humeral Shaft, Left
use Humeral Shaft, Right

Medial malleolus
use Tibia, Left
use Tibia, Right

Medial meniscus
use Joint, Knee, Left
use Joint, Knee, Right

Medial plantar artery
use Artery, Foot, Left
use Artery, Foot, Right

Medial plantar nerve
use Nerve, Tibial

Medial popliteal nerve
use Nerve, Tibial

Medial rectus muscle
use Muscle, Extraocular, Left
use Muscle, Extraocular, Right

Medial sural cutaneous nerve
use Nerve, Tibial

Median antebrachial vein
use Vein, Basilic, Left
use Vein, Basilic, Right

Median cubital vein
use Vein, Basilic, Left
use Vein, Basilic, Right

Median sacral artery
use Aorta, Abdominal

Mediastinal lymph node
use Lymphatic, Thorax

Mediastinoscopy 0WJC4ZZ

Medication Management GZ3ZZZZ
For substance abuse
Antabuse **HZ83ZZZ**
Bupropion **HZ87ZZZ**
Clonidine **HZ86ZZZ**
Levo-alpha-acetyl-methadol (LAAM) **HZ82ZZZ**
Methadone Maintenance **HZ81ZZZ**
Naloxone **HZ85ZZZ**
Naltrexone **HZ84ZZZ**
Nicotine Replacement **HZ80ZZZ**
Other Replacement Medication **HZ89ZZZ**
Psychiatric Medication **HZ88ZZZ**

Meditation 8E0ZXY5

Medtronic Endurant® II AAA stent graft system
use Intraluminal Device

Meissner's (submucous) plexus
use Nerve, Abdominal Sympathetic

Melody® transcatheter pulmonary valve
use Zooplastic Tissue in Heart and Great Vessels

Membranous urethra
use Urethra

Meningeorrhaphy
see Repair, Cerebral Meninges **00Q1**-
see Repair, Spinal Meninges **00QT**-

Meniscectomy, knee
see Excision, Joint, Knee, Left **0SBD**-
see Excision, Joint, Knee, Right **0SBC**-

Mental foramen
use Mandible, Left
use Mandible, Right

Mentalis muscle
use Muscle, Facial

Mentoplasty *see* Alteration, Jaw, Lower **0W05**-

Mesenterectomy *see* Excision, Mesentery **0DBV**-

Mesenteriorrhaphy, mesenterorrhaphy *see* Repair, Mesentery **0DQV**-

Mesenteriplication *see* Repair, Mesentery **0DQV**-

Mesoappendix
  use Mesentery
Mesocolon
  use Mesentery
Metacarpal ligament
  use Bursa and Ligament, Hand, Left
  use Bursa and Ligament, Hand, Right
Metacarpophalangeal ligament
  use Bursa and Ligament, Hand, Left
  use Bursa and Ligament, Hand, Right
Metal on metal bearing surface
  use Synthetic Substitute, Metal in **OSR-**
Metatarsal ligament
  use Bursa and Ligament, Foot, Left
  use Bursa and Ligament, Foot, Right
Metatarsectomy
  see Excision, Lower Bones **0QB-**
  see Resection, Lower Bones **0QT-**
Metatarsophalangeal (MTP) joint
  use Joint, Metatarsal-Phalangeal, Left
  use Joint, Metatarsal-Phalangeal, Right
Metatarsophalangeal ligament
  use Bursa and Ligament, Foot, Left
  use Bursa and Ligament, Foot, Right
Metathalamus
  use Thalamus
Micro-Driver stent (RX) (OTW)
  use Intraluminal Device
MicroMed HeartAssist
  use Implantable Heart Assist System in Heart and Great Vessels
Micrus CERECYTE microcoil
  use Intraluminal Device, Bioactive in Upper Arteries
Midcarpal joint
  use Joint, Carpal, Left
  use Joint, Carpal, Right
Middle cardiac nerve
  use Nerve, Thoracic Sympathetic
Middle cerebral artery
  use Artery, Intracranial
Middle cerebral vein
  use Vein, Intracranial
Middle colic vein
  use Vein, Colic
Middle genicular artery
  use Artery, Popliteal, Left
  use Artery, Popliteal, Right
Middle hemorrhoidal vein
  use Vein, Hypogastric, Left
  use Vein, Hypogastric, Right
Middle rectal artery
  use Artery, Internal Iliac, Left
  use Artery, Internal Iliac, Right
Middle suprarenal artery
  use Aorta, Abdominal
Middle temporal artery
  use Artery, Temporal, Left
  use Artery, Temporal, Right
Middle turbinate
  use Turbinate, Nasal
MIRODERM™ Biologic Wound Matrix
  use Skin Substitute, Porcine Liver Derived in New Technology
MitraClip valve repair system
  use Synthetic Substitute
Mitral annulus
  use Valve, Mitral
Mitroflow® Aortic Pericardial Heart Valve
  use Zooplastic Tissue in Heart and Great Vessels
Mobilization, adhesions *see* Release
Molar gland
  use Buccal Mucosa

Monitoring
  Arterial
    Flow
      Coronary **4A13-**
      Peripheral **4A13-**
      Pulmonary **4A13-**
    Pressure
      Coronary **4A13-**
      Peripheral **4A13-**
      Pulmonary **4A13-**
    Pulse
      Coronary **4A13-**
      Peripheral **4A13-**
      Pulmonary **4A13-**
    Saturation, Peripheral **4A13-**
    Sound, Peripheral **4A13-**
  Cardiac
    Electrical Activity **4A12-**
      Ambulatory **4A12X45**
      No Qualifier **4A12X4Z**
    Output **4A12-**
    Rate **4A12-**
    Rhythm **4A12-**
    Sound **4A12-**
    Total Activity, Stress **4A12XM4**
    Vascular Perfusion, Indocyanine Green Dye **4A12XSH**
  Central Nervous
    Conductivity **4A10-**
    Electrical Activity
      Intraoperative **4A10-**
      No Qualifier **4A10-**
    Pressure **4A100BZ**
      Intracranial **4A10-**
    Saturation, Intracranial **4A10-**
    Temperature, Intracranial **4A10-**
  Gastrointestinal
    Motility **4A1B-**
    Pressure **4A1B-**
    Secretion **4A1B-**
    Vascular Perfusion, Indocyanine Green Dye **4A1BXSH**
  Intraoperative Knee Replacement Sensor **XR2-**
  Lymphatic
    Flow **4A16-**
    Pressure **4A16-**
  Peripheral Nervous
    Conductivity
      Motor **4A11-**
      Sensory **4A11-**
    Electrical Activity
      Intraoperative **4A11-**
      No Qualifier **4A11-**
  Products of Conception
    Cardiac
      Electrical Activity **4A1H-**
      Rate **4A1H-**
      Rhythm **4A1H-**
      Sound **4A1H-**
    Nervous
      Conductivity **4A1J-**
      Electrical Activity **4A1J-**
      Pressure **4A1J-**
  Respiratory
    Capacity **4A19-**
    Flow **4A19-**
    Rate **4A19-**
    Resistance **4A19-**
    Volume **4A19-**
  Skin and Breast
    Vascular Perfusion, Indocyanine Green Dye **4A1GXSH**
  Sleep **4A1ZXQZ**
  Temperature **4A1Z-**
  Urinary
    Contractility **4A1D73Z**
    Flow **4A1D75Z**
    Pressure **4A1D7BZ**
    Resistance **4A1D7DZ**
    Volume **4A1D7LZ**

Monitoring — *continued*
  Venous
    Flow
      Central **4A14-**
      Peripheral **4A14-**
      Portal **4A14-**
      Pulmonary **4A14-**
    Pressure
      Central **4A14-**
      Peripheral **4A14-**
      Portal **4A14-**
      Pulmonary **4A14-**
    Pulse
      Central **4A14-**
      Peripheral **4A14-**
      Portal **4A14-**
      Pulmonary **4A14-**
    Saturation
      Central **4A14-**
      Portal **4A14-**
      Pulmonary **4A14-**
Monitoring Device, Hemodynamic
  Abdomen **0JH8-**
  Chest **0JH6-**
Mosaic Bioprosthesis (aortic) (mitral) valve
  use Zooplastic Tissue in Heart and Great Vessels
Motor Function Assessment F01-
Motor Treatment F07-
MR Angiography
  see Magnetic Resonance Imaging (MRI), Heart **B23-**
  see Magnetic Resonance Imaging (MRI), Lower Arteries **B43-**
  see Magnetic Resonance Imaging (MRI), Upper Arteries **B33-**
MULTI-LINK (VISION) (MINI-VISION) (ULTRA) Coronary Stent System
  use Intraluminal Device
Multiple sleep latency test 4A0ZXQZ
Musculocutaneous nerve
  use Nerve, Brachial Plexus
Musculopexy
  see Repair, Muscles **0KQ-**
  see Reposition, Muscles **0KS-**
Musculophrenic artery
  use Artery, Internal Mammary, Left
  use Artery, Internal Mammary, Right
Musculoplasty
  see Repair, Muscles **0KQ-**
  see Supplement, Muscles **0KU-**
Musculorrhaphy *see* Repair, Muscles **0KQ-**
Musculospiral nerve
  use Nerve, Radial
Myectomy
  see Excision, Muscles **0KB-**
  see Resection, Muscles **0KT-**
Myelencephalon
  use Medulla Oblongata
Myelogram
  CT *see* Computerized Tomography (CT Scan), Central Nervous System **B02-**
  MRI *see* Magnetic Resonance Imaging (MRI), Central Nervous System **B03-**
Myenteric (Auerbach's) plexus
  use Nerve, Abdominal Sympathetic
Myomectomy *see* Excision, Female Reproductive System **0UB-**
Myometrium
  use Uterus
Myopexy
  see Repair, Muscles **0KQ-**
  see Reposition, Muscles **0KS-**

Myoplasty
  see Repair, Muscles **0KQ-**
  see Supplement, Muscles **0KU-**
Myorrhaphy *see* Repair, Muscles **0KQ-**
Myoscopy *see* Inspection, Muscles **0KJ-**
Myotomy
  see Division, Muscles **0K8-**
  see Drainage, Muscles **0K9-**
Myringectomy
  see Excision, Ear, Nose, Sinus **09B-**
  see Resection, Ear, Nose, Sinus **09T-**
Myringoplasty
  see Repair, Ear, Nose, Sinus **09Q-**
  see Replacement, Ear, Nose, Sinus **09R-**
  see Supplement, Ear, Nose, Sinus **09U-**
Myringostomy *see* Drainage, Ear, Nose, Sinus **099-**
Myringotomy *see* Drainage, Ear, Nose, Sinus **099-**

PROCEDURE INDEX

N

Nail bed
use Finger Nail
use Toe Nail

Nail plate
use Finger Nail
use Toe Nail

nanoLOCK™ interbody fusion device
use Interbody Fusion Device, Nanotextured Surface in New Technology

Narcosynthesis GZGZZZZ

Nasal cavity
use Nose

Nasal concha
use Turbinate, Nasal

Nasalis muscle
use Muscle, Facial

Nasolacrimal duct
use Duct, Lacrimal, Left
use Duct, Lacrimal, Right

Nasopharyngeal airway (NPA)
use Intraluminal Device, Airway in Ear, Nose, Sinus

Navicular bone
use Tarsal, Left
use Tarsal, Right

Near Infrared Spectroscopy, Circulatory System 8E023DZ

Neck of femur
use Femur, Upper, Left
use Femur, Upper, Right

Neck of humerus (anatomical) (surgical)
use Humeral Head, Left
use Humeral Head, Right

Nephrectomy
see Excision, Urinary System 0TB-
see Resection, Urinary System 0TT-

Nephrolithotomy *see* Extirpation, Urinary System 0TC-

Nephrolysis *see* Release, Urinary System 0TN-

Nephropexy
see Repair, Urinary System 0TQ-
see Reposition, Urinary System 0TS-

Nephroplasty
see Repair, Urinary System 0TQ-
see Supplement, Urinary System 0TU-

Nephropyeloureterostomy
see Bypass, Urinary System 0T1-
see Drainage, Urinary System 0T9-

Nephrorrhaphy *see* Repair, Urinary System 0TQ-

Nephroscopy, transurethral 0TJ58ZZ

Nephrostomy
see Bypass, Urinary System 0T1-
see Drainage, Urinary System 0T9-

Nephrotomography
see Fluoroscopy, Urinary System BT1-
see Plain Radiography, Urinary System BT0-

Nephrotomy
see Drainage, Urinary System 0T9-
see Division, Urinary System 0T8-

Nerve conduction study
see Measurement, Central Nervous 4A00-
see Measurement, Peripheral Nervous 4A01-

Nerve Function Assessment F01-

Nerve to the stapedius
use Nerve, Facial

Nesiritide
use Human B-type Natriuretic Peptide

Neurectomy
see Excision, Central Nervous System 00B-
see Excision, Peripheral Nervous System 01B-

Neurexeresis
see Extraction, Central Nervous System 00D-
see Extraction, Peripheral Nervous System 01D-

Neurohypophysis
use Gland, Pituitary

Neurolysis
see Release, Central Nervous System 00N-
see Release, Peripheral Nervous System 01N-

Neuromuscular electrical stimulation (NEMS) lead
use Stimulator Lead in Muscles

Neurophysiologic monitoring *see* Monitoring, Central Nervous 4A10-

Neuroplasty
see Repair, Central Nervous System 00Q-
see Repair, Peripheral Nervous System 01Q-
see Supplement, Central Nervous System 00U-
see Supplement, Peripheral Nervous System 01U-

Neurorrhaphy
see Repair, Central Nervous System 00Q-
see Repair, Peripheral Nervous System 01Q-

Neurostimulator Generator
Insertion of device in, Skull 0NH00NZ
Removal of device from, Skull 0NP00NZ
Revision of device in, Skull 0NW00NZ

Neurostimulator generator, multiple channel
use Stimulator Generator, Multiple Array in 0JH

Neurostimulator generator, multiple channel rechargeable
use Stimulator Generator, Multiple Array Rechargeable in 0JH

Neurostimulator generator, single channel
use Stimulator Generator, Single Array in 0JH

Neurostimulator generator, single channel rechargeable
use Stimulator Generator, Single Array Rechargeable in 0JH

Neurostimulator Lead
Insertion of device in
Brain 00H0-
Cerebral Ventricle 00H6-
Nerve
Cranial 00HE-
Peripheral 01HY-
Spinal Canal 00HU-
Spinal Cord 00HV-
Vein
Azygos 05H0-
Innominate
Left 05H4-
Right 05H3-
Removal of device from
Brain 00P0-
Cerebral Ventricle 00P6-
Nerve
Cranial 00PE-
Peripheral 01PY-
Spinal Canal 00PU-
Spinal Cord 00PV-
Vein
Azygos 05P0-
Innominate
Left 05P4-
Right 05P3-
Revision of device in
Brain 00W0-
Cerebral Ventricle 00W6-
Nerve
Cranial 00WE-
Peripheral 01WY-
Spinal Canal 00WU-
Spinal Cord 00WV-
Vein
Azygos 05W0-
Innominate
Left 05W4-
Right 05W3-

Neurotomy
see Division, Central Nervous System 008-
see Division, Peripheral Nervous System 018-

Neurotripsy
see Destruction, Central Nervous System 005-
see Destruction, Peripheral Nervous System 015-

Neutralization plate
use Internal Fixation Device in Head and Facial Bones
use Internal Fixation Device in Lower Bones
use Internal Fixation Device in Upper Bones

New Technology
Andexanet Alfa, Factor Xa Inhibitor Reversal Agent XW0-
Blinatumomab antineoplastic immunotherapy XW0-
Ceftazidime-avibactam anti-infective XW0-
Cerebral Embolic Filtration, Dual Filter X2A5312
Defibrotide Sodium Anticoagulant XW0-
Fusion
Cervical Vertebral
2 or more, Interbody Fusion Device, Nanotextured Surface XRG2092
Interbody Fusion Device, Nanotextured Surface XRG1092
Cervicothoracic Vertebral, Interbody Fusion Device, Nanotextured Surface XRG4092
Lumbar Vertebral
2 or more, Interbody Fusion Device, Nanotextured Surface XRGC092
Interbody Fusion Device, Nanotextured Surface XRGB092
Lumbosacral, Interbody Fusion Device, Nanotextured Surface XRGD092
Occipital-cervical, Interbody Fusion Device, Nanotextured Surface XRG0092
Thoracic Vertebral
2 to 7, Interbody Fusion Device, Nanotextured Surface XRG7092
8 or more, Interbody Fusion Device, Nanotextured Surface XRG8092
Interbody Fusion Device, Nanotextured Surface XRG6092
Thoracolumbar Vertebral, Interbody Fusion Device, Nanotextured Surface XRGA092
Idarucizumab, Dabigatran reversal agent XW0-
Intraoperative knee replacement sensor XR2-
Isavuconazole anti-infective XW0-
Orbital atherectomy technology X2C-
Replacement
Skin Substitute, Porcine Liver Derived XHRPXL2
Zooplastic Tissue, Rapid Deployment Technique X2RF-
Reposition
Cervical, Magnetically Controlled Growth Rod(s) XNS3-
Lumbar, Magnetically Controlled Growth Rod(s) XNS0-
Thoracic, Magnetically Controlled Growth Rod(s) XNS4-
Uridine Triacetate XW0DX82

Ninth cranial nerve
use Nerve, Glossopharyngeal

Nitinol framed polymer mesh
use Synthetic Substitute

Non-tunneled central venous catheter
use Infusion Device

PROCEDURE INDEX

Nonimaging Nuclear Medicine Assay
Bladder, Kidneys and Ureters **CT63**-
Blood **C763**-
Kidneys, Ureters and Bladder **CT63**-
Lymphatics and Hematologic System **C76YYZZ**
Ureters, Kidneys and Bladder **CT63**-
Urinary System **CT6YYZZ**
Nonimaging Nuclear Medicine Probe
Abdomen **CW50**-
Abdomen and Chest **CW54**-
Abdomen and Pelvis **CW51**-
Brain **C050**-
Central Nervous System **C05YYZZ**
Chest **CW53**-
Chest and Abdomen **CW54**-
Chest and Neck **CW56**-
Extremity
Lower **CP5PZZZ**
Upper **CP5NZZZ**
Head and Neck **CW5B**-
Heart **C25YYZZ**
Right and Left **C256**-
Lymphatics
Head **C75J**-
Head and Neck **C755**-
Lower Extremity **C75P**-
Neck **C75K**-
Pelvic **C75D**-
Trunk **C75M**-
Upper Chest **C75L**-
Upper Extremity **C75N**-
Lymphatics and Hematologic System **C75YYZZ**
Musculoskeletal System, Other **CP5YYZZ**
Neck and Chest **CW56**-
Neck and Head **CW5B**-
Pelvic Region **CW5J**-
Pelvis and Abdomen **CW51**-
Spine **CP55ZZZ**
Nonimaging Nuclear Medicine Uptake
Endocrine System **CG4YYZZ**
Gland, Thyroid **CG42**-
Nostril
use Nose
Novacor Left Ventricular Assist Device
use Implantable Heart Assist System in Heart and Great Vessels
Novation® Ceramic AHS® (Articulation Hip System)
use Synthetic Substitute, Ceramic in **0SR**-
Nuclear medicine
see Nonimaging Nuclear Medicine Assay
see Nonimaging Nuclear Medicine Probe
see Nonimaging Nuclear Medicine Uptake
see Planar Nuclear Medicine Imaging
see Positron Emission Tomographic (PET) Imaging
see Systemic Nuclear Medicine Therapy
see Tomographic (Tomo) Nuclear Medicine Imaging
Nuclear scintigraphy *see* Nuclear Medicine
Nutrition, concentrated substances
Enteral infusion **3E0**G36Z
Parenteral (peripheral) infusion *see* Introduction of Nutritional Substance

O

Obliteration *see* Destruction
Obturator artery
use Artery, Internal Iliac, Left
use Artery, Internal Iliac, Right
Obturator lymph node
use Lymphatic, Pelvis
Obturator muscle
use Muscle, Hip, Left
use Muscle, Hip, Right
Obturator nerve
use Nerve, Lumbar Plexus
Obturator vein
use Vein, Hypogastric, Left
use Vein, Hypogastric, Right
Obtuse margin
use Heart, Left
Occipital artery
use Artery, External Carotid, Left
use Artery, External Carotid, Right
Occipital lobe
use Cerebral Hemisphere
Occipital lymph node
use Lymphatic, Neck, Left
use Lymphatic, Neck, Right
Occipitofrontalis muscle
use Muscle, Facial
Occlusion
Ampulla of Vater **0FLC**-
Anus **0DLQ**-
Aorta, Abdominal **04L0**-
Artery
Anterior Tibial
Left **04LQ**-
Right **04LP**-
Axillary
Left **03L6**-
Right **03L5**-
Brachial
Left **03L8**-
Right **03L7**-
Celiac **04L1**-
Colic
Left **04L7**-
Middle **04L8**-
Right **04L6**-
Common Carotid
Left **03LJ**-
Right **03LH**-
Common Iliac
Left **04LD**-
Right **04LC**-
External Carotid
Left **03LN**-
Right **03LM**-
External Iliac
Left **04LJ**-
Right **04LH**-
Face **03LR**-
Femoral
Left **04LL**-
Right **04LK**-
Foot
Left **04LW**-
Right **04LV**-
Gastric **04L2**-
Hand
Left **03LF**-
Right **03LD**-
Hepatic **04L3**-
Inferior Mesenteric **04LB**-
Innominate **03L2**-
Internal Carotid
Left **03LL**-
Right **03LK**-
Internal Iliac
Left, **04LF**-
Right, **04LE**-

Occlusion — *continued*
Artery — *continued*
Internal Mammary
Left **03L1**-
Right **03L0**-
Intracranial **03LG**-
Lower **04LY**-
Peroneal
Left **04LU**-
Right **04LT**-
Popliteal
Left **04LN**-
Right **04LM**-
Posterior Tibial
Left **04LS**-
Right **04LR**-
Pulmonary, Left **02LR**-
Radial
Left **03LC**-
Right **03LB**-
Renal
Left **04LA**-
Right **04L9**-
Splenic **04L4**-
Subclavian
Left **03L4**-
Right **03L3**-
Superior Mesenteric **04L5**-
Temporal
Left **03LT**-
Right **03LS**-
Thyroid
Left **03LV**-
Right **03LU**-
Ulnar
Left **03LA**-
Right **03L9**-
Upper **03LY**-
Vertebral
Left **03LQ**-
Right **03LP**-
Atrium, Left **02L7**-
Bladder **0TLB**-
Bladder Neck **0TLC**-
Bronchus
Lingula **0BL9**-
Lower Lobe
Left **0BLB**-
Right **0BL6**-
Main
Left **0BL7**-
Right **0BL3**-
Middle Lobe, Right **0BL5**-
Upper Lobe
Left **0BL8**-
Right **0BL4**-
Carina **0BL2**-
Cecum **0DLH**-
Cisterna Chyli **07LL**-
Colon
Ascending **0DLK**-
Descending **0DLM**-
Sigmoid **0DLN**-
Transverse **0DLL**-
Cord
Bilateral **0VLH**-
Left **0VLG**-
Right **0VLF**-
Cul-de-sac **0ULF**-
Duct
Common Bile **0FL9**-
Cystic **0FL8**-
Hepatic
Left **0FL6**-
Right **0FL5**-
Lacrimal
Left **08LY**-
Right **08LX**-
Pancreatic **0FLD**-
Accessory **0FLF**-
Parotid
Left **0CLC**-
Right **0CLB**-

Occlusion — *continued*
Duodenum **0DL9**-
Esophagogastric Junction **0DL4**-
Esophagus **0DL5**-
Lower **0DL3**-
Middle **0DL2**-
Upper **0DL1**-
Fallopian Tube
Left **0UL6**-
Right **0UL5**-
Fallopian Tubes, Bilateral **0UL7**-
Ileocecal Valve **0DLC**-
Ileum **0DLB**-
Intestine
Large **0DLE**-
Left **0DLG**-
Right **0DLF**-
Small **0DL8**-
Jejunum **0DLA**-
Kidney Pelvis
Left **0TL4**-
Right **0TL3**-
Left atrial appendage (LAA) *see* Occlusion, Atrium, Left **02L7**-
Lymphatic
Aortic **07LD**-
Axillary
Left **07L6**-
Right **07L5**-
Head **07L0**-
Inguinal
Left **07LJ**-
Right **07LH**-
Internal Mammary
Left **07L9**-
Right **07L8**-
Lower Extremity
Left **07LG**-
Right **07LF**-
Mesenteric **07LB**-
Neck
Left **07L2**-
Right **07L1**-
Pelvis **07LC**-
Thoracic Duct **07LK**-
Thorax **07L7**-
Upper Extremity
Left **07L4**-
Right **07L3**-
Rectum **0DLP**-
Stomach **0DL6**-
Pylorus **0DL7**-
Trachea **0BL1**-
Ureter
Left **0TL7**-
Right **0TL6**-
Urethra **0TLD**-
Vagina **0ULG**-
Valve, Pulmonary **02LH**-
Vas Deferens
Bilateral **0VLQ**-
Left **0VLP**-
Right **0VLN**-
Vein
Axillary
Left **05L8**-
Right **05L7**-
Azygos **05L0**-
Basilic
Left **05LC**-
Right **05LB**-
Brachial
Left **05LA**-
Right **05L9**-
Cephalic
Left **05LF**-
Right **05LD**-
Colic **06L7**-
Common Iliac
Left **06LD**-
Right **06LC**-

PROCEDURE INDEX

PROCEDURE INDEX

Occlusion — *continued*
  Vein — *continued*
    Esophageal **06L3**-
    External Iliac
      Left **06LG**-
      Right **06LF**-
    External Jugular
      Left **05LQ**-
      Right **05LP**-
    Face
      Left **05LV**-
      Right **05LT**-
    Femoral
      Left **06LN**-
      Right **06LM**-
    Foot
      Left **06LV**-
      Right **06LT**-
    Gastric **06L2**-
    Greater Saphenous
      Left **06LQ**-
      Right **06LP**-
    Hand
      Left **05LH**-
      Right **05LG**-
    Hemiazygos **05L1**-
    Hepatic **06L4**-
    Hypogastric
      Left **06LJ**-
      Right **06LH**-
    Inferior Mesenteric **06L6**-
    Innominate
      Left **05L4**-
      Right **05L3**-
    Internal Jugular
      Left **05LN**-
      Right **05LM**-
    Intracranial **05LL**-
    Lesser Saphenous
      Left **06LS**-
      Right **06LR**-
    Lower **06LY**-
    Portal **06L8**-
    Pulmonary
      Left **02LT**-
      Right **02LS**-
    Renal
      Left **06LB**-
      Right **06L9**-
    Splenic **06L1**-
    Subclavian
      Left **05L6**-
      Right **05L5**-
    Superior Mesenteric **06L5**-
    Upper **05LY**-
    Vertebral
      Left **05LS**-
      Right **05LR**-
  Vena Cava
    Inferior **06L0**-
    Superior **02LV**-
Occupational therapy *see* Activities of Daily Living Treatment, Rehabilitation **F08**-
Odentectomy
  see Excision, Mouth and Throat **0CB**-
  see Resection, Mouth and Throat **0CT**-
Olecranon bursa
  use Bursa and Ligament, Elbow, Left
  use Bursa and Ligament, Elbow, Right
Olecranon process
  use Ulna, Left
  use Ulna, Right
Olfactory bulb
  use Nerve, Olfactory

Omentectomy, omentumectomy
  see Excision, Gastrointestinal System **0DB**-
  see Resection, Gastrointestinal System **0DT**-
Omentofixation *see* Repair, Gastrointestinal System **0DQ**-
Omentoplasty
  see Repair, Gastrointestinal System **0DQ**-
  see Replacement, Gastrointestinal System **0DR**-
  see Supplement, Gastrointestinal System **0DU**-
Omentorrhaphy *see* Repair, Gastrointestinal System **0DQ**-
Omentotomy *see* Drainage, Gastrointestinal System **0D9**-
Omnilink Elite Vascular Balloon Expandable Stent System
  use Intraluminal Device
Onychectomy
  see Excision, Skin and Breast **0HB**-
  see Resection, Skin and Breast **0HT**-
Onychoplasty
  see Repair, Skin and Breast **0HQ**-
  see Replacement, Skin and Breast **0HR**-
Onychotomy *see* Drainage, Skin and Breast **0H9**-
Oophorectomy
  see Excision, Female Reproductive System **0UB**-
  see Resection, Female Reproductive System **0UT**-
Oophoropexy
  see Repair, Female Reproductive System **0UQ**-
  see Reposition, Female Reproductive System **0US**-
Oophoroplasty
  see Repair, Female Reproductive System **0UQ**-
  see Supplement, Female Reproductive System **0UU**-
Oophororrhaphy *see* Repair, Female Reproductive System **0UQ**-
Oophorostomy *see* Drainage, Female Reproductive System **0U9**-
Oophorotomy
  see Drainage, Female Reproductive System **0U9**-
  see Division, Female Reproductive System **0U8**-
Oophorrhaphy *see* Repair, Female Reproductive System **0UQ**-
Open Pivot Aortic Valve Graft (AVG)
  use Synthetic Substitute
Open Pivot (mechanical) valve
  use Synthetic Substitute
Ophthalmic artery
  use Intracranial Artery
Ophthalmic nerve
  use Nerve, Trigeminal
Ophthalmic vein
  use Vein, Intracranial
Opponensplasty
  Tendon replacement *see* Replacement, Tendons **0LR**-
  Tendon transfer *see* Transfer, Tendons **0LX**-
Optic chiasma
  use Nerve, Optic
Optic disc
  use Retina, Left
  use Retina, Right
Optic foramen
  use Bone, Sphenoid, Left
  use Bone, Sphenoid, Right

Optical coherence tomography, intravascular *see* Computerized Tomography (CT Scan)
Optimizer™ III implantable pulse generator
  use Contractility Modulation Device in **0JH**-
Orbicularis oculi muscle
  use Eyelid, Upper, Left
  use Eyelid, Upper, Right
Orbicularis oris muscle
  use Muscle, Facial
Orbital atherectomy technology X2C-
Orbital fascia
  use Subcutaneous Tissue and Fascia, Face
Orbital portion of ethmoid bone
  use Orbit, Left
  use Orbit, Right
Orbital portion of frontal bone
  use Orbit, Left
  use Orbit, Right
Orbital portion of lacrimal bone
  use Orbit, Left
  use Orbit, Right
Orbital portion of maxilla
  use Orbit, Left
  use Orbit, Right
Orbital portion of palatine bone
  use Orbit, Left
  use Orbit, Right
Orbital portion of sphenoid bone
  use Orbit, Left
  use Orbit, Right
Orbital portion of zygomatic bone
  use Orbit, Left
  use Orbit, Right
Orchectomy, orchidectomy, orchiectomy
  see Excision, Male Reproductive System **0VB**-
  see Resection, Male Reproductive System **0VT**-
Orchidoplasty, orchioplasty
  see Repair, Male Reproductive System **0VQ**-
  see Replacement, Male Reproductive System **0VR**-
  see Supplement, Male Reproductive System **0VU**-
Orchidorrhaphy, orchiorrhaphy
  see Repair, Male Reproductive System **0VQ**-
Orchidotomy, orchiotomy, orchotomy *see* Drainage, Male Reproductive System **0V9**-
Orchiopexy
  see Repair, Male Reproductive System **0VQ**-
  see Reposition, Male Reproductive System **0VS**-
Oropharyngeal airway (OPA)
  use Intraluminal Device, Airway in Mouth and Throat
Oropharynx
  use Pharynx
Ossiculectomy
  see Excision, Ear, Nose, Sinus **09B**-
  see Resection, Ear, Nose, Sinus **09T**-
Ossiculotomy *see* Drainage, Ear, Nose, Sinus **099**-

Ostectomy
  see Excision, Head and Facial Bones **0NB**-
  see Excision, Lower Bones **0QB**-
  see Excision, Upper Bones **0PB**-
  see Resection, Head and Facial Bones **0NT**-
  see Resection, Lower Bones **0QT**-
  see Resection, Upper Bones **0PT**-
Osteoclasis
  see Division, Head and Facial Bones **0N8**-
  see Division, Lower Bones **0Q8**-
  see Division, Upper Bones **0P8**-
Osteolysis
  see Release, Head and Facial Bones **0NN**-
  see Release, Lower Bones **0QN**-
  see Release, Upper Bones **0PN**-
Osteopathic Treatment
  Abdomen **7W09X**-
  Cervical **7W01X**-
  Extremity
    Lower **7W06X**-
    Upper **7W07X**-
  Head **7W00X**-
  Lumbar **7W03X**-
  Pelvis **7W05X**-
  Rib Cage **7W08X**-
  Sacrum **7W04X**-
  Thoracic **7W02X**-
Osteopexy
  see Repair, Head and Facial Bones **0NQ**-
  see Repair, Lower Bones **0QQ**-
  see Repair, Upper Bones **0PQ**-
  see Reposition, Head and Facial Bones **0NS**-
  see Reposition, Lower Bones **0QS**-
  see Reposition, Upper Bones **0PS**-
Osteoplasty
  see Repair, Head and Facial Bones **0NQ**-
  see Repair, Lower Bones **0QQ**-
  see Repair, Upper Bones **0PQ**-
  see Replacement, Head and Facial Bones **0NR**-
  see Replacement, Lower Bones **0QR**-
  see Replacement, Upper Bones **0PR**-
  see Supplement, Head and Facial Bones **0NU**-
  see Supplement, Lower Bones **0QU**-
  see Supplement, Upper Bones **0PU**-
Osteorrhaphy
  see Repair, Head and Facial Bones **0NQ**-
  see Repair, Lower Bones **0QQ**-
  see Repair, Upper Bones **0PQ**-
Osteotomy, ostotomy
  see Division, Head and Facial Bones **0N8**-
  see Division, Lower Bones **0Q8**-
  see Division, Upper Bones **0P8**-
  see Drainage, Head and Facial Bones **0N9**-
  see Drainage, Lower Bones **0Q9**-
  see Drainage, Upper Bones **0P9**-
Otic ganglion
  use Nerve, Head and Neck Sympathetic
Otoplasty
  see Repair, Ear, Nose, Sinus **09Q**-
  see Replacement, Ear, Nose, Sinus **09R**-
  see Supplement, Ear, Nose, Sinus **09U**-
Otoscopy *see* Inspection, Ear, Nose, Sinus **09J**-

P

Oval window
 use Ear, Middle, Left
 use Ear, Middle, Right
Ovarian artery
 use Aorta, Abdominal
Ovarian ligament
 use Uterine Supporting Structure
Ovariectomy
 see Excision, Female Reproductive System 0UB-
 see Resection, Female Reproductive System 0UT-
Ovariocentesis see Drainage, Female Reproductive System 0U9-
Ovariopexy
 see Repair, Female Reproductive System 0UQ-
 see Reposition, Female Reproductive System 0US-
Ovariotomy
 see Drainage, Female Reproductive System 0U9-
 see Division, Female Reproductive System 0U8-
Ovatio™ CRT-D
 use Cardiac Resynchronization Defibrillator Pulse Generator in 0JH-
Oversewing
 Gastrointestinal ulcer see Repair, Gastrointestinal System 0DQ-
 Pleural bleb see Repair, Respiratory System 0BQ-
Oviduct
 use Fallopian Tube, Left
 use Fallopian Tube, Right
Oxidized zirconium ceramic hip bearing surface
 use Synthetic Substitute, Ceramic on Polyethylene in 0SR-
Oximetry, Fetal pulse 10H073Z
Oxygenation
 Extracorporeal membrane (ECMO) see Performance, Circulatory 5A15-
 Hyperbaric see Assistance, Circulatory 5A05-
 Supersaturated see Assistance, Circulatory 5A05-

Pacemaker
 Dual Chamber
 Abdomen 0JH8-
 Chest 0JH6-
 Intracardiac
 Insertion of device in
 Atrium
 Left 02H7-
 Right 02H6-
 Vein, Coronary 02H4-
 Ventricle
 Left 02HL-
 Right 02HK-
 Removal of device from, Heart 02PA-
 Revision of device in, Heart 02WA-
 Single Chamber
 Abdomen 0JH8-
 Chest 0JH6-
 Single Chamber Rate Responsive
 Abdomen 0JH8-
 Chest 0JH6-
Packing
 Abdominal Wall 2W43X5Z
 Anorectal 2Y43X5Z
 Arm
 Lower
 Left 2W4DX5Z
 Right 2W4CX5Z
 Upper
 Left 2W4BX5Z
 Right 2W4AX5Z
 Back 2W45X5Z
 Chest Wall 2W44X5Z
 Ear 2Y42X5Z
 Extremity
 Lower
 Left 2W4MX5Z
 Right 2W4LX5Z
 Upper
 Left 2W49X5Z
 Right 2W48X5Z
 Face 2W41X5Z
 Finger
 Left 2W4KX5Z
 Right 2W4JX5Z
 Foot
 Left 2W4TX5Z
 Right 2W4SX5Z
 Genital Tract, Female 2Y44X5Z
 Hand
 Left 2W4FX5Z
 Right 2W4EX5Z
 Head 2W40X5Z
 Inguinal Region
 Left 2W47X5Z
 Right 2W46X5Z
 Leg
 Lower
 Left 2W4RX5Z
 Right 2W4QX5Z
 Upper
 Left 2W4PX5Z
 Right 2W4NX5Z
 Mouth and Pharynx 2Y40X5Z
 Nasal 2Y41X5Z
 Neck 2W42X5Z
 Thumb
 Left 2W4HX5Z
 Right 2W4GX5Z
 Toe
 Left 2W4VX5Z
 Right 2W4UX5Z
 Urethra 2Y45X5Z

Paclitaxel-eluting coronary stent
 use Intraluminal Device, Drug-eluting in Heart and Great Vessels
Paclitaxel-eluting peripheral stent
 use Intraluminal Device, Drug-eluting in Lower Arteries
 use Intraluminal Device, Drug-eluting in Upper Arteries
Palatine gland
 use Buccal Mucosa
Palatine tonsil
 use Tonsils
Palatine uvula
 use Uvula
Palatoglossal muscle
 use Muscle, Tongue, Palate, Pharynx
Palatopharyngeal muscle
 use Muscle, Tongue, Palate, Pharynx
Palatoplasty
 see Repair, Mouth and Throat 0CQ-
 see Replacement, Mouth and Throat 0CR-
 see Supplement, Mouth and Throat 0CU-
Palatorrhaphy see Repair, Mouth and Throat 0CQ-
Palmar (volar) digital vein
 use Vein, Hand, Left
 use Vein, Hand, Right
Palmar (volar) metacarpal vein
 use Vein, Hand, Left
 use Vein, Hand, Right
Palmar cutaneous nerve
 use Nerve, Median
 use Nerve, Radial
Palmar fascia (aponeurosis)
 use Subcutaneous Tissue and Fascia, Hand, Left
 use Subcutaneous Tissue and Fascia, Hand, Right
Palmar interosseous muscle
 use Muscle, Hand, Left
 use Muscle, Hand, Right
Palmar ulnocarpal ligament
 use Bursa and Ligament, Wrist, Left
 use Bursa and Ligament, Wrist, Right
Palmaris longus muscle
 use Muscle, Lower Arm and Wrist, Left
 use Muscle, Lower Arm and Wrist, Right
Pancreatectomy
 see Excision, Pancreas 0FBG-
 see Resection, Pancreas 0FTG-
Pancreatic artery
 use Artery, Splenic
Pancreatic plexus
 use Nerve, Abdominal Sympathetic
Pancreatic vein
 use Vein, Splenic
Pancreaticoduodenostomy see Bypass, Hepatobiliary System and Pancreas 0F1-
Pancreaticosplenic lymph node
 use Lymphatic, Aortic
Pancreatogram, endoscopic retrograde see Fluoroscopy, Pancreatic Duct BF18-
Pancreatolithotomy see Extirpation, Pancreas 0FCG-
Pancreatotomy
 see Drainage, Pancreas 0F9G-
 see Division, Pancreas 0F8G-
Panniculectomy
 see Excision, Abdominal Wall 0WBF-
 see Excision, Skin, Abdomen 0HB7-
Paraaortic lymph node
 use Lymphatic, Aortic

Paracentesis
 Eye see Drainage, Eye 089-
 Peritoneal Cavity see Drainage, Peritoneal Cavity 0W9G-
 Tympanum see Drainage, Ear, Nose, Sinus 099-
Pararectal lymph node
 use Lymphatic, Mesenteric
Parasternal lymph node
 use Lymphatic, Thorax
Parathyroidectomy
 see Excision, Endocrine System 0GB-
 see Resection, Endocrine System 0GT-
Paratracheal lymph node
 use Lymphatic, Thorax
Paraurethral (Skene's) gland
 use Gland, Vestibular
Parenteral nutrition, total see Introduction of Nutritional Substance
Parietal lobe
 use Cerebral Hemisphere
Parotid lymph node
 use Lymphatic, Head
Parotid plexus
 use Nerve, Facial
Parotidectomy
 see Excision, Mouth and Throat 0CB-
 see Resection, Mouth and Throat 0CT-
Pars flaccida
 use Tympanic Membrane, Left
 use Tympanic Membrane, Right
Partial joint replacement
 Hip see Replacement, Lower Joints 0SR-
 Knee see Replacement, Lower Joints 0SR-
 Shoulder see Replacement, Upper Joints 0RR-
Partially absorbable mesh
 use Synthetic Substitute
Patch, blood, spinal 3E0S3GC
Patellapexy
 see Repair, Lower Bones 0QQ-
 see Reposition, Lower Bones 0QS-
Patellaplasty
 see Repair, Lower Bones 0QQ-
 see Replacement, Lower Bones 0QR-
 see Supplement, Lower Bones 0QU-
Patellar ligament
 use Bursa and Ligament, Knee, Left
 use Bursa and Ligament, Knee, Right
Patellar tendon
 use Tendon, Knee, Left
 use Tendon, Knee, Right
Patellectomy
 see Excision, Lower Bones 0QB-
 see Resection, Lower Bones 0QT-
Patellofemoral joint
 use Joint, Knee, Left
 use Joint, Knee, Right
 use Joint, Knee, Left, Femoral Surface
 use Joint, Knee, Right, Femoral Surface
Pectineus muscle
 use Muscle, Upper Leg, Left
 use Muscle, Upper Leg, Right
Pectoral (anterior) lymph node
 use Lymphatic, Axillary, Left
 use Lymphatic, Axillary, Right
Pectoral fascia
 use Subcutaneous Tissue and Fascia, Chest
Pectoralis major muscle
 use Muscle, Thorax, Left
 use Muscle, Thorax, Right
Pectoralis minor muscle
 use Muscle, Thorax, Left
 use Muscle, Thorax, Right

PROCEDURE INDEX

Pedicle-based dynamic stabilization device
use Spinal Stabilization Device, Pedicle-Based in **0RH**-
use Spinal Stabilization Device, Pedicle-Based in **0SH**-

PEEP (positive end expiratory pressure) *see* Assistance, Respiratory **5A09**-

PEG (percutaneous endoscopic gastrostomy) 0DH63UZ

PEJ (percutaneous endoscopic jejunostomy) 0DHA3UZ

Pelvic splanchnic nerve
use Nerve, Abdominal Sympathetic
use Nerve, Sacral Sympathetic

Penectomy
see Excision, Male Reproductive System **0VB**-
see Resection, Male Reproductive System **0VT**-

Penile urethra
use Urethra

Perceval sutureless valve
use Zooplastic Tissue, Rapid Deployment Technique in New Technology

Percutaneous endoscopic gastrojejunostomy (PEG/J) tube
use Feeding Device in Gastrointestinal System

Percutaneous endoscopic gastrostomy (PEG) tube
use Feeding Device in Gastrointestinal System

Percutaneous nephrostomy catheter
use Drainage Device

Percutaneous transluminal coronary angioplasty (PTCA)
see Dilation, Heart and Great Vessels **027**-

Performance
Biliary
Multiple, Filtration **5A1C60Z**
Single, Filtration **5A1C00Z**
Cardiac
Continuous
Output **5A1221Z**
Pacing **5A1223Z**
Intermittent, Pacing **5A1213Z**
Single, Output, Manual **5A12012**
Circulatory, Continuous, Oxygenation, Membrane **5A15223**
Respiratory
24-96 Consecutive Hours, Ventilation **5A1945Z**
Greater than 96 Consecutive Hours, Ventilation **5A1955Z**
Less than 24 Consecutive Hours, Ventilation **5A1935Z**
Single, Ventilation, Nonmechanical **5A19054**
Urinary
Multiple, Filtration **5A1D60Z**
Single, Filtration **5A1D00Z**

Perfusion *see* Introduction of substance in or on

Perfusion, donor organ
Heart **6AB50BZ**
Kidney(s) **6ABT0BZ**
Liver **6ABF0BZ**
Lung(s) **6ABB0BZ**

Pericardiectomy
see Excision, Pericardium **02BN**-
see Resection, Pericardium **02TN**-

Pericardiocentesis *see* Drainage, Pericardial Cavity **0W9D**-

Pericardiolysis *see* Release, Pericardium **02NN**-

Pericardiophrenic artery
use Artery, Internal Mammary, Left
use Artery, Internal Mammary, Right

Pericardioplasty
see Repair, Pericardium **02QN**-
see Replacement, Pericardium **02RN**-
see Supplement, Pericardium **02UN**-

Pericardiorrhaphy *see* Repair, Pericardium **02QN**-

Pericardiostomy *see* Drainage, Pericardial Cavity **0W9D**-

Pericardiotomy *see* Drainage, Pericardial Cavity **0W9D**-

Perimetrium
use Uterus

Peripheral parenteral nutrition
see Introduction of Nutritional Substance

Peripherally inserted central catheter (PICC)
use Infusion Device

Peritoneal dialysis 3E1M39Z

Peritoneocentesis
see Drainage, Peritoneal Cavity **0W9G**-
see Drainage, Peritoneum **0D9W**-

Peritoneoplasty
see Repair, Peritoneum **0DQW**-
see Replacement, Peritoneum **0DRW**-
see Supplement, Peritoneum **0DUW**-

Peritoneoscopy 0DJW4ZZ

Peritoneotomy *see* Drainage, Peritoneum **0D9W**-

Peritoneumectomy *see* Excision, Peritoneum **0DBW**-

Peroneus brevis muscle
use Muscle, Lower Leg, Left
use Muscle, Lower Leg, Right

Peroneus longus muscle
use Muscle, Lower Leg, Left
use Muscle, Lower Leg, Right

Pessary ring
use Intraluminal Device, Pessary in Female Reproductive System

PET scan *see* Positron Emission Tomographic (PET) Imaging

Petrous part of temporal bone
use Bone, Temporal, Left
use Bone, Temporal, Right

Phacoemulsification, lens
With IOL implant *see* Replacement, Eye **08R**-
Without IOL implant *see* Extraction, Eye **08D**-

Phalangectomy
see Excision, Lower Bones **0QB**-
see Excision, Upper Bones **0PB**-
see Resection, Lower Bones **0QT**-
see Resection, Upper Bones **0PT**-

Phallectomy
see Excision, Penis **0VBS**-
see Resection, Penis **0VTS**-

Phalloplasty
see Repair, Penis **0VQS**-
see Supplement, Penis **0VUS**-

Phallotomy *see* Drainage, Penis **0V9S**-

Pharmacotherapy, for substance abuse
Antabuse **HZ93ZZZ**
Bupropion **HZ97ZZZ**
Clonidine **HZ96ZZZ**
Levo-alpha-acetyl-methadol (LAAM) **HZ92ZZZ**
Methadone Maintenance **HZ91ZZZ**
Naloxone **HZ95ZZZ**
Naltrexone **HZ94ZZZ**
Nicotine Replacement **HZ90ZZZ**
Psychiatric Medication **HZ98ZZZ**
Replacement Medication, Other **HZ99ZZZ**

Pharyngeal constrictor muscle
use Muscle, Tongue, Palate, Pharynx

Pharyngeal plexus
use Nerve, Vagus

Pharyngeal recess
use Nasopharynx

Pharyngeal tonsil
use Adenoids

Pharyngogram *see* Fluoroscopy, Pharynix **B91G**-

Pharyngoplasty
see Repair, Mouth and Throat **0CQ**-
see Replacement, Mouth and Throat **0CR**-
see Supplement, Mouth and Throat **0CU**-

Pharyngorrhaphy *see* Repair, Mouth and Throat **0CQ**-

Pharyngotomy *see* Drainage, Mouth and Throat **0C9**-

Pharyngotympanic tube
use Eustachian Tube, Left
use Eustachian Tube, Right

Pheresis
Erythrocytes **6A55**-
Leukocytes **6A55**-
Plasma **6A55**-
Platelets **6A55**-
Stem Cells
Cord Blood **6A55**-
Hematopoietic **6A55**-

Phlebectomy
see Excision, Lower Veins **06B**-
see Excision, Upper Veins **05B**-
see Extraction, Lower Veins **06D**-
see Extraction, Upper Veins **05D**-

Phlebography
see Plain Radiography, Veins **B50**-
Impedance **4A04X51**

Phleborrhaphy
see Repair, Lower Veins **06Q**-
see Repair, Upper Veins **05Q**-

Phlebotomy
see Drainage, Lower Veins **069**-
see Drainage, Upper Veins **059**-

Photocoagulation
for Destruction *see* Destruction
for Repair *see* Repair

Photopheresis, therapeutic *see* Phototherapy, Circulatory **6A65**-

Phototherapy
Circulatory **6A65**-
Skin **6A60**-

Phrenectomy, phrenoneurectomy *see* Excision, Nerve, Phrenic **01B2**-

Phrenemphraxis *see* Destruction, Nerve, Phrenic **0152**-

Phrenic nerve stimulator generator
use Stimulator Generator in Subcutaneous Tissue and Fascia

Phrenic nerve stimulator lead
use Diaphragmatic Pacemaker Lead in Respiratory System

Phreniclasis *see* Destruction, Nerve, Phrenic **0152**-

Phrenicoexeresis *see* Extraction, Nerve, Phrenic **01D2**-

Phrenicotomy *see* Division, Nerve, Phrenic **0182**-

Phrenicotripsy *see* Destruction, Nerve, Phrenic **0152**-

Phrenoplasty
see Repair, Respiratory System **0BQ**-
see Supplement, Respiratory System **0BU**-

Phrenotomy *see* Drainage, Respiratory System **0B9**-

Physiatry *see* Motor Treatment, Rehabilitation **F07**-

Physical medicine *see* Motor Treatment, Rehabilitation **F07**-

Physical therapy *see* Motor Treatment, Rehabilitation **F07**-

PHYSIOMESH™ Flexible Composite Mesh
use Synthetic Substitute

Pia mater, intracranial
use Cerebral Meninges

Pia mater, spinal
use Spinal Meninges

Pinealectomy
see Excision, Pineal Body **0GB1**-
see Resection, Pineal Body **0GT1**-

Pinealoscopy 0GJ14ZZ

Pinealotomy *see* Drainage, Pineal Body **0G91**-

Pinna
use Ear, External, Bilateral
use Ear, External, Left
use Ear, External, Right

Pipeline™ Embolization device (PED)
use Intraluminal Device

Piriform recess (sinus)
use Pharynx

Piriformis muscle
use Muscle, Hip, Left
use Muscle, Hip, Right

Pisiform bone
use Carpal, Left
use Carpal, Right

Pisohamate ligament
use Bursa and Ligament, Hand, Left
use Bursa and Ligament, Hand, Right

Pisometacarpal ligament
use Bursa and Ligament, Hand, Left
use Bursa and Ligament, Hand, Right

Pituitectomy
see Excision, Gland, Pituitary **0GB0**-
see Resection, Gland, Pituitary **0GT0**-

Plain film radiology *see* Plain
      Radiography
Plain Radiography
   Abdomen **BW0**0ZZZ
   Abdomen and Pelvis **BW0**1ZZZ
   Abdominal Lymphatic
      Bilateral **B70**1-
      Unilateral **B70**0-
   Airway, Upper **BB0**DZZZ
   Ankle
      Left **BQ0**H-
      Right **BQ0**G-
   Aorta
      Abdominal **B40**0-
      Thoracic **B30**0-
      Thoraco-Abdominal **B30**P-
   Aorta and Bilateral Lower Extremity
         Arteries **B40**D-
   Arch
      Bilateral **BN0**DZZZ
      Left **BN0**CZZZ
      Right **BN0**BZZZ
   Arm
      Left **BP0**FZZZ
      Right **BP0**EZZZ
   Artery
      Brachiocephalic-Subclavian, Right
         B301-
      Bronchial **B30**L-
      Bypass Graft, Other **B20**F-
      Cervico-Cerebral Arch **B30**Q-
      Common Carotid
         Bilateral **B30**5-
         Left **B30**4-
         Right **B30**3-
      Coronary
         Bypass Graft
            Multiple **B20**3-
            Single **B20**2-
         Multiple **B20**1-
         Single **B20**0-
      External Carotid
         Bilateral **B30**C-
         Left **B30**B-
         Right **B30**9-
      Hepatic **B40**2-
      Inferior Mesenteric **B40**5-
      Intercostal **B30**L-
      Internal Carotid
         Bilateral **B30**8-
         Left **B30**7-
         Right **B30**6-
      Internal Mammary Bypass Graft
         Left **B20**8-
         Right **B20**7-
      Intra-Abdominal, Other **B40**B-
      Intracranial **B30**R-
      Lower, Other **B40**J-
      Lower Extremity
         Bilateral and Aorta **B40**D-
         Left **B40**G-
         Right **B40**F-
      Lumbar **B40**9-
      Pelvic **B40**C-
      Pulmonary
         Left **B30**T-
         Right **B30**S-
      Renal
         Bilateral **B40**8-
         Left **B40**7-
         Right **B40**6-
         Transplant **B40**M-
      Spinal **B30**M-
      Splenic **B40**3-
      Subclavian, Left **B30**2-
      Superior Mesenteric **B40**4-
      Upper, Other **B30**N-
      Upper Extremity
         Bilateral **B30**K-
         Left **B30**J-
         Right **B30**H-

Plain Radiography — *continued*
   Artery — *continued*
      Vertebral
         Bilateral **B30**G-
         Left **B30**F-
         Right **B30**D-
   Bile Duct **BF0**0-
   Bile Duct and Gallbladder **BF0**3-
   Bladder **BT0**0-
      Kidney and Ureter **BT0**4-
   Bladder and Urethra **BT0**B-
   Bone
      Facial **BN0**5ZZZ
      Nasal **BN0**4ZZZ
   Bones, Long, All **BW0**BZZZ
   Breast
      Bilateral **BH0**2ZZZ
      Left **BH0**1ZZZ
      Right **BH0**0ZZZ
   Calcaneus
      Left **BQ0**KZZZ
      Right **BQ0**JZZZ
   Chest **BW0**3ZZZ
   Clavicle
      Left **BP0**5ZZZ
      Right **BP0**4ZZZ
   Coccyx **BR0**FZZZ
   Corpora Cavernosa **BV0**0-
   Dialysis Fistula **B50**W-
   Dialysis Shunt **B50**W-
   Disc
      Cervical **BR0**1-
      Lumbar **BR0**3-
      Thoracic **BR0**2-
   Duct
      Lacrimal
         Bilateral **B80**2-
         Left **B80**1-
         Right **B80**0-
      Mammary
         Multiple
            Left **BH0**6-
            Right **BH0**5-
         Single
            Left **BH0**4-
            Right **BH0**3-
   Elbow
      Left **BP0**H-
      Right **BP0**G-
   Epididymis
      Left **BV0**2-
      Right **BV0**1-
   Extremity
      Lower **BW0**CZZZ
      Upper **BW0**JZZZ
   Eye
      Bilateral **B80**7ZZZ
      Left **B80**6ZZZ
      Right **B80**5ZZZ
   Facet Joint
      Cervical **BR0**4-
      Lumbar **BR0**6-
      Thoracic **BR0**5-
   Fallopian Tube
      Bilateral **BU0**2-
      Left **BU0**1-
      Right **BU0**0-
   Fallopian Tube and Uterus **BU0**8-
   Femur
      Left, Densitometry **BQ0**4ZZ1
      Right, Densitometry **BQ0**3ZZ1
   Finger
      Left **BP0**SZZZ
      Right **BP0**RZZZ
   Foot
      Left **BQ0**MZZZ
      Right **BQ0**LZZZ
   Forearm
      Left **BP0**KZZZ
      Right **BP0**JZZZ

Plain Radiography — *continued*
   Gallbladder and Bile Duct **BF0**3-
   Gland
      Parotid
         Bilateral **B90**6-
         Left **B90**5-
         Right **B90**4-
      Salivary
         Bilateral **B90**D-
         Left **B90**C-
         Right **B90**B-
      Submandibular
         Bilateral **B90**9-
         Left **B90**8-
         Right **B90**7-
   Hand
      Left **BP0**PZZZ
      Right **BP0**NZZZ
   Heart
      Left **B20**5-
      Right **B20**4-
      Right and Left **B20**6-
   Hepatobiliary System, All **BF0**C-
   Hip
      Left **BQ0**1-
         Densitometry **BQ0**1ZZ1
      Right **BQ0**0-
         Densitometry **BQ0**0ZZ1
   Humerus
      Left **BP0**BZZZ
      Right **BP0**AZZZ
   Ileal Diversion Loop **BT0**C-
   Intracranial Sinus **B50**2-
   Joint
      Acromioclavicular, Bilateral
         BP03ZZZ
      Finger
         Left **BP0**D-
         Right **BP0**C-
      Foot
         Left **BQ0**Y-
         Right **BQ0**X-
      Hand
         Left **BP0**D-
         Right **BP0**C-
      Lumbosacral **BR0**BZZZ
      Sacroiliac **BR0**D-
      Sternoclavicular
         Bilateral **BP0**2ZZZ
         Left **BP0**1ZZZ
         Right **BP0**0ZZZ
      Temporomandibular
         Bilateral **BN0**9-
         Left **BN0**8-
         Right **BN0**7-
      Thoracolumbar **BR0**8ZZZ
      Toe
         Left **BQ0**Y-
         Right **BQ0**X-
   Kidney
      Bilateral **BT0**3-
      Left **BT0**2-
      Right **BT0**1-
      Ureter and Bladder **BT0**4-
   Knee
      Left **BQ0**8-
      Right **BQ0**7-
   Leg
      Left **BQ0**FZZZ
      Right **BQ0**DZZZ
   Lymphatic
      Head **B70**4-
      Lower Extremity
         Bilateral **B70**B-
         Left **B70**9-
         Right **B70**8-
      Neck **B70**4-
      Pelvic **B70**C-
      Upper Extremity
         Bilateral **B70**7-
         Left **B70**6-
         Right **B70**5-

Plain Radiography — *continued*
   Mandible **BN0**6ZZZ
   Mastoid **B90**HZZZ
   Nasopharynx **B90**FZZZ
   Optic Foramina
      Left **B80**4ZZZ
      Right **B80**3ZZZ
   Orbit
      Bilateral **BN0**3ZZZ
      Left **BN0**2ZZZ
      Right **BN0**1ZZZ
   Oropharynx **B90**FZZZ
   Patella
      Left **BQ0**WZZZ
      Right **BQ0**VZZZ
   Pelvis **BR0**CZZZ
   Pelvis and Abdomen **BW0**1ZZZ
   Prostate **BV0**3-
   Retroperitoneal Lymphatic
      Bilateral **B70**1-
      Unilateral **B70**0-
   Ribs
      Left **BP0**YZZZ
      Right **BP0**XZZZ
   Sacrum **BR0**FZZZ
   Scapula
      Left **BP0**7ZZZ
      Right **BP0**6ZZZ
   Shoulder
      Left **BP0**9-
      Right **BP0**8-
   Sinus
      Intracranial **B50**2-
      Paranasal **B90**2ZZZ
   Skull **BN0**0ZZZ
   Spinal Cord **B00**B-
   Spine
      Cervical, Densitometry **BR0**0ZZ1
      Lumbar, Densitometry **BR0**9ZZ1
      Thoracic, Densitometry **BR0**7ZZ1
      Whole, Densitometry **BR0**GZZ1
   Sternum **BR0**HZZZ
   Teeth
      All **BN0**JZZZ
      Multiple **BN0**HZZZ
   Testicle
      Left **BV0**6-
      Right **BV0**5-
   Toe
      Left **BQ0**QZZZ
      Right **BQ0**PZZZ
   Tooth, Single **BN0**GZZZ
   Tracheobronchial Tree
      Bilateral **BB0**9YZZ
      Left **BB0**8YZZ
      Right **BB0**7YZZ
   Ureter
      Bilateral **BT0**8-
      Kidney and Bladder **BT0**4-
      Left **BT0**7-
      Right **BT0**6-
   Urethra **BT0**5-
   Urethra and Bladder **BT0**B-
   Uterus **BU0**6-
   Uterus and Fallopian Tube **BU0**8-
   Vagina **BU0**9-
   Vasa Vasorum **BV0**8-
   Vein
      Cerebellar **B50**1-
      Cerebral **B50**1-
      Epidural **B50**0-
      Jugular
         Bilateral **B50**5-
         Left **B50**4-
         Right **B50**3-
      Lower Extremity
         Bilateral **B50**D-
         Left **B50**C-
         Right **B50**B-
         Other **B50**V-

© 2016 Channel Publishing, Ltd.

Plain Radiography — *continued*
Vein — *continued*
Pelvic (Iliac)
Bilateral **B50H**-
Left **B50G**-
Right **B50F**-
Portal **B50T**-
Pulmonary
Bilateral **B50S**-
Left **B50R**-
Right **B50Q**-
Renal
Bilateral **B50L**-
Left **B50K**-
Right **B50J**-
Spanchnic **B50T**-
Subclavian
Left **B507**-
Right **B506**-
Upper Extremity
Bilateral **B50P**-
Left **B50N**-
Right **B50M**-
Vena Cava
Inferior **B509**-
Superior **B508**-
Whole Body **BW0KZZZ**
Infant **BW0MZZZ**
Whole Skeleton **BW0LZZZ**
Wrist
Left **BP0M**-
Right **BP0L**-
Planar Nuclear Medicine Imaging
Abdomen **CW10**-
Abdomen and Chest **CW14**-
Abdomen and Pelvis **CW11**-
Anatomical Region, Other **CW1ZZZZ**
Anatomical Regions, Multiple **CW1YYZZ**
Bladder and Ureters **CT1H**-
Bladder, Kidneys and Ureters **CT13**-
Blood **C713**-
Bone Marrow **C710**-
Brain **C010**-
Breast **CH1YYZZ**
Bilateral **CH12**-
Left **CH11**-
Right **CH10**-
Bronchi and Lungs **CB12**-
Central Nervous System **C01YYZZ**
Cerebrospinal Fluid **C015**-
Chest **CW13**-
Chest and Abdomen **CW14**-
Chest and Neck **CW16**-
Digestive System **CD1YYZZ**
Ducts, Lacrimal, Bilateral **C819**-
Ear, Nose, Mouth and Throat **C91YYZZ**
Endocrine System **CG1YYZZ**
Extremity
Lower **CW1D**-
Bilateral **CP1F**-
Left **CP1D**-
Right **CP1C**-
Upper **CW1M**-
Bilateral **CP1B**-
Left **CP19**-
Right **CP18**-
Eye **C81YYZZ**
Gallbladder **CF14**-
Gastrointestinal Tract **CD17**-
Upper **CD15**-

Planar Nuclear Medicine Imaging — *continued*
Gland
Adrenal, Bilateral **CG14**-
Parathyroid **CG11**-
Thyroid **CG12**-
Glands, Salivary, Bilateral **C91B**-
Head and Neck **CW1B**-
Heart **C21YYZZ**
Right and Left **C216**-
Hepatobiliary System, All **CF1C**-
Hepatobiliary System and Pancreas **CF1YYZZ**
Kidneys, Ureters and Bladder **CT13**-
Liver **CF15**-
Liver and Spleen **CF16**-
Lungs and Bronchi **CB12**-
Lymphatics
Head **C71J**-
Head and Neck **C715**-
Lower Extremity **C71P**-
Neck **C71K**-
Pelvic **C71D**-
Trunk **C71M**-
Upper Chest **C71L**-
Upper Extremity **C71N**-
Lymphatics and Hematologic System **C71YYZZ**
Musculoskeletal System
All **CP1Z**-
Other **CP1YYZZ**-
Myocardium **C21G**-
Neck and Chest **CW16**-
Neck and Head **CW1B**-
Pancreas and Hepatobiliary System **CF1YYZZ**
Pelvic Region **CW1J**-
Pelvis **CP16**-
Pelvis and Abdomen **CW11**-
Pelvis and Spine **CP17**-
Reproductive System, Male **CV1YYZZ**
Respiratory System **CB1YYZZ**
Skin **CH1YYZZ**
Skull **CP11**-
Spine **CP15**-
Spine and Pelvis **CP17**-
Spleen **C712**-
Spleen and Liver **CF16**-
Subcutaneous Tissue **CH1YYZZ**
Testicles, Bilateral **CV19**-
Thorax **CP14**-
Ureters, Kidneys and Bladder **CT13**-
Ureters and Bladder **CT1H**-
Urinary System **CT1YYZZ**
Veins **C51YYZZ**
Central **C51R**-
Lower Extremity
Bilateral **C51D**-
Left **C51C**-
Right **C51B**-
Upper Extremity
Bilateral **C51Q**-
Left **C51P**-
Right **C51N**-
Whole Body **CW1N**-

Plantar digital vein
use Vein, Foot, Left
use Vein, Foot, Right
Plantar fascia (aponeurosis)
use Subcutaneous Tissue and Fascia, Foot, Left
use Subcutaneous Tissue and Fascia, Foot, Right

Plantar metatarsal vein
use Vein, Foot, Left
use Vein, Foot, Right
Plantar venous arch
use Vein, Foot, Left
use Vein, Foot, Right
Plaque Radiation
Abdomen **DWY3FZZ**
Adrenal Gland **DGY2FZZ**
Anus **DDY8FZZ**
Bile Ducts **DFY2FZZ**
Bladder **DTY2FZZ**
Bone, Other **DPYCFZZ**
Bone Marrow **D7Y0FZZ**
Brain **D0Y0FZZ**
Brain Stem **D0Y1FZZ**
Breast
Left **DMY0FZZ**
Right **DMY1FZZ**
Bronchus **DBY1FZZ**
Cervix **DUY1FZZ**
Chest **DWY2FZZ**
Chest Wall **DBY7FZZ**
Colon **DDY5FZZ**
Diaphragm **DBY8FZZ**
Duodenum **DDY2FZZ**
Ear **D9Y0FZZ**
Esophagus **DDY0FZZ**
Eye **D8Y0FZZ**
Femur **DPY9FZZ**
Fibula **DPYBFZZ**
Gallbladder **DFY1FZZ**
Gland
Adrenal **DGY2FZZ**
Parathyroid **DGY4FZZ**
Pituitary **DGY0FZZ**
Thyroid **DGY5FZZ**
Glands, Salivary **D9Y6FZZ**
Head and Neck **DWY1FZZ**
Hemibody **DWY4FZZ**
Humerus **DPY6FZZ**
Ileum **DDY4FZZ**
Jejunum **DDY3FZZ**
Kidney **DTY0FZZ**
Larynx **D9YBFZZ**
Liver **DFY0FZZ**
Lung **DBY2FZZ**
Lymphatics
Abdomen **D7Y6FZZ**
Axillary **D7Y4FZZ**
Inguinal **D7Y8FZZ**
Neck **D7Y3FZZ**
Pelvis **D7Y7FZZ**
Thorax **D7Y5FZZ**
Mandible **DPY3FZZ**
Maxilla **DPY2FZZ**
Mediastinum **DBY6FZZ**
Mouth **D9Y4FZZ**
Nasopharynx **D9YDFZZ**
Neck and Head **DWY1FZZ**
Nerve, Peripheral **D0Y7FZZ**
Nose **D9Y1FZZ**
Ovary **DUY0FZZ**
Palate
Hard **D9Y8FZZ**
Soft **D9Y9FZZ**
Pancreas **DFY3FZZ**
Parathyroid Gland **DGY4FZZ**
Pelvic Bones **DPY8FZZ**
Pelvic Region **DWY6FZZ**
Pharynx **D9YCFZZ**
Pineal Body **DGY1FZZ**
Pituitary Gland **DGY0FZZ**
Pleura **DBY5FZZ**
Prostate **DVY0FZZ**

Plaque Radiation — *continued*
Radius **DPY7FZZ**
Rectum **DDY7FZZ**
Rib **DPY5FZZ**
Sinuses **D9Y7FZZ**
Skin
Abdomen **DHY8FZZ**
Arm **DHY4FZZ**
Back **DHY7FZZ**
Buttock **DHY9FZZ**
Chest **DHY6FZZ**
Face **DHY2FZZ**
Foot **DHYCFZZ**
Hand **DHY5FZZ**
Leg **DHYBFZZ**
Neck **DHY3FZZ**
Skull **DPY0FZZ**
Spinal Cord **D0Y6FZZ**
Spleen **D7Y2FZZ**
Sternum **DPY4FZZ**
Stomach **DDY1FZZ**
Testis **DVY1FZZ**
Thymus **D7Y1FZZ**
Thyroid Gland **DGY5FZZ**
Tibia **DPYBFZZ**
Tongue **D9Y5FZZ**
Trachea **DBY0FZZ**
Ulna **DPY7FZZ**
Ureter **DTY1FZZ**
Urethra **DTY3FZZ**
Uterus **DUY2FZZ**
Whole Body **DWY5FZZ**
Plasmapheresis, therapeutic 6A550Z3
Plateletpheresis, therapeutic 6A550Z2
Platysma muscle
use Muscle, Neck, Left
use Muscle, Neck, Right
Pleurectomy
see Excision, Respiratory System **0BB**-
see Resection, Respiratory System **0BT**-
Pleurocentesis *see* Drainage, Anatomical Regions, General **0W9**-
Pleurodesis, pleurosclerosis
Chemical injection *see* Introduction of substance in or on, Pleural Cavity **3E0L**-
Surgical *see* Destruction, Respiratory System **0B5**-
Pleurolysis *see* Release, Respiratory System **0BN**-
Pleuroscopy 0BJQ4ZZ
Pleurotomy *see* Drainage, Respiratory System **0B9**-
Plica semilunaris
use Conjunctiva, Left
use Conjunctiva, Right
Plication *see* Restriction
Pneumectomy
see Excision, Respiratory System **0BB**-
see Resection, Respiratory System **0BT**-
Pneumocentesis *see* Drainage, Respiratory System **0B9**-
Pneumogastric nerve
use Nerve, Vagus
Pneumolysis *see* Release, Respiratory System **0BN**-
Pneumonectomy
see Resection, Respiratory System **0BT**-
Pneumonolysis *see* Release, Respiratory System **0BN**-

Pneumonopexy
  see Repair, Respiratory System **0BQ**-
  see Reposition, Respiratory System **0BS**-
Pneumonorrhaphy *see* Repair, Respiratory System **0BQ**-
Pneumonotomy *see* Drainage, Respiratory System **0B9**-
Pneumotaxic center
  use Pons
Pneumotomy *see* Drainage, Respiratory System **0B9**-
Pollicization *see* Transfer, Anatomical Regions, Upper Extremities **0XX**-
Polyethylene socket
  use Synthetic Substitute, Polyethylene in **0SR**-
Polymethylmethacrylate (PMMA)
  use Synthetic Substitute
Polypectomy, gastrointestinal *see* Excision, Gastrointestinal System **0DB**-
Polypropylene mesh
  use Synthetic Substitute
Polysomnogram 4A1ZXQZ
Pontine tegmentum
  use Pons
Popliteal ligament
  use Bursa and Ligament, Knee, Left
  use Bursa and Ligament, Knee, Right
Popliteal lymph node
  use Lymphatic, Lower Extremity, Left
  use Lymphatic, Lower Extremity, Right
Popliteal vein
  use Vein, Femoral, Left
  use Vein, Femoral, Right
Popliteus muscle
  use Muscle, Lower Leg, Left
  use Muscle, Lower Leg, Right
Porcine (bioprosthetic) valve
  use Zooplastic Tissue in Heart and Great Vessels
Positive end expiratory pressure
  see Performance, Respiratory **5A19**-
Positron Emission Tomographic (PET) Imaging
  Brain **C030**-
  Bronchi and Lungs **CB32**-
  Central Nervous System **C03YYZZ**
  Heart **C23YYZZ**
  Lungs and Bronchi **CB32**-
  Myocardium **C23G**-
  Respiratory System **CB3YYZZ**
  Whole Body **CW3NYZZ**
Positron emission tomography *see* Positron Emission Tomographic (PET) Imaging
Postauricular (mastoid) lymph node
  use Lymphatic, Neck, Left
  use Lymphatic, Neck, Right
Postcava
  use Vena Cava, Inferior
Posterior (subscapular) lymph node
  use Lymphatic, Axillary, Left
  use Lymphatic, Axillary, Right
Posterior auricular artery
  use Artery, External Carotid, Left
  use Artery, External Carotid, Right
Posterior auricular nerve
  use Nerve, Facial
Posterior auricular vein
  use Vein, External Jugular, Left
  use Vein, External Jugular, Right

Posterior cerebral artery
  use Artery, Intracranial
Posterior chamber
  use Eye, Left
  use Eye, Right
Posterior circumflex humeral artery
  use Artery, Axillary, Left
  use Artery, Axillary, Right
Posterior communicating artery
  use Artery, Intracranial
Posterior cruciate ligament (PCL)
  use Bursa and Ligament, Knee, Left
  use Bursa and Ligament, Knee, Right
Posterior facial (retromandibular) vein
  use Vein, Face, Left
  use Vein, Face, Right
Posterior femoral cutaneous nerve
  use Nerve, Sacral Plexus
Posterior inferior cerebellar artery (PICA)
  use Artery, Intracranial
Posterior interosseous nerve
  use Nerve, Radial
Posterior labial nerve
  use Nerve, Pudendal
Posterior scrotal nerve
  use Nerve, Pudendal
Posterior spinal artery
  use Artery, Vertebral, Left
  use Artery, Vertebral, Right
Posterior tibial recurrent artery
  use Artery, Anterior Tibial, Left
  use Artery, Anterior Tibial, Right
Posterior ulnar recurrent artery
  use Artery, Ulnar, Left
  use Artery, Ulnar, Right
Posterior vagal trunk
  use Nerve, Vagus
PPN (peripheral parenteral nutrition) *see* Introduction of Nutritional Substance
Preauricular lymph node
  use Lymphatic, Head
Precava
  use Vena Cava, Superior
Prepatellar bursa
  use Bursa and Ligament, Knee, Left
  use Bursa and Ligament, Knee, Right
Preputiotomy *see* Drainage, Male Reproductive System **0V9**-
Pressure support ventilation *see* Performance, Respiratory **5A19**-
PRESTIGE® Cervical Disc
  use Synthetic Substitute
Pretracheal fascia
  use Subcutaneous Tissue and Fascia, Neck, Anterior
Prevertebral fascia
  use Subcutaneous Tissue and Fascia, Neck, Posterior
PrimeAdvanced neurostimulator (SureScan) (MRI Safe)
  use Stimulator Generator, Multiple Array in **0JH**-
Princeps pollicis artery
  use Artery, Hand, Left
  use Artery, Hand, Right
Probing, duct
  Diagnostic *see* Inspection
  Dilation *see* Dilation
PROCEED™ Ventral Patch
  use Synthetic Substitute

Procerus muscle
  use Muscle, Facial
Proctectomy
  see Excision, Rectum **0DBP**-
  see Resection, Rectum **0DTP**-
Proctoclysis *see* Introduction of substance in or on, Gastrointestinal Tract, Lower **3E0H**-
Proctocolectomy
  see Excision, Gastrointestinal System **0DB**-
  see Resection, Gastrointestinal System **0DT**-
Proctocolpoplasty
  see Repair, Gastrointestinal System **0DQ**-
  see Supplement, Gastrointestinal System **0DU**-
Proctoperineoplasty
  see Repair, Gastrointestinal System **0DQ**-
  see Supplement, Gastrointestinal System **0DU**-
Proctoperineorrhaphy *see* Repair, Gastrointestinal System **0DQ**-
Proctopexy
  see Repair, Rectum **0DQP**-
  see Reposition, Rectum **0DSP**-
Proctoplasty
  see Repair, Rectum **0DQP**-
  see Supplement, Rectum **0DUP**-
Proctorrhaphy *see* Repair, Rectum **0DQP**-
Proctoscopy 0DJD8ZZ
Proctosigmoidectomy
  see Excision, Gastrointestinal System **0DB**-
  see Resection, Gastrointestinal System **0DT**-
Proctosigmoidoscopy 0DJD8ZZ
Proctostomy *see* Drainage, Rectum **0D9P**-
Proctotomy *see* Drainage, Rectum **0D9P**-
Prodisc-C
  use Synthetic Substitute
Prodisc-L
  use Synthetic Substitute
Production, atrial septal defect *see* Excision, Septum, Atrial **02B5**-
Profunda brachii
  use Artery, Brachial, Left
  use Artery, Brachial, Right
Profunda femoris (deep femoral) vein
  use Vein, Femoral, Left
  use Vein, Femoral, Right
PROLENE Polypropylene Hernia System (PHS)
  use Synthetic Substitute
Pronator quadratus muscle
  use Muscle, Lower Arm and Wrist, Left
  use Muscle, Lower Arm and Wrist, Right
Pronator teres muscle
  use Muscle, Lower Arm and Wrist, Left
  use Muscle, Lower Arm and Wrist, Right
Prostatectomy
  see Excision, Prostate **0VB0**-
  see Resection, Prostate **0VT0**-
Prostatic urethra
  use Urethra
Prostatomy, prostatotomy *see* Drainage, Prostate **0V90**-

Protecta XT CRT-D
  use Cardiac Resynchronization Defibrillator Pulse Generator in **0JH**-
Protecta XT DR (XT VR)
  use Defibrillator Generator in **0JH**-
Protégé® RX Carotid Stent System
  use Intraluminal Device
Proximal radioulnar joint
  use Joint, Elbow, Left
  use Joint, Elbow, Right
Psoas muscle
  use Muscle, Hip, Left
  use Muscle, Hip, Right
PSV (pressure support ventilation) *see* Performance, Respiratory **5A19**-
Psychoanalysis GZ54ZZZ
Psychological Tests
  Cognitive Status **GZ14ZZZ**
  Developmental **GZ10ZZZ**
  Intellectual and Psychoeducational **GZ12ZZZ**
  Neurobehavioral Status **GZ14ZZZ**
  Neuropsychological **GZ13ZZZ**
  Personality and Behavioral **GZ11ZZZ**
Psychotherapy
  Family, Mental Health Services **GZ72ZZZ**
  Group **GZHZZZZ**
    Mental Health Services **GZHZZZZ**
  Individual
    see Psychotherapy, Individual, Mental Health Services
  For substance abuse
    12-Step **HZ53ZZZ**
    Behavioral **HZ51ZZZ**
    Cognitive **HZ50ZZZ**
    Cognitive-Behavioral **HZ52ZZZ**
    Confrontational **HZ58ZZZ**
    Interactive **HZ55ZZZ**
    Interpersonal **HZ54ZZZ**
    Motivational Enhancement **HZ57ZZZ**
    Psychoanalysis **HZ5BZZZ**
    Psychodynamic **HZ5CZZZ**
    Psychoeducation **HZ56ZZZ**
    Psychophysiological **HZ5DZZZ**
    Supportive **HZ59ZZZ**
  Mental Health Services
    Behavioral **GZ51ZZZ**
    Cognitive **GZ52ZZZ**
    Cognitive-Behavioral **GZ58ZZZ**
    Interactive **GZ50ZZZ**
    Interpersonal **GZ53ZZZ**
    Psychoanalysis **GZ54ZZZ**
    Psychodynamic **GZ55ZZZ**
    Psychophysiological **GZ59ZZZ**
    Supportive **GZ56ZZZ**
PTCA (percutaneous transluminal coronary angioplasty) *see* Dilation, Heart and Great Vessels **027**-
Pterygoid muscle
  use Muscle, Head
Pterygoid process
  use Bone, Sphenoid, Left
  use Bone, Sphenoid, Right
Pterygopalatine (sphenopalatine) ganglion
  use Nerve, Head and Neck Sympathetic
Pubic ligament
  use Bursa and Ligament, Trunk, Left
  use Bursa and Ligament, Trunk, Right
Pubis
  use Bone, Pelvic, Left
  use Bone, Pelvic, Right

P
R
O
C
E
D
U
R
E

I
N
D
E
X

Pubofemoral ligament
   use Bursa and Ligament, Hip, Left
   use Bursa and Ligament, Hip, Right
Pudendal nerve
   use Nerve, Sacral Plexus
Pull-through, rectal *see* Resection,
   Rectum 0DTP-
Pulmoaortic canal
   use Artery, Pulmonary, Left
Pulmonary annulus
   use Valve, Pulmonary
Pulmonary artery wedge
   monitoring *see* Monitoring,
   Arterial 4A13-
Pulmonary plexus
   use Nerve, Thoracic Sympathetic
   use Nerve, Vagus
Pulmonic valve
   use Valve, Pulmonary
Pulpectomy *see* Excision, Mouth and
   Throat 0CB-
Pulverization *see* Fragmentation
Pulvinar
   use Thalamus
Pump reservoir
   use Infusion Device, Pump in
   Subcutaneous Tissue and Fascia
Punch biopsy *see* Excision with
   qualifier Diagnostic
Puncture *see* Drainage
Puncture, lumbar *see* Drainage,
   Spinal Canal 009U-
Pyelography
   see Fluoroscopy, Urinary System BT1-
   see Plain Radiography, Urinary
   System BT0-
Pyeloileostomy, urinary diversion
   see Bypass, Urinary System 0T1-
Pyeloplasty
   see Repair, Urinary System 0TQ-
   see Replacement, Urinary System
   0TR-
   see Supplement, Urinary System 0TU-
Pyelorrhaphy *see* Repair, Urinary
   System 0TQ-
Pyeloscopy 0TJ58ZZ
Pyelostomy
   see Drainage, Urinary System 0T9-
   see Bypass, Urinary System 0T1-
Pyelotomy *see* Drainage, Urinary
   System 0T9-
Pylorectomy
   see Excision, Stomach, Pylorus 0DB7-
   see Resection, Stomach, Pylorus
   0DT7-
Pyloric antrum
   use Stomach, Pylorus
Pyloric canal
   use Stomach, Pylorus
Pyloric sphincter
   use Stomach, Pylorus
Pylorodiosis *see* Dilation, Stomach,
   Pylorus 0D77-
Pylorogastrectomy
   see Excision, Gastrointestinal System
   0DB-
   see Resection, Gastrointestinal System
   0DT-
Pyloroplasty
   see Repair, Stomach, Pylorus 0DQ7-
   see Supplement, Stomach, Pylorus
   0DU7-
Pyloroscopy 0DJ68ZZ
Pylorotomy *see* Drainage, Stomach,
   Pylorus 0D97-
Pyramidalis muscle
   use Muscle, Abdomen, Left
   use Muscle, Abdomen, Right

Q

Quadrangular cartilage
   use Septum, Nasal
Quadrant resection of breast *see*
   Excision, Skin and Breast 0HB-
Quadrate lobe
   use Liver
Quadratus femoris muscle
   use Muscle, Hip, Left
   use Muscle, Hip, Right
Quadratus lumborum muscle
   use Muscle, Trunk, Left
   use Muscle, Trunk, Right
Quadratus plantae muscle
   use Muscle, Foot, Left
   use Muscle, Foot, Right
Quadriceps (femoris)
   use Muscle, Upper Leg, Left
   use Muscle, Upper Leg, Right
Quarantine 8E0ZXY6

R

Radial collateral carpal ligament
use Bursa and Ligament, Wrist, Left
use Bursa and Ligament, Wrist, Right
Radial collateral ligament
use Bursa and Ligament, Elbow, Left
use Bursa and Ligament, Elbow, Right
Radial notch
use Ulna, Left
use Ulna, Right
Radial recurrent artery
use Artery, Radial, Left
use Artery, Radial, Right
Radial vein
use Vein, Brachial, Left
use Vein, Brachial, Right
Radialis indicis
use Artery, Hand, Left
use Artery, Hand, Right
Radiation Therapy
see Beam Radiation
see Brachytherapy
see Stereotactic Radiosurgery
Radiation treatment see Radiation Therapy
Radiocarpal joint
use Joint, Wrist, Left
use Joint, Wrist, Right
Radiocarpal ligament
use Bursa and Ligament, Wrist, Left
use Bursa and Ligament, Wrist, Right
Radiography see Plain Radiography
Radiology, analog see Plain Radiography
Radiology, diagnostic see Imaging, Diagnostic
Radioulnar ligament
use Bursa and Ligament, Wrist, Left
use Bursa and Ligament, Wrist, Right
Range of motion testing see Motor Function Assessment, Rehabilitation F01-
REALIZE® Adjustable Gastric Band
use Extraluminal Device

Reattachment
Abdominal Wall 0WMF0ZZ
Ampulla of Vater 0FMC-
Ankle Region
  Left 0YML0ZZ
  Right 0YMK0ZZ
Arm
  Lower
    Left 0XMF0ZZ
    Right 0XMD0ZZ
  Upper
    Left 0XM90ZZ
    Right 0XM80ZZ
Axilla
  Left 0XM50ZZ
  Right 0XM40ZZ
Back
  Lower 0WML0ZZ
  Upper 0WMK0ZZ
Bladder 0TMB-
Bladder Neck 0TMC-
Breast
  Bilateral 0HMVXZZ
  Left 0HMUXZZ
  Right 0HMTXZZ
Bronchus
  Lingula 0BM90ZZ
  Lower Lobe
    Left 0BMB0ZZ
    Right 0BM60ZZ
  Main
    Left 0BM70ZZ
    Right 0BM30ZZ
  Middle Lobe, Right 0BM50ZZ
  Upper Lobe
    Left 0BM80ZZ
    Right 0BM40ZZ

Reattachment — continued
Bursa and Ligament
  Abdomen
    Left 0MMJ-
    Right 0MMH-
  Ankle
    Left 0MMR-
    Right 0MMQ-
  Elbow
    Left 0MM4-
    Right 0MM3-
  Foot
    Left 0MMT-
    Right 0MMS-
  Hand
    Left 0MM8-
    Right 0MM7-
  Head and Neck 0MM0-
  Hip
    Left 0MMM-
    Right 0MML-
  Knee
    Left 0MMP-
    Right 0MMN-
  Lower Extremity
    Left 0MMW-
    Right 0MMV-
  Perineum 0MMK-
  Shoulder
    Left 0MM2-
    Right 0MM1-
  Thorax
    Left 0MMG-
    Right 0MMF-
  Trunk
    Left 0MMD-
    Right 0MMC-
  Upper Extremity
    Left 0MMB-
    Right 0MM9-
  Wrist
    Left 0MM6-
    Right 0MM5-
Buttock
  Left 0YM10ZZ
  Right 0YM00ZZ
Carina 0BM20ZZ
Cecum 0DMH-
Cervix 0UMC-
Chest Wall 0WM80ZZ
Clitoris 0UMJXZZ
Colon
  Ascending 0DMK-
  Descending 0DMM-
  Sigmoid 0DMN-
  Transverse 0DML-
Cord
  Bilateral 0VMH-
  Left 0VMG-
  Right 0VMF-
Cul-de-sac 0UMF-
Diaphragm
  Left 0BMS0ZZ
  Right 0BMR0ZZ
Duct
  Common Bile 0FM9-
  Cystic 0FM8-
  Hepatic
    Left 0FM6-
    Right 0FM5-
  Pancreatic 0FMD-
    Accessory 0FMF-
Duodenum 0DM9-
Ear
  Left 09M1XZZ
  Right 09M0XZZ
Elbow Region
  Left 0XMC0ZZ
  Right 0XMB0ZZ
Esophagus 0DM5-

Reattachment — continued
Extremity
  Lower
    Left 0YMB0ZZ
    Right 0YM90ZZ
  Upper
    Left 0XM70ZZ
    Right 0XM60ZZ
Eyelid
  Lower
    Left 08MRXZZ
    Right 08MQXZZ
  Upper
    Left 08MPXZZ
    Right 08MNXZZ
Face 0WM20ZZ
Fallopian Tube
  Left 0UM6-
  Right 0UM5-
Fallopian Tubes, Bilateral 0UM7-
Femoral Region
  Left 0YM80ZZ
  Right 0YM70ZZ
Finger
  Index
    Left 0XMP0ZZ
    Right 0XMN0ZZ
  Little
    Left 0XMW0ZZ
    Right 0XMV0ZZ
  Middle
    Left 0XMR0ZZ
    Right 0XMQ0ZZ
  Ring
    Left 0XMT0ZZ
    Right 0XMS0ZZ
Foot
  Left 0YMN0ZZ
  Right 0YMM0ZZ
Forequarter
  Left 0XM10ZZ
  Right 0XM00ZZ
Gallbladder 0FM4
Gland
  Left 0GM2-
  Right 0GM3-
Hand
  Left 0XMK0ZZ
  Right 0XMJ0ZZ
Hindquarter
  Bilateral 0YM40ZZ
  Left 0YM30ZZ
  Right 0YM20ZZ
Hymen 0UMK-
Ileum 0DMB-
Inguinal Region
  Left 0YM60ZZ
  Right 0YM50ZZ
Intestine
  Large 0DME-
    Left 0DMG-
    Right 0DMF-
  Small 0DM8-
Jaw
  Lower 0WM50ZZ
  Upper 0WM40ZZ
Jejunum 0DMA-
Kidney
  Left 0TM1-
  Right 0TM0-
Kidney Pelvis
  Left 0TM4-
  Right 0TM3-
Kidneys, Bilateral 0TM2-
Knee Region
  Left 0YMG0ZZ
  Right 0YMF0ZZ
Leg
  Lower
    Left 0YMJ0ZZ
    Right 0YMH0ZZ

Reattachment — continued
Leg — continued
  Upper
    Left 0YMD0ZZ
    Right 0YMC0ZZ
Lip
  Lower 0CM10ZZ
  Upper 0CM00ZZ
Liver 0FM0-
  Left Lobe 0FM2-
  Right Lobe 0FM1-
Lung
  Left 0BML0ZZ
  Lower Lobe
    Left 0BMJ0ZZ
    Right 0BMF0ZZ
  Middle Lobe, Right 0BMD0ZZ
  Right 0BMK0ZZ
  Upper Lobe
    Left 0BMG0ZZ
    Right 0BMC0ZZ
Lung Lingula 0BMH0ZZ
Muscle
  Abdomen
    Left 0KML-
    Right 0KMK-
  Facial 0KM1-
  Foot
    Left 0KMW-
    Right 0KMV-
  Hand
    Left 0KMD-
    Right 0KMC-
  Head 0KM0-
  Hip
    Left 0KMP-
    Right 0KMN-
  Lower Arm and Wrist
    Left 0KMB-
    Right 0KM9-
  Lower Leg
    Left 0KMT-
    Right 0KMS-
  Neck
    Left 0KM3-
    Right 0KM2-
  Perineum 0KMM-
  Shoulder
    Left 0KM6-
    Right 0KM5-
  Thorax
    Left 0KMJ-
    Right 0KMH-
  Tongue, Palate, Pharynx 0KM4-
  Trunk
    Left 0KMG-
    Right 0KMF-
  Upper Arm
    Left 0KM8-
    Right 0KM7-
  Upper Leg
    Left 0KMR-
    Right 0KMQ-
Neck 0WM60ZZ
Nipple
  Left 0HMXXZZ
  Right 0HMWXZZ
Nose 09MKXZZ
Ovary
  Bilateral 0UM2-
  Left 0UM1-
  Right 0UM0-
Palate, Soft 0CM30ZZ
Pancreas 0FMG-
Parathyroid Gland 0GMR-
  Inferior
    Left 0GMP-
    Right 0GMN-
  Multiple 0GMQ-
  Superior
    Left 0GMM-
    Right 0GML-

PROCEDURE INDEX

PROCEDURE INDEX

Reattachment — *continued*
Penis **0VMSXZZ**
Perineum
  Female **0WMN0ZZ**
  Male **0WMM0ZZ**
Rectum **0DMP-**
Scrotum **0VM5XZZ**
Shoulder Region
  Left **0XM30ZZ**
  Right **0XM20ZZ**
Skin
  Abdomen **0HM7XZZ**
  Back **0HM6XZZ**
  Buttock **0HM8XZZ**
  Chest **0HM5XZZ**
  Ear
    Left **0HM3XZZ**
    Right **0HM2XZZ**
  Face **0HM1XZZ**
  Foot
    Left **0HMNXZZ**
    Right **0HMMXZZ**
  Genitalia **0HMAXZZ**
  Hand
    Left **0HMGXZZ**
    Right **0HMFXZZ**
  Lower Arm
    Left **0HMEXZZ**
    Right **0HMDXZZ**
  Lower Leg
    Left **0HMLXZZ**
    Right **0HMKXZZ**
  Neck **0HM4XZZ**
  Perineum **0HM9XZZ**
  Scalp **0HM0XZZ**
  Upper Arm
    Left **0HMCXZZ**
    Right **0HMBXZZ**
  Upper Leg
    Left **0HMJXZZ**
    Right **0HMHXZZ**
Stomach **0DM6-**
Tendon
  Abdomen
    Left **0LMG-**
    Right **0LMF-**
  Ankle
    Left **0LMT-**
    Right **0LMS-**
  Foot
    Left **0LMW-**
    Right **0LMV-**
  Hand
    Left **0LM8-**
    Right **0LM7-**
  Head and Neck **0LM0-**
  Hip
    Left **0LMK-**
    Right **0LMJ-**
  Knee
    Left **0LMR-**
    Right **0LMQ-**
  Lower Arm and Wrist
    Left **0LM6-**
    Right **0LM5-**
  Lower Leg
    Left **0LMP-**
    Right **0LMN-**
  Perineum **0LMH-**
  Shoulder
    Left **0LM2-**
    Right **0LM1-**
  Thorax
    Left **0LMD-**
    Right **0LMC-**
  Trunk
    Left **0LMB-**
    Right **0LM9-**
  Upper Arm
    Left **0LM4-**
    Right **0LM3-**
  Upper Leg
    Left **0LMM-**
    Right **0LML-**

Reattachment — *continued*
Testis
  Bilateral **0VMC-**
  Left **0VMB-**
  Right **0VM9-**
Thumb
  Left **0XMM0ZZ**
  Right **0XML0ZZ**
Thyroid Gland
  Left Lobe **0GMG-**
  Right Lobe **0GMH-**
Toe
  1st
    Left **0YMQ0ZZ**
    Right **0YMP0ZZ**
  2nd
    Left **0YMS0ZZ**
    Right **0YMR0ZZ**
  3rd
    Left **0YMU0ZZ**
    Right **0YMT0ZZ**
  4th
    Left **0YMW0ZZ**
    Right **0YMV0ZZ**
  5th
    Left **0YMY0ZZ**
    Right **0YMX0ZZ**
Tongue **0CM70ZZ**
Tooth
  Lower **0CMX-**
  Upper **0CMW-**
Trachea **0BM10ZZ**
Tunica Vaginalis
  Left **0VM7-**
  Right **0VM6-**
Ureter
  Left **0TM7-**
  Right **0TM6-**
Ureters, Bilateral **0TM8-**
Urethra **0TMD-**
Uterine Supporting Structure **0UM4-**
Uterus **0UM9-**
Uvula **0CMN0ZZ**
Vagina **0UMG-**
Vulva **0UMMXZZ**
Wrist Region
  Left **0XMH0ZZ**
  Right **0XMG0ZZ**
Rebound HRD® (Hernia Repair Device)
  use Synthetic Substitute
Recession
  see Repair
  see Reposition
Reclosure, disrupted abdominal wall 0WQFXZZ
Reconstruction
  see Repair
  see Replacement
  see Supplement
Rectectomy
  see Excision, Rectum **0DBP-**
  see Resection, Rectum **0DTP-**
Rectocele repair
  see Repair, Subcutaneous Tissue and Fascia, Pelvic Region **0JQC-**
Rectopexy
  see Repair, Gastrointestinal System **0DQ-**
  see Reposition, Gastrointestinal System **0DS-**
Rectoplasty
  see Repair, Gastrointestinal System **0DQ-**
  see Supplement, Gastrointestinal System **0DU-**

Rectorrhaphy *see* Repair, Gastrointestinal System **0DQ-**
Rectoscopy 0DJD8ZZ
Rectosigmoid junction
  use Colon, Sigmoid
Rectosigmoidectomy
  see Excision, Gastrointestinal System **0DB-**
  see Resection, Gastrointestinal System **0DT-**
Rectostomy *see* Drainage, Rectum **0D9P-**
Rectotomy *see* Drainage, Rectum **0D9P-**
Rectus abdominis muscle
  use Muscle, Abdomen, Left
  use Muscle, Abdomen, Right
Rectus femoris muscle
  use Muscle, Upper Leg, Left
  use Muscle, Upper Leg, Right
Recurrent laryngeal nerve
  use Nerve, Vagus
Reduction
  Dislocation *see* Reposition
  Fracture *see* Reposition
  Intussusception, intestinal *see* Reposition, Gastrointestinal System **0DS-**
  Mammoplasty *see* Excision, Skin and Breast **0HB-**
  Prolapse *see* Reposition
  Torsion *see* Reposition
  Volvulus, gastrointestinal *see* Reposition, Gastrointestinal System **0DS-**
Refusion *see* Fusion
Rehabilitation
  see Activities of Daily Living Assessment, Rehabilitation **F02-**
  see Activities of Daily Living Treatment, Rehabilitation **F08-**
  see Caregiver Training, Rehabilitation **F0F-**
  see Cochlear Implant Treatment, Rehabilitation **F0B-**
  see Device Fitting, Rehabilitation **F0D-**
  see Hearing Treatment, Rehabilitation **F09-**
  see Motor Function Assessment, Rehabilitation **F01-**
  see Motor Treatment, Rehabilitation **F07-**
  see Speech Assessment, Rehabilitation **F00-**
  see Speech Treatment, Rehabilitation **F06-**
  see Vestibular Treatment, Rehabilitation **F0C-**
Reimplantation
  see Reattachment
  see Reposition
  see Transfer
Reinforcement
  see Repair
  see Supplement
Relaxation, scar tissue *see* Release
Release
Acetabulum
  Left **0QN5-**
  Right **0QN4-**
Adenoids **0CNQ-**
Ampulla of Vater **0FNC-**
Anal Sphincter **0DNR-**
Anterior Chamber
  Left **08N33ZZ**
  Right **08N23ZZ**

Release — *continued*
Anus **0DNQ-**
Aorta
  Abdominal **04N0-**
  Thoracic
    Ascending/Arch **02NX-**
    Descending **02NW-**
Aortic Body **0GND-**
Appendix **0DNJ-**
Artery
  Anterior Tibial
    Left **04NQ-**
    Right **04NP-**
  Axillary
    Left **03N6-**
    Right **03N5-**
  Brachial
    Left **03N8-**
    Right **03N7-**
  Celiac **04N1-**
  Colic
    Left **04N7-**
    Middle **04N8-**
    Right **04N6-**
  Common Carotid
    Left **03NJ-**
    Right **03NH-**
  Common Iliac
    Left **04ND-**
    Right **04NC-**
  External Carotid
    Left **03NN-**
    Right **03NM-**
  External Iliac
    Left **04NJ-**
    Right **04NH-**
  Face **03NR-**
  Femoral
    Left **04NL-**
    Right **04NK-**
  Foot
    Left **04NW-**
    Right **04NV-**
  Gastric **04N2-**
  Hand
    Left **03NF-**
    Right **03ND-**
  Hepatic **04N3-**
  Inferior Mesenteric **04NB-**
  Innominate **03N2-**
  Internal Carotid
    Left **03NL-**
    Right **03NK-**
  Internal Iliac
    Left **04NF-**
    Right **04NE-**
  Internal Mammary
    Left **03N1-**
    Right **03N0-**
  Intracranial **03NG-**
  Lower **04NY-**
  Peroneal
    Left **04NU-**
    Right **04NT-**
  Popliteal
    Left **04NN-**
    Right **04NM-**
  Posterior Tibial
    Left **04NS-**
    Right **04NR-**
  Pulmonary
    Left **02NR-**
    Right **02NQ-**
  Pulmonary Trunk **02NP-**
  Radial
    Left **03NC-**
    Right **03NB-**
  Renal
    Left **04NA-**
    Right **04N9-**

Release — *continued*
  Artery — *continued*
    Splenic **04N**4-
    Subclavian
      Left **03N**4-
      Right **03N**3-
    Superior Mesenteric **04N**5-
    Temporal
      Left **03N**T-
      Right **03N**S-
    Thyroid
      Left **03N**V-
      Right **03N**U-
    Ulnar
      Left **03N**A-
      Right **03N**9-
    Upper **03N**Y-
    Vertebral
      Left **03N**Q-
      Right **03N**P-
  Atrium
    Left **02N**7-
    Right **02N**6-
  Auditory Ossicle
    Left **09N**A0ZZ
    Right **09N**90ZZ
  Basal Ganglia **00N**8-
  Bladder **0TN**B-
  Bladder Neck **0TN**C-
  Bone
    Ethmoid
      Left **0NN**G-
      Right **0NN**F-
    Frontal
      Left **0NN**2-
      Right **0NN**1-
    Hyoid **0NN**X-
    Lacrimal
      Left **0NN**J-
      Right **0NN**H-
    Nasal **0NN**B-
    Occipital
      Left **0NN**8-
      Right **0NN**7-
    Palatine
      Left **0NN**L-
      Right **0NN**K-
    Parietal
      Left **0NN**4-
      Right **0NN**3-
    Pelvic
      Left **0QN**3-
      Right **0QN**2-
    Sphenoid
      Left **0NN**D-
      Right **0NN**C-
    Temporal
      Left **0NN**6-
      Right **0NN**5-
    Zygomatic
      Left **0NN**N-
      Right **0NN**M-
  Brain **00N**0-
  Breast
    Bilateral **0HN**V-
    Left **0HN**U-
    Right **0HN**T-
  Bronchus
    Lingula **0BN**9-
    Lower Lobe
      Left **0BN**B-
      Right **0BN**6-
    Main
      Left **0BN**7-
      Right **0BN**3-
    Middle Lobe, Right **0BN**5-
    Upper Lobe
      Left **0BN**8-
      Right **0BN**4-
  Buccal Mucosa **0CN**4-

Release — *continued*
  Bursa and Ligament
    Abdomen
      Left **0MN**J-
      Right **0MN**H-
    Ankle
      Left **0MN**R-
      Right **0MN**Q-
    Elbow
      Left **0MN**4-
      Right **0MN**3-
    Foot
      Left **0MN**T-
      Right **0MN**S-
    Hand
      Left **0MN**8-
      Right **0MN**7-
    Head and Neck **0MN**0-
    Hip
      Left **0MN**M-
      Right **0MN**L-
    Knee
      Left **0MN**P-
      Right **0MN**N-
    Lower Extremity
      Left **0MN**W-
      Right **0MN**V-
    Perineum **0MN**K-
    Shoulder
      Left **0MN**2-
      Right **0MN**1-
    Thorax
      Left **0MN**G-
      Right **0MN**F-
    Trunk
      Left **0MN**D-
      Right **0MN**C-
    Upper Extremity
      Left **0MN**B-
      Right **0MN**9-
    Wrist
      Left **0MN**6-
      Right **0MN**5-
  Carina **0BN**2-
  Carotid Bodies, Bilateral **0GN**8-
  Carotid Body
    Left **0GN**6-
    Right **0GN**7-
  Carpal
    Left **0PN**N-
    Right **0PN**M-
  Cecum **0DN**H-
  Cerebellum **00N**C-
  Cerebral Hemisphere **00N**7-
  Cerebral Meninges **00N**1-
  Cerebral Ventricle **00N**6-
  Cervix **0UN**C-
  Chordae Tendineae **02N**9-
  Choroid
    Left **08N**B-
    Right **08N**A-
  Cisterna Chyli **07N**L-
  Clavicle
    Left **0PN**B-
    Right **0PN**9-
  Clitoris **0UN**J-
  Coccygeal Glomus **0GN**B-
  Coccyx **0QN**S-
  Colon
    Ascending **0DN**K-
    Descending **0DN**M-
    Sigmoid **0DN**N-
    Transverse **0DN**L-
  Conduction Mechanism **02N**8-
  Conjunctiva
    Left **08N**TXZZ
    Right **08N**SXZZ
  Cord
    Bilateral **0VN**H-
    Left **0VN**G-
    Right **0VN**F-

Release — *continued*
  Cornea
    Left **08N**9XZZ
    Right **08N**8XZZ
  Cul-de-sac **0UN**F-
  Diaphragm
    Left **0BN**S-
    Right **0BN**R-
  Disc
    Cervical Vertebral **0RN**3-
    Cervicothoracic Vertebral **0RN**5-
    Lumbar Vertebral **0SN**2-
    Lumbosacral **0SN**4-
    Thoracic Vertebral **0RN**9-
    Thoracolumbar Vertebral **0RN**B-
  Duct
    Common Bile **0FN**9-
    Cystic **0FN**8-
    Hepatic
      Left **0FN**6-
      Right **0FN**5-
    Lacrimal
      Left **08N**Y-
      Right **08N**X-
    Pancreatic **0FN**D-
      Accessory **0FN**F-
    Parotid
      Left **0CN**C-
      Right **0CN**B-
  Duodenum **0DN**9-
  Dura Mater **00N**2-
  Ear
    External
      Left **09N**1-
      Right **09N**0-
    External Auditory Canal
      Left **09N**4-
      Right **09N**3-
    Inner
      Left **09N**E0ZZ
      Right **09N**D0ZZ
    Middle
      Left **09N**60ZZ
      Right **09N**50ZZ
  Epididymis
    Bilateral **0VN**L-
    Left **0VN**K-
    Right **0VN**J-
  Epiglottis **0CN**R-
  Esophagogastric Junction **0DN**4-
  Esophagus **0DN**5-
    Lower **0DN**3-
    Middle **0DN**2-
    Upper **0DN**1-
  Eustachian Tube
    Left **09N**G-
    Right **09N**F-
  Eye
    Left **08N**1XZZ
    Right **08N**0XZZ
  Eyelid
    Lower
      Left **08N**R-
      Right **08N**Q-
    Upper
      Left **08N**P-
      Right **08N**N-
  Fallopian Tube
    Left **0UN**6-
    Right **0UN**5-
  Fallopian Tubes, Bilateral **0UN**7-
  Femoral Shaft
    Left **0QN**9-
    Right **0QN**8-
  Femur
    Lower
      Left **0QN**C-
      Right **0QN**B-
    Upper
      Left **0QN**7-
      Right **0QN**6-

Release — *continued*
  Fibula
    Left **0QN**K-
    Right **0QN**J-
  Finger Nail **0HN**QXZZ
  Gallbladder **0FN**4-
  Gingiva
    Lower **0CN**6-
    Upper **0CN**5-
  Gland
    Adrenal
      Bilateral **0GN**4-
      Left **0GN**2-
      Right **0GN**3-
    Lacrimal
      Left **08N**W-
      Right **08N**V-
    Minor Salivary **0CN**J-
    Parotid
      Left **0CN**9-
      Right **0CN**8-
    Pituitary **0GN**0-
    Sublingual
      Left **0CN**F-
      Right **0CN**D-
    Submaxillary
      Left **0CN**H-
      Right **0CN**G-
    Vestibular **0UN**L-
  Glenoid Cavity
    Left **0PN**8-
    Right **0PN**7-
  Glomus Jugulare **0GN**C-
  Humeral Head
    Left **0PN**D-
    Right **0PN**C-
  Humeral Shaft
    Left **0PN**G-
    Right **0PN**F-
  Hymen **0UN**K-
  Hypothalamus **00N**A-
  Ileocecal Valve **0DN**C-
  Ileum **0DN**B-
  Intestine
    Large **0DN**E-
      Left **0DN**G-
      Right **0DN**F-
    Small **0DN**8-
  Iris
    Left **08N**D3ZZ
    Right **08N**C3ZZ
  Jejunum **0DN**A-
  Joint
    Acromioclavicular
      Left **0RN**H-
      Right **0RN**G-
    Ankle
      Left **0SN**G-
      Right **0SN**F-
    Carpal
      Left **0RN**R-
      Right **0RN**Q-
    Cervical Vertebral **0RN**1-
    Cervicothoracic Vertebral **0RN**4-
    Coccygeal **0SN**6-
    Elbow
      Left **0RN**M-
      Right **0RN**L-
    Finger Phalangeal
      Left **0RN**X-
      Right **0RN**W-
    Hip
      Left **0SN**B-
      Right **0SN**9-
    Knee
      Left **0SN**D-
      Right **0SN**C-
    Lumbar Vertebral **0SN**0-
    Lumbosacral **0SN**3-

Release — continued
Joint — continued
Metacarpocarpal
Left 0RNT-
Right 0RNS-
Metacarpophalangeal
Left 0RNV-
Right 0RNU-
Metatarsal-Phalangeal
Left 0SNN-
Right 0SNM-
Metatarsal-Tarsal
Left 0SNL-
Right 0SNK-
Occipital-cervical 0RN0-
Sacrococcygeal 0SN5-
Sacroiliac
Left 0SN8-
Right 0SN7-
Shoulder
Left 0RNK-
Right 0RNJ-
Sternoclavicular
Left 0RNF-
Right 0RNE-
Tarsal
Left 0SNJ-
Right 0SNH-
Temporomandibular
Left 0RND-
Right 0RNC-
Thoracic Vertebral 0RN6-
Thoracolumbar Vertebral 0RNA-
Toe Phalangeal
Left 0SNQ-
Right 0SNP-
Wrist
Left 0RNP-
Right 0RNN-
Kidney
Left 0TN1-
Right 0TN0-
Kidney Pelvis
Left 0TN4-
Right 0TN3-
Larynx 0CNS-
Lens
Left 08NK3ZZ
Right 08NJ3ZZ
Lip
Lower 0CN1-
Upper 0CN0-
Liver 0FN0-
Left Lobe 0FN2-
Right Lobe 0FN1-
Lung
Bilateral 0BNM-
Left 0BNL-
Lower Lobe
Left 0BNJ-
Right 0BNF-
Middle Lobe, Right 0BND-
Right 0BNK-
Upper Lobe
Left 0BNG-
Right 0BNC-
Lung Lingula 0BNH-
Lymphatic
Aortic 07ND-
Axillary
Left 07N6-
Right 07N5-
Head 07N0-
Inguinal
Left 07NJ-
Right 07NH-
Internal Mammary
Left 07N9-
Right 07N8-
Lower Extremity
Left 07NG-
Right 07NF-

Release — continued
Lymphatic — continued
Mesenteric 07NB-
Neck
Left 07N2-
Right 07N1-
Pelvis 07NC-
Thoracic Duct 07NK-
Thorax 07N7-
Upper Extremity
Left 07N4-
Right 07N3-
Mandible
Left 0NNV-
Right 0NNT-
Maxilla
Left 0NNS-
Right 0NNR-
Medulla Oblongata 00ND-
Mesentery 0DNV-
Metacarpal
Left 0PNQ-
Right 0PNP-
Metatarsal
Left 0QNP-
Right 0QNN-
Muscle
Abdomen
Left 0KNL-
Right 0KNK-
Extraocular
Left 08NM-
Right 08NL-
Facial 0KN1-
Foot
Left 0KNW-
Right 0KNV-
Hand
Left 0KND-
Right 0KNC-
Head 0KN0-
Hip
Left 0KNP-
Right 0KNN-
Lower Arm and Wrist
Left 0KNB-
Right 0KN9-
Lower Leg
Left 0KNT-
Right 0KNS-
Neck
Left 0KN3-
Right 0KN2-
Papillary 02ND-
Perineum 0KNM-
Shoulder
Left 0KN6-
Right 0KN5-
Thorax
Left 0KNJ-
Right 0KNH-
Tongue, Palate, Pharynx 0KN4-
Trunk
Left 0KNG-
Right 0KNF-
Upper Arm
Left 0KN8-
Right 0KN7-
Upper Leg
Left 0KNR-
Right 0KNQ-
Nasopharynx 09NN-
Nerve
Abdominal Sympathetic 01NM-
Abducens 00NL-
Accessory 00NR-
Acoustic 00NN-
Brachial Plexus 01N3-
Cervical 01N1-
Cervical Plexus 01N0-
Facial 00NM-
Femoral 01ND-

Release — continued
Nerve — continued
Glossopharyngeal 00NP-
Head and Neck Sympathetic 01NK-
Hypoglossal 00NS-
Lumbar 01NB-
Lumbar Plexus 01N9-
Lumbar Sympathetic 01NN-
Lumbosacral Plexus 01NA-
Median 01N5-
Oculomotor 00NH-
Olfactory 00NF-
Optic 00NG-
Peroneal 01NH-
Phrenic 01N2-
Pudendal 01NC-
Radial 01N6-
Sacral 01NR-
Sacral Plexus 01NQ-
Sacral Sympathetic 01NP-
Sciatic 01NF-
Thoracic 01N8-
Thoracic Sympathetic 01NL -
Tibial 01NG-
Trigeminal 00NK-
Trochlear 00NJ-
Ulnar 01N4-
Vagus 00NQ-
Nipple
Left 0HNX-
Right 0HNW-
Nose 09NK-
Omentum
Greater 0DNS-
Lesser 0DNT-
Orbit
Left 0NNQ-
Right 0NNP-
Ovary
Bilateral 0UN2-
Left 0UN1-
Right 0UN0-
Palate
Hard 0CN2-
Soft 0CN3-
Pancreas 0FNG-
Para-aortic Body 0GN9-
Paraganglion Extremity 0GNF-
Parathyroid Gland 0GNR-
Inferior
Left 0GNP-
Right 0GNN-
Multiple 0GNQ-
Superior
Left 0GNM-
Right 0GNL-
Patella
Left 0QNF-
Right 0QND-
Penis 0VNS-
Pericardium 02NN-
Peritoneum 0DNW-
Phalanx
Finger
Left 0PNV-
Right 0PNT-
Thumb
Left 0PNS-
Right 0PNR-
Toe
Left 0QNR-
Right 0QNQ-
Pharynx 0CNM-
Pineal Body 0GN1-
Pleura
Left 0BNP-
Right 0BNN-
Pons 00NB-
Prepuce 0VNT-
Prostate 0VN0-

Release — continued
Radius
Left 0PNJ-
Right 0PNH-
Rectum 0DNP-
Retina
Left 08NF3ZZ
Right 08NE3ZZ
Retinal Vessel
Left 08NH3ZZ
Right 08NG3ZZ
Rib
Left 0PN2-
Right 0PN1-
Sacrum 0QN1-
Scapula
Left 0PN6-
Right 0PN5-
Sclera
Left 08N7XZZ
Right 08N6XZZ
Scrotum 0VN5-
Septum
Atrial 02N5-
Nasal 09NM-
Ventricular 02NM-
Sinus
Accessory 09NP-
Ethmoid
Left 09NV-
Right 09NU-
Frontal
Left 09NT-
Right 09NS-
Mastoid
Left 09NC-
Right 09NB-
Maxillary
Left 09NR-
Right 09NQ-
Sphenoid
Left 09NX-
Right 09NW-
Skin
Abdomen 0HN7XZZ
Back 0HN6XZZ
Buttock 0HN8XZZ
Chest 0HN5XZZ
Ear
Left 0HN3XZZ
Right 0HN2XZZ
Face 0HN1XZZ
Foot
Left 0HNNXZZ
Right 0HNMXZZ
Genitalia 0HNAXZZ
Hand
Left 0HNGXZZ
Right 0HNFXZZ
Lower Arm
Left 0HNEXZZ
Right 0HNDXZZ
Lower Leg
Left 0HNLXZZ
Right 0HNKXZZ
Neck 0HN4XZZ
Perineum 0HN9XZZ
Scalp 0HN0XZZ
Upper Arm
Left 0HNCXZZ
Right 0HNBXZZ
Upper Leg
Left 0HNJXZZ
Right 0HNHXZZ
Spinal Cord
Cervical 00NW-
Lumbar 00NY-
Thoracic 00NX-
Spinal Meninges 00NT-
Spleen 07NP-
Sternum 0PN0-
Stomach 0DN6-
Pylorus 0DN7-

PROCEDURE INDEX

Release — *continued*
Subcutaneous Tissue and Fascia
  Abdomen **0JN8-**
  Back **0JN7-**
  Buttock **0JN9-**
  Chest **0JN6-**
  Face **0JN1-**
  Foot
    Left **0JNR-**
    Right **0JNQ-**
  Hand
    Left **0JNK-**
    Right **0JNJ-**
  Lower Arm
    Left **0JNH-**
    Right **0JNG-**
  Lower Leg
    Left **0JNP-**
    Right **0JNN-**
  Neck
    Anterior **0JN4-**
    Posterior **0JN5-**
  Pelvic Region **0JNC-**
  Perineum **0JNB-**
  Scalp **0JN0-**
  Upper Arm
    Left **0JNF-**
    Right **0JND-**
  Upper Leg
    Left **0JNM-**
    Right **0JNL-**
Tarsal
  Left **0QNM-**
  Right **0QNL-**
Tendon
  Abdomen
    Left **0LNG-**
    Right **0LNF-**
  Ankle
    Left **0LNT-**
    Right **0LNS-**
  Foot
    Left **0LNW-**
    Right **0LNV-**
  Hand
    Left **0LN8-**
    Right **0LN7-**
  Head and Neck **0LN0-**
  Hip
    Left **0LNK-**
    Right **0LNJ-**
  Knee
    Left **0LNR-**
    Right **0LNQ-**
  Lower Arm and Wrist
    Left **0LN6-**
    Right **0LN5-**
  Lower Leg
    Left **0LNP-**
    Right **0LNN-**
  Perineum **0LNH-**
  Shoulder
    Left **0LN2-**
    Right **0LN1-**
  Thorax
    Left **0LND-**
    Right **0LNC-**
  Trunk
    Left **0LNB-**
    Right **0LN9-**
  Upper Arm
    Left **0LN4-**
    Right **0LN3-**
  Upper Leg
    Left **0LNM-**
    Right **0LNL-**
Testis
  Bilateral **0VNC-**
  Left **0VNB-**
  Right **0VN9-**

Release — *continued*
Thalamus **00N9-**
Thymus **07NM-**
Thyroid Gland **0GNK-**
  Left Lobe **0GNG-**
  Right Lobe **0GNH-**
Tibia
  Left **0QNH-**
  Right **0QNG-**
Toe Nail **0HNRXZZ**
Tongue **0CN7-**
Tonsils **0CNP-**
Tooth
  Lower **0CNX-**
  Upper **0CNW-**
Trachea **0BN1-**
Tunica Vaginalis
  Left **0VN7-**
  Right **0VN6-**
Turbinate, Nasal **09NL-**
Tympanic Membrane
  Left **09N8-**
  Right **09N7-**
Ulna
  Left **0PNL-**
  Right **0PNK-**
Ureter
  Left **0TN7-**
  Right **0TN6-**
Urethra **0TND-**
Uterine Supporting Structure **0UN4-**
Uterus **0UN9-**
Uvula **0CNN-**
Vagina **0UNG-**
Valve
  Aortic **02NF-**
  Mitral **02NG-**
  Pulmonary **02NH-**
  Tricuspid **02NJ-**
Vas Deferens
  Bilateral **0VNQ-**
  Left **0VNP-**
  Right **0VNN-**
Vein
  Axillary
    Left **05N8-**
    Right **05N7-**
  Azygos **05N0-**
  Basilic
    Left **05NC-**
    Right **05NB-**
  Brachial
    Left **05NA-**
    Right **05N9-**
  Cephalic
    Left **05NF-**
    Right **05ND-**
  Colic **06N7-**
  Common Iliac
    Left **06ND-**
    Right **06NC-**
  Coronary **02N4-**
  Esophageal **06N3-**
  External Iliac
    Left **06NG-**
    Right **06NF-**
  External Jugular
    Left **05NQ-**
    Right **05NP-**
  Face
    Left **05NV-**
    Right **05NT-**
  Femoral
    Left **06NN-**
    Right **06NM-**
  Foot
    Left **06NV-**
    Right **06NT-**
  Gastric **06N2-**

Release — *continued*
Vein — *continued*
  Greater Saphenous
    Left **06NQ-**
    Right **06NP-**
  Hand
    Left **05NH-**
    Right **05NG-**
  Hemiazygos **05N1-**
  Hepatic **06N4-**
  Hypogastric
    Left **06NJ-**
    Right **06NH-**
  Inferior Mesenteric **06N6-**
  Innominate
    Left **05N4-**
    Right **05N3-**
  Internal Jugular
    Left **05NN-**
    Right **05NM-**
  Intracranial **05NL-**
  Lesser Saphenous
    Left **06NS-**
    Right **06NR-**
  Lower **06NY-**
  Portal **06N8-**
  Pulmonary
    Left **02NT-**
    Right **02NS-**
  Renal
    Left **06NB-**
    Right **06N9-**
  Splenic **06N1-**
  Subclavian
    Left **05N6-**
    Right **05N5-**
  Superior Mesenteric **06N5-**
  Upper **05NY-**
  Vertebral
    Left **05NS-**
    Right **05NR-**
Vena Cava
  Inferior **06N0-**
  Superior **02NV-**
Ventricle
  Left **02NL-**
  Right **02NK-**
Vertebra
  Cervical **0PN3-**
  Lumbar **0QN0-**
  Thoracic **0PN4-**
Vesicle
  Bilateral **0VN3-**
  Left **0VN2-**
  Right **0VN1-**
Vitreous
  Left **08N53ZZ**
  Right **08N43ZZ**
Vocal Cord
  Left **0CNV-**
  Right **0CNT-**
Vulva **0UNM-**
Relocation *see* Reposition
Removal
Abdominal Wall **2W53X-**
Anorectal **2Y53X5Z**
Arm
  Lower
    Left **2W5DX-**
    Right **2W5CX-**
  Upper
    Left **2W5BX-**
    Right **2W5AX-**
Back **2W55X-**
Chest Wall **2W54X-**
Ear **2Y52X5Z**
Extremity
  Lower
    Left **2W5MX-**
    Right **2W5LX-**
  Upper
    Left **2W59X-**
    Right **2W58X-**

Removal — *continued*
Face **2W51X-**
Finger
  Left **2W5KX-**
  Right **2W5JX-**
Foot
  Left **2W5TX-**
  Right **2W5SX-**
Genital Tract, Female **2Y54X5Z**
Hand
  Left **2W5FX-**
  Right **2W5EX-**
Head **2W50X-**
Inguinal Region
  Left **2W57X-**
  Right **2W56X-**
Leg
  Lower
    Left **2W5RX-**
    Right **2W5QX-**
  Upper
    Left **2W5PX-**
    Right **2W5NX-**
Mouth and Pharynx **2Y50X5Z**
Nasal **2Y51X5Z**
Neck **2W52X-**
Thumb
  Left **2W5HX-**
  Right **2W5GX-**
Toe
  Left **2W5VX-**
  Right **2W5UX-**
Urethra **2Y55X5Z**
Removal of device from
Abdominal Wall **0WPF-**
Acetabulum
  Left **0QP5-**
  Right **0QP4-**
Anal Sphincter **0DPR-**
Anus **0DPQ-**
Artery
  Lower **04PY-**
  Upper **03PY-**
Back
  Lower **0WPL-**
  Upper **0WPK-**
Bladder **0TPB-**
Bone
  Facial **0NPW-**
  Lower **0QPY-**
  Nasal **0NPB-**
  Pelvic
    Left **0QP3-**
    Right **0QP2-**
  Upper **0PPY-**
Bone Marrow **07PT-**
Brain **00P0-**
Breast
  Left **0HPU-**
  Right **0HPT-**
Bursa and Ligament
  Lower **0MPY-**
  Upper **0MPX-**
Carpal
  Left **0PPN-**
  Right **0PPM-**
Cavity, Cranial **0WP1-**
Cerebral Ventricle **00P6-**
Chest Wall **0WP8-**
Cisterna Chyli **07PL-**
Clavicle
  Left **0PPB-**
  Right **0PP9-**
Coccyx **0QPS-**
Diaphragm **0BPT-**
Disc
  Cervical Vertebral **0RP3-**
  Cervicothoracic Vertebral **0RP5-**
  Lumbar Vertebral **0SP2-**
  Lumbosacral **0SP4-**
  Thoracic Vertebral **0RP9-**
  Thoracolumbar Vertebral **0RPB-**

PROCEDURE INDEX

Removal of device from — *continued*
Duct
 Hepatobiliary **0FPB-**
 Pancreatic **0FPD-**
Ear
 Inner
  Left **09PE-**
  Right **09PD-**
 Left **09PJ-**
 Right **09PH-**
Epididymis and Spermatic Cord **0VPM-**
Esophagus **0DP5-**
Extremity
 Lower
  Left **0YPB-**
  Right **0YP9-**
 Upper
  Left **0XP7-**
  Right **0XP6-**
Eye
 Left **08P1-**
 Right **08P0-**
Face **0WP2-**
Fallopian Tube **0UP8-**
Femoral Shaft
 Left **0QP9-**
 Right **0QP8-**
Femur
 Lower
  Left **0QPC-**
  Right **0QPB-**
 Upper
  Left **0QP7-**
  Right **0QP6-**
Fibula
 Left **0QPK-**
 Right **0QPJ-**
Finger Nail **0HPQX-**
Gallbladder **0FP4-**
Gastrointestinal Tract **0WPP-**
Genitourinary Tract **0WPR-**
Gland
 Adrenal **0GP5-**
 Endocrine **0GPS-**
 Pituitary **0GP0-**
 Salivary **0CPA-**
Glenoid Cavity
 Left **0PP8-**
 Right **0PP7-**
Great Vessel **02PY-**
Hair **0HPSX-**
Head **0WP0-**
Heart **02PA-**
Humeral Head
 Left **0PPD-**
 Right **0PPC-**
Humeral Shaft
 Left **0PPG-**
 Right **0PPF-**
Intestinal Tract
 Lower **0DPD-**
 Upper **0DP0-**
Jaw
 Lower **0WP5-**
 Upper **0WP4-**
Joint
 Acromioclavicular
  Left **0RPH-**
  Right **0RPG-**
 Ankle
  Left **0SPG-**
  Right **0SPF-**
 Carpal
  Left **0RPR-**
  Right **0RPQ-**
 Cervical Vertebral **0RP1-**
 Cervicothoracic Vertebral **0RP4-**
 Coccygeal **0SP6-**
 Elbow
  Left **0RPM-**
  Right **0RPL-**

Removal of device from — *continued*
Joint — *continued*
 Finger Phalangeal
  Left **0RPX-**
  Right **0RPW-**
 Hip
  Left **0SPB-**
   Acetabular Surface **0SPE-**
   Femoral Surface **0SPS-**
  Right **0SP9-**
   Acetabular Surface **0SPA-**
   Femoral Surface **0SPR-**
 Knee
  Left **0SPD-**
   Femoral Surface **0SPU-**
   Tibial Surface **0SPW-**
  Right **0SPC-**
   Femoral Surface **0SPT-**
   Tibial Surface **0SPV-**
 Lumbar Vertebral **0SP0-**
 Lumbosacral **0SP3-**
 Metacarpocarpal
  Left **0RPT-**
  Right **0RPS-**
 Metacarpophalangeal
  Left **0RPV-**
  Right **0RPU-**
 Metatarsal-Phalangeal
  Left **0SPN-**
  Right **0SPM-**
 Metatarsal-Tarsal
  Left **0SPL-**
  Right **0SPK-**
 Occipital-cervical **0RP0-**
 Sacrococcygeal **0SP5-**
 Sacroiliac
  Left **0SP8-**
  Right **0SP7-**
 Shoulder
  Left **0RPK-**
  Right **0RPJ-**
 Sternoclavicular
  Left **0RPF-**
  Right **0RPE-**
 Tarsal
  Left **0SPJ-**
  Right **0SPH-**
 Temporomandibular
  Left **0RPD-**
  Right **0RPC-**
 Thoracic Vertebral **0RP6-**
 Thoracolumbar Vertebral **0RPA-**
 Toe Phalangeal
  Left **0SPQ-**
  Right **0SPP-**
 Wrist
  Left **0RPP-**
  Right **0RPN-**
Kidney **0TP5-**
Larynx **0CPS-**
Lens
 Left **08PK3JZ**
 Right **08PJ3JZ**
Liver **0FP0-**
Lung
 Left **0BPL-**
 Right **0BPK-**
Lymphatic **07PN-**
 Thoracic Duct **07PK-**
Mediastinum **0WPC-**
Mesentery **0DPV-**
Metacarpal
 Left **0PPQ-**
 Right **0PPP-**
Metatarsal
 Left **0QPP-**
 Right **0QPN-**
Mouth and Throat **0CPY-**

Removal of device from — *continued*
Muscle
 Extraocular
  Left **08PM-**
  Right **08PL-**
 Lower **0KPY-**
 Upper **0KPX-**
Neck **0WP6-**
Nerve
 Cranial **00PE-**
 Peripheral **01PY-**
Nose **09PK-**
Omentum **0DPU-**
Ovary **0UP3-**
Pancreas **0FPG-**
Parathyroid Gland **0GPR-**
Patella
 Left **0QPF-**
 Right **0QPD-**
Pelvic Cavity **0WPJ-**
Penis **0VPS-**
Pericardial Cavity **0WPD-**
Perineum
 Female **0WPN-**
 Male **0WPM-**
Peritoneal Cavity **0WPG-**
Peritoneum **0DPW-**
Phalanx
 Finger
  Left **0PPV-**
  Right **0PPT-**
 Thumb
  Left **0PPS-**
  Right **0PPR-**
 Toe
  Left **0QPR-**
  Right **0QPQ-**
Pineal Body **0GP1-**
Pleura **0BPQ-**
Pleural Cavity
 Left **0WPB-**
 Right **0WP9-**
Products of Conception **10P0-**
Prostate and Seminal Vesicles **0VP4-**
Radius
 Left **0PPJ-**
 Right **0PPH-**
Rectum **0DPP-**
Respiratory Tract **0WPQ-**
Retroperitoneum **0WPH-**
Rib
 Left **0PP2-**
 Right **0PP1-**
Sacrum **0QP1-**
Scapula
 Left **0PP6-**
 Right **0PP5-**
Scrotum and Tunica Vaginalis **0VP8-**
Sinus **09PY-**
Skin **0HPPX-**
Skull **0NP0-**
Spinal Canal **00PU-**
Spinal Cord **00PV-**
Spleen **07PP-**
Sternum **0PP0-**
Stomach **0DP6-**
Subcutaneous Tissue and Fascia
 Head and Neck **0JPS-**
 Lower Extremity **0JPW-**
 Trunk **0JPT-**
 Upper Extremity **0JPV-**
Tarsal
 Left **0QPM-**
 Right **0QPL-**
Tendon
 Lower **0LPY-**
 Upper **0LPX-**
Testis **0VPD-**

Removal of device from — *continued*
Thymus **07PM-**
Thyroid Gland **0GPK-**
Tibia
 Left **0QPH-**
 Right **0QPG-**
Toe Nail **0HPRX-**
Trachea **0BP1-**
Tracheobronchial Tree **0BP0-**
Tympanic Membrane
 Left **09P8-**
 Right **09P7-**
Ulna
 Left **0PPL-**
 Right **0PPK-**
Ureter **0TP9-**
Urethra **0TPD-**
Uterus and Cervix **0UPD-**
Vagina and Cul-de-sac **0UPH-**
Vas Deferens **0VPR-**
Vein
 Azygos **05P0-**
 Innominate
  Left **05P4-**
  Right **05P3-**
 Lower **06PY-**
 Upper **05PY-**
Vertebra
 Cervical **0PP3-**
 Lumbar **0QP0-**
 Thoracic **0PP4-**
Vulva **0UPM-**
Renal calyx
 use Kidney
 use Kidneys, Bilateral
 use Kidney, Left
 use Kidney, Right
Renal capsule
 use Kidney
 use Kidneys, Bilateral
 use Kidney, Left
 use Kidney, Right
Renal cortex
 use Kidney
 use Kidneys, Bilateral
 use Kidney, Left
 use Kidney, Right
Renal dialysis *see* Performance, Urinary **5A1D-**
Renal plexus
 use Nerve, Abdominal Sympathetic
Renal segment
 use Kidney
 use Kidney, Left
 use Kidney, Right
 use Kidneys, Bilateral
Renal segmental artery
 use Artery, Renal, Left
 use Artery, Renal, Right
Reopening, operative site
 Control of bleeding *see* Control bleeding in
 Inspection only *see* Inspection
Repair
 Abdominal Wall **0WQF-**
 Acetabulum
  Left **0QQ5-**
  Right **0QQ4-**
 Adenoids **0CQQ-**
 Ampulla of Vater **0FQC-**
 Anal Sphincter **0DQR-**
 Ankle Region
  Left **0YQL-**
  Right **0YQK-**
 Anterior Chamber
  Left **08Q33ZZ**
  Right **08Q23ZZ**
 Anus **0DQQ-**
 Aorta
  Abdominal **04Q0-**
  Thoracic
   Ascending/Arch **02QX-**
   Descending **02QW-**

Repair — *continued*
Aortic Body **0GQ**D-
Appendix **0DQ**J-
Arm
　Lower
　　Left **0XQ**F-
　　Right **0XQ**D-
　Upper
　　Left **0XQ**9-
　　Right **0XQ**8-
Artery
　Anterior Tibial
　　Left **04Q**Q-
　　Right **04Q**P-
　Axillary
　　Left **03Q**6-
　　Right **03Q**5-
　Brachial
　　Left **03Q**8-
　　Right **03Q**7-
　Celiac **04Q**1-
　Colic
　　Left **04Q**7-
　　Middle **04Q**8-
　　Right **04Q**6-
　Common Carotid
　　Left **03Q**J-
　　Right **03Q**H-
　Common Iliac
　　Left **04Q**D-
　　Right **04Q**C-
　Coronary
　　Four or More Arteries **02Q**3-
　　One Artery **02Q**0-
　　Three Arteries **02Q**2-
　　Two Arteries **02Q**1-
　External Carotid
　　Left **03Q**N-
　　Right **03Q**M-
　External Iliac
　　Left **04Q**J-
　　Right **04Q**H-
　Face **03Q**R-
　Femoral
　　Left **04Q**L-
　　Right **04Q**K-
　Foot
　　Left **04Q**W-
　　Right **04Q**V-
　Gastric **04Q**2-
　Hand
　　Left **03Q**F-
　　Right **03Q**D-
　Hepatic **04Q**3-
　Inferior Mesenteric **04Q**B-
　Innominate **03Q**2-
　Internal Carotid
　　Left **03Q**L-
　　Right **03Q**K-
　Internal Iliac
　　Left **04Q**F-
　　Right **04Q**E-
　Internal Mammary
　　Left **03Q**1-
　　Right **03Q**0-
　Intracranial **03Q**G-
　Lower **04Q**Y-
　Peroneal
　　Left **04Q**U-
　　Right **04Q**T-
　Popliteal
　　Left **04Q**N-
　　Right **04Q**M-
　Posterior Tibial
　　Left **04Q**S-
　　Right **04Q**R-
　Pulmonary
　　Left **02Q**R-
　　Right **02Q**Q-
　Pulmonary Trunk **02Q**P-

Repair — *continued*
Artery — *continued*
　Radial
　　Left **03Q**C-
　　Right **03Q**B-
　Renal
　　Left **04Q**A-
　　Right **04Q**9-
　Splenic **04Q**4-
　Subclavian
　　Left **03Q**4-
　　Right **03Q**3-
　Superior Mesenteric **04Q**5-
　Temporal
　　Left **03Q**T-
　　Right **03Q**S-
　Thyroid
　　Left **03Q**V-
　　Right **03Q**U-
　Ulnar
　　Left **03Q**A-
　　Right **03Q**9-
　Upper **03Q**Y-
　Vertebral
　　Left **03Q**Q-
　　Right **03Q**P-
Atrium
　Left **02Q**7-
　Right **02Q**6-
Auditory Ossicle
　Left **09Q**A0ZZ
　Right **09Q**90ZZ
Axilla
　Left **0XQ**5-
　Right **0XQ**4-
Back
　Lower **0WQ**L-
　Upper **0WQ**K-
Basal Ganglia **00Q**8-
Bladder **0TQ**B-
Bladder Neck **0TQ**C-
Bone
　Ethmoid
　　Left **0NQ**G-
　　Right **0NQ**F-
　Frontal
　　Left **0NQ**2-
　　Right **0NQ**1-
　Hyoid **0NQ**X-
　Lacrimal
　　Left **0NQ**J-
　　Right **0NQ**H-
　Nasal **0NQ**B-
　Occipital
　　Left **0NQ**8-
　　Right **0NQ**7-
　Palatine
　　Left **0NQ**L-
　　Right **0NQ**K-
　Parietal
　　Left **0NQ**4-
　　Right **0NQ**3-
　Pelvic
　　Left **0QQ**3-
　　Right **0QQ**2-
　Sphenoid
　　Left **0NQ**D-
　　Right **0NQ**C-
　Temporal
　　Left **0NQ**6-
　　Right **0NQ**5-
　Zygomatic
　　Left **0NQ**N-
　　Right **0NQ**M-
Brain **00Q**0-
Breast
　Bilateral **0HQ**V-
　Left **0HQ**U-
　Right **0HQ**T-
　Supernumerary **0HQ**Y-

Repair — *continued*
Bronchus
　Lingula **0BQ**9-
　Lower Lobe
　　Left **0BQ**B-
　　Right **0BQ**6-
　Main
　　Left **0BQ**7-
　　Right **0BQ**3-
　Middle Lobe, Right **0BQ**5-
　Upper Lobe
　　Left **0BQ**8-
　　Right **0BQ**4-
Buccal Mucosa **0CQ**4-
Bursa and Ligament
　Abdomen
　　Left **0MQ**J-
　　Right **0MQ**H-
　Ankle
　　Left **0MQ**R-
　　Right **0MQ**Q-
　Elbow
　　Left **0MQ**4-
　　Right **0MQ**3-
　Foot
　　Left **0MQ**T-
　　Right **0MQ**S-
　Hand
　　Left **0MQ**8-
　　Right **0MQ**7-
　Head and Neck **0MQ**0-
　Hip
　　Left **0MQ**M-
　　Right **0MQ**L-
　Knee
　　Left **0MQ**P-
　　Right **0MQ**N-
　Lower Extremity
　　Left **0MQ**W-
　　Right **0MQ**V-
　Perineum **0MQ**K-
　Shoulder
　　Left **0MQ**2-
　　Right **0MQ**1-
　Thorax
　　Left **0MQ**G-
　　Right **0MQ**F-
　Trunk
　　Left **0MQ**D-
　　Right **0MQ**C-
　Upper Extremity
　　Left **0MQ**B-
　　Right **0MQ**9-
　Wrist
　　Left **0MQ**6-
　　Right **0MQ**5-
Buttock
　Left **0YQ**1-
　Right **0YQ**0-
Carina **0BQ**2
Carotid Bodies, Bilateral **0GQ**8-
Carotid Body
　Left **0GQ**6-
　Right **0GQ**7-
Carpal
　Left **0PQ**N-
　Right **0PQ**M-
Cecum **0DQ**H-
Cerebellum **00Q**C-
Cerebral Hemisphere **00Q**7-
Cerebral Meninges **00Q**1-
Cerebral Ventricle **00Q**6-
Cervix **0UQ**C-
Chest Wall **0WQ**8-
Chordae Tendineae **02Q**9-
Choroid
　Left **08Q**B-
　Right **08Q**A-
Cisterna Chyli **07Q**L-

Repair — *continued*
Clavicle
　Left **0PQ**B-
　Right **0PQ**9-
Clitoris **0UQ**J-
Coccygeal Glomus **0GQ**B-
Coccyx **0QQ**S-
Colon
　Ascending **0DQ**K-
　Descending **0DQ**M-
　Sigmoid **0DQ**N-
　Transverse **0DQ**L-
Conduction Mechanism **02Q**8-
Conjunctiva
　Left **08Q**TXZZ
　Right **08Q**SXZZ
Cord
　Bilateral **0VQ**H-
　Left **0VQ**G-
　Right **0VQ**F-
Cornea
　Left **08Q**9XZZ
　Right **08Q**8XZZ
Cul-de-sac **0UQ**F-
Diaphragm
　Left **0BQ**S-
　Right **0BQ**R-
Disc
　Cervical Vertebral **0RQ**3-
　Cervicothoracic Vertebral **0RQ**5-
　Lumbar Vertebral **0SQ**2-
　Lumbosacral **0SQ**4-
　Thoracic Vertebral **0RQ**9-
　Thoracolumbar Vertebral **0RQ**B-
Duct
　Common Bile **0FQ**9-
　Cystic **0FQ**8-
　Hepatic
　　Left **0FQ**6-
　　Right **0FQ**5-
　Lacrimal
　　Left **08Q**Y-
　　Right **08Q**X-
　Pancreatic **0FQ**D-
　　Accessory **0FQ**F-
　Parotid
　　Left **0CQ**C-
　　Right **0CQ**B-
Duodenum **0DQ**9-
Dura Mater **00Q**2-
Ear
　External
　　Bilateral **09Q**2-
　　Left **09Q**1-
　　Right **09Q**0-
　External Auditory Canal
　　Left **09Q**4-
　　Right **09Q**3-
　Inner
　　Left **09Q**E0ZZ
　　Right **09Q**D0ZZ
　Middle
　　Left **09Q**60ZZ
　　Right **09Q**50ZZ
Elbow Region
　Left **0XQ**C-
　Right **0XQ**B-
Epididymis
　Bilateral **0VQ**L-
　Left **0VQ**K-
　Right **0VQ**J-
Epiglottis **0CQ**R-
Esophagogastric Junction **0DQ**4-
Esophagus **0DQ**5-
　Lower **0DQ**3-
　Middle **0DQ**2-
　Upper **0DQ**1-
Eustachian Tube
　Left **09Q**G-
　Right **09Q**F-

PROCEDURE INDEX

Repair — *continued*
Extremity
Lower
Left **0YQ**B-
Right **0YQ**9-
Upper
Left **0XQ**7-
Right **0XQ**6-
Eye
Left **08Q**1XZZ
Right **08Q**0XZZ
Eyelid
Lower
Left **08Q**R-
Right **08Q**Q-
Upper
Left **08Q**P-
Right **08Q**N-
Face **0WQ**2-
Fallopian Tube
Left **0UQ**6-
Right **0UQ**5-
Fallopian Tubes, Bilateral **0UQ**7-
Femoral Region
Bilateral **0YQ**E-
Left **0YQ**8-
Right **0YQ**7-
Femoral Shaft
Left **0QQ**9-
Right **0QQ**8-
Femur
Lower
Left **0QQ**C-
Right **0QQ**B-
Upper
Left **0QQ**7-
Right **0QQ**6-
Fibula
Left **0QQ**K-
Right **0QQ**J-
Finger
Index
Left **0XQ**P-
Right **0XQ**N-
Little
Left **0XQ**W-
Right **0XQ**V-
Middle
Left **0XQ**R-
Right **0XQ**Q-
Ring
Left **0XQ**T-
Right **0XQ**S-
Finger Nail **0HQ**QXZZ
Foot
Left **0YQ**N-
Right **0YQ**M-
Gallbladder **0FQ**4-
Gingiva
Lower **0CQ**6-
Upper **0CQ**5-
Gland
Adrenal
Bilateral **0GQ**4-
Left **0GQ**2-
Right **0GQ**3-
Lacrimal
Left **08Q**W-
Right **08Q**V-
Minor Salivary **0CQ**J-
Parotid
Left **0CQ**9-
Right **0CQ**8-
Pituitary **0GQ**0-
Sublingual
Left **0CQ**F-
Right **0CQ**D-
Submaxillary
Left **0CQ**H-
Right **0CQ**G-
Vestibular **0UQ**L-

Repair — *continued*
Glenoid Cavity
Left **0PQ**8-
Right **0PQ**7-
Glomus Jugulare **0GQ**C-
Hand
Left **0XQ**K-
Right **0XQ**J-
Head **0WQ**0-
Heart **02Q**A-
Left **02Q**C-
Right **02Q**B-
Humeral Head
Left **0PQ**D-
Right **0PQ**C-
Humeral Shaft
Left **0PQ**G-
Right **0PQ**F-
Hymen **0UQ**K-
Hypothalamus **00Q**A-
Ileocecal Valve **0DQ**C-
Ileum **0DQ**B-
Inguinal Region
Bilateral **0YQ**A-
Left **0YQ**6-
Right **0YQ**5-
Intestine
Large **0DQ**E-
Left **0DQ**G-
Right **0DQ**F-
Small **0DQ**8-
Iris
Left **08Q**D3ZZ
Right **08Q**C3ZZ
Jaw
Lower **0WQ**5-
Upper **0WQ**4-
Jejunum **0DQ**A-
Joint
Acromioclavicular
Left **0RQ**H-
Right **0RQ**G-
Ankle
Left **0SQ**G-
Right **0SQ**F-
Carpal
Left **0RQ**R-
Right **0RQ**Q-
Cervical Vertebral **0RQ**1-
Cervicothoracic Vertebral **0RQ**4-
Coccygeal **0SQ**6-
Elbow
Left **0RQ**M-
Right **0RQ**L-
Finger Phalangeal
Left **0RQ**X-
Right **0RQ**W-
Hip
Left **0SQ**B-
Right **0SQ**9-
Knee
Left **0SQ**D-
Right **0SQ**C-
Lumbar Vertebral **0SQ**0-
Lumbosacral **0SQ**3-
Metacarpocarpal
Left **0RQ**T-
Right **0RQ**S-
Metacarpophalangeal
Left **0RQ**V-
Right **0RQ**U-
Metatarsal-Phalangeal
Left **0SQ**N-
Right **0SQ**M-
Metatarsal-Tarsal
Left **0SQ**L-
Right **0SQ**K-
Occipital-cervical **0RQ**0-
Sacrococcygeal **0SQ**5-

Repair — *continued*
Joint — *continued*
Sacroiliac
Left **0SQ**8-
Right **0SQ**7-
Shoulder
Left **0RQ**K-
Right **0RQ**J-
Sternoclavicular
Left **0RQ**F-
Right **0RQ**E-
Tarsal
Left **0SQ**J-
Right **0SQ**H-
Temporomandibular
Left **0RQ**D-
Right **0RQ**C-
Thoracic Vertebral **0RQ**6-
Thoracolumbar Vertebral **0RQ**A-
Toe Phalangeal
Left **0SQ**Q-
Right **0SQ**P
Wrist
Left **0RQ**P-
Right **0RQ**N-
Kidney
Left **0TQ**1-
Right **0TQ**0-
Kidney Pelvis
Left **0TQ**4-
Right **0TQ**3-
Knee Region
Left **0YQ**G-
Right **0YQ**F-
Larynx **0CQ**S-
Leg
Lower
Left **0YQ**J-
Right **0YQ**H-
Upper
Left **0YQ**D-
Right **0YQ**C-
Lens
Left **08Q**K3ZZ
Right **08Q**J3ZZ
Lip
Lower **0CQ**1-
Upper **0CQ**0-
Liver **0FQ**0-
Left Lobe **0FQ**2-
Right Lobe **0FQ**1-
Lung
Bilateral **0BQ**M-
Left **0BQ**L-
Lower Lobe
Left **0BQ**J-
Right **0BQ**F-
Middle Lobe, Right **0BQ**D-
Right **0BQ**K-
Upper Lobe
Left **0BQ**G-
Right **0BQ**C-
Lung Lingula **0BQ**H-
Lymphatic
Aortic **07Q**D-
Axillary
Left **07Q**6-
Right **07Q**5-
Head **07Q**0-
Inguinal
Left **07Q**J-
Right **07Q**H-
Internal Mammary
Left **07Q**9-
Right **07Q**8-
Lower Extremity
Left **07Q**G-
Right **07Q**F-
Mesenteric **07Q**B-
Neck
Left **07Q**2-
Right **07Q**1-
Pelvis **07Q**C-

Repair — *continued*
Lymphatic — *continued*
Thoracic Duct **07Q**K-
Thorax **07Q**7-
Upper Extremity
Left **07Q**4-
Right **07Q**3-
Mandible
Left **0NQ**V-
Right **0NQ**T-
Maxilla
Left **0NQ**S-
Right **0NQ**R-
Mediastinum **0WQ**C-
Medulla Oblongata **00Q**D-
Mesentery **0DQ**V-
Metacarpal
Left **0PQ**Q-
Right **0PQ**P-
Metatarsal
Left **0QQ**P-
Right **0QQ**N-
Muscle
Abdomen
Left **0KQ**L-
Right **0KQ**K-
Extraocular
Left **08Q**M-
Right **08Q**L-
Facial **0KQ**1-
Foot
Left **0KQ**W-
Right **0KQ**V-
Hand
Left **0KQ**D-
Right **0KQ**C-
Head **0KQ**0-
Hip
Left **0KQ**P-
Right **0KQ**N-
Lower Arm and Wrist
Left **0KQ**B-
Right **0KQ**9-
Lower Leg
Left **0KQ**T-
Right **0KQ**S-
Neck
Left **0KQ**3-
Right **0KQ**2-
Papillary **02Q**D-
Perineum **0KQ**M-
Shoulder
Left **0KQ**6-
Right **0KQ**5-
Thorax
Left **0KQ**J-
Right **0KQ**H-
Tongue, Palate, Pharynx **0KQ**4-
Trunk
Left **0KQ**G-
Right **0KQ**F-
Upper Arm
Left **0KQ**8-
Right **0KQ**7-
Upper Leg
Left **0KQ**R-
Right **0KQ**Q-
Nasopharynx **09Q**N-
Neck **0WQ**6-
Nerve
Abdominal Sympathetic **01Q**M-
Abducens **00Q**L-
Accessory **00Q**R-
Acoustic **00Q**N-
Brachial Plexus **01Q**3-
Cervical **01Q**1-
Cervical Plexus **01Q**0-
Facial **00Q**M-
Femoral **01Q**D-
Glossopharyngeal **00Q**P-
Head and Neck Sympathetic **01Q**K-
Hypoglossal **00Q**S-

Repair — *continued*
  Nerve — *continued*
    Lumbar **01Q**B-
    Lumbar Plexus **01Q**9-
    Lumbar Sympathetic **01Q**N-
    Lumbosacral Plexus **01Q**A-
    Median **01Q**5-
    Oculomotor **00Q**H-
    Olfactory **00Q**F-
    Optic **00Q**G-
    Peroneal **01Q**H-
    Phrenic **01Q**2-
    Pudendal **01Q**C-
    Radial **01Q**6-
    Sacral **01Q**R-
    Sacral Plexus **01Q**Q-
    Sacral Sympathetic **01Q**P-
    Sciatic **01Q**F-
    Thoracic **01Q**8-
    Thoracic Sympathetic **01Q**L-
    Tibial **01Q**G-
    Trigeminal **00Q**K-
    Trochlear **00Q**J-
    Ulnar **01Q**4-
    Vagus **00Q**Q-
  Nipple
    Left **0HQ**X-
    Right **0HQ**W-
  Nose **09Q**K-
  Omentum
    Greater **0DQ**S-
    Lesser **0DQ**T-
  Orbit
    Left **0NQ**Q-
    Right **0NQ**P-
  Ovary
    Bilateral **0UQ**2-
    Left **0UQ**1-
    Right **0UQ**0-
  Palate
    Hard **0CQ**2-
    Soft **0CQ**3-
  Pancreas **0FQ**G-
  Para-aortic Body **0GQ**9-
  Paraganglion Extremity **0GQ**F-
  Parathyroid Gland **0GQ**R-
    Inferior
      Left **0GQ**P-
      Right **0GQ**N-
    Multiple **0GQ**Q-
    Superior
      Left **0GQ**M-
      Right **0GQ**L-
  Patella
    Left **0QQ**F-
    Right **0QQ**D-
  Penis **0VQ**S-
  Pericardium **02Q**N-
  Perineum
    Female **0WQ**N-
    Male **0WQ**M-
  Peritoneum **0DQ**W-
  Phalanx
    Finger
      Left **0PQ**V-
      Right **0PQ**T-
    Thumb
      Left **0PQ**S-
      Right **0PQ**R-
    Toe
      Left **0QQ**R-
      Right **0QQ**Q-
  Pharynx **0CQ**M-
  Pineal Body **0GQ**1-
  Pleura
    Left **0BQ**P-
    Right **0BQ**N-
  Pons **00Q**B-
  Prepuce **0VQ**T-
  Products of Conception **10Q**0-
  Prostate **0VQ**0-

Repair — *continued*
  Radius
    Left **0PQ**J-
    Right **0PQ**H-
  Rectum **0DQ**P-
  Retina
    Left **08Q**F3ZZ
    Right **08Q**E3ZZ
  Retinal Vessel
    Left **08Q**H3ZZ
    Right **08Q**G3ZZ
  Rib
    Left **0PQ**2-
    Right **0PQ**1-
  Sacrum **0QQ**1-
  Scapula
    Left **0PQ**6-
    Right **0PQ**5-
  Sclera
    Left **08Q**7XZZ
    Right **08Q**6XZZ
  Scrotum **0VQ**5-
  Septum
    Atrial **02Q**5-
    Nasal **09Q**M-
    Ventricular **02Q**M-
  Shoulder Region
    Left **0XQ**3-
    Right **0XQ**2-
  Sinus
    Accessory **09Q**P-
    Ethmoid
      Left **09Q**V-
      Right **09Q**U-
    Frontal
      Left **09Q**T-
      Right **09Q**S-
    Mastoid
      Left **09Q**C-
      Right **09Q**B-
    Maxillary
      Left **09Q**R-
      Right **09Q**Q-
    Sphenoid
      Left **09Q**X-
      Right **09Q**W-
  Skin
    Abdomen **0HQ**7XZZ
    Back **0HQ**6XZZ
    Buttock **0HQ**8XZZ
    Chest **0HQ**5XZZ
    Ear
      Left **0HQ**3XZZ
      Right **0HQ**2XZZ
    Face **0HQ**1XZZ
    Foot
      Left **0HQ**NXZZ
      Right **0HQ**MXZZ
    Genitalia **0HQ**AXZZ
    Hand
      Left **0HQ**GXZZ
      Right **0HQ**FXZZ
    Lower Arm
      Left **0HQ**EXZZ
      Right **0HQ**DXZZ
    Lower Leg
      Left **0HQ**LXZZ
      Right **0HQ**KXZZ
    Neck **0HQ**4XZZ
    Perineum **0HQ**9XZZ
    Scalp **0HQ**0XZZ
    Upper Arm
      Left **0HQ**CXZZ
      Right **0HQ**BXZZ
    Upper Leg
      Left **0HQ**JXZZ
      Right **0HQ**HXZZ
  Skull **0NQ**0-
  Spinal Cord
    Cervical **00Q**W-
    Lumbar **00Q**Y-
    Thoracic **00Q**X-

Repair — *continued*
  Spinal Meninges **00Q**T-
  Spleen **07Q**P-
  Sternum **0PQ**0-
  Stomach **0DQ**6-
    Pylorus **0DQ**7-
  Subcutaneous Tissue and Fascia
    Abdomen **0JQ**8-
    Back **0JQ**7-
    Buttock **0JQ**9-
    Chest **0JQ**6-
    Face **0JQ**1-
    Foot
      Left **0JQ**R-
      Right **0JQ**Q-
    Hand
      Left **0JQ**K-
      Right **0JQ**J-
    Lower Arm
      Left **0JQ**H-
      Right **0JQ**G-
    Lower Leg
      Left **0JQ**P-
      Right **0JQ**N-
    Neck
      Anterior **0JQ**4-
      Posterior **0JQ**5-
    Pelvic Region **0JQ**C-
    Perineum **0JQ**B-
    Scalp **0JQ**0-
    Upper Arm
      Left **0JQ**F-
      Right **0JQ**D-
    Upper Leg
      Left **0JQ**M-
      Right **0JQ**L-
  Tarsal
    Left **0QQ**M-
    Right **0QQ**L-
  Tendon
    Abdomen
      Left **0LQ**G-
      Right **0LQ**F-
    Ankle
      Left **0LQ**T-
      Right **0LQ**S-
    Foot
      Left **0LQ**W-
      Right **0LQ**V-
    Hand
      Left **0LQ**8-
      Right **0LQ**7-
    Head and Neck **0LQ**0-
    Hip
      Left **0LQ**K-
      Right **0LQ**J-
    Knee
      Left **0LQ**R-
      Right **0LQ**Q-
    Lower Arm and Wrist
      Left **0LQ**6-
      Right **0LQ**5-
    Lower Leg
      Left **0LQ**P-
      Right **0LQ**N-
    Perineum **0LQ**H-
    Shoulder
      Left **0LQ**2-
      Right **0LQ**1-
    Thorax
      Left **0LQ**D-
      Right **0LQ**C-
    Trunk
      Left **0LQ**B-
      Right **0LQ**9-
    Upper Arm
      Left **0LQ**4-
      Right **0LQ**3-
    Upper Leg
      Left **0LQ**M-
      Right **0LQ**L-

Repair — *continued*
  Testis
    Bilateral **0VQ**C-
    Left **0VQ**B-
    Right **0VQ**9-
  Thalamus **00Q**9-
  Thumb
    Left **0XQ**M-
    Right **0XQ**L-
  Thymus **07Q**M-
  Thyroid Gland **0GQ**K-
    Left Lobe **0GQ**G-
    Right Lobe **0GQ**H-
  Thyroid Gland Isthmus **0GQ**J-
  Tibia
    Left **0QQ**H-
    Right **0QQ**G-
  Toe
    1st
      Left **0YQ**Q-
      Right **0YQ**P-
    2nd
      Left **0YQ**S-
      Right **0YQ**R-
    3rd
      Left **0YQ**U-
      Right **0YQ**T-
    4th
      Left **0YQ**W-
      Right **0YQ**V-
    5th
      Left **0YQ**Y-
      Right **0YQ**X-
  Toe Nail **0HQ**RXZZ
  Tongue **0CQ**7-
  Tonsils **0CQ**P-
  Tooth
    Lower **0CQ**X-
    Upper **0CQ**W-
  Trachea **0BQ**1-
  Tunica Vaginalis
    Left **0VQ**7-
    Right **0VQ**6-
  Turbinate, Nasal **09Q**L-
  Tympanic Membrane
    Left **09Q**8-
    Right **09Q**7-
  Ulna
    Left **0PQ**L-
    Right **0PQ**K-
  Ureter
    Left **0TQ**7-
    Right **0TQ**6-
  Urethra **0TQ**D-
  Uterine Supporting Structure **0UQ**4-
  Uterus **0UQ**9-
  Uvula **0CQ**N-
  Vagina **0UQ**G-
  Valve
    Aortic **02Q**F-
    Mitral **02Q**G-
    Pulmonary **02Q**H-
    Tricuspid **02Q**J-
  Vas Deferens
    Bilateral **0VQ**Q-
    Left **0VQ**P-
    Right **0VQ**N-
  Vein
    Axillary
      Left **05Q**8-
      Right **05Q**7-
    Azygos **05Q**0-
    Basilic
      Left **05Q**C-
      Right **05Q**B-
    Brachial
      Left **05Q**A-
      Right **05Q**9-
    Cephalic
      Left **05Q**F-
      Right **05Q**D-

PROCEDURE INDEX

Repair — *continued*
  Vein — *continued*
    Colic 06Q7-
    Common Iliac
      Left 06QD-
      Right 06QC-
    Coronary 02Q4-
    Esophageal 06Q3-
    External Iliac
      Left 06QG-
      Right 06QF-
    External Jugular
      Left 05QQ-
      Right 05QP-
    Face
      Left 05QV-
      Right 05QT-
    Femoral
      Left 06QN-
      Right 06QM-
    Foot
      Left 06QV-
      Right 06QT-
    Gastric 06Q2-
    Greater Saphenous
      Left 06QQ-
      Right 06QP-
    Hand
      Left 05QH-
      Right 05QG-
    Hemiazygos 05Q1-
    Hepatic 06Q4-
    Hypogastric
      Left 06QJ-
      Right 06QH-
    Inferior Mesenteric 06Q6-
    Innominate
      Left 05Q4-
      Right 05Q3-
    Internal Jugular
      Left 05QN-
      Right 05QM-
    Intracranial 05QL-
    Lesser Saphenous
      Left 06QS-
      Right 06QR-
    Lower 06QY-
    Portal 06Q8-
    Pulmonary
      Left 02QT-
      Right 02QS-
    Renal
      Left 06QB-
      Right 06Q9-
    Splenic 06Q1-
    Subclavian
      Left 05Q6-
      Right 05Q5-
    Superior Mesenteric 06Q5-
    Upper 05QY-
    Vertebral
      Left 05QS-
      Right 05QR-
  Vena Cava
    Inferior 06Q0-
    Superior 02QV-
  Ventricle
    Left 02QL-
    Right 02QK-
  Vertebra
    Cervical 0PQ3-
    Lumbar 0QQ0-
    Thoracic 0PQ4-
  Vesicle
    Bilateral 0VQ3-
    Left 0VQ2-
    Right 0VQ1-
  Vitreous
    Left 08Q53ZZ
    Right 08Q43ZZ

Repair — *continued*
  Vocal Cord
    Left 0CQV-
    Right 0CQT-
  Vulva 0UQM-
  Wrist Region
    Left 0XQH-
    Right 0XQG-
Repair, obstetric laceration, periurethral 0UQMXZZ
Replacement
  Acetabulum
    Left 0QR5-
    Right 0QR4
  Ampulla of Vater 0FRC-
  Anal Sphincter 0DRR-
  Aorta
    Abdominal 04R0-
    Thoracic
      Ascending/Arch 02RX-
      Descending 02RW-
  Artery
    Anterior Tibial
      Left 04RQ-
      Right 04RP-
    Axillary
      Left 03R6-
      Right 03R5-
    Brachial
      Left 03R8-
      Right 03R7-
    Celiac 04R1-
    Colic
      Left 04R7-
      Middle 04R8-
      Right 04R6-
    Common Carotid
      Left 03RJ-
      Right 03RH-
    Common Iliac
      Left 04RD-
      Right 04RC-
    External Carotid
      Left 03RN-
      Right 03RM-
    External Iliac
      Left 04RJ-
      Right 04RH-
    Face 03RR-
    Femoral
      Left 04RL-
      Right 04RK-
    Foot
      Left 04RW-
      Right 04RV-
    Gastric 04R2-
    Hand
      Left 03RF-
      Right 03RD-
    Hepatic 04R3-
    Inferior Mesenteric 04RB-
    Innominate 03R2-
    Internal Carotid
      Left 03RL-
      Right 03RK-
    Internal Iliac
      Left 04RF-
      Right 04RE-
    Internal Mammary
      Left 03R1-
      Right 03R0-
    Intracranial 03RG-
    Lower 04RY-
    Peroneal
      Left 04RU-
      Right 04RT-
    Popliteal
      Left 04RN-
      Right 04RM-
    Posterior Tibial
      Left 04RS-
      Right 04RR-

Replacement — *continued*
  Artery — *continued*
    Pulmonary
      Left 02RR-
      Right 02RQ-
    Pulmonary Trunk 02RP-
    Radial
      Left 03RC-
      Right 03RB-
    Renal
      Left 04RA-
      Right 04R9-
    Splenic 04R4-
    Subclavian
      Left 03R4-
      Right 03R3-
    Superior Mesenteric 04R5-
    Temporal
      Left 03RT-
      Right 03RS-
    Thyroid
      Left 03RV-
      Right 03RU-
    Ulnar
      Left 03RA-
      Right 03R9-
    Upper 03RY-
    Vertebral
      Left 03RQ-
      Right 03RP-
  Atrium
    Left 02R7-
    Right 02R6-
  Auditory Ossicle
    Left 09RA0-
    Right 09R90-
  Bladder 0TRB-
  Bladder Neck 0TRC-
  Bone
    Ethmoid
      Left 0NRG-
      Right 0NRF-
    Frontal
      Left 0NR2-
      Right 0NR1-
    Hyoid 0NRX-
    Lacrimal
      Left 0NRJ-
      Right 0NRH-
    Nasal 0NRB-
    Occipital
      Left 0NR8-
      Right 0NR7-
    Palatine
      Left 0NRL-
      Right 0NRK-
    Parietal
      Left 0NR4-
      Right 0NR3-
    Pelvic
      Left 0QR3-
      Right 0QR2-
    Sphenoid
      Left 0NRD-
      Right 0NRC-
    Temporal
      Left 0NR6-
      Right 0NR5-
    Zygomatic
      Left 0NRN-
      Right 0NRM-
  Breast
    Bilateral 0HRV-
    Left 0HRU-
    Right 0HRT-
  Buccal Mucosa 0CR4-
  Carpal
    Left 0PRN-
    Right 0PRM-
  Chordae Tendineae 02R9-

Replacement — *continued*
  Choroid
    Left 08RB-
    Right 08RA-
  Clavicle
    Left 0PRB-
    Right 0PR9-
  Coccyx 0QRS-
  Conjunctiva
    Left 08RTX-
    Right 08RSX-
  Cornea
    Left 08R9-
    Right 08R8-
  Disc
    Cervical Vertebral 0RR30-
    Cervicothoracic Vertebral 0RR50-
    Lumbar Vertebral 0SR20-
    Lumbosacral 0SR40-
    Thoracic Vertebral 0RR90-
    Thoracolumbar Vertebral 0RRB0-
  Duct
    Common Bile 0FR9-
    Cystic 0FR8-
    Hepatic
      Left 0FR6-
      Right 0FR5-
    Lacrimal
      Left 08RY-
      Right 08RX-
    Pancreatic 0FRD-
      Accessory 0FRF-
    Parotid
      Left 0CRC-
      Right 0CRB-
  Ear
    External
      Bilateral 09R2-
      Left 09R1-
      Right 09R0-
    Inner
      Left 09RE0-
      Right 09RD0-
    Middle
      Left 09R60-
      Right 09R50-
  Epiglottis 0CRR-
  Esophagus 0DR5-
  Eye
    Left 08R1-
    Right 08R0-
  Eyelid
    Lower
      Left 08RR-
      Right 08RQ-
    Upper
      Left 08RP-
      Right 08RN-
  Femoral Shaft
    Left 0QR9-
    Right 0QR8-
  Femur
    Lower
      Left 0QRC-
      Right 0QRB-
    Upper
      Left 0QR7-
      Right 0QR6-
  Fibula
    Left 0QRK-
    Right 0QRJ-
  Finger Nail 0HRQX-
  Gingiva
    Lower 0CR6-
    Upper 0CR5-
  Glenoid Cavity
    Left 0PR8-
    Right 0PR7-
  Hair 0HRSX-
  Humeral Head
    Left 0PRD-
    Right 0PRC-

Replacement — *continued*
Humeral Shaft
 Left **OPR**G-
 Right **OPR**F
Iris
 Left **08R**D3-
 Right **08R**C3-
Joint
 Acromioclavicular
  Left **ORR**H0-
  Right **ORR**G0-
 Ankle
  Left **OSR**G-
  Right **OSR**F-
 Carpal
  Left **ORR**R0-
  Right **ORR**Q0-
 Cervical Vertebral **ORR**10-
 Cervicothoracic Vertebral **ORR**40-
 Coccygeal **OSR**60-
 Elbow
  Left **ORR**M0-
  Right **ORR**L0-
 Finger Phalangeal
  Left **ORR**X0-
  Right **ORR**W0-
 Hip
  Left **OSR**B-
   Acetabular Surface **OSR**E-
   Femoral Surface **OSR**S-
  Right **OSR**9-
   Acetabular Surface **OSR**A-
   Femoral Surface **OSR**R-
 Knee
  Left **OSR**D-
   Femoral Surface **OSR**U-
   Tibial Surface **OSR**W-
  Right **OSR**C-
   Femoral Surface **OSR**T-
   Tibial Surface **OSR**V-
 Lumbar Vertebral **OSR**00-
 Lumbosacral **OSR**30-
 Metacarpocarpal
  Left **ORR**T0-
  Right **ORR**S0-
 Metacarpophalangeal
  Left **ORR**V0-
  Right **ORR**U0-
 Metatarsal-Phalangeal
  Left **OSR**N0-
  Right **OSR**M0-
 Metatarsal-Tarsal
  Left **OSR**L0-
  Right **OSR**K0-
 Occipital-cervical **ORR**00-
 Sacrococcygeal **OSR**50-
 Sacroiliac
  Left **OSR**80-
  Right **OSR**70-
 Shoulder
  Left **ORR**K-
  Right **ORR**J-
 Sternoclavicular
  Left **ORR**F0-
  Right **ORR**E0-
 Tarsal
  Left **OSR**J0-
  Right **OSR**H0-
 Temporomandibular
  Left **ORR**D0-
  Right **ORR**C0-
 Thoracic Vertebral **ORR**60-
 Thoracolumbar Vertebral **ORR**A0-
 Toe Phalangeal
  Left **OSR**Q0-
  Right **OSR**P0-
 Wrist
  Left **ORR**P0-
  Right **ORR**N0-

Replacement — *continued*
Kidney Pelvis
 Left **OTR**4-
 Right **OTR**3-
Larynx **OCR**S-
Lens
 Left **08R**K30Z
 Right **08R**J30Z
Lip
 Lower **OCR**1-
 Upper **OCR**0-
Mandible
 Left **ONR**V-
 Right **ONR**T-
Maxilla
 Left **ONR**S-
 Right **ONR**R-
Mesentery **ODR**V-
Metacarpal
 Left **OPR**Q-
 Right **OPR**P-
Metatarsal
 Left **OQR**P-
 Right **OQR**N-
Muscle, Papillary **02R**D-
Nasopharynx **09R**N-
Nipple
 Left **OHR**X-
 Right **OHR**W-
Nose **09R**K-
Omentum
 Greater **ODR**S-
 Lesser **ODR**T-
Orbit
 Left **ONR**Q-
 Right **ONR**P-
Palate
 Hard **OCR**2-
 Soft **OCR**3-
Patella
 Left **OQR**F-
 Right **OQR**D-
Pericardium **02R**N-
Peritoneum **ODR**W-
Phalanx
 Finger
  Left **OPR**V-
  Right **OPR**T-
 Thumb
  Left **OPR**S-
  Right **OPR**R-
 Toe
  Left **OQR**R-
  Right **OQR**Q-
Pharynx **OCR**M-
Radius
 Left **OPR**J-
 Right **OPR**H-
Retinal Vessel
 Left **08R**H3-
 Right **08R**G3-
Rib
 Left **OPR**2-
 Right **OPR**1-
Sacrum **OQR**1-
Scapula
 Left **OPR**6-
 Right **OPR**5-
Sclera
 Left **08R**7X-
 Right **08R**6X-
Septum
 Atrial **02R**5-
 Nasal **09R**M-
 Ventricular **02R**M-

Replacement — *continued*
Skin
 Abdomen **OHR**7-
 Back **OHR**6-
 Buttock **OHR**8-
 Chest **OHR**5-
 Ear
  Left **OHR**3-
  Right **OHR**2-
 Face **OHR**1-
 Foot
  Left **OHR**N-
  Right **OHR**M-
 Genitalia **OHR**A-
 Hand
  Left **OHR**G-
  Right **OHR**F-
 Lower Arm
  Left **OHR**E-
  Right **OHR**D-
 Lower Leg
  Left **OHR**L-
  Right **OHR**K-
 Neck **OHR**4-
 Perineum **OHR**9-
 Scalp **OHR**0-
 Upper Arm
  Left **OHR**C-
  Right **OHR**B-
 Upper Leg
  Left **OHR**J-
  Right **OHR**H-
Skin Substitute, Porcine Liver Derived **XHR**PXL2
Skull **ONR**0-
Sternum **OPR**0-
Subcutaneous Tissue and Fascia
 Abdomen **OJR**8-
 Back **OJR**7-
 Buttock **OJR**9-
 Chest **OJR**6-
 Face **OJR**1-
 Foot
  Left **OJR**R-
  Right **OJR**Q-
 Hand
  Left **OJR**K-
  Right **OJR**J-
 Lower Arm
  Left **OJR**H-
  Right **OJR**G-
 Lower Leg
  Left **OJR**P-
  Right **OJR**N-
 Neck
  Anterior **OJR**4-
  Posterior **OJR**5-
 Pelvic Region **OJR**C-
 Perineum **OJR**B-
 Scalp **OJR**0-
 Upper Arm
  Left **OJR**F-
  Right **OJR**D-
 Upper Leg
  Left **OJR**M-
  Right **OJR**L-
Tarsal
 Left **OQR**M-
 Right **OQR**L-
Tendon
 Abdomen
  Left **OLR**G-
  Right **OLR**F-
 Ankle
  Left **OLR**T-
  Right **OLR**S-
 Foot
  Left **OLR**W-
  Right **OLR**V-
 Hand
  Left **OLR**8-
  Right **OLR**7-

Replacement — *continued*
Tendon — *continued*
 Head and Neck **OLR**0-
 Hip
  Left **OLR**K-
  Right **OLR**J-
 Knee
  Left **OLR**R-
  Right **OLR**Q-
 Lower Arm and Wrist
  Left **OLR**6-
  Right **OLR**5-
 Lower Leg
  Left **OLR**P-
  Right **OLR**N-
 Perineum **OLR**H-
 Shoulder
  Left **OLR**2-
  Right **OLR**1-
 Thorax
  Left **OLR**D-
  Right **OLR**C-
 Trunk
  Left **OLR**B-
  Right **OLR**9-
 Upper Arm
  Left **OLR**4-
  Right **OLR**3-
 Upper Leg
  Left **OLR**M-
  Right **OLR**L-
Testis
 Bilateral **OVR**C0JZ
 Left **OVR**B0JZ
 Right **OVR**90JZ
Thumb
 Left **OXR**M-
 Right **OXR**L-
Tibia
 Left **OQR**H-
 Right **OQR**G-
Toe Nail **OHR**RX-
Tongue **OCR**7-
Tooth
 Lower **OCR**X-
 Upper **OCR**W-
Turbinate, Nasal **09R**L-
Tympanic Membrane
 Left **09R**8-
 Right **09R**7-
Ulna
 Left **OPR**L-
 Right **OPR**K-
Ureter
 Left **OTR**7-
 Right **OTR**6-
Urethra **OTR**D-
Uvula **OCR**N-
Valve
 Aortic **02R**F-
 Mitral **02R**G-
 Pulmonary **02R**H-
 Tricuspid **02R**J-
Vein
 Axillary
  Left **05R**8-
  Right **05R**7-
 Azygos **05R**0-
 Basilic
  Left **05R**C-
  Right **05R**B-
 Brachial
  Left **05R**A-
  Right **05R**9-
 Cephalic
  Left **05R**F-
  Right **05R**D-
 Colic **06R**7-
 Common Iliac
  Left **06R**D-
  Right **06R**C-

PROCEDURE INDEX

PROCEDURE INDEX

Reposition — continued
Ear
  Bilateral 09S2-
  Left 09S1-
  Right 09S0-
Epiglottis 0CSR-
Esophagus 0DS5-
Eustachian Tube
  Left 09SG-
  Right 09SF-
Eyelid
  Lower
    Left 08SR-
    Right 08SQ-
  Upper
    Left 08SP-
    Right 08SN-
Fallopian Tube
  Left 0US6-
  Right 0US5-
Fallopian Tubes, Bilateral 0US7-
Femoral Shaft
  Left 0QS9-
  Right 0QS8-
Femur
  Lower
    Left 0QSC-
    Right 0QSB-
  Upper
    Left 0QS7-
    Right 0QS6-
Fibula
  Left 0QSK-
  Right 0QSJ-
Gallbladder 0FS4-
Gland
  Adrenal
    Left 0GS2-
    Right 0GS3-
  Lacrimal
    Left 08SW-
    Right 08SV-
Glenoid Cavity
  Left 0PS8-
  Right 0PS7-
Hair 0HSSXZZ
Humeral Head
  Left 0PSD-
  Right 0PSC-
Humeral Shaft
  Left 0PSG-
  Right 0PSF-
Ileum 0DSB-
Iris
  Left 08SD3ZZ
  Right 08SC3ZZ
Jejunum 0DSA-
Joint
  Acromioclavicular
    Left 0RSH-
    Right 0RSG-
  Ankle
    Left 0SSG-
    Right 0SSF-
  Carpal
    Left 0RSR-
    Right 0RSQ-
  Cervical Vertebral 0RS1-
  Cervicothoracic Vertebral 0RS4-
  Coccygeal 0SS6-
  Elbow
    Left 0RSM-
    Right 0RSL-
  Finger Phalangeal
    Left 0RSX-
    Right 0RSW-
  Hip
    Left 0SSB-
    Right 0SS9-
  Knee
    Left 0SSD-
    Right 0SSC-

Reposition — continued
Joint — continued
  Lumbar Vertebral 0SS0-
  Lumbosacral 0SS3-
  Metacarpocarpal
    Left 0RST-
    Right 0RSS-
  Metacarpophalangeal
    Left 0RSV-
    Right 0RSU-
  Metatarsal-Phalangeal
    Left 0SSN-
    Right 0SSM-
  Metatarsal-Tarsal
    Left 0SSL-
    Right 0SSK-
  Occipital-cervical 0RS0-
  Sacrococcygeal 0SS5-
  Sacroiliac
    Left 0SS8-
    Right 0SS7-
  Shoulder
    Left 0RSK-
    Right 0RSJ-
  Sternoclavicular
    Left 0RSF-
    Right 0RSE-
  Tarsal
    Left 0SSJ-
    Right 0SSH-
  Temporomandibular
    Left 0RSD-
    Right 0RSC-
  Thoracic Vertebral 0RS6-
  Thoracolumbar Vertebral 0RSA-
  Toe Phalangeal
    Left 0SSQ-
    Right 0SSP-
  Wrist
    Left 0RSP-
    Right 0RSN-
Kidney
  Left 0TS1-
  Right 0TS0-
Kidney Pelvis
  Left 0TS4-
  Right 0TS3-
Kidneys, Bilateral 0TS2-
Lens
  Left 08SK3ZZ
  Right 08SJ3ZZ
Lip
  Lower 0CS1-
  Upper 0CS0-
Liver 0FS0-
Lung
  Left 0BSL0ZZ
  Lower Lobe
    Left 0BSJ0ZZ
    Right 0BSF0ZZ
  Middle Lobe, Right 0BSD0ZZ
  Right 0BSK0ZZ
  Upper Lobe
    Left 0BSG0ZZ
    Right 0BSC0ZZ
Lung Lingula 0BSH0ZZ
Mandible
  Left 0NSV-
  Right 0NST-
Maxilla
  Left 0NSS-
  Right 0NSR-
Metacarpal
  Left 0PSQ-
  Right 0PSP-
Metatarsal
  Left 0QSP-
  Right 0QSN-

Reposition — continued
Muscle
  Abdomen
    Left 0KSL-
    Right 0KSK-
  Extraocular
    Left 08SM-
    Right 08SL-
  Facial 0KS1-
  Foot
    Left 0KSW-
    Right 0KSV-
  Hand
    Left 0KSD-
    Right 0KSC-
  Head 0KS0-
  Hip
    Left 0KSP-
    Right 0KSN-
  Lower Arm and Wrist
    Left 0KSB-
    Right 0KS9-
  Lower Leg
    Left 0KST-
    Right 0KSS-
  Neck
    Left 0KS3-
    Right 0KS2-
  Perineum 0KSM-
  Shoulder
    Left 0KS6-
    Right 0KS5-
  Thorax
    Left 0KSJ-
    Right 0KSH-
  Tongue, Palate, Pharynx 0KS4-
  Trunk
    Left 0KSG-
    Right 0KSF-
  Upper Arm
    Left 0KS8-
    Right 0KS7-
  Upper Leg
    Left 0KSR-
    Right 0KSQ-
Nerve
  Abducens 00SL-
  Accessory 00SR-
  Acoustic 00SN-
  Brachial Plexus 01S3-
  Cervical 01S1-
  Cervical Plexus 01S0-
  Facial 00SM-
  Femoral 01SD-
  Glossopharyngeal 00SP-
  Hypoglossal 00SS-
  Lumbar 01SB-
  Lumbar Plexus 01S9-
  Lumbosacral Plexus 01SA-
  Median 01S5-
  Oculomotor 00SH-
  Olfactory 00SF-
  Optic 00SG-
  Peroneal 01SH-
  Phrenic 01S2-
  Pudendal 01SC-
  Radial 01S6-
  Sacral 01SR-
  Sacral Plexus 01SQ-
  Sciatic 01SF-
  Thoracic 01S8-
  Tibial 01SG-
  Trigeminal 00SK-
  Trochlear 00SJ-
  Ulnar 01S4-
  Vagus 00SQ-
Nipple
  Left 0HSXXZZ
  Right 0HSWXZZ
Nose 09SK-

Reposition — continued
Orbit
  Left 0NSQ-
  Right 0NSP-
Ovary
  Bilateral 0US2-
  Left 0US1-
  Right 0US0-
Palate
  Hard 0CS2-
  Soft 0CS3-
Pancreas 0FSG-
Parathyroid Gland 0GSR-
  Inferior
    Left 0GSP-
    Right 0GSN-
  Multiple 0GSQ-
  Superior
    Left 0GSM-
    Right 0GSL-
Patella
  Left 0QSF-
  Right 0QSD-
Phalanx
  Finger
    Left 0PSV-
    Right 0PST-
  Thumb
    Left 0PSS-
    Right 0PSR-
  Toe
    Left 0QSR-
    Right 0QSQ-
Products of Conception 10S0-
  Ectopic 10S2-
Radius
  Left 0PSJ-
  Right 0PSH-
Rectum 0DSP-
Retinal Vessel
  Left 08SH3ZZ
  Right 08SG3ZZ
Rib
  Left 0PS2-
  Right 0PS1-
Sacrum 0QS1-
Scapula
  Left 0PS6-
  Right 0PS5-
Septum, Nasal 09SM-
Skull 0NS0-
Spinal Cord
  Cervical 00SW-
  Lumbar 00SY-
  Thoracic 00SX-
Spleen 07SP0ZZ
Sternum 0PS0-
Stomach 0DS6-
Tarsal
  Left 0QSM-
  Right 0QSL-
Tendon
  Abdomen
    Left 0LSG-
    Right 0LSF-
  Ankle
    Left 0LST-
    Right 0LSS-
  Foot
    Left 0LSW-
    Right 0LSV-
  Hand
    Left 0LS8-
    Right 0LS7-
  Head and Neck 0LS0-
  Hip
    Left 0LSK-
    Right 0LSJ-
  Knee
    Left 0LSR-
    Right 0LSQ-

PROCEDURE INDEX

PROCEDURE INDEX

Reposition — continued
Tendon — continued
Lower Arm and Wrist
Left 0LS6-
Right 0LS5-
Lower Leg
Left 0LSP-
Right 0LSN-
Perineum 0LSH-
Shoulder
Left 0LS2-
Right 0LS1-
Thorax
Left 0LSD-
Right 0LSC-
Trunk
Left 0LSB-
Right 0LS9-
Upper Arm
Left 0LS4-
Right 0LS3-
Upper Leg
Left 0LSM-
Right 0LSL-
Testis
Bilateral 0VSC-
Left 0VSB-
Right 0VS9-
Thymus 07SM0ZZ
Thyroid Gland
Left Lobe 0GSG-
Right Lobe 0GSH-
Tibia
Left 0QSH-
Right 0QSG-
Tongue 0CS7-
Tooth
Lower 0CSX-
Upper 0CSW-
Trachea 0BS10ZZ
Turbinate, Nasal 09SL-
Tympanic Membrane
Left 09S8-
Right 09S7-
Ulna
Left 0PSL-
Right 0PSK-
Ureter
Left 0TS7-
Right 0TS6-
Ureters, Bilateral 0TS8-
Urethra 0TSD-
Uterine Supporting Structure 0US4-
Uterus 0US9-
Uvula 0CSN-
Vagina 0USG-
Vein
Axillary
Left 05S8-
Right 05S7-
Azygos 05S0-
Basilic
Left 05SC-
Right 05SB-
Brachial
Left 05SA-
Right 05S9-
Cephalic
Left 05SF-
Right 05SD-
Colic 06S7-
Common Iliac
Left 06SD-
Right 06SC-
Esophageal 06S3-
External Iliac
Left 06SG-
Right 06SF-
External Jugular
Left 05SQ-
Right 05SP-

Reposition — continued
Vein — continued
Face
Left 05SV-
Right 05ST-
Femoral
Left 06SN-
Right 06SM-
Foot
Left 06SV-
Right 06ST-
Gastric 06S2-
Greater Saphenous
Left 06SQ-
Right 06SP-
Hand
Left 05SH-
Right 05SG-
Hemiazygos 05S1-
Hepatic 06S4-
Hypogastric
Left 06SJ-
Right 06SH-
Inferior Mesenteric 06S6-
Innominate
Left 05S4-
Right 05S3-
Internal Jugular
Left 05SN-
Right 05SM-
Intracranial 05SL-
Lesser Saphenous
Left 06SS-
Right 06SR-
Lower 06SY-
Portal 06S8-
Pulmonary
Left 02ST0ZZ
Right 02SS0ZZ
Renal
Left 06SB-
Right 06S9-
Splenic 06S1-
Subclavian
Left 05S6-
Right 05S5-
Superior Mesenteric 06S5-
Upper 05SY-
Vertebral
Left 05SS-
Right 05SR-
Vena Cava
Inferior 06S0-
Superior 02SV0ZZ
Vertebra
Cervical 0PS3-
Magnetically Controlled Growth Rod(s) XNS3-
Lumbar 0QS0-
Magnetically Controlled Growth Rod(s) XNS0-
Thoracic 0PS4-
Magnetically Controlled Growth Rod(s) XNS4-
Vocal Cord
Left 0CSV-
Right 0CST-

Resection
Acetabulum
Left 0QT50ZZ
Right 0QT40ZZ
Adenoids 0CTQ-
Ampulla of Vater 0FTC-
Anal Sphincter 0DTR-
Anus 0DTQ-
Aortic Body 0GTD-
Appendix 0DTJ-
Auditory Ossicle
Left 09TA0ZZ
Right 09T90ZZ
Bladder 0TTB-
Bladder Neck 0TTC-

Resection — continued
Bone
Ethmoid
Left 0NTG0ZZ
Right 0NTF0ZZ
Frontal
Left 0NT20ZZ
Right 0NT10ZZ
Hyoid 0NTX0ZZ
Lacrimal
Left 0NTJ0ZZ
Right 0NTH0ZZ
Nasal 0NTB0ZZ
Occipital
Left 0NT80ZZ
Right 0NT70ZZ
Palatine
Left 0NTL0ZZ
Right 0NTK0ZZ
Parietal
Left 0NT40ZZ
Right 0NT30ZZ
Pelvic
Left 0QT30ZZ
Right 0QT20ZZ
Sphenoid
Left 0NTD0ZZ
Right 0NTC0ZZ
Temporal
Left 0NT60ZZ
Right 0NT50ZZ
Zygomatic
Left 0NTN0ZZ
Right 0NTM0ZZ
Breast
Bilateral 0HTV0ZZ
Left 0HTU0ZZ
Right 0HTT0ZZ
Supernumerary 0HTY0ZZ
Bronchus
Lingula 0BT9-
Lower Lobe
Left 0BTB-
Right 0BT6-
Main
Left 0BT7-
Right 0BT3-
Middle Lobe, Right 0BT5-
Upper Lobe
Left 0BT8-
Right 0BT4-
Bursa and Ligament
Abdomen
Left 0MTJ-
Right 0MTH-
Ankle
Left 0MTR-
Right 0MTQ-
Elbow
Left 0MT4-
Right 0MT3-
Foot
Left 0MTT-
Right 0MTS-
Hand
Left 0MT8-
Right 0MT7-
Head and Neck 0MT0-
Hip
Left 0MTM-
Right 0MTL-
Knee
Left 0MTP-
Right 0MTN-
Lower Extremity
Left 0MTW-
Right 0MTV-
Perineum 0MTK-
Shoulder
Left 0MT2-
Right 0MT1-

Resection — continued
Bursa and Ligament — continued
Thorax
Left 0MTG-
Right 0MTF-
Trunk
Left 0MTD-
Right 0MTC-
Upper Extremity
Left 0MTB-
Right 0MT9-
Wrist
Left 0MT6-
Right 0MT5-
Carina 0BT2-
Carotid Bodies, Bilateral 0GT8-
Carotid Body
Left 0GT6-
Right 0GT7-
Carpal
Left 0PTN0ZZ
Right 0PTM0ZZ
Cecum 0DTH-
Cerebral Hemisphere 00T7-
Cervix 0UTC-
Chordae Tendineae 02T9-
Cisterna Chyli 07TL-
Clavicle
Left 0PTB0ZZ
Right 0PT90ZZ
Clitoris 0UTJ-
Coccygeal Glomus 0GTB-
Coccyx 0QTS0ZZ
Colon
Ascending 0DTK-
Descending 0DTM-
Sigmoid 0DTN-
Transverse 0DTL-
Conduction Mechanism 02T8-
Cord
Bilateral 0VTH-
Left 0VTG-
Right 0VTF-
Cornea
Left 08T9XZZ
Right 08T8XZZ
Cul-de-sac 0UTF-
Diaphragm
Left 0BTS-
Right 0BTR-
Disc
Cervical Vertebral 0RT30ZZ
Cervicothoracic Vertebral 0RT50ZZ
Lumbar Vertebral 0ST20ZZ
Lumbosacral 0ST40ZZ
Thoracic Vertebral 0RT90ZZ
Thoracolumbar Vertebral 0RTB0ZZ
Duct
Common Bile 0FT9-
Cystic 0FT8-
Hepatic
Left 0FT6-
Right 0FT5-
Lacrimal
Left 08TY-
Right 08TX-
Pancreatic 0FTD-
Accessory 0FTF-
Parotid
Left 0CTC0ZZ
Right 0CTB0ZZ
Duodenum 0DT9-
Ear
External
Left 09T1-
Right 09T0-
Inner
Left 09TE0ZZ
Right 09TD0ZZ
Middle
Left 09T60ZZ
Right 09T50ZZ

Resection — *continued*
Epididymis
  Bilateral **0VTL**-
  Left **0VTK**-
  Right **0VTJ**-
Epiglottis **0CTR**-
Esophagogastric Junction **0DT4**-
Esophagus **0DT5**-
  Lower **0DT3**-
  Middle **0DT2**-
  Upper **0DT1**-
Eustachian Tube
  Left **09TG**-
  Right **09TF**-
Eye
  Left **08T1**XZZ
  Right **08T0**XZZ
Eyelid
  Lower
    Left **08TR**-
    Right **08TQ**-
  Upper
    Left **08TP**-
    Right **08TN**-
Fallopian Tube
  Left **0UT6**-
  Right **0UT5**-
Fallopian Tubes, Bilateral **0UT7**-
Femoral Shaft
  Left **0QT90**ZZ
  Right **0QT80**ZZ
Femur
  Lower
    Left **0QTC0**ZZ
    Right **0QTB0**ZZ
  Upper
    Left **0QT70**ZZ
    Right **0QT60**ZZ
Fibula
  Left **0QTK0**ZZ
  Right **0QTJ0**ZZ
Finger Nail **0HTQ**XZZ
Gallbladder **0FT4**-
Gland
  Adrenal
    Bilateral **0GT4**-
    Left **0GT2**-
    Right **0GT3**-
  Lacrimal
    Left **08TW**-
    Right **08TV**-
  Minor Salivary **0CTJ0**ZZ
  Parotid
    Left **0CT90**ZZ
    Right **0CT80**ZZ
  Pituitary **0GT0**-
  Sublingual
    Left **0CTF0**ZZ
    Right **0CTD0**ZZ
  Submaxillary
    Left **0CTH0**ZZ
    Right **0CTG0**ZZ
  Vestibular **0UTL**-
Glenoid Cavity
  Left **0PT80**ZZ
  Right **0PT70**ZZ
Glomus Jugulare **0GTC**-
Humeral Head
  Left **0PTD0**ZZ
  Right **0PTC0**ZZ
Humeral Shaft
  Left **0PTG0**ZZ
  Right **0PTF0**ZZ
Hymen **0UTK**-
Ileocecal Valve **0DTC**-
Ileum **0DTB**-
Intestine
  Large **0DTE**-
    Left **0DTG**-
    Right **0DTF**-
  Small **0DT8**-

Resection — *continued*
Iris
  Left **08TD3**ZZ
  Right **08TC3**ZZ
Jejunum **0DTA**-
Joint
  Acromioclavicular
    Left **0RTH0**ZZ
    Right **0RTG0**ZZ
  Ankle
    Left **0STG0**ZZ
    Right **0STF0**ZZ
  Carpal
    Left **0RTR0**ZZ
    Right **0RTQ0**ZZ
  Cervicothoracic Vertebral **0RT40**ZZ
  Coccygeal **0ST60**ZZ
  Elbow
    Left **0RTM0**ZZ
    Right **0RTL0**ZZ
  Finger Phalangeal
    Left **0RTX0**ZZ
    Right **0RTW0**ZZ
  Hip
    Left **0STB0**ZZ
    Right **0ST90**ZZ
  Knee
    Left **0STD0**ZZ
    Right **0STC0**ZZ
  Metacarpocarpal
    Left **0RTT0**ZZ
    Right **0RTS0**ZZ
  Metacarpophalangeal
    Left **0RTV0**ZZ
    Right **0RTU0**ZZ
  Metatarsal-Phalangeal
    Left **0STN0**ZZ
    Right **0STM0**ZZ
  Metatarsal-Tarsal
    Left **0STL0**ZZ
    Right **0STK0**ZZ
  Sacrococcygeal **0ST50**ZZ
  Sacroiliac
    Left **0ST80**ZZ
    Right **0ST70**ZZ
  Shoulder
    Left **0RTK0**ZZ
    Right **0RTJ0**ZZ
  Sternoclavicular
    Left **0RTF0**ZZ
    Right **0RTE0**ZZ
  Tarsal
    Left **0STJ0**ZZ
    Right **0STH0**ZZ
  Temporomandibular
    Left **0RTD0**ZZ
    Right **0RTC0**ZZ
  Toe Phalangeal
    Left **0STQ0**ZZ
    Right **0STP0**ZZ
  Wrist
    Left **0RTP0**ZZ
    Right **0RTN0**ZZ
Kidney
  Left **0TT1**-
  Right **0TT0**-
Kidney Pelvis
  Left **0TT4**-
  Right **0TT3**-
Kidneys, Bilateral **0TT2**-
Larynx **0CTS**-
Lens
  Left **08TK3**ZZ
  Right **08TJ3**ZZ
Lip
  Lower **0CT1**-
  Upper **0CT0**-
Liver **0FT0**-
  Left Lobe **0FT2**-
  Right Lobe **0FT1**-

Resection — *continued*
Lung
  Bilateral **0BTM**-
  Left **0BTL**-
  Lower Lobe
    Left **0BTJ**-
    Right **0BTF**-
  Middle Lobe, Right **0BTD**-
  Right **0BTK**-
  Upper Lobe
    Left **0BTG**-
    Right **0BTC**-
Lung Lingula **0BTH**-
Lymphatic
  Aortic **07TD**-
  Axillary
    Left **07T6**-
    Right **07T5**-
  Head **07T0**-
  Inguinal
    Left **07TJ**-
    Right **07TH**-
  Internal Mammary
    Left **07T9**-
    Right **07T8**-
  Lower Extremity
    Left **07TG**-
    Right **07TF**-
  Mesenteric **07TB**-
  Neck
    Left **07T2**-
    Right **07T1**-
  Pelvis **07TC**-
  Thoracic Duct **07TK**-
  Thorax **07T7**-
  Upper Extremity
    Left **07T4**-
    Right **07T3**-
Mandible
  Left **0NTV0**ZZ
  Right **0NTT0**ZZ
Maxilla
  Left **0NTS0**ZZ
  Right **0NTR0**ZZ
Metacarpal
  Left **0PTQ0**ZZ
  Right **0PTP0**ZZ
Metatarsal
  Left **0QTP0**ZZ
  Right **0QTN0**ZZ
Muscle
  Abdomen
    Left **0KTL**-
    Right **0KTK**-
  Extraocular
    Left **08TM**-
    Right **08TL**-
  Facial **0KT1**-
  Foot
    Left **0KTW**-
    Right **0KTV**-
  Hand
    Left **0KTD**-
    Right **0KTC**-
  Head **0KT0**-
  Hip
    Left **0KTP**-
    Right **0KTN**-
  Lower Arm and Wrist
    Left **0KTB**-
    Right **0KT9**-
  Lower Leg
    Left **0KTT**-
    Right **0KTS**-
  Neck
    Left **0KT3**-
    Right **0KT2**-
  Papillary **02TD**-
  Perineum **0KTM**-

Resection — *continued*
Muscle — *continued*
  Shoulder
    Left **0KT6**-
    Right **0KT5**-
  Thorax
    Left **0KTJ**-
    Right **0KTH**-
  Tongue, Palate, Pharynx **0KT4**-
  Trunk
    Left **0KTG**-
    Right **0KTF**-
  Upper Arm
    Left **0KT8**-
    Right **0KT7**-
  Upper Leg
    Left **0KTR**-
    Right **0KTQ**-
Nasopharynx **09TN**-
Nipple
  Left **0HTX**XZZ
  Right **0HTW**XZZ
Nose **09TK**-
Omentum
  Greater **0DTS**-
  Lesser **0DTT**-
Orbit
  Left **0NTQ0**ZZ
  Right **0NTP0**ZZ
Ovary
  Bilateral **0UT2**-
  Left **0UT1**-
  Right **0UT0**-
Palate
  Hard **0CT2**-
  Soft **0CT3**-
Pancreas **0FTG**-
Para-aortic Body **0GT9**-
Paraganglion Extremity **0GTF**-
Parathyroid Gland **0GTR**-
  Inferior
    Left **0GTP**-
    Right **0GTN**-
  Multiple **0GTQ**-
  Superior
    Left **0GTM**-
    Right **0GTL**-
Patella
  Left **0QTF0**ZZ
  Right **0QTD0**ZZ
Penis **0VTS**-
Pericardium **02TN**-
Phalanx
  Finger
    Left **0PTV0**ZZ
    Right **0PTT0**ZZ
  Thumb
    Left **0PTS0**ZZ
    Right **0PTR0**ZZ
  Toe
    Left **0QTR0**ZZ
    Right **0QTQ0**ZZ
Pharynx **0CTM**-
Pineal Body **0GT1**-
Prepuce **0VTT**-
Products of Conception, Ectopic **10T2**-
Prostate **0VT0**-
Radius
  Left **0PTJ0**ZZ
  Right **0PTH0**ZZ
Rectum **0DTP**-
Rib
  Left **0PT20**ZZ
  Right **0PT10**ZZ
Scapula
  Left **0PT60**ZZ
  Right **0PT50**ZZ
Scrotum **0VT5**-
Septum
  Atrial **02T5**-
  Nasal **09TM**-
  Ventricular **02TM**-

PROCEDURE INDEX

PROCEDURE INDEX

Resection — *continued*
Sinus
  Accessory **09T**P-
  Ethmoid
    Left **09T**V-
    Right **09T**U-
  Frontal
    Left **09T**T-
    Right **09T**S-
  Mastoid
    Left **09T**C-
    Right **09T**B-
  Maxillary
    Left **09T**R-
    Right **09T**Q-
  Sphenoid
    Left **09T**X-
    Right **09T**W-
Spleen **07T**P-
Sternum **0PT**00ZZ
Stomach **0DT**6-
  Pylorus **0DT**7-
Tarsal
  Left **0QT**M0ZZ
  Right **0QT**L0ZZ
Tendon
  Abdomen
    Left **0LT**G-
    Right **0LT**F-
  Ankle
    Left **0LT**T-
    Right **0LT**S-
  Foot
    Left **0LT**W-
    Right **0LT**V-
  Hand
    Left **0LT**8-
    Right **0LT**7-
  Head and Neck **0LT**0-
  Hip
    Left **0LT**K-
    Right **0LT**J-
  Knee
    Left **0LT**R-
    Right **0LT**Q-
  Lower Arm and Wrist
    Left **0LT**6-
    Right **0LT**5-
  Lower Leg
    Left **0LT**P-
    Right **0LT**N-
  Perineum **0LT**H-
  Shoulder
    Left **0LT**2-
    Right **0LT**1-
  Thorax
    Left **0LT**D-
    Right **0LT**C-
  Trunk
    Left **0LT**B-
    Right **0LT**9-
  Upper Arm
    Left **0LT**4-
    Right **0LT**3-
  Upper Leg
    Left **0LT**M-
    Right **0LT**L-
Testis
  Bilateral **0VT**C-
  Left **0VT**B-
  Right **0VT**9-
Thymus **07T**M-
Thyroid Gland **0GT**K-
  Left Lobe **0GT**G-
  Right Lobe **0GT**H-
Tibia
  Left **0QT**H0ZZ
  Right **0QT**G0ZZ
Toe Nail **0HT**RXZZ
Tongue **0CT**7-
Tonsils **0CT**P-

Resection — *continued*
Tooth
  Lower **0CT**X0Z-
  Upper **0CT**W0Z-
Trachea **0BT**1-
Tunica Vaginalis
  Left **0VT**7-
  Right **0VT**6-
Turbinate, Nasal **09T**L-
Tympanic Membrane
  Left **09T**8-
  Right **09T**7-
Ulna
  Left **0PT**L0ZZ
  Right **0PT**K0ZZ
Ureter
  Left **0TT**7-
  Right **0TT**6-
Urethra **0TT**D-
Uterine Supporting Structure **0UT**4-
Uterus **0UT**9-
Uvula **0CT**N-
Vagina **0UT**G-
Valve, Pulmonary **02T**H-
Vas Deferens
  Bilateral **0VT**Q-
  Left **0VT**P-
  Right **0VT**N-
Vesicle
  Bilateral **0VT**3-
  Left **0VT**2-
  Right **0VT**1-
Vitreous
  Left **08T**53ZZ
  Right **08T**43ZZ
Vocal Cord
  Left **0CT**V-
  Right **0CT**T-
Vulva **0UT**M-

Restoration, Cardiac, Single, Rhythm 5A2204Z
RestoreAdvanced neurostimulator (SureScan) (MRI Safe)
  use Stimulator Generator, Multiple Array Rechargeable in **0JH**-
RestoreSensor neurostimulator (SureScan) (MRI Safe)
  use Stimulator Generator, Multiple Array Rechargeable in **0JH**-
RestoreUltra neurostimulator (SureScan) (MRI Safe)
  use Stimulator Generator, Multiple Array Rechargeable in **0JH**-

Restriction
Ampulla of Vater **0FV**C-
Anus **0DV**Q-
Aorta
  Abdominal **04V**0-
    Intraluminal Device, Branched or Fenestrated **04V**0-
  Thoracic
    Ascending/Arch, Intraluminal Device, Branched or Fenestrated **02V**X-
    Descending, Intraluminal Device, Branched or Fenestrated **02V**W-
Artery
  Anterior Tibial
    Left **04V**Q-
    Right **04V**P-
  Axillary
    Left **03V**6-
    Right **03V**5-
  Brachial
    Left **03V**8-
    Right **03V**7-
  Celiac **04V**1-
  Colic
    Left **04V**7-
    Middle **04V**8-
    Right **04V**6-

Restriction — *continued*
Artery — *continued*
  Common Carotid
    Left **03V**J-
    Right **03V**H-
  Common Iliac
    Left, Intraluminal Device, Branched or Fenestrated **04V**D-
    Right, Intraluminal Device, Branched or Fenestrated **04V**C-
  External Carotid
    Left **03V**N-
    Right **03V**M-
  External Iliac
    Left **04V**J-
    Right **04V**H-
  Face **03V**R-
  Femoral
    Left **04V**L-
    Right **04V**K-
  Foot
    Left **04V**W-
    Right **04V**V-
  Gastric **04V**2-
  Hand
    Left **03V**F-
    Right **03V**D-
  Hepatic **04V**3-
  Inferior Mesenteric **04V**B-
  Innominate **03V**2-
  Internal Carotid
    Left **03V**L-
    Right **03V**K-
  Internal Iliac
    Left **04V**F-
    Right **04V**E-
  Internal Mammary
    Left **03V**1-
    Right **03V**0-
  Intracranial **03V**G-
  Lower **04V**Y-
  Peroneal
    Left **04V**U-
    Right **04V**T-
  Popliteal
    Left **04V**N-
    Right **04V**M-
  Posterior Tibial
    Left **04V**S-
    Right **04V**R-
  Pulmonary
    Left **02V**R-
    Right **02V**Q-
  Pulmonary Trunk **02V**P-
  Radial
    Left **03V**C-
    Right **03V**B-
  Renal
    Left **04V**A-
    Right **04V**9-
  Splenic **04V**4-
  Subclavian
    Left **03V**4-
    Right **03V**3-
  Superior Mesenteric **04V**5-
  Temporal
    Left **03V**T-
    Right **03V**S-
  Thyroid
    Left **03V**V-
    Right **03V**U-
  Ulnar
    Left **03V**A-
    Right **03V**9-
  Upper **03V**Y-
  Vertebral
    Left **03V**Q-
    Right **03V**P-

Restriction — *continued*
Bladder **0TV**B-
Bladder Neck **0TV**C-
Bronchus
  Lingula **0BV**9-
  Lower Lobe
    Left **0BV**B-
    Right **0BV**6-
  Main
    Left **0BV**7-
    Right **0BV**3-
  Middle Lobe, Right **0BV**5-
  Upper Lobe
    Left **0BV**8-
    Right **0BV**4-
Carina **0BV**2-
Cecum **0DV**H-
Cervix **0UV**C-
Cisterna Chyli **07V**L-
Colon
  Ascending **0DV**K-
  Descending **0DV**M-
  Sigmoid **0DV**N-
  Transverse **0DV**L-
Duct
  Common Bile **0FV**9-
  Cystic **0FV**8-
  Hepatic
    Left **0FV**6-
    Right **0FV**5-
  Lacrimal
    Left **08V**Y-
    Right **08V**X-
  Pancreatic **0FV**D-
    Accessory **0FV**F-
  Parotid
    Left **0CV**C-
    Right **0CV**B-
Duodenum **0DV**9-
Esophagogastric Junction **0DV**4-
Esophagus **0DV**5-
  Lower **0DV**3-
  Middle **0DV**2-
  Upper **0DV**1-
Heart **02V**A-
Ileocecal Valve **0DV**C-
Ileum **0DV**B-
Intestine
  Large **0DV**E-
    Left **0DV**G-
    Right **0DV**F-
  Small **0DV**8-
Jejunum **0DV**A-
Kidney Pelvis
  Left **0TV**4-
  Right **0TV**3-
Lymphatic
  Aortic **07V**D-
  Axillary
    Left **07V**6-
    Right **07V**5-
  Head **07V**0-
  Inguinal
    Left **07V**J-
    Right **07V**H-
  Internal Mammary
    Left **07V**9-
    Right **07V**8-
  Lower Extremity
    Left **07V**G-
    Right **07V**F-
  Mesenteric **07V**B-
  Neck
    Left **07V**2-
    Right **07V**1-
  Pelvis **07V**C-
  Thoracic Duct **07V**K-
  Thorax **07V**3-
  Upper Extremity
    Left **07V**4-
    Right **07V**3-

Restriction — *continued*
Rectum **0DV**P-
Stomach **0DV**6-
Pylorus **0DV**7-
Trachea **0BV**1-
Ureter
Left **0TV**7-
Right **0TV**6-
Urethra **0TV**D-
Vein
Axillary
Left **05V**8-
Right **05V**7-
Azygos **05V**0-
Basilic
Left **05V**C-
Right **05V**B-
Brachial
Left **05V**A-
Right **05V**9-
Cephalic
Left **05V**F-
Right **05V**D-
Colic **06V**7-
Common Iliac
Left **06V**D-
Right **06V**C-
Esophageal **06V**3-
External Iliac
Left **06V**G-
Right **06V**F-
External Jugular
Left **05V**Q-
Right **05V**P-
Face
Left **05V**V-
Right **05V**T-
Femoral
Left **06V**N-
Right **06V**M-
Foot
Left **06V**V-
Right **06V**T-
Gastric **06V**2-
Greater Saphenous
Left **06V**Q-
Right **06V**P-
Hand
Left **05V**H-
Right **05V**G-
Hemiazygos **05V**1-
Hepatic **06V**4-
Hypogastric
Left **06V**J-
Right **06V**H-
Inferior Mesenteric **06V**6-
Innominate
Left **05V**4-
Right **05V**3-
Internal Jugular
Left **05V**N-
Right **05V**M-
Intracranial **05V**L-
Lesser Saphenous
Left **06V**S-
Right **06V**R-
Lower **06V**Y-
Portal **06V**8-
Pulmonary
Left **02V**T-
Right **02V**S-
Renal
Left **06V**B-
Right **06V**9-
Splenic **06V**1-
Subclavian
Left **05V**6-
Right **05V**5-
Superior Mesenteric **06V**5-

Restriction — *continued*
Vein — *continued*
Upper **05V**Y-
Vertebral
Left **05V**S-
Right **05V**R-
Vena Cava
Inferior **06V**0-
Superior **02V**V-
Resurfacing Device
Removal of device from
Hip joint
Left **0SP**B0BZ
Right **0SP**90BZ
Revision of device in
Hip joint
Left **0SW**B0BZ
Right **0SW**90BZ
Supplement
Hip joint
Left **0SU**B0BZ
Acetabular Surface **0SU**E0BZ
Femoral Surface **0SU**S0BZ
Right **0SU**90BZ
Acetabular Surface **0SU**A0BZ
Femoral Surface **0SU**R0BZ
Resuscitation
Cardiopulmonary *see* Assistance, Cardiac **5A0**2-
Cardioversion **5A2**204Z
Defibrillation **5A2**204Z
Endotracheal intubation *see* Insertion of device in, Trachea **0BH**1-
External chest compression **5A1**2012
Pulmonary **5A1**9054
Resuture, Heart valve prosthesis
see Revision of device in, Heart and Great Vessels **02W**-
Retraining
Cardiac *see* Motor Treatment, Rehabilitation **F07**-
Vocational *see* Activities of Daily Living Treatment, Rehabilitation **F08**-
Retrogasserian rhizotomy *see* Division, Nerve, Trigeminal **008**K-
Retroperitoneal lymph node
use Lymphatic, Aortic
Retroperitoneal space
use Retroperitoneum
Retropharyngeal lymph node
use Lymphatic, Neck, Left
use Lymphatic, Neck, Right
Retropubic space
use Pelvic Cavity
Reveal (DX) (XT)
use Monitoring Device
Reverse total shoulder replacement *see* Replacement, Upper Joints **0RR**-
Reverse® Shoulder Prosthesis
use Synthetic Substitute, Reverse Ball and Socket in **0RR**-
Revision
Correcting a portion of existing device *see* Revision of device in
Removal of device without replacement *see* Removal of device from
Replacement of existing device *see* Removal of device from
see Root operation to place new device, e.g., Insertion, Replacement, Supplement
Revision of device in
Abdominal Wall **0WW**F-
Acetabulum
Left **0QW**5-
Right **0QW**4-
Anal Sphincter **0DW**R-
Anus **0DW**Q-

Revision of device in — *continued*
Artery
Lower **04W**Y-
Upper **03W**Y-
Auditory Ossicle
Left **09W**A-
Right **09W**9-
Back
Lower **0WW**L-
Upper **0WW**K-
Bladder **0TW**B-
Bone
Facial **0NW**W-
Lower **0QW**Y-
Nasal **0NW**B-
Pelvic
Left **0QW**3-
Right **0QW**2-
Upper **0PW**Y-
Bone Marrow **07W**T-
Brain **00W**0-
Breast
Left **0HW**U-
Right **0HW**T-
Bursa and Ligament
Lower **0MW**Y-
Upper **0MW**X-
Carpal
Left **0PW**N-
Right **0PW**M-
Cavity, Cranial **0WW**1-
Cerebral Ventricle **00W**6-
Chest Wall **0WW**8-
Cisterna Chyli **07W**L-
Clavicle
Left **0PW**B-
Right **0PW**9-
Coccyx **0QW**S-
Diaphragm **0BW**T-
Disc
Cervical Vertebral **0RW**3-
Cervicothoracic Vertebral **0RW**5-
Lumbar Vertebral **0SW**2-
Lumbosacral **0SW**4-
Thoracic Vertebral **0RW**9-
Thoracolumbar Vertebral **0RW**B-
Duct
Hepatobiliary **0FW**B-
Pancreatic **0FW**D-
Ear
Inner
Left **09W**E-
Right **09W**D-
Left **09W**J-
Right **09W**H-
Epididymis and Spermatic Cord **0VW**M-
Esophagus **0DW**5-
Extremity
Lower
Left **0YW**B-
Right **0YW**9-
Upper
Left **0XW**7-
Right **0XW**6-
Eye
Left **08W**1-
Right **08W**0-
Face **0WW**2-
Fallopian Tube **0UW**8-
Femoral Shaft
Left **0QW**9-
Right **0QW**8-
Femur
Lower
Left **0QW**C-
Right **0QW**B-
Upper
Left **0QW**7-
Right **0QW**6-

Revision of device in — *continued*
Fibula
Left **0QW**K-
Right **0QW**J-
Finger Nail **0HW**QX-
Gallbladder **0FW**4-
Gastrointestinal Tract **0WW**P-
Genitourinary Tract **0WW**R-
Gland
Adrenal **0GW**5-
Endocrine **0GW**S-
Pituitary **0GW**0-
Salivary **0CW**A-
Glenoid Cavity
Left **0PW**8-
Right **0PW**7-
Great Vessel **02W**Y-
Hair **0HW**SX-
Head **0WW**0-
Heart **02W**A-
Humeral Head
Left **0PW**D-
Right **0PW**C-
Humeral Shaft
Left **0PW**G-
Right **0PW**F-
Intestinal Tract
Lower **0DW**D-
Upper **0DW**0-
Intestine
Large **0DW**E-
Small **0DW**8-
Jaw
Lower **0WW**5-
Upper **0WW**4-
Joint
Acromioclavicular
Left **0RW**H-
Right **0RW**G-
Ankle
Left **0SW**G-
Right **0SW**F-
Carpal
Left **0RW**R-
Right **0RW**Q-
Cervical Vertebral **0RW**1-
Cervicothoracic Vertebral **0RW**4-
Coccygeal **0SW**6-
Elbow
Left **0RW**M-
Right **0RW**L-
Finger Phalangeal
Left **0RW**X-
Right **0RW**W-
Hip
Left **0SW**B-
Acetabular Surface **0SW**E-
Femoral Surface **0SW**S-
Right **0SW**9-
Acetabular Surface **0SW**A-
Femoral Surface **0SW**R-
Knee
Left **0SW**D-
Femoral Surface **0SW**U-
Tibial Surface **0SW**W-
Right **0SW**C-
Femoral Surface **0SW**T-
Tibial Surface **0SW**V-
Lumbar Vertebral **0SW**0-
Lumbosacral **0SW**3-
Metacarpocarpal
Left **0RW**T-
Right **0RW**S-
Metacarpophalangeal
Left **0RW**V-
Right **0RW**U-
Metatarsal-Phalangeal
Left **0SW**N-
Right **0SW**M-
Metatarsal-Tarsal
Left **0SW**L-
Right **0SW**K-

PROCEDURE INDEX

Revision of device in — *continued*
Joint — *continued*
  Occipital-cervical **0RW0-**
  Sacrococcygeal **0SW5-**
  Sacroiliac
    Left **0SW8-**
    Right **0SW7-**
  Shoulder
    Left **0RWK-**
    Right **0RWJ-**
  Sternoclavicular
    Left **0RWF-**
    Right **0RWE-**
  Tarsal
    Left **0SWJ-**
    Right **0SWH-**
  Temporomandibular
    Left **0RWD-**
    Right **0RWC-**
  Thoracic Vertebral **0RW6-**
  Thoracolumbar Vertebral **0RWA-**
  Toe Phalangeal
    Left **0SWQ-**
    Right **0SWP-**
  Wrist
    Left **0RWP-**
    Right **0RWN-**
Kidney **0TW5-**
Larynx **0CWS-**
Lens
  Left **08WK-**
  Right **08WJ-**
Liver **0FW0-**
Lung
  Left **0BWL-**
  Right **0BWK-**
Lymphatic **07WN-**
  Thoracic Duct **07WK-**
Mediastinum **0WWC-**
Mesentery **0DWV-**
Metacarpal
  Left **0PWQ-**
  Right **0PWP-**
Metatarsal
  Left **0QWP-**
  Right **0QWN-**
Mouth and Throat **0CWY-**
Muscle
  Extraocular
    Left **08WM-**
    Right **08WL-**
  Lower **0KWY-**
  Upper **0KWX-**
Neck **0WW6-**
Nerve
  Cranial **00WE-**
  Peripheral **01WY-**
Nose **09WK-**
Omentum **0DWU-**
Ovary **0UW3-**
Pancreas **0FWG-**
Parathyroid Gland **0GWR-**
Patella
  Left **0QWF-**
  Right **0QWD-**
Pelvic Cavity **0WWJ-**
Penis **0VWS-**
Pericardial Cavity **0WWD-**
Perineum
  Female **0WWN-**
  Male **0WWM-**
Peritoneal Cavity **0WWG-**
Peritoneum **0DWW-**

Revision of device in — *continued*
Phalanx
  Finger
    Left **0PWV-**
    Right **0PWT-**
  Thumb
    Left **0PWS-**
    Right **0PWR-**
  Toe
    Left **0QWR-**
    Right **0QWQ-**
Pineal Body **0GW1-**
Pleura **0BWQ-**
Pleural Cavity-
  Left **0WWB-**
  Right **0WW9-**
Prostate and Seminal Vesicles **0VW4-**
Radius
  Left **0PWJ-**
  Right **0PWH-**
Respiratory Tract **0WWQ-**
Retroperitoneum **0WWH-**
Rib
  Left **0PW2-**
  Right **0PW1-**
Sacrum **0QW1-**
Scapula
  Left **0PW6-**
  Right **0PW5-**
Scrotum and Tunica Vaginalis **0VW8-**
Septum
  Atrial **02W5-**
  Ventricular **02WM-**
Sinus **09WY-**
Skin **0HWPX-**
Skull **0NW0-**
Spinal Canal **00WU-**
Spinal Cord **00WV-**
Spleen **07WP-**
Sternum **0PW0-**
Stomach **0DW6-**
Subcutaneous Tissue and Fascia
  Head and Neck **0JWS-**
  Lower Extremity **0JWW-**
  Trunk **0JWT-**
  Upper Extremity **0JWV-**
Tarsal
  Left **0QWM-**
  Right **0QWL-**
Tendon
  Lower **0LWY-**
  Upper **0LWX-**
Testis **0VWD-**
Thymus **07WM-**
Thyroid Gland **0GWK-**
Tibia
  Left **0QWH-**
  Right **0QWG-**
Toe Nail **0HWRX-**
Trachea **0BW1-**
Tracheobronchial Tree **0BW0-**
Tympanic Membrane
  Left **09W8-**
  Right **09W7-**
Ulna
  Left **0PWL-**
  Right **0PWK-**
Ureter **0TW9-**
Urethra **0TWD-**
Uterus and Cervix **0UWD-**
Vagina and Cul-de-sac **0UWH-**
Valve
  Aortic **02WF-**
  Mitral **02WG-**
  Pulmonary **02WH-**
  Tricuspid **02WJ-**
Vas Deferens **0VWR-**
Vein
  Azygos **05W0-**
  Innominate
    Left **05W4-**
    Right **05W3-**
  Lower **06WY-**
  Upper **05WY-**

Revision of device in — *continued*
Vertebra
  Cervical **0PW3-**
  Lumbar **0QW0-**
  Thoracic **0PW4-**
Vulva **0UWM-**
Revo MRI™ SureScan® pacemaker
  use Pacemaker, Dual Chamber in **0JH-**
rhBMP-2
  use Recombinant Bone Morphogenetic Protein
Rheos® System device
  use Stimulator Generator in Subcutaneous Tissue and Fascia
Rheos® System lead
  use Stimulator Lead in Upper Arteries
Rhinopharynx
  use Nasopharynx
Rhinoplasty
  see Alteration, Nose **090K-**
  see Repair, Nose **09QK-**
  see Replacement, Nose **09RK-**
  see Supplement, Nose **09UK-**
Rhinorrhaphy *see* Repair, Nose **09QK-**
Rhinoscopy 09JKXZZ
Rhizotomy
  see Division, Central Nervous System **008-**
  see Division, Peripheral Nervous System **018-**
Rhomboid major muscle
  use Muscle, Trunk, Left
  use Muscle, Trunk, Right
Rhomboid minor muscle
  use Muscle, Trunk, Left
  use Muscle, Trunk, Right
Rhythm electrocardiogram *see* Measurement, Cardiac **4A02-**
Rhytidectomy *see* Face lift
Right ascending lumbar vein
  use Vein, Azygos
Right atrioventricular valve
  use Valve, Tricuspid
Right auricular appendix
  use Atrium, Right
Right colic vein
  use Vein, Colic
Right coronary sulcus
  use Heart, Right
Right gastric artery
  use Artery, Gastric
Right gastroepiploic vein
  use Vein, Superior Mesenteric
Right inferior phrenic vein
  use Vena Cava, Inferior
Right inferior pulmonary vein
  use Vein, Pulmonary, Right
Right jugular trunk
  use Lymphatic, Neck, Right
Right lateral ventricle
  use Cerebral Ventricle
Right lymphatic duct
  use Lymphatic, Neck, Right
Right ovarian vein
  use Vena Cava, Inferior
Right second lumbar vein
  use Vena Cava, Inferior
Right subclavian trunk
  use Lymphatic, Neck, Right
Right subcostal vein
  use Vein, Azygos
Right superior pulmonary vein
  use Vein, Pulmonary, Right
Right suprarenal vein
  use Vena Cava, Inferior
Right testicular vein
  use Vena Cava, Inferior
Rima glottidis
  use Larynx

Risorius muscle
  use Muscle, Facial
RNS System lead
  use Neurostimulator Lead in Central Nervous System
RNS system neurostimulator generator
  use Neurostimulator Generator in Head and Facial Bones
Robotic Assisted Procedure
  Extremity
    Lower **8E0Y-**
    Upper **8E0X-**
  Head and Neck Region **8E09-**
  Trunk Region **8E0W-**
Rotation of fetal head
  Forceps **10S07ZZ**
  Manual **10S0XZZ**
Round ligament of uterus
  use Uterine Supporting Structure
Round window
  use Ear, Inner, Left
  use Ear, Inner, Right
Roux-en-Y operation
  see Bypass, Gastrointestinal System **0D1-**
  see Bypass, Hepatobiliary System and Pancreas **0F1-**
Rupture
  Adhesions *see* Release
  Fluid collection *see* Drainage

S

Sacral ganglion
  use Nerve, Sacral Sympathetic
Sacral lymph node
  use Lymphatic, Pelvis
Sacral nerve modulation (SNM) lead
  use Stimulator Lead in Urinary System
Sacral neuromodulation lead
  use Stimulator Lead in Urinary System
Sacral splanchnic nerve
  use Nerve, Sacral Sympathetic
Sacrectomy *see* Excision, Lower Bones **0QB-**
Sacrococcygeal ligament
  use Bursa and Ligament, Trunk, Left
  use Bursa and Ligament, Trunk, Right
Sacrococcygeal symphysis
  use Joint, Sacrococcygeal
Sacroiliac ligament
  use Bursa and Ligament, Trunk, Left
  use Bursa and Ligament, Trunk, Right
Sacrospinous ligament
  use Bursa and Ligament, Trunk, Left
  use Bursa and Ligament, Trunk, Right
Sacrotuberous ligament
  use Bursa and Ligament, Trunk, Left
  use Bursa and Ligament, Trunk, Right
Salpingectomy
  see Excision, Female Reproductive System **0UB-**
  see Resection, Female Reproductive System **0UT-**
Salpingolysis *see* Release, Female Reproductive System **0UN-**
Salpingopexy
  see Repair, Female Reproductive System **0UQ-**
  see Reposition, Female Reproductive System **0US-**
Salpingopharyngeus muscle
  use Muscle, Tongue, Palate, Pharynx
Salpingoplasty
  see Repair, Female Reproductive System **0UQ-**
  see Supplement, Female Reproductive System **0UU-**
Salpingorrhaphy *see* Repair, Female Reproductive System **0UQ-**
Salpingoscopy 0UJ88ZZ
Salpingostomy *see* Drainage, Female Reproductive System **0U9-**
Salpingotomy *see* Drainage, Female Reproductive System **0U9-**
Salpinx
  use Fallopian Tube, Left
  use Fallopian Tube, Right
Saphenous nerve
  use Nerve, Femoral
SAPIEN transcatheter aortic valve
  use Zooplastic Tissue in Heart and Great Vessels
Sartorius muscle
  use Muscle, Upper Leg, Left
  use Muscle, Upper Leg, Right
Scalene muscle
  use Muscle, Neck, Left
  use Muscle, Neck, Right
Scan
  Computerized Tomography (CT) *see* Computerized Tomography (CT Scan)
  Radioisotope *see* Planar Nuclear Medicine Imaging

Scaphoid bone
  use Carpal, Left
  use Carpal, Right
Scapholunate ligament
  use Bursa and Ligament, Hand, Left
  use Bursa and Ligament, Hand, Right
Scaphotrapezium ligament
  use Bursa and Ligament, Hand, Left
  use Bursa and Ligament, Hand, Right
Scapulectomy
  see Excision, Upper Bones **0PB-**
  see Resection, Upper Bones **0PT-**
Scapulopexy
  see Repair, Upper Bones **0PQ-**
  see Reposition, Upper Bones **0PS-**
Scarpa's (vestibular) ganglion
  use Nerve, Acoustic
Sclerectomy *see* Excision, Eye **08B-**
Sclerotherapy, mechanical *see* Destruction
Sclerotomy *see* Drainage, Eye **089-**
Scrotectomy
  see Excision, Male Reproductive System **0VB-**
  see Resection, Male Reproductive System **0VT-**
Scrotoplasty
  see Repair, Male Reproductive System **0VQ-**
  see Supplement, Male Reproductive System **0VU-**
Scrotorrhaphy *see* Repair, Male Reproductive System **0VQ-**
Scrototomy *see* Drainage, Male Reproductive System **0V9-**
Sebaceous gland
  use Skin
Second cranial nerve
  use Nerve, Optic
Section, cesarean *see* Extraction, Pregnancy **10D-**
Secura (DR) (VR)
  use Defibrillator Generator in **0JH-**
Sella Turcica
  use Bone, Sphenoid, Left
  use Bone, Sphenoid, Right
Semicircular canal
  use Ear, Inner, Left
  use Ear, Inner, Right
Semimembranosus muscle
  use Muscle, Upper Leg, Left
  use Muscle, Upper Leg, Right
Semitendinosus muscle
  use Muscle, Upper Leg, Left
  use Muscle, Upper Leg, Right
Seprafilm
  use Adhesion Barrier
Septal cartilage
  use Septum, Nasal
Septectomy
  see Excision, Ear, Nose, Sinus **09B-**
  see Excision, Heart and Great Vessels **02B-**
  see Resection, Ear, Nose, Sinus **09T-**
  see Resection, Heart and Great Vessels **02T-**
Septoplasty
  see Repair, Ear, Nose, Sinus **09Q-**
  see Repair, Heart and Great Vessels **02Q-**
  see Replacement, Ear, Nose, Sinus **09R-**
  see Replacement, Heart and Great Vessels **02R-**
  see Reposition, Ear, Nose, Sinus **09S-**
  see Supplement, Ear, Nose, Sinus **09U-**
  see Supplement, Heart and Great Vessels **02U-**

Septotomy *see* Drainage, Ear, Nose, Sinus **099-**
Sequestrectomy, bone *see* Extirpation
Serratus anterior muscle
  use Muscle, Thorax, Left
  use Muscle, Thorax, Right
Serratus posterior muscle
  use Muscle, Trunk, Left
  use Muscle, Trunk, Right
Seventh cranial nerve
  use Nerve, Facial
Sheffield hybrid external fixator
  use External Fixation Device, Hybrid in **0PH-**
  use External Fixation Device, Hybrid in **0PS-**
  use External Fixation Device, Hybrid in **0QH-**
  use External Fixation Device, Hybrid in **0QS-**
Sheffield ring external fixator
  use External Fixation Device, Ring in **0PH-**
  use External Fixation Device, Ring in **0PS-**
  use External Fixation Device, Ring in **0QH-**
  use External Fixation Device, Ring in **0QS-**
Shirodkar cervical cerclage 0UVC7ZZ
Shock Wave Therapy, Musculoskeletal 6A93-
Short gastric artery
  use Artery, Splenic
Shortening
  see Excision
  see Repair
  see Reposition
Shunt creation *see* Bypass
Sialoadenectomy
  Complete *see* Resection, Mouth and Throat **0CT-**
  Partial *see* Excision, Mouth and Throat **0CB-**
Sialodochoplasty
  see Repair, Mouth and Throat **0CQ-**
  see Replacement, Mouth and Throat **0CR-**
  see Supplement, Mouth and Throat **0CU-**
Sialoectomy
  see Excision, Mouth and Throat **0CB-**
  see Resection, Mouth and Throat **0CT-**
Sialography *see* Plain Radiography, Ear, Nose, Mouth and Throat **B90-**
Sialolithotomy *see* Extirpation, Mouth and Throat **0CC-**
Sigmoid artery
  use Artery, Inferior Mesenteric
Sigmoid flexure
  use Colon, Sigmoid
Sigmoid vein
  use Vein, Inferior Mesenteric
Sigmoidectomy
  see Excision, Gastrointestinal System **0DB-**
  see Resection, Gastrointestinal System **0DT-**
Sigmoidorrhaphy *see* Repair, Gastrointestinal System **0DQ-**
Sigmoidoscopy 0DJD8ZZ
Sigmoidotomy *see* Drainage, Gastrointestinal System **0D9-**

Single lead pacemaker (atrium) (ventricle)
  use Pacemaker, Single Chamber in **0JH-**
Single lead rate responsive pacemaker (atrium) (ventricle)
  use Pacemaker, Single Chamber Rate Responsive in **0JH-**
Sinoatrial node
  use Conduction Mechanism
Sinogram
  Abdominal Wall *see* Fluoroscopy, Abdomen and Pelvis **BW11-**
  Chest Wall *see* Plain Radiography, Chest **BW03-**
  Retroperitoneum *see* Fluoroscopy, Abdomen and Pelvis **BW11-**
Sinus venosus
  use Atrium, Right
Sinusectomy
  see Excision, Ear, Nose, Sinus **09B-**
  see Resection, Ear, Nose, Sinus **09T-**
Sinusoscopy 09JY4ZZ
Sinusotomy *see* Drainage, Ear, Nose, Sinus **099-**
Sirolimus-eluting coronary stent
  use Intraluminal Device, Drug-eluting in Heart and Great Vessels
Sixth cranial nerve
  use Nerve, Abducens
Size reduction, breast *see* Excision, Skin and Breast **0HB-**
SJM Biocor® Stented Valve System
  use Zooplastic Tissue in Heart and Great Vessels
Skene's (paraurethral) gland
  use Gland, Vestibular
Skin substitute, porcine liver derived, replacement XHRPXL2
Sling
  Fascial, orbicularis muscle (mouth) *see* Supplement, Muscle, Facial **0KU1-**
  Levator muscle, for urethral suspension *see* Reposition, Bladder Neck **0TSC-**
  Pubococcygeal, for urethral suspension *see* Reposition, Bladder Neck **0TSC-**
  Rectum *see* Reposition, Rectum **0DSP-**
Small bowel series *see* Fluoroscopy, Bowel, Small **BD13-**
Small saphenous vein
  use Vein, Lesser Saphenous, Left
  use Vein, Lesser Saphenous, Right
Snaring, polyp, colon *see* Excision, Gastrointestinal System **0DB-**
Solar (celiac) plexus
  use Nerve, Abdominal Sympathetic
Soleus muscle
  use Muscle, Lower Leg, Left
  use Muscle, Lower Leg, Right
Spacer
  Insertion of device in
    Disc
      Lumbar Vertebral **0SH2-**
      Lumbosacral **0SH4-**
    Joint
      Acromioclavicular
        Left **0RHH-**
        Right **0RHG-**
      Ankle
        Left **0SHG-**
        Right **0SHF-**
      Carpal
        Left **0RHR-**
        Right **0RHQ-**

PROCEDURE INDEX

Spacer — *continued*
Insertion of device in — *continued*
Joint — *continued*
Cervical Vertebral **0RH**1-
Cervicothoracic Vertebral **0RH**4-
Coccygeal **0SH**6-
Elbow
Left **0RH**M-
Right **0RH**L-
Finger Phalangeal
Left **0RH**X-
Right **0RH**W-
Hip
Left **0SH**B-
Right **0SH**9-
Knee
Left **0SH**D-
Right **0SH**C-
Lumbar Vertebral **0SH**0-
Lumbosacral **0SH**3-
Metacarpocarpal
Left **0RH**T-
Right **0RH**S-
Metacarpophalangeal
Left **0RH**V-
Right **0RH**U-
Metatarsal-Phalangeal
Left **0SH**N-
Right **0SH**M-
Metatarsal-Tarsal
Left **0SH**L-
Right **0SH**K-
Occipital-cervical **0RH**0-
Sacrococcygeal **0SH**5-
Sacroiliac
Left **0SH**8-
Right **0SH**7-
Shoulder
Left **0RH**K-
Right **0RH**J-
Sternoclavicular
Left **0RH**F-
Right **0RH**E-
Tarsal
Left **0SH**J-
Right **0SH**H-
Temporomandibular
Left **0RH**D-
Right **0RH**C-
Thoracic Vertebral **0RH**6-
Thoracolumbar Vertebral **0RH**A-
Toe Phalangeal
Left **0SH**Q-
Right **0SH**P-
Wrist
Left **0RH**P-
Right **0RH**N-
Removal of device from
Acromioclavicular
Left **0RP**H-
Right **0RP**G-
Ankle
Left **0SP**G-
Right **0SP**F-
Carpal
Left **0RP**R-
Right **0RP**Q-
Cervical Vertebral **0RP**1-
Cervicothoracic Vertebral **0RP**4-
Coccygeal **0SP**6-
Elbow
Left **0RP**M -
Right **0RP**L-
Finger Phalangeal
Left **0RP**X-
Right **0RP**W-
Hip
Left **0SP**B-
Right **0SP**9-

Spacer — *continued*
Removal of device from — *continued*
Knee
Left **0SP**D-
Right **0SP**C-
Lumbar Vertebral **0SP**0-
Lumbosacral **0SP**3-
Metacarpocarpal
Left **0RP**T-
Right **0RP**S-
Metacarpophalangeal
Left **0RP**V-
Right **0RP**U-
Metatarsal-Phalangeal
Left **0SP**N-
Right **0SP**M-
Metatarsal-Tarsal
Left **0SP**L-
Right **0SP**K-
Occipital-cervical **0RP**0-
Sacrococcygeal **0SP**5-
Sacroiliac
Left **0SP**8-
Right **0SP**7-
Shoulder
Left **0RP**K-
Right **0RP**J-
Sternoclavicular
Left **0RP**F-
Right **0RP**E-
Tarsal
Left **0SP**J-
Right **0SP**H-
Temporomandibular
Left **0RP**D-
Right **0RP**C-
Thoracic Vertebral **0RP**6-
Thoracolumbar Vertebral **0RP**A-
Toe Phalangeal
Left **0SP**Q-
Right **0SP**P-
Wrist
Left **0RP**P-
Right **0RP**N-
Revision of device in
Acromioclavicular
Left **0RW**H-
Right **0RW**G-
Ankle
Left **0SW**G-
Right **0SW**F-
Carpal
Left **0RW**R-
Right **0RW**Q-
Cervical Vertebral **0RW**1-
Cervicothoracic Vertebral **0RW**4-
Coccygeal **0SW**6-
Elbow
Left **0RW**M-
Right **0RW**L-
Finger Phalangeal
Left **0RW**X-
Right **0RW**W-
Hip
Left **0SW**B-
Right **0SW**9-
Knee
Left **0SW**D-
Right **0SW**C-
Lumbar Vertebral **0SW**0-
Lumbosacral **0SW**3-
Metacarpocarpal
Left **0RW**T-
Right **0RW**S-

Spacer — *continued*
Revision of device in — *continued*
Metacarpophalangeal
Left **0RW**V-
Right **0RW**U-
Metatarsal-Phalangeal
Left **0SW**N-
Right **0SW**M-
Metatarsal-Tarsal
Left **0SW**L-
Right **0SW**K-
Occipital-cervical **0RW**0-
Sacrococcygeal **0SW**5-
Sacroiliac
Left **0SW**8-
Right **0SW**7-
Shoulder
Left **0RW**K-
Right **0RW**J-
Sternoclavicular
Left **0RW**F-
Right **0RW**E-
Tarsal
Left **0SW**J-
Right **0SW**H-
Temporomandibular
Left **0RW**D-
Right **0RW**C-
Thoracic Vertebral **0RW**6-
Thoracolumbar Vertebral **0RW**A-
Toe Phalangeal
Left **0SW**Q-
Right **0SW**P-
Wrist
Left **0RW**P-
Right **0RW**N-
Spectroscopy
Intravascular **8E0**23DZ
Near infrared **8E0**23DZ
Speech Assessment F00-
Speech therapy *see* Speech
Treatment, Rehabilitation **F06**-
Speech Treatment F06-
Sphenoidectomy
see Excision, Ear, Nose, Sinus **09B**-
see Excision, Head and Facial Bones **0NB**-
see Resection, Ear, Nose, Sinus **09T**-
see Resection, Head and Facial Bones **0NT**-
Sphenoidotomy *see* Drainage, Ear, Nose, Sinus **099**-
Sphenomandibular ligament
use Bursa and Ligament, Head and Neck
Sphenopalatine (pterygopalatine) ganglion
use Nerve, Head and Neck Sympathetic
Sphincterorrhaphy, anal *see* Repair, Anal Sphincter **0DQR**-
Sphincterotomy, anal
see Division, Anal Sphincter **0D8R**-
see Drainage, Anal Sphincter **0D9R**-
Spinal cord neurostimulator lead
use Neurostimulator Lead in Central Nervous System
Spinal growth rods, magnetically controlled
use Magnetically Controlled Growth Rod(s) in New Technology
Spinal nerve, cervical
use Nerve, Cervical
Spinal nerve, lumbar
use Nerve, Lumbar
Spinal nerve, sacral
use Nerve, Sacral
Spinal nerve, thoracic
use Nerve, Thoracic

Spinal Stabilization Device
Facet Replacement
Cervical Vertebral **0RH**1-
Cervicothoracic Vertebral **0RH**4-
Lumbar Vertebral **0SH**0-
Lumbosacral **0SH**3-
Occipital-cervical **0RH**0-
Thoracic Vertebral **0RH**6-
Thoracolumbar Vertebral **0RH**A-
Interspinous Process
Cervical Vertebral **0RH**1-
Cervicothoracic Vertebral **0RH**4-
Lumbar Vertebral **0SH**0-
Lumbosacral **0SH**3-
Occipital-cervical **0RH**0-
Thoracic Vertebral **0RH**6-
Thoracolumbar Vertebral **0RH**A-
Pedicle-Based
Cervical Vertebral **0RH**1-
Cervicothoracic Vertebral **0RH**4-
Lumbar Vertebral **0SH**0-
Lumbosacral **0SH**3-
Occipital-cervical **0RH**0-
Thoracic Vertebral **0RH**6-
Thoracolumbar Vertebral **0RH**A-
Spinous process
use Vertebra, Cervical
use Vertebra, Lumbar
use Vertebra, Thoracic
Spiral ganglion
use Nerve, Acoustic
Spiration IBV™ Valve System
use Intraluminal Device, Endobronchial Valve in Respiratory System
Splenectomy
see Excision, Lymphatic and Hemic Systems **07B**-
see Resection, Lymphatic and Hemic Systems **07T**-
Splenic flexure
use Colon, Transverse
Splenic plexus
use Nerve, Abdominal Sympathetic
Splenius capitis muscle
use Muscle, Head
Splenius cervicis muscle
use Muscle, Neck, Left
use Muscle, Neck, Right
Splenolysis *see* Release, Lymphatic and Hemic Systems **07N**-
Splenopexy
see Repair, Lymphatic and Hemic Systems **07Q**-
see Reposition, Lymphatic and Hemic Systems **07S**-
Splenoplasty *see* Repair, Lymphatic and Hemic Systems **07Q**-
Splenorrhaphy *see* Repair, Lymphatic and Hemic Systems **07Q**-
Splenotomy *see* Drainage, Lymphatic and Hemic Systems **079**-
Splinting, musculoskeletal *see* Immobilization, Anatomical Regions **2W3**-
SPY system intravascular fluorescence angiography *see* Monitoring, Physiological Systems **4A1**-
Stapedectomy
see Excision, Ear, Nose, Sinus **09B**-
see Resection, Ear, Nose, Sinus **09T**-
Stapediolysis *see* Release, Ear, Nose, Sinus **09N**-
Stapedioplasty
see Repair, Ear, Nose, Sinus **09Q**-
see Replacement, Ear, Nose, Sinus **09R**-
see Supplement, Ear, Nose, Sinus **09U**-

Stapedotomy *see* Drainage, Ear, Nose, Sinus **099-**

Stapes
  use Auditory Ossicle, Left
  use Auditory Ossicle, Right

Stellate ganglion
  use Nerve, Head and Neck Sympathetic

Stem cell transplant *see* Transfusion, Circulatory **302-**

Stensen's duct
  use Duct, Parotid, Left
  use Duct, Parotid, Right

Stent, intraluminal (cardiovascular) (gastrointestinal) (hepatobiliary) (urinary)
  use Intraluminal Device

Stented tissue valve
  use Zooplastic Tissue in Heart and Great Vessels

Stereotactic Radiosurgery
Abdomen **DW23-**
Adrenal Gland **DG22-**
Bile Ducts **DF22-**
Bladder **DT22-**
Bone Marrow **D720-**
Brain **D020-**
Brain Stem **D021-**
Breast
  Left **DM20-**
  Right **DM21-**
Bronchus **DB21-**
Cervix **DU21-**
Chest **DW22-**
Chest Wall **DB27-**
Colon **DD25-**
Diaphragm **DB28-**
Duodenum **DD22-**
Ear **D920-**
Esophagus **DD20-**
Eye **D820-**
Gallbladder **DF21-**
Gamma Beam
  Abdomen **DW23JZZ**
  Adrenal Gland **DG22JZZ**
  Bile Ducts **DF22JZZ**
  Bladder **DT22JZZ**
  Bone Marrow **D720JZZ**
  Brain **D020JZZ**
  Brain Stem **D021JZZ**
  Breast
    Left **DM20JZZ**
    Right **DM21JZZ**
  Bronchus **DB21JZZ**
  Cervix **DU21JZZ**
  Chest **DW22JZZ**
  Chest Wall **DB27JZZ**
  Colon **DD25JZZ**
  Diaphragm **DB28JZZ**
  Duodenum **DD22JZZ**
  Ear **D920JZZ**
  Esophagus **DD20JZZ**
  Eye **D820JZZ**
  Gallbladder **DF21JZZ**
  Gland
    Adrenal **DG22JZZ**
    Parathyroid **DG24JZZ**
    Pituitary **DG20JZZ**
    Thyroid **DG25JZZ**
  Glands, Salivary **D926JZZ**
  Head and Neck **DW21JZZ**
  Ileum **DD24JZZ**
  Jejunum **DD23JZZ**
  Kidney **DT20JZZ**
  Larynx **D92BJZZ**
  Liver **DF20JZZ**
  Lung **DB22JZZ**

Stereotactic Radiosurgery — *continued*
Gamma Beam — *continued*
  Lymphatics
    Abdomen **D726JZZ**
    Axillary **D724JZZ**
    Inguinal **D728JZZ**
    Neck **D723JZZ**
    Pelvis **D727JZZ**
    Thorax **D725JZZ**
  Mediastinum **DB26JZZ**
  Mouth **D924JZZ**
  Nasopharynx **D92DJZZ**
  Neck and Head **DW21JZZ**
  Nerve, Peripheral **D027JZZ**
  Nose **D921JZZ**
  Ovary **DU20JZZ**
  Palate
    Hard **D928JZZ**
    Soft **D929JZZ**
  Pancreas **DF23JZZ**
  Parathyroid Gland **DG24JZZ**
  Pelvic Region **DW26JZZ**
  Pharynx **D92CJZZ**
  Pineal Body **DG21JZZ**
  Pituitary Gland **DG20JZZ**
  Pleura **DB25JZZ**
  Prostate **DV20JZZ**
  Rectum **DD27JZZ**
  Sinuses **D927JZZ**
  Spinal Cord **D026JZZ**
  Spleen **D722JZZ**
  Stomach **DD21JZZ**
  Testis **DV21JZZ**
  Thymus **D721JZZ**
  Thyroid Gland **DG25JZZ**
  Tongue **D925JZZ**
  Trachea **DB20JZZ**
  Ureter **DT21JZZ**
  Urethra **DT23JZZ**
  Uterus **DU22JZZ**
Gland
  Adrenal **DG22-**
  Parathyroid **DG24-**
  Pituitary **DG20-**
  Thyroid **DG25-**
Glands, Salivary **D926-**
Head and Neck **DW21-**
Ileum **DD24-**
Jejunum **DD23-**
Kidney **DT20-**
Larnyx **D92B-**
Liver **DF20-**
Lung **DB22-**
Lymphatics
  Abdomen **D726-**
  Axillary **D724-**
  Inguinal **D728-**
  Neck **D723-**
  Pelvis **D727-**
  Thorax **D725-**
Mediastinum **DB26-**
Mouth **D924-**
Nasopharynx **D92D-**
Neck and Head **DW21-**
Nerve, Peripheral **D027-**
Nose **D921-**
Other Photon
  Abdomen **DW23DZZ**
  Adrenal Gland **DG22DZZ**
  Bile Ducts **DF22DZZ**
  Bladder **DT22DZZ**
  Bone Marrow **D720DZZ**
  Brain **D020DZZ**
  Brain Stem **D021DZZ**
  Breast
    Left **DM20DZZ**
    Right **DM21DZZ**
  Bronchus **DB21DZZ**
  Cervix **DU21DZZ**
  Chest **DW22DZZ**
  Chest Wall **DB27DZZ**
  Colon **DD25DZZ**

Stereotactic Radiosurgery — *continued*
Other Photon — *continued*
  Diaphragm **DB28DZZ**
  Duodenum **DD22DZZ**
  Ear **D920DZZ**
  Esophagus **DD20DZZ**
  Eye **D820DZZ**
  Gallbladder **DF21DZZ**
  Gland
    Adrenal **DG22DZZ**
    Parathyroid **DG24DZZ**
    Pituitary **DG20DZZ**
    Thyroid **DG25DZZ**
  Glands, Salivary **D926DZZ**
  Head and Neck **DW21DZZ**
  Ileum **DD24DZZ**
  Jejunum **DD23DZZ**
  Kidney **DT20DZZ**
  Larynx **D92BDZZ**
  Liver **DF20DZZ**
  Lung **DB22DZZ**
  Lymphatics
    Abdomen **D726DZZ**
    Axillary **D724DZZ**
    Inguinal **D728DZZ**
    Neck **D723DZZ**
    Pelvis **D727DZZ**
    Thorax **D725DZZ**
  Mediastinum **DB26DZZ**
  Mouth **D924DZZ**
  Nasopharynx **D92DDZZ**
  Neck and Head **DW21DZZ**
  Nerve, Peripheral **D027DZZ**
  Nose **D921DZZ**
  Ovary **DU20DZZ**
  Palate
    Hard **D928DZZ**
    Soft **D929DZZ**
  Pancreas **DF23DZZ**
  Parathyroid Gland **DG24DZZ**
  Pelvic Region **DW26DZZ**
  Pharynx **D92CDZZ**
  Pineal Body **DG21DZZ**
  Pituitary Gland **DG20DZZ**
  Pleura **DB25DZZ**
  Prostate **DV20DZZ**
  Rectum **DD27DZZ**
  Sinuses **D927DZZ**
  Spinal Cord **D026DZZ**
  Spleen **D722DZZ**
  Stomach **DD21DZZ**
  Testis **DV21DZZ**
  Thymus **D721DZZ**
  Thyroid Gland **DG25DZZ**
  Tongue **D925DZZ**
  Trachea **DB20DZZ**
  Ureter **DT21DZZ**
  Urethra **DT23DZZ**
  Uterus **DU22DZZ**
Ovary **DU20-**
Palate
  Hard **D928-**
  Soft **D929-**
Pancreas **DF23-**
Parathyroid Gland **DG24-**
Particulate
  Abdomen **DW23HZZ**
  Adrenal Gland **DG22HZZ**
  Bile Ducts **DF22HZZ**
  Bladder **DT22HZZ**
  Bone Marrow **D720HZZ**
  Brain **D020HZZ**
  Brain Stem **D021HZZ**
  Breast
    Left **DM20HZZ**
    Right **DM21HZZ**
  Bronchus **DB21HZZ**
  Cervix **DU21HZZ**
  Chest **DW22HZZ**
  Chest Wall **DB27HZZ**
  Colon **DD25HZZ**

Stereotactic Radiosurgery — *continued*
Particulate — *continued*
  Diaphragm **DB28HZZ**
  Duodenum **DD22HZZ**
  Ear **D920HZZ**
  Esophagus **DD20HZZ**
  Eye **D820HZZ**
  Gallbladder **DF21HZZ**
  Gland
    Adrenal **DG22HZZ**
    Parathyroid **DG24HZZ**
    Pituitary **DG20HZZ**
    Thyroid **DG25HZZ**
  Glands, Salivary **D926HZZ**
  Head and Neck **DW21HZZ**
  Ileum **DD24HZZ**
  Jejunum **DD23HZZ**
  Kidney **DT20HZZ**
  Larynx **D92BHZZ**
  Liver **DF20HZZ**
  Lung **DB22HZZ**
  Lymphatics
    Abdomen **D726HZZ**
    Axillary **D724HZZ**
    Inguinal **D728HZZ**
    Neck **D723HZZ**
    Pelvis **D727HZZ**
    Thorax **D725HZZ**
  Mediastinum **DB26HZZ**
  Mouth **D924HZZ**
  Nasopharynx **D92DHZZ**
  Neck and Head **DW21HZZ**
  Nerve, Peripheral **D027HZZ**
  Nose **D921HZZ**
  Ovary **DU20HZZ**
  Palate
    Hard **D928HZZ**
    Soft **D929HZZ**
  Pancreas **DF23HZZ**
  Parathyroid Gland **DG24HZZ**
  Pelvic Region **DW26HZZ**
  Pharynx **D92CHZZ**
  Pineal Body **DG21HZZ**
  Pituitary Gland **DG20HZZ**
  Pleura **DB25HZZ**
  Prostate **DV20HZZ**
  Rectum **DD27HZZ**
  Sinuses **D927HZZ**
  Spinal Cord **D026HZZ**
  Spleen **D722HZZ**
  Stomach **DD21HZZ**
  Testis **DV21HZZ**
  Thymus **D721HZZ**
  Thyroid Gland **DG25HZZ**
  Tongue **D925HZZ**
  Trachea **DB20HZZ**
  Ureter **DT21HZZ**
  Urethra **DT23HZZ**
  Uterus **DU22HZZ**
Pelvic Region **DW26-**
Pharynx **D92C-**
Pineal Body **DG21-**
Pituitary Gland **DG20-**
Pleura **DB25-**
Prostate **DV20-**
Rectum **DD27-**
Sinuses **D927-**
Spinal Cord **D026-**
Spleen **D722-**
Stomach **DD21-**
Testis **DV21-**
Thymus **D721-**
Thyroid Gland **DG25-**
Tongue **D925-**
Trachea **DB20-**
Ureter **DT21-**
Urethra **DT23-**
Uterus **DU22-**

Sternoclavicular ligament
  use Bursa and Ligament, Shoulder, Left
  use Bursa and Ligament, Shoulder, Right
Sternocleidomastoid artery
  use Artery, Thyroid, Left
  use Artery, Thyroid, Right
Sternocleidomastoid muscle
  use Muscle, Neck, Left
  use Muscle, Neck, Right
Sternocostal ligament
  use Bursa and Ligament, Thorax, Left
  use Bursa and Ligament, Thorax, Right
Sternotomy
  see Division, Sternum 0P80-
  see Drainage, Sternum 0P90-
Stimulation, cardiac
  Cardioversion 5A2204Z
  Electrophysiologic testing *see* Measurement, Cardiac 4A02-
Stimulator Generator
  Insertion of device in
    Abdomen 0JH8-
    Back 0JH7-
    Chest 0JH6-
  Multiple Array
    Abdomen 0JH8-
    Back 0JH7-
    Chest 0JH6-
  Multiple Array Rechargeable
    Abdomen 0JH8-
    Back 0JH7-
    Chest 0JH6-
  Removal of device from, Subcutaneous Tissue and Fascia, Trunk 0JPT-
  Revision of device in, Subcutaneous Tissue and Fascia, Trunk 0JWT-
  Single Array
    Abdomen 0JH8-
    Back 0JH7-
    Chest 0JH6-
  Single Array Rechargeable
    Abdomen 0JH8-
    Back 0JH7-
    Chest 0JH6-
Stimulator Lead
  Insertion of device in
    Anal Sphincter 0DHR-
    Artery
      Left 03HL-
      Right 03HK-
    Bladder 0THB-
    Muscle
      Lower 0KHY-
      Upper 0KHX-
    Stomach 0DH6-
    Ureter 0TH9-
  Removal of device from
    Anal Sphincter 0DPR-
    Artery, Upper 03PY-
    Bladder 0TPB-
    Muscle
      Lower 0KPY-
      Upper 0KPX-
    Stomach 0DP6-
    Ureter 0TP9-
  Revision of device in
    Anal Sphincter 0DWR-
    Artery, Upper 03WY-
    Bladder 0TWB-
    Muscle
      Lower 0KWY-
      Upper 0KWX-
    Stomach 0DW6-
    Ureter 0TW9-

Stoma
  Excision
    Abdominal Wall 0WBFXZ2
    Neck 0WB6XZ2
  Repair
    Abdominal Wall 0WQFXZ2
    Neck 0WQ6XZ2
Stomatoplasty
  see Repair, Mouth and Throat 0CQ-
  see Replacement, Mouth and Throat 0CR-
  see Supplement, Mouth and Throat 0CU-
Stomatorrhaphy *see* Repair, Mouth and Throat 0CQ-
Stratos LV
  use Cardiac Resynchronization Pacemaker Pulse Generator in 0JH-
Stress test
  4A02XM4
  4A12XM4
Stripping *see* Extraction
Study
  Electrophysiologic stimulation, cardiac *see* Measurement, Cardiac 4A02-
  Ocular motility 4A07X7Z
  Pulmonary airway flow measurement *see* Measurement, Respiratory 4A09-
  Visual acuity 4A07X0Z
Styloglossus muscle
  use Muscle, Tongue, Palate, Pharynx
Stylomandibular ligament
  use Bursa and Ligament, Head and Neck
Stylopharyngeus muscle
  use Muscle, Tongue, Palate, Pharynx
Subacromial bursa
  use Bursa and Ligament, Shoulder, Left
  use Bursa and Ligament, Shoulder, Right
Subaortic (common iliac) lymph node
  use Lymphatic, Pelvis
Subarachnoid space, intracranial
  use Subarachnoid Space
Subarachnoid space, spinal
  use Spinal Canal
Subclavicular (apical) lymph node
  use Lymphatic, Axillary, Left
  use Lymphatic, Axillary, Right
Subclavius muscle
  use Muscle, Thorax, Left
  use Muscle, Thorax, Right
Subclavius nerve
  use Nerve, Brachial Plexus
Subcostal artery
  use Upper Artery
Subcostal muscle
  use Muscle, Thorax, Left
  use Muscle, Thorax, Right
Subcostal nerve
  use Nerve, Thoracic
Subcutaneous injection reservoir, port
  use Vascular Access Device, Reservoir in Subcutaneous Tissue and Fascia
Subcutaneous injection reservoir, pump
  use Infusion Device, Pump in Subcutaneous Tissue and Fascia
Subdermal progesterone implant
  use Contraceptive Device in Subcutaneous Tissue and Fascia

Subdural space, intracranial
  use Subdural Space
Subdural space, spinal
  use Spinal Canal
Submandibular ganglion
  use Nerve, Facial
  use Nerve, Head and Neck Sympathetic
Submandibular gland
  use Gland, Submaxillary, Left
  use Gland, Submaxillary, Right
Submandibular lymph node
  use Lymphatic, Head
Submaxillary ganglion
  use Nerve, Head and Neck Sympathetic
Submaxillary lymph node
  use Lymphatic, Head
Submental artery
  use Artery, Face
Submental lymph node
  use Lymphatic, Head
Submucous (Meissner's) plexus
  use Nerve, Abdominal Sympathetic
Suboccipital nerve
  use Nerve, Cervical
Suboccipital venous plexus
  use Vein, Vertebral, Left
  use Vein, Vertebral, Right
Subparotid lymph node
  use Lymphatic, Head
Subscapular (posterior) lymph node
  use Lymphatic, Axillary, Left
  use Lymphatic, Axillary, Right
Subscapular aponeurosis
  use Subcutaneous Tissue and Fascia, Upper Arm, Left
  use Subcutaneous Tissue and Fascia, Upper Arm, Right
Subscapular artery
  use Artery, Axillary, Left
  use Artery, Axillary, Right
Subscapularis muscle
  use Muscle, Shoulder, Left
  use Muscle, Shoulder, Right
Substance Abuse Treatment
  Counseling
    Family, for substance abuse, Other Family Counseling HZ63ZZZ
    Group
      12-Step HZ43ZZZ
      Behavioral HZ41ZZZ
      Cognitive HZ40ZZZ
      Cognitive-Behavioral HZ42ZZZ
      Confrontational HZ48ZZZ
      Continuing Care HZ49ZZZ
      Infectious Disease
        Post-Test HZ4CZZZ
        Pre-Test HZ4CZZZ
      Interpersonal HZ44ZZZ
      Motivational Enhancement HZ47ZZZ
      Psychoeducation HZ46ZZZ
      Spiritual HZ4BZZZ
      Vocational HZ45ZZZ
    Individual
      12-Step HZ33ZZZ
      Behavioral HZ31ZZZ
      Cognitive HZ30ZZZ
      Cognitive-Behavioral HZ32ZZZ
      Confrontational HZ38ZZZ
      Continuing Care HZ39ZZZ
      Infectious Disease
        Post-Test HZ3CZZZ
        Pre-Test HZ3CZZZ
      Interpersonal HZ34ZZZ
      Motivational Enhancement HZ37ZZZ
      Psychoeducation HZ36ZZZ
      Spiritual HZ3BZZZ
      Vocational HZ35ZZZ

Substance Abuse Treatment — continued
  Detoxification Services, for substance abuse HZ2ZZZZ
  Medication Management
    Antabuse HZ83ZZZ
    Bupropion HZ87ZZZ
    Clonidine HZ86ZZZ
    Levo-alpha-acetyl-methadol (LAAM) HZ82ZZZ
    Methadone Maintenance HZ81ZZZ
    Naloxone HZ85ZZZ
    Naltrexone HZ84ZZZ
    Nicotine Replacement HZ80ZZZ
    Other Replacement Medication HZ89ZZZ
    Psychiatric Medication HZ88ZZZ
  Pharmacotherapy
    Antabuse HZ93ZZZ
    Bupropion HZ97ZZZ
    Clonidine HZ96ZZZ
    Levo-alpha-acetyl-methadol (LAAM) HZ92ZZZ
    Methadone Maintenance HZ91ZZZ
    Naloxone HZ95ZZZ
    Naltrexone HZ94ZZZ
    Nicotine Replacement HZ90ZZZ
    Psychiatric Medication HZ98ZZZ
    Replacement Medication, Other HZ99ZZZ
  Psychotherapy
    12-Step HZ53ZZZ
    Behavioral HZ51ZZZ
    Cognitive HZ50ZZZ
    Cognitive-Behavioral HZ52ZZZ
    Confrontational HZ58ZZZ
    Interactive HZ55ZZZ
    Interpersonal HZ54ZZZ
    Motivational Enhancement HZ57ZZZ
    Psychoanalysis HZ5BZZZ
    Psychodynamic HZ5CZZZ
    Psychoeducation HZ56ZZZ
    Psychophysiological HZ5DZZZ
    Supportive HZ59ZZZ
Substantia nigra
  use Basal Ganglia
Subtalar (talocalcaneal) joint
  use Joint, Tarsal, Left
  use Joint, Tarsal, Right
Subtalar ligament
  use Bursa and Ligament, Foot, Left
  use Bursa and Ligament, Foot, Right
Subthalamic nucleus
  use Basal Ganglia
Suction curettage (D&C), nonobstetric *see* Extraction, Endometrium 0UDB-
Suction curettage, obstetric post-delivery *see* Extraction, Products of Conception, Retained 10D1-
Superficial circumflex iliac vein
  use Vein, Greater Saphenous, Left
  use Vein, Greater Saphenous, Right
Superficial epigastric artery
  use Artery, Femoral, Left
  use Artery, Femoral, Right
Superficial epigastric vein
  use Vein, Greater Saphenous, Left
  use Vein, Greater Saphenous, Right
Superficial Inferior Epigastric Artery Flap
  Bilateral 0HRV078
  Left 0HRU078
  Right 0HRT078
Superficial palmar arch
  use Artery, Hand, Left
  use Artery, Hand, Right
Superficial palmar venous arch
  use Vein, Hand, Left
  use Vein, Hand, Right

Superficial temporal artery
  use Artery, Temporal, Left
  use Artery, Temporal, Right
Superficial transverse perineal muscle
  use Muscle, Perineum
Superior cardiac nerve
  use Nerve, Thoracic Sympathetic
Superior cerebellar vein
  use Vein, Intracranial
Superior cerebral vein
  use Vein, Intracranial
Superior clunic (cluneal) nerve
  use Nerve, Lumbar
Superior epigastric artery
  use Artery, Internal Mammary, Left
  use Artery, Internal Mammary, Right
Superior genicular artery
  use Artery, Popliteal, Left
  use Artery, Popliteal, Right
Superior gluteal artery
  use Artery, Internal Iliac, Left
  use Artery, Internal Iliac, Right
Superior gluteal nerve
  use Nerve, Lumbar Plexus
Superior hypogastric plexus
  use Nerve, Abdominal Sympathetic
Superior labial artery
  use Artery, Face
Superior laryngeal artery
  use Artery, Thyroid, Left
  use Artery, Thyroid, Right
Superior laryngeal nerve
  use Nerve, Vagus
Superior longitudinal muscle
  use Muscle, Tongue, Palate, Pharynx
Superior mesenteric ganglion
  use Nerve, Abdominal Sympathetic
Superior mesenteric lymph node
  use Lymphatic, Mesenteric
Superior mesenteric plexus
  use Nerve, Abdominal Sympathetic
Superior oblique muscle
  use Muscle, Extraocular, Left
  use Muscle, Extraocular, Right
Superior olivary nucleus
  use Pons
Superior rectal artery
  use Artery, Inferior Mesenteric
Superior rectal vein
  use Vein, Inferior Mesenteric
Superior rectus muscle
  use Muscle, Extraocular, Left
  use Muscle, Extraocular, Right
Superior tarsal plate
  use Eyelid, Upper, Left
  use Eyelid, Upper, Right
Superior thoracic artery
  use Artery, Axillary, Left
  use Artery, Axillary, Right
Superior thyroid artery
  use Artery, External Carotid, Left
  use Artery, External Carotid, Right
  use Artery, Thyroid, Left
  use Artery, Thyroid, Right
Superior turbinate
  use Turbinate, Nasal
Superior ulnar collateral artery
  use Artery, Brachial, Left
  use Artery, Brachial, Right
Supplement
  Abdominal Wall **0WUF**-
  Acetabulum
    Left **0QU5**-
    Right **0QU4**-
  Ampulla of Vater **0FUC**-
  Anal Sphincter **0DUR**-
  Ankle Region
    Left **0YUL**-
    Right **0YUK**-

Supplement — *continued*
Anus **0DUQ**-
Aorta
  Abdominal **04U0**-
  Thoracic
    Ascending/Arch **02UX**-
    Descending **02UW**-
Arm
  Lower
    Left **0XUF**-
    Right **0XUD**-
  Upper
    Left **0XU9**-
    Right **0XU8**-
Artery
  Anterior Tibial
    Left **04UQ**-
    Right **04UP**-
  Axillary
    Left **03U6**-
    Right **03U5**-
  Brachial
    Left **03U8**-
    Right **03U7**-
  Celiac **04U1**-
  Colic
    Left **04U7**-
    Middle **04U8**-
    Right **04U6**-
  Common Carotid
    Left **03UJ**-
    Right **03UH**-
  Common Iliac
    Left **04UD**-
    Right **04UC**-
  External Carotid
    Left **03UN**-
    Right **03UM**-
  External Iliac
    Left **04UJ**-
    Right **04UH**-
  Face **03UR**-
  Femoral
    Left **04UL**-
    Right **04UK**-
  Foot
    Left **04UW**-
    Right **04UV**-
  Gastric **04U2**-
  Hand
    Left **03UF**-
    Right **03UD**-
  Hepatic **04U3**-
  Inferior Mesenteric **04UB**-
  Innominate **03U2**-
  Internal Carotid
    Left **03UL**-
    Right **03UK**-
  Internal Iliac
    Left **04UF**-
    Right **04UE**-
  Internal Mammary
    Left **03U1**-
    Right **03U0**-
  Intracranial **03UG**-
  Lower **04UY**-
  Peroneal
    Left **04UU**-
    Right **04UT**-
  Popliteal
    Left **04UN**-
    Right **04UM**-
  Posterior Tibial
    Left **04US**-
    Right **04UR**-
  Pulmonary
    Left **02UR**-
    Right **02UQ**-
  Pulmonary Trunk **02UP**-
  Radial
    Left **03UC**-
    Right **03UB**-

Supplement — *continued*
Artery — *continued*
  Renal
    Left **04UA**-
    Right **04U9**-
  Splenic **04U4**-
  Subclavian
    Left **03U4**-
    Right **03U3**-
  Superior Mesenteric **04U5**-
  Temporal
    Left **03UT**-
    Right **03US**-
  Thyroid
    Left **03UV**-
    Right **03UU**-
  Ulnar
    Left **03UA**-
    Right **03U9**-
  Upper **03UY**-
  Vertebral
    Left **03UQ**-
    Right **03UP**-
Atrium
  Left **02U7**-
  Right **02U6**-
Auditory Ossicle
  Left **09UA0**-
  Right **09U90**-
Axilla
  Left **0XU5**-
  Right **0XU4**-
Back
  Lower **0WUL**-
  Upper **0WUK**-
Bladder **0TUB**-
Bladder Neck **0TUC**-
Bone
  Ethmoid
    Left **0NUG**-
    Right **0NUF**-
  Frontal
    Left **0NU2**-
    Right **0NU1**-
  Hyoid **0NUX**-
  Lacrimal
    Left **0NUJ**-
    Right **0NUH**-
  Nasal **0NUB**-
  Occipital
    Left **0NU8**-
    Right **0NU7**-
  Palatine
    Left **0NUL**-
    Right **0NUK**-
  Parietal
    Left **0NU4**-
    Right **0NU3**-
  Pelvic
    Left **0QU3**-
    Right **0QU2**-
  Sphenoid
    Left **0NUD**-
    Right **0NUC**-
  Temporal
    Left **0NU6**-
    Right **0NU5**-
  Zygomatic
    Left **0NUN**-
    Right **0NUM**-
Breast
  Bilateral **0HUV**-
  Left **0HUU**-
  Right **0HUT**-
Bronchus
  Lingula **0BU9**-
  Lower Lobe
    Left **0BUB**-
    Right **0BU6**-
  Main
    Left **0BU7**-
    Right **0BU3**-

Supplement — *continued*
Bronchus — *continued*
  Middle Lobe, Right **0BU5**-
  Upper Lobe
    Left **0BU8**-
    Right **0BU4**-
Buccal Mucosa **0CU4**-
Bursa and Ligament
  Abdomen
    Left **0MUJ**-
    Right **0MUH**-
  Ankle
    Left **0MUR**-
    Right **0MUQ**-
  Elbow
    Left **0MU4**-
    Right **0MU3**-
  Foot
    Left **0MUT**-
    Right **0MUS**-
  Hand
    Left **0MU8**-
    Right **0MU7**-
  Head and Neck **0MU0**-
  Hip
    Left **0MUM**-
    Right **0MUL**-
  Knee
    Left **0MUP**-
    Right **0MUN**-
  Lower Extremity
    Left **0MUW**-
    Right **0MUV**-
  Perineum **0MUK**-
  Shoulder
    Left **0MU2**-
    Right **0MU1**-
  Thorax
    Left **0MUG**-
    Right **0MUF**-
  Trunk
    Left **0MUD**-
    Right **0MUC**-
  Upper Extremity
    Left **0MUB**-
    Right **0MU9**-
  Wrist
    Left **0MU6**-
    Right **0MU5**-
Buttock
  Left **0YU1**-
  Right **0YU0**-
Carina **0BU2**-
Carpal
  Left **0PUN**-
  Right **0PUM**-
Cecum **0DUH**-
Cerebral Meninges **00U1**-
Chest Wall **0WU8**-
Chordae Tendineae **02U9**-
Cisterna Chyli **07UL**-
Clavicle
  Left **0PUB**-
  Right **0PU9**-
Clitoris **0UUJ**-
Coccyx **0QUS**-
Colon
  Ascending **0DUK**-
  Descending **0DUM**-
  Sigmoid **0DUN**-
  Transverse **0DUL**-
Cord
  Bilateral **0VUH**-
  Left **0VUG**-
  Right **0VUF**-
Cornea
  Left **08U9**-
  Right **08U8**-
Cul-de-sac **0UUF**-
Diaphragm
  Left **0BUS**-
  Right **0BUR**-

Supplement — *continued*
Disc
  Cervical Vertebral **0RU**3-
  Cervicothoracic Vertebral **0RU**5-
  Lumbar Vertebral **0SU**2-
  Lumbosacral **0SU**4-
  Thoracic Vertebral **0RU**9-
  Thoracolumbar Vertebral **0RU**B-
Duct
  Common Bile **0FU**9-
  Cystic **0FU**8-
  Hepatic
    Left **0FU**6-
    Right **0FU**5-
  Lacrimal
    Left **08U**Y-
    Right **08U**X-
  Pancreatic **0FU**D-
    Accessory **0FU**F-
Duodenum **0DU**9-
Dura Mater **00U**2-
Ear
  External
    Bilateral **09U**2-
    Left **09U**1-
    Right **09U**0-
  Inner
    Left **09U**E0-
    Right **09U**D0-
  Middle
    Left **09U**60-
    Right **09U**50-
Elbow Region
  Left **0XU**C-
  Right **0XU**B-
Epididymis
  Bilateral **0VU**L-
  Left **0VU**K-
  Right **0VU**J-
Epiglottis **0CU**R-
Esophagogastric Junction **0DU**4-
Esophagus **0DU**5-
  Lower **0DU**3-
  Middle **0DU**2-
  Upper **0DU**1-
Extremity
  Lower
    Left **0YU**B-
    Right **0YU**9-
  Upper
    Left **0XU**7-
    Right **0XU**6-
Eye
  Left **08U**1-
  Right **08U**0-
Eyelid
  Lower
    Left **08U**R-
    Right **08U**Q-
  Upper
    Left **08U**P-
    Right **08U**N-
Face **0WU**2-
Fallopian Tube
  Left **0UU**6-
  Right **0UU**5-
Fallopian Tubes, Bilateral **0UU**7-
Femoral Region
  Bilateral **0YU**E-
  Left **0YU**8-
  Right **0YU**7-
Femoral Shaft
  Left **0QU**9-
  Right **0QU**8-
Femur
  Lower
    Left **0QU**C-
    Right **0QU**B-
  Upper
    Left **0QU**7-
    Right **0QU**6-

Supplement — *continued*
Fibula
  Left **0QU**K-
  Right **0QU**J-
Finger
  Index
    Left **0XU**P-
    Right **0XU**N-
  Little
    Left **0XU**W-
    Right **0XU**V-
  Middle
    Left **0XU**R-
    Right **0XU**Q-
  Ring
    Left **0XU**T-
    Right **0XU**S-
Foot
  Left **0YU**N-
  Right **0YU**M-
Gingiva
  Lower **0CU**6-
  Upper **0CU**5-
Glenoid Cavity
  Left **0PU**8-
  Right **0PU**7-
Hand
  Left **0XU**K-
  Right **0XU**J-
Head **0WU**0-
Heart **02U**A-
Humeral Head
  Left **0PU**D-
  Right **0PU**C-
Humeral Shaft
  Left **0PU**G-
  Right **0PU**F-
Hymen **0UU**K-
Ileocecal Valve **0DU**C-
Ileum **0DU**B-
Inguinal Region
  Bilateral **0YU**A-
  Left **0YU**6-
  Right **0YU**5-
Intestine
  Large **0DU**E-
    Left **0DU**G-
    Right **0DU**F-
  Small **0DU**8-
Iris
  Left **08U**D-
  Right **08U**C-
Jaw
  Lower **0WU**5-
  Upper **0WU**4-
Jejunum **0DU**A-
Joint
  Acromioclavicular
    Left **0RU**H-
    Right **0RU**G-
  Ankle
    Left **0SU**G-
    Right **0SU**F-
  Carpal
    Left **0RU**R-
    Right **0RU**Q-
  Cervical Vertebral **0RU**1-
  Cervicothoracic Vertebral **0RU**4-
  Coccygeal **0SU**6-
  Elbow
    Left **0RU**M-
    Right **0RU**L-
  Finger Phalangeal
    Left **0RU**X-
    Right **0RU**W-
  Hip
    Left **0SU**B-
      Acetabular Surface **0SU**E-
      Femoral Surface **0SU**S-
    Right **0SU**9-
      Acetabular Surface **0SU**A-
      Femoral Surface **0SU**R-

Supplement — *continued*
Joint — *continued*
  Knee
    Left **0SU**D-
      Femoral Surface **0SU**U09Z
      Tibial Surface **0SU**W09Z
    Right **0SU**C-
      Femoral Surface **0SU**T09Z
      Tibial Surface **0SU**V09Z
  Lumbar Vertebral **0SU**0-
  Lumbosacral **0SU**3-
  Metacarpocarpal
    Left **0RU**T-
    Right **0RU**S-
  Metacarpophalangeal
    Left **0RU**V-
    Right **0RU**U-
  Metatarsal-Phalangeal
    Left **0SU**N-
    Right **0SU**M-
  Metatarsal-Tarsal
    Left **0SU**L-
    Right **0SU**K-
  Occipital-cervical **0RU**0-
  Sacrococcygeal **0SU**5-
  Sacroiliac
    Left **0SU**8-
    Right **0SU**7-
  Shoulder
    Left **0RU**K-
    Right **0RU**J-
  Sternoclavicular
    Left **0RU**F-
    Right **0RU**E-
  Tarsal
    Left **0SU**J-
    Right **0SU**H-
  Temporomandibular
    Left **0RU**D-
    Right **0RU**C-
  Thoracic Vertebral **0RU**6-
  Thoracolumbar Vertebral **0RU**A-
  Toe Phalangeal
    Left **0SU**Q-
    Right **0SU**P-
  Wrist
    Left **0RU**P-
    Right **0RU**N-
Kidney Pelvis
  Left **0TU**4-
  Right **0TU**3-
Knee Region
  Left **0YU**G-
  Right **0YU**F-
Larynx **0CU**S-
Leg
  Lower
    Left **0YU**J-
    Right **0YU**H-
  Upper
    Left **0YU**D-
    Right **0YU**C-
Lip
  Lower **0CU**1-
  Upper **0CU**0-
Lymphatic
  Aortic **07U**D-
  Axillary
    Left **07U**6-
    Right **07U**5-
  Head **07U**0-
  Inguinal
    Left **07U**J-
    Right **07U**H-
  Internal Mammary
    Left **07U**9-
    Right **07U**8-
  Lower Extremity
    Left **07U**G-
    Right **07U**F-
  Mesenteric **07U**B-

Supplement — *continued*
Lymphatic — *continued*
  Neck
    Left **07U**2-
    Right **07U**1-
  Pelvis **07U**C-
  Thoracic Duct **07U**K-
  Thorax **07U**7-
  Upper Extremity
    Left **07U**4-
    Right **07U**3-
Mandible
  Left **0NU**V-
  Right **0NU**T-
Maxilla
  Left **0NU**S-
  Right **0NU**R-
Mediastinum **0WU**C-
Mesentery **0DU**V-
Metacarpal
  Left **0PU**Q-
  Right **0PU**P-
Metatarsal
  Left **0QU**P-
  Right **0QU**N-
Muscle
  Abdomen
    Left **0KU**L-
    Right **0KU**K-
  Extraocular
    Left **08U**M-
    Right **08U**L-
  Facial **0KU**1-
  Foot
    Left **0KU**W-
    Right **0KU**V-
  Hand
    Left **0KU**D-
    Right **0KU**C-
  Head **0KU**0-
  Hip
    Left **0KU**P-
    Right **0KU**N-
  Lower Arm and Wrist
    Left **0KU**B-
    Right **0KU**9-
  Lower Leg
    Left **0KU**T-
    Right **0KU**S-
  Neck
    Left **0KU**3-
    Right **0KU**2-
  Papillary **02U**D-
  Perineum **0KU**M-
  Shoulder
    Left **0KU**6-
    Right **0KU**5-
  Thorax
    Left **0KU**J-
    Right **0KU**H-
  Tongue, Palate, Pharynx **0KU**4-
  Trunk
    Left **0KU**G-
    Right **0KU**F-
  Upper Arm
    Left **0KU**8-
    Right **0KU**7-
  Upper Leg
    Left **0KU**R-
    Right **0KU**Q-
Nasopharynx **09U**N-
Neck **0WU**6-
Nerve
  Abducens **00U**L-
  Accessory **00U**R-
  Acoustic **00U**N-
  Cervical **01U**1-
  Facial **00U**M-
  Femoral **01U**D-
  Glossopharyngeal **00U**P-
  Hypoglossal **00U**S-
  Lumbar **01U**B-

P R O C E D U R E   I N D E X

Suprarenal gland
  use Gland, Adrenal
  use Gland, Adrenal, Bilateral
  use Gland, Adrenal, Left
  use Gland, Adrenal, Right
Suprarenal plexus
  use Nerve, Abdominal Sympathetic
Suprascapular nerve
  use Nerve, Brachial Plexus
Supraspinatus fascia
  use Subcutaneous Tissue and Fascia,
    Upper Arm, Left
  use Subcutaneous Tissue and Fascia,
    Upper Arm, Right
Supraspinatus muscle
  use Muscle, Shoulder, Left
  use Muscle, Shoulder, Right
Supraspinous ligament
  use Bursa and Ligament, Trunk, Left
  use Bursa and Ligament, Trunk, Right
Suprasternal notch
  use Sternum
Supratrochlear lymph node
  use Lymphatic, Upper Extremity, Left
  use Lymphatic, Upper Extremity, Right
Sural artery
  use Artery, Popliteal, Left
  use Artery, Popliteal, Right
Suspension
  Bladder Neck *see* Reposition, Bladder
    Neck 0TSC-
  Kidney *see* Reposition, Urinary System
    0TS-
  Urethra *see* Reposition, Urinary
    System 0TS-
  Urethrovesical *see* Reposition, Bladder
    Neck 0TSC-
  Uterus *see* Reposition, Uterus 0US9-
  Vagina *see* Reposition, Vagina 0USG-
Suture
  Laceration repair *see* Repair
  Ligation *see* Occlusion
Suture Removal
  Extremity
    Lower 8E0YXY8
    Upper 8E0XXY8
  Head and Neck Region 8E09XY8
  Trunk Region 8E0WXY8
Sutureless valve, Perceval
  use Zooplastic Tissue, Rapid
    Deployment Technique in New
    Technology
Sweat gland
  use Skin
Sympathectomy *see* Excision,
    Peripheral Nervous System 01B-
SynCardia Total Artificial Heart
  use Synthetic Substitute
Synchra CRT-P
  use Cardiac Resynchronization
    Pacemaker Pulse Generator in
    0JH-
SynchroMed pump
  use Infusion Device, Pump in
    Subcutaneous Tissue and Fascia
Synechiotomy, iris *see* Release, Eye
    08N-
Synovectomy
  Lower joint *see* Excision, Lower Joints
    0SB-
  Upper joint *see* Excision, Upper Joints
    0RB-
Systemic Nuclear Medicine
    Therapy
  Abdomen CW70-
  Anatomical Regions, Multiple
    CW7YYZZ
  Chest CW73-
  Thyroid CW7G-
  Whole Body CW7N-

T

Takedown
  Arteriovenous shunt *see* Removal of
    device from, Upper Arteries 03P-
  Arteriovenous shunt, with creation of
    new shunt *see* Bypass, Upper
    Arteries 031-
  Stoma *see* Repair
Talent® Converter
  use Intraluminal Device
Talent® Occluder
  use Intraluminal Device
Talent® Stent Graft (abdominal)
    (thoracic)
  use Intraluminal Device
Talocalcaneal (subtalar) joint
  use Joint, Tarsal, Left
  use Joint, Tarsal, Right
Talocalcaneal ligament
  use Bursa and Ligament, Foot, Left
  use Bursa and Ligament, Foot, Right
Talocalcaneonavicular joint
  use Joint, Tarsal, Left
  use Joint, Tarsal, Right
Talocalcaneonavicular ligament
  use Bursa and Ligament, Foot, Left
  use Bursa and Ligament, Foot, Right
Talocrural joint
  use Joint, Ankle, Left
  use Joint, Ankle, Right
Talofibular ligament
  use Bursa and Ligament, Ankle, Left
  use Bursa and Ligament, Ankle, Right
Talus bone
  use Tarsal, Left
  use Tarsal, Right
TandemHeart® System
  use External Heart Assist System in
    Heart and Great Vessels
Tarsectomy
  see Excision, Lower Bones 0QB-
  see Resection, Lower Bones 0QT-
Tarsometatarsal joint
  use Joint, Metatarsal-Tarsal, Left
  use Joint, Metatarsal-Tarsal, Right
Tarsometatarsal ligament
  use Bursa and Ligament, Foot, Left
  use Bursa and Ligament, Foot, Right
Tarsorrhaphy *see* Repair, Eye 08Q-
Tattooing
  Cornea 3E0CXMZ
  Skin *see* Introduction of substance in
    or on, Skin 3E00-
TAXUS® Liberté® Paclitaxel-eluting
    Coronary Stent System
  use Intraluminal Device, Drug-eluting
    in Heart and Great Vessels
TBNA (transbronchial needle
    aspiration) *see* Drainage,
    Respiratory System 0B9-
Telemetry 4A12X4Z
  Ambulatory 4A12X45
Temperature gradient study
    4A0ZXKZ
Temporal lobe
  use Cerebral Hemisphere
Temporalis muscle
  use Muscle, Head
Temporoparietalis muscle
  use Muscle, Head
Tendolysis *see* Release, Tendons 0LN-
Tendonectomy
  see Excision, Tendons 0LB-
  see Resection, Tendons 0LT-
Tendonoplasty, tenoplasty
  see Repair, Tendons 0LQ-
  see Replacement, Tendons 0LR-
  see Supplement, Tendons 0LU-

Tendorrhaphy *see* Repair, Tendons
    0LQ-
Tendototomy
  see Division, Tendons 0L8-
  see Drainage, Tendons 0L9-
Tenectomy, tenonectomy
  see Excision, Tendons 0LB-
  see Resection, Tendons 0LT-
Tenolysis *see* Release, Tendons 0LN-
Tenontorrhaphy *see* Repair, Tendons
    0LQ-
Tenontotomy
  see Division, Tendons 0L8-
  see Drainage, Tendons 0L9-
Tenorrhaphy *see* Repair, Tendons
    0LQ-
Tenosynovectomy
  see Excision, Tendons 0LB-
  see Resection, Tendons 0LT-
Tenotomy
  see Division, Tendons 0L8-
  see Drainage, Tendons 0L9-
Tensor fasciae latae muscle
  use Muscle, Hip, Left
  use Muscle, Hip, Right
Tensor veli palatini muscle
  use Muscle, Tongue, Palate, Pharynx
Tenth cranial nerve
  use Nerve, Vagus
Tentorium cerebelli
  use Dura Mater
Teres major muscle
  use Muscle, Shoulder, Left
  use Muscle, Shoulder, Right
Teres minor muscle
  use Muscle, Shoulder, Left
  use Muscle, Shoulder, Right
Termination of pregnancy
  Aspiration curettage 10A07ZZ
  Dilation and curettage 10A07ZZ
  Hysterotomy 10A00ZZ
  Intra-amniotic injection 10A03ZZ
  Laminaria 10A07ZW
  Vacuum 10A07Z6
Testectomy
  see Excision, Male Reproductive
    System 0VB-
  see Resection, Male Reproductive
    System 0VT-
Testicular artery
  use Aorta, Abdominal
Testing
  Glaucoma 4A07XBZ
  Hearing *see* Hearing Assessment,
    Diagnostic Audiology F13-
  Mental health *see* Psychological Tests
  Muscle function, electromyography
    (EMG) *see* Measurement,
    Musculoskeletal 4A0F-
  Muscle function, manual *see* Motor
    Function Assessment,
    Rehabilitation F01-
  Neurophysiologic monitoring, intra-
    operative *see* Monitoring,
    Physiological Systems 4A1-
  Range of motion *see* Motor Function
    Assessment, Rehabilitation F01-
  Vestibular function *see* Vestibular
    Assessment, Diagnostic Audiology
    F15-
Thalamectomy *see* Excision,
    Thalamus 00B9-
Thalamotomy *see* Drainage,
    Thalamus 0099-
Thenar muscle
  use Muscle, Hand, Left
  use Muscle, Hand, Right
Therapeutic Massage
  Musculoskeletal System 8E0KX1Z
  Reproductive System
    Prostate 8E0VX1C
    Rectum 8E0VX1D

Therapeutic occlusion coil(s)
  use Intraluminal Device
Thermography 4A0ZXKZ
Thermotherapy, prostate *see*
    Destruction, Prostate 0V50-
Third cranial nerve
  use Nerve, Oculomotor
Third occipital nerve
  use Nerve, Cervical
Third ventricle
  use Cerebral Ventricle
Thoracectomy *see* Excision,
    Anatomical Regions, General 0WB-
Thoracentesis *see* Drainage,
    Anatomical Regions, General 0W9-
Thoracic aortic plexus
  use Nerve, Thoracic Sympathetic
Thoracic esophagus
  use Esophagus, Middle
Thoracic facet joint
  use Joint, Thoracic Vertebral
Thoracic ganglion
  use Nerve, Thoracic Sympathetic
Thoracoacromial artery
  use Artery, Axillary, Left
  use Artery, Axillary, Right
Thoracocentesis *see* Drainage,
    Anatomical Regions, General 0W9-
Thoracolumbar facet joint
  use Joint, Thoracolumbar Vertebral
Thoracoplasty
  see Repair, Anatomical Regions,
    General 0WQ-
  see Supplement, Anatomical Regions,
    General 0WU-
Thoracostomy tube
  use Drainage Device
Thoracostomy, for lung collapse
  see Drainage, Respiratory System
    0B9-
Thoracotomy *see* Drainage,
    Anatomical Regions, General 0W9-
Thoratec IVAD (Implantable
    Ventricular Assist Device)
  use Implantable Heart Assist System
    in Heart and Great Vessels
Thoratec Paracorporeal
    Ventricular Assist Device
  use External Heart Assist System in
    Heart and Great Vessels
Thrombectomy *see* Extirpation
Thymectomy
  see Excision, Lymphatic and Hemic
    Systems 07B-
  see Resection, Lymphatic and Hemic
    Systems 07T-
Thymopexy
  see Repair, Lymphatic and Hemic
    Systems 07Q-
  see Reposition, Lymphatic and Hemic
    Systems 07S-
Thymus gland
  use Thymus
Thyroarytenoid muscle
  use Muscle, Neck, Left
  use Muscle, Neck, Right
Thyrocervical trunk
  use Artery, Thyroid, Left
  use Artery, Thyroid, Right
Thyroid cartilage
  use Larynx
Thyroidectomy
  see Excision, Endocrine System 0GB-
  see Resection, Endocrine System 0GT-
Thyroidorrhaphy *see* Repair,
    Endocrine System 0GQ-
Thyroidoscopy 0GJK4ZZ
Thyroidotomy *see* Drainage,
    Endocrine System 0G9-

Tibial insert
  use Liner in Lower Joints
Tibialis anterior muscle
  use Muscle, Lower Leg, Left
  use Muscle, Lower Leg, Right
Tibialis posterior muscle
  use Muscle, Lower Leg, Left
  use Muscle, Lower Leg, Right
Tibiofemoral joint
  use Joint, Knee, Left
  use Joint, Knee, Right
  use Joint, Knee, Left, Tibial Surface
  use Joint, Knee, Right, Tibial Surface
TigerPaw® system for closure of left atrial appendage
  use Extraluminal Device
Tissue bank graft
  use Nonautologous Tissue Substitute
Tissue Expander
  Insertion of device in
    Breast
      Bilateral **0HH**V-
      Left **0HH**U-
      Right **0HH**T-
    Nipple
      Left **0HH**X-
      Right **0HH**W-
    Subcutaneous Tissue and Fascia
      Abdomen **0JH**8-
      Back **0JH**7-
      Buttock **0JH**9-
      Chest **0JH**6-
      Face **0JH**1-
      Foot
        Left **0JH**R-
        Right **0JH**Q-
      Hand
        Left **0JH**K-
        Right **0JH**J-
      Lower Arm
        Left **0JH**H-
        Right **0JH**G-
      Lower Leg
        Left **0JH**P-
        Right **0JH**N-
      Neck
        Anterior **0JH**4-
        Posterior **0JH**5-
      Pelvic Region **0JH**C-
      Perineum **0JH**B-
      Scalp **0JH**0-
      Upper Arm
        Left **0JH**F-
        Right **0JH**D-
      Upper Leg
        Left **0JH**M-
        Right **0JH**L-
  Removal of device from
    Breast
      Left **0HP**U-
      Right **0HP**T-
    Subcutaneous Tissue and Fascia
      Head and Neck **0JP**S-
      Lower Extremity **0JP**W-
      Trunk **0JP**T-
      Upper Extremity **0JP**V-
  Revision of device in
    Breast
      Left **0HW**U-
      Right **0HW**T-
    Subcutaneous Tissue and Fascia
      Head and Neck **0JW**S-
      Lower Extremity **0JW**W-
      Trunk **0JW**T-
      Upper Extremity **0JW**V-
Tissue expander (inflatable) (injectable)
  use Tissue Expander in Skin and Breast
  use Tissue Expander in Subcutaneous Tissue and Fascia

Tissue Plasminogen Activator (tPA) (r-tPA)
  use Thrombolytic, Other
Titanium Sternal Fixation System (TSFS)
  use Internal Fixation Device, Rigid Plate in **0PS**-
  use Internal Fixation Device, Rigid Plate in **0PH**-
Tomographic (Tomo) Nuclear Medicine Imaging
  Abdomen **CW2**0-
  Abdomen and Chest **CW2**4-
  Abdomen and Pelvis **CW2**1-
  Anatomical Regions, Multiple **CW2**YYZZ
  Bladder, Kidneys and Ureters **CT2**3-
  Brain **C02**0-
  Breast **CH2**YYZZ
    Bilateral **CH2**2-
    Left **CH2**1-
    Right **CH2**0-
  Bronchi and Lungs **CB2**2-
  Central Nervous System **C02**YYZZ
  Cerebrospinal Fluid **C02**5-
  Chest **CW2**3-
  Chest and Abdomen **CW2**4-
  Chest and Neck **CW2**6-
  Digestive System **CD2**YYZZ
  Endocrine System **CG2**YYZZ
  Extremity
    Lower **CW2**D-
      Bilateral **CP2**F-
      Left **CP2**D-
      Right **CP2**C-
    Upper **CW2**M-
      Bilateral **CP2**B-
      Left **CP2**9-
      Right **CP2**8-
  Gallbladder **CF2**4-
  Gastrointestinal Tract **CD2**7-
  Gland, Parathyroid **CG2**1-
  Head and Neck **CW2**B-
  Heart **C22**YYZZ
    Right and Left **C22**6-
  Hepatobiliary System and Pancreas **CF2**YYZZ
  Kidneys, Ureters and Bladder **CT2**3-
  Liver **CF2**5-
  Liver and Spleen **CF2**6-
  Lungs and Bronchi **CB2**2-
  Lymphatics and Hematologic System **C72**YYZZ
  Musculoskeletal System, Other **CP2**YYZZ
  Myocardium **C22**G-
  Neck and Chest **CW2**6-
  Neck and Head **CW2**B-
  Pancreas and Hepatobiliary System **CF2**YYZZ
  Pelvic Region **CW2**J-
  Pelvis **CP2**6-
  Pelvis and Abdomen **CW2**1-
  Pelvis and Spine **CP2**7-
  Respiratory System **CB2**YYZZ
  Skin **CH2**YYZZ
  Skull **CP2**1-
  Skull and Cervical Spine **CP2**3-
  Spine
    Cervical **CP2**2-
    Cervical and Skull **CP2**3-
    Lumbar **CP2**H-
    Thoracic **CP2**G-
    Thoracolumbar **CP2**J-
  Spine and Pelvis **CP2**7-
  Spleen **C72**2-
  Spleen and Liver **CF2**6-
  Subcutaneous Tissue **CH2**YYZZ
  Thorax **CP2**4-
  Ureters, Kidneys and Bladder **CT2**3-
  Urinary System **CT2**YYZZ

Tomography, computerized *see* Computerized Tomography (CT Scan)
Tongue, base of
  use Pharynx
Tonometry 4A07XBZ
Tonsillectomy
  see Excision, Mouth and Throat **0CB**-
  see Resection, Mouth and Throat **0CT**-
Tonsillotomy *see* Drainage, Mouth and Throat **0C9**-
Total anomalous pulmonary venous return (TAPVR) repair
  see Bypass, Atrium **0217**-
  see Bypass, Vena Cava, Superior **021**V-
Total artificial (replacement) heart
  use Synthetic Substitute
Total parenteral nutrition (TPN)
  see Introduction of Nutritional Substance
Trachectomy
  see Excision, Trachea **0BB**1-
  see Resection, Trachea **0BT**1-
Trachelectomy
  see Excision, Cervix **0UB**C-
  see Resection, Cervix **0UT**C-
Trachelopexy
  see Repair, Cervix **0UQ**C-
  see Reposition, Cervix **0US**C-
Tracheloplasty *see* Repair, Cervix **0UQ**C-
Trachelorrhaphy *see* Repair, Cervix **0UQ**C-
Trachelotomy *see* Drainage, Cervix **0U9**C-
Tracheobronchial lymph node
  use Lymphatic, Thorax
Tracheoesophageal fistulization 0B110D6
Tracheolysis *see* Release, Respiratory System **0BN**-
Tracheoplasty
  see Repair, Respiratory System **0BQ**-
  see Supplement, Respiratory System **0BU**-
Tracheorrhaphy *see* Repair, Respiratory System **0BQ**-
Tracheoscopy 0BJ18ZZ
Tracheostomy *see* Bypass, Respiratory System **0B1**-
Tracheostomy Device
  Bypass, Trachea **0B11**-
  Change device in, Trachea **0B21**XFZ
  Removal of device from, Trachea **0BP**1-
  Revision of device in, Trachea **0BW**1-
Tracheostomy tube
  use Tracheostomy Device in Respiratory System
Tracheotomy *see* Drainage, Respiratory System **0B9**-
Traction
  Abdominal Wall **2W63**X-
  Arm
    Lower
      Left **2W6**DX-
      Right **2W6**CX-
    Upper
      Left **2W6**BX-
      Right **2W6**AX-
  Back **2W65**X-
  Chest Wall **2W64**X-
  Extremity
    Lower
      Left **2W6**MX-
      Right **2W6**LX-
    Upper
      Left **2W69**X-
      Right **2W68**X-

Traction — *continued*
  Face **2W61**X-
  Finger
    Left **2W6**KX-
    Right **2W6**JX-
  Foot
    Left **2W6**TX-
    Right **2W6**SX-
  Hand
    Left **2W6**FX-
    Right **2W6**EX-
  Head **2W60**X-
  Inguinal Region
    Left **2W6**7X-
    Right **2W6**6X-
  Leg
    Lower
      Left **2W6**RX-
      Right **2W6**QX-
    Upper
      Left **2W6**PX-
      Right **2W6**NX-
  Neck **2W62**X-
  Thumb
    Left **2W6**HX-
    Right **2W6**GX-
  Toe
    Left **2W6**VX-
    Right **2W6**UX-
Tractotomy *see* Division, Central Nervous System **008**-
Tragus
  use Ear, External, Bilateral
  use Ear, External, Left
  use Ear, External, Right
Training, caregiver *see* Caregiver Training
TRAM (transverse rectus abdominis myocutaneous) flap reconstruction
  Free *see* Replacement, Skin and Breast **0HR**-
  Pedicled *see* Transfer, Muscles **0KX**-
Transection *see* Division
Transfer
  Buccal Mucosa **0CX**4-
  Bursa and Ligament
    Abdomen
      Left **0MX**J-
      Right **0MX**H-
    Ankle
      Left **0MX**R-
      Right **0MX**Q-
    Elbow
      Left **0MX**4-
      Right **0MX**3-
    Foot
      Left **0MX**T-
      Right **0MX**S-
    Hand
      Left **0MX**8-
      Right **0MX**7-
    Head and Neck **0MX**0-
    Hip
      Left **0MX**M-
      Right **0MX**L-
    Knee
      Left **0MX**P-
      Right **0MX**N-
    Lower Extremity
      Left **0MX**W-
      Right **0MX**V-
    Perineum **0MX**K-
    Shoulder
      Left **0MX**2-
      Right **0MX**1-
    Thorax
      Left **0MX**G-
      Right **0MX**F-

PROCEDURE INDEX (side tab)

Transplantation — *continued*
  Liver **0FY00Z-**
  Lung
    Bilateral **0BYM0Z-**
    Left **0BYL0Z-**
    Lower Lobe
      Left **0BYJ0Z-**
      Right **0BYF0Z-**
    Middle Lobe, Right **0BYD0Z-**
    Right **0BYK0Z-**
    Upper Lobe
      Left **0BYG0Z-**
      Right **0BYC0Z-**
  Lung Lingula **0BYH0Z-**
  Ovary
    Left **0UY10Z-**
    Right **0UY00Z-**
  Pancreas **0FYG0Z-**
  Products of Conception **10Y0-**
  Spleen **07YP0Z-**
  Stem cell *see* Transfusion, Circulatory **302-**
  Stomach **0DY60Z-**
  Thymus **07YM0Z-**
Transposition
  see Reposition
  see Transfer
Transversalis fascia
  use Subcutaneous Tissue and Fascia, Trunk
Transverse (cutaneous) cervical nerve
  use Nerve, Cervical Plexus
Transverse acetabular ligament
  use Bursa and Ligament, Hip, Left
  use Bursa and Ligament, Hip, Right
Transverse facial artery
  use Artery, Temporal, Left
  use Artery, Temporal, Right
Transverse humeral ligament
  use Bursa and Ligament, Shoulder, Left
  use Bursa and Ligament, Shoulder, Right
Transverse ligament of atlas
  use Bursa and Ligament, Head and Neck
Transverse Rectus Abdominis Myocutaneous Flap
  Replacement
    Bilateral **0HRV076**
    Left **0HRU076**
    Right **0HRT076**
  Transfer
    Left **0KXL-**
    Right **0KXK-**
Transverse scapular ligament
  use Bursa and Ligament, Shoulder, Left
  use Bursa and Ligament, Shoulder, Right
Transverse thoracis muscle
  use Muscle, Thorax, Left
  use Muscle, Thorax, Right
Transversospinalis muscle
  use Muscle, Trunk, Left
  use Muscle, Trunk, Right
Transversus abdominis muscle
  use Muscle, Abdomen, Left
  use Muscle, Abdomen, Right
Trapezium bone
  use Carpal, Left
  use Carpal, Right
Trapezius muscle
  use Muscle, Trunk, Left
  use Muscle, Trunk, Right
Trapezoid bone
  use Carpal, Left
  use Carpal, Right

Triceps brachii muscle
  use Muscle, Upper Arm, Left
  use Muscle, Upper Arm, Right
Tricuspid annulus
  use Valve, Tricuspid
Trifacial nerve
  use Nerve, Trigeminal
Trifecta™ Valve (aortic)
  use Zooplastic Tissue in Heart and Great Vessels
Trigone of bladder
  use Bladder
Trimming, excisional *see* Excision
Triquetral bone
  use Carpal, Left
  use Carpal, Right
Trochanteric bursa
  use Bursa and Ligament, Hip, Left
  use Bursa and Ligament, Hip, Right
TUMT (Transurethral microwave thermotherapy of prostate) **0V507ZZ**
TUNA (transurethral needle ablation of prostate) **0V507ZZ**
Tunneled central venous catheter
  use Vascular Access Device in Subcutaneous Tissue and Fascia
Tunneled spinal (intrathecal) catheter
  use Infusion Device
Turbinectomy
  see Excision, Ear, Nose, Sinus **09B-**
  see Resection, Ear, Nose, Sinus **09T-**
Turbinoplasty
  see Repair, Ear, Nose, Sinus **09Q-**
  see Replacement, Ear, Nose, Sinus **09R-**
  see Supplement, Ear, Nose, Sinus **09U-**
Turbinotomy
  see Drainage, Ear, Nose, Sinus **099-**
  see Division, Ear, Nose, Sinus **098-**
TURP (transurethral resection of prostate)
  see Excision, Prostate **0VB0-**
  see Resection, Prostate **0VT0-**
Twelfth cranial nerve
  use Nerve, Hypoglossal
Two lead pacemaker
  use Pacemaker, Dual Chamber in **0JH-**
Tympanic cavity
  use Ear, Middle, Left
  use Ear, Middle, Right
Tympanic nerve
  use Nerve, Glossopharyngeal
Tympanic part of temporal bone
  use Bone, Temporal, Left
  use Bone, Temporal, Right
Tympanogram *see* Hearing Assessment, Diagnostic Audiology **F13-**
Tympanoplasty
  see Repair, Ear, Nose, Sinus **09Q-**
  see Replacement, Ear, Nose, Sinus **09R-**
  see Supplement, Ear, Nose, Sinus **09U-**
Tympanosympathectomy *see* Excision, Nerve, Head and Neck Sympathetic **01BK-**
Tympanotomy *see* Drainage, Ear, Nose, Sinus **099-**

U

Ulnar collateral carpal ligament
  use Bursa and Ligament, Wrist, Left
  use Bursa and Ligament, Wrist, Right
Ulnar collateral ligament
  use Bursa and Ligament, Elbow, Left
  use Bursa and Ligament, Elbow, Right
Ulnar notch
  use Radius, Left
  use Radius, Right
Ulnar vein
  use Vein, Brachial, Left
  use Vein, Brachial, Right
Ultrafiltration
  Hemodialysis *see* Performance, Urinary **5A1D-**
  Therapeutic plasmapheresis *see* Pheresis, Circulatory **6A55-**
Ultraflex™ Precision Colonic Stent System
  use Intraluminal Device
ULTRAPRO Hernia System (UHS)
  use Synthetic Substitute
ULTRAPRO Partially Absorbable Lightweight Mesh
  use Synthetic Substitute
ULTRAPRO Plug
  use Synthetic Substitute
Ultrasonic osteogenic stimulator
  use Bone Growth Stimulator in Head and Facial Bones
  use Bone Growth Stimulator in Lower Bones
  use Bone Growth Stimulator in Upper Bones
Ultrasonography
  Abdomen **BW40ZZZ**
  Abdomen and Pelvis **BW41ZZZ**
  Abdominal Wall **BH49ZZZ**
  Aorta
    Abdominal, Intravascular **B440ZZ3**
    Thoracic, Intravascular **B340ZZ3**
  Appendix **BD48ZZZ**
  Artery
    Brachiocephalic-Subclavian, Right, Intravascular **B341ZZ3**
    Celiac and Mesenteric, Intravascular **B44KZZ3**
    Common Carotid
      Bilateral, Intravascular **B345ZZ3**
      Left, Intravascular **B344ZZ3**
      Right, Intravascular **B343ZZ3**
    Coronary
      Multiple **B241YZZ**
        Intravascular **B241ZZ3**
        Transesophageal **B241ZZ4**
      Single **B240YZZ**
        Intravascular **B240ZZ3**
        Transesophageal **B240ZZ4**
    Femoral, Intravascular **B44LZZ3**
    Inferior Mesenteric, Intravascular **B445ZZ3**
    Internal Carotid
      Bilateral, Intravascular **B348ZZ3**
      Left, Intravascular **B347ZZ3**
      Right, Intravascular **B346ZZ3**
    Intra-Abdominal, Other, Intravascular **B44BZZ3**
    Intracranial, Intravascular **B34RZZ3**
    Lower Extremity
      Bilateral, Intravascular **B44HZZ3**
      Left, Intravascular **B44GZZ3**
      Right, Intravascular **B44FZZ3**
    Mesenteric and Celiac, Intravascular **B44KZZ3**
    Ophthalmic, Intravascular **B34VZZ3**
    Penile, Intravascular **B44NZZ3**

Ultrasonography — *continued*
  Artery — *continued*
    Pulmonary
      Left, Intravascular **B34TZZ3**
      Right, Intravascular **B34SZZ3**
    Renal
      Bilateral, Intravascular **B448ZZ3**
      Left, Intravascular **B447ZZ3**
      Right, Intravascular **B446ZZ3**
    Subclavian, Left, Intravascular **B342ZZ3**
    Superior Mesenteric, Intravascular **B444ZZ3**
    Upper Extremity
      Bilateral, Intravascular **B34KZZ3**
      Left, Intravascular **B34JZZ3**
      Right, Intravascular **B34HZZ3**
  Bile Duct **BF40ZZZ**
  Bile Duct and Gallbladder **BF43ZZZ**
  Bladder **BT40ZZZ**
    and Kidney **BT4JZZZ**
  Brain **B040ZZZ**
  Breast
    Bilateral **BH42ZZZ**
    Left **BH41ZZZ**
    Right **BH40ZZZ**
  Chest Wall **BH4BZZZ**
  Coccyx **BR4FZZZ**
  Connective Tissue
    Lower Extremity **BL41ZZZ**
    Upper Extremity **BL40ZZZ**
  Duodenum **BD49ZZZ**
  Elbow
    Left, Densitometry **BP4HZZ1**
    Right, Densitometry **BP4GZZ1**
  Esophagus **BD41ZZZ**
  Extremity
    Lower **BH48ZZZ**
    Upper **BH47ZZZ**
  Eye
    Bilateral **B847ZZZ**
    Left **B846ZZZ**
    Right **B845ZZZ**
  Fallopian Tube
    Bilateral **BU42-**
    Left **BU41-**
    Right **BU40-**
  Fetal Umbilical Cord **BY47ZZZ**
  Fetus
    First Trimester, Multiple Gestation **BY4BZZZ**
    Second Trimester, Multiple Gestation **BY4DZZZ**
    Single
      First Trimester **BY49ZZZ**
      Second Trimester **BY4CZZZ**
      Third Trimester **BY4FZZZ**
    Third Trimester, Multiple Gestation **BY4GZZZ**
  Gallbladder **BF42ZZZ**
  Gallbladder and Bile Duct **BF43ZZZ**
  Gastrointestinal Tract **BD47ZZZ**
  Gland
    Adrenal
      Bilateral **BG42ZZZ**
      Left **BG41ZZZ**
      Right **BG40ZZZ**
    Parathyroid **BG43ZZZ**
    Thyroid **BG44ZZZ**
  Hand
    Left, Densitometry **BP4PZZ1**
    Right, Densitometry **BP4NZZ1**
  Head and Neck **BH4CZZZ**

Ultrasonography — *continued*
Heart
  Left **B245**YZZ
    Intravascular **B245**ZZ3
    Transesophageal **B245**ZZ4
  Pediatric **B24D**YZZ
    Intravascular **B24D**ZZ3
    Transesophageal **B24D**ZZ4
  Right **B244**YZZ
    Intravascular **B244**ZZ3
    Transesophageal **B244**ZZ4
  Right and Left **B246**YZZ
    Intravascular **B246**ZZ3
    Transesophageal **B246**ZZ4
Heart with Aorta **B24B**YZZ
  Intravascular **B24B**ZZ3
  Transesophageal **B24B**ZZ4
Hepatobiliary System, All **BF4C**ZZZ
Hip
  Bilateral **BQ42**ZZZ
  Left **BQ41**ZZZ
  Right **BQ40**ZZZ
Kidney
  and Bladder **BT4J**ZZZ
  Bilateral **BT43**ZZZ
  Left **BT42**ZZZ
  Right **BT41**ZZZ
  Transplant **BT49**ZZZ
Knee
  Bilateral **BQ49**ZZZ
  Left **BQ48**ZZZ
  Right **BQ47**ZZZ
Liver **BF45**ZZZ
Liver and Spleen **BF46**ZZZ
Mediastinum **BB4C**ZZZ
Neck **BW4F**ZZZ
Ovary
  Bilateral **BU45**-
  Left **BU44**-
  Right **BU43**-
Ovary and Uterus **BU4C**-
Pancreas **BF47**ZZZ
Pelvic Region **BW4G**ZZZ
Pelvis and Abdomen **BW41**ZZZ
Penis **BV4B**ZZZ
Pericardium **B24C**YZZ
  Intravascular **B24C**ZZ3
  Transesophageal **B24C**ZZ4
Placenta **BY48**ZZZ
Pleura **BB4B**ZZZ
Prostate and Seminal Vesicle
  BV49ZZZ
Rectum **BD4C**ZZZ
Sacrum **BR4F**ZZZ
Scrotum **BV44**ZZZ
Seminal Vesicle and Prostate
  BV49ZZZ
Shoulder
  Left, Densitometry **BP49**ZZ1
  Right, Densitometry **BP48**ZZ1
Spinal Cord **B04B**ZZZ
Spine
  Cervical **BR40**ZZZ
  Lumbar **BR49**ZZZ
  Thoracic **BR47**ZZZ
Spleen and Liver **BF46**ZZZ
Stomach **BD42**ZZZ
Tendon
  Lower Extremity **BL43**ZZZ
  Upper Extremity **BL42**ZZZ
Ureter
  Bilateral **BT48**ZZZ
  Left **BT47**ZZZ
  Right **BT46**ZZZ
Urethra **BT45**ZZZ
Uterus **BU46**-
Uterus and Ovary **BU4C**-

Ultrasonography — *continued*
Vein
  Jugular
    Left, Intravascular **B544**ZZ3
    Right, Intravascular **B543**ZZ3
  Lower Extremity
    Bilateral, Intravascular **B54D**ZZ3
    Left, Intravascular **B54C**ZZ3
    Right, Intravascular **B54B**ZZ3
  Portal, Intravascular **B54T**ZZ3
  Renal
    Bilateral, Intravascular **B54L**ZZ3
    Left, Intravascular **B54K**ZZ3
    Right, Intravascular **B54J**ZZ3
  Spanchnic, Intravascular **B54T**ZZ3
  Subclavian
    Left, Intravascular **B547**ZZ3
    Right, Intravascular **B546**ZZ3
  Upper Extremity
    Bilateral, Intravascular **B54P**ZZ3
    Left, Intravascular **B54N**ZZ3
    Right, Intravascular **B54M**ZZ3
  Vena Cava
    Inferior, Intravascular **B549**ZZ3
    Superior, Intravascular **B548**ZZ3
Wrist
  Left, Densitometry **BP4M**ZZ1
  Right, Densitometry **BP4L**ZZ1

Ultrasound bone healing system
  use Bone Growth Stimulator in Head
    and Facial Bones
  use Bone Growth Stimulator in Lower
    Bones
  use Bone Growth Stimulator in Upper
    Bones

Ultrasound Therapy
  Heart **6A75**-
  No Qualifier **6A75**-
  Vessels
    Head and Neck **6A75**-
    Other **6A75**-
    Peripheral **6A75**-

Ultraviolet Light Therapy, Skin
  6A80-

Umbilical artery
  use Artery, Internal Iliac, Left
  use Artery, Internal Iliac, Right

Uniplanar external fixator
  use External Fixation Device,
    Monoplanar in **0PH**-
  use External Fixation Device,
    Monoplanar in **0PS**-
  use External Fixation Device,
    Monoplanar in **0QH**-
  use External Fixation Device,
    Monoplanar in **0QS**-

Upper GI series *see* Fluoroscopy,
  Gastrointestinal, Upper **BD15**-

Ureteral orifice
  use Ureter
  use Ureter, Left
  use Ureter, Right
  use Ureters, Bilateral

Ureterectomy
  see Excision, Urinary System **0TB**-
  see Resection, Urinary System **0TT**-

Ureterocolostomy *see* Bypass,
  Urinary System **0T1**-

Ureterocystostomy *see* Bypass,
  Urinary System **0T1**-

Ureteroenterostomy *see* Bypass,
  Urinary System **0T1**-

Ureteroileostomy *see* Bypass,
  Urinary System **0T1**-

Ureterolithotomy *see* Extirpation,
  Urinary System **0TC**-

Ureterolysis *see* Release, Urinary
  System **0TN**-

Ureteroneocystostomy
  see Bypass, Urinary System **0T1**-
  see Reposition, Urinary System **0TS**-

Ureteropelvic junction (UPJ)
  use Kidney Pelvis, Left
  use Kidney Pelvis, Right

Ureteropexy
  see Repair, Urinary System **0TQ**-
  see Reposition, Urinary System **0TS**-

Ureteroplasty
  see Repair, Urinary System **0TQ**-
  see Replacement, Urinary System
    0TR-
  see Supplement, Urinary System **0TU**-

Ureteroplication *see* Restriction,
  Urinary System **0TV**-

Ureteropyelography *see*
  Fluoroscopy, Urinary System **BT1**-

Ureterorrhaphy *see* Repair, Urinary
  System **0TQ**-

Ureteroscopy 0TJ98ZZ

Ureterostomy
  see Bypass, Urinary System **0T1**-
  see Drainage, Urinary System **0T9**-

Ureterotomy *see* Drainage, Urinary
  System **0T9**-

Ureteroureterostomy *see* Bypass,
  Urinary System **0T1**-

Ureterovesical orifice
  use Ureter
  use Ureter, Left
  use Ureter, Right
  use Ureters, Bilateral

**Urethral catheterization,
indwelling 0T9B70Z**

Urethrectomy
  see Excision, Urethra **0TBD**-
  see Resection, Urethra **0TTD**-

Urethrolithotomy *see* Extirpation,
  Urethra **0TCD**-

Urethrolysis *see* Release, Urethra
  0TND-

Urethropexy
  see Repair, Urethra **0TQD**-
  see Reposition, Urethra **0TSD**-

Urethroplasty
  see Repair, Urethra **0TQD**-
  see Replacement, Urethra **0TRD**-
  see Supplement, Urethra **0TUD**-

Urethrorrhaphy *see* Repair, Urethra
  0TQD-

Urethroscopy 0TJD8ZZ

Urethrotomy *see* Drainage, Urethra
  0T9D-

Uridine triacetate XW0DX82

**Urinary incontinence stimulator
lead**
  use Stimulator Lead in Urinary System

Urography *see* Fluoroscopy, Urinary
  System **BT1**-

Uterine Artery
  use Artery, Internal Iliac, Left
  use Artery, Internal Iliac, Right

Uterine artery embolization (UAE)
  see Occlusion, Lower Arteries **04L**-

Uterine cornu
  use Uterus

Uterine tube
  use Fallopian Tube, Left
  use Fallopian Tube, Right

Uterine vein
  use Vein, Hypogastric, Left
  use Vein, Hypogastric, Right

Uvulectomy
  see Excision, Uvula **0CBN**-
  see Resection, Uvula **0CTN**-

Uvulorrhaphy *see* Repair, Uvula
  0CQN-

Uvulotomy *see* Drainage, Uvula
  0C9N-

V

Vaccination *see* Introduction of Serum,
  Toxoid, and Vaccine

Vacuum extraction, obstetric
  10D07Z6

Vaginal artery
  use Artery, Internal Iliac, Left
  use Artery, Internal Iliac, Right

Vaginal pessary
  use Intraluminal Device, Pessary in
    Female Reproductive System

Vaginal vein
  use Vein, Hypogastric, Left
  use Vein, Hypogastric, Right

Vaginectomy
  see Excision, Vagina **0UBG**-
  see Resection, Vagina **0UTG**-

Vaginofixation
  see Repair, Vagina **0UQG**-
  see Reposition, Vagina **0USG**-

Vaginoplasty
  see Repair, Vagina **0UQG**-
  see Supplement, Vagina **0UUG**-

Vaginorrhaphy *see* Repair, Vagina
  0UQG-

Vaginoscopy 0UJH8ZZ

Vaginotomy *see* Drainage, Female
  Reproductive System **0U9**-

Vagotomy *see* Division, Nerve, Vagus
  008Q-

Valiant Thoracic Stent Graft
  use Intraluminal Device

Valvotomy, valvulotomy
  see Division, Heart and Great Vessels
    028-
  see Release, Heart and Great Vessels
    02N-

Valvuloplasty
  see Repair, Heart and Great Vessels
    02Q-
  see Replacement, Heart and Great
    Vessels **02R**-
  see Supplement, Heart and Great
    Vessels **02U**-

Vascular Access Device
  Insertion of device in
    Abdomen **0JH8**-
    Chest **0JH6**-
    Lower Arm
      Left **0JHH**-
      Right **0JHG**-
    Lower Leg
      Left **0JHP**-
      Right **0JHN**-
    Upper Arm
      Left **0JHF**-
      Right **0JHD**-
    Upper Leg
      Left **0JHM**-
      Right **0JHL**-
  Removal of device from
    Lower Extremity **0JPW**-
    Trunk **0JPT**-
    Upper Extremity **0JPV**-
  Reservoir
    Insertion of device in
      Abdomen **0JH8**-
      Chest **0JH6**-
      Lower Arm
        Left **0JHH**-
        Right **0JHG**-
      Lower Leg
        Left **0JHP**-
        Right **0JHN**-
      Upper Arm
        Left **0JHF**-
        Right **0JHD**-
      Upper Leg
        Left **0JHM**-
        Right **0JHL**-

Vascular Access Device —
continued
Reservoir — *continued*
Removal of device from
Lower Extremity **0JPW**-
Trunk **0JPT**-
Upper Extremity **0JPV**-
Revision of device in
Lower Extremity **0JWW**-
Trunk **0JWT**-
Upper Extremity **0JWV**-
Revision of device in
Lower Extremity **0JWW**-
Trunk **0JWT**-
Upper Extremity **0JWV**
Vasectomy *see* Excision, Male
Reproductive System **0VB**-
Vasography
see Fluoroscopy, Male Reproductive
System **BV1**-
see Plain Radiography, Male
Reproductive System **BV0**-
Vasoligation *see* Occlusion, Male
Reproductive System **0VL**-
Vasorrhaphy *see* Repair, Male
Reproductive System **0VQ**-
Vasostomy *see* Bypass, Male
Reproductive System **0V1**-
Vasotomy
Drainage *see* Drainage, Male
Reproductive System **0V9**-
With ligation *see* Occlusion, Male
Reproductive System **0VL**-
Vasovasostomy *see* Repair, Male
Reproductive System **0VQ**-
Vastus intermedius muscle
use Muscle, Upper Leg, Left
use Muscle, Upper Leg, Right
Vastus lateralis muscle
use Muscle, Upper Leg, Left
use Muscle, Upper Leg, Right
Vastus medialis muscle
use Muscle, Upper Leg, Left
use Muscle, Upper Leg, Right
VCG (vectorcardiogram) *see*
Measurement, Cardiac **4A02**-
Vectra® Vascular Access Graft
use Vascular Access Device in
Subcutaneous Tissue and Fascia
Venectomy
see Excision, Lower Veins **06B**-
see Excision, Upper Veins **05B**-
Venography
see Fluoroscopy, Veins **B51**-
see Plain Radiography, Veins **B50**-
Venorrhaphy
see Repair, Lower Veins **06Q**-
see Repair, Upper Veins **05Q**-
Venotripsy
see Occlusion, Lower Veins **06L**-
see Occlusion, Upper Veins **05L**-
Ventricular fold
use Larynx
Ventriculoatriostomy *see* Bypass,
Central Nervous System **001**-
Ventriculocisternostomy *see*
Bypass, Central Nervous System
001-
Ventriculogram, cardiac
Combined left and right heart *see*
Fluoroscopy, Heart, Right and Left
B216-
Left ventricle *see* Fluoroscopy, Heart,
Left **B215**-
Right ventricle *see* Fluoroscopy, Heart,
Right **B214**-
**Ventriculopuncture, through
previously implanted catheter**
8C01X6J
Ventriculoscopy 00J04ZZ

Ventriculostomy
External drainage *see* Drainage,
Cerebral Ventricle **0096**-
Internal shunt *see* Bypass, Cerebral
Ventricle **0016**-
Ventriculovenostomy *see* Bypass,
Cerebral Ventricle **0016**-
Ventrio™ Hernia Patch
use Synthetic Substitute
VEP (visual evoked potential)
4A07X0Z
Vermiform appendix
use Appendix
Vermilion border
use Lip, Lower
use Lip, Upper
Versa
use Pacemaker, Dual chamber in
0JH-
Version, obstetric
External **10S0XZZ**
Internal **10S07ZZ**
Vertebral arch
use Vertebra, Cervical
use Vertebra, Lumbar
use Vertebra, Thoracic
Vertebral canal
use Spinal Canal
Vertebral foramen
use Vertebra, Cervical
use Vertebra, Lumbar
use Vertebra, Thoracic
Vertebral lamina
use Vertebra, Cervical
use Vertebra, Lumbar
use Vertebra, Thoracic
Vertebral pedicle
use Vertebra, Cervical
use Vertebra, Lumbar
use Vertebra, Thoracic
Vesical vein
use Vein, Hypogastric, Left
use Vein, Hypogastric, Right
Vesicotomy *see* Drainage, Urinary
System **0T9**-
Vesiculectomy
see Excision, Male Reproductive
System **0VB**-
see Resection, Male Reproductive
System **0VT**-
Vesiculogram, seminal *see* Plain
Radiography, Male Reproductive
System **BV0**-
Vesiculotomy *see* Drainage, Male
Reproductive System **0V9**-
Vestibular (Scarpa's) ganglion
use Nerve, Acoustic
Vestibular Assessment F15Z-
Vestibular nerve
use Nerve, Acoustic
Vestibular Treatment F0C-
Vestibulocochlear nerve
use Nerve, Acoustic
**VH-IVUS (virtual histology
intravascular ultrasound)**
see Ultrasonography, Heart **B24**-
**Virchow's (supraclavicular) lymph
node**
use Lymphatic, Neck, Left
use Lymphatic, Neck, Right
Virtuoso (II) (DR) (VR)
use Defibrillator Generator in **0JH**-
Vistogard®
use Uridine Triacetate
Vitrectomy
see Excision, Eye **08B**-
see Resection, Eye **08T**-
Vitreous body
use Vitreous, Left
use Vitreous, Right
Viva (XT) (S)
use Cardiac Resynchronization
Defibrillator Pulse Generator in
0JH-

Vocal fold
use Vocal Cord, Left
use Vocal Cord, Right
Vocational
Assessment *see* Activities of Daily
Living Assessment, Rehabilitation
F02-
Retraining *see* Activities of Daily Living
Treatment, Rehabilitation **F08**-
Volar (palmar) digital vein
use Vein, Hand, Left
use Vein, Hand, Right
Volar (palmar) metacarpal vein
use Vein, Hand, Left
use Vein, Hand, Right
Vomer bone
use Septum, Nasal
Vomer of nasal septum
use Bone, Nasal
Voraxaze
use Glucarpidase
Vulvectomy
see Excision, Female Reproductive
System **0UB**-
see Resection, Female Reproductive
System **0UT**-

W

WALLSTENT® Endoprosthesis
use Intraluminal Device
Washing *see* Irrigation
Wedge resection, pulmonary *see*
Excision, Respiratory System **0BB**-
Window *see* Drainage
Wiring, dental 2W31X9Z

PROCEDURE INDEX

X

Xact Carotid Stent System
use Intraluminal Device
X-ray *see* Plain Radiography
X-STOP® Spacer
use Spinal Stabilization Device, Interspinous Process in **0RH-**
use Spinal Stabilization Device, Interspinous Process in **0SH-**
Xenograft
use Zooplastic Tissue in Heart and Great Vessels
XIENCE Everolimus Eluting Coronary Stent System
use Intraluminal Device, Drug-eluting in Heart and Great Vessels
Xiphoid process
use Sternum
XLIF® System
use Interbody Fusion Device in Lower Joints

Y

Yoga Therapy 8E0ZXY4

Z

Z-plasty, skin for scar contracture
see Release, Skin and Breast **0HN-**
Zenith AAA Endovascular Graft
use Intraluminal Device
use Intraluminal Device, Branched or Fenestrated, One or Two Arteries **04V-**
use Intraluminal Device, Branched or Fenestrated, Three or More Arteries **04V-**
Zenith Flex® AAA Endovascular Graft
use Intraluminal Device
Zenith TX2® TAA Endovascular Graft
use Intraluminal Device
Zenith® Renu™ AAA Ancillary Graft
use Intraluminal Device
Zilver® PTX® (paclitaxel) Drug-Eluting Peripheral Stent
use Intraluminal Device, Drug-eluting in Lower Arteries
use Intraluminal Device, Drug-eluting in Upper Arteries
Zimmer® NexGen® LPS Mobile Bearing Knee
use Synthetic Substitute
Zimmer® NexGen® LPS-Flex Mobile Knee
use Synthetic Substitute
Zonule of Zinn
use Lens, Left
use Lens, Right
Zooplastic tissue, rapid deployment technique, replacement X2RF-
Zotarolimus-eluting coronary stent
use Intraluminal Device, Drug-eluting in Heart and Great Vessels
Zygomatic process of frontal bone
use Bone, Frontal, Left
use Bone, Frontal, Right
Zygomatic process of temporal bone
use Bone, Temporal, Left
use Bone, Temporal, Right
Zygomaticus muscle
use Muscle, Facial
Zyvox
use Oxazolidinones

Educational Annotations | 0 – Central Nervous System

Body System Specific Educational Annotations for the Central Nervous System include:

- Anatomy and Physiology Review
- Anatomical Illustrations
- Definitions of Common Procedures
- AHA Coding Clinic® Reference Notations
- Body Part Key Listings
- Device Key Listings
- Device Aggregation Table Listings
- Coding Notes

Anatomy and Physiology Review of Central Nervous System

BODY PART VALUES – 0 - CENTRAL NERVOUS SYSTEM

Abducens Nerve – The sixth (VI) cranial nerve that innervates the lateral rectus muscles of the eye.

Accessory Nerve – The eleventh (XI) cranial nerve that innervates the sternocleidomastoideus and trapezius muscles.

Acoustic Nerve – The cochlear (hearing) portion of the eighth (VIII) cranial nerve (also known as the vestibulocochlear or auditory nerve).

Basal Ganglia – ANATOMY – The basal ganglia are masses of gray matter located deep within the cerebral hemispheres, including the globus pallidus. The corpus striatum consists of 2 of the basal ganglia, the caudate and lentiform nuclei. PHYSIOLOGY – The basal ganglia function as relay stations for motor impulses.

Brain – ANATOMY – The brain is the largest and most complex part of the nervous system, and is located in the cranial cavity. The cerebrum is the largest part of the brain, and is divided sagittally (front and back through the center) into 2 hemispheres. The corpus callosum lies below and connects the 2 hemispheres. The frontal lobe forms the anterior portion of each cerebral hemisphere. The temporal lobes lie below the frontal lobe on the lateral side of each cerebral hemisphere. The parietal lobe forms the superior portion of the cerebrum, lying posterior to the frontal lobe. The occipital lobe forms the posterior portion of each cerebral hemisphere. The brain stem connects the upper end of the spinal cord with the cerebrum. It contains the pons, cerebral peduncle, medulla oblongata, and midbrain. The tapetum is a layer of fibers from the corpus callosum forming the roof and lateral walls of the lateral ventricles. PHYSIOLOGY – The cerebrum, including its lobes and cerebral cortex, is concerned with the higher brain functions, such as memory, learning, thought, reasoning, hearing, vision, speech, language, and voluntary muscle control.

Cerebellum – ANATOMY – The cerebellum is the second largest portion of the brain, located below the occipital lobe and behind the brain stem. PHYSIOLOGY – The cerebellum functions primarily as a reflex center in the coordination of skeletal muscle movements and the maintenance of equilibrium.

Cerebral Hemisphere – ANATOMY – The cerebrum is the largest portion of the brain and is symmetrically divided into left and right cerebral hemispheres that are linked by the corpus callosum. PHYSIOLOGY – Although both hemispheres are involved in most brain functions, the left hemisphere generally controls the right half of the body, and the right hemisphere generally controls the left half of the body.

Cerebral Meninges – ANATOMY – The cerebral meninges are continuous with the spinal meninges, completely enclosing the brain (and spinal cord), and consist of three layers: Dura mater, arachnoid mater, and pia mater. The dura mater is the outermost tough, fibroelastic tissue layer. The arachnoid mater is the thin, transparent middle layer. The pia mater is the thin, delicate layer that adheres to the brain and spinal cord tissues. PHYSIOLOGY – The spinal meninges function to protect the spinal cord and contain the cerebrospinal fluid. The subarachnoid space is the cerebrospinal fluid-filled space between the arachnoid and the pia mater.

Cerebral Ventricle – ANATOMY – The ventricles are a series of four interconnected cavities of the brain and are continuous with the central canal of the spinal cord, which are filled with the cerebrospinal fluid. The tapetum is a layer of fibers from the corpus callosum forming the roof and lateral walls of the lateral ventricles. PHYSIOLOGY – The ventricles produce and are filled by continuously replaced cerebrospinal fluid which serves to protect the brain by absorbing shocks and removing any waste substances. It also provides a stable ionic concentration in the central nervous system, which is important for maximum nerve impulse transfers.

Cervical Spinal Cord – That portion within the cervical vertebral column.

Cranial Nerve – ANATOMY – The 12 pairs of nerves arising from the brain stem and cerebrum. PHYSIOLOGY – The cranial nerves serve the various specific organs of the head and neck, with some being mostly sensory (olfactory, optic), others being mostly motor (abducens), and most being of mixed sensory and motor nerve fibers and function.

Continued on next page

Educational Annotations | 0 – Central Nervous System

Anatomy and Physiology Review of Central Nervous System

BODY PART VALUES – 0 - CENTRAL NERVOUS SYSTEM

Continued from previous page

Dura Mater – ANATOMY – The dura mater is the outermost cerebral and spinal cord layer comprised of tough, fibroelastic tissue. PHYSIOLOGY – The dura mater protects the brain and spinal cord from injury, pathogens, and any contaminates.

Epidural Space – The space inside the vertebral column and outside of the dura mater spinal meninges layer.

Facial Nerve – The seventh (VII) cranial nerve that innervates a significant number of structures both motor and sensory including facial expression and sensation, salivary glands, taste sense from the anterior portion of the tongue, and the oral and nasal cavities.

Glossopharyngeal Nerve – The ninth (IX) cranial nerve that innervates most of the motor and sensory structures of the tongue and pharynx.

Hypoglossal Nerve – The twelfth (XII) cranial nerve that innervates the musculature of the tongue and pharynx.

Hypothalamus – ANATOMY – The hypothalamus lies above the brain stem and forms the floor of the third ventricle. PHYSIOLOGY – The hypothalamus functions to control homeostasis by regulation of the heart rate, arterial blood pressure, body temperature, body weight, and sleep, and controls the anterior pituitary gland.

Lumbar Spinal Cord – That portion within the lumbar vertebral column.

Medulla Oblongata – ANATOMY – The cone-shaped part of the brainstem that is situated between the pons and the spinal cord. PHYSIOLOGY – The medulla oblongata connects the higher levels of the cerebrum to the spinal cord and transmits ascending and descending impulses. The medulla oblongata helps regulate breathing, heart rate, blood pressure, digestion, sneezing, and swallowing.

Oculomotor Nerve – The third (III) cranial nerve that innervates most of the motor function of the eye, both somatic and autonomic.

Olfactory Nerve – The first (I) cranial nerve that innervates the olfactory epithelium (sense of smell).

Optic Nerve – The second (II) cranial nerve that innervates the retina.

Pons – ANATOMY – The pons is part of the brainstem that is situated between the midbrain and above the medulla oblongata. PHYSIOLOGY – The pons transmits impulses between the cerebrum and cerebellum and other parts of the nervous system.

Spinal Canal – The spinal canal is the round space in the vertebrae through which the spinal cord passes.

Spinal Cord – ANATOMY – The spinal cord is a long cylindrical structure of nervous tissue that runs the length of the vertebral column from the medulla oblongata to the lumbar vertebral column. There are two consecutive rows of nerve roots that form 31 pairs of spinal nerves that emerge on each side. PHYSIOLOGY – The spinal cord is the nervous system link between the brain and most of the body through sensory, autonomic, and motor pathways.

Spinal Meninges – ANATOMY – The spinal meninges are continuous with the cerebral meninges, completely enclosing the spinal cord (and brain), and consist of three layers: Dura mater, arachnoid mater, and pia mater. The dura mater is the outermost tough, fibroelastic tissue layer. The arachnoid mater is the thin, transparent middle layer. The pia mater is the thin, delicate layer that adheres to the brain and spinal cord tissues. PHYSIOLOGY – The spinal meninges function to protect the spinal cord and contain the cerebrospinal fluid. The subarachnoid space is the cerebrospinal fluid-filled space between the arachnoid and the pia mater.

Subarachnoid Space – The subarachnoid space is the cerebrospinal fluid-filled space between the arachnoid and the pia mater.

Subdural Space – The potential space between the dura mater and the subarachnoid mater. Any actual space may develop due to illness or trauma.

Thalamus – ANATOMY – The thalamus lies below the corpus callosum on either side of the third ventricle. PHYSIOLOGY – The thalamus functions as a central relay station for sensory impulses and regulation of motor functions. It also functions to regulate the states of sleep and consciousness.

Continued on next page

Educational Annotations | 0 – Central Nervous System

Anatomy and Physiology Review of Central Nervous System – *continued*

BODY PART VALUES – 0 - CENTRAL NERVOUS SYSTEM
Continued from previous page

Thoracic Spinal Cord – That portion within the thoracic vertebral column.

Trigeminal Nerve – The fifth (V) cranial nerve that innervates a large number of structures, both motor and sensory, including touch, pain, and temperature of the face, nose, and mouth.

Trochlear Nerve – The fourth (IV) cranial nerve that innervates the superior oblique muscle of the orbit.

Vagus Nerve – The tenth (X) cranial nerve that innervates a large number of parasympathetic nerves of the heart, lungs, and digestive tract and controls the muscles of swallowing.

Anatomical Illustrations of Central Nervous System

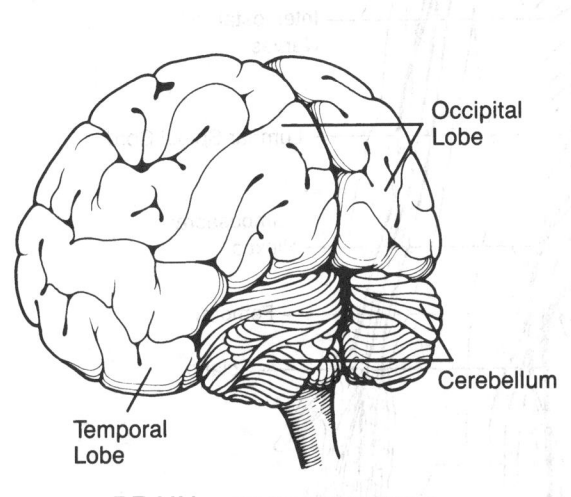

BRAIN — POSTERIOR VIEW

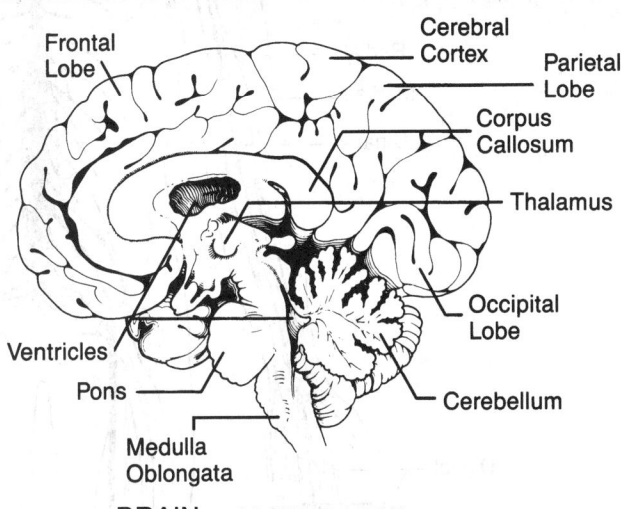

BRAIN — SAGITTAL VIEW

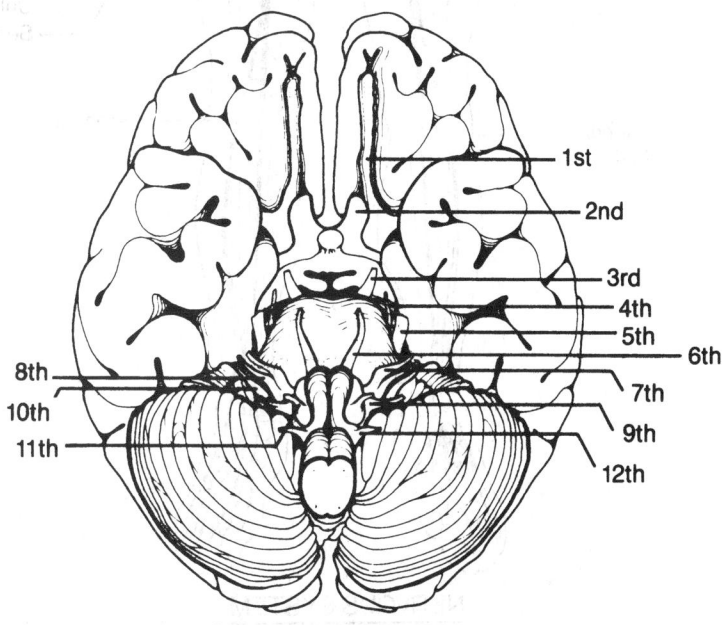

CRANIAL NERVES

Continued on next page

CENTRAL NERVOUS 0 0

Educational Annotations | 0 – Central Nervous System

Continued from previous page

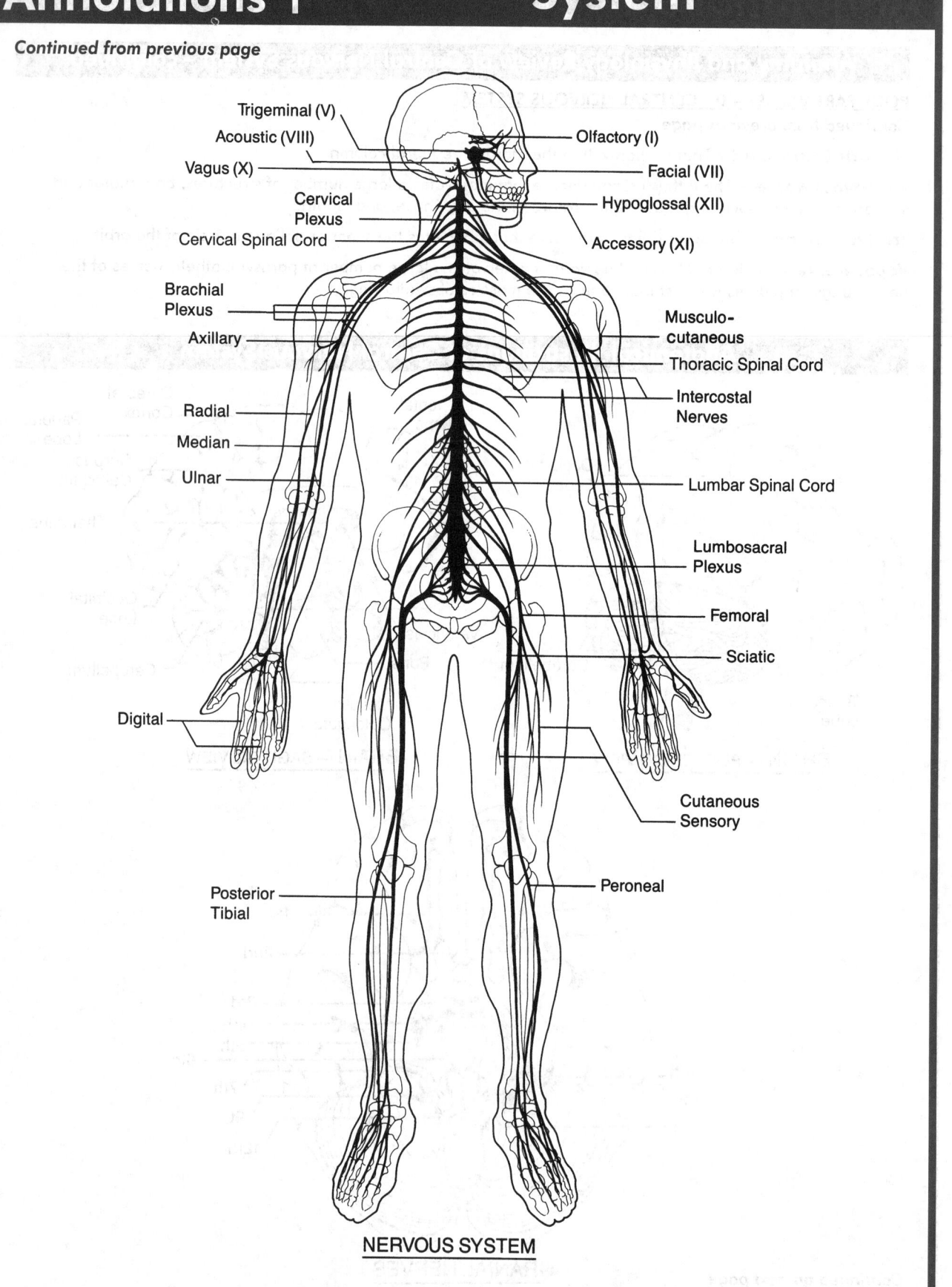

Trigeminal (V)
Acoustic (VIII)
Vagus (X)
Cervical Plexus
Cervical Spinal Cord
Brachial Plexus
Axillary
Radial
Median
Ulnar
Digital
Posterior Tibial

Olfactory (I)
Facial (VII)
Hypoglossal (XII)
Accessory (XI)
Musculo-cutaneous
Thoracic Spinal Cord
Intercostal Nerves
Lumbar Spinal Cord
Lumbosacral Plexus
Femoral
Sciatic
Cutaneous Sensory
Peroneal

NERVOUS SYSTEM

Educational Annotations | 0 – Central Nervous System

Definitions of Common Procedures of Central Nervous System

Anterior temporal lobectomy – The surgical removal of a portion of the temporal lobe of the brain to treat medically intractable temporal lobe epilepsy.

Brain biopsy – The removal of brain tissue for microscopic examination that is performed through a small hole (burr hole) drilled into the skull, often using the stereotactic navigation system.

Chiari decompression – The surgical procedure to reduce or eliminate the pressure on the spinal cord by removal of a portion of the base of the skull that creates space at the level of the foramen magnum and is often accompanied by durotomy/duraplasty.

Gasserian ganglionectomy – The surgical removal of gasserian ganglion of the trigeminal nerve.

Lumbar puncture (spinal tap) – The insertion of a needle into the lumbar subarachnoid space to withdraw cerebrospinal fluid, usually for diagnostic reasons.

Ventriculoperitoneal shunt – The shunting redirection of excessive cerebrospinal fluid (hydrocephalus) by placing a catheter into a cerebral ventricle and tunneling it under the skin and into the peritoneal cavity.

AHA Coding Clinic® Reference Notations of Central Nervous System

ROOT OPERATION SPECIFIC - 0 - CENTRAL NERVOUS SYSTEM

BYPASS - 1
Ventriculoperitoneal shunt (VP) with laparoscopic assistance ....AHA 13:2Q:p36

CHANGE - 2

DESTRUCTION - 5

DIVISION - 8

DRAINAGE - 9
Aspiration via a lumbar drain port ....AHA 14:1Q:p8
Burr hole drainage of hydrocephalus with catheter placement ....AHA 15:3Q:p12
Drainage of (fluid) subdural hematoma ....AHA 15:3Q:p10
Diagnostic lumbar tap ....AHA 14:1Q:p8
Percutaneous burr hole drainage of (fluid) chronic subdural hematoma ....AHA 15:3Q:p11
Shunting (drainage) of spinal syrinx ....AHA 15:2Q:p30
Subdural drainage using subdural evacuation portal system (SEPS) ....AHA 15:3Q:p12

EXCISION - B
Amygdalohippocampectomy ....AHA 16:2Q:p18
Brain biopsy...AHA 15:1Q:p12
Excision of spinal cord lipoma ....AHA 14:3Q:p24
Infratemporal fossa malignancy with nerve excision ....AHA 16:2Q:p12
Resection of brain tumor ....AHA 14:4Q:p34

EXTIRPATION - C
Burr hole evacuation of solid intracerebral hematoma ....AHA 15:3Q:p13
Decompressive craniectomy ....AHA 16:2Q:p29
Evacuation of brain hematoma...AHA 15:1Q:p12
Extirpation of (solid) subdural hematoma ....AHA 15:3Q:p10

EXTRACTION - D
Nonexcisional debridement of dura mater ....AHA 15:3Q:p13

FRAGMENTATION - F

INSERTION - H
Replacement of Baclofen medication pump/spinal canal catheter ....AHA 14:3Q:p19

INSPECTION - J

MAP - K

RELEASE - N
Decompressive cervical laminectomy at multiple sites ....AHA 15:2Q:p21
Decompressive craniectomy ....AHA 16:2Q:p29
Laminoplasty to expand spinal canal space..AHA 15:2Q:p20
Release of tethered spinal cord ....AHA 14:3Q:p24

REMOVAL - P
Replacement of Baclofen medication pump/spinal canal catheter ....AHA 14:3Q:p19

Continued on next page

Educational Annotations | 0 – Central Nervous System

AHA Coding Clinic® Reference Notations of Central Nervous System

Continued from previous page

REPAIR - Q
Dural rent repair ....AHA 13:3Q:p25
....AHA 14:3Q:p7
REPOSITION - S
Reimplantation of transected facial nerve into muscle ....AHA 14:4Q:p35
RESECTION - T
SUPPLEMENT - U
Dural patch graft with Durepair® ....AHA 14:3Q:p24
Dural patch graft with Durepair® clarification ....AHA 15:4Q:p39
REVISION - W
TRANSFER - X

Body Part Key Listings of Central Nervous System

See also Body Part Key in Appendix C

Anterior vagal trunk..*use* Vagus Nerve
Apneustic center ....*use* Pons
Aqueduct of Sylvius ....*use* Cerebral Ventricle
Arachnoid mater, intracranial ....*use* Cerebral Meninges
Arachnoid mater, spinal......................................*use* Spinal Meninges
Basal nuclei ....*use* Basal Ganglia
Basis pontis ....*use* Pons
Carotid sinus nerve ....*use* Glossopharyngeal Nerve
Cauda equina ....*use* Lumbar Spinal Cord
Cerebral aqueduct (Sylvius) ....*use* Cerebral Ventricle
Cerebrum...*use* Brain
Chorda tympani ....*use* Facial Nerve
Choroid plexus..*use* Cerebral Ventricle
Claustrum ....*use* Basal Ganglia
Cochlear nerve..*use* Acoustic Nerve
Conus medullaris..*use* Lumbar Spinal Cord
Corpus callosum ....*use* Brain
Corpus striatum ....*use* Basal Ganglia
Culmen ....*use* Cerebellum
Denticulate (dentate) ligament...........................*use* Spinal Meninges
Diaphragma sellae ....*use* Dura Mater
Dura mater, intracranial ....*use* Dura Mater
Dura mater, spinal ....*use* Spinal Meninges
Eighth cranial nerve..*use* Acoustic Nerve
Eleventh cranial nerve ....*use* Accessory Nerve
Encephalon ....*use* Brain
Ependyma ....*use* Cerebral Ventricle
Epidural space, intracranial ....*use* Epidural Space
Epidural space, spinal ....*use* Spinal Canal
Epithalamus ....*use* Thalamus
Extradural space, intracranial ....*use* Epidural Space
Extradural space, spinal......................................*use* Spinal Canal
Extradural space ....*use* Epidural Space
Falx cerebri ....*use* Dura Mater
Fifth cranial nerve ....*use* Trigeminal Nerve
Filum terminale ....*use* Spinal Meninges

Continued on next page

Educational Annotations | 0 – Central Nervous System

Body Part Key Listings of Central Nervous System

Continued from previous page

First cranial nerve	*use* Olfactory Nerve
Foramen of Monro (intraventricular)	*use* Cerebral Ventricle
Fourth cranial nerve	*use* Trochlear Nerve
Fourth ventricle	*use* Cerebral Ventricle
Frontal lobe	*use* Cerebral Hemisphere
Gasserian ganglion	*use* Trigeminal Nerve
Geniculate ganglion	*use* Facial Nerve
Geniculate nucleus	*use* Thalamus
Globus pallidus	*use* Basal Ganglia
Greater superficial petrosal nerve	*use* Facial Nerve
Interventricular foramen (Monro)	*use* Cerebral Ventricle
Left lateral ventricle	*use* Cerebral Ventricle
Leptomeninges, intracranial	*use* Cerebral Meninges
Leptomeninges, spinal	*use* Spinal Meninges
Locus ceruleus	*use* Pons
Mammillary body	*use* Hypothalamus
Mandibular nerve	*use* Trigeminal Nerve
Maxillary nerve	*use* Trigeminal Nerve
Metathalamus	*use* Thalamus
Myelencephalon	*use* Medulla Oblongata
Nerve to the stapedius	*use* Facial Nerve
Ninth cranial nerve	*use* Glossopharyngeal Nerve
Occipital lobe	*use* Cerebral Hemisphere
Olfactory bulb	*use* Olfactory Nerve
Ophthalmic nerve	*use* Trigeminal Nerve
Optic chiasma	*use* Optic Nerve
Parietal lobe	*use* Cerebral Hemisphere
Parotid plexus	*use* Facial Nerve
Pharyngeal plexus	*use* Vagus Nerve
Pia mater, intracranial	*use* Cerebral Meninges
Pia mater, spinal	*use* Spinal Meninges
Pneumogastric nerve	*use* Vagus Nerve
Pneumotaxic center	*use* Pons
Pontine tegmentum	*use* Pons
Posterior auricular nerve	*use* Facial Nerve
Posterior vagal trunk	*use* Vagus Nerve
Pulmonary plexus	*use* Vagus Nerve/Thoracic Sympathetic Nerve
Pulvinar	*use* Thalamus
Recurrent laryngeal nerve	*use* Vagus Nerve
Right lateral ventricle	*use* Cerebral Ventricle
Scarpa's (vestibular) ganglion	*use* Acoustic Nerve
Second cranial nerve	*use* Optic Nerve
Seventh cranial nerve	*use* Facial Nerve
Sixth cranial nerve	*use* Abducens Nerve
Spiral ganglion	*use* Acoustic Nerve
Subarachnoid space, intracranial	*use* Subarchnoid Space
Subarachnoid space, spinal	*use* Spinal Canal
Subdural space, intracranial	*use* Subdural Space
Subdural space, spinal	*use* Spinal Canal

Continued on next page

Educational Annotations | 0 – Central Nervous System

Body Part Key Listings of Central Nervous System

Continued from previous page

Submandibular ganglion	*use* Facial Nerve
Substantia nigra	*use* Basal Ganglia
Subthalamic nucleus	*use* Basal Ganglia
Superior laryngeal nerve	*use* Vagus Nerve
Superior olivary nucleus	*use* Pons
Temporal lobe	*use* Cerebral Hemisphere
Tenth cranial nerve	*use* Vagus Nerve
Tentorium cerebelli	*use* Dura Mater
Third cranial nerve	*use* Oculomotor Nerve
Third ventricle	*use* Cerebral Ventricle
Trifacial nerve	*use* Trigeminal Nerve
Twelfth cranial nerve	*use* Hypoglossal Nerve
Tympanic nerve	*use* Glossopharyngeal Nerve
Vertebral canal	*use* Spinal Canal
Vestibular (Scarpa's) ganglion	*use* Acoustic Nerve
Vestibular nerve	*use* Acoustic Nerve
Vestibulocochlear nerve	*use* Acoustic Nerve

Device Key Listings of Central Nervous System

See also Device Key in Appendix D

Ascenda Intrathecal Catheter	*use* Infusion Device
Autograft	*use* Autologous Tissue Substitute
Cortical strip neurostimulator lead	*use* Neurostimulator Lead in Central Nervous System
DBS lead	*use* Neurostimulator Lead in Central Nervous System
Deep brain neurostimulator lead	*use* Neurostimulator Lead in Central Nervous System
Holter valve ventricular shunt	*use* Synthetic Substitute
InDura, intrathecal catheter (1P) (spinal)	*use* Infusion Device
RNS System lead	*use* Neurostimulator Lead in Central Nervous System
Spinal cord neurostimulator lead	*use* Neurostimulator Lead in Central Nervous System
Tissue bank graft	*use* Nonautologous Tissue Substitute
Tunneled spinal (intrathecal) catheter	*use* Infusion Device

Device Aggregation Table Listings of Central Nervous System

See also Device Aggregation Table in Appendix E

Specific Device	For Operation	In Body System	General Device
None Listed in Device Aggregation Table for this Body System			

Coding Notes of Central Nervous System

Body System Specific PCS Reference Manual Exercises

PCS CODE	0 – CENTRAL NERVOUS SYSTEM EXERCISES
0 0 1 6 0 J 6	Shunting of intrathecal cerebrospinal fluid to peritoneal cavity using synthetic shunt.
0 0 1 6 3 J 6	Percutaneous placement of ventriculoperitoneal shunt for treatment of hydrocephalus.
0 0 2 0 X 0 Z	Exchange of cerebral ventriculostomy drainage tube.
0 0 9 6 3 0 Z	External ventricular CSF drainage catheter placement via burr hole.
0 0 K 0 0 Z Z	Intraoperative whole brain mapping via craniotomy.
0 0 K 7 4 Z Z	Mapping of left cerebral hemisphere, percutaneous endoscopic.
0 0 K 8 3 Z Z	Percutaneous mapping of basal ganglia.
0 0 X K 4 Z M	Trigeminal to facial nerve transfer, percutaneous endoscopic.

TUBULAR GROUP: Bypass, (Dilation), (Occlusion), (Restriction)
Root Operations that alter the diameter/route of a tubular body part.

1ST - **0** Medical and Surgical

2ND - **0** Central Nervous System

3RD - **1 BYPASS**

EXAMPLE: Ventriculoperitoneal shunt | CMS Ex: Coronary artery bypass

BYPASS: Altering the route of passage of the contents of a tubular body part.

EXPLANATION: Rerouting contents to a downstream part ...

Body Part – 4TH	Approach – 5TH	Device – 6TH	Qualifier – 7TH
6 Cerebral Ventricle	0 Open 3 Percutaneous	7 Autologous tissue substitute J Synthetic substitute K Nonautologous tissue substitute	0 Nasopharynx 1 Mastoid sinus 2 Atrium 3 Blood vessel 4 Pleural cavity 5 Intestine 6 Peritoneal cavity 7 Urinary tract 8 Bone marrow B Cerebral cisterns
U Spinal Canal	0 Open 3 Percutaneous	7 Autologous tissue substitute J Synthetic substitute K Nonautologous tissue substitute	4 Pleural cavity 6 Peritoneal cavity 7 Urinary tract 9 Fallopian tube

DEVICE GROUP: Change, Insertion, Removal, (Replacement), Revision, Supplement
Root Operations that always involve a device.

1ST - **0** Medical and Surgical

2ND - **0** Central Nervous System

3RD - **2 CHANGE**

EXAMPLE: Exchange ventriculostomy tube | CMS Ex: Change urinary cath

CHANGE: Taking out or off a device from a body part and putting back an identical or similar device in or on the same body part without cutting or puncturing the skin or a mucous membrane.

EXPLANATION: ALL Changes use EXTERNAL approach only...

Body Part – 4TH	Approach – 5TH	Device – 6TH	Qualifier – 7TH
0 Brain E Cranial Nerve U Spinal Canal	X External	0 Drainage device Y Other device	Z No qualifier

EXCISION GROUP: Excision, Resection, Destruction, Extraction, (Detachment)
Root Operations that take out some or all of a body part.

1ST – **0** Medical and Surgical	EXAMPLE: Ablation trigeminal nerve CMS Ex: Fulguration polyp
2ND – **0** Central Nervous System	**DESTRUCTION:** Physical eradication of all or a portion of a body part by the direct use of energy, force, or a destructive agent.
3RD – **5 DESTRUCTION**	EXPLANATION: None of the body part is physically taken out

Body Part – 4TH		Approach – 5TH	Device – 6TH	Qualifier – 7TH
0 Brain	J Trochlear Nerve	0 Open	Z No device	Z No qualifier
1 Cerebral Meninges	K Trigeminal Nerve	3 Percutaneous		
2 Dura Mater	L Abducens Nerve	4 Percutaneous		
6 Cerebral Ventricle	M Facial Nerve	endoscopic		
7 Cerebral Hemisphere	N Acoustic Nerve			
8 Basal Ganglia	P Glossopharyngeal Nerve			
9 Thalamus	Q Vagus Nerve			
A Hypothalamus	R Accessory Nerve			
B Pons	S Hypoglossal Nerve			
C Cerebellum	T Spinal Meninges			
D Medulla Oblongata	W Cervical Spinal Cord			
F Olfactory Nerve	X Thoracic Spinal Cord			
G Optic Nerve	Y Lumbar Spinal Cord			
H Oculomotor Nerve				

DIVISION GROUP: Division, Release
Root Operations involving cutting or separation only.

1ST – **0** Medical and Surgical	EXAMPLE: Bisection facial nerve CMS Ex: Osteotomy
2ND – **0** Central Nervous System	**DIVISION:** Cutting into a body part without draining fluids and/or gases from the body part in order to separate or transect a body part.
3RD – **8 DIVISION**	EXPLANATION: Separated into two or more portions ...

Body Part – 4TH	Approach – 5TH	Device – 6TH	Qualifier – 7TH
0 Brain	0 Open	Z No device	Z No qualifier
7 Cerebral Hemisphere	3 Percutaneous		
8 Basal Ganglia	4 Percutaneous		
F Olfactory Nerve	endoscopic		
G Optic Nerve			
H Oculomotor Nerve			
J Trochlear Nerve			
K Trigeminal Nerve			
L Abducens Nerve			
M Facial Nerve			
N Acoustic Nerve			
P Glossopharyngeal Nerve			
Q Vagus Nerve			
R Accessory Nerve			
S Hypoglossal Nerve			
W Cervical Spinal Cord			
X Thoracic Spinal Cord			
Y Lumbar Spinal Cord			

DRAINAGE GROUP: Drainage, Extirpation, Fragmentation
Root Operations that take out solids/fluids/gases from a body part.

1ST - 0 Medical and Surgical	EXAMPLE: Lumbar puncture	CMS Ex: Thoracentesis

2ND - 0 Central Nervous System

3RD - 9 DRAINAGE

DRAINAGE: Taking or letting out fluids and/or gases from a body part.

EXPLANATION: Qualifier "X Diagnostic" indicates biopsy ...

Body Part – 4TH		Approach – 5TH	Device – 6TH	Qualifier – 7TH
0 Brain	H Oculomotor Nerve	0 Open	0 Drainage device	Z No qualifier
1 Cerebral Meninges	J Trochlear Nerve	3 Percutaneous		
2 Dura Mater	K Trigeminal Nerve	4 Percutaneous endoscopic		
3 Epidural Space	L Abducens Nerve			
4 Subdural Space	M Facial Nerve			
5 Subarachnoid Space	N Acoustic Nerve			
6 Cerebral Ventricle	P Glossopharyngeal Nerve			
7 Cerebral Hemisphere	Q Vagus Nerve			
8 Basal Ganglia	R Accessory Nerve			
9 Thalamus	S Hypoglossal Nerve			
A Hypothalamus	T Spinal Meninges			
B Pons	U Spinal Canal			
C Cerebellum	W Cervical Spinal Cord			
D Medulla Oblongata	X Thoracic Spinal Cord			
F Olfactory Nerve	Y Lumbar Spinal Cord			
G Optic Nerve				
0 Brain	H Oculomotor Nerve	0 Open	Z No device	X Diagnostic
1 Cerebral Meninges	J Trochlear Nerve	3 Percutaneous		Z No qualifier
2 Dura Mater	K Trigeminal Nerve	4 Percutaneous endoscopic		
3 Epidural Space	L Abducens Nerve			
4 Subdural Space	M Facial Nerve			
5 Subarachnoid Space	N Acoustic Nerve			
6 Cerebral Ventricle	P Glossopharyngeal Nerve			
7 Cerebral Hemisphere	Q Vagus Nerve			
8 Basal Ganglia	R Accessory Nerve			
9 Thalamus	S Hypoglossal Nerve			
A Hypothalamus	T Spinal Meninges			
B Pons	U Spinal Canal			
C Cerebellum	W Cervical Spinal Cord			
D Medulla Oblongata	X Thoracic Spinal Cord			
F Olfactory Nerve	Y Lumbar Spinal Cord			
G Optic Nerve				

CENTRAL NERVOUS 009

EXCISION GROUP: Excision, Resection, Destruction, Extraction, (Detachment)
Root Operations that take out some or all of a body part.

1ST – 0 Medical and Surgical	EXAMPLE: Stereotactic thalamic biopsy CMS Ex: Liver biopsy
2ND – 0 Central Nervous System	**EXCISION:** Cutting out or off, without replacement, a portion of a body part.
3RD – B EXCISION	EXPLANATION: Qualifier "X Diagnostic" indicates biopsy …

Body Part – 4TH		Approach – 5TH	Device – 6TH	Qualifier – 7TH
0 Brain	J Trochlear Nerve	0 Open	Z No device	X Diagnostic
1 Cerebral Meninges	K Trigeminal Nerve	3 Percutaneous		Z No qualifier
2 Dura Mater	L Abducens Nerve	4 Percutaneous endoscopic		
6 Cerebral Ventricle	M Facial Nerve			
7 Cerebral Hemisphere	N Acoustic Nerve			
8 Basal Ganglia	P Glossopharyngeal Nerve			
9 Thalamus	Q Vagus Nerve			
A Hypothalamus	R Accessory Nerve			
B Pons	S Hypoglossal Nerve			
C Cerebellum	T Spinal Meninges			
D Medulla Oblongata	W Cervical Spinal Cord			
F Olfactory Nerve	X Thoracic Spinal Cord			
G Optic Nerve	Y Lumbar Spinal Cord			
H Oculomotor Nerve				

DRAINAGE GROUP: Drainage, Extirpation, Fragmentation
Root Operations that take out solids/fluids/gases from a body part.

1ST – 0 Medical and Surgical	EXAMPLE: Removal FB lumbar spinal cord CMS Ex: Choledocholithotomy
2ND – 0 Central Nervous System	**EXTIRPATION:** Taking or cutting out solid matter from a body part.
3RD – C EXTIRPATION	EXPLANATION: Abnormal byproduct or foreign body …

Body Part – 4TH		Approach – 5TH	Device – 6TH	Qualifier – 7TH
0 Brain	H Oculomotor Nerve	0 Open	Z No device	Z No qualifier
1 Cerebral Meninges	J Trochlear Nerve	3 Percutaneous		
2 Dura Mater	K Trigeminal Nerve	4 Percutaneous endoscopic		
3 Epidural Space	L Abducens Nerve			
4 Subdural Space	M Facial Nerve			
5 Subarachnoid Space	N Acoustic Nerve			
6 Cerebral Ventricle	P Glossopharyngeal Nerve			
7 Cerebral Hemisphere	Q Vagus Nerve			
8 Basal Ganglia	R Accessory Nerve			
9 Thalamus	S Hypoglossal Nerve			
A Hypothalamus	T Spinal Meninges			
B Pons	W Cervical Spinal Cord			
C Cerebellum	X Thoracic Spinal Cord			
D Medulla Oblongata	Y Lumbar Spinal Cord			
F Olfactory Nerve				
G Optic Nerve				

EXCISION GROUP: Excision, Resection, Destruction, Extraction, (Detachment)
Root Operations that take out some or all of a body part.

1ST - **0** Medical and Surgical

2ND - **0** Central Nervous System

3RD - **D EXTRACTION**

EXAMPLE: Extraction vagus nerve segment   CMS Ex: D&C

EXTRACTION: Pulling or stripping out or off all or a portion of a body part by the use of force.

EXPLANATION: None for this Body System

Body Part – 4TH		Approach – 5TH	Device – 6TH	Qualifier – 7TH
1 Cerebral Meninges	M Facial Nerve	0 Open	Z No device	Z No qualifier
2 Dura Mater	N Acoustic Nerve	3 Percutaneous		
F Olfactory Nerve	P Glossopharyngeal Nerve	4 Percutaneous endoscopic		
G Optic Nerve	Q Vagus Nerve			
H Oculomotor Nerve	R Accessory Nerve			
J Trochlear Nerve	S Hypoglossal Nerve			
K Trigeminal Nerve	T Spinal Meninges			
L Abducens Nerve				

DRAINAGE GROUP: Drainage, Extirpation, Fragmentation
Root Operations that take out solids/fluids/gases from a body part.

1ST - **0** Medical and Surgical

2ND - **0** Central Nervous System

3RD - **F FRAGMENTATION**

EXAMPLE: Fragmentation foreign body   CMS Ex: ESWL

FRAGMENTATION: Breaking solid matter in a body part into pieces.

EXPLANATION: Pieces are not taken out during procedure ...

Body Part – 4TH	Approach – 5TH	Device – 6TH	Qualifier – 7TH
3 Epidural Space	0 Open	Z No device	Z No qualifier
4 Subdural Space	3 Percutaneous		
5 Subarachnoid Space	4 Percutaneous endoscopic		
6 Cerebral Ventricle	X External NC*		
U Spinal Canal			

NC* – Some procedures are considered non-covered by Medicare. See current Medicare Code Editor for details.

DEVICE GROUP: Change, Insertion, Removal, (Replacement), Revision, Supplement
Root Operations that always involve a device.

1ST - **0** Medical and Surgical

2ND - **0** Central Nervous System

3RD - **H INSERTION**

EXAMPLE: Intrathecal spinal cord cath   CMS Ex: Central venous catheter

INSERTION: Putting in a nonbiological appliance that monitors, assists, performs, or prevents a physiological function but does not physically take the place of a body part.

EXPLANATION: None

Body Part – 4TH	Approach – 5TH	Device – 6TH	Qualifier – 7TH
0 Brain	0 Open	2 Monitoring device	Z No qualifier
6 Cerebral Ventricle	3 Percutaneous	3 Infusion device	
E Cranial Nerve	4 Percutaneous endoscopic	M Neurostimulator lead	
U Spinal Canal			
V Spinal Cord			

EXAMINATION GROUP: Inspection, Map
Root Operations involving examination only.

1ST - 0 Medical and Surgical	EXAMPLE: Examination cranial nerve	CMS Ex: Colonoscopy
2ND - 0 Central Nervous System	INSPECTION: Visually and/or manually exploring a body part.	
3RD - J INSPECTION	EXPLANATION: Direct or instrumental visualization ...	

Body Part – 4TH	Approach – 5TH	Device – 6TH	Qualifier – 7TH
0 Brain E Cranial Nerve U Spinal Canal V Spinal Cord	0 Open 3 Percutaneous 4 Percutaneous endoscopic	Z No device	Z No qualifier

EXAMINATION GROUP: Inspection, Map
Root Operations involving examination only.

1ST - 0 Medical and Surgical	EXAMPLE: Mapping of basal ganglia	CMS Ex: Cardiac mapping
2ND - 0 Central Nervous System	MAP: Locating the route of passage of electrical impulses and/or locating functional areas in a body part.	
3RD - K MAP	EXPLANATION: Limited to cardiac and nervous systems...	

Body Part – 4TH	Approach – 5TH	Device – 6TH	Qualifier – 7TH
0 Brain 7 Cerebral Hemisphere 8 Basal Ganglia 9 Thalamus A Hypothalamus B Pons C Cerebellum D Medulla Oblongata	0 Open 3 Percutaneous 4 Percutaneous endoscopic	Z No device	Z No qualifier

C E N T R A L   N E R V O U S   0 0 J

DIVISION GROUP: Division, Release
Root Operations involving cutting or separation only.

| EXAMPLE: Lysis acoustic nerve scar tissue | CMS Ex: Carpal tunnel release |

1ST - 0 Medical and Surgical

2ND - 0 Central Nervous System

3RD - N RELEASE

RELEASE: Freeing a body part from an abnormal physical constraint by cutting or by the use of force.

EXPLANATION: None of the body part is taken out ...

Body Part – 4TH		Approach – 5TH	Device – 6TH	Qualifier – 7TH
0 Brain	J Trochlear Nerve	0 Open	Z No device	Z No qualifier
1 Cerebral Meninges	K Trigeminal Nerve	3 Percutaneous		
2 Dura Mater	L Abducens Nerve	4 Percutaneous endoscopic		
6 Cerebral Ventricle	M Facial Nerve			
7 Cerebral Hemisphere	N Acoustic Nerve			
8 Basal Ganglia	P Glossopharyngeal Nerve			
9 Thalamus	Q Vagus Nerve			
A Hypothalamus	R Accessory Nerve			
B Pons	S Hypoglossal Nerve			
C Cerebellum	T Spinal Meninges			
D Medulla Oblongata	W Cervical Spinal Cord			
F Olfactory Nerve	X Thoracic Spinal Cord			
G Optic Nerve	Y Lumbar Spinal Cord			
H Oculomotor Nerve				

DEVICE GROUP: Change, Insertion, Removal, (Replacement), Revision, Supplement
Root Operations that always involve a device.

1ST - 0 Medical and Surgical	EXAMPLE: Removal neurostimulator lead	CMS Ex: Chest tube removal

2ND - 0 Central Nervous System

3RD - P REMOVAL

REMOVAL: Taking out or off a device from a body part.

EXPLANATION: Removal device without reinsertion …

Body Part – 4TH	Approach – 5TH	Device – 6TH	Qualifier – 7TH
0 Brain V Spinal Cord	0 Open 3 Percutaneous 4 Percutaneous endoscopic	0 Drainage device 2 Monitoring device 3 Infusion device 7 Autologous tissue substitute J Synthetic substitute K Nonautologous tissue substitute M Neurostimulator lead	Z No qualifier
0 Brain V Spinal Cord	X External	0 Drainage device 2 Monitoring device 3 Infusion device M Neurostimulator lead	Z No qualifier
6 Cerebral Ventricle U Spinal Canal	0 Open 3 Percutaneous 4 Percutaneous endoscopic	0 Drainage device 2 Monitoring device 3 Infusion device J Synthetic substitute M Neurostimulator lead	Z No qualifier
6 Cerebral Ventricle U Spinal Canal	X External	0 Drainage device 2 Monitoring device 3 Infusion device M Neurostimulator lead	Z No qualifier
E Cranial Nerve	0 Open 3 Percutaneous 4 Percutaneous endoscopic	0 Drainage device 2 Monitoring device 3 Infusion device 7 Autologous tissue substitute M Neurostimulator lead	Z No qualifier
E Cranial Nerve	X External	0 Drainage device 2 Monitoring device 3 Infusion device M Neurostimulator lead	Z No qualifier

---

OTHER REPAIRS GROUP: (Control), Repair
Root Operations that define other repairs.

1ST - 0	Medical and Surgical	EXAMPLE: Cerebral meningeorrhaphy	CMS Ex: Suture laceration
2ND - 0	Central Nervous System	**REPAIR:** Restoring, to the extent possible, a body part to its normal anatomic structure and function.	
3RD - Q REPAIR			
		EXPLANATION: Only when no other root operation applies ...	

Body Part – 4TH		Approach – 5TH	Device – 6TH	Qualifier – 7TH
0 Brain	J Trochlear Nerve	0 Open	Z No device	Z No qualifier
1 Cerebral Meninges	K Trigeminal Nerve	3 Percutaneous		
2 Dura Mater	L Abducens Nerve	4 Percutaneous endoscopic		
6 Cerebral Ventricle	M Facial Nerve			
7 Cerebral Hemisphere	N Acoustic Nerve			
8 Basal Ganglia	P Glossopharyngeal Nerve			
9 Thalamus	Q Vagus Nerve			
A Hypothalamus	R Accessory Nerve			
B Pons	S Hypoglossal Nerve			
C Cerebellum	T Spinal Meninges			
D Medulla Oblongata	W Cervical Spinal Cord			
F Olfactory Nerve	X Thoracic Spinal Cord			
G Optic Nerve	Y Lumbar Spinal Cord			
H Oculomotor Nerve				

MOVE GROUP: (Reattachment), Reposition, Transfer, (Transplantation)
Root Operations that put in/put back or move some/all of a body part.

1ST - 0	Medical and Surgical	EXAMPLE: Relocation hypoglossal nerve	CMS Ex: Fracture reduction
2ND - 0	Central Nervous System	**REPOSITION:** Moving to its normal location, or other suitable location, all or a portion of a body part.	
3RD - S REPOSITION			
		EXPLANATION: May or may not be cut to be moved ...	

Body Part – 4TH		Approach – 5TH	Device – 6TH	Qualifier – 7TH
F Olfactory Nerve	P Glossopharyngeal Nerve	0 Open	Z No device	Z No qualifier
G Optic Nerve	Q Vagus Nerve	3 Percutaneous		
H Oculomotor Nerve	R Accessory Nerve	4 Percutaneous endoscopic		
J Trochlear Nerve	S Hypoglossal Nerve			
K Trigeminal Nerve	W Cervical Spinal Cord			
L Abducens Nerve	X Thoracic Spinal Cord			
M Facial Nerve	Y Lumbar Spinal Cord			
N Acoustic Nerve				

EXCISION GROUP: Excision, Resection, Destruction, Extraction, (Detachment)
Root Operations that take out some or all of a body part.

1ST - 0 Medical and Surgical	EXAMPLE: Cerebral hemispherectomy	CMS Ex: Cholecystectomy
2ND - 0 Central Nervous System 3RD - T **RESECTION**	**RESECTION:** Cutting out or off, without replacement, all of a body part.	
	EXPLANATION: None	

Body Part – 4TH	Approach – 5TH	Device – 6TH	Qualifier – 7TH
7 Cerebral Hemisphere	0 Open 3 Percutaneous 4 Percutaneous endoscopic	Z No device	Z No qualifier

DEVICE GROUP: Change, Insertion, Removal, (Replacement), Revision, Supplement
Root Operations that always involve a device.

1ST - 0 Medical and Surgical	EXAMPLE: Dural patch graft	CMS Ex: Hernia repair with mesh
2ND - 0 Central Nervous System 3RD - U **SUPPLEMENT**	**SUPPLEMENT:** Putting in or on biological or synthetic material that physically reinforces and/or augments the function of a portion of a body part.	
	EXPLANATION: Biological material from same individual ...	

Body Part – 4TH	Approach – 5TH	Device – 6TH	Qualifier – 7TH
1 Cerebral Meninges 2 Dura Mater T Spinal Meninges	0 Open 3 Percutaneous 4 Percutaneous endoscopic	7 Autologous tissue substitute J Synthetic substitute K Nonautologous tissue substitute	Z No qualifier
F Olfactory Nerve M Facial Nerve G Optic Nerve N Acoustic Nerve H Oculomotor Nerve P Glossopharyngeal Nerve J Trochlear Nerve Q Vagus Nerve K Trigeminal Nerve R Accessory Nerve L Abducens Nerve S Hypoglossal Nerve	0 Open 3 Percutaneous 4 Percutaneous endoscopic	7 Autologous tissue substitute	Z No qualifier

DEVICE GROUP: Change, Insertion, Removal, (Replacement), Revision, Supplement
Root Operations that always involve a device.

1ST - 0 Medical and Surgical	EXAMPLE: Reposition neurostimulator lead	CMS Ex: Adjust pacemaker lead
2ND - 0 Central Nervous System	**REVISION:** Correcting, to the extent possible, a portion of a malfunctioning device or the position of a displaced device.	
3RD - W REVISION	EXPLANATION: May replace components of a device ...	

Body Part – 4TH	Approach – 5TH	Device – 6TH	Qualifier – 7TH
0 Brain V Spinal Cord	0 Open 3 Percutaneous 4 Percutaneous endoscopic X External	0 Drainage device 2 Monitoring device 3 Infusion device 7 Autologous tissue substitute J Synthetic substitute K Nonautologous tissue substitute M Neurostimulator lead	Z No qualifier
6 Cerebral Ventricle U Spinal Canal	0 Open 3 Percutaneous 4 Percutaneous endoscopic X External	0 Drainage device 2 Monitoring device 3 Infusion device J Synthetic substitute M Neurostimulator lead	Z No qualifier
E Cranial Nerve	0 Open 3 Percutaneous 4 Percutaneous endoscopic X External	0 Drainage device 2 Monitoring device 3 Infusion device 7 Autologous tissue substitute M Neurostimulator lead	Z No qualifier

MOVE GROUP: (Reattachment), **Reposition, Transfer,** (Transplantation)
Root Operations that put in/put back or move some/all of a body part.

1ST - **0** Medical and Surgical	**EXAMPLE:** Transfer trigeminal to facial nerve	**CMS Ex:** Tendon transfer
2ND - **0** Central Nervous System	**TRANSFER:** Moving, without taking out, all or a portion of a body part to another location to take over the function of all or a portion of a body part.	
3RD - **X TRANSFER**	**EXPLANATION:** The body part remains connected ...	

Body Part – 4TH	Approach – 5TH	Device – 6TH	Qualifier – 7TH
F Olfactory Nerve G Optic Nerve H Oculomotor Nerve J Trochlear Nerve K Trigeminal Nerve L Abducens Nerve M Facial Nerve N Acoustic Nerve P Glossopharyngeal Nerve Q Vagus Nerve R Accessory Nerve S Hypoglossal Nerve	0 Open 4 Percutaneous endoscopic	Z No device	F Olfactory Nerve G Optic Nerve H Oculomotor Nerve J Trochlear Nerve K Trigeminal Nerve L Abducens Nerve M Facial Nerve N Acoustic Nerve P Glossopharyngeal Nerve Q Vagus Nerve R Accessory Nerve S Hypoglossal Nerve

Educational Annotations | 1 – Peripheral Nervous System

Body System Specific Educational Annotations for the Peripheral Nervous System include:

- Anatomy and Physiology Review
- Anatomical Illustrations
- Definitions of Common Procedures
- AHA Coding Clinic® Reference Notations
- Body Part Key Listings
- Device Key Listings
- Device Aggregation Table Listings
- Coding Notes

Anatomy and Physiology Review of Peripheral Nervous System

BODY PART VALUES – 1 - PERIPHERAL NERVOUS SYSTEM

Abdominal Sympathetic Nerve – The autonomic nervous system sympathetic nerve trunk portion that innervates the smooth muscles, glands, and organs of the abdominal region.

Brachial Plexus – A branching network of the last four cervical spinal nerves and the first thoracic spinal nerve (C5-C8, T1) that primarily innervates the skin and muscles of the upper limbs.

Cervical Nerve – One of eight pairs of spinal nerves emerging from the cervical vertebrae.

Cervical Plexus – A branching network of the first four cervical spinal nerves (C1-C4) that primarily innervates the skin and muscles of the head and neck.

Femoral Nerve – The femoral nerve is the major nerve that innervates the muscles and skin of the thigh and leg.

Head and Neck Sympathetic Nerve – The autonomic nervous system sympathetic nerve trunk portion that innervates the smooth muscles, glands, and organs of the head and neck region.

Lumbar Nerve – One of five pairs of spinal nerves emerging from the lumbar vertebrae.

Lumbar Plexus – A branching network of the first four lumbar spinal nerves and the last thoracic spinal nerve (L1-L4, T12) that primarily innervates the skin and muscles of the lower abdomen and upper legs.

Lumbar Sympathetic Nerve – The autonomic nervous system sympathetic nerve trunk portion that innervates the smooth muscles, glands, and organs of the lower abdominal and pelvic regions.

Lumbosacral Plexus – A branching network of the lumbar spinal nerves, the last thoracic spinal nerve (L1-L5, T12), the sacral plexus (S1-S3), and pudendal plexus (S4-S5 and coccygeal nerve) that primarily innervates the skin and muscles of the lower abdomen and legs.

Median Nerve – The median nerve is one of the three major upper limb nerves that innervates the muscles and skin of the forearm and hand.

Peripheral Nerve – ANATOMY – A nerve outside of the brain and spinal cord. PHYSIOLOGY – The peripheral nervous system consists of a network of nerves that coordinates its voluntary and involuntary actions and communication among its parts.

Peroneal Nerve – The peroneal nerve is a division of the sciatic nerve that innervates the muscles and skin of the lower leg.

Phrenic Nerve – The phrenic nerve is the major nerve that innervates the muscles of the diaphragm and is the nerve responsible for the hiccough reflex.

Pudendal Nerve – The pudendal nerve is the major nerve that innervates the perineum, external genitalia, and anus.

Radial Nerve – The radial nerve is one of the three major upper limb nerves that innervates the muscles and skin of the arm (specifically the triceps muscle), wrist, and hand.

Sacral Nerve – One of five pairs of spinal nerves emerging from the sacrum.

Sacral Plexus – A branching network of the sacral nerves (S1-S5) and coccygeal nerve that primarily innervates the skin and muscles of the legs.

Sacral Sympathetic Nerve – The autonomic nervous system sympathetic nerve trunk portion that innervates the smooth muscles, glands, and organs of the pelvic region.

Sciatic Nerve – The sciatic nerve is the major nerve that innervates the muscles and skin of the thighs, lower legs, and feet.

Thoracic Nerve – One of twelve pairs of spinal nerves emerging from the thoracic vertebrae.

Continued on next page

Educational Annotations | 1 – Peripheral Nervous System

Anatomy and Physiology Review of Peripheral Nervous System

BODY PART VALUES – 1 - PERIPHERAL NERVOUS SYSTEM
Continued from previous page

Thoracic Sympathetic Nerve – The autonomic nervous system sympathetic nerve trunk portion that innervates the smooth muscles, glands, and organs of the thoracic region.

Tibial Nerve – The tibial nerve is a division of the sciatic nerve that innervates the muscles and skin of the lower legs and feet.

Ulnar Nerve – The ulnar nerve is one of the three major upper limb nerves that innervates the muscles and skin of the arm, hand, little finger, and half of the ring finger.

Anatomical Illustrations of Peripheral Nervous System

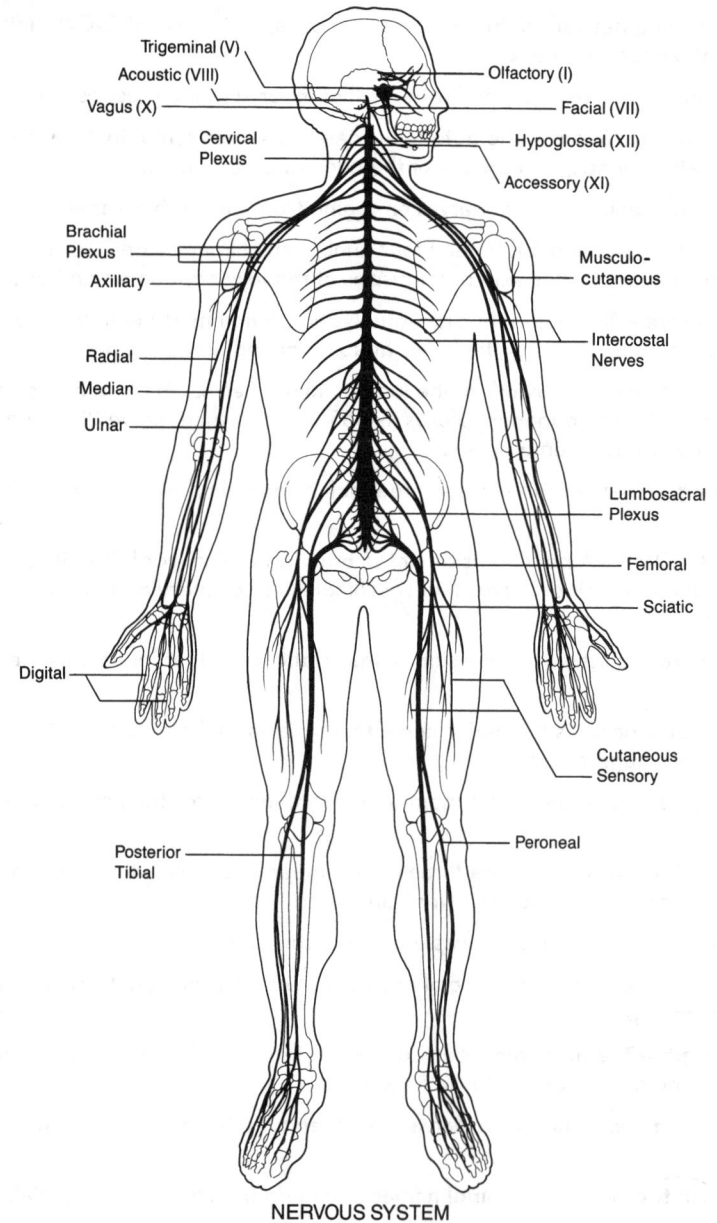

NERVOUS SYSTEM

Educational Annotations | 1 – Peripheral Nervous System

Definitions of Common Procedures of Peripheral Nervous System

Carpal tunnel release – The surgical relief from pain and weakness of the hand due to compression of the median nerve at the wrist by dividing the transverse carpal ligament causing the compression.

Free nerve graft – The surgical repair of a damaged nerve to restore nerve function using a harvested nerve section to connect both ends of the damaged nerve.

Nerve transfer – The surgical dissection to free a viable redundant nerve branch to connect to the damaged nerve in order to restore movement or sensory function.

Thoracic sympathectomy – The surgical excision or destruction of the thoracic sympathetic nerve chain ganglia to alleviate the symptoms of hyperhidrosis, sweaty palms, or Raynaud's disease.

AHA Coding Clinic® Reference Notations of Peripheral Nervous System

ROOT OPERATION SPECIFIC - 1 - PERIPHERAL NERVOUS SYSTEM
CHANGE - 2
DESTRUCTION - 5
DIVISION - 8
DRAINAGE - 9
EXCISION - B
EXTIRPATION - C
EXTRACTION - D
INSERTION - H
INSPECTION - J
RELEASE - N
    Carpal tunnel release ....AHA 14:3Q:p33
    Cervical neural foraminal decompression................................AHA 16:2Q:p17
    Complete release of brachial plexus......................................AHA 16:2Q:p23
    Discectomy with decompressive foraminotomy/laminectomy.....................AHA 16:2Q:p16
REMOVAL - P
REPAIR - Q
REPOSITION - S
SUPPLEMENT - U
REVISION - W
TRANSFER - X

Body Part Key Listings of Peripheral Nervous System

See also Body Part Key in Appendix C
Abdominal aortic plexus ....*use* Abdominal Sympathetic Nerve
Accessory obturator nerve ....*use* Lumbar Plexus
Accessory phrenic nerve ....*use* Phrenic Nerve
Ansa cervicalis ....*use* Cervical Plexus
Anterior crural nerve ....*use* Femoral Nerve
Anterior interosseous nerve ....*use* Median Nerve
Auerbach's (myenteric) plexus ....*use* Abdominal Sympathetic Nerve
Axillary nerve...............................*use* Brachial Plexus
Cardiac plexus ....*use* Thoracic Sympathetic Nerve
Cavernous plexus.............................*use* Head and Neck Sympathetic Nerve
Continued on next page

Educational Annotations | 1 – Peripheral Nervous System

Body Part Key Listings of Peripheral Nervous System

Continued from previous page

Celiac ganglion	*use* Abdominal Sympathetic Nerve
Celiac (solar) plexus	*use* Abdominal Sympathetic Nerve
Cervical ganglion	*use* Head and Neck Sympathetic Nerve
Ciliary ganglion	*use* Head and Neck Sympathetic Nerve
Common fibular nerve	*use* Peroneal Nerve
Common peroneal nerve	*use* Peroneal Nerve
Cubital nerve	*use* Ulnar Nerve
Cutaneous (transverse) cervical nerve	*use* Cervical Plexus
Dorsal digital nerve	*use* Radial Nerve
Dorsal scapular nerve	*use* Brachial Plexus
Esophageal plexus	*use* Thoracic Sympathetic Nerve
External popliteal nerve	*use* Peroneal Nerve
First intercostal nerve	*use* Brachial Plexus
Ganglion impar (ganglion of Walther)	*use* Sacral Sympathetic Nerve
Gastric plexus	*use* Abdominal Sympathetic Nerve
Genitofemoral nerve	*use* Lumbar Plexus
Great auricular nerve	*use* Cervical Plexus
Greater occipital nerve	*use* Cervical Nerve
Greater splanchnic nerve	*use* Thoracic Sympathetic Nerve
Hepatic plexus	*use* Abdominal Sympathetic Nerve
Iliohypogastric nerve	*use* Lumbar Plexus
Ilioinguinal nerve	*use* Lumbar Plexus
Inferior cardiac nerve	*use* Thoracic Sympathetic Nerve
Inferior gluteal nerve	*use* Sacral Plexus
Inferior hypogastric plexus	*use* Abdominal Sympathetic Nerve
Inferior mesenteric ganglion	*use* Abdominal Sympathetic Nerve
Inferior mesenteric plexus	*use* Abdominal Sympathetic Nerve
Intercostal nerve	*use* Thoracic Nerve
Intercostobrachial nerve	*use* Thoracic Nerve
Internal carotid plexus	*use* Head and Neck Sympathetic Nerve
Ischiatic nerve	*use* Sciatic Nerve
Lateral femoral cutaneous nerve	*use* Lumbar Plexus
Lateral plantar nerve	*use* Tibial Nerve
Lateral sural cutaneous nerve	*use* Peroneal Nerve
Least splanchnic nerve	*use* Thoracic Sympathetic Nerve
Lesser occipital nerve	*use* Cervical Plexus
Lesser splanchnic nerve	*use* Thoracic Sympathetic Nerve
Long thoracic nerve	*use* Brachial Plexus
Lumbar ganglion	*use* Lumbar Sympathetic Nerve
Lumbar splanchnic nerve	*use* Lumbar Sympathetic Nerve
Lumbosacral trunk	*use* Lumbar Nerve
Medial plantar nerve	*use* Tibial Nerve
Medial popliteal nerve	*use* Tibial Nerve
Medial sural cutaneous nerve	*use* Tibial Nerve
Meissner's (submucous) plexus	*use* Abdominal Sympathetic Nerve
Middle cardiac nerve	*use* Thoracic Sympathetic Nerve
Musculocutaneous nerve	*use* Brachial Plexus
Musculospiral nerve	*use* Radial Nerve

Continued on next page

Educational Annotations | 1 – Peripheral Nervous System

Body Part Key Listings of Peripheral Nervous System

Continued from previous page

Myenteric (Auerbach's) plexus ....*use* Abdominal Sympathetic Nerve
Obturator nerve..*use* Lumbar Plexus
Otic ganglion..*use* Head and Neck Sympathetic Nerve
Palmar cutaneous nerve ....*use* Median Nerve, Radial Nerve
Pancreatic plexus ....*use* Abdominal Sympathetic Nerve
Pelvic splanchnic nerve ....*use* Abdominal Sympathetic Nerve
....*use* Sacral Sympathetic Nerve
Posterior femoral cutaneous nerve ....*use* Sacral Plexus
Posterior interosseous nerve ....*use* Radial Nerve
Posterior labial nerve ....*use* Pudendal Nerve
Posterior scrotal nerve ....*use* Pudendal Nerve
Pterygopalatine (sphenopalatine) ganglion ......*use* Head and Neck Sympathetic Nerve
Pudendal nerve ....*use* Sacral Plexus
Pulmonary plexus..*use* Vagus Nerve/Thoracic Sympathetic Nerve
Renal plexus...*use* Abdominal Sympathetic Nerve
Sacral ganglion ....*use* Sacral Sympathetic Nerve
Sacral splanchnic nerve ....*use* Sacral Sympathetic Nerve
Saphenous nerve ....*use* Femoral Nerve
Solar (celiac) plexus ....*use* Abdominal Sympathetic Nerve
Sphenopalatine (pterygopalatine) ganglion ....*use* Head and Neck Sympathetic Nerve
Spinal nerve, cervical..*use* Cervical Nerve
Spinal nerve, lumbar ....*use* Lumbar Nerve
Spinal nerve, sacral ....*use* Sacral Nerve
Spinal nerve, thoracic ....*use* Thoracic Nerve
Splenic plexus ....*use* Abdominal Sympathetic Nerve
Stellate ganglion ....*use* Head and Neck Sympathetic Nerve
Subclavius nerve ....*use* Brachial Plexus
Subcostal nerve ....*use* Thoracic Nerve
Submandibular ganglion ....*use* Head and Neck Sympathetic Nerve
Submaxillary ganglion ....*use* Head and Neck Sympathetic Nerve
Submucous (Meissner's) plexus ....*use* Abdominal Sympathetic Nerve
Suboccipital nerve ....*use* Cervical Nerve
Superior cardiac nerve......................................*use* Thoracic Sympathetic Nerve
Superior clunic (cluneal) nerve ....*use* Lumbar Nerve
Superior gluteal nerve ....*use* Lumbar Plexus
Superior hypogastric plexus.............................*use* Abdominal Sympathetic Nerve
Superior mesenteric ganglion ....*use* Abdominal Sympathetic Nerve
Superior mesenteric plexus ....*use* Abdominal Sympathetic Nerve
Supraclavicular nerve ....*use* Cervical Plexus
Suprascapular nerve ....*use* Brachial Plexus
Suprarenal plexus ....*use* Abdominal Sympathetic Nerve
Third occipital nerve..*use* Cervical Nerve
Thoracic aortic plexus ....*use* Thoracic Sympathetic Nerve
Thoracic ganglion ....*use* Thoracic Sympathetic Nerve
Transverse (cutaneous) cervical nerve ....*use* Cervical Plexus

PERIPHERAL NERVOUS 01

Educational Annotations | 1 – Peripheral Nervous System

Device Key Listings of Peripheral Nervous System

See also Device Key in Appendix D
Autograft ....*use* Autologous Tissue Substitute
InterStim® Therapy lead ....*use* Neurostimulator Lead in Peripheral Nervous System

Device Aggregation Table Listings of Peripheral Nervous System

See also Device Aggregation Table in Appendix E

Specific Device	For Operation	In Body System	General Device
None Listed in Device Aggregation Table for this Body System			

Coding Notes of Peripheral Nervous System

Body System Relevant Coding Guidelines

Branches of body parts
B4.2

Where a specific branch of a body part does not have its own body part value in PCS, the body part is typically coded to the closest proximal branch that has a specific body part value. In the cardiovascular body systems, if a general body part is available in the correct root operation table, and coding to a proximal branch would require assigning a code in a different body system, the procedure is coded using the general body part value.
Examples: A procedure performed on the mandibular branch of the trigeminal nerve is coded to the trigeminal nerve body part value.
Occlusion of the bronchial artery is coded to the body part value Upper Artery in the body system Upper Arteries, and not to the body part value Thoracic Aorta, Descending in the body system Heart and Great Vessels.

Body System Specific PCS Reference Manual Exercises

PCS CODE	1 – PERIPHERAL NERVOUS SYSTEM EXERCISES
0 1 8 R 3 Z Z	Sacral rhizotomy for pain control, percutaneous.
0 1 N G 0 Z Z	Open posterior tarsal tunnel release. (The nerve released in the posterior tarsal tunnel is the tibial nerve.)
0 1 P Y 0 M Z	Open removal of lumbar sympathetic neurostimulator.
0 1 Q 6 0 Z Z	Suture repair of left radial nerve laceration. (The approach value is Open, though the surgical exposure may have been created by the wound itself.)
0 1 S 4 0 Z Z	Open transposition of ulnar nerve.
0 1 U 5 4 7 Z	Autograft nerve graft to right median nerve, percutaneous endoscopic (graft harvest not coded for this exercise example).
0 1 X 6 4 Z 5	Endoscopic radial to median nerve transfer.

DEVICE GROUP: Change, Insertion, Removal, (Replacement), Revision, Supplement
Root Operations that always involve a device.

1ST - **0** Medical and Surgical

2ND - **1** Peripheral Nervous System

3RD - **2 CHANGE**

EXAMPLE: Exchange ulnar nerve drain tube | CMS Ex: Change urinary cath

CHANGE: Taking out or off a device from a body part and putting back an identical or similar device in or on the same body part without cutting or puncturing the skin or a mucous membrane.

EXPLANATION: ALL Changes use EXTERNAL approach only...

Body Part – 4TH	Approach – 5TH	Device – 6TH	Qualifier – 7TH
Y Peripheral Nerve	X External	0 Drainage device Y Other device	Z No qualifier

EXCISION GROUP: Excision, Resection, Destruction, Extraction, (Detachment)
Root Operations that take out some or all of a body part.

1ST - **0** Medical and Surgical

2ND - **1** Peripheral Nervous System

3RD - **5 DESTRUCTION**

EXAMPLE: Cryoablation nerve lesion | CMS Ex: Fulguration polyp

DESTRUCTION: Physical eradication of all or a portion of a body part by the direct use of energy, force, or a destructive agent.

EXPLANATION: None of the body part is physically taken out

Body Part – 4TH		Approach – 5TH	Device – 6TH	Qualifier – 7TH
0 Cervical Plexus	F Sciatic Nerve	0 Open	Z No device	Z No qualifier
1 Cervical Nerve	G Tibial Nerve	3 Percutaneous		
2 Phrenic Nerve	H Peroneal Nerve	4 Percutaneous endoscopic		
3 Brachial Plexus	K Head and Neck Sympathetic Nerve			
4 Ulnar Nerve	L Thoracic Sympathetic Nerve			
5 Median Nerve	M Abdominal Sympathetic Nerve			
6 Radial Nerve	N Lumbar Sympathetic Nerve			
8 Thoracic Nerve	P Sacral Sympathetic Nerve			
9 Lumbar Plexus	Q Sacral Plexus			
A Lumbosacral Plexus	R Sacral Nerve			
B Lumbar Nerve				
C Pudendal Nerve				
D Femoral Nerve				

DIVISION GROUP: Division, Release

Root Operations involving cutting or separation only.

1ST - 0 Medical and Surgical	**EXAMPLE:** Sacral nerve rhizotomy **CMS Ex:** Osteotomy
2ND - 1 Peripheral Nervous System	**DIVISION:** Cutting into a body part without draining fluids and/or gases from the body part in order to separate or transect a body part.
3RD - 8 DIVISION	**EXPLANATION:** Separated into two or more portions …

Body Part – 4TH		Approach – 5TH	Device – 6TH	Qualifier – 7TH
0 Cervical Plexus	F Sciatic Nerve	0 Open	Z No device	Z No qualifier
1 Cervical Nerve	G Tibial Nerve	3 Percutaneous		
2 Phrenic Nerve	H Peroneal Nerve	4 Percutaneous		
3 Brachial Plexus	K Head and Neck	endoscopic		
4 Ulnar Nerve	Sympathetic Nerve			
5 Median Nerve	L Thoracic Sympathetic Nerve			
6 Radial Nerve	M Abdominal Sympathetic			
8 Thoracic Nerve	Nerve			
9 Lumbar Plexus	N Lumbar Sympathetic Nerve			
A Lumbosacral Plexus	P Sacral Sympathetic Nerve			
B Lumbar Nerve	Q Sacral Plexus			
C Pudendal Nerve	R Sacral Nerve			
D Femoral Nerve				

DRAINAGE GROUP: Drainage, Extirpation, (Fragmentation)
Root Operations that take out solids/fluids/gases from a body part.

1ST - **0** Medical and Surgical	EXAMPLE: Aspiration nerve abscess CMS Ex: Thoracentesis
2ND - **1** Peripheral Nervous System	**DRAINAGE:** Taking or letting out fluids and/or gases from a body part.
3RD - **9 DRAINAGE**	EXPLANATION: Qualifier "X Diagnostic" indicates biopsy ...

Body Part – 4TH		Approach – 5TH	Device – 6TH	Qualifier – 7TH
0 Cervical Plexus 1 Cervical Nerve 2 Phrenic Nerve 3 Brachial Plexus 4 Ulnar Nerve 5 Median Nerve 6 Radial Nerve 8 Thoracic Nerve 9 Lumbar Plexus A Lumbosacral Plexus B Lumbar Nerve C Pudendal Nerve D Femoral Nerve	F Sciatic Nerve G Tibial Nerve H Peroneal Nerve K Head and Neck Sympathetic Nerve L Thoracic Sympathetic Nerve M Abdominal Sympathetic Nerve N Lumbar Sympathetic Nerve P Sacral Sympathetic Nerve Q Sacral Plexus R Sacral Nerve	0 Open 3 Percutaneous 4 Percutaneous endoscopic	0 Drainage device	Z No qualifier
0 Cervical Plexus 1 Cervical Nerve 2 Phrenic Nerve 3 Brachial Plexus 4 Ulnar Nerve 5 Median Nerve 6 Radial Nerve 8 Thoracic Nerve 9 Lumbar Plexus A Lumbosacral Plexus B Lumbar Nerve C Pudendal Nerve D Femoral Nerve	F Sciatic Nerve G Tibial Nerve H Peroneal Nerve K Head and Neck Sympathetic Nerve L Thoracic Sympathetic Nerve M Abdominal Sympathetic Nerve N Lumbar Sympathetic Nerve P Sacral Sympathetic Nerve Q Sacral Plexus R Sacral Nerve	0 Open 3 Percutaneous 4 Percutaneous endoscopic	Z No device	X Diagnostic Z No qualifier

---

EXCISION GROUP: Excision, Resection, Destruction, Extraction, (Detachment)
Root Operations that take out some or all of a body part.

1ST - 0 Medical and Surgical

2ND - 1 Peripheral Nervous System

3RD - B EXCISION

EXAMPLE: Biopsy of lumbosacral plexus   CMS Ex: Liver biopsy

<u>EXCISION:</u> Cutting out or off, without replacement, a portion of a body part.

EXPLANATION: Qualifier "X Diagnostic" indicates biopsy ...

Body Part – 4TH		Approach – 5TH	Device – 6TH	Qualifier – 7TH
0 Cervical Plexus	F Sciatic Nerve	0 Open	Z No device	X Diagnostic
1 Cervical Nerve	G Tibial Nerve	3 Percutaneous		Z No qualifier
2 Phrenic Nerve	H Peroneal Nerve	4 Percutaneous		
3 Brachial Plexus	K Head and Neck	endoscopic		
4 Ulnar Nerve	Sympathetic Nerve			
5 Median Nerve	L Thoracic Sympathetic Nerve			
6 Radial Nerve	M Abdominal Sympathetic			
8 Thoracic Nerve	Nerve			
9 Lumbar Plexus	N Lumbar Sympathetic Nerve			
A Lumbosacral Plexus	P Sacral Sympathetic Nerve			
B Lumbar Nerve	Q Sacral Plexus			
C Pudendal Nerve	R Sacral Nerve			
D Femoral Nerve				

DRAINAGE GROUP: Drainage, Extirpation, (Fragmentation)
Root Operations that take out solids/fluids/gases from a body part.

1ST - 0 Medical and Surgical

2ND - 1 Peripheral Nervous System

3RD - C EXTIRPATION

EXAMPLE: Removal FB cervical plexus   CMS Ex: Choledocholithotomy

<u>EXTIRPATION:</u> Taking or cutting out solid matter from a body part.

EXPLANATION: Abnormal byproduct or foreign body ...

Body Part – 4TH		Approach – 5TH	Device – 6TH	Qualifier – 7TH
0 Cervical Plexus	F Sciatic Nerve	0 Open	Z No device	Z No qualifier
1 Cervical Nerve	G Tibial Nerve	3 Percutaneous		
2 Phrenic Nerve	H Peroneal Nerve	4 Percutaneous		
3 Brachial Plexus	K Head and Neck	endoscopic		
4 Ulnar Nerve	Sympathetic Nerve			
5 Median Nerve	L Thoracic Sympathetic Nerve			
6 Radial Nerve	M Abdominal Sympathetic			
8 Thoracic Nerve	Nerve			
9 Lumbar Plexus	N Lumbar Sympathetic Nerve			
A Lumbosacral Plexus	P Sacral Sympathetic Nerve			
B Lumbar Nerve	Q Sacral Plexus			
C Pudendal Nerve	R Sacral Nerve			
D Femoral Nerve				

EXCISION GROUP: Excision, Resection, Destruction, Extraction, (Detachment)
Root Operations that take out some or all of a body part.

1ST - 0 Medical and Surgical

2ND - 1 Peripheral Nervous System

3RD - D EXTRACTION

EXAMPLE: Neurexeresis radial nerve | CMS Ex: D&C

EXTRACTION: Pulling or stripping out or off all or a portion of a body part by the use of force.

EXPLANATION: None for this Body System

Body Part – 4TH	Approach – 5TH	Device – 6TH	Qualifier – 7TH
0 Cervical Plexus F Sciatic Nerve 1 Cervical Nerve G Tibial Nerve 2 Phrenic Nerve H Peroneal Nerve 3 Brachial Plexus K Head and Neck 4 Ulnar Nerve Sympathetic Nerve 5 Median Nerve L Thoracic Sympathetic Nerve 6 Radial Nerve M Abdominal Sympathetic 8 Thoracic Nerve Nerve 9 Lumbar Plexus N Lumbar Sympathetic Nerve A Lumbosacral Plexus P Sacral Sympathetic Nerve B Lumbar Nerve Q Sacral Plexus C Pudendal Nerve R Sacral Nerve D Femoral Nerve	0 Open 3 Percutaneous 4 Percutaneous endoscopic	Z No device	Z No qualifier

---

DEVICE GROUP: Change, Insertion, Removal, (Replacement), Revision, Supplement
Root Operations that always involve a device.

1ST - 0 Medical and Surgical

2ND - 1 Peripheral Nervous System

3RD - H INSERTION

EXAMPLE: Insertion neurostimulator lead | CMS Ex: Central venous catheter

INSERTION: Putting in a nonbiological appliance that monitors, assists, performs, or prevents a physiological function but does not physically take the place of a body part.

EXPLANATION: None

Body Part – 4TH	Approach – 5TH	Device – 6TH	Qualifier – 7TH
Y Peripheral Nerve	0 Open 3 Percutaneous 4 Percutaneous endoscopic	2 Monitoring device M Neurostimulator lead	Z No qualifier

EXAMINATION GROUP: Inspection, (Map)
Root Operations involving examination only.

1ST - 0 Medical and Surgical	EXAMPLE: Examination injured nerve	CMS Ex: Colonoscopy
2ND - 1 Peripheral Nervous System	INSPECTION: Visually and/or manually exploring a body part.	
3RD - J INSPECTION	EXPLANATION: Direct or instrumental visualization ...	

Body Part – 4TH	Approach – 5TH	Device – 6TH	Qualifier – 7TH
Y Peripheral Nerve	0 Open 3 Percutaneous 4 Percutaneous endoscopic	Z No device	Z No qualifier

DIVISION GROUP: Division, Release
Root Operations involving cutting or separation only.

1ST - 0 Medical and Surgical	EXAMPLE: Carpal tunnel release	CMS Ex: Carpal tunnel release
2ND - 1 Peripheral Nervous System	RELEASE: Freeing a body part from an abnormal physical constraint by cutting or by the use of force.	
3RD - N RELEASE	EXPLANATION: None of the body part is taken out ...	

Body Part – 4TH	Approach – 5TH	Device – 6TH	Qualifier – 7TH
0 Cervical Plexus F Sciatic Nerve 1 Cervical Nerve G Tibial Nerve 2 Phrenic Nerve H Peroneal Nerve 3 Brachial Plexus K Head and Neck 4 Ulnar Nerve Sympathetic Nerve 5 Median Nerve L Thoracic Sympathetic Nerve 6 Radial Nerve M Abdominal Sympathetic 8 Thoracic Nerve Nerve 9 Lumbar Plexus N Lumbar Sympathetic Nerve A Lumbosacral Plexus P Sacral Sympathetic Nerve B Lumbar Nerve Q Sacral Plexus C Pudendal Nerve R Sacral Nerve D Femoral Nerve	0 Open 3 Percutaneous 4 Percutaneous endoscopic	Z No device	Z No qualifier

DEVICE GROUP: Change, Insertion, Removal, (Replacement), Revision, Supplement
Root Operations that always involve a device.

1ST - **0** Medical and Surgical

2ND - **1** Peripheral Nervous System

3RD - **P REMOVAL**

EXAMPLE: Removal neurostimulator lead | CMS Ex: Chest tube removal

REMOVAL: Taking out or off a device from a body part.

EXPLANATION: Removal device without reinsertion ...

Body Part – 4TH	Approach – 5TH	Device – 6TH	Qualifier – 7TH
Y Peripheral Nerve	0 Open 3 Percutaneous 4 Percutaneous endoscopic	0 Drainage device 2 Monitoring device 7 Autologous tissue substitute M Neurostimulator lead	Z No qualifier
Y Peripheral Nerve	X External	0 Drainage device 2 Monitoring device M Neurostimulator lead	Z No qualifier

OTHER REPAIRS GROUP: (Control), Repair
Root Operations that define other repairs.

1ST - **0** Medical and Surgical

2ND - **1** Peripheral Nervous System

3RD - **Q REPAIR**

EXAMPLE: Microsurgical repair nerve | CMS Ex: Suture laceration

REPAIR: Restoring, to the extent possible, a body part to its normal anatomic structure and function.

EXPLANATION: Only when no other root operation applies ...

Body Part – 4TH	Approach – 5TH	Device – 6TH	Qualifier – 7TH
0 Cervical Plexus 1 Cervical Nerve 2 Phrenic Nerve 3 Brachial Plexus 4 Ulnar Nerve 5 Median Nerve 6 Radial Nerve 8 Thoracic Nerve 9 Lumbar Plexus A Lumbosacral Plexus B Lumbar Nerve C Pudendal Nerve D Femoral Nerve F Sciatic Nerve G Tibial Nerve H Peroneal Nerve K Head and Neck Sympathetic Nerve L Thoracic Sympathetic Nerve M Abdominal Sympathetic Nerve N Lumbar Sympathetic Nerve P Sacral Sympathetic Nerve Q Sacral Plexus R Sacral Nerve	0 Open 3 Percutaneous 4 Percutaneous endoscopic	Z No device	Z No qualifier

MOVE GROUP: (Reattachment), **Reposition, Transfer,** (Transplantation)
Root Operations that put in/put back or move some/all of a body part.

1ST - **0** Medical and Surgical

2ND - **1** Peripheral Nervous System

3RD - **S REPOSITION**

EXAMPLE: Relocation femoral nerve	CMS Ex: Fracture reduction

REPOSITION: Moving to its normal location, or other suitable location, all or a portion of a body part.

EXPLANATION: May or may not be cut to be moved ...

Body Part – 4TH		Approach – 5TH	Device – 6TH	Qualifier – 7TH
0 Cervical Plexus	A Lumbosacral Plexus	0 Open	Z No device	Z No qualifier
1 Cervical Nerve	B Lumbar Nerve	3 Percutaneous		
2 Phrenic Nerve	C Pudendal Nerve	4 Percutaneous endoscopic		
3 Brachial Plexus	D Femoral Nerve			
4 Ulnar Nerve	F Sciatic Nerve			
5 Median Nerve	G Tibial Nerve			
6 Radial Nerve	H Peroneal Nerve			
8 Thoracic Nerve	Q Sacral Plexus			
9 Lumbar Plexus	R Sacral Nerve			

DEVICE GROUP: Change, Insertion, Removal, (Replacement), **Revision, Supplement**
Root Operations that always involve a device.

1ST - **0** Medical and Surgical

2ND - **1** Peripheral Nervous System

3RD - **U SUPPLEMENT**

EXAMPLE: Free nerve autograft	CMS Ex: Hernia repair with mesh

SUPPLEMENT: Putting in or on biological or synthetic material that physically reinforces and/or augments the function of a portion of a body part.

EXPLANATION: Biological material from same individual ...

Body Part – 4TH		Approach – 5TH	Device – 6TH	Qualifier – 7TH
1 Cervical Nerve	C Pudendal Nerve	0 Open	7 Autologous tissue substitute	Z No qualifier
2 Phrenic Nerve	D Femoral Nerve	3 Percutaneous		
4 Ulnar Nerve	F Sciatic Nerve	4 Percutaneous endoscopic		
5 Median Nerve	G Tibial Nerve			
6 Radial Nerve	H Peroneal Nerve			
8 Thoracic Nerve	R Sacral Nerve			
B Lumbar Nerve				

PERIPHERAL NERVOUS 0 1 S

DEVICE GROUP: Change, Insertion, Removal, (Replacement), Revision, Supplement
Root Operations that always involve a device.

1ST – 0 Medical and Surgical

2ND – 1 Peripheral Nervous System

3RD – W REVISION

EXAMPLE: Reposition neurostimulator lead | CMS Ex: Adjust pacemaker lead

REVISION: Correcting, to the extent possible, a portion of a malfunctioning device or the position of a displaced device.

EXPLANATION: May replace components of a device …

Body Part – 4TH	Approach – 5TH	Device – 6TH	Qualifier – 7TH
Y Peripheral Nerve	0 Open 3 Percutaneous 4 Percutaneous endoscopic X External	0 Drainage device 2 Monitoring device 7 Autologous tissue substitute M Neurostimulator lead	Z No qualifier

MOVE GROUP: (Reattachment), Reposition, Transfer, (Transplantation)
Root Operations that put in/put back or move some/all of a body part.

1ST – 0 Medical and Surgical

2ND – 1 Peripheral Nervous System

3RD – X TRANSFER

EXAMPLE: Radial to median nerve transfer | CMS Ex: Tendon transfer

TRANSFER: Moving, without taking out, all or a portion of a body part to another location to take over the function of all or a portion of a body part.

EXPLANATION: The body part remains connected …

Body Part – 4TH	Approach – 5TH	Device – 6TH	Qualifier – 7TH
1 Cervical Nerve 2 Phrenic Nerve	0 Open 4 Percutaneous endoscopic	Z No device	1 Cervical Nerve 2 Phrenic Nerve
4 Ulnar Nerve 5 Median Nerve 6 Radial Nerve	0 Open 4 Percutaneous endoscopic	Z No device	4 Ulnar Nerve 5 Median Nerve 6 Radial Nerve
8 Thoracic Nerve	0 Open 4 Percutaneous endoscopic	Z No device	8 Thoracic Nerve
B Lumbar Nerve C Pudendal Nerve	0 Open 4 Percutaneous endoscopic	Z No device	B Lumbar Nerve C Perineal Nerve
D Femoral Nerve F Sciatic Nerve G Tibial Nerve H Peroneal Nerve	0 Open 4 Percutaneous endoscopic	Z No device	D Femoral Nerve F Sciatic Nerve G Tibial Nerve H Peroneal Nerve

NOTES

PERIPHERAL NERVOUS 01

Educational Annotations | 2 – Heart and Great Vessels

Body System Specific Educational Annotations for the Heart and Great Vessels include:

- Anatomy and Physiology Review
- Anatomical Illustrations
- Definitions of Common Procedures
- AHA Coding Clinic® Reference Notations
- Body Part Key Listings
- Device Key Listings
- Device Aggregation Table Listings
- Coding Notes

Anatomy and Physiology Review of Heart and Great Vessels

BODY PART VALUES – 2 - HEART AND GREAT VESSELS

Aortic Valve – ANATOMY – The aortic valve has three cusps and is located between the outlet of the left ventricle and the base of the aorta. PHYSIOLOGY – The aortic valve prevents backflow of blood into the left ventricle from the aorta via its one-way valve function.

Atrial Septum – The strong tissue wall that separates the left and right atria.

Atrium, Left – ANATOMY – One of the two smaller chambers of the heart's four chambers. PHYSIOLOGY – The left atrium receives and pools the oxygenated blood from the lungs briefly before the tricuspid valve opens and the blood flows into the left ventricle.

Atrium, Right – ANATOMY – One of the two smaller chambers of the heart's four chambers. PHYSIOLOGY – The right atrium receives and pools the deoxygenated blood from the inferior vena cava and the superior vena cava briefly before the pulmonary valve opens and the blood flows into the right ventricle.

Chordae Tendineae – The very strong tendinous cord attaching a papillary muscle to a valve leaflet.

Conduction Mechanism – The electrical signal transmission system that controls the rhythmical heart beat through various structures and fibers including the sinoatrial node (the heart's pacemaker), the atrioventricular node, and the Bundle of HIS.

Coronary Artery – Coronary arteries supply oxygenated blood to the heart.

Coronary Vein – Coronary veins remove the deoxygenated blood from the heart muscle and return it to the right atrium.

Great Vessel – The major vessels associated with the heart that lie within the thoracic cavity including: Thoracic aorta, pulmonary arteries, pulmonary veins, and the superior vena cava and thoracic portion of the inferior vena cava.

Heart – ANATOMY – The heart is the 4 chambered, muscular, blood pumping organ behind the mediastinum in the thorax, and is approximately 5.5 inches (14 cm) long and 3.5 inches (9 cm) wide. The heart has 3 layers: The endocardium, myocardium, and pericardium. The endocardium is the interior lining of endothelium. The myocardium is the thick muscular layer. The pericardium is the double-layered serous membrane protecting the heart from friction as it beats. The heart has 4 valves and 4 chambers: The tricuspid valve, mitral valve, aortic valve, the pulmonary valve, right and left atria, and right and left ventricles. The mediastinum is the mass of tissue between the sternum and vertebral column which divides the thoracic cavity. PHYSIOLOGY – The heart functions to pump and maintain sufficient pressure of the blood to constantly meet the needs of the body cells. The venous blood is returned from the body via the inferior and superior vena cava to the right atrium where it is pooled momentarily before the tricuspid valve opens and allows the venous blood to enter the right ventricle. The right ventricle then contracts forcing the blood through the pulmonary valve to the lungs. The lungs return the reoxygenated blood to the left atrium where it is pooled momentarily before the mitral valve opens and allows the venous blood to enter the left ventricle. The left ventricle then contracts, forcing the blood through the aortic valve to all the tissues of the body.

Heart, Left – ANATOMY – The portion of the heart that includes the left atria and left ventricle. PHYSIOLOGY – The left heart receives the reoxygenated blood from the lungs and pumps it out to the body.

Heart, Right – ANATOMY – The portion of the heart that includes the right atria and right ventricle. PHYSIOLOGY – The right heart receives the venous blood and pumps it to the lungs for reoxygenation.

Mitral Valve – ANATOMY – The mitral valve (also known as the bicuspid valve) has two cusps and is located between the left atrium and the left ventricle. PHYSIOLOGY – The mitral valve prevents backflow of blood from the left ventricle back into the left atrium via its one-way valve function. The mitral valve's closure is strengthened by the papillary muscles and their chordae tendineae during the left ventricle's forceful contraction.

Continued on next page

Educational Annotations | 2 – Heart and Great Vessels

Anatomy and Physiology Review of Heart and Great Vessels

BODY PART VALUES – 2 - HEART AND GREAT VESSELS
Continued from previous page

Papillary Muscle – ANATOMY – The intraventricular muscles that connect with the mitral and tricuspid valves via a chordae tendineae. PHYSIOLOGY – The papillary muscles contract at the same time as the ventricle, thus reinforcing the closure of the atrial inlet valve.

Pericardium – The pericardium is the double-layered serous membrane protecting the heart from friction as it beats.

Pulmonary Artery, Left – The major blood vessel transporting deoxygenated blood from the right ventricle to the left lobes of the lungs. Blood vessels with blood flow going away from the heart are termed arteries. Pulmonary arteries carry venous blood, the opposite of the rest of the arteries.

Pulmonary Artery, Right – The major blood vessel transporting deoxygenated blood from the right ventricle to the right lobes of the lungs. Blood vessels with blood flow going away from the heart are termed arteries. Pulmonary arteries carry venous blood, the opposite of the rest of the arteries.

Pulmonary Trunk – The short, large blood vessel connecting the right ventricle to the right and left pulmonary arteries.

Pulmonary Valve – ANATOMY – The pulmonary valve has three cusps and is located between the outlet of the right ventricle and the base of the pulmonary artery. PHYSIOLOGY – The pulmonary valve prevents backflow of blood into the right ventricle from the pulmonary artery via its one-way valve function.

Pulmonary Vein, Left – The major blood vessel transporting oxygenated blood from the left lobes of the lungs to the left atrium. Blood vessels with blood flow going to the heart are termed veins. Pulmonary veins carry arterial blood, the opposite of the rest of the veins.

Pulmonary Vein, Right – The major blood vessel transporting oxygenated blood from the right lobes of the lungs to the left atrium. Blood vessels with blood flow going to the heart are termed veins. Pulmonary veins carry arterial blood, the opposite of the rest of the veins.

Superior Vena Cava – The major vein transporting deoxygenated blood from the upper body and head that empties into the right atrium.

Thoracic Aorta – The uppermost portion of the aorta that lies within the thoracic cavity.

Tricuspid Valve – ANATOMY – The tricuspid valve has three cusps and is located between the right atrium and the right ventricle. PHYSIOLOGY – The tricuspid valve prevents backflow of blood from the right ventricle back into the right atrium via its one-way valve function. The tricuspid valve's closure is strengthened by the papillary muscles and their chordae tendineae during the right ventricle's forceful contraction.

Ventricle, Left – ANATOMY – One of the two large chambers of the heart's four chambers. PHYSIOLOGY – The left ventricle pumps oxygenated blood from the heart into the aorta to be carried throughout the body.

Ventricle, Right – ANATOMY – One of the two large chambers of the heart's four chambers. PHYSIOLOGY – The right ventricle pumps deoxygenated blood from the heart to the lungs through the pulmonary arteries.

Ventricular Septum – The strong tissue wall that separates the left and right ventricles.

Educational Annotations | 2 – Heart and Great Vessels

Anatomical Illustrations of Heart and Great Vessels

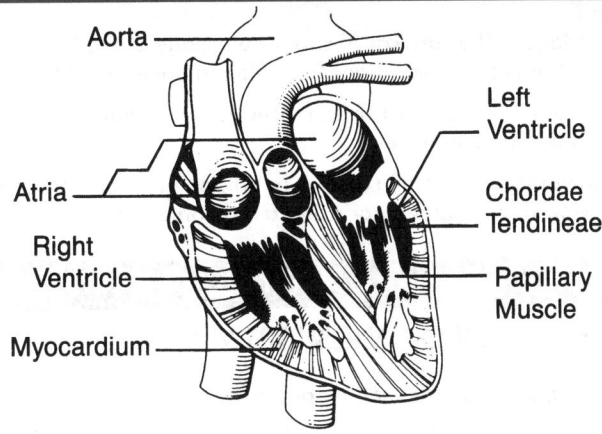

HEART — ANTERIOR (CUT-AWAY) VIEW

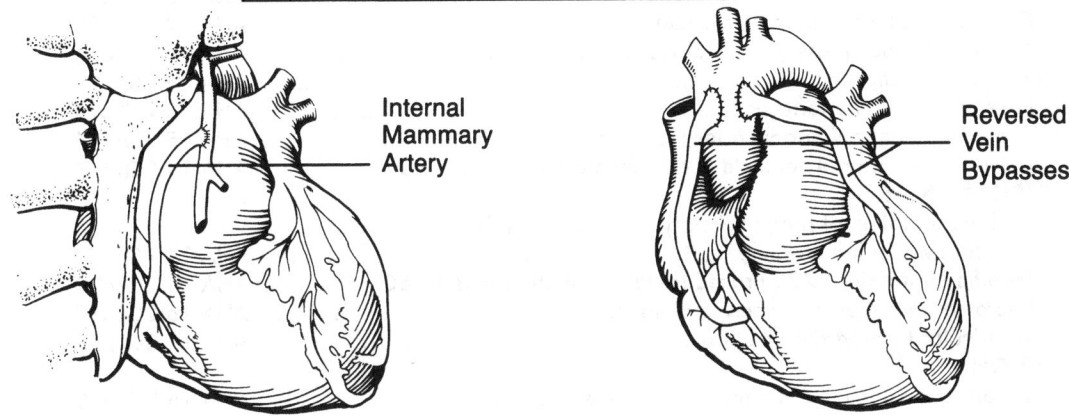

INTERNAL MAMMARY-CORONARY BYPASS   DOUBLE AORTOCORONARY BYPASS

HEART & GREAT V. 02

Definitions of Common Procedures of Heart and Great Vessels

Aortocoronary artery bypass – The restoration of coronary artery blood flow by using a tubular graft (usually a saphenous vein) to bring blood from the aorta to the coronary artery that is distal to the blocked site.

Coronary artery stent – The widening of the coronary artery lumen by placing a stent (tubular supporting device) in the narrowed arterial site. The stent may or may not be coated in a drug-eluting substance.

Heart transplant – The removal of the end-staged diseased heart and replacement with a donor heart.

Internal mammary artery coronary artery bypass – The restoration of coronary artery blood flow by using the direct connection of an internal mammary artery to the coronary artery that is distal to the blocked site.

Intra-aortic balloon pump (IABP) – The computer-controlled inflatable circulatory assist device that is placed in the descending thoracic aorta. The balloon is inflated during diastole (heart not contracting and filling with blood) to increase cardiac output pressure and increase coronary blood flow.

MAZE procedure (Cox-MAZE) – The surgical cutting or destruction of atrial tissue to disrupt the electrical pathways and re-direct them through a maze-like pattern that creates only one path that the electrical impulse can take from the SA node to the AV node, which prevents the irregular electrical impulses of atrial fibrillation.

Continued on next page

Educational Annotations | 2 – Heart and Great Vessels

Definitions of Common Procedures of Heart and Great Vessels

Continued from previous page

Occlusion of left atrial appendage – The surgical closure or blockage of the left atrial appendage (small pouch in muscle wall of the left atrium) to prevent blood clot formation in patients with atrial fibrillation.

Valve replacement – The replacement of a heart valve (aortic, mitral, pulmonary, or tricuspid) using a mechanical or bioprosthetic valve that replaces the entire valve.

Valvuloplasty – The restoration of the heart valve (aortic, mitral, pulmonary, or tricuspid) anatomy and/or function using a tissue graft or synthetic material, or using a balloon catheter.

AHA Coding Clinic® Reference Notations of Heart and Great Vessels

ROOT OPERATION SPECIFIC - 2 - HEART AND GREAT VESSELS

BYPASS - 1

Coronary artery bypass graft, using greater saphenous vein	AHA 14:3Q:p20
	AHA 14:1Q:p10
Coronary artery bypass graft, using internal mammary artery	AHA 14:3Q:p8,20
Coronary bypass from internal mammary and aorta	AHA 16:1Q:p27
Fontan completion stage II procedure	AHA 14:3Q:p29
Modified Blalock-Taussig shunt procedure	AHA 14:3Q:p3
Rastelli operation	AHA 15:4Q:p22
Repair of truncus arteriosus	AHA 15:4Q:p24
Replacement of pulmonary artery conduit	AHA 15:3Q:p16
Replacement of right ventricle (RV) to pulmonary artery conduit	AHA 14:3Q:p30

DESTRUCTION - 5

Catheter ablation of peripulmonary veins to target the conduction pathway of left atrium	AHA 14:4Q:p47
Modified left atrial MAZE procedure using ablation and AtrioClip®	AHA 14:3Q:p20
Photodynamic therapy of pericardium	AHA 16:2Q:p17
Ventricular tachycardia ablation	AHA 14:3Q:p19

DILATION - 7

Coronary angioplasty with unsuccessful stent placement	AHA 15:3Q:p10
Distinct coronary lesion sites treated	AHA 15:2Q:p3-5
Orbital atherectomy and drug-eluting balloon angioplasty of coronary artery	AHA 15:4Q:p13
Placement of pulmonary artery stent	AHA 15:3Q:p16
Pulmonary valvotomy with commisurotomies	AHA 16:1Q:p16
Restenosis of saphenous vein coronary artery bypass graft using a stent	AHA 14:2Q:p4

DIVISION - 8

EXCISION - B

Wedge resection of mitral valve leaflet	AHA 15:2Q:p.23

EXTIRPATION - C

Decalcification of mitral valve	AHA 16:2Q:p24

FRAGMENTATION - F

Continued on next page

Educational Annotations | 2 – Heart and Great Vessels

AHA Coding Clinic® Reference Notations of Heart and Great Vessels

Continued from previous page

INSERTION - H

Exchange of tunneled hemodialysis catheter with chest port ....AHA 15:4Q:p31

Insertion of central venous catheter though jugluar vein into superior
vena cava ....AHA 15:4Q:p28

Insertion of central venous line ending in the cavoatrial junction...............AHA 15:4Q:p28

Insertion of dialysis catheter ending in the cavoatrial junction ....AHA 15:4Q:p29

Insertion of dual-lumen PICC line ending in the right atrial junction ....AHA 15:4Q:p29

Insertion of infusion device into superior vena cava ....AHA 15:2Q:p.33

Insertion of infusion device into superior vena cava ....AHA 15:4Q:p14

Insertion of leadless pacemaker ....AHA 15:2Q:p.31

Insertion of Swan Ganz catheter for pressure monitoring ....AHA 15:3Q:p35

Insertion of tunneled hemodialysis catheter into superior vena cava
with port chest pocket ....AHA 15:4Q:p30

Placement of peripherally inserted central catheter (PICC line) into
superior vena cava ....AHA 13:3Q:p18

Removal with new insertion of jugular tunneled catheter in right atrium ....AHA 16:2Q:p15

INSPECTION - J

MAP - K

OCCLUSION - L

Closure of patent ductus arteriosus ....AHA 15:4Q:p23

Modified left atrial MAZE procedure using ablation and AtrioClip® ....AHA 14:3Q:p20

Occlusion of right pulmonary artery ....AHA 16:2Q:p26

RELEASE - N

Widening of right ventricular outflow tract ....AHA 14:3Q:p16

REMOVAL - P

Exchange of tunneled hemodialysis catheter with chest port ....AHA 15:4Q:p31

Removal of cardiac lead..AHA 15:3Q:p33

Removal with new insertion of jugular tunneled catheter in right atrium ....AHA 16:2Q:p15

REPAIR - Q

Division (repair) of double aortic arch...AHA 15:3Q:p16

Repair of atrial septal defect..AHA 15:4Q:p23

Thoracic aortic valve repair (TAVR) ....AHA 13:3Q:p26

REPLACEMENT - R

Graft repair of thoracic aortic arch aneurysm ....AHA 14:1Q:p10

REPOSITION - S

Correction surgery for transposition of great arteries ....AHA 15:4Q:p23

RESECTION - T

SUPPLEMENT - U

Aortic root enlargement ....AHA 16:2Q:p26

Closure of ventricular septal defect with Goretex® patch ....AHA 14:3Q:p16

Enlargement of pulmonary artery and trunk ....AHA 16:2Q:p23

Mitral valve ring annuloplasty ....AHA 15:2Q:p.23

Pulmonary artery patch allograft ....AHA 15:3Q:p16

Rastelli operation ....AHA 15:4Q:p22

Repair of truncal valve ....AHA 15:4Q:p24

Repair of ventricular septal defect...AHA 15:4Q:p24

RESTRICTION - V

REVISION - W

Closure of paravalvular leak ....AHA 14:3Q:p31

Reposition of dislocated pacemaker lead ....AHA 15:3Q:p32

TRANSPLANTATION - Y

Heart transplant..AHA 13:3Q:p18

Educational Annotations | 2 – Heart and Great Vessels

Body Part Key Listings of Heart and Great Vessels

See also Body Part Key in Appendix C

Aortic annulus	*use* Aortic Valve
Aortic arch	*use* Thoracic Aorta, Ascending/Arch
Arterial canal (duct)	*use* Pulmonary Artery, Left
Ascending aorta	*use* Thoracic Aorta, Ascending/Arch
Atrioventricular node	*use* Conduction Mechanism
Atrium dextrum cordis	*use* Atrium, Right
Atrium pulmonale	*use* Atrium, Left
Bicuspid valve	*use* Mitral Valve
Botallo's duct	*use* Pulmonary Artery, Left
Bundle of His	*use* Conduction Mechanism
Bundle of Kent	*use* Conduction Mechanism
Conus arteriosus	*use* Ventricle, Right
Interatrial septum	*use* Atrial Septum
Interventricular septum	*use* Ventricular Septum
Left atrioventricular valve	*use* Mitral Valve
Left auricular appendix	*use* Atrium, Left
Left coronary sulcus	*use* Heart, Left
Left inferior pulmonary vein	*use* Pulmonary Vein, Left
Left superior pulmonary vein	*use* Pulmonary Vein, Left
Mitral annulus	*use* Mitral Valve
Obtuse margin	*use* Heart, Left
Precava	*use* Superior Vena Cava
Pulmoaortic canal	*use* Pulmonary Artery, Left
Pulmonary annulus	*use* Pulmonary Valve
Pulmonic valve	*use* Pulmonary Valve
Right atrioventricular valve	*use* Tricuspid Valve
Right auricular appendix	*use* Atrium, Right
Right coronary sulcus	*use* Heart, Right
Right inferior pulmonary vein	*use* Pulmonary Vein, Right
Right superior pulmonary vein	*use* Pulmonary Vein, Right
Sinoatrial node	*use* Conduction Mechanism
Sinus venosus	*use* Atrium, Right
Tricuspid annulus	*use* Tricuspid Valve

HEART & GREAT V. 02

© 2016 Channel Publishing, Ltd.

Educational Annotations | 2 – Heart and Great Vessels

Device Key Listings of Heart and Great Vessels

See also Device Key in Appendix D

3f (Aortic) Bioprosthesis valve ....*use* Zooplastic Tissue in Heart and Great Vessels

AbioCor® Total Replacement Heart...........................*use* Synthetic Substitute

ACUITY™ Steerable Lead ....*use* Cardiac Lead, Pacemaker for Insertion in Heart and Great Vessels

....*use* Cardiac Lead, Defibrillator for Insertion in Heart and Great Vessels

AMPLATZER® Muscular VSD Occluder ....*use* Synthetic Substitute

Annuloplasty ring ....*use* Synthetic Substitute

Attain Ability® lead ....*use* Cardiac Lead, Pacemaker for Insertion in Heart and Great Vessels

....*use* Cardiac Lead, Defibrillator for Insertion in Heart and Great Vessels

Attain StarFix® (OTW) lead......................................*use* Cardiac Lead, Pacemaker for Insertion in Heart and Great Vessels

....*use* Cardiac Lead, Defibrillator for Insertion in Heart and Great Vessels

Autograft..*use* Autologous Tissue Substitute

Autologous artery graft ....*use* Autologous Arterial Tissue in Heart and Great Vessels

Autologous vein graft ....*use* Autologous Venous Tissue in Heart and Great Vessels

Berlin Heart Ventricular Assist Device ....*use* Implantable Heart Assist System in Heart and Great Vessels

Biventricular external heart assist system ....*use* External Heart Assist System in Heart and Great Vessels

Bovine pericardial valve...*use* Zooplastic Tissue in Heart and Great Vessels

Bovine pericardium graft ....*use* Zooplastic Tissue in Heart and Great Vessels

BVS 5000 Ventricular Assist Device ....*use* External Heart Assist System in Heart and Great Vessels

Cardiac contractility modulation lead ....*use* Cardiac Lead in Heart and Great Vessels

Cardiac event recorder ....*use* Monitoring Device

Cardiac resynchronization therapy (CRT) lead ....*use* Cardiac Lead, Pacemaker for Insertion in Heart and Great Vessels

....*use* Cardiac Lead, Defibrillator for Insertion in Heart and Great Vessels

CardioMEMS® pressure sensor ....*use* Monitoring Device, Pressure Sensor for Insertion in Heart and Great Vessels

Centrimag® Blood Pump...*use* External Heart Assist System in Heart and Great Vessels

CoAxia NeuroFlo catheter ....*use* Intraluminal Device

Contegra Pulmonary Valved Conduit ....*use* Zooplastic Tissue in Heart and Great Vessels

CoreValve transcatheter aortic valve......................*use* Zooplastic Tissue in Heart and Great Vessels

Corox OTW (Bipolar) Lead ....*use* Cardiac Lead, Pacemaker for Insertion in Heart and Great Vessels

....*use* Cardiac Lead, Defibrillator for Insertion in Heart and Great Vessels

CYPHER® Stent ....*use* Intraluminal Device, Drug-eluting in Heart and Great Vessels

DeBakey Left Ventricular Assist Device ....*use* Implantable Heart Assist System in Heart and Great Vessels

Driver stent (RX) (OTW)..*use* Intraluminal Device

DuraHeart Left Ventricular Assist System ....*use* Implantable Heart Assist System in Heart and Great Vessels

Durata® Defibrillation Lead ....*use* Cardiac Lead, Defibrillator for Insertion in Heart and Great Vessels

Endeavor® (III) (IV) (Sprint) Zotarolimus-eluting

Coronary Stent System ....*use* Intraluminal Device, Drug-eluting in Heart and Great Vessels

EndoSure® sensor ....*use* Monitoring Device, Pressure Sensor for Insertion in Heart and Great Vessels

ENDOTAK RELIANCE® (G) Defibrillation Lead ....*use* Cardiac Lead, Defibrillator for Insertion in Heart and Great Vessels

Epic™ Stented Tissue Valve (aortic)...........................*use* Zooplastic Tissue in Heart and Great Vessels

Everolimus-eluting coronary stent ....*use* Intraluminal Device, Drug-eluting in Heart and Great Vessels

Freestyle (Stentless) Aortic Root Bioprosthesis ....*use* Zooplastic Tissue in Heart and Great Vessels

Hancock Bioprosthesis (aortic) (mitral) valve ....*use* Zooplastic Tissue in Heart and Great Vessels

Hancock Bioprosthetic Valved Conduit ....*use* Zooplastic Tissue in Heart and Great Vessels

HeartMate II® Left Ventricular Assist Device (LVAD)*use* Implantable Heart Assist System in Heart and Great Vessels

HeartMate XVE® Left Ventricular Assist Device (LVAD) ......*use* Implantable Heart Assist System in Heart and Great Vessels

Melody® transcatheter pulmonary valve ....*use* Zooplastic Tissue in Heart and Great Vessels

Continued on next page

Educational Annotations | 2 – Heart and Great Vessels

HEART & GREAT V. 02

Device Key Listings of Heart and Great Vessels

Continued from previous page

Micro-Driver stent (RX) (OTW) ....*use* Intraluminal Device

MicroMed HeartAssist ....*use* Implantable Heart Assist System in Heart and Great Vessels

MitraClip valve repair system ....*use* Synthetic Substitute

Mitroflow® Aortic Pericardial Heart Valve ....*use* Zooplastic Tissue in Heart and Great Vessels

Mosaic Bioprosthesis (aortic) (mitral) valve.............*use* Zooplastic Tissue in Heart and Great Vessels

MULTI-LINK (VISION) (MINI-VISION) (ULTRA)
    Coronary Stent System ....*use* Intraluminal Device

Novacor Left Ventricular Assist Device......................*use* Implantable Heart Assist System in Heart and Great Vessels

Open Pivot Aortic Valve Graft (AVG) ....*use* Synthetic Substitute

Open Pivot (mechanical) valve ....*use* Synthetic Substitute

Paclitaxel-eluting coronary stent ....*use* Intraluminal Device, Drug-eluting in Heart and Great Vessels

Peripherally inserted central catheter (PICC) ....*use* Infusion Device

Porcine (bioprosthetic) valve ....*use* Zooplastic Tissue in Heart and Great Vessels

SAPIEN transcatheter aortic valve............................*use* Zooplastic Tissue in Heart and Great Vessels

Sirolimus-eluting coronary stent ....*use* Intraluminal Device, Drug-eluting in Heart and Great Vessels

SJM Biocor® Stented Valve System ....*use* Zooplastic Tissue in Heart and Great Vessels

Stent, intraluminal (cardiovascular)
    (gastrointestinal) (hepatobiliary) (urinary) ......*use* Intraluminal Device

Stented tissue valve ....*use* Zooplastic Tissue in Heart and Great Vessels

SynCardia Total Artificial Heart ....*use* Synthetic Substitute

TandemHeart® System...*use* External Heart Assist System in Heart and Great Vessels

TAXUS® Liberté® Paclitaxel-eluting Coronary
    Stent System ....*use* Intraluminal Device, Drug-eluting in Heart and Great Vessels

Thoratec IVAD (Implantable Ventricular Assist
Device) ....*use* Implantable Heart Assist System in Heart and Great Vessels

Thoratec Paracorporeal Ventricular Assist Device ..*use* External Heart Assist System in Heart and Great Vessels

TigerPaw® system for closure of left atrial
    appendage ....*use* Extraluminal Device

Tissue bank graft ....*use* Nonautologous Tissue Substitute

Total artificial (replacement) heart ....*use* Synthetic Substitute

Trifecta™ Valve (aortic) ....*use* Zooplastic Tissue in Heart and Great Vessels

Valiant Thoracic Stent Graft ....*use* Intraluminal Device

Xenograft..*use* Zooplastic Tissue in Heart and Great Vessels

XIENCE Everolimus Eluting Coronary Stent System *use* Intraluminal Device, Drug-eluting in Heart and Great Vessels

Zenith TX2® TAA Endovascular Graft ....*use* Intraluminal Device

Zotarolimus-eluting coronary stent ....*use* Intraluminal Device, Drug-eluting in Heart and Great Vessels

Educational Annotations | 2 – Heart and Great Vessels

Device Aggregation Table Listings of Heart and Great Vessels

See also Device Aggregation Table in Appendix E

Specific Device	For Operation	In Body System		General Device
Autologous Arterial Tissue	All applicable	Heart and Great Vessels	7	Autologous Tissue Substitute
Autologous Venous Tissue	All applicable	Heart and Great Vessels	7	Autologous Tissue Substitute
Cardiac Lead, Defibrillator	Insertion	Heart and Great Vessels	M	Cardiac Lead
Cardiac Lead, Pacemaker	Insertion	Heart and Great Vessels	M	Cardiac Lead
Intraluminal Device, Branched or Fenestrated, One or Two Arteries	All applicable	Heart and Great Vessels	D	Intraluminal Device
Intraluminal Device, Branched or Fenestrated, Three or More Arteries	All applicable	Heart and Great Vessels	D	Intraluminal Device
Intraluminal Device, Drug-eluting	All applicable	Heart and Great Vessels	D	Intraluminal Device
Intraluminal Device, Drug-eluting, Four or More	All applicable	Heart and Great Vessels	D	Intraluminal Device
Intraluminal Device, Drug-eluting, Three	All applicable	Heart and Great Vessels	D	Intraluminal Device
Intraluminal Device, Drug-eluting, Two	All applicable	Heart and Great Vessels	D	Intraluminal Device
Intraluminal Device, Four or More	All applicable	Heart and Great Vessels	D	Intraluminal Device
Intraluminal Device, Radioactive	All applicable	Heart and Great Vessels	D	Intraluminal Device
Intraluminal Device, Three	All applicable	Heart and Great Vessels	D	Intraluminal Device
Intraluminal Device, Two	All applicable	Heart and Great Vessels	D	Intraluminal Device
Monitoring Device, Pressure Sensor	Insertion	Heart and Great Vessels	2	Monitoring Device

Coding Notes of Heart and Great Vessels

Body System Relevant Coding Guidelines

Bypass procedures
B3.6b

~~Coronary arteries are classified by number of distinct sites treated, rather than number of coronary arteries or anatomic name of a coronary artery (e.g., left anterior descending).~~ Coronary artery bypass procedures are coded differently than other bypass procedures as described in the previous guideline. Rather than identifying the body part bypassed from, the body part identifies the number of coronary artery sites bypassed to, and the qualifier specifies the vessel bypassed from.

Example: Aortocoronary artery bypass of ~~one site on~~ the left anterior descending coronary artery and ~~one site on~~ the obtuse marginal coronary artery is classified in the body part axis of classification as two coronary ~~artery sites~~ arteries and the qualifier specifies the aorta as the body part bypassed from.

B3.6c

If multiple coronary ~~artery sites~~ arteries are bypassed, a separate procedure is coded for each coronary artery ~~site~~ that uses a different device and/or qualifier.

Example: Aortocoronary artery bypass and internal mammary coronary artery bypass are coded separately.

B4.4

The coronary arteries are classified as a single body part that is further specified by number of ~~sites~~ arteries treated. ~~and not by name or number of arteries.~~ One procedure code specifying multiple arteries is used when the same procedure is performed, including the same device and qualifier values. ~~Separate body part values are used to specify the number of sites treated when the same procedure is performed on multiple sites in the coronary arteries.~~

Examples: Angioplasty of two distinct ~~sites in the left anterior descending coronary artery~~ coronary arteries with placement of two stents is coded as Dilation of Coronary Arteries, Two ~~Sites~~ Arteries, with Two Intraluminal Devices.

Angioplasty of two distinct ~~sites in the left anterior descending coronary artery~~ coronary arteries, one with stent placed and one without, is coded separately as Dilation of Coronary Artery, One ~~Site~~ Artery with Intraluminal Device, and Dilation of Coronary Artery, One ~~Site~~ Artery with no device.

Continued on next page

Educational Annotations | 2 – Heart and Great Vessels

Coding Notes of Heart and Great Vessels

Continued from previous page

Body System Specific PCS Reference Manual Exercises

PCS CODE	2 – HEART AND GREAT VESSELS EXERCISES
0 2 1 0 0 Z 9	CABG of LAD using left internal mammary artery, open off-bypass.
0 2 1 0 3 D 4	PICVA (Percutaneous in-situ coronary venous arterialization) of single coronary artery.
0 2 5 8 3 Z Z	Left heart catheterization with laser destruction of arrhythmogenic focus, A-V node.
0 2 7 0 3 D Z	PTCA of two coronary arteries, LAD with stent placement, RCA with no stent.
0 2 7 0 3 Z Z	(A separate procedure is coded for each artery dilated, since the device value differs for each artery.)
0 2 8 8 3 Z Z	Left heart catheterization with division of bundle of HIS.
0 2 F N 0 Z Z	Thoracotomy with crushing of pericardial calcifications.
0 2 H 7 3 J Z	Percutaneous replacement of broken pacemaker lead in left atrium. (Taking out the broken pacemaker lead is coded separately to the root operation Removal.)
0 2 H P 3 2 Z	Percutaneous placement of Swan-Ganz catheter in pulmonary trunk. The Swan-Ganz catheter is coded to the device value Monitoring Device because it monitors pulmonary artery output.)
0 2 K 8 0 Z Z	Intraoperative cardiac mapping during open heart surgery.
0 2 K 8 3 Z Z	Heart catheterization with cardiac mapping.
0 2 L 7 0 C K	Open occlusion of left atrial appendage, using extraluminal pressure clips.
0 2 L 7 3 Z K	Percutaneous suture exclusion of left atrial appendage, via femoral artery access.
0 2 N G 0 Z Z	Mitral valvulotomy for release of fused leaflets, open approach.
0 2 P Y X 2 Z	Non-incisional removal of Swan-Ganz catheter from right pulmonary artery.
0 2 R G 0 8 Z	Mitral valve replacement using porcine valve, open.
0 2 R H 3 8 Z	Transcatheter replacement of pulmonary valve using a bovine jugular vein valve.
0 2 T D 0 Z Z	Open resection of papillary muscle. (The papillary muscle refers to the heart and is found in the Heart and Great Vessels body system.)
0 2 U A 0 J Z	Implantation of CorCap cardiac support device, open approach.
0 2 U F 0 J Z	Aortic valve annuloplasty using ring, open.
0 2 H V 3 3 Z	Percutaneous placement of venous central line in right internal jugular, with tip in superior vena cava.
0 2 V R 0 C Z	Thoracotomy with banding of left pulmonary artery using extraluminal device.
0 2 V W 3 D J	Catheter-based temporary restriction of blood flow in descending aorta for treatment of cerebral ischemia.
0 2 W A 3 M Z	Adjustment of position, pacemaker lead in left ventricle, percutaneous.
0 2 Y A 0 Z 2	Orthotopic heart transplant using porcine heart. (The donor heart comes from an animal (pig), so the qualifier value is Zooplastic.)

HEART & GREAT V. 02

TUBULAR GROUP: Bypass, Dilation, Occlusion, Restriction
Root Operations that alter the diameter/route of a tubular body part.

1ST - 0 Medical and Surgical

2ND - 2 Heart and Great Vessels

3RD - 1 BYPASS

EXAMPLE: Coronary artery bypass	CMS Ex: Coronary artery bypass

BYPASS: Altering the route of passage of the contents of a tubular body part.

EXPLANATION: Rerouting contents to a downstream part ...

Body Part – 4TH	Approach – 5TH	Device – 6TH	Qualifier – 7TH
0 Coronary Artery, One Artery 1 Coronary Artery, Two Arteries 2 Coronary Artery, Three Arteries 3 Coronary Artery, Four or More Arteries	0 Open	8 Zooplastic tissue 9 Autologous venous tissue A Autologous arterial tissue J Synthetic substitute K Nonautologous tissue substitute	3 Coronary Artery 8 Internal Mammary, Right 9 Internal Mammary, Left C Thoracic Artery F Abdominal Artery W Aorta
0 Coronary Artery, One Artery 1 Coronary Artery, Two Arteries 2 Coronary Artery, Three Arteries 3 Coronary Artery, Four or More Arteries	0 Open	Z No device	3 Coronary Artery 8 Internal Mammary, Right 9 Internal Mammary, Left C Thoracic Artery F Abdominal Artery
0 Coronary Artery, One Artery 1 Coronary Artery, Two Arteries 2 Coronary Artery, Three Arteries 3 Coronary Artery, Four or More Arteries	3 Percutaneous	4 Drug-eluting intraluminal device D Intraluminal device	4 Coronary Vein
0 Coronary Artery, One Artery 1 Coronary Artery, Two Arteries 2 Coronary Artery, Three Arteries 3 Coronary Artery, Four or More Arteries	4 Percutaneous endoscopic	4 Drug-eluting intraluminal device D Intraluminal device	4 Coronary Vein

HEART & GREAT V. **021**

c o n t i n u e d ⇨

0   2   1   BYPASS – continued

Body Part – 4TH	Approach – 5TH	Device – 6TH	Qualifier – 7TH
0 Coronary Artery, One Artery 1 Coronary Artery, Two Arteries 2 Coronary Artery, Three Arteries 3 Coronary Artery, Four or More Arteries	4 Percutaneous endoscopic	8 Zooplastic tissue 9 Autologous venous tissue A Autologous arterial tissue J Synthetic substitute K Nonautologous tissue substitute	3 Coronary Artery 8 Internal Mammary, Right 9 Internal Mammary, Left C Thoracic Artery F Abdominal Artery W Aorta
0 Coronary Artery, One Artery 1 Coronary Artery, Two Arteries 2 Coronary Artery, Three Arteries 3 Coronary Artery, Four or More Arteries	4 Percutaneous endoscopic	Z No device	3 Coronary Artery 8 Internal Mammary, Right 9 Internal Mammary, Left C Thoracic Artery F Abdominal Artery
6 Atrium, Right	0 Open 4 Percutaneous endoscopic	8 Zooplastic tissue 9 Autologous venous tissue A Autologous arterial tissue J Synthetic substitute K Nonautologous tissue substitute	P Pulmonary Trunk Q Pulmonary Artery, Right R Pulmonary Artery, Left
6 Atrium, Right	0 Open 4 Percutaneous endoscopic	Z No device	7 Atrium, Left P Pulmonary Trunk Q Pulmonary Artery, Right R Pulmonary Artery, Left
7 Atrium, Left V Superior Vena Cava	0 Open 4 Percutaneous endoscopic	8 Zooplastic tissue 9 Autologous venous tissue A Autologous arterial tissue J Synthetic substitute K Nonautologous tissue substitute Z No device	P Pulmonary Trunk Q Pulmonary Artery, Right R Pulmonary Artery, Left S Pulmonary Vein, Right T Pulmonary Vein, Left U Pulmonary Vein, Confluence

c o n t i n u e d ⇨

0	2	1	BYPASS – *continued*

Body Part – 4TH	Approach – 5TH	Device – 6TH	Qualifier – 7TH
K Ventricle, Right L Ventricle, Left	0 Open 4 Percutaneous endoscopic	8 Zooplastic tissue 9 Autologous venous tissue A Autologous arterial tissue J Synthetic substitute K Nonautologous tissue substitute	P Pulmonary Trunk Q Pulmonary Artery, Right R Pulmonary Artery, Left
K Ventricle, Right L Ventricle, Left	0 Open 4 Percutaneous endoscopic	Z No device	5 Coronary Circulation 8 Internal Mammary, Right 9 Internal Mammary, Left C Thoracic Artery F Abdominal Artery P Pulmonary Trunk Q Pulmonary Artery, Right R Pulmonary Artery, Left W Aorta
P Pulmonary Trunk Q Pulmonary Artery, Right R Pulmonary Artery, Left	0 Open 4 Percutaneous endoscopic	8 Zooplastic tissue 9 Autologous venous tissue A Autologous arterial tissue J Synthetic substitute K Nonautologous tissue substitute Z No device	A Innominate Artery B Subclavian D Carotid
W Thoracic Aorta, Descending X Thoracic Aorta, Ascending/Arch	0 Open 4 Percutaneous endoscopic	8 Zooplastic tissue 9 Autologous venous tissue A Autologous arterial tissue J Synthetic substitute K Nonautologous tissue substitute Z No device	B Subclavian D Carotid P Pulmonary Trunk Q Pulmonary Artery, Right R Pulmonary Artery, Left

HEART & GREAT V. **021**

OTHER OBJECTIVES GROUP: (Alteration), Creation, (Fusion)
Root Operations that define other objectives.

1ST - 0 Medical and Surgical	EXAMPLE: Creation aortic valve	CMS Ex: Creation vagina in male
2ND - 2 Heart and Great Vessels	**CREATION:** Putting in or on biological or synthetic material to form a new body part that to the extent possible replicates the anatomic structure or function of an absent body part.	
3RD - 4 CREATION	EXPLANATION: Gender reassignment, anomaly correction	

Body Part – 4TH	Approach – 5TH	Device – 6TH	Qualifier – 7TH
F Aortic Valve	0 Open	7 Autologous tissue substitute 8 Zooplastic tissue J Synthetic substitute K Nonautologous tissue substitute	J Truncal Valve
G Mitral Valve J Tricuspid Valve	0 Open	7 Autologous tissue substitute 8 Zooplastic tissue J Synthetic substitute K Nonautologous tissue substitute	2 Common Atrioventricular Valve

EXCISION GROUP: Excision, Resection, Destruction, (Extraction), (Detachment)
Root Operations that take out some or all of a body part.

1ST - 0 Medical and Surgical	EXAMPLE: Atrioventricular node ablation	CMS Ex: Fulguration polyp
2ND - 2 Heart and Great Vessels	**DESTRUCTION:** Physical eradication of all or a portion of a body part by the direct use of energy, force, or a destructive agent.	
3RD - 5 DESTRUCTION	EXPLANATION: None of the body part is physically taken out	

Body Part – 4TH	Approach – 5TH	Device – 6TH	Qualifier – 7TH
4 Coronary Vein 5 Atrial Septum 6 Atrium, Right 8 Conduction Mechanism 9 Chordae Tendineae D Papillary Muscle F Aortic Valve G Mitral Valve H Pulmonary Valve J Tricuspid Valve K Ventricle, Right L Ventricle, Left M Ventricular Septum N Pericardium P Pulmonary Trunk Q Pulmonary Artery, Right R Pulmonary Artery, Left S Pulmonary Vein, Right T Pulmonary Vein, Left V Superior Vena Cava W Thoracic Aorta, Descending X Thoracic Aorta, Ascending/Arch	0 Open 3 Percutaneous 4 Percutaneous endoscopic	Z No device	Z No qualifier
7 Atrium, Left	0 Open 3 Percutaneous 4 Percutaneous endoscopic	Z No device	K Left Atrial Appendage Z No qualifier

© 2016 Channel Publishing, Ltd.

TUBULAR GROUP: Bypass, Dilation, Occlusion, Restriction
Root Operations that alter the diameter/route of a tubular body part.

1ST - 0 Medical and Surgical

2ND - 2 Heart and Great Vessels

3RD - 7 DILATION

EXAMPLE: PTCA coronary artery | CMS Ex: Transluminal angioplasty

DILATION: Expanding an orifice or the lumen of a tubular body part.

EXPLANATION: By force (stretching) or cutting ...

Body Part – 4TH	Approach – 5TH	Device – 6TH	Qualifier – 7TH
0 Coronary Artery, One Artery 1 Coronary Artery, Two Arteries 2 Coronary Artery, Three Arteries 3 Coronary Artery, Four or More Arteries	0 Open 3 Percutaneous 4 Percutaneous endoscopic	4 Drug-eluting intraluminal device 5 Drug-eluting intraluminal device, two 6 Drug-eluting intraluminal device, three 7 Drug-eluting intraluminal device, four or more D Intraluminal device E Intraluminal device, two F Intraluminal device, three G Intraluminal device, four or more T Intraluminal device, radioactive Z No device	6 Bifurcation Z No qualifier
F Aortic Valve S Pulmonary Vein, Right G Mitral Valve T Pulmonary Vein, Left H Pulmonary Valve V Superior Vena Cava J Tricuspid Valve W Thoracic Aorta, Descending K Ventricle, Right P Pulmonary Trunk X Thoracic Aorta, Ascending/Arch Q Pulmonary Artery, Right	0 Open 3 Percutaneous 4 Percutaneous endoscopic	4 Drug-eluting intraluminal device D Intraluminal device Z No device	Z No qualifier
R Pulmonary Artery, Left	0 Open 3 Percutaneous 4 Percutaneous endoscopic	4 Drug-eluting intraluminal device D Intraluminal device Z No device	T Ductus Arteriosus Z No qualifier

HEART & GREAT V. 027

DIVISION GROUP: Division, Release
Root Operations involving cutting or separation only.

1ST - 0 Medical and Surgical	EXAMPLE: Division bundle of HIS	CMS Ex: Osteotomy

2ND - 2 Heart and Great Vessels

3RD - 8 DIVISION

DIVISION: Cutting into a body part without draining fluids and/or gases from the body part in order to separate or transect a body part.

EXPLANATION: Separated into two or more portions ...

Body Part – 4TH	Approach – 5TH	Device – 6TH	Qualifier – 7TH
8 Conduction Mechanism 9 Chordae Tendineae D Papillary Muscle	0 Open 3 Percutaneous 4 Percutaneous endoscopic	Z No device	Z No qualifier

EXCISION GROUP: Excision, Resection, Destruction, (Extraction), (Detachment)
Root Operations that take out some or all of a body part.

1ST - 0 Medical and Surgical	EXAMPLE: Pericardial biopsy	CMS Ex: Liver biopsy

2ND - 2 Heart and Great Vessels

3RD - B EXCISION

EXCISION: Cutting out or off, without replacement, a portion of a body part.

EXPLANATION: Qualifier "X Diagnostic" indicates biopsy ...

Body Part – 4TH	Approach – 5TH	Device – 6TH	Qualifier – 7TH
4 Coronary Vein 5 Atrial Septum 6 Atrium, Right 8 Conduction Mechanism 9 Chordae Tendineae D Papillary Muscle F Aortic Valve G Mitral Valve H Pulmonary Valve J Tricuspid Valve K Ventricle, Right NC* L Ventricle, Left NC* M Ventricular Septum N Pericardium P Pulmonary Trunk Q Pulmonary Artery, Right R Pulmonary Artery, Left S Pulmonary Vein, Right T Pulmonary Vein, Left V Superior Vena Cava W Thoracic Aorta, Descending X Thoracic Aorta, Ascending/Arch	0 Open 3 Percutaneous 4 Percutaneous endoscopic	Z No device	X Diagnostic Z No qualifier
7 Atrium, Left	0 Open 3 Percutaneous 4 Percutaneous endoscopic	Z No device	K Left Atrial Appendage X Diagnostic Z No qualifier

NC* – Some procedures are considered non-covered by Medicare. See current Medicare Code Editor for details.

DRAINAGE GROUP: (Drainage), Extirpation, Fragmentation
Root Operations that take out solids/fluids/gases from a body part.

1ST – 0 Medical and Surgical	EXAMPLE: Pulmonary artery thrombectomy	CMS Ex: Choledocholithotomy

2ND – 2 Heart and Great Vessels

3RD – C EXTIRPATION

EXTIRPATION: Taking or cutting out solid matter from a body part.

EXPLANATION: Abnormal byproduct or foreign body ...

Body Part – 4TH		Approach – 5TH	Device – 6TH	Qualifier – 7TH
0 Coronary Artery, One Artery 1 Coronary Artery, Two Arteries 2 Coronary Artery, Three Arteries 3 Coronary Artery, Four or More Arteries		0 Open 3 Percutaneous 4 Percutaneous endoscopic	Z No device	6 Bifurcation Z No qualifier
4 Coronary Vein 5 Atrial Septum 6 Atrium, Right 7 Atrium, Left 8 Conduction Mechanism 9 Chordae Tendineae D Papillary Muscle F Aortic Valve G Mitral Valve H Pulmonary Valve J Tricuspid Valve K Ventricle, Right L Ventricle, Left	M Ventricular Septum N Pericardium P Pulmonary Trunk Q Pulmonary Artery, Right R Pulmonary Artery, Left S Pulmonary Vein, Right T Pulmonary Vein, Left V Superior Vena Cava W Thoracic Aorta, Descending X Thoracic Aorta, Ascending/Arch	0 Open 3 Percutaneous 4 Percutaneous endoscopic	Z No device	Z No qualifier

DRAINAGE GROUP: (Drainage), Extirpation, Fragmentation
Root Operations that take out solids/fluids/gases from a body part.

1ST – 0 Medical and Surgical	EXAMPLE: Pulverization pericardial calcifications	CMS Ex: ESWL

2ND – 2 Heart and Great Vessels

3RD – F FRAGMENTATION

FRAGMENTATION: Breaking solid matter in a body part into pieces.

EXPLANATION: Pieces are not taken out during procedure ...

Body Part – 4TH	Approach – 5TH	Device – 6TH	Qualifier – 7TH
N Pericardium	0 Open 3 Percutaneous 4 Percutaneous endoscopic X External NC*	Z No device	Z No qualifier

NC* – Non-covered by Medicare. See current Medicare Code Editor for details.

DEVICE GROUP: (Change), Insertion, Removal, Replacement, Revision, Supplement
Root Operations that always involve a device.

1ST - **0** Medical and Surgical

2ND - **2** Heart and Great Vessels

3RD - **H INSERTION**

EXAMPLE: Insertion pacemaker lead   **CMS Ex:** Central venous catheter

INSERTION: Putting in a nonbiological appliance that monitors, assists, performs, or prevents a physiological function but does not physically take the place of a body part.

EXPLANATION: None

Body Part – 4TH	Approach – 5TH	Device – 6TH	Qualifier – 7TH
4 Coronary Vein 6 Atrium, Right 7 Atrium, Left K Ventricle, Right L Ventricle, Left	0 Open 3 Percutaneous 4 Percutaneous endoscopic	0 Monitoring device, pressure sensor 2 Monitoring device 3 Infusion device D Intraluminal device J Cardiac lead, pacemaker K Cardiac lead, defibrillator M Cardiac lead N Intracardiac pacemaker	Z No qualifier
A Heart NC*LC*	0 Open 3 Percutaneous 4 Percutaneous endoscopic	Q Implantable heart assist system	Z No qualifier
A Heart	0 Open 3 Percutaneous 4 Percutaneous endoscopic	R External heart assist system	S Biventricular Z No qualifier
N Pericardium	0 Open 3 Percutaneous 4 Percutaneous endoscopic	0 Monitoring device, pressure sensor 2 Monitoring device J Cardiac lead, pacemaker K Cardiac lead, defibrillator M Cardiac lead	Z No qualifier
P Pulmonary Trunk Q Pulmonary Artery, Right R Pulmonary Artery, Left S Pulmonary Vein, Right T Pulmonary Vein, Left V Superior Vena Cava W Thoracic Aorta, Descending X Thoracic Aorta, Ascending/Arch	0 Open 3 Percutaneous 4 Percutaneous endoscopic	0 Monitoring device, pressure sensor 2 Monitoring device 3 Infusion device D Intraluminal device	Z No qualifier

NC*LC* – Some procedures are considered non-covered or limited coverage by Medicare. See current Medicare Code Editor for details.

HEART & GREAT V. 02H

1ST – 0 Medical and Surgical	**EXAMPLE:** Thoracoscopic visualization heart	**CMS Ex:** Colonoscopy
2ND – 2 Heart and Great Vessels	**INSPECTION:** Visually and/or manually exploring a body part.	
3RD – J INSPECTION	**EXPLANATION:** Direct or instrumental visualization ...	

Body Part – 4TH	Approach – 5TH	Device – 6TH	Qualifier – 7TH
A Heart Y Great Vessel	0 Open 3 Percutaneous 4 Percutaneous endoscopic	Z No device	Z No qualifier

1ST – 0 Medical and Surgical	**EXAMPLE:** Cardiac mapping	**CMS Ex:** Cardiac mapping
2ND – 2 Heart and Great Vessels	**MAP:** Locating the route of passage of electrical impulses and/or locating functional areas in a body part.	
3RD – K MAP	**EXPLANATION:** Limited to cardiac and nervous systems...	

Body Part – 4TH	Approach – 5TH	Device – 6TH	Qualifier – 7TH
8 Conduction Mechanism	0 Open 3 Percutaneous 4 Percutaneous endoscopic	Z No device	Z No qualifier

TUBULAR GROUP: Bypass, Dilation, Occlusion, Restriction
Root Operations that alter the diameter/route of a tubular body part.

1ST - 0 Medical and Surgical

2ND - 2 Heart and Great Vessels

3RD - L OCCLUSION

EXAMPLE: Suture closure of LAA | CMS Ex: Fallopian tube ligation

OCCLUSION: Completely closing an orifice or lumen of a tubular body part.

EXPLANATION: Natural or artificially created orifice …

Body Part – 4TH	Approach – 5TH	Device – 6TH	Qualifier – 7TH
7 Atrium, Left	0 Open 3 Percutaneous 4 Percutaneous endoscopic	C Extraluminal device D Intraluminal device Z No device	K Left Atrial Appendage
H Pulmonary Valve S Pulmonary Vein, Right T Pulmonary Vein, Left V Superior Vena Cava	0 Open 3 Percutaneous 4 Percutaneous endoscopic	C Extraluminal device D Intraluminal device Z No device	Z No qualifier
R Pulmonary Artery, Left	0 Open 3 Percutaneous 4 Percutaneous endoscopic	C Extraluminal device D Intraluminal device Z No device	T Ductus Arteriosus

DIVISION GROUP: Division, Release
Root Operations involving cutting or separation only.

1ST - 0 Medical and Surgical

2ND - 2 Heart and Great Vessels

3RD - N RELEASE

EXAMPLE: Mitral valvulotomy of fused leaflets | CMS Ex: Carpal tunnel

RELEASE: Freeing a body part from an abnormal physical constraint by cutting or by the use of force.

EXPLANATION: None of the body part is taken out …

Body Part – 4TH	Approach – 5TH	Device – 6TH	Qualifier – 7TH
4 Coronary Vein 5 Atrial Septum 6 Atrium, Right 7 Atrium, Left 8 Conduction Mechanism 9 Chordae Tendineae D Papillary Muscle F Aortic Valve G Mitral Valve H Pulmonary Valve J Tricuspid Valve K Ventricle, Right L Ventricle, Left M Ventricular Septum N Pericardium P Pulmonary Trunk Q Pulmonary Artery, Right R Pulmonary Artery, Left S Pulmonary Vein, Right T Pulmonary Vein, Left V Superior Vena Cava W Thoracic Aorta, Descending X Thoracic Aorta, Ascending/Arch	0 Open 3 Percutaneous 4 Percutaneous endoscopic	Z No device	Z No qualifier

DEVICE GROUP: (Change), Insertion, Removal, Replacement, Revision, Supplement
Root Operations that always involve a device.

1ST - **0** Medical and Surgical

2ND - **2** Heart and Great Vessels

3RD - **P** REMOVAL

EXAMPLE: Removal of Swan Ganz catheter | CMS Ex: Chest tube removal

REMOVAL: Taking out or off a device from a body part.

EXPLANATION: Removal device without reinsertion ...

Body Part – 4TH	Approach – 5TH	Device – 6TH	Qualifier – 7TH
A Heart	0 Open 3 Percutaneous 4 Percutaneous endoscopic	2 Monitoring device 3 Infusion device 7 Autologous tissue substitute 8 Zooplastic tissue C Extraluminal device D Intraluminal device J Synthetic substitute K Nonautologous tissue substitute M Cardiac lead N Intracardiac pacemaker Q Implantable heart assist system R External heart assist system	Z No qualifier
A Heart	X External	2 Monitoring device 3 Infusion device D Intraluminal device M Cardiac lead	Z No qualifier
Y Great Vessel	0 Open 3 Percutaneous 4 Percutaneous endoscopic	2 Monitoring device 3 Infusion device 7 Autologous tissue substitute 8 Zooplastic tissue C Extraluminal device D Intraluminal device J Synthetic substitute K Nonautologous tissue substitute	Z No qualifier
Y Great Vessel	X External	2 Monitoring device 3 Infusion device D Intraluminal device	Z No qualifier

HEART & GREAT V. 0 2 P

OTHER REPAIRS GROUP: (Control), **Repair**	
Root Operations that define other repairs.	

1ST - 0 Medical and Surgical	EXAMPLE: Suture pericardial injury CMS Ex: Suture laceration
2ND - 2 Heart and Great Vessels	**REPAIR:** Restoring, to the extent possible, a body part to its normal anatomic structure and function.
3RD - Q REPAIR	EXPLANATION: Only when no other root operation applies …

Body Part – 4TH		Approach – 5TH	Device – 6TH	Qualifier – 7TH
0 Coronary Artery, One Artery 1 Coronary Artery, Two Arteries 2 Coronary Artery, Three Arteries 3 Coronary Artery, Four or More Arteries 4 Coronary Vein 5 Atrial Septum 6 Atrium, Right 7 Atrium, Left 8 Conduction Mechanism 9 Chordae Tendineae A Heart B Heart, Right C Heart, Left	D Papillary Muscle H Pulmonary Valve K Ventricle, Right L Ventricle, Left M Ventricular Septum N Pericardium P Pulmonary Trunk Q Pulmonary Artery, Right R Pulmonary Artery, Left S Pulmonary Vein, Right T Pulmonary Vein, Left V Superior Vena Cava W Thoracic Aorta, Descending X Thoracic Aorta, Ascending/Arch	0 Open 3 Percutaneous 4 Percutaneous endoscopic	Z No device	Z No qualifier
F Aortic Valve		0 Open 3 Percutaneous 4 Percutaneous endoscopic	Z No device	J Truncal valve Z No qualifier
G Mitral Valve		0 Open 3 Percutaneous 4 Percutaneous endoscopic	Z No device	E Atrioventricular valve, left Z No qualifier
J Tricuspid Valve		0 Open 3 Percutaneous 4 Percutaneous endoscopic	Z No device	G Atrioventricular valve, right Z No qualifier

HEART & GREAT V. 02Q

DEVICE GROUP: (Change), Insertion, Removal, Replacement, Revision, Supplement
Root Operations that always involve a device.

1ST - **0** Medical and Surgical

2ND - **2** Heart and Great Vessels

3RD - **R REPLACEMENT**

EXAMPLE: Mitral valve replacement   CMS Ex: Total hip

REPLACEMENT: Putting in or on a biological or synthetic material that physically takes the place and/or function of all or a portion of a body part.

EXPLANATION: Includes taking out body part, or eradication...

Body Part – 4TH	Approach – 5TH	Device – 6TH	Qualifier – 7TH
5 Atrial Septum 6 Atrium, Right 7 Atrium, Left 9 Chordae Tendineae D Papillary Muscle J Tricuspid Valve K Ventricle, Right NC*LC* L Ventricle, Left NC*LC* M Ventricular Septum N Pericardium P Pulmonary Trunk Q Pulmonary Artery, Right R Pulmonary Artery, Left S Pulmonary Vein, Right T Pulmonary Vein, Left V Superior Vena Cava W Thoracic Aorta, Descending X Thoracic Aorta, Ascending/Arch	0 Open 4 Percutaneous endoscopic	7 Autologous tissue substitute 8 Zooplastic tissue J Synthetic substitute K Nonautologous tissue substitute	Z No qualifier
F Aortic Valve G Mitral Valve H Pulmonary Valve	0 Open 4 Percutaneous endoscopic	7 Autologous tissue substitute 8 Zooplastic tissue J Synthetic substitute K Nonautologous tissue substitute	Z No qualifier
F Aortic Valve G Mitral Valve H Pulmonary Valve	3 Percutaneous	7 Autologous tissue substitute 8 Zooplastic tissue J Synthetic substitute K Nonautologous tissue substitute	H Transapical Z No qualifier

NC*LC* – Some procedures are considered non-covered or limited coverage by Medicare. See current Medicare Code Editor for details.

MOVE GROUP: (Reattachment), Reposition, (Transfer), Transplantation
Root Operations that put in/put back or move some/all of a body part.

1ST - **0** Medical and Surgical

2ND - **2** Heart and Great Vessels

3RD - **S REPOSITION**

EXAMPLE: Relocation pulmonary vein   CMS Ex: Fracture reduction

REPOSITION: Moving to its normal location, or other suitable location, all or a portion of a body part.

EXPLANATION: May or may not be cut to be moved ...

Body Part – 4TH	Approach – 5TH	Device – 6TH	Qualifier – 7TH
0 Coronary Artery, One Artery 1 Coronary Artery, Two Arteries P Pulmonary Trunk Q Pulmonary Artery, Right R Pulmonary Artery, Left S Pulmonary Vein, Right T Pulmonary Vein, Left V Superior Vena Cava W Thoracic Aorta, Descending X Thoracic Aorta, Ascending/Arch	0 Open	Z No device	Z No qualifier

<u>**EXCISION GROUP:** Excision, Resection, Destruction,</u> (Extraction), (Detachment)
Root Operations that take out some or all of a body part.

1ST - **0** Medical and Surgical	**EXAMPLE:** Atrial septectomy — **CMS Ex:** Cholecystectomy
2ND - **2** Heart and Great Vessels	<u>**RESECTION:**</u> Cutting out or off, without replacement, all of a body part.
3RD - **T RESECTION**	**EXPLANATION:** None

Body Part – 4TH		Approach – 5TH	Device – 6TH	Qualifier – 7TH
5 Atrial Septum	H Pulmonary Valve	0 Open	Z No device	Z No qualifier
8 Conduction Mechanism	M Ventricular Septum	3 Percutaneous		
9 Chordae Tendineae	N Pericardium	4 Percutaneous endoscopic		
D Papillary Muscle				

DEVICE GROUP: (Change), Insertion, Removal, Replacement, Revision, Supplement
Root Operations that always involve a device.

1ST - 0 Medical and Surgical

2ND - 2 Heart and Great Vessels

3RD - U SUPPLEMENT

EXAMPLE: Valve graft annuloplasty | CMS Ex: Hernia repair with mesh

SUPPLEMENT: Putting in or on biological or synthetic material that physically reinforces and/or augments the function of a portion of a body part.

EXPLANATION: Biological material from same individual ...

Body Part – 4TH	Approach – 5TH	Device – 6TH	Qualifier – 7TH
5 Atrial Septum 6 Atrium, Right 7 Atrium, Left 9 Chordae Tendineae A Heart D Papillary Muscle H Pulmonary Valve K Ventricle, Right L Ventricle, Left M Ventricular Septum N Pericardium P Pulmonary Trunk Q Pulmonary Artery, Right R Pulmonary Artery, Left S Pulmonary Vein, Right T Pulmonary Vein, Left V Superior Vena Cava W Thoracic Aorta, Descending X Thoracic Aorta, Ascending/Arch	0 Open 3 Percutaneous 4 Percutaneous endoscopic	7 Autologous tissue substitute 8 Zooplastic tissue J Synthetic substitute K Nonautologous tissue substitute	Z No qualifier
F Aortic Valve	0 Open 3 Percutaneous 4 Percutaneous endoscopic	7 Autologous tissue substitute 8 Zooplastic tissue J Synthetic substitute K Nonautologous tissue substitute	J Truncal valve Z No qualifier
G Mitral Valve	0 Open 3 Percutaneous 4 Percutaneous endoscopic	7 Autologous tissue substitute 8 Zooplastic tissue J Synthetic substitute K Nonautologous tissue substitute	E Atrioventricular valve, left Z No qualifier
J Tricuspid Valve	0 Open 3 Percutaneous 4 Percutaneous endoscopic	7 Autologous tissue substitute 8 Zooplastic tissue J Synthetic substitute K Nonautologous tissue substitute	G Atrioventricular valve, right Z No qualifier

HEART & GREAT V. 0 2 U

TUBULAR GROUP: Bypass, Dilation, Occlusion, Restriction			
Root Operations that alter the diameter/route of a tubular body part.			

1ST - 0 Medical and Surgical

2ND - 2 Heart and Great Vessels

3RD - V RESTRICTION

EXAMPLE: Banding left pulmonary artery | CMS Ex: Cervical cerclage

RESTRICTION: Partially closing an orifice or the lumen of a tubular body part.

EXPLANATION: Natural or artificially created orifice ...

Body Part – 4TH	Approach – 5TH	Device – 6TH	Qualifier – 7TH
A Heart	0 Open 3 Percutaneous 4 Percutaneous endoscopic	C Extraluminal device Z No device	Z No qualifier
P Pulmonary Trunk Q Pulmonary Artery, Right S Pulmonary Vein, Right T Pulmonary Vein, Left V Superior Vena Cava	0 Open 3 Percutaneous 4 Percutaneous endoscopic	C Extraluminal device D Intraluminal device Z No device	Z No qualifier
R Pulmonary Artery, Left	0 Open 3 Percutaneous 4 Percutaneous endoscopic	C Extraluminal device D Intraluminal device Z No device	T Ductus Arteriosus Z No qualifier
W Thoracic Aorta, Descending X Thoracic Aorta, Ascending/Arch	0 Open 3 Percutaneous 4 Percutaneous endoscopic	C Extraluminal device D Intraluminal device E Intraluminal device, branched or fenestrated, one or two arteries F Intraluminal device, branched or fenestrated, three or more arteries Z No device	Z No qualifier

DEVICE GROUP: (Change), **Insertion, Removal, Replacement, Revision, Supplement**
Root Operations that always involve a device.

1ST - 0	Medical and Surgical	EXAMPLE: Reposition cardiac lead	CMS Ex: Adjustment pacemaker lead

2ND - 2 Heart and Great Vessels

3RD - W REVISION

REVISION: Correcting, to the extent possible, a portion of a malfunctioning device or the position of a displaced device.

EXPLANATION: May replace components of a device ...

Body Part – 4TH	Approach – 5TH	Device – 6TH	Qualifier – 7TH
5 Atrial Septum M Ventricular Septum	0 Open 4 Percutaneous endoscopic	J Synthetic substitute	Z No qualifier
A Heart	0 Open 3 Percutaneous 4 Percutaneous endoscopic X External	2 Monitoring device 3 Infusion device 7 Autologous tissue substitute 8 Zooplastic tissue C Extraluminal device D Intraluminal device J Synthetic substitute LC* K Nonautologous tissue substitute M Cardiac lead N Intracardiac pacemaker Q Implantable heart assist system NC*LC* R External heart assist system	Z No qualifier
F Aortic Valve G Mitral Valve H Pulmonary Valve J Tricuspid Valve	0 Open 4 Percutaneous endoscopic	7 Autologous tissue substitute 8 Zooplastic tissue J Synthetic substitute K Nonautologous tissue substitute	Z No qualifier
Y Great Vessel	0 Open 3 Percutaneous 4 Percutaneous endoscopic X External	2 Monitoring device 3 Infusion device 7 Autologous tissue substitute 8 Zooplastic tissue C Extraluminal device D Intraluminal device J Synthetic substitute K Nonautologous tissue substitute	Z No qualifier

HEART & GREAT V. 0 2 W

NC*LC* – Some procedures are considered non-covered or limited coverage by Medicare. See current Medicare Code Editor for details.

MOVE GROUP: (Reattachment), Reposition, (Transfer), Transplantation			
Root Operations that put in/put back or move some/all of a body part.			

1ST - 0 Medical and Surgical

2ND - 2 Heart and Great Vessels

3RD - Y TRANSPLANTATION

EXAMPLE: Heart transplant   **CMS Ex:** Kidney transplant

TRANSPLANTATION: Putting in or on all or a portion of a living body part taken from another individual or animal to physically take the place and/or function of all or a portion of a similar body part.

EXPLANATION: May take over all or part of its function ...

Body Part – 4TH	Approach – 5TH	Device – 6TH	Qualifier – 7TH
A Heart LC*	0 Open	Z No device	0 Allogeneic 1 Syngeneic 2 Zooplastic

LC* – Some procedures are considered limited coverage by Medicare. See current Medicare Code Editor for details.

HEART & GREAT V. 02Y

Educational Annotations | 3 – Upper Arteries

Body System Specific Educational Annotations for the Upper Arteries include:

- Anatomy and Physiology Review
- Anatomical Illustrations
- Definitions of Common Procedures
- AHA Coding Clinic® Reference Notations
- Body Part Key Listings
- Device Key Listings
- Device Aggregation Table Listings
- Coding Notes

Anatomy and Physiology Review of Upper Arteries

BODY PART VALUES – 3 - UPPER ARTERIES

Artery – Blood vessels that carry oxygenated (arterial) blood away from the heart and to the organs and tissues of the body. Arteries have a higher blood pressure than other parts of the circulatory system in order to adequately perfuse all the tissues with oxygenated red blood cells.

Axillary Artery – The axillary artery branches from the subclavian artery and serves the lateral thorax and upper limb.

Brachial Artery – The brachial artery branches from the axillary artery and serves the upper limb.

Common Carotid Artery – The left common carotid artery branches from the aortic arch and serves the head and brain. The right common carotid artery branches from the innominate artery (also known as the brachiocephalic artery) and serves the head and brain.

External Carotid Artery – The external carotid artery branches from the common carotid artery and serves the head.

Face Artery – Any of the smaller arterial branches that serves the face.

Hand Artery – Any of the smaller arterial branches that serves the hand.

Innominate Artery – The innominate artery (also known as the brachiocephalic artery) branches from the aortic arch and branches to the right common carotid artery, the internal mammary artery, and the subclavian artery.

Internal Carotid Artery – The internal carotid artery branches from the common carotid artery and serves primarily the brain.

Internal Mammary Artery – The internal mammary artery branches from the innominate artery and serves the anterior chest wall and breasts.

Intracranial Artery – Any of the smaller arterial branches that lies within the skull.

Radial Artery – The radial artery branches from the brachial artery and serves the forearm, wrist, and hand.

Subclavian Artery – The left subclavian artery branches from the aortic arch and serves the thorax, head, and left upper limb. The right subclavian artery branches from the innominate artery (also known as the brachiocephalic artery) and serves the thorax, head, and right upper limb.

Temporal Artery – The temporal artery branches from the external carotid artery and serves the head.

Thyroid Artery – The thyroid artery branches from the thyrocervical trunk of the subclavian artery and serves the thyroid gland.

Ulnar Artery – The ulnar artery branches from the brachial artery and serves the forearm and wrist.

Upper Artery – The arteries located above the diaphragm (see Coding Guideline B2.1b).

Vertebral Artery – The vertebral artery branches from the subclavian artery and serves the brain.

Educational Annotations | 3 – Upper Arteries

Anatomical Illustrations of Upper Arteries

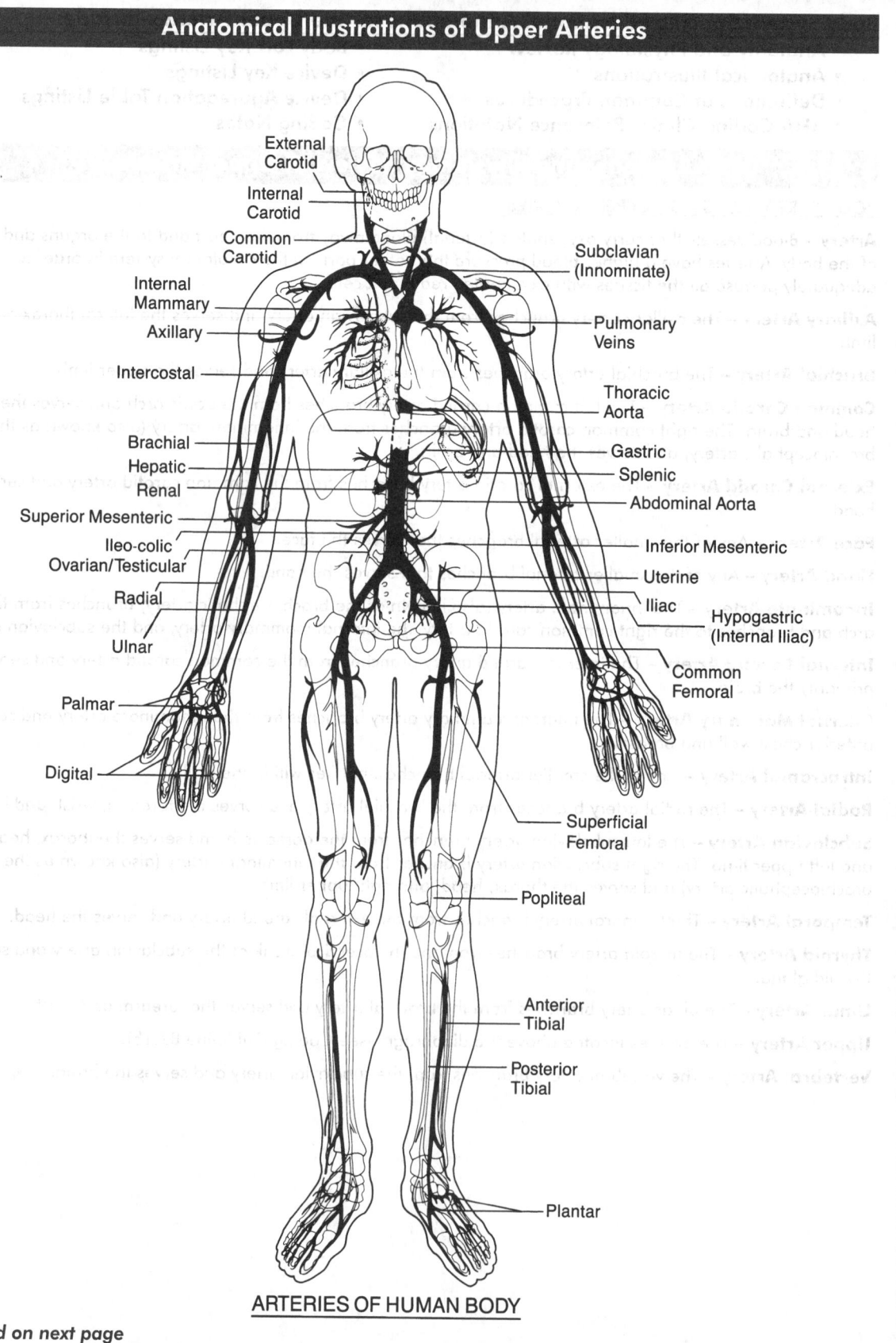

- External Carotid
- Internal Carotid
- Common Carotid
- Internal Mammary
- Axillary
- Intercostal
- Brachial
- Hepatic
- Renal
- Superior Mesenteric
- Ileo-colic
- Ovarian/Testicular
- Radial
- Ulnar
- Palmar
- Digital
- Subclavian (Innominate)
- Pulmonary Veins
- Thoracic Aorta
- Gastric
- Splenic
- Abdominal Aorta
- Inferior Mesenteric
- Uterine
- Iliac
- Hypogastric (Internal Iliac)
- Common Femoral
- Superficial Femoral
- Popliteal
- Anterior Tibial
- Posterior Tibial
- Plantar

ARTERIES OF HUMAN BODY

Continued on next page

UPPER ARTERIES 0 3

Educational Annotations | 3 – Upper Arteries

Anatomical Illustrations of Upper Arteries

Continued from previous page

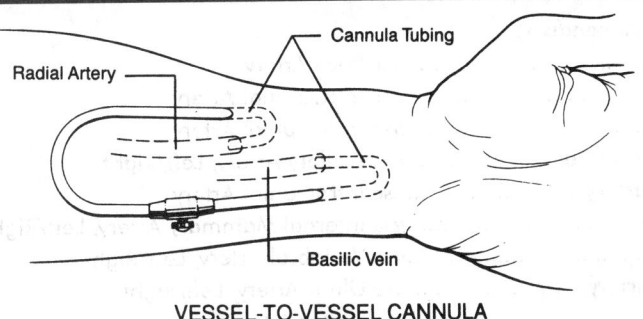

Cannula Tubing

Radial Artery

Basilic Vein

VESSEL-TO-VESSEL CANNULA

Definitions of Common Procedures of Upper Arteries

Balloon angioplasty – The surgical restoration of a narrowed arterial lumen using a balloon-dilating catheter.

Carotid artery to vertebral artery bypass – The restoration of vertebral artery blood flow by using a tubular graft (tissue or synthetic) from a carotid artery to bypass the diseased section of a vertebral artery.

Carotid endarterectomy – The surgical removal of lumen-reducing plaque from a carotid artery to increase the blood flow to the head and reduce the risk of stroke.

Creation of arteriovenous (AV) fistula – The surgical re-routing of an artery in the forearm directly into a vein in the forearm to create an easy and reliable access for repeated hemodialysis.

AHA Coding Clinic® Reference Notations of Upper Arteries

ROOT OPERATION SPECIFIC - 3 - UPPER ARTERIES
BYPASS - 1
Anastomosis between an artery and a vein for hemodialysis access ....AHA 13:1Q:p27
Arteriovenous anastomosis of brachial artery ....AHA 13:4Q:p125
DESTRUCTION - 5
DILATION - 7
DRAINAGE - 9
EXCISION - B
Infratemporal fossa malignancy with excision of carotid artery ....AHA 16:2Q:p12
EXTIRPATION - C
Carotid endarterectomy with patch angioplasty ....AHA 16:2Q:p11
INSERTION - H
Arterial line placement...AHA 16:2Q:p32
INSPECTION - J
Discontinued carotid artery procedure ....AHA 15:1Q:p29
OCCLUSION - L
Clipping occlusion of cerebral artery aneurysm...AHA 16:2Q:p30
Endovascular Onyx-18 liquid embolization ....AHA 14:4Q:p37
RELEASE - N
REMOVAL - P
REPAIR - Q
Epistaxis control using sutures ....AHA 14:4Q:p20
REPLACEMENT - R
REPOSITION - S
Creation of superficial temporal artery cuff..AHA 15:3Q:p27
SUPPLEMENT - U
Carotid endarterectomy with patch angioplasty ....AHA 16:2Q:p11
RESTRICTION - V
Stent assisted coil embolization of carotid artery......................................AHA 16:1Q:p19
REVISION - W
Stent to trap herniated/migrated coil in basilar artery ....AHA 15:1Q:p32

Educational Annotations | 3 – Upper Arteries

Body Part Key Listings of Upper Arteries

See also Body Part Key in Appendix C

Angular artery	*use* Face Artery
Anterior cerebral artery	*use* Intracranial Artery
Anterior choroidal artery	*use* Intracranial Artery
Anterior circumflex humeral artery	*use* Axillary Artery, Left/Right
Anterior communicating artery	*use* Intracranial Artery
Anterior intercostal artery	*use* Internal Mammary Artery, Left/Right
Anterior spinal artery	*use* Vertebral Artery, Left/Right
Anterior ulnar recurrent artery	*use* Ulnar Artery, Left/Right
Aortic intercostal artery	*use* Upper Artery
Ascending palatine artery	*use* Face Artery
Ascending pharyngeal artery	*use* External Carotid Artery, Left/Right
Basilar artery	*use* Intracranial Artery
Brachiocephalic artery	*use* Innominate Artery
Brachiocephalic trunk	*use* Innominate Artery
Bronchial artery	*use* Upper Artery
Caroticotympanic artery	*use* Internal Carotid Artery, Left/Right
Carotid sinus	*use* Internal Carotid Artery, Left/Right
Circle of Willis	*use* Intracranial Artery
Common interosseous artery	*use* Ulnar Artery, Left/Right
Costocervical trunk	*use* Subclavian Artery, Left/Right
Cricothyroid artery	*use* Thyroid Artery, Left/Right
Deep palmar arch	*use* Hand Artery, Left/Right
Dorsal scapular artery	*use* Subclavian Artery, Left/Right
Esophageal artery	*use* Upper Artery
External maxillary artery	*use* Face Artery
Facial artery	*use* Face Artery
Hyoid artery	*use* Thyroid Artery, Left/Right
Inferior labial artery	*use* Face Artery
Inferior ulnar collateral artery	*use* Brachial Artery, Left/Right
Internal carotid artery, intracranial portion	*use* Intracranial Artery
Internal maxillary artery	*use* External Carotid Artery, Left/Right
Internal thoracic artery	*use* Internal Mammary Artery, Left/Right
	use Subclavian Artery, Left/Right
Lateral thoracic artery	*use* Axillary Artery, Left/Right
Lingual artery	*use* External Carotid Artery, Left/Right
Maxillary artery	*use* External Carotid Artery, Left/Right
Middle cerebral artery	*use* Intracranial Artery
Middle temporal artery	*use* Temporal Artery, Left/Right
Musculophrenic artery	*use* Internal Mammary Artery, Left/Right
Occipital artery	*use* External Carotid Artery, Left/Right
Ophthalmic artery	*use* Intracranial Artery
Pericardiophrenic artery	*use* Internal Mammary Artery, Left/Right
Posterior auricular artery	*use* External Carotid Artery, Left/Right
Posterior cerebral artery	*use* Intracranial Artery
Posterior circumflex humeral artery	*use* Axillary Artery, Left/Right
Posterior communicating artery	*use* Intracranial Artery
Posterior inferior cerebellar artery (PICA)	*use* Intracranial Artery
Posterior spinal artery	*use* Vertebral Artery, Left/Right
Posterior ulnar recurrent artery	*use* Ulnar Artery, Left/Right

Continued on next page

UPPER ARTERIES 03

Educational Annotations | 3 – Upper Arteries

Body Part Key Listings of Upper Arteries

Continued from previous page

Princeps pollicis artery ....*use* Hand Artery, Left/Right
Profunda brachii ....*use* Brachial Artery, Left/Right
Radial recurrent artery....................................*use* Radial Artery, Left/Right
Radialis indicis ....*use* Hand Artery, Left/Right
Sternocleidomastoid artery ....*use* Thyroid Artery, Left/Right
Subcostal artery ....*use* Upper Artery
Submental artery ....*use* Face Artery
Subscapular artery...*use* Axillary Artery, Left/Right
Superficial palmar arch ....*use* Hand Artery, Left/Right
Superficial temporal artery ....*use* Temporal Artery, Left/Right
Superior epigastric artery ....*use* Internal Mammary Artery, Left/Right
Superior labial artery.......................................*use* Face Artery
Superior laryngeal artery.................................*use* Thyroid Artery, Left/Right
Superior thoracic artery ....*use* Axillary Artery, Left/Right
Superior thyroid artery....................................*use* External Carotid Artery, Left/Right
                                    ....*use* Thyroid Artery, Left/Right
Superior ulnar collateral artery ....*use* Brachial Artery, Left/Right
Thoracoacromial artery ....*use* Axillary Artery, Left/Right
Thyrocervical trunk ....*use* Thyroid Artery, Left/Right
Transverse facial artery ....*use* Temporal Artery, Left/Right

Device Key Listings of Upper Arteries

See also Device Key in Appendix D

Absolute Pro Vascular (OTW) Self-Expanding Stent
    System ....*use* Intraluminal Device
Acculink (RX) Carotid Stent System ....*use* Intraluminal Device
AneuRx® AAA Advantage® ....*use* Intraluminal Device
Autograft..*use* Autologous Tissue Substitute
Autologous artery graft ....*use* Autologous Arterial Tissue in Upper Arteries
Autologous vein graft ....*use* Autologous Venous Tissue in Upper Arteries
Baroreflex Activation Therapy® (BAT®) ....*use* Stimulator Lead in Upper Arteries
Bioactive embolization coil(s) ....*use* Intraluminal Device, Bioactive in Upper Arteries
Carotid (artery) sinus (baroreceptor) lead...............*use* Stimulator Lead in Upper Arteries
Carotid WALLSTENT® Monorail® Endoprosthesis ....*use* Intraluminal Device
Embolization coil(s) ....*use* Intraluminal Device
FLAIR® Endovascular Stent Graft............................*use* Intraluminal Device
GORE TAG® Thoracic Endoprosthesis......................*use* Intraluminal Device
Micrus CERECYTE microcoil ....*use* Intraluminal Device, Bioactive in Upper Arteries
Paclitaxel-eluting peripheral stent ....*use* Intraluminal Device, Drug-eluting in Upper Arteries, Lower
                                Arteries
Pipeline™ Embolization device (PED) ....*use* Intraluminal Device
Protégé® RX Carotid Stent System ....*use* Intraluminal Device
Rheos® System lead...*use* Stimulator Lead in Upper Arteries
Stent, intraluminal (cardiovascular)
    (gastrointestinal) (hepatobiliary) (urinary) ......*use* Intraluminal Device
Talent® Converter...*use* Intraluminal Device
Talent® Occluder ....*use* Intraluminal Device
Talent® Stent Graft (abdominal) (thoracic)..............*use* Intraluminal Device

Continued on next page

UPPER ARTERIES 03

Educational Annotations | 3 – Upper Arteries

Device Key Listings of Upper Arteries

Continued from previous page

Therapeutic occlusion coil(s) .... *use* Intraluminal Device

Tissue bank graft .... *use* Nonautologous Tissue Substitute

WALLSTENT® Endoprosthesis .... *use* Intraluminal Device

Xact Carotid Stent System .... *use* Intraluminal Device

Zilver® PTX® (paclitaxel) Drug-Eluting Peripheral Stent .... *use* Intraluminal Device, Drug-eluting in Upper Arteries, Lower Arteries

Device Aggregation Table Listings of Upper Arteries

See also Device Aggregation Table in Appendix E

Specific Device	For Operation	In Body System		General Device
Autologous Arterial Tissue	All applicable	Upper Arteries	7	Autologous Tissue Substitute
Autologous Venous Tissue	All applicable	Upper Arteries	7	Autologous Tissue Substitute
Intraluminal Device, Bioactive	All applicable	Upper Arteries	D	Intraluminal Device
Intraluminal Device, Drug-eluting	All applicable	Upper Arteries	D	Intraluminal Device
Intraluminal Device, Drug-eluting, Four or More	All applicable	Heart and Great Vessels	D	Intraluminal Device
Intraluminal Device, Drug-eluting, Three	All applicable	Heart and Great Vessels	D	Intraluminal Device
Intraluminal Device, Drug-eluting, Two	All applicable	Heart and Great Vessels	D	Intraluminal Device
Intraluminal Device, Four or More	All applicable	Heart and Great Vessels	D	Intraluminal Device
Intraluminal Device, Three	All applicable	Heart and Great Vessels	D	Intraluminal Device
Intraluminal Device, Two	All applicable	Heart and Great Vessels	D	Intraluminal Device

Coding Notes of Upper Arteries

Body System Relevant Coding Guidelines

General Guidelines

B2.1b

Where the general body part values "upper" and "lower" are provided as an option in the Upper Arteries, Lower Arteries, Upper Veins, Lower Veins, Muscles and Tendons body systems, "upper" and "lower" specifies body parts located above or below the diaphragm respectively.

Example: Vein body parts above the diaphragm are found in the Upper Veins body system; vein body parts below the diaphragm are found in the Lower Veins body system.

Branches of body parts

B4.2

Where a specific branch of a body part does not have its own body part value in PCS, the body part is typically coded to the closest proximal branch that has a specific body part value. In the cardiovascular body systems, if a general body part is available in the correct root operation table, and coding to a proximal branch would require assigning a code in a different body system, the procedure is coded using the general body part value.

Examples: A procedure performed on the mandibular branch of the trigeminal nerve is coded to the trigeminal nerve body part value.

Occlusion of the bronchial artery is coded to the body part value Upper Artery in the body system Upper Arteries, and not to the body part value Thoracic Aorta, Descending in the body system Heart and Great Vessels.

Body System Specific PCS Reference Manual Exercises

PCS CODE	3 – UPPER ARTERIES EXERCISES
0 3 1 S 0 J G	Right temporal artery to intracranial artery bypass using goretex graft, open.
0 3 7 7 3 Z Z	PTA of right brachial artery stenosis.
0 3 C 8 3 Z Z	Percutaneous mechanical thrombectomy, left brachial artery.
0 3 C H 0 Z Z	Right common carotid endarterectomy, open.
0 3 L 8 0 Z Z	Open suture ligation of failed AV graft, left brachial artery.
0 3 L G 3 D Z	Percutaneous embolization of vascular supply, intracranial meningioma.
0 3 L L 3 D Z	Percutaneous embolization of left internal carotid-cavernous fistula.
0 3 V G 0 C Z	Craniotomy with clipping of cerebral aneurysm. (A clip is placed lengthwise on the outside wall of the widened portion of the vessel.)

TUBULAR GROUP: Bypass, Dilation, Occlusion, Restriction
Root Operations that alter the diameter/route of a tubular body part.

1ST - **0** Medical and Surgical

2ND - **3** Upper Arteries

3RD - **1 BYPASS**

EXAMPLE: Arteriovenous hemodialysis fistula | CMS Ex: Coronary bypass

BYPASS: Altering the route of passage of the contents of a tubular body part.

EXPLANATION: Rerouting contents to a downstream part …

Body Part – 4TH	Approach – 5TH	Device – 6TH	Qualifier – 7TH
2 Innominate Artery 5 Axillary Artery, Right 6 Axillary Artery, Left	0 Open	9 Autologous venous tissue A Autologous arterial tissue J Synthetic substitute K Nonautologous tissue substitute Z No device	0 Upper Arm Artery, Right 1 Upper Arm Artery, Left 2 Upper Arm Artery, Bilateral 3 Lower Arm Artery, Right 4 Lower Arm Artery, Left 5 Lower Arm Artery, Bilateral 6 Upper Leg Artery, Right 7 Upper Leg Artery, Left 8 Upper Leg Artery, Bilateral 9 Lower Leg Artery, Right B Lower Leg Artery, Left C Lower Leg Artery, Bilateral D Upper Arm Vein F Lower Arm Vein J Extracranial Artery, Right K Extracranial Artery, Left
3 Subclavian Artery, Right 4 Subclavian Artery, Left	0 Open	9 Autologous venous tissue A Autologous arterial tissue J Synthetic substitute K Nonautologous tissue substitute Z No device	0 Upper Arm Artery, Right 1 Upper Arm Artery, Left 2 Upper Arm Artery, Bilateral 3 Lower Arm Artery, Right 4 Lower Arm Artery, Left 5 Lower Arm Artery, Bilateral 6 Upper Leg Artery, Right 7 Upper Leg Artery, Left 8 Upper Leg Artery, Bilateral 9 Lower Leg Artery, Right B Lower Leg Artery, Left C Lower Leg Artery, Bilateral D Upper Arm Vein F Lower Arm Vein J Extracranial Artery, Right K Extracranial Artery, Left M Pulmonary Artery, Right N Pulmonary Artery, Left

UPPER ARTERIES 031

continued ⇨

0	3	1	BYPASS – *continued*

Body Part – 4TH	Approach – 5TH	Device – 6TH	Qualifier – 7TH
7 Brachial Artery, Right	0 Open	9 Autologous venous tissue A Autologous arterial tissue J Synthetic substitute K Nonautologous tissue substitute Z No device	0 Upper Arm Artery, Right 3 Lower Arm Artery, Right D Upper Arm Vein F Lower Arm Vein
8 Brachial Artery, Left	0 Open	9 Autologous venous tissue A Autologous arterial tissue J Synthetic substitute K Nonautologous tissue substitute Z No device	1 Upper Arm Artery, Left 4 Lower Arm Artery, Left D Upper Arm Vein F Lower Arm Vein
9 Ulnar Artery, Right B Radial Artery, Right	0 Open	9 Autologous venous tissue A Autologous arterial tissue J Synthetic substitute K Nonautologous tissue substitute Z No device	3 Lower Arm Artery, Right F Lower Arm Vein
A Ulnar Artery, Left C Radial Artery, Left	0 Open	9 Autologous venous tissue A Autologous arterial tissue J Synthetic substitute K Nonautologous tissue substitute Z No device	4 Lower Arm Artery, Left F Lower Arm Vein
G Intracranial Artery S Temporal Artery, Right NC* T Temporal Artery, Left NC*	0 Open	9 Autologous venous tissue A Autologous arterial tissue J Synthetic substitute K Nonautologous tissue substitute Z No device	G Intracranial Artery

continued ⇨

UPPER ARTERIES 031

0 3 1   BYPASS – *continued*

Body Part – 4TH	Approach – 5TH	Device – 6TH	Qualifier – 7TH
H Common Carotid Artery, Right	0 Open	9 Autologous venous tissue A Autologous arterial tissue J Synthetic substitute K Nonautologous tissue substitute Z No device	G Intracranial Artery NC* J Extracranial Artery, Right
J Common Carotid Artery, Left	0 Open	9 Autologous venous tissue A Autologous arterial tissue J Synthetic substitute K Nonautologous tissue substitute Z No device	G Intracranial Artery NC* K Extracranial Artery, Left
K Internal Carotid Artery, Right M External Carotid Artery, Right	0 Open	9 Autologous venous tissue A Autologous arterial tissue J Synthetic substitute K Nonautologous tissue substitute Z No device	J Extracranial Artery, Right
L Internal Carotid Artery, Left N External Carotid Artery, Left	0 Open	9 Autologous venous tissue A Autologous arterial tissue J Synthetic substitute K Nonautologous tissue substitute Z No device	K Extracranial Artery, Left

NC* – Non-covered by Medicare. See current Medicare Code Editor for details.

UPPER ARTERIES 031

EXCISION GROUP: Excision, (Resection), Destruction, (Extraction), (Detachment)
Root Operations that take out some or all of a body part.

1ST - 0 Medical and Surgical	EXAMPLE: Fulguration arterial lesion	CMS Ex: Fulguration polyp

2ND - 3 Upper Arteries

3RD - 5 DESTRUCTION

DESTRUCTION: Physical eradication of all or a portion of a body part by the direct use of energy, force, or a destructive agent.

EXPLANATION: None of the body part is physically taken out

Body Part – 4TH	Approach – 5TH	Device – 6TH	Qualifier – 7TH
0 Internal Mammary Artery, Right 1 Internal Mammary Artery, Left 2 Innominate Artery 3 Subclavian Artery, Right 4 Subclavian Artery, Left 5 Axillary Artery, Right 6 Axillary Artery, Left 7 Brachial Artery, Right 8 Brachial Artery, Left 9 Ulnar Artery, Right A Ulnar Artery, Left B Radial Artery, Right C Radial Artery, Left D Hand Artery, Right F Hand Artery, Left G Intracranial Artery H Common Carotid Artery, Right J Common Carotid Artery, Left K Internal Carotid Artery, Right L Internal Carotid Artery, Left M External Carotid Artery, Right N External Carotid Artery, Left P Vertebral Artery, Right Q Vertebral Artery, Left R Face Artery S Temporal Artery, Right T Temporal Artery, Left U Thyroid Artery, Right V Thyroid Artery, Left Y Upper Artery	0 Open 3 Percutaneous 4 Percutaneous endoscopic	Z No device	Z No qualifier

TUBULAR GROUP: Bypass, Dilation, Occlusion, Restriction
Root Operations that alter the diameter/route of a tubular body part.

1ST - **0** Medical and Surgical

2ND - **3** Upper Arteries

3RD - **7 DILATION**

EXAMPLE: PTA common carotid | CMS Ex: Transluminal angioplasty

DILATION: Expanding an orifice or the lumen of a tubular body part.

EXPLANATION: By force (stretching) or cutting ...

Body Part – 4TH		Approach – 5TH	Device – 6TH	Qualifier – 7TH
0 Internal Mammary Artery, Right	J Common Carotid Artery, Left	0 Open	4 Drug-eluting intraluminal device	6 Bifurcation
1 Internal Mammary Artery, Left	K Internal Carotid Artery, Right	3 Percutaneous	5 Drug-eluting intraluminal device, two	Z No qualifier
2 Innominate Artery	L Internal Carotid Artery, Left	4 Percutaneous endoscopic	6 Drug-eluting intraluminal device, three	
3 Subclavian Artery, Right	M External Carotid Artery, Right		7 Drug-eluting intraluminal device, four or more	
4 Subclavian Artery, Left	N External Carotid Artery, Left		D Intraluminal device	
5 Axillary Artery, Right	P Vertebral Artery, Right		E Intraluminal device, two	
6 Axillary Artery, Left	Q Vertebral Artery, Left		F Intraluminal device, three	
7 Brachial Artery, Right	R Face Artery		G Intraluminal device, four or more	
8 Brachial Artery, Left	S Temporal Artery, Right		Z No device	
9 Ulnar Artery, Right	T Temporal Artery, Left			
A Ulnar Artery, Left	U Thyroid Artery, Right			
B Radial Artery, Right	V Thyroid Artery, Left			
C Radial Artery, Left	Y Upper Artery			
D Hand Artery, Right				
F Hand Artery, Left				
G Intracranial Artery NC*				
H Common Carotid Artery, Right				

NC* – Some procedures are considered non-covered by Medicare. See current Medicare Code Editor for details.

UPPER ARTERIES 037

DRAINAGE GROUP: Drainage, Extirpation, (Fragmentation)
Root Operations that take out solids/fluids/gases from a body part.

1ST – **0** Medical and Surgical	**EXAMPLE:** Aspiration arterial abscess **CMS Ex:** Thoracentesis
2ND – **3** Upper Arteries	**DRAINAGE:** Taking or letting out fluids and/or gases from a body part.
3RD – **9 DRAINAGE**	**EXPLANATION:** Qualifier "X Diagnostic" indicates biopsy …

Body Part – 4TH		Approach – 5TH	Device – 6TH	Qualifier – 7TH
0 Internal Mammary Artery, Right	J Common Carotid Artery, Left	0 Open	0 Drainage device	Z No qualifier
1 Internal Mammary Artery, Left	K Internal Carotid Artery, Right	3 Percutaneous		
2 Innominate Artery	L Internal Carotid Artery, Left	4 Percutaneous endoscopic		
3 Subclavian Artery, Right				
4 Subclavian Artery, Left	M External Carotid Artery, Right			
5 Axillary Artery, Right				
6 Axillary Artery, Left	N External Carotid Artery, Left			
7 Brachial Artery, Right				
8 Brachial Artery, Left	P Vertebral Artery, Right			
9 Ulnar Artery, Right	Q Vertebral Artery, Left			
A Ulnar Artery, Left	R Face Artery			
B Radial Artery, Right	S Temporal Artery, Right			
C Radial Artery, Left	T Temporal Artery, Left			
D Hand Artery, Right	U Thyroid Artery, Right			
F Hand Artery, Left	V Thyroid Artery, Left			
G Intracranial Artery	Y Upper Artery			
H Common Carotid Artery, Right				
0 Internal Mammary Artery, Right	J Common Carotid Artery, Left	0 Open	Z No device	X Diagnostic
1 Internal Mammary Artery, Left	K Internal Carotid Artery, Right	3 Percutaneous		Z No qualifier
2 Innominate Artery	L Internal Carotid Artery, Left	4 Percutaneous endoscopic		
3 Subclavian Artery, Right				
4 Subclavian Artery, Left	M External Carotid Artery, Right			
5 Axillary Artery, Right				
6 Axillary Artery, Left	N External Carotid Artery, Left			
7 Brachial Artery, Right				
8 Brachial Artery, Left	P Vertebral Artery, Right			
9 Ulnar Artery, Right	Q Vertebral Artery, Left			
A Ulnar Artery, Left	R Face Artery			
B Radial Artery, Right	S Temporal Artery, Right			
C Radial Artery, Left	T Temporal Artery, Left			
D Hand Artery, Right	U Thyroid Artery, Right			
F Hand Artery, Left	V Thyroid Artery, Left			
G Intracranial Artery	Y Upper Artery			
H Common Carotid Artery, Right				

EXCISION GROUP: Excision, (Resection), **Destruction,** (Extraction), (Detachment)	
Root Operations that take out some or all of a body part.	

1ST - 0 Medical and Surgical	EXAMPLE: Temporal artery biopsy	CMS Ex: Liver biopsy
2ND - 3 Upper Arteries	**EXCISION:** Cutting out or off, without replacement, a portion of a body part.	
3RD - B EXCISION	EXPLANATION: Qualifier "X Diagnostic" indicates biopsy ...	

Body Part – 4TH		Approach – 5TH	Device – 6TH	Qualifier – 7TH
0 Internal Mammary Artery, Right	J Common Carotid Artery, Left	0 Open	Z No device	X Diagnostic
1 Internal Mammary Artery, Left	K Internal Carotid Artery, Right	3 Percutaneous		Z No qualifier
2 Innominate Artery	L Internal Carotid Artery, Left	4 Percutaneous endoscopic		
3 Subclavian Artery, Right				
4 Subclavian Artery, Left	M External Carotid Artery, Right			
5 Axillary Artery, Right	N External Carotid Artery, Left			
6 Axillary Artery, Left				
7 Brachial Artery, Right	P Vertebral Artery, Right			
8 Brachial Artery, Left	Q Vertebral Artery, Left			
9 Ulnar Artery, Right	R Face Artery			
A Ulnar Artery, Left	S Temporal Artery, Right			
B Radial Artery, Right	T Temporal Artery, Left			
C Radial Artery, Left	U Thyroid Artery, Right			
D Hand Artery, Right	V Thyroid Artery, Left			
F Hand Artery, Left	Y Upper Artery			
G Intracranial Artery				
H Common Carotid Artery, Right				

UPPER ARTERIES

0 3 B

DRAINAGE GROUP: Drainage, Extirpation, (Fragmentation)
Root Operations that take out solids/fluids/gases from a body part.

1ST - **0** Medical and Surgical	EXAMPLE: Carotid artery endarterectomy	CMS Ex: Choledocholithotomy

2ND - **3** Upper Arteries

3RD - **C EXTIRPATION**

EXTIRPATION: Taking or cutting out solid matter from a body part.

EXPLANATION: Abnormal byproduct or foreign body ...

Body Part – 4TH		Approach – 5TH	Device – 6TH	Qualifier – 7TH
0 Internal Mammary Artery, Right	J Common Carotid Artery, Left	0 Open	Z No device	6 Bifurcation
1 Internal Mammary Artery, Left	K Internal Carotid Artery, Right	3 Percutaneous		Z No qualifier
2 Innominate Artery	L Internal Carotid Artery, Left	4 Percutaneous endoscopic		
3 Subclavian Artery, Right	M External Carotid Artery, Right			
4 Subclavian Artery, Left				
5 Axillary Artery, Right	N External Carotid Artery, Left			
6 Axillary Artery, Left	P Vertebral Artery, Right			
7 Brachial Artery, Right	Q Vertebral Artery, Left			
8 Brachial Artery, Left	R Face Artery			
9 Ulnar Artery, Right	S Temporal Artery, Right			
A Ulnar Artery, Left	T Temporal Artery, Left			
B Radial Artery, Right	U Thyroid Artery, Right			
C Radial Artery, Left	V Thyroid Artery, Left			
D Hand Artery, Right	Y Upper Artery			
F Hand Artery, Left				
G Intracranial Artery				
H Common Carotid Artery, Right				

DEVICE GROUP: (Change), Insertion, Removal, Replacement, Revision, Supplement
Root Operations that always involve a device.

1ST - 0 Medical and Surgical	EXAMPLE: Carotid artery stimulator lead	CMS Ex: Central venous cath
2ND - 3 Upper Arteries	**INSERTION:** Putting in a nonbiological appliance that monitors, assists, performs, or prevents a physiological function but does not physically take the place of a body part.	
3RD - H INSERTION	EXPLANATION: None	

Body Part – 4TH		Approach – 5TH	Device – 6TH	Qualifier – 7TH
0 Internal Mammary Artery, Right 1 Internal Mammary Artery, Left 2 Innominate Artery 3 Subclavian Artery, Right 4 Subclavian Artery, Left 5 Axillary Artery, Right 6 Axillary Artery, Left 7 Brachial Artery, Right 8 Brachial Artery, Left 9 Ulnar Artery, Right A Ulnar Artery, Left B Radial Artery, Right C Radial Artery, Left D Hand Artery, Right F Hand Artery, Left	G Intracranial Artery H Common Carotid Artery, Right J Common Carotid Artery, Left M External Carotid Artery, Right N External Carotid Artery, Left P Vertebral Artery, Right Q Vertebral Artery, Left R Face Artery S Temporal Artery, Right T Temporal Artery, Left U Thyroid Artery, Right V Thyroid Artery, Left	0 Open 3 Percutaneous 4 Percutaneous endoscopic	3 Infusion device D Intraluminal device	Z No qualifier
K Internal Carotid Artery, Right L Internal Carotid Artery, Left		0 Open 3 Percutaneous 4 Percutaneous endoscopic	3 Infusion device D Intraluminal device M Stimulator lead	Z No qualifier
Y Upper Artery		0 Open 3 Percutaneous 4 Percutaneous endoscopic	2 Monitoring device 3 Infusion device D Intraluminal device	Z No qualifier

UPPER ARTERIES 03J

EXAMINATION GROUP: Inspection, (Map)
Root Operations involving examination only.

1ST - 0 Medical and Surgical	EXAMPLE: Exploration arterial cath removal site	CMS Ex: Colonoscopy
2ND - 3 Upper Arteries	**INSPECTION:** Visually and/or manually exploring a body part.	
3RD - J INSPECTION	EXPLANATION: Direct or instrumental visualization ...	

Body Part – 4TH	Approach – 5TH	Device – 6TH	Qualifier – 7TH
Y Upper Artery	0 Open 3 Percutaneous 4 Percutaneous endoscopic X External	Z No device	Z No qualifier

TUBULAR GROUP: Bypass, Dilation, Occlusion, Restriction
Root Operations that alter the diameter/route of a tubular body part.

1ST - 0 Medical and Surgical	EXAMPLE: Embolization carotid fistula	CMS Ex: Fallopian tube ligation
2ND - 3 Upper Arteries	OCCLUSION: Completely closing an orifice or lumen of a tubular body part.	
3RD - L OCCLUSION	EXPLANATION: Natural or artificially created orifice ...	

Body Part – 4TH		Approach – 5TH	Device – 6TH	Qualifier – 7TH
0 Internal Mammary Artery, Right 1 Internal Mammary Artery, Left 2 Innominate Artery 3 Subclavian Artery, Right 4 Subclavian Artery, Left 5 Axillary Artery, Right 6 Axillary Artery, Left 7 Brachial Artery, Right 8 Brachial Artery, Left 9 Ulnar Artery, Right	A Ulnar Artery, Left B Radial Artery, Right C Radial Artery, Left D Hand Artery, Right F Hand Artery, Left R Face Artery S Temporal Artery, Right T Temporal Artery, Left U Thyroid Artery, Right V Thyroid Artery, Left Y Upper Artery	0 Open 3 Percutaneous 4 Percutaneous endoscopic	C Extraluminal device D Intraluminal device Z No device	Z No qualifier
G Intracranial Artery H Common Carotid Artery, Right J Common Carotid Artery, Left K Internal Carotid Artery, Right L Internal Carotid Artery, Left M External Carotid Artery, Right N External Carotid Artery, Left P Vertebral Artery, Right Q Vertebral Artery, Left		0 Open 3 Percutaneous 4 Percutaneous endoscopic	B Bioactive intraluminal device C Extraluminal device D Intraluminal device Z No device	Z No qualifier

DIVISION GROUP: (Division), Release
Root Operations involving cutting or separation only.

1ST - **0**   Medical and Surgical

2ND - **3**   Upper Arteries

3RD - **N RELEASE**

EXAMPLE: Arterial adhesiolysis   CMS Ex: Carpal tunnel release

RELEASE: Freeing a body part from an abnormal physical constraint by cutting or by the use of force.

EXPLANATION: None of the body part is taken out ...

Body Part – 4TH	Approach – 5TH	Device – 6TH	Qualifier – 7TH
0 Internal Mammary Artery, Right 1 Internal Mammary Artery, Left 2 Innominate Artery 3 Subclavian Artery, Right 4 Subclavian Artery, Left 5 Axillary Artery, Right 6 Axillary Artery, Left 7 Brachial Artery, Right 8 Brachial Artery, Left 9 Ulnar Artery, Right A Ulnar Artery, Left B Radial Artery, Right C Radial Artery, Left D Hand Artery, Right F Hand Artery, Left G Intracranial Artery H Common Carotid Artery, Right J Common Carotid Artery, Left K Internal Carotid Artery, Right L Internal Carotid Artery, Left M External Carotid Artery, Right N External Carotid Artery, Left P Vertebral Artery, Right Q Vertebral Artery, Left R Face Artery S Temporal Artery, Right T Temporal Artery, Left U Thyroid Artery, Right V Thyroid Artery, Left Y Upper Artery	0 Open 3 Percutaneous 4 Percutaneous endoscopic	Z No device	Z No qualifier

DEVICE GROUP: (Change), Insertion, Removal, Replacement, Revision, Supplement			
Root Operations that always involve a device.			

1ST - 0 Medical and Surgical	EXAMPLE: Removal vascular clip		CMS Ex: Chest tube removal
2ND - 3 Upper Arteries	REMOVAL: Taking out or off a device from a body part.		
3RD - P REMOVAL	EXPLANATION: Removal device without reinsertion ...		

Body Part – 4TH	Approach – 5TH	Device – 6TH	Qualifier – 7TH
Y Upper Artery	0 Open 3 Percutaneous 4 Percutaneous endoscopic	0 Drainage device 2 Monitoring device 3 Infusion device 7 Autologous tissue substitute C Extraluminal device D Intraluminal device J Synthetic substitute K Nonautologous tissue substitute M Stimulator lead	Z No qualifier
Y Upper Artery	X External	0 Drainage device 2 Monitoring device 3 Infusion device D Intraluminal device M Stimulator lead	Z No qualifier

OTHER REPAIRS GROUP: (Control), **Repair**
Root Operations that define other repairs.

1ST - **0** Medical and Surgical	EXAMPLE: Suture arterial laceration CMS Ex: Suture laceration
2ND - **3** Upper Arteries	**REPAIR:** Restoring, to the extent possible, a body part to its normal anatomic structure and function.
3RD - **Q REPAIR**	EXPLANATION: Only when no other root operation applies ...

Body Part – 4TH		Approach – 5TH	Device – 6TH	Qualifier – 7TH
0 Internal Mammary Artery, Right	J Common Carotid Artery, Left	0 Open	Z No device	Z No qualifier
1 Internal Mammary Artery, Left	K Internal Carotid Artery, Right	3 Percutaneous		
2 Innominate Artery	L Internal Carotid Artery, Left	4 Percutaneous endoscopic		
3 Subclavian Artery, Right				
4 Subclavian Artery, Left	M External Carotid Artery, Right			
5 Axillary Artery, Right	N External Carotid Artery, Left			
6 Axillary Artery, Left				
7 Brachial Artery, Right	P Vertebral Artery, Right			
8 Brachial Artery, Left	Q Vertebral Artery, Left			
9 Ulnar Artery, Right	R Face Artery			
A Ulnar Artery, Left	S Temporal Artery, Right			
B Radial Artery, Right	T Temporal Artery, Left			
C Radial Artery, Left	U Thyroid Artery, Right			
D Hand Artery, Right	V Thyroid Artery, Left			
F Hand Artery, Left	Y Upper Artery			
G Intracranial Artery				
H Common Carotid Artery, Right				

UPPER ARTERIES

03Q

DEVICE GROUP: (Change), **Insertion, Removal, Replacement, Revision, Supplement**
Root Operations that always involve a device.

1ST – **0** Medical and Surgical

2ND – **3** Upper Arteries

3RD – **R REPLACEMENT**

EXAMPLE: Reconstruction artery using graft   CMS Ex: Total hip

REPLACEMENT: Putting in or on a biological or synthetic material that physically takes the place and/or function of all or a portion of a body part.

EXPLANATION: Includes taking out body part, or eradication...

Body Part – 4TH	Approach – 5TH	Device – 6TH	Qualifier – 7TH
0 Internal Mammary Artery, Right	0 Open	7 Autologous tissue substitute	Z No qualifier
1 Internal Mammary Artery, Left	4 Percutaneous endoscopic	J Synthetic substitute	
2 Innominate Artery		K Nonautologous tissue substitute	
3 Subclavian Artery, Right			
4 Subclavian Artery, Left			
5 Axillary Artery, Right			
6 Axillary Artery, Left			
7 Brachial Artery, Right			
8 Brachial Artery, Left			
9 Ulnar Artery, Right			
A Ulnar Artery, Left			
B Radial Artery, Right			
C Radial Artery, Left			
D Hand Artery, Right			
F Hand Artery, Left			
G Intracranial Artery			
H Common Carotid Artery, Right			
J Common Carotid Artery, Left			
K Internal Carotid Artery, Right			
L Internal Carotid Artery, Left			
M External Carotid Artery, Right			
N External Carotid Artery, Left			
P Vertebral Artery, Right			
Q Vertebral Artery, Left			
R Face Artery			
S Temporal Artery, Right			
T Temporal Artery, Left			
U Thyroid Artery, Right			
V Thyroid Artery, Left			
Y Upper Artery			

MOVE GROUP: (Reattachment), **Reposition,** (Transfer), (Transplantation)
Root Operations that put in/put back or move some/all of a body part.

1ST - 0 Medical and Surgical

2ND - 3 Upper Arteries

3RD - S REPOSITION

EXAMPLE: Relocation ulnar artery	CMS Ex: Fracture reduction

REPOSITION: Moving to its normal location, or other suitable location, all or a portion of a body part.

EXPLANATION: May or may not be cut to be moved ...

Body Part – 4TH		Approach – 5TH	Device – 6TH	Qualifier – 7TH
0 Internal Mammary Artery, Right	J Common Carotid Artery, Left	0 Open	Z No device	Z No qualifier
1 Internal Mammary Artery, Left	K Internal Carotid Artery, Right	3 Percutaneous		
2 Innominate Artery	L Internal Carotid Artery, Left	4 Percutaneous endoscopic		
3 Subclavian Artery, Right				
4 Subclavian Artery, Left	M External Carotid Artery, Right			
5 Axillary Artery, Right	N External Carotid Artery, Left			
6 Axillary Artery, Left				
7 Brachial Artery, Right	P Vertebral Artery, Right			
8 Brachial Artery, Left	Q Vertebral Artery, Left			
9 Ulnar Artery, Right	R Face Artery			
A Ulnar Artery, Left	S Temporal Artery, Right			
B Radial Artery, Right	T Temporal Artery, Left			
C Radial Artery, Left	U Thyroid Artery, Right			
D Hand Artery, Right	V Thyroid Artery, Left			
F Hand Artery, Left	Y Upper Artery			
G Intracranial Artery				
H Common Carotid Artery, Right				

U P P E R   A R T E R I E S

0 3 S

DEVICE GROUP: (Change), Insertion, Removal, Replacement, Revision, Supplement
Root Operations that always involve a device.

1ST - 0 Medical and Surgical

2ND - 3 Upper Arteries

3RD - U SUPPLEMENT

EXAMPLE: Bovine patch angioplasty	CMS Ex: Hernia repair with mesh

SUPPLEMENT: Putting in or on biological or synthetic material that physically reinforces and/or augments the function of a portion of a body part.

EXPLANATION: Biological material from same individual ...

Body Part – 4TH		Approach – 5TH	Device – 6TH	Qualifier – 7TH
0 Internal Mammary Artery, Right 1 Internal Mammary Artery, Left 2 Innominate Artery 3 Subclavian Artery, Right 4 Subclavian Artery, Left 5 Axillary Artery, Right 6 Axillary Artery, Left 7 Brachial Artery, Right 8 Brachial Artery, Left 9 Ulnar Artery, Right A Ulnar Artery, Left B Radial Artery, Right C Radial Artery, Left D Hand Artery, Right F Hand Artery, Left G Intracranial Artery H Common Carotid Artery, Right	J Common Carotid Artery, Left K Internal Carotid Artery, Right L Internal Carotid Artery, Left M External Carotid Artery, Right N External Carotid Artery, Left P Vertebral Artery, Right Q Vertebral Artery, Left R Face Artery S Temporal Artery, Right T Temporal Artery, Left U Thyroid Artery, Right V Thyroid Artery, Left Y Upper Artery	0 Open 3 Percutaneous 4 Percutaneous endoscopic	7 Autologous tissue substitute J Synthetic substitute K Nonautologous tissue substitute	Z No qualifier

TUBULAR GROUP: Bypass, Dilation, Occlusion, Restriction
Root Operations that alter the diameter/route of a tubular body part.

1ST - 0 Medical and Surgical	EXAMPLE: Clipping cerebral aneurysm	CMS Ex: Cervical cerclage

2ND - 3 Upper Arteries

3RD - V RESTRICTION

RESTRICTION: Partially closing an orifice or the lumen of a tubular body part.

EXPLANATION: Natural or artificially created orifice ...

Body Part – 4TH		Approach – 5TH	Device – 6TH	Qualifier – 7TH
0 Internal Mammary Artery, Right 1 Internal Mammary Artery, Left 2 Innominate Artery 3 Subclavian Artery, Right 4 Subclavian Artery, Left 5 Axillary Artery, Right 6 Axillary Artery, Left 7 Brachial Artery, Right 8 Brachial Artery, Left 9 Ulnar Artery, Right	A Ulnar Artery, Left B Radial Artery, Right C Radial Artery, Left D Hand Artery, Right F Hand Artery, Left R Face Artery S Temporal Artery, Right T Temporal Artery, Left U Thyroid Artery, Right V Thyroid Artery, Left Y Upper Artery	0 Open 3 Percutaneous 4 Percutaneous endoscopic	C Extraluminal device D Intraluminal device Z No device	Z No qualifier
G Intracranial Artery H Common Carotid Artery, Right J Common Carotid Artery, Left K Internal Carotid Artery, Right L Internal Carotid Artery, Left M External Carotid Artery, Right N External Carotid Artery, Left P Vertebral Artery, Right Q Vertebral Artery, Left		0 Open 3 Percutaneous 4 Percutaneous endoscopic	B Bioactive intraluminal device C Extraluminal device D Intraluminal device Z No device	Z No qualifier

UPPER ARTERIES 0 3 V

DEVICE GROUP: (Change), **Insertion, Removal, Replacement, Revision, Supplement**
Root Operations that always involve a device.

1ST - **0** Medical and Surgical	EXAMPLE: Repair ruptured graft CMS Ex: Adjustment pacemaker lead
2ND - **3** Upper Arteries	**REVISION:** Correcting, to the extent possible, a portion of a malfunctioning device or the position of a displaced device.
3RD - **W REVISION**	EXPLANATION: May replace components of a device ...

Body Part – 4TH	Approach – 5TH	Device – 6TH	Qualifier – 7TH
Y Upper Artery	0 Open 3 Percutaneous 4 Percutaneous endoscopic X External	0 Drainage device 2 Monitoring device 3 Infusion device 7 Autologous tissue substitute C Extraluminal device D Intraluminal device J Synthetic substitute K Nonautologous tissue substitute M Stimulator lead	Z No qualifier

UPPER ARTERIES 03W

Educational Annotations | 4 – Lower Arteries

Body System Specific Educational Annotations for the Lower Arteries include:

- **Anatomy and Physiology Review**
- **Anatomical Illustrations**
- **Definitions of Common Procedures**
- **AHA Coding Clinic® Reference Notations**
- **Body Part Key Listings**
- **Device Key Listings**
- **Device Aggregation Table Listings**
- **Coding Notes**

Anatomy and Physiology Review of Lower Arteries

BODY PART VALUES – 4 - LOWER ARTERIES

Abdominal Aorta – The abdominal aorta is continuous from the thoracic aorta artery and ends by branching into the right and left common iliac arteries. Many abdominal arteries branch off from the abdominal aorta.

Anterior Tibial Artery – The anterior tibial artery branches from the popliteal artery and serves the anterior portion of the lower leg and dorsal portion of the foot.

Artery – Blood vessels that carry oxygenated (arterial) blood away from the heart and to the organs and tissues of the body. Arteries have a higher blood pressure than other parts of the circulatory system in order to adequately perfuse all the tissues with oxygenated red blood cells.

Celiac Artery – The celiac artery (also known as the celiac trunk) branches from the abdominal aorta and then almost immediately (1-2cm) branches into the common hepatic artery, the splenic artery, and left gastric artery.

Colic Artery – The colic artery branches from the superior mesenteric artery and serves the colon, ileum, appendix.

Common Iliac Artery – The common iliac artery branches from the aortic bifurcation of the abdominal aorta and branch almost immediately (4 cm in length) into the internal and external iliac arteries.

External Iliac Artery – The external iliac artery branches from the common iliac artery and serves the legs.

Femoral Artery – The femoral artery branches from the external iliac artery and serves the legs.

Foot Artery – Any of the smaller arterial branches that serve the foot.

Gastric Artery – The gastric artery branches from the celiac artery and serves the stomach and esophagus.

Hepatic Artery – The hepatic artery branches from the celiac artery and serves the gallbladder, liver, duodenum, pylorus, and pancreas.

Inferior Mesenteric Artery – The inferior mesenteric artery branches from the abdominal aorta and serves the descending colon, part of the transverse colon, sigmoid colon, and the upper part of the rectum.

Internal Iliac Artery – The internal iliac artery branches from the common iliac artery and serves the pelvic viscera, buttocks, and reproductive organs.

Lower Artery – The arteries located below the diaphragm (see Coding Guideline B2.1b).

Peroneal Artery – The peroneal artery (also known as the fibular artery) branches from the posterior tibial artery and serves the lateral portion of the leg.

Popliteal Artery – The popliteal artery branches from the femoral artery and serves the knee and lower leg.

Posterior Tibial Artery – The posterior tibial artery branches from the popliteal artery and serves the posterior portion of the lower leg and the plantar portion of the foot.

Renal Artery – The renal artery branches from the abdominal aorta and serves the kidney.

Splenic Artery – The splenic artery branches from the celiac artery and serves the spleen.

Superior Mesenteric Artery – The superior mesenteric artery branches from the abdominal aorta and serves the duodenum, ascending colon, part of the transverse colon, and pancreas.

Uterine Artery – The uterine artery branches from the internal iliac artery and serves the uterus.

Educational Annotations | 4 – Lower Arteries

Anatomical Illustrations of Lower Arteries

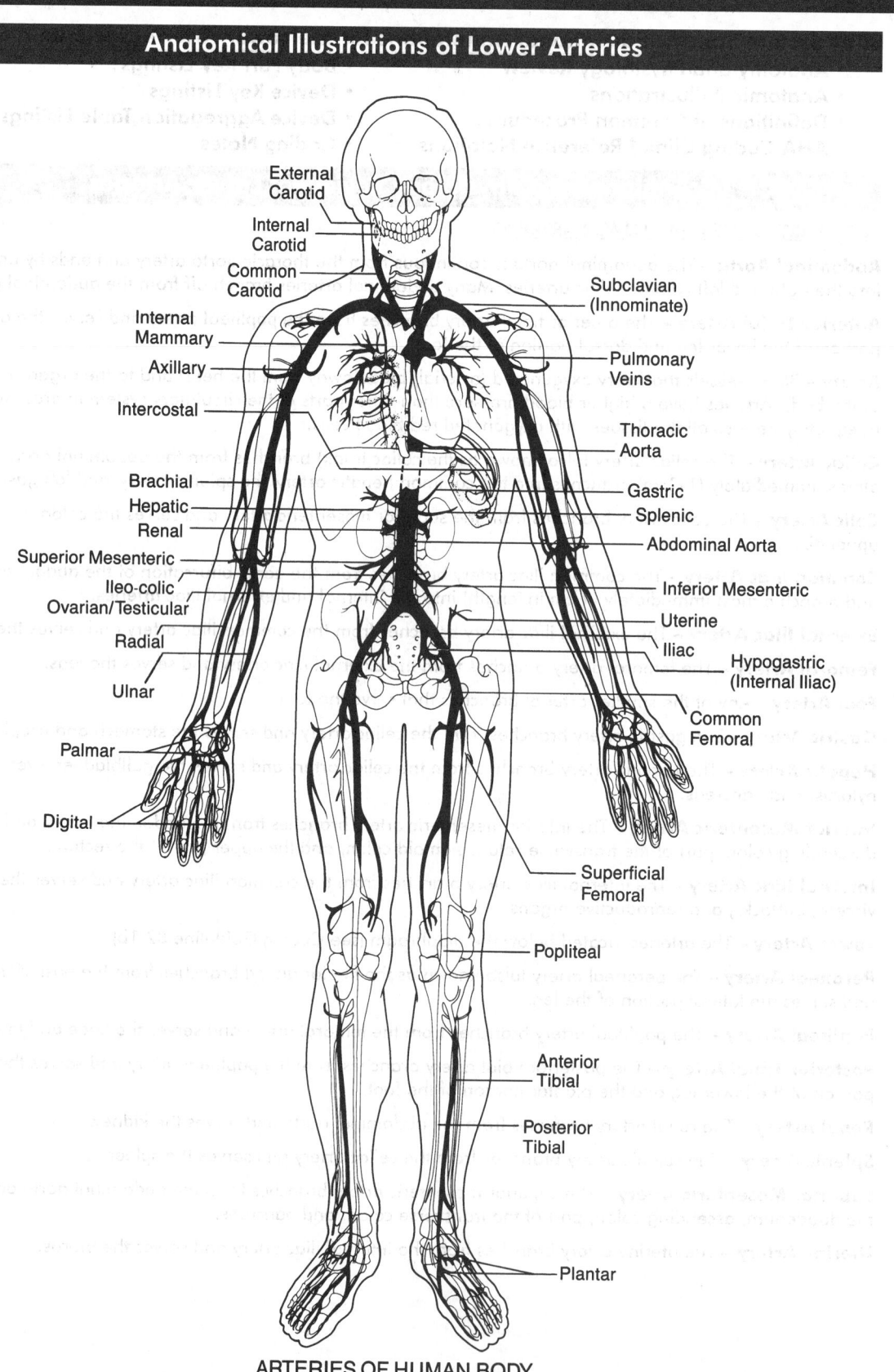

External Carotid
Internal Carotid
Common Carotid
Internal Mammary
Axillary
Intercostal
Brachial
Hepatic
Renal
Superior Mesenteric
Ileo-colic
Ovarian/Testicular
Radial
Ulnar
Palmar
Digital

Subclavian (Innominate)
Pulmonary Veins
Thoracic Aorta
Gastric
Splenic
Abdominal Aorta
Inferior Mesenteric
Uterine
Iliac
Hypogastric (Internal Iliac)
Common Femoral
Superficial Femoral
Popliteal
Anterior Tibial
Posterior Tibial
Plantar

ARTERIES OF HUMAN BODY

Continued on next page

Educational Annotations | 4 – Lower Arteries

Anatomical Illustrations of Lower Arteries

Continued from previous page

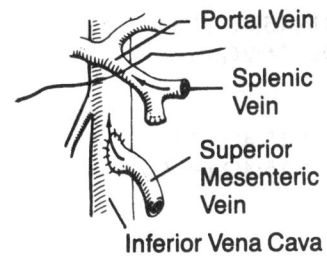

MESOCAVAL SHUNT

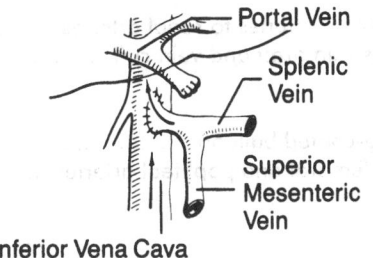

PORTACAVAL ANASTOMOSIS

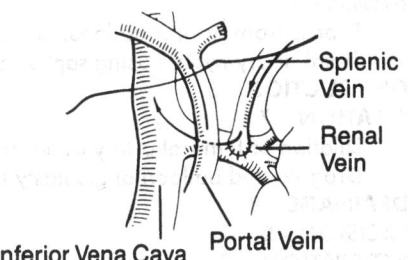

SPLENORENAL SHUNT

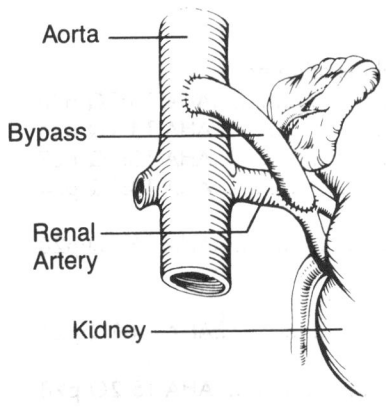
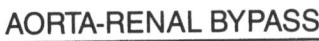

AORTA-RENAL BYPASS

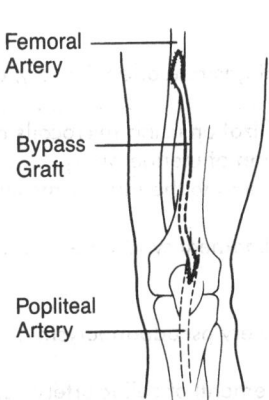

FEMORAL-POPLITEAL BYPASS

Definitions of Common Procedures of Lower Arteries

Aorto-bifemoral bypass – The restoration of blood flow to the legs by replacing the aortic-femoral bifurcation with a replacement graft that is usually synthetic, or the addition of a bypass graft sewn to the distal aorta and to the femoral arteries distal to the blockage site(s).

Abdominal aortic aneurysmectomy – The resection of an enlarged abdominal aortic wall protrusion and replacement with a graft that is usually synthetic. An endovascular version inserts a synthetic graft intravascularly to reinforce the weakened section without resecting any of the native aorta.

Femoral-popliteal bypass – The restoration of blood flow to the popliteal artery by using a bypass graft from the femoral artery.

Percutaneous mechanical thrombectomy – A minimally invasive approach to remove an acute thrombus in a lower extremity artery or graft by an endovascular approach using attachments to break up and remove the clot.

Educational Annotations | 4 – Lower Arteries

AHA Coding Clinic® Reference Notations of Lower Arteries

ROOT OPERATION SPECIFIC - 4 - LOWER ARTERIES

BYPASS - 1
    Bypass from gastroduodenal and splenic arteries to renal arteries..............AHA 15:3Q:p28
    Tibial artery bypass using saphenous vein graft and vein cuff ....AHA 16:2Q:p18

DESTRUCTION - 5

DILATION - 7
    Dilation of femoral artery using drug-coated balloon ....AHA 15:4Q:p15
    Drug-coated balloon angioplasty in femoral and popliteal arteries ....AHA 15:4Q:p4-7

DRAINAGE - 9

EXCISION - B

EXTIRPATION - C
    Iliofemoral endarterectomy with bovine patch repair ....AHA 16:1Q:p31
    Thrombectomy of femoral popliteal bypass graft......................................AHA 15:1Q:p36

INSERTION - H

INSPECTION - J

OCCLUSION - L
    Coil embolization of gastroduodenal artery, and chemoembolization of
        hepatic artery ....AHA 14:3Q:p26
    Endovascular embolization using microcoils of colic artery ....AHA 14:1Q:p24
    Gelfoam embolization of uterine artery ....AHA 15:2Q:p27
    Microbead embolization to the inferior mesenteric artery ....AHA 14:1Q:p24

RELEASE - N
    Release of arcuate ligament syndrome ....AHA 15:2Q:p28

REMOVAL - P

REPAIR - Q
    Repair of femoral artery pseudoaneurysm ....AHA 14:1Q:p21

REPLACEMENT - R
    Bypass graft (replacement) of celiac artery ....AHA 15:2Q:p28

REPOSITION - S

SUPPLEMENT - U
    Bovine patch arterioplasty of femoral artery ....AHA 14:4Q:p37
    Iliofemoral endarterectomy with bovine patch repair ....AHA 16:1Q:p31
    Placement of stent graft in saphenous vein graft....................................AHA 14:1Q:p22
    Tibial artery bypass using saphenous vein graft and vein cuff ....AHA 16:2Q:p18

RESTRICTION - V
    Stent graft repair of abdominal aortic aneurysm......................................AHA 14:1Q:p9

REVISION - W
    Reanastomosed femoral popliteal bypass graft ....AHA 15:1Q:p36
    Reattachment of abdominal aortic stent graft ....AHA 14:1Q:p9
    Repair of ruptured femoral-popliteal bypass graft...................................AHA 14:1Q:p22

LOWER ARTERIES 04

Educational Annotations | 4 – Lower Arteries

Body Part Key Listings of Lower Arteries

See also Body Part Key in Appendix C

Anterior lateral malleolar artery	*use* Anterior Tibial Artery, Left/Right
Anterior medial malleolar artery	*use* Anterior Tibial Artery, Left/Right
Anterior tibial recurrent artery	*use* Anterior Tibial Artery, Left/Right
Arcuate artery	*use* Foot Artery, Left/Right
Celiac trunk	*use* Celiac Artery
Circumflex iliac artery	*use* Femoral Artery, Left/Right
Common hepatic artery	*use* Hepatic Artery
Deep circumflex iliac artery	*use* External Iliac Artery, Left/Right
Deep femoral artery	*use* Femoral Artery, Left/Right
Deferential artery	*use* Internal Iliac Artery, Left/Right
Descending genicular artery	*use* Femoral Artery, Left/Right
Dorsal metatarsal artery	*use* Foot Artery, Left/Right
Dorsalis pedis artery	*use* Anterior Tibial Artery, Left/Right
External pudendal artery	*use* Femoral Artery, Left/Right
Fibular artery	*use* Peroneal Artery, Left/Right
Gastroduodenal artery	*use* Hepatic Artery
Hepatic artery proper	*use* Hepatic Artery
Hypogastric artery	*use* Internal Iliac Artery, Left/Right
Ileal artery	*use* Superior Mesenteric Artery
Ileocolic artery	*use* Superior Mesenteric Artery
Iliolumbar artery	*use* Internal Iliac Artery, Left/Right
Inferior epigastric artery	*use* External Iliac Artery, Left/Right
Inferior genicular artery	*use* Popliteal Artery, Left/Right
Inferior gluteal artery	*use* Internal Iliac Artery, Left/Right
Inferior pancreaticoduodenal artery	*use* Superior Mesenteric Artery
Inferior phrenic artery	*use* Abdominal Aorta
Inferior suprarenal artery	*use* Renal Artery, Left/Right
Inferior vesical artery	*use* Internal Iliac Artery, Left/Right
Internal pudendal artery	*use* Internal Iliac Artery, Left/Right
Internal thoracic artery	*use* Internal Mammary Artery, Left/Right
....	*use* Subclavian Artery, Left/Right
Jejunal artery	*use* Superior Mesenteric Artery
Lateral plantar artery	*use* Foot Artery, Left/Right
Lateral sacral artery	*use* Internal Iliac Artery, Left/Right
Lateral tarsal artery	*use* Foot Artery, Left/Right
Left gastric artery	*use* Gastric Artery
Left gastroepiploic artery	*use* Splenic Artery
Lumbar artery	*use* Abdominal Aorta
Medial plantar artery	*use* Foot Artery, Left/Right
Median sacral artery	*use* Abdominal Aorta
Middle genicular artery	*use* Popliteal Artery, Left/Right
Middle rectal artery	*use* Internal Iliac Artery, Left/Right
Middle suprarenal artery	*use* Abdominal Aorta
Obturator artery	*use* Internal Iliac Artery, Left/Right
Ovarian artery	*use* Abdominal Aorta

Continued on next page

LOWER ARTERIES 0 4

Educational Annotations | 4 – Lower Arteries

Body Part Key Listings of Lower Arteries

Continued from previous page

Pancreatic artery	*use* Splenic Artery
Posterior tibial recurrent artery	*use* Anterior Tibial Artery, Left/Right
Renal segmental artery	*use* Renal Artery, Left/Right
Right gastric artery	*use* Gastric Artery
Short gastric artery	*use* Splenic Artery
Sigmoid artery	*use* Inferior Mesenteric Artery
Superficial epigastric artery	*use* Femoral Artery, Left/Right
Superior genicular artery	*use* Popliteal Artery, Left/Right
Superior gluteal artery	*use* Internal Iliac Artery, Left/Right
Superior rectal artery	*use* Inferior Mesenteric Artery
Sural artery	*use* Popliteal Artery, Left/Right
Testicular artery	*use* Abdominal Aorta
Umbilical artery	*use* Internal Iliac Artery, Left/Right
Uterine artery	*use* Internal Iliac Artery, Left/Right
Vaginal artery	*use* Internal Iliac Artery, Left/Right

Device Key Listings of Lower Arteries

See also Device Key in Appendix D

Absolute Pro Vascular (OTW) Self-Expanding Stent System *use* Intraluminal Device

AFX® Endovascular AAA System *use* Intraluminal Device

AneuRx® AAA Advantage® *use* Intraluminal Device

Assurant (Cobalt) stent *use* Intraluminal Device

Autograft *use* Autologous Tissue Substitute

Autologous artery graft *use* Autologous Arterial Tissue in Lower Arteries

Autologous vein graft *use* Autologous Venous Tissue in Lower Arteries

Brachytherapy seeds *use* Radioactive Element

CoAxia NeuroFlo catheter *use* Intraluminal Device

Complete (SE) stent *use* Intraluminal Device

Cook Zenith AAA Endovascular Graft *use* Intraluminal Device; Intraluminal Device, Branched or Fenestrated, One or Two Arteries for Restriction in Lower Arteries; Intraluminal Device, Branched or Fenestrated, Three or More Arteries for Restriction in Lower Arteries

E-Luminexx™ (Biliary) (Vascular) Stent *use* Intraluminal Device

Embolization coil(s) *use* Intraluminal Device

Endologix AFX® Endovascular AAA System *use* Intraluminal Device

Endurant® II AAA stent graft system *use* Intraluminal Device

Endurant® Endovascular Stent Graft *use* Intraluminal Device

EXCLUDER® AAA Endoprothesis *use* Intraluminal Device; Intraluminal Device, Branched or Fenestrated, One or Two Arteries for Restriction in Lower Arteries; Intraluminal Device, Branched or Fenestrated, Three or More Arteries for Restriction in Lower Arteries

EXCLUDER® IBE Endoprothesis *use* Intraluminal Device; Intraluminal Device, Branched or Fenestrated, One or Two Arteries for Restriction in Lower Arteries

Express® (LD) Premounted Stent System *use* Intraluminal Device

Express® Biliary SD Monorail® Premounted Stent System *use* Intraluminal Device

Express® SD Renal Monorail® Premounted Stent System *use* Intraluminal Device

Formula™ Balloon-Expandable Renal Stent System *use* Intraluminal Device

Continued on next page

Educational Annotations | 4 – Lower Arteries

Device Key Listings of Lower Arteries

Continued from previous page

GORE EXCLUDER® AAA Endoprothesis ....*use* Intraluminal Device; Intraluminal Device, Branched or Fenestrated, One or Two Arteries for Restriction in Lower Arteries; Intraluminal Device, Branched or Fenestrated, Three or More Arteries for Restriction in Lower Arteries

GORE EXCLUDER® IBE Endoprothesis........................*use* Intraluminal Device, Branched or Fenestrated, One or Two Arteries for Restriction in Lower Arteries

Herculink (RX) Elite Renal Stent System ....*use* Intraluminal Device

LifeStent® (Flexstar) (XL) Vascular Stent System ......*use* Intraluminal Device

Medtronic Endurant® II AAA stent graft system ......*use* Intraluminal Device

Omnilink Elite Vascular Balloon Expandable Stent System ....*use* Intraluminal Device

Paclitaxel-eluting peripheral stent ....*use* Intraluminal Device, Drug-eluting in Upper Arteries, Lower Arteries

Stent, intraluminal (cardiovascular) (gastrointestinal) (hepatobiliary) (urinary) ......*use* Intraluminal Device

Talent® Converter...*use* Intraluminal Device

Talent® Occluder ....*use* Intraluminal Device

Talent® Stent Graft (abdominal) (thoracic)................*use* Intraluminal Device

Tissue bank graft ....*use* Nonautologous Tissue Substitute

Zenith AAA Endovascular Graft ....*use* Intraluminal Device; Intraluminal Device, Branched or Fenestrated, One or Two Arteries for Restriction in Lower Arteries; Intraluminal Device, Branched or Fenestrated, Three or More Arteries for Restriction in Lower Arteries

Zenith Flex® AAA Endovascular Graft ....*use* Intraluminal Device

Zenith® Renu™ AAA Ancillary Graft ....*use* Intraluminal Device

Zilver® PTX® (paclitaxel) Drug-Eluting Peripheral Stent ....*use* Intraluminal Device, Drug-eluting in Upper Arteries, Lower Arteries

LOWER ARTERIES 04

Educational Annotations | 4 – Lower Arteries

Device Aggregation Table Listings of Lower Arteries

See also Device Aggregation Table in Appendix E

Specific Device	For Operation	In Body System		General Device
Autologous Arterial Tissue	All applicable	Lower Arteries	7	Autologous Tissue Substitute
Autologous Venous Tissue	All applicable	Lower Arteries	7	Autologous Tissue Substitute
Intraluminal Device, Branched or Fenestrated, One or Two Arteries	All applicable	Heart and Great Vessels	D	Intraluminal Device
Intraluminal Device, Branched or Fenestrated, Three or More Arteries	All applicable	Heart and Great Vessels	D	Intraluminal Device
Intraluminal Device, Drug-eluting	All applicable	Lower Arteries	D	Intraluminal Device
Intraluminal Device, Drug-eluting, Four or More	All applicable	Heart and Great Vessels	D	Intraluminal Device
Intraluminal Device, Drug-eluting, Three	All applicable	Heart and Great Vessels	D	Intraluminal Device
Intraluminal Device, Drug-eluting, Two	All applicable	Heart and Great Vessels	D	Intraluminal Device
Intraluminal Device, Four or More	All applicable	Heart and Great Vessels	D	Intraluminal Device
Intraluminal Device, Three	All applicable	Heart and Great Vessels	D	Intraluminal Device
Intraluminal Device, Two	All applicable	Heart and Great Vessels	D	Intraluminal Device

Coding Notes of Lower Arteries

Body System Relevant Coding Guidelines

General Guidelines

B2.1b

Where the general body part values "upper" and "lower" are provided as an option in the Upper Arteries, Lower Arteries, Upper Veins, Lower Veins, Muscles and Tendons body systems, "upper" and "lower" specifies body parts located above or below the diaphragm respectively.

Example: Vein body parts above the diaphragm are found in the Upper Veins body system; vein body parts below the diaphragm are found in the Lower Veins body system.

Branches of body parts

B4.2

Where a specific branch of a body part does not have its own body part value in PCS, the body part is typically coded to the closest proximal branch that has a specific body part value. In the cardiovascular body systems, if a general body part is available in the correct root operation table, and coding to a proximal branch would require assigning a code in a different body system, the procedure is coded using the general body part value.

Examples: A procedure performed on the mandibular branch of the trigeminal nerve is coded to the trigeminal nerve body part value.

Occlusion of the bronchial artery is coded to the body part value Upper Artery in the body system Upper Arteries, and not to the body part value Thoracic Aorta, Descending in the body system Heart and Great Vessels.

Body System Specific PCS Reference Manual Exercises

PCS CODE	4 – LOWER ARTERIES EXERCISES
0 4 1 L 0 K L	Open left femoral-popliteal artery bypass using cadaver vein graft.
0 4 7 L 0 Z Z	Open dilation of old anastomosis, left femoral artery.
0 4 L E 3 D T	Percutaneous embolization of right uterine artery, using coils.
0 4 R 0 0 J Z	Excision of abdominal aorta with goretex graft replacement, open.
0 4 W Y 0 J Z	Trimming and reanastomosis of stenosed femorofemoral synthetic bypass graft, open.

TUBULAR GROUP: Bypass, Dilation, Occlusion, Restriction			
Root Operations that alter the diameter/route of a tubular body part.			

		EXAMPLE: Aorto-bifemoral bypass	CMS Ex: Coronary artery bypass
1ST - 0 Medical and Surgical		BYPASS: Altering the route of passage of the contents of a tubular body part.	
2ND - 4 Lower Arteries			
3RD - 1 BYPASS		EXPLANATION: Rerouting contents to a downstream part ...	

Body Part – 4TH	Approach – 5TH	Device – 6TH	Qualifier – 7TH
0 Abdominal Aorta C Common Iliac Artery, Right D Common Iliac Artery, Left	0 Open 4 Percutaneous endoscopic	9 Autologous venous tissue A Autologous arterial tissue J Synthetic substitute K Nonautologous tissue substitute Z No device	0 Abdominal Aorta 1 Celiac Artery 2 Mesenteric Artery 3 Renal Artery, Right 4 Renal Artery, Left 5 Renal Artery, Bilateral 6 Common Iliac Artery, Right 7 Common Iliac Artery, Left 8 Common Iliac Arteries, Bilateral 9 Internal Iliac Artery, Right B Internal Iliac Artery, Left C Internal Iliac Arteries, Bilateral D External Iliac Artery, Right F External Iliac Artery, Left G External Iliac Arteries, Bilateral H Femoral Artery, Right J Femoral Artery, Left K Femoral Arteries, Bilateral Q Lower Extremity Artery R Lower Artery
4 Splenic Artery	0 Open 4 Percutaneous endoscopic	9 Autologous venous tissue A Autologous arterial tissue J Synthetic substitute K Nonautologous tissue substitute Z No device	3 Renal Artery, Right 4 Renal Artery, Left 5 Renal Artery, Bilateral
E Internal Iliac Artery, Right F Internal Iliac Artery, Left H External Iliac Artery, Right J External Iliac Artery, Left	0 Open 4 Percutaneous endoscopic	9 Autologous venous tissue A Autologous arterial tissue J Synthetic substitute K Nonautologous tissue substitute Z No device	9 Internal Iliac Artery, Right B Internal Iliac Artery, Left C Internal Iliac Arteries, Bilateral D External Iliac Artery, Right F External Iliac Artery, Left G External Iliac Arteries, Bilateral H Femoral Artery, Right J Femoral Artery, Left K Femoral Arteries, Bilateral P Foot Artery Q Lower Extremity Artery

LOWER ARTERIES 041

c o n t i n u e d ⇨

0 4 1   BYPASS – continued

Body Part – 4TH	Approach – 5TH	Device – 6TH	Qualifier – 7TH
K Femoral Artery, Right L Femoral Artery, Left	0 Open 4 Percutaneous endoscopic	9 Autologous venous tissue A Autologous arterial tissue J Synthetic substitute K Nonautologous tissue substitute Z No device	H Femoral Artery, Right J Femoral Artery, Left K Femoral Arteries, Bilateral L Popliteal Artery M Peroneal Artery N Posterior Tibial Artery P Foot Artery Q Lower Extremity Artery S Lower Extremity Vein
M Popliteal Artery, Right N Popliteal Artery, Left	0 Open 4 Percutaneous endoscopic	9 Autologous venous tissue A Autologous arterial tissue J Synthetic substitute K Nonautologous tissue substitute Z No device	L Popliteal Artery M Peroneal Artery P Foot Artery Q Lower Extremity Artery S Lower Extremity Vein

LOWER ARTERIES 041

EXCISION GROUP: Excision, (Resection), Destruction, (Extraction), (Detachment)
Root Operations that take out some or all of a body part.

1ST - 0   Medical and Surgical

2ND - 4   Lower Arteries

3RD - 5   DESTRUCTION

EXAMPLE: Fulguration arterial lesion   **CMS Ex:** Fulguration polyp

DESTRUCTION: Physical eradication of all or a portion of a body part by the direct use of energy, force, or a destructive agent.

EXPLANATION: None of the body part is physically taken out

Body Part – 4TH		Approach – 5TH	Device – 6TH	Qualifier – 7TH
0 Abdominal Aorta 1 Celiac Artery 2 Gastric Artery 3 Hepatic Artery 4 Splenic Artery 5 Superior Mesenteric Artery 6 Colic Artery, Right 7 Colic Artery, Left 8 Colic Artery, Middle 9 Renal Artery, Right A Renal Artery, Left B Inferior Mesenteric Artery C Common Iliac Artery, Right D Common Iliac Artery, Left E Internal Iliac Artery, Right F Internal Iliac Artery, Left	H External Iliac Artery, Right J External Iliac Artery, Left K Femoral Artery, Right L Femoral Artery, Left M Popliteal Artery, Right N Popliteal Artery, Left P Anterior Tibial Artery, Right Q Anterior Tibial Artery, Left R Posterior Tibial Artery, Right S Posterior Tibial Artery, Left T Peroneal Artery, Right U Peroneal Artery, Left V Foot Artery, Right W Foot Artery, Left Y Lower Artery	0 Open 3 Percutaneous 4 Percutaneous endoscopic	Z No device	Z No qualifier

TUBULAR GROUP: Bypass, Dilation, Occlusion, Restriction
Root Operations that alter the diameter/route of a tubular body part.

1ST - 0 Medical and Surgical	EXAMPLE: PTA femoral artery CMS Ex: Transluminal angioplasty
2ND - 4 Lower Arteries	**DILATION:** Expanding an orifice or the lumen of a tubular body part.
3RD - 7 DILATION	EXPLANATION: By force (stretching) or cutting ...

Body Part – 4TH		Approach – 5TH	Device – 6TH	Qualifier – 7TH
0 Abdominal Aorta 1 Celiac Artery 2 Gastric Artery 3 Hepatic Artery 4 Splenic Artery 5 Superior Mesenteric Artery 6 Colic Artery, Right 7 Colic Artery, Left 8 Colic Artery, Middle 9 Renal Artery, Right A Renal Artery, Left B Inferior Mesenteric Artery C Common Iliac Artery, Right D Common Iliac Artery, Left	E Internal Iliac Artery, Right F Internal Iliac Artery, Left H External Iliac Artery, Right J External Iliac Artery, Left P Anterior Tibial Artery, Right Q Anterior Tibial Artery, Left R Posterior Tibial Artery, Right S Posterior Tibial Artery, Left T Peroneal Artery, Right U Peroneal Artery, Left V Foot Artery, Right W Foot Artery, Left Y Lower Artery	0 Open 3 Percutaneous 4 Percutaneous endoscopic	4 Drug-eluting intraluminal device 5 Drug-eluting intraluminal device, two 6 Drug-eluting intraluminal device, three 7 Drug-eluting intraluminal device, four or more D Intraluminal device E Intraluminal device, two F Intraluminal device, three G Intraluminal device, four or more Z No device	6 Bifurcation Z No qualifier
K Femoral Artery, Right L Femoral Artery, Left M Popliteal Artery, Right N Popliteal Artery, Left		0 Open 3 Percutaneous 4 Percutaneous endoscopic	4 Drug-eluting intraluminal device D Intraluminal device Z No device	1 Drug-coated balloon 6 Bifurcation Z No qualifier
K Femoral Artery, Right L Femoral Artery, Left M Popliteal Artery, Right N Popliteal Artery, Left		0 Open 3 Percutaneous 4 Percutaneous endoscopic	5 Drug-eluting intraluminal device, two 6 Drug-eluting intraluminal device, three 7 Drug-eluting intraluminal device, four or more E Intraluminal device, two F Intraluminal device, three G Intraluminal device, four or more	6 Bifurcation Z No qualifier

LOWER ARTERIES 047

DRAINAGE GROUP: Drainage, Extirpation, (Fragmentation)
Root Operations that take out solids/fluids/gases from a body part.

1ST - **0** Medical and Surgical

2ND - **4** Lower Arteries

3RD - **9 DRAINAGE**

EXAMPLE: Aspiration arterial abscess   CMS Ex: Thoracentesis

DRAINAGE: Taking or letting out fluids and/or gases from a body part.

EXPLANATION: Qualifier "X Diagnostic" indicates biopsy ...

Body Part – 4TH		Approach – 5TH	Device – 6TH	Qualifier – 7TH
0 Abdominal Aorta	H External Iliac Artery, Right	0 Open	0 Drainage device	Z No qualifier
1 Celiac Artery	J External Iliac Artery, Left	3 Percutaneous		
2 Gastric Artery	K Femoral Artery, Right	4 Percutaneous endoscopic		
3 Hepatic Artery	L Femoral Artery, Left			
4 Splenic Artery	M Popliteal Artery, Right			
5 Superior Mesenteric Artery	N Popliteal Artery, Left			
	P Anterior Tibial Artery, Right			
6 Colic Artery, Right				
7 Colic Artery, Left	Q Anterior Tibial Artery, Left			
8 Colic Artery, Middle				
9 Renal Artery, Right	R Posterior Tibial Artery, Right			
A Renal Artery, Left				
B Inferior Mesenteric Artery	S Posterior Tibial Artery, Left			
C Common Iliac Artery, Right	T Peroneal Artery, Right			
	U Peroneal Artery, Left			
D Common Iliac Artery, Left	V Foot Artery, Right			
	W Foot Artery, Left			
E Internal Iliac Artery, Right	Y Lower Artery			
F Internal Iliac Artery, Left				
0 Abdominal Aorta	H External Iliac Artery, Right	0 Open	Z No device	X Diagnostic
1 Celiac Artery	J External Iliac Artery, Left	3 Percutaneous		Z No qualifier
2 Gastric Artery	K Femoral Artery, Right	4 Percutaneous endoscopic		
3 Hepatic Artery	L Femoral Artery, Left			
4 Splenic Artery	M Popliteal Artery, Right			
5 Superior Mesenteric Artery	N Popliteal Artery, Left			
	P Anterior Tibial Artery, Right			
6 Colic Artery, Right				
7 Colic Artery, Left	Q Anterior Tibial Artery, Left			
8 Colic Artery, Middle				
9 Renal Artery, Right	R Posterior Tibial Artery, Right			
A Renal Artery, Left				
B Inferior Mesenteric Artery	S Posterior Tibial Artery, Left			
C Common Iliac Artery, Right	T Peroneal Artery, Right			
	U Peroneal Artery, Left			
D Common Iliac Artery, Left	V Foot Artery, Right			
	W Foot Artery, Left			
E Internal Iliac Artery, Right	Y Lower Artery			
F Internal Iliac Artery, Left				

EXCISION GROUP: Excision, (Resection), **Destruction**, (Extraction), (Detachment)
Root Operations that take out some or all of a body part.

1ST - **0** Medical and Surgical

2ND - **4** Lower Arteries

3RD - **B EXCISION**

EXAMPLE: Femoral artery biopsy

CMS Ex: Liver biopsy

EXCISION: Cutting out or off, without replacement, a portion of a body part.

EXPLANATION: Qualifier "X Diagnostic" indicates biopsy ...

Body Part – 4TH		Approach – 5TH	Device – 6TH	Qualifier – 7TH
0 Abdominal Aorta	H External Iliac Artery, Right	0 Open	Z No device	X Diagnostic
1 Celiac Artery	J External Iliac Artery, Left	3 Percutaneous		Z No qualifier
2 Gastric Artery	K Femoral Artery, Right	4 Percutaneous endoscopic		
3 Hepatic Artery	L Femoral Artery, Left			
4 Splenic Artery	M Popliteal Artery, Right			
5 Superior Mesenteric Artery	N Popliteal Artery, Left			
6 Colic Artery, Right	P Anterior Tibial Artery, Right			
7 Colic Artery, Left	Q Anterior Tibial Artery, Left			
8 Colic Artery, Middle	R Posterior Tibial Artery, Right			
9 Renal Artery, Right	S Posterior Tibial Artery, Left			
A Renal Artery, Left	T Peroneal Artery, Right			
B Inferior Mesenteric Artery	U Peroneal Artery, Left			
C Common Iliac Artery, Right	V Foot Artery, Right			
D Common Iliac Artery, Left	W Foot Artery, Left			
E Internal Iliac Artery, Right	Y Lower Artery			
F Internal Iliac Artery, Left				

LOWER ARTERIES 04B

DRAINAGE GROUP: Drainage, Extirpation, (Fragmentation)
Root Operations that take out solids/fluids/gases from a body part.

1ST - **0** Medical and Surgical

2ND - **4** Lower Arteries

3RD - **C EXTIRPATION**

EXAMPLE: Iliac artery thrombectomy	CMS Ex: Choledocholithotomy

EXTIRPATION: Taking or cutting out solid matter from a body part.

EXPLANATION: Abnormal byproduct or foreign body ...

Body Part – 4TH		Approach – 5TH	Device – 6TH	Qualifier – 7TH
0 Abdominal Aorta	H External Iliac Artery, Right	0 Open	Z No device	6 Bifurcation
1 Celiac Artery	J External Iliac Artery, Left	3 Percutaneous		Z No qualifier
2 Gastric Artery	K Femoral Artery, Right	4 Percutaneous endoscopic		
3 Hepatic Artery	L Femoral Artery, Left			
4 Splenic Artery	M Popliteal Artery, Right			
5 Superior Mesenteric Artery	N Popliteal Artery, Left			
6 Colic Artery, Right	P Anterior Tibial Artery, Right			
7 Colic Artery, Left	Q Anterior Tibial Artery, Left			
8 Colic Artery, Middle	R Posterior Tibial Artery, Right			
9 Renal Artery, Right	S Posterior Tibial Artery, Left			
A Renal Artery, Left	T Peroneal Artery, Right			
B Inferior Mesenteric Artery	U Peroneal Artery, Left			
C Common Iliac Artery, Right	V Foot Artery, Right			
D Common Iliac Artery, Left	W Foot Artery, Left			
E Internal Iliac Artery, Right	Y Lower Artery			
F Internal Iliac Artery, Left				

LOWER ARTERIES 04C

DEVICE GROUP: (Change), Insertion, Removal, Replacement, Revision, Supplement
Root Operations that always involve a device.

1ST - 0 Medical and Surgical

2ND - 4 Lower Arteries

3RD - H INSERTION

EXAMPLE: Arterial infusion catheter | **CMS Ex:** Central venous catheter

INSERTION: Putting in a nonbiological appliance that monitors, assists, performs, or prevents a physiological function but does not physically take the place of a body part.

EXPLANATION: None

Body Part – 4TH	Approach – 5TH	Device – 6TH	Qualifier – 7TH
0 Abdominal Aorta Y Lower Artery	0 Open 3 Percutaneous 4 Percutaneous endoscopic	2 Monitoring device 3 Infusion device D Intraluminal device	Z No qualifier
1 Celiac Artery 2 Gastric Artery 3 Hepatic Artery 4 Splenic Artery 5 Superior Mesenteric Artery 6 Colic Artery, Right 7 Colic Artery, Left 8 Colic Artery, Middle 9 Renal Artery, Right A Renal Artery, Left B Inferior Mesenteric Artery C Common Iliac Artery, Right D Common Iliac Artery, Left E Internal Iliac Artery, Right F Internal Iliac Artery, Left H External Iliac Artery, Right J External Iliac Artery, Left K Femoral Artery, Right L Femoral Artery, Left M Popliteal Artery, Right N Popliteal Artery, Left P Anterior Tibial Artery, Right Q Anterior Tibial Artery, Left R Posterior Tibial Artery, Right S Posterior Tibial Artery, Left T Peroneal Artery, Right U Peroneal Artery, Left V Foot Artery, Right W Foot Artery, Left	0 Open 3 Percutaneous 4 Percutaneous endoscopic	3 Infusion device D Intraluminal device	Z No qualifier

LOWER ARTERIES 0 4 H

EXAMINATION GROUP: Inspection, (Map)
Root Operations involving examination only.

1ST – 0 Medical and Surgical	EXAMPLE: Exploration arterial cath removal site	CMS Ex: Colonoscopy
2ND – 4 Lower Arteries	**INSPECTION:** Visually and/or manually exploring a body part.	
3RD – J **INSPECTION**		
	EXPLANATION: Direct or instrumental visualization …	

Body Part – 4TH	Approach – 5TH	Device – 6TH	Qualifier – 7TH
Y Lower Artery	0 Open 3 Percutaneous 4 Percutaneous endoscopic X External	Z No device	Z No qualifier

TUBULAR GROUP: Bypass, Dilation, Occlusion, Restriction
Root Operations that alter the diameter/route of a tubular body part.

1ST – 0 Medical and Surgical	EXAMPLE: Renal artery embolization	CMS Ex: Fallopian tube ligation
2ND – 4 Lower Arteries	**OCCLUSION:** Completely closing an orifice or lumen of a tubular body part.	
3RD – L **OCCLUSION**		
	EXPLANATION: Natural or artificially created orifice …	

Body Part – 4TH	Approach – 5TH	Device – 6TH	Qualifier – 7TH
0 Abdominal Aorta 1 Celiac Artery 2 Gastric Artery 3 Hepatic Artery 4 Splenic Artery 5 Superior Mesenteric Artery 6 Colic Artery, Right 7 Colic Artery, Left 8 Colic Artery, Middle 9 Renal Artery, Right A Renal Artery, Left B Inferior Mesenteric Artery C Common Iliac Artery, Right D Common Iliac Artery, Left H External Iliac Artery, Right J External Iliac Artery, Left K Femoral Artery, Right L Femoral Artery, Left M Popliteal Artery, Right N Popliteal Artery, Left P Anterior Tibial Artery, Right Q Anterior Tibial Artery, Left R Posterior Tibial Artery, Right S Posterior Tibial Artery, Left T Peroneal Artery, Right U Peroneal Artery, Left V Foot Artery, Right W Foot Artery, Left Y Lower Artery	0 Open 3 Percutaneous 4 Percutaneous endoscopic	C Extraluminal device D Intraluminal device Z No device	Z No qualifier
E Internal Iliac Artery, Right	0 Open 3 Percutaneous 4 Percutaneous endoscopic	C Extraluminal device D Intraluminal device Z No device	T Uterine artery, right ♀ Z No qualifier
F Internal Iliac Artery, Left	0 Open 3 Percutaneous 4 Percutaneous endoscopic	C Extraluminal device D Intraluminal device Z No device	U Uterine artery, left ♀ Z No qualifier

DIVISION GROUP: (Division), Release
Root Operations involving cutting or separation only.

1ST - 0 Medical and Surgical

2ND - 4 Lower Arteries

3RD - N RELEASE

EXAMPLE: Arterial adhesiolysis

CMS Ex: Carpal tunnel release

RELEASE: Freeing a body part from an abnormal physical constraint by cutting or by the use of force.

EXPLANATION: None of the body part is taken out ...

Body Part – 4TH		Approach – 5TH	Device – 6TH	Qualifier – 7TH
0 Abdominal Aorta	H External Iliac Artery, Right	0 Open	Z No device	Z No qualifier
1 Celiac Artery	J External Iliac Artery, Left	3 Percutaneous		
2 Gastric Artery	K Femoral Artery, Right	4 Percutaneous endoscopic		
3 Hepatic Artery	L Femoral Artery, Left			
4 Splenic Artery	M Popliteal Artery, Right			
5 Superior Mesenteric Artery	N Popliteal Artery, Left			
6 Colic Artery, Right	P Anterior Tibial Artery, Right			
7 Colic Artery, Left	Q Anterior Tibial Artery, Left			
8 Colic Artery, Middle	R Posterior Tibial Artery, Right			
9 Renal Artery, Right	S Posterior Tibial Artery, Left			
A Renal Artery, Left	T Peroneal Artery, Right			
B Inferior Mesenteric Artery	U Peroneal Artery, Left			
C Common Iliac Artery, Right	V Foot Artery, Right			
D Common Iliac Artery, Left	W Foot Artery, Left			
E Internal Iliac Artery, Right	Y Lower Artery			
F Internal Iliac Artery, Left				

DEVICE GROUP: (Change), **Insertion, Removal, Replacement, Revision, Supplement**
Root Operations that always involve a device.

1ST - **0** Medical and Surgical	EXAMPLE: Removal arterial catheter — CMS Ex: Chest tube removal
2ND - **4** Lower Arteries	**REMOVAL:** Taking out or off a device from a body part.
3RD - **P REMOVAL**	EXPLANATION: Removal device without reinsertion ...

Body Part – 4TH	Approach – 5TH	Device – 6TH	Qualifier – 7TH
Y Lower Artery	0 Open 3 Percutaneous 4 Percutaneous endoscopic	0 Drainage device 2 Monitoring device 3 Infusion device 7 Autologous tissue substitute C Extraluminal device D Intraluminal device J Synthetic substitute K Nonautologous tissue substitute	Z No qualifier
Y Lower Artery	X External	0 Drainage device 1 Radioactive element 2 Monitoring device 3 Infusion device D Intraluminal device	Z No qualifier

LOWER ARTERIES 04P

OTHER REPAIRS GROUP: (Control), Repair
Root Operations that define other repairs.

1ST - 0 Medical and Surgical	EXAMPLE: Repair arterial injury	CMS Ex: Suture laceration

2ND - 4 Lower Arteries

3RD - Q REPAIR

REPAIR: Restoring, to the extent possible, a body part to its normal anatomic structure and function.

EXPLANATION: Only when no other root operation applies ...

Body Part – 4TH		Approach – 5TH	Device – 6TH	Qualifier – 7TH
0 Abdominal Aorta	H External Iliac Artery, Right	0 Open	Z No device	Z No qualifier
1 Celiac Artery	J External Iliac Artery, Left	3 Percutaneous		
2 Gastric Artery	K Femoral Artery, Right	4 Percutaneous endoscopic		
3 Hepatic Artery	L Femoral Artery, Left			
4 Splenic Artery	M Popliteal Artery, Right			
5 Superior Mesenteric Artery	N Popliteal Artery, Left			
6 Colic Artery, Right	P Anterior Tibial Artery, Right			
7 Colic Artery, Left	Q Anterior Tibial Artery, Left			
8 Colic Artery, Middle	R Posterior Tibial Artery, Right			
9 Renal Artery, Right	S Posterior Tibial Artery, Left			
A Renal Artery, Left	T Peroneal Artery, Right			
B Inferior Mesenteric Artery	U Peroneal Artery, Left			
C Common Iliac Artery, Right	V Foot Artery, Right			
D Common Iliac Artery, Left	W Foot Artery, Left			
E Internal Iliac Artery, Right	Y Lower Artery			
F Internal Iliac Artery, Left				

LOWER ARTERIES 04Q

DEVICE GROUP: (Change), **Insertion, Removal, Replacement, Revision, Supplement**
Root Operations that always involve a device.

1ST - **0** Medical and Surgical	EXAMPLE: Reconstruction artery using graft	CMS Ex: Total hip

2ND - **4** Lower Arteries

3RD - **R REPLACEMENT**

REPLACEMENT: Putting in or on a biological or synthetic material that physically takes the place and/or function of all or a portion of a body part.

EXPLANATION: Includes taking out body part, or eradication...

Body Part – 4TH		Approach – 5TH	Device – 6TH	Qualifier – 7TH
0 Abdominal Aorta	H External Iliac Artery, Right	0 Open	7 Autologous tissue substitute	Z No qualifier
1 Celiac Artery	J External Iliac Artery, Left	4 Percutaneous endoscopic	J Synthetic substitute	
2 Gastric Artery	K Femoral Artery, Right		K Nonautologous tissue substitute	
3 Hepatic Artery	L Femoral Artery, Left			
4 Splenic Artery	M Popliteal Artery, Right			
5 Superior Mesenteric Artery	N Popliteal Artery, Left			
6 Colic Artery, Right	P Anterior Tibial Artery, Right			
7 Colic Artery, Left	Q Anterior Tibial Artery, Left			
8 Colic Artery, Middle	R Posterior Tibial Artery, Right			
9 Renal Artery, Right	S Posterior Tibial Artery, Left			
A Renal Artery, Left	T Peroneal Artery, Right			
B Inferior Mesenteric Artery	U Peroneal Artery, Left			
C Common Iliac Artery, Right	V Foot Artery, Right			
D Common Iliac Artery, Left	W Foot Artery, Left			
E Internal Iliac Artery, Right	Y Lower Artery			
F Internal Iliac Artery, Left				

LOWER ARTERIES 0 4 R

MOVE GROUP: (Reattachment), **Reposition,** (Transfer), (Transplantation)
Root Operations that put in/put back or move some/all of a body part.

1ST - 0 Medical and Surgical

2ND - 4 Lower Arteries

3RD - S REPOSITION

EXAMPLE: Relocation peroneal artery	CMS Ex: Fracture reduction

REPOSITION: Moving to its normal location, or other suitable location, all or a portion of a body part.

EXPLANATION: May or may not be cut to be moved ...

Body Part – 4TH		Approach – 5TH	Device – 6TH	Qualifier – 7TH
0 Abdominal Aorta	H External Iliac Artery, Right	0 Open	Z No device	Z No qualifier
1 Celiac Artery	J External Iliac Artery, Left	3 Percutaneous		
2 Gastric Artery	K Femoral Artery, Right	4 Percutaneous endoscopic		
3 Hepatic Artery	L Femoral Artery, Left			
4 Splenic Artery	M Popliteal Artery, Right			
5 Superior Mesenteric Artery	N Popliteal Artery, Left			
6 Colic Artery, Right	P Anterior Tibial Artery, Right			
7 Colic Artery, Left	Q Anterior Tibial Artery, Left			
8 Colic Artery, Middle	R Posterior Tibial Artery, Right			
9 Renal Artery, Right	S Posterior Tibial Artery, Left			
A Renal Artery, Left				
B Inferior Mesenteric Artery	T Peroneal Artery, Right			
C Common Iliac Artery, Right	U Peroneal Artery, Left			
D Common Iliac Artery, Left	V Foot Artery, Right			
E Internal Iliac Artery, Right	W Foot Artery, Left			
F Internal Iliac Artery, Left	Y Lower Artery			

LOWER ARTERIES

0 4 S

DEVICE GROUP: (Change), **Insertion, Removal, Replacement, Revision, Supplement**	
Root Operations that always involve a device.	

1ST - 0 Medical and Surgical

2ND - 4 Lower Arteries

3RD - U SUPPLEMENT

EXAMPLE: Bovine patch angioplasty | CMS Ex: Hernia repair with mesh

SUPPLEMENT: Putting in or on biological or synthetic material that physically reinforces and/or augments the function of a portion of a body part.

EXPLANATION: Biological material from same individual ...

Body Part – 4TH		Approach – 5TH	Device – 6TH	Qualifier – 7TH
0 Abdominal Aorta	H External Iliac Artery, Right	0 Open	7 Autologous tissue substitute	Z No qualifier
1 Celiac Artery	J External Iliac Artery, Left	3 Percutaneous	J Synthetic substitute	
2 Gastric Artery	K Femoral Artery, Right	4 Percutaneous endoscopic	K Nonautologous tissue substitute	
3 Hepatic Artery	L Femoral Artery, Left			
4 Splenic Artery	M Popliteal Artery, Right			
5 Superior Mesenteric Artery	N Popliteal Artery, Left			
6 Colic Artery, Right	P Anterior Tibial Artery, Right			
7 Colic Artery, Left	Q Anterior Tibial Artery, Left			
8 Colic Artery, Middle	R Posterior Tibial Artery, Right			
9 Renal Artery, Right	S Posterior Tibial Artery, Left			
A Renal Artery, Left	T Peroneal Artery, Right			
B Inferior Mesenteric Artery	U Peroneal Artery, Left			
C Common Iliac Artery, Right	V Foot Artery, Right			
D Common Iliac Artery, Left	W Foot Artery, Left			
E Internal Iliac Artery, Right	Y Lower Artery			
F Internal Iliac Artery, Left				

LOWER ARTERIES 0 4 U

TUBULAR GROUP: Bypass, Dilation, Occlusion, Restriction
Root Operations that alter the diameter/route of a tubular body part.

1ST - 0 Medical and Surgical	EXAMPLE: Stent graft repair aneurysm	CMS Ex: Cervical cerclage
2ND - 4 Lower Arteries	**RESTRICTION:** Partially closing an orifice or the lumen of a tubular body part.	
3RD - V RESTRICTION	EXPLANATION: Natural or artificially created orifice ...	

Body Part – 4TH	Approach – 5TH	Device – 6TH	Qualifier – 7TH
0 Abdominal Aorta	0 Open 3 Percutaneous 4 Percutaneous endoscopic	C Extraluminal device E Intraluminal device, branched or fenestrated, one or two arteries F Intraluminal device, branched or fenestrated, three or more arteries Z No device	6 Bifurcation Z No qualifier
0 Abdominal Aorta	0 Open 3 Percutaneous 4 Percutaneous endoscopic	D Intraluminal device	6 Bifurcation J Temporary Z No qualifier
1 Celiac Artery 2 Gastric Artery 3 Hepatic Artery 4 Splenic Artery 5 Superior Mesenteric Artery 6 Colic Artery, Right 7 Colic Artery, Left 8 Colic Artery, Middle 9 Renal Artery, Right A Renal Artery, Left B Inferior Mesenteric Artery E Internal Iliac Artery, Right F Internal Iliac Artery, Left H External Iliac Artery, Right J External Iliac Artery, Left K Femoral Artery, Right L Femoral Artery, Left M Popliteal Artery, Right N Popliteal Artery, Left P Anterior Tibial Artery, Right Q Anterior Tibial Artery, Left R Posterior Tibial Artery, Right S Posterior Tibial Artery, Left T Peroneal Artery, Right U Peroneal Artery, Left V Foot Artery, Right W Foot Artery, Left Y Lower Artery	0 Open 3 Percutaneous 4 Percutaneous endoscopic	C Extraluminal device D Intraluminal device Z No device	Z No qualifier

LOWER ARTERIES 0 4 V

continued ⇨

0   4   V   RESTRICTION – continued

Body Part – 4TH	Approach – 5TH	Device – 6TH	Qualifier – 7TH
C Common Iliac Artery, Right D Common Iliac Artery, Left	0 Open 3 Percutaneous 4 Percutaneous endoscopic	C Extraluminal device D Intraluminal device E Intraluminal device, branched or fenestrated, one or two arteries F Intraluminal device, branched or fenestrated, three or more arteries Z No device	Z No qualifier

DEVICE GROUP: (Change), Insertion, Removal, Replacement, Revision, Supplement
Root Operations that always involve a device.

1ST – 0 Medical and Surgical	EXAMPLE: Repair ruptured graft	CMS Ex: Adjustment pacemaker lead
2ND – 4 Lower Arteries 3RD – W REVISION	**REVISION:** Correcting, to the extent possible, a portion of a malfunctioning device or the position of a displaced device.	
	EXPLANATION: May replace components of a device ...	

Body Part – 4TH	Approach – 5TH	Device – 6TH	Qualifier – 7TH
Y Lower Artery	0 Open 3 Percutaneous 4 Percutaneous endoscopic X External	0 Drainage device 2 Monitoring device 3 Infusion device 7 Autologous tissue substitute C Extraluminal device D Intraluminal device J Synthetic substitute K Nonautologous tissue substitute	Z No qualifier

Educational Annotations | 5 – Upper Veins

Body System Specific Educational Annotations for the Upper Veins include:

- **Anatomy and Physiology Review**
- **Anatomical Illustrations**
- **Definitions of Common Procedures**
- **AHA Coding Clinic® Reference Notations**
- **Body Part Key Listings**
- **Device Key Listings**
- **Device Aggregation Table Listings**
- **Coding Notes**

Anatomy and Physiology Review of Upper Veins

BODY PART VALUES – 5 - UPPER VEINS

Axillary Vein – The axillary vein drains to the subclavian vein and drains blood from the axilla, lateral thorax, and upper limb.

Azygos Vein – The azygos vein drains to the superior vena cava and drains blood from the right side of the posterior thorax.

Basilic Vein – The basilic vein drains to the axillary vein and drains blood from the hand and forearm.

Brachial Vein – The brachial vein drains to the axillary vein and drains blood from the upper limb.

Cephalic Vein – The cephalic vein drains to the axillary vein and drains blood from the hand.

External Jugular Vein – The external jugular vein drains to the subclavian vein and drains blood from the head and face.

Face Vein – Any of the smaller vein branches that drains the blood from the face.

Hand Vein – Any of the smaller vein branches that drains the blood from the hand.

Hemiazygos Vein – The hemiazygos vein drains to the azygos vein and drains blood from the left side of the posterior thorax.

Innominate Vein – The innominate vein drains to the superior vena cava and drains blood from the internal jugular vein and subclavian vein.

Internal Jugular Vein – The internal jugular vein drains to the subclavian vein and drains blood from the brain and face.

Intracranial Vein – Any of the smaller vein branches that drains the blood from within the skull.

Subclavian Vein – The subclavian vein drains to the innominate vein and drains blood from the axillary vein and external jugular vein.

Upper Vein – The veins located above the diaphragm (see Coding Guideline B2.1b).

Vein – Blood vessels that carry de-oxygenated (venous) blood away from the organs and tissues of the body and to the heart. Most veins have one-way valves to prevent backflow of venous blood and to assist the lower-pressure venous blood back to the heart.

Vertebral Vein – The vertebral vein drains to the innominate vein and drains blood from the neck.

UPPER VEINS

0 5

Educational Annotations | 5 – Upper Veins

Anatomical Illustrations of Upper Veins

External Jugular
Internal Jugular
Superior Vena Cava
Pulmonary Arteries
Intercostal
Portal
Renal
Azygos
Superior Mesenteric
Ileo-colic
Ulnar
Radial
Digital

Subclavian
Axillary
Internal Mammary
Brachial
Cephalic
Splenic
Inferior Mesenteric
Inferior Vena Cava
Ovarian/Testicular
Uterine
Iliac
Hypogastric (Internal Iliac)
Common Femoral
Superficial Femoral
Saphenous
Popliteal
Anterior Tibial
Posterior Tibial
Plantar

VEINS OF HUMAN BODY

Educational Annotations | 5 – Upper Veins

Definitions of Common Procedures of Upper Veins

Excision of damaged vein – The surgical removal of a damaged vein segment.

Mobilization/superficialization of vein – The surgical elevation of a vein to a location just under the skin from a deeper tissue location for easier and safer cannulation access.

Superior vena cava filter – The placement of a wire filter device in the superior vena cava to prevent pulmonary emboli (PE) from upper-extremity deep vein thrombosis.

AHA Coding Clinic® Reference Notations of Upper Veins

ROOT OPERATION SPECIFIC - 5 - UPPER VEINS
BYPASS - 1
DESTRUCTION - 5
DILATION - 7
DRAINAGE - 9
EXCISION - B
   Infratemporal fossa malignancy with excision of jugular vein ....AHA 16:2Q:p12
EXTIRPATION - C
EXTRACTION - D
INSERTION - H
INSPECTION - J
OCCLUSION - L
RELEASE - N
REMOVAL - P
REPAIR - Q
REPLACEMENT - R
REPOSITION - S
   Superficialization of cephalic vein...AHA 13:4Q:p125
SUPPLEMENT - U
RESTRICTION - V
REVISION - W

UPPER VEINS 05

Educational Annotations | 5 – Upper Veins

Body Part Key Listings of Upper Veins

See also Body Part Key in Appendix C

Accessory cephalic vein	*use* Cephalic Vein, Left/Right
Angular vein	*use* Face Vein, Left/Right
Anterior cerebral vein	*use* Intracranial Vein
Anterior facial vein	*use* Face Vein, Left/Right
Basal (internal) cerebral vein	*use* Intracranial Vein
Brachiocephalic vein	*use* Innominate Vein, Left/Right
Common facial vein	*use* Face Vein, Left/Right
Deep cervical vein	*use* Vertebral Vein, Left/Right
Deep facial vein	*use* Face Vein, Left/Right
Dorsal metacarpal vein	*use* Hand Vein, Left/Right
Dural venous sinus	*use* Intracranial Vein
Frontal vein	*use* Face Vein, Left/Right
Great cerebral vein	*use* Intracranial Vein
Inferior cerebellar vein	*use* Intracranial Vein
Inferior cerebral vein	*use* Intracranial Vein
Inferior thyroid vein	*use* Innominate Vein, Left/Right
Internal (basal) cerebral vein	*use* Intracranial Vein
Left ascending lumbar vein	*use* Hemiazygos Vein
Left subcostal vein	*use* Hemiazygos Vein
Median antebrachial vein	*use* Basilic Vein, Left/Right
Median cubital vein	*use* Basilic Vein, Left/Right
Middle cerebral vein	*use* Intracranial Vein
Ophthalmic vein	*use* Intracranial Vein
Palmar (volar) digital vein	*use* Hand Vein, Left/Right
Palmar (volar) metacarpal vein	*use* Hand Vein, Left/Right
Posterior auricular vein	*use* External Jugular Vein, Left/Right
Posterior facial (retromandibular) vein	*use* Face Vein, Left/Right
Radial vein	*use* Brachial Vein, Left/Right
Right ascending lumbar vein	*use* Azygos Vein
Right subcostal vein	*use* Azygos Vein
Suboccipital venous plexus	*use* Vertebral Vein, Left/Right
Superficial palmar venous arch	*use* Hand Vein, Left/Right
Superior cerebellar vein	*use* Intracranial Vein
Superior cerebral vein	*use* Intracranial Vein
Supraorbital vein	*use* Face Vein, Left/Right
Ulnar vein	*use* Brachial Vein, Left/Right
Volar (palmar) digital vein	*use* Hand Vein, Left/Right
Volar (palmar) metacarpal vein	*use* Hand Vein, Left/Right

Device Key Listings of Upper Veins

See also Device Key in Appendix D

Autograft	*use* Autologous Tissue Substitute
Autologous artery graft	*use* Autologous Arterial Tissue in Upper Veins
Autologous vein graft	*use* Autologous Venous Tissue in Upper Veins
Non-tunneled central venous catheter	*use* Infusion Device
Peripherally inserted central catheter (PICC)	*use* Infusion Device
Tissue bank graft	*use* Nonautologous Tissue Substitute

Educational Annotations | 5 – Upper Veins

Device Aggregation Table Listings of Upper Veins

See also Device Aggregation Table in Appendix E

Specific Device	For Operation	In Body System	General Device
Autologous Arterial Tissue	All applicable	Upper Veins	7 Autologous Tissue Substitute
Autologous Venous Tissue	All applicable	Upper Veins	7 Autologous Tissue Substitute

Coding Notes of Upper Veins

Body System Relevant Coding Guidelines

General Guidelines
B2.1b

Where the general body part values "upper" and "lower" are provided as an option in the Upper Arteries, Lower Arteries, Upper Veins, Lower Veins, Muscles and Tendons body systems, "upper" and "lower" specifies body parts located above or below the diaphragm respectively.

Example: Vein body parts above the diaphragm are found in the Upper Veins body system; vein body parts below the diaphragm are found in the Lower Veins body system.

Branches of body parts
B4.2

Where a specific branch of a body part does not have its own body part value in PCS, the body part is typically coded to the closest proximal branch that has a specific body part value. In the cardiovascular body systems, if a general body part is available in the correct root operation table, and coding to a proximal branch would require assigning a code in a different body system, the procedure is coded using the general body part value.

Examples: A procedure performed on the mandibular branch of the trigeminal nerve is coded to the trigeminal nerve body part value.

Occlusion of the bronchial artery is coded to the body part value Upper Artery in the body system Upper Arteries, and not to the body part value Thoracic Aorta, Descending in the body system Heart and Great Vessels.

Body System Specific PCS Reference Manual Exercises

PCS CODE	5 – UPPER VEINS EXERCISES
0 5 9 C 3 Z Z	Phlebotomy of left median cubital vein for polycythemia vera. (The median cubital vein is a branch of the basilic vein.)

Educational Annotations | 5 – Upper Veins

NOTES

TUBULAR GROUP: Bypass, Dilation, Occlusion, Restriction
Root Operations that alter the diameter/route of a tubular body part.

1ST - 0 Medical and Surgical

2ND - 5 Upper Veins

3RD - 1 BYPASS

EXAMPLE: Bypass damaged subclavian | CMS Ex: Coronary artery bypass

BYPASS: Altering the route of passage of the contents of a tubular body part.

EXPLANATION: Rerouting contents to a downstream part ...

Body Part – 4TH		Approach – 5TH	Device – 6TH	Qualifier – 7TH
0 Azygos Vein	H Hand Vein, Left	0 Open	7 Autologous tissue substitute	Y Upper Vein
1 Hemiazygos Vein	L Intracranial Vein	4 Percutaneous endoscopic	9 Autologous venous tissue	
3 Innominate Vein, Right	M Internal Jugular Vein, Right		A Autologous arterial tissue	
4 Innominate Vein, Left	N Internal Jugular Vein, Left		J Synthetic substitute	
5 Subclavian Vein, Right	P External Jugular Vein, Right		K Nonautologous tissue substitute	
6 Subclavian Vein, Left	Q External Jugular Vein, Left		Z No device	
7 Axillary Vein, Right	R Vertebral Vein, Right			
8 Axillary Vein, Left	S Vertebral Vein, Left			
9 Brachial Vein, Right	T Face Vein, Right			
A Brachial Vein, Left	V Face Vein, Left			
B Basilic Vein, Right				
C Basilic Vein, Left				
D Cephalic Vein, Right				
F Cephalic Vein, Left				
G Hand Vein, Right				

EXCISION GROUP: Excision, (Resection), Destruction, Extraction, (Detachment)
Root Operations that take out some or all of a body part.

1ST - 0 Medical and Surgical

2ND - 5 Upper Veins

3RD - 5 DESTRUCTION

EXAMPLE: Fulguration venous lesion | CMS Ex: Fulguration polyp

DESTRUCTION: Physical eradication of all or a portion of a body part by the direct use of energy, force, or a destructive agent.

EXPLANATION: None of the body part is physically taken out

Body Part – 4TH		Approach – 5TH	Device – 6TH	Qualifier – 7TH
0 Azygos Vein	H Hand Vein, Left	0 Open	Z No device	Z No qualifier
1 Hemiazygos Vein	L Intracranial Vein	3 Percutaneous		
3 Innominate Vein, Right	M Internal Jugular Vein, Right	4 Percutaneous endoscopic		
4 Innominate Vein, Left	N Internal Jugular Vein, Left			
5 Subclavian Vein, Right	P External Jugular Vein, Right			
6 Subclavian Vein, Left	Q External Jugular Vein, Left			
7 Axillary Vein, Right	R Vertebral Vein, Right			
8 Axillary Vein, Left	S Vertebral Vein, Left			
9 Brachial Vein, Right	T Face Vein, Right			
A Brachial Vein, Left	V Face Vein, Left			
B Basilic Vein, Right	Y Upper Vein			
C Basilic Vein, Left				
D Cephalic Vein, Right				
F Cephalic Vein, Left				
G Hand Vein, Right				

TUBULAR GROUP: Bypass, Dilation, Occlusion, Restriction
Root Operations that alter the diameter/route of a tubular body part.

1ST - 0 Medical and Surgical	EXAMPLE: Balloon dilation axillary vein	CMS Ex: Transluminal angioplasty
2ND - 5 Upper Veins	DILATION: Expanding an orifice or the lumen of a tubular body part.	
3RD - 7 DILATION	EXPLANATION: By force (stretching) or cutting ...	

Body Part – 4TH	Approach – 5TH	Device – 6TH	Qualifier – 7TH
0 Azygos Vein H Hand Vein, Left 1 Hemiazygos Vein L Intracranial Vein NC* 3 Innominate Vein, Right M Internal Jugular Vein, Right 4 Innominate Vein, Left N Internal Jugular Vein, Left 5 Subclavian Vein, Right 6 Subclavian Vein, Left P External Jugular Vein, Right 7 Axillary Vein, Right 8 Axillary Vein, Left Q External Jugular Vein, Left 9 Brachial Vein, Right A Brachial Vein, Left R Vertebral Vein, Right B Basilic Vein, Right S Vertebral Vein, Left C Basilic Vein, Left T Face Vein, Right D Cephalic Vein, Right V Face Vein, Left F Cephalic Vein, Left Y Upper Vein G Hand Vein, Right	0 Open 3 Percutaneous 4 Percutaneous endoscopic	D Intraluminal device Z No device	Z No qualifier

NC* – Some procedures are considered non-covered by Medicare. See current Medicare Code Editor for details.

DRAINAGE GROUP: Drainage, Extirpation, (Fragmentation)
Root Operations that take out solids/fluids/gases from a body part.

1ST - 0 Medical and Surgical	EXAMPLE: Phlebotomy basilic vein	CMS Ex: Thoracentesis

2ND - 5 Upper Veins

3RD - 9 DRAINAGE

DRAINAGE: Taking or letting out fluids and/or gases from a body part.

EXPLANATION: Qualifier "X Diagnostic" indicates biopsy ...

Body Part – 4TH		Approach – 5TH	Device – 6TH	Qualifier – 7TH
0 Azygos Vein 1 Hemiazygos Vein 3 Innominate Vein, Right 4 Innominate Vein, Left 5 Subclavian Vein, Right 6 Subclavian Vein, Left 7 Axillary Vein, Right 8 Axillary Vein, Left 9 Brachial Vein, Right A Brachial Vein, Left B Basilic Vein, Right C Basilic Vein, Left D Cephalic Vein, Right F Cephalic Vein, Left G Hand Vein, Right	H Hand Vein, Left L Intracranial Vein M Internal Jugular Vein, Right N Internal Jugular Vein, Left P External Jugular Vein, Right Q External Jugular Vein, Left R Vertebral Vein, Right S Vertebral Vein, Left T Face Vein, Right V Face Vein, Left Y Upper Vein	0 Open 3 Percutaneous 4 Percutaneous endoscopic	0 Drainage device	Z No qualifier
0 Azygos Vein 1 Hemiazygos Vein 3 Innominate Vein, Right 4 Innominate Vein, Left 5 Subclavian Vein, Right 6 Subclavian Vein, Left 7 Axillary Vein, Right 8 Axillary Vein, Left 9 Brachial Vein, Right A Brachial Vein, Left B Basilic Vein, Right C Basilic Vein, Left D Cephalic Vein, Right F Cephalic Vein, Left G Hand Vein, Right	H Hand Vein, Left L Intracranial Vein M Internal Jugular Vein, Right N Internal Jugular Vein, Left P External Jugular Vein, Right Q External Jugular Vein, Left R Vertebral Vein, Right S Vertebral Vein, Left T Face Vein, Right V Face Vein, Left Y Upper Vein	0 Open 3 Percutaneous 4 Percutaneous endoscopic	Z No device	X Diagnostic Z No qualifier

UPPER VEINS

059

EXCISION GROUP: Excision, (Resection), Destruction, Extraction, (Detachment)
Root Operations that take out some or all of a body part.

1ST - 0 Medical and Surgical	EXAMPLE: Harvest brachial vein	CMS Ex: Liver biopsy

2ND - 5 Upper Veins

3RD - B EXCISION

EXCISION: Cutting out or off, without replacement, a portion of a body part.

EXPLANATION: Qualifier "X Diagnostic" indicates biopsy ...

Body Part – 4TH		Approach – 5TH	Device – 6TH	Qualifier – 7TH
0 Azygos Vein	H Hand Vein, Left	0 Open	Z No device	X Diagnostic
1 Hemiazygos Vein	L Intracranial Vein	3 Percutaneous		Z No qualifier
3 Innominate Vein, Right	M Internal Jugular Vein, Right	4 Percutaneous endoscopic		
4 Innominate Vein, Left				
5 Subclavian Vein, Right	N Internal Jugular Vein, Left			
6 Subclavian Vein, Left				
7 Axillary Vein, Right	P External Jugular Vein, Right			
8 Axillary Vein, Left				
9 Brachial Vein, Right	Q External Jugular Vein, Left			
A Brachial Vein, Left				
B Basilic Vein, Right	R Vertebral Vein, Right			
C Basilic Vein, Left	S Vertebral Vein, Left			
D Cephalic Vein, Right	T Face Vein, Right			
F Cephalic Vein, Left	V Face Vein, Left			
G Hand Vein, Right	Y Upper Vein			

DRAINAGE GROUP: Drainage, Extirpation, (Fragmentation)
Root Operations that take out solids/fluids/gases from a body part.

1ST - 0 Medical and Surgical	EXAMPLE: Mechanical thrombectomy	CMS Ex: Choledocholithotomy

2ND - 5 Upper Veins

3RD - C EXTIRPATION

EXTIRPATION: Taking or cutting out solid matter from a body part.

EXPLANATION: Abnormal byproduct or foreign body ...

Body Part – 4TH		Approach – 5TH	Device – 6TH	Qualifier – 7TH
0 Azygos Vein	H Hand Vein, Left	0 Open	Z No device	Z No qualifier
1 Hemiazygos Vein	L Intracranial Vein	3 Percutaneous		
3 Innominate Vein, Right	M Internal Jugular Vein, Right	4 Percutaneous endoscopic		
4 Innominate Vein, Left				
5 Subclavian Vein, Right	N Internal Jugular Vein, Left			
6 Subclavian Vein, Left				
7 Axillary Vein, Right	P External Jugular Vein, Right			
8 Axillary Vein, Left				
9 Brachial Vein, Right	Q External Jugular Vein, Left			
A Brachial Vein, Left				
B Basilic Vein, Right	R Vertebral Vein, Right			
C Basilic Vein, Left	S Vertebral Vein, Left			
D Cephalic Vein, Right	T Face Vein, Right			
F Cephalic Vein, Left	V Face Vein, Left			
G Hand Vein, Right	Y Upper Vein			

EXCISION GROUP: Excision, (Resection), Destruction, Extraction, (Detachment)
Root Operations that take out some or all of a body part.

1ST - 0 Medical and Surgical

2ND - 5 Upper Veins

3RD - D EXTRACTION

EXAMPLE: Vein ligation and stripping

CMS Ex: D&C

EXTRACTION: Pulling or stripping out or off all or a portion of a body part by the use of force.

EXPLANATION: None for this Body System

Body Part – 4TH		Approach – 5TH	Device – 6TH	Qualifier – 7TH
9 Brachial Vein, Right A Brachial Vein, Left B Basilic Vein, Right C Basilic Vein, Left	D Cephalic Vein, Right F Cephalic Vein, Left G Hand Vein, Right H Hand Vein, Left Y Upper Vein	0 Open 3 Percutaneous	Z No device	Z No qualifier

---

DEVICE GROUP: (Change), Insertion, Removal, Replacement, Revision, Supplement
Root Operations that always involve a device.

1ST - 0 Medical and Surgical

2ND - 5 Upper Veins

3RD - H INSERTION

EXAMPLE: Insertion central venous line

CMS Ex: Insertion CVP cath

INSERTION: Putting in a nonbiological appliance that monitors, assists, performs, or prevents a physiological function but does not physically take the place of a body part.

EXPLANATION: None

Body Part – 4TH		Approach – 5TH	Device – 6TH	Qualifier – 7TH
0 Azygos Vein		0 Open 3 Percutaneous 4 Percutaneous endoscopic	2 Monitoring device 3 Infusion device D Intraluminal device M Neurostimulator lead	Z No qualifier
1 Hemiazygos Vein 5 Subclavian Vein, Right 6 Subclavian Vein, Left 7 Axillary Vein, Right 8 Axillary Vein, Left 9 Brachial Vein, Right A Brachial Vein, Left B Basilic Vein, Right C Basilic Vein, Left D Cephalic Vein, Right F Cephalic Vein, Left G Hand Vein, Right H Hand Vein, Left	L Intracranial Vein M Internal Jugular Vein, Right N Internal Jugular Vein, Left P External Jugular Vein, Right Q External Jugular Vein, Left R Vertebral Vein, Right S Vertebral Vein, Left T Face Vein, Right V Face Vein, Left	0 Open 3 Percutaneous 4 Percutaneous endoscopic	3 Infusion device D Intraluminal device	Z No qualifier
3 Innominate Vein, Right 4 Innominate Vein, Left		0 Open 3 Percutaneous 4 Percutaneous endoscopic	3 Infusion device D Intraluminal device M Neurostimulator lead	Z No qualifier
Y Upper Vein		0 Open 3 Percutaneous 4 Percutaneous endoscopic	2 Monitoring device 3 Infusion device D Intraluminal device	Z No qualifier

EXAMINATION GROUP: Inspection, (Map)
Root Operations involving examination only.

1ST – 0 Medical and Surgical	EXAMPLE: Open intracranial vein examination	CMS Ex: Colonoscopy

2ND – 5 Upper Veins

3RD – J INSPECTION

INSPECTION: Visually and/or manually exploring a body part.

EXPLANATION: Direct or instrumental visualization ...

Body Part – 4TH	Approach – 5TH	Device – 6TH	Qualifier – 7TH
Y Upper Vein	0 Open 3 Percutaneous 4 Percutaneous endoscopic X External	Z No device	Z No qualifier

---

TUBULAR GROUP: Bypass, Dilation, Occlusion, Restriction
Root Operations that alter the diameter/route of a tubular body part.

1ST – 0 Medical and Surgical

EXAMPLE: Ligation jugular vein | CMS Ex: Fallopian tube ligation

2ND – 5 Upper Veins

3RD – L OCCLUSION

OCCLUSION: Completely closing an orifice or lumen of a tubular body part.

EXPLANATION: Natural or artificially created orifice ...

Body Part – 4TH	Approach – 5TH	Device – 6TH	Qualifier – 7TH
0 Azygos Vein 1 Hemiazygos Vein 3 Innominate Vein, Right 4 Innominate Vein, Left 5 Subclavian Vein, Right 6 Subclavian Vein, Left 7 Axillary Vein, Right 8 Axillary Vein, Left 9 Brachial Vein, Right A Brachial Vein, Left B Basilic Vein, Right C Basilic Vein, Left D Cephalic Vein, Right F Cephalic Vein, Left G Hand Vein, Right H Hand Vein, Left L Intracranial Vein M Internal Jugular Vein, Right N Internal Jugular Vein, Left P External Jugular Vein, Right Q External Jugular Vein, Left R Vertebral Vein, Right S Vertebral Vein, Left T Face Vein, Right V Face Vein, Left Y Upper Vein	0 Open 3 Percutaneous 4 Percutaneous endoscopic	C Extraluminal device D Intraluminal device Z No device	Z No qualifier

---

DIVISION GROUP: (Division), Release

Root Operations involving cutting or separation only.

1ST - 0 Medical and Surgical	EXAMPLE: Adhesiolysis brachial vein CMS Ex: Carpal tunnel release
2ND - 5 Upper Veins	**RELEASE:** Freeing a body part from an abnormal physical constraint by cutting or by the use of force.
3RD - N RELEASE	EXPLANATION: None of the body part is taken out ...

Body Part – 4TH		Approach – 5TH	Device – 6TH	Qualifier – 7TH
0 Azygos Vein	H Hand Vein, Left	0 Open	Z No device	Z No qualifier
1 Hemiazygos Vein	L Intracranial Vein	3 Percutaneous		
3 Innominate Vein, Right	M Internal Jugular Vein, Right	4 Percutaneous endoscopic		
4 Innominate Vein, Left				
5 Subclavian Vein, Right	N Internal Jugular Vein, Left			
6 Subclavian Vein, Left				
7 Axillary Vein, Right	P External Jugular Vein, Right			
8 Axillary Vein, Left				
9 Brachial Vein, Right	Q External Jugular Vein, Left			
A Brachial Vein, Left				
B Basilic Vein, Right	R Vertebral Vein, Right			
C Basilic Vein, Left	S Vertebral Vein, Left			
D Cephalic Vein, Right	T Face Vein, Right			
F Cephalic Vein, Left	V Face Vein, Left			
G Hand Vein, Right	Y Upper Vein			

DEVICE GROUP: (Change), Insertion, Removal, Replacement, Revision, Supplement
Root Operations that always involve a device.

1ST - **0** Medical and Surgical 2ND - **5** Upper Veins 3RD - **P REMOVAL**		

EXAMPLE: Removal central venous line	CMS Ex: Chest tube removal

REMOVAL: Taking out or off a device from a body part.

EXPLANATION: Removal device without reinsertion ...

Body Part – 4TH	Approach – 5TH	Device – 6TH	Qualifier – 7TH
0 Azygos Vein	0 Open 3 Percutaneous 4 Percutaneous endoscopic X External	2 Monitoring device M Neurostimulator lead	Z No qualifier
3 Innominate Vein, Right 4 Innominate Vein, Left	0 Open 3 Percutaneous 4 Percutaneous endoscopic X External	M Neurostimulator lead	Z No qualifier
Y Upper Vein	0 Open 3 Percutaneous 4 Percutaneous endoscopic	0 Drainage device 2 Monitoring device 3 Infusion device 7 Autologous tissue substitute C Extraluminal device D Intraluminal device J Synthetic substitute K Nonautologous tissue substitute	Z No qualifier
Y Upper Vein	X External	0 Drainage device 2 Monitoring device 3 Infusion device D Intraluminal device	Z No qualifier

OTHER REPAIRS GROUP: (Control), Repair
Root Operations that define other repairs.

1ST - 0 Medical and Surgical

2ND - 5 Upper Veins

3RD - Q REPAIR

EXAMPLE: Suture lacerated cephalic vein | CMS Ex: Suture laceration

REPAIR: Restoring, to the extent possible, a body part to its normal anatomic structure and function.

EXPLANATION: Only when no other root operation applies ...

Body Part – 4TH		Approach – 5TH	Device – 6TH	Qualifier – 7TH
0 Azygos Vein	H Hand Vein, Left	0 Open	Z No device	Z No qualifier
1 Hemiazygos Vein	L Intracranial Vein	3 Percutaneous		
3 Innominate Vein, Right	M Internal Jugular Vein, Right	4 Percutaneous endoscopic		
4 Innominate Vein, Left	N Internal Jugular Vein, Left			
5 Subclavian Vein, Right	P External Jugular Vein, Right			
6 Subclavian Vein, Left	Q External Jugular Vein, Left			
7 Axillary Vein, Right	R Vertebral Vein, Right			
8 Axillary Vein, Left	S Vertebral Vein, Left			
9 Brachial Vein, Right	T Face Vein, Right			
A Brachial Vein, Left	V Face Vein, Left			
B Basilic Vein, Right	Y Upper Vein			
C Basilic Vein, Left				
D Cephalic Vein, Right				
F Cephalic Vein, Left				
G Hand Vein, Right				

DEVICE GROUP: (Change), Insertion, Removal, Replacement, Revision, Supplement
Root Operations that always involve a device.

1ST - 0 Medical and Surgical

2ND - 5 Upper Veins

3RD - R REPLACEMENT

EXAMPLE: Spiral jugular vein replacement graft | CMS Ex: Total hip

REPLACEMENT: Putting in or on a biological or synthetic material that physically takes the place and/or function of all or a portion of a body part.

EXPLANATION: Includes taking out body part, or eradication...

Body Part – 4TH		Approach – 5TH	Device – 6TH	Qualifier – 7TH
0 Azygos Vein	H Hand Vein, Left	0 Open	7 Autologous tissue substitute	Z No qualifier
1 Hemiazygos Vein	L Intracranial Vein	4 Percutaneous endoscopic	J Synthetic substitute	
3 Innominate Vein, Right	M Internal Jugular Vein, Right		K Nonautologous tissue substitute	
4 Innominate Vein, Left	N Internal Jugular Vein, Left			
5 Subclavian Vein, Right	P External Jugular Vein, Right			
6 Subclavian Vein, Left	Q External Jugular Vein, Left			
7 Axillary Vein, Right	R Vertebral Vein, Right			
8 Axillary Vein, Left	S Vertebral Vein, Left			
9 Brachial Vein, Right	T Face Vein, Right			
A Brachial Vein, Left	V Face Vein, Left			
B Basilic Vein, Right	Y Upper Vein			
C Basilic Vein, Left				
D Cephalic Vein, Right				
F Cephalic Vein, Left				
G Hand Vein, Right				

UPPER VEINS 0 5 R

MOVE GROUP: (Reattachment), **Reposition,** (Transfer), (Transplantation)
Root Operations that put in/put back or move some/all of a body part.

1ST - **0** Medical and Surgical

2ND - **5** Upper Veins

3RD - **S REPOSITION**

EXAMPLE: Superficialization cephalic vein   CMS Ex: Fracture reduction

REPOSITION: Moving to its normal location, or other suitable location, all or a portion of a body part.

EXPLANATION: May or may not be cut to be moved ...

Body Part – 4TH		Approach – 5TH	Device – 6TH	Qualifier – 7TH
0 Azygos Vein	H Hand Vein, Left	0 Open	Z No device	Z No qualifier
1 Hemiazygos Vein	L Intracranial Vein	3 Percutaneous		
3 Innominate Vein, Right	M Internal Jugular Vein, Right	4 Percutaneous endoscopic		
4 Innominate Vein, Left				
5 Subclavian Vein, Right	N Internal Jugular Vein, Left			
6 Subclavian Vein, Left				
7 Axillary Vein, Right	P External Jugular Vein, Right			
8 Axillary Vein, Left				
9 Brachial Vein, Right	Q External Jugular Vein, Left			
A Brachial Vein, Left				
B Basilic Vein, Right	R Vertebral Vein, Right			
C Basilic Vein, Left	S Vertebral Vein, Left			
D Cephalic Vein, Right	T Face Vein, Right			
F Cephalic Vein, Left	V Face Vein, Left			
G Hand Vein, Right	Y Upper Vein			

DEVICE GROUP: (Change), **Insertion, Removal, Replacement, Revision, Supplement**
Root Operations that always involve a device.

1ST - **0** Medical and Surgical

2ND - **5** Upper Veins

3RD - **U SUPPLEMENT**

EXAMPLE: Patch graft venoplasty   CMS Ex: Hernia repair with mesh

SUPPLEMENT: Putting in or on biological or synthetic material that physically reinforces and/or augments the function of a portion of a body part.

EXPLANATION: Biological material from same individual ...

Body Part – 4TH		Approach – 5TH	Device – 6TH	Qualifier – 7TH
0 Azygos Vein	H Hand Vein, Left	0 Open	7 Autologous tissue substitute	Z No qualifier
1 Hemiazygos Vein	L Intracranial Vein	3 Percutaneous		
3 Innominate Vein, Right	M Internal Jugular Vein, Right	4 Percutaneous endoscopic	J Synthetic substitute	
4 Innominate Vein, Left				
5 Subclavian Vein, Right	N Internal Jugular Vein, Left		K Nonautologous tissue substitute	
6 Subclavian Vein, Left				
7 Axillary Vein, Right	P External Jugular Vein, Right			
8 Axillary Vein, Left				
9 Brachial Vein, Right	Q External Jugular Vein, Left			
A Brachial Vein, Left				
B Basilic Vein, Right	R Vertebral Vein, Right			
C Basilic Vein, Left	S Vertebral Vein, Left			
D Cephalic Vein, Right	T Face Vein, Right			
F Cephalic Vein, Left	V Face Vein, Left			
G Hand Vein, Right	Y Upper Vein			

TUBULAR GROUP: Bypass, Dilation, Occlusion, Restriction
Root Operations that alter the diameter/route of a tubular body part.

1ST - **0** Medical and Surgical	EXAMPLE: Restrictive venous stent — CMS Ex: Cervical cerclage
2ND - **5** Upper Veins	**RESTRICTION:** Partially closing an orifice or the lumen of a tubular body part.
3RD - **V RESTRICTION**	EXPLANATION: Natural or artificially created orifice ...

Body Part – 4TH		Approach – 5TH	Device – 6TH	Qualifier – 7TH
0 Azygos Vein	H Hand Vein, Left	0 Open	C Extraluminal device	Z No qualifier
1 Hemiazygos Vein	L Intracranial Vein	3 Percutaneous	D Intraluminal device	
3 Innominate Vein, Right	M Internal Jugular Vein, Right	4 Percutaneous endoscopic	Z No device	
4 Innominate Vein, Left	N Internal Jugular Vein, Left			
5 Subclavian Vein, Right	P External Jugular Vein, Right			
6 Subclavian Vein, Left	Q External Jugular Vein, Left			
7 Axillary Vein, Right	R Vertebral Vein, Right			
8 Axillary Vein, Left	S Vertebral Vein, Left			
9 Brachial Vein, Right	T Face Vein, Right			
A Brachial Vein, Left	V Face Vein, Left			
B Basilic Vein, Right	Y Upper Vein			
C Basilic Vein, Left				
D Cephalic Vein, Right				
F Cephalic Vein, Left				
G Hand Vein, Right				

UPPER VEINS

0 5 V

DEVICE GROUP: (Change), **Insertion, Removal, Replacement, Revision, Supplement**
Root Operations that always involve a device.

1ST - 0	Medical and Surgical
2ND - 5	Upper Veins
3RD - W	REVISION

EXAMPLE: Reposition central line line | **CMS Ex:** Adjust pacemaker lead

REVISION: Correcting, to the extent possible, a portion of a malfunctioning device or the position of a displaced device.

EXPLANATION: May replace components of a device ...

Body Part – 4TH	Approach – 5TH	Device – 6TH	Qualifier – 7TH
0 Azygos Vein	0 Open 3 Percutaneous 4 Percutaneous endoscopic X External	2 Monitoring device M Neurostimulator lead	Z No qualifier
3 Innominate Vein, Right 4 Innominate Vein, Left	0 Open 3 Percutaneous 4 Percutaneous endoscopic X External	M Neurostimulator lead	Z No qualifier
Y Upper Vein	0 Open 3 Percutaneous 4 Percutaneous endoscopic X External	0 Drainage device 2 Monitoring device 3 Infusion device 7 Autologous tissue substitute C Extraluminal device D Intraluminal device J Synthetic substitute K Nonautologous tissue substitute	Z No qualifier

UPPER VEINS 0 5 W

Educational Annotations | 6 – Lower Veins

Body System Specific Educational Annotations for the Lower Veins include:

- Anatomy and Physiology Review
- Anatomical Illustrations
- Definitions of Common Procedures
- AHA Coding Clinic® Reference Notations
- Body Part Key Listings
- Device Key Listings
- Device Aggregation Table Listings
- Coding Notes

Anatomy and Physiology Review of Lower Veins

BODY PART VALUES – 6 - LOWER VEINS

Colic Vein – The colic vein drains to the superior mesenteric vein and drains blood from the colon.

Common Iliac Vein – The common iliac vein drains to the inferior vena cava and drains blood from the external and hypogastric (also known as the internal iliac vein) veins.

Esophageal Vein – The esophageal vein drains to the azygos vein and drains blood from the esophagus.

External Iliac Vein – The external iliac vein drains to the common iliac vein and drains blood from the femoral veins.

Femoral Vein – The femoral vein drains to the external iliac vein and drains blood from the lower limb.

Foot Vein – Any of the smaller vein branches that drains the blood from the foot.

Gastric Vein – The gastric vein drains to the portal vein and drains blood from the stomach.

Greater Saphenous Vein – The greater saphenous vein drains to the femoral vein and drains blood from the lower limb including the plantar portion of the foot.

Hepatic Vein – The hepatic vein drains to the inferior vena cava and drains blood from the liver, pancreas, and small intestine.

Hypogastric Vein – The hypogastric vein (also known as the internal iliac vein) drains to the common iliac vein and drains blood from the pelvic viscera and reproductive organs.

Inferior Mesenteric Vein – The inferior mesenteric vein drains to the splenic vein and drains blood from the large intestine.

Inferior Vena Cava – The inferior vena cava drains to the right atrium of the heart and drains blood from the common iliac veins.

Lesser Saphenous Vein – The lesser saphenous vein drains to the popliteal vein and drains blood from the dorsal portion of the foot.

Lower Vein – The veins located below the diaphragm (see Coding Guideline B2.1b).

Portal Vein – The portal vein drains to the hepatic vein and drains blood from the gastrointestinal tract and liver.

Renal Vein – The renal vein drains to the inferior vena cava and drains blood from the kidney.

Splenic Vein – The splenic vein drains to the portal vein and drains blood from the spleen and pancreas.

Superior Mesenteric Vein – The superior mesenteric vein drains to the portal vein and drains blood from the small intestine.

Vein – Blood vessels that carry de-oxygenated (venous) blood away from the organs and tissues of the body and to the heart. Most veins have one-way valves to prevent backflow of venous blood and to assist the lower-pressure venous blood back to the heart.

Educational Annotations | 6 – Lower Veins

Anatomical Illustrations of Lower Veins

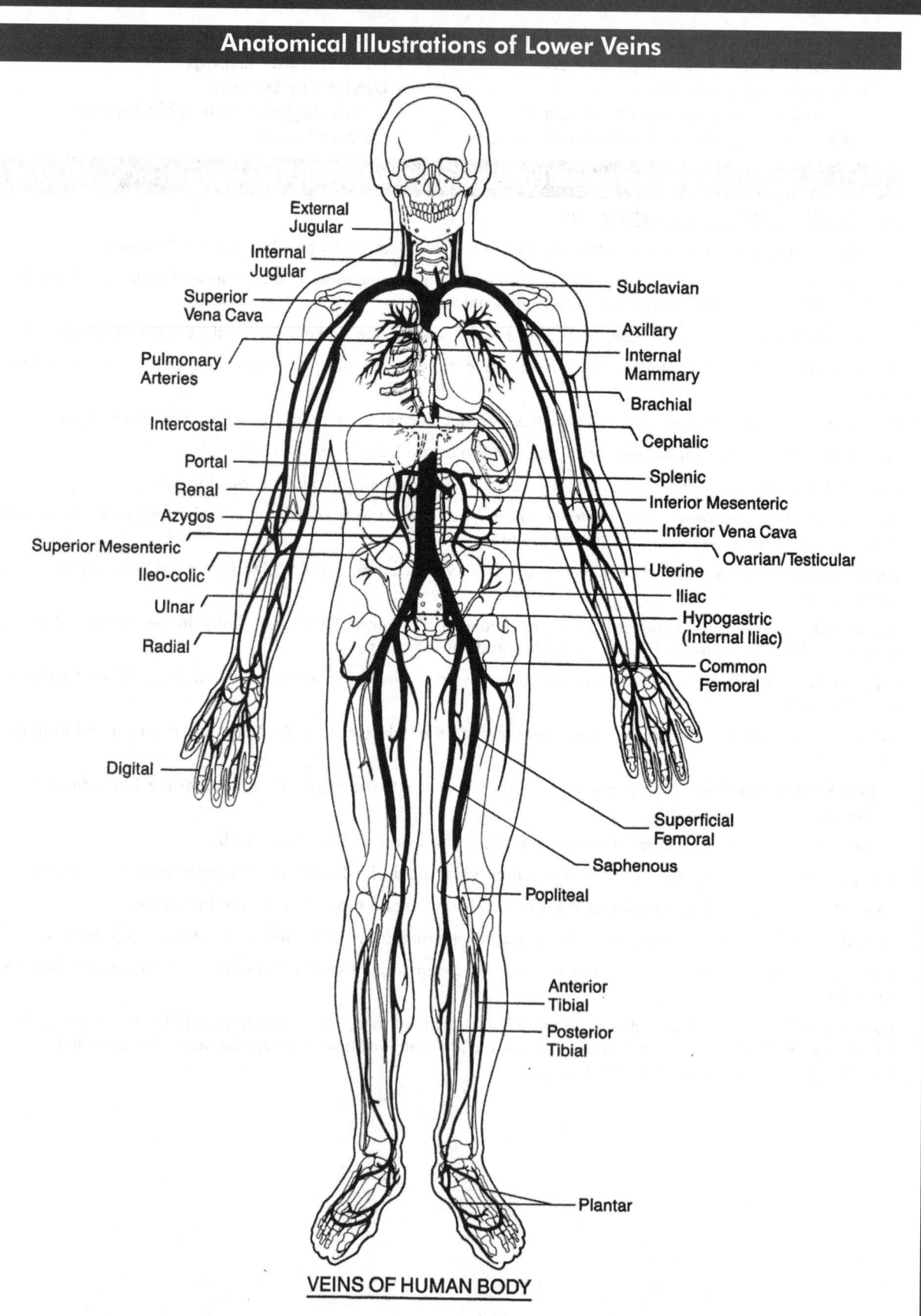

VEINS OF HUMAN BODY

Educational Annotations | 6 – Lower Veins

Definitions of Common Procedures of Lower Veins

Endovenous laser vein ablation – The placement of a laser-tipped catheter into the targeted vein, using the laser energy to destroy the vein by causing it to collapse and seal shut without removing it.

External light laser treatment of varicose veins – The use of an external laser to send strong bursts of light to small, superficial varicose veins and spider veins that make the veins slowly fade away.

Harvesting of saphenous vein – The surgical removal of a segment of a saphenous vein to be used as a vessel graft (e.g., coronary artery bypass, femoral-popliteal bypass).

Inferior vena cava filter – The placement of a wire filter device in the inferior vena cava to prevent pulmonary emboli (PE) from lower-extremity deep vein thrombosis.

Ligation and stripping of varicose veins – The surgical removal of enlarged, painful lower leg veins that is performed by making small incisions at the distal and proximal locations and using an attached endovenous wire to pull the vein out of the leg.

AHA Coding Clinic® Reference Notations of Lower Veins

ROOT OPERATION SPECIFIC - 6 - LOWER VEINS
BYPASS - 1
DESTRUCTION - 5
DILATION - 7
DIVISION - 8
EXCISION - B
    Coronary artery bypass graft, using greater saphenous vein ....AHA 14:3Q:p20
    ....AHA 14:1Q:p10
    Tibial artery bypass using saphenous vein graft and vein cuff ....AHA 16:2Q:p18
    Unspecified saphenous vein harvested ....AHA 14:3Q:p8
EXTIRPATION - C
    Pharmacomechanical thrombolysis of femoral venous thrombus ....AHA 13:4Q:p115
EXTRACTION - D
INSERTION - H
    Insertion of a Mahurkar catheter into inferior vena cava (IVC)....................AHA 13:3Q:p18
INSPECTION - J
OCCLUSION - L
    Endoscopic ligation of esophageal varices using bands ....AHA 13:4Q:p112
RELEASE - N
REMOVAL - P
REPAIR - Q
REPLACEMENT - R
REPOSITION - S
SUPPLEMENT - U
RESTRICTION - T
REVISION - W
    Removal of clots from transjugular intrahepatic portosystemic shunt (TIPS) AHA 14:3Q:p25

Educational Annotations | 6 – Lower Veins

Body Part Key Listings of Lower Veins

See also Body Part Key in Appendix C

Common digital vein	*use* Foot Vein, Left/Right
Deep femoral (profunda femoris) vein	*use* Femoral Vein, Left/Right
Dorsal metatarsal vein	*use* Foot Vein, Left/Right
Dorsal venous arch	*use* Foot Vein, Left/Right
External pudendal vein	*use* Greater Saphenous Vein, Left/Right
Gluteal vein	*use* Hypogastric Vein, Left/Right
Great saphenous vein	*use* Greater Saphenous Vein, Left/Right
Hepatic portal vein	*use* Portal Vein
Ileocolic vein	*use* Colic Vein
Internal iliac vein	*use* Hypogastric Vein, Left/Right
Internal pudendal vein	*use* Hypogastric Vein, Left/Right
Lateral sacral vein	*use* Hypogastric Vein, Left/Right
Left colic vein	*use* Colic Vein
Left gastroepiploic vein	*use* Splenic Vein
Left inferior phrenic vein	*use* Renal Vein, Left
Left ovarian vein	*use* Renal Vein, Left
Left second lumbar vein	*use* Renal Vein, Left
Left suprarenal vein	*use* Renal Vein, Left
Left testicular vein	*use* Renal Vein, Left
Middle colic vein	*use* Colic Vein
Middle hemorrhoidal vein	*use* Hypogastric Vein, Left/Right
Obturator vein	*use* Hypogastric Vein, Left/Right
Pancreatic vein	*use* Splenic Vein
Plantar digital vein	*use* Foot Vein, Left/Right
Plantar metatarsal vein	*use* Foot Vein, Left/Right
Plantar venous arch	*use* Foot Vein, Left/Right
Popliteal vein	*use* Femoral Vein, Left/Right
Postcava	*use* Inferior Vena Cava
Profunda femoris (deep femoral) vein	*use* Femoral Vein, Left/Right
Right colic vein	*use* Colic Vein
Right gastroepiploic vein	*use* Superior Mesenteric Vein
Right inferior phrenic vein	*use* Inferior Vena Cava
Right ovarian vein	*use* Inferior Vena Cava
Right second lumbar vein	*use* Inferior Vena Cava
Right suprarenal vein	*use* Inferior Vena Cava
Right testicular vein	*use* Inferior Vena Cava
Sigmoid vein	*use* Inferior Mesenteric Vein
Small saphenous vein	*use* Lesser Saphenous Vein, Left/Right
Superficial circumflex iliac vein	*use* Greater Saphenous Vein, Left/Right
Superficial epigastric vein	*use* Greater Saphenous Vein, Left/Right
Superior rectal vein	*use* Inferior Mesenteric Vein
Uterine vein	*use* Hypogastric Vein, Left/Right
Vaginal vein	*use* Hypogastric Vein, Left/Right
Vesical vein	*use* Hypogastric Vein, Left/Right

Educational Annotations | 6 – Lower Veins

Device Key Listings of Lower Veins

See also Device Key in Appendix D

Autograft ....*use* Autologous Tissue Substitute

Autologous artery graft ....*use* Autologous Arterial Tissue in Lower Veins

Autologous vein graft ....*use* Autologous Venous Tissue in Lower Veins

Non-tunneled central venous catheter ....*use* Infusion Device

Tissue bank graft ....*use* Nonautologous Tissue Substitute

Device Aggregation Table Listings of Lower Veins

See also Device Aggregation Table in Appendix E

Specific Device	For Operation	In Body System	General Device	
Autologous Arterial Tissue	All applicable	Lower Veins	7	Autologous Tissue Substitute
Autologous Venous Tissue	All applicable	Lower Veins	7	Autologous Tissue Substitute

Coding Notes of Lower Veins

Body System Relevant Coding Guidelines

General Guidelines

B2.1b

Where the general body part values "upper" and "lower" are provided as an option in the Upper Arteries, Lower Arteries, Upper Veins, Lower Veins, Muscles and Tendons body systems, "upper" and "lower" specifies body parts located above or below the diaphragm respectively.

Example: Vein body parts above the diaphragm are found in the Upper Veins body system; vein body parts below the diaphragm are found in the Lower Veins body system.

Branches of body parts

B4.2

Where a specific branch of a body part does not have its own body part value in PCS, the body part is typically coded to the closest proximal branch that has a specific body part value. In the cardiovascular body systems, if a general body part is available in the correct root operation table, and coding to a proximal branch would require assigning a code in a different body system, the procedure is coded using the general body part value.

Examples: A procedure performed on the mandibular branch of the trigeminal nerve is coded to the trigeminal nerve body part value.

Occlusion of the bronchial artery is coded to the body part value Upper Artery in the body system Upper Arteries, and not to the body part value Thoracic Aorta, Descending in the body system Heart and Great Vessels.

Body System Specific PCS Reference Manual Exercises

PCS CODE	6 – LOWER VEINS EXERCISES
0 6 5 Y 3 Z Z	Cautery of oozing varicose vein, left calf. (The approach is coded "Percutaneous" because that is the normal route to a vein. No mention is made of approach, because likely the skin has eroded at that spot.)
0 6 D Y 3 Z Z	Microincisional phlebectomy of spider veins, right lower leg.
0 6 H 0 3 D Z	Percutaneous insertion of Greenfield IVC filter.
0 6 L 3 3 Z Z	Percutaneous ligation of esophageal vein.

Educational Annotations | 6 – Lower Veins

NOTES

TUBULAR GROUP: Bypass, Dilation, Occlusion, Restriction
Root Operations that alter the diameter/route of a tubular body part.

1ST - 0 Medical and Surgical	EXAMPLE: Bypass damaged splenic vein	CMS Ex: Coronary artery bypass

1ST - 0 Medical and Surgical

2ND - 6 Lower Veins

3RD - 1 BYPASS

BYPASS: Altering the route of passage of the contents of a tubular body part.

EXPLANATION: Rerouting contents to a downstream part ...

Body Part – 4TH		Approach – 5TH	Device – 6TH	Qualifier – 7TH
0 Inferior Vena Cava		0 Open 4 Percutaneous endoscopic	7 Autologous tissue substitute 9 Autologous venous tissue A Autologous arterial tissue J Synthetic substitute K Nonautologous tissue substitute Z No device	5 Superior Mesenteric Vein 6 Inferior Mesenteric Vein Y Lower Vein
1 Splenic Vein		0 Open 4 Percutaneous endoscopic	7 Autologous tissue substitute 9 Autologous venous tissue A Autologous arterial tissue J Synthetic substitute K Nonautologous tissue substitute Z No device	9 Renal Vein, Right B Renal Vein, Left Y Lower Vein
2 Gastric Vein 3 Esophageal Vein 4 Hepatic Vein 5 Superior Mesenteric Vein 6 Inferior Mesenteric Vein 7 Colic Vein 9 Renal Vein, Right B Renal Vein, Left C Common Iliac Vein, Right D Common Iliac Vein, Left F External Iliac Vein, Right G External Iliac Vein, Left H Hypogastric Vein, Right J Hypogastric Vein, Left	M Femoral Vein, Right N Femoral Vein, Left P Greater Saphenous Vein, Right Q Greater Saphenous Vein, Left R Lesser Saphenous Vein, Right S Lesser Saphenous Vein, Left T Foot Vein, Right V Foot Vein, Left	0 Open 4 Percutaneous endoscopic	7 Autologous tissue substitute 9 Autologous venous tissue A Autologous arterial tissue J Synthetic substitute K Nonautologous tissue substitute Z No device	Y Lower Vein

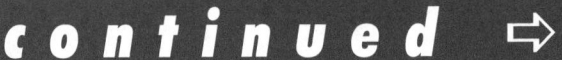
continued ⇨

LOWER VEINS 061

0   6   1   BYPASS – *continued*

Body Part – 4TH	Approach – 5TH	Device – 6TH	Qualifier – 7TH
8 Portal Vein	0 Open	7 Autologous tissue substitute 9 Autologous venous tissue A Autologous arterial tissue J Synthetic substitute K Nonautologous tissue substitute Z No device	9 Renal Vein, Right B Renal Vein, Left Y Lower Vein
8 Portal Vein	3 Percutaneous	D Intraluminal device	Y Lower Vein
8 Portal Vein	4 Percutaneous endoscopic	7 Autologous tissue substitute 9 Autologous venous tissue A Autologous arterial tissue J Synthetic substitute K Nonautologous tissue substitute Z No device	9 Renal Vein, Right B Renal Vein, Left Y Lower Vein
8 Portal Vein	4 Percutaneous endoscopic	D Intraluminal device	Y Lower Vein

LOWER VEINS 061

EXCISION GROUP: Excision, (Resection), Destruction, Extraction, (Detachment)
Root Operations that take out some or all of a body part.

1ST - 0 Medical and Surgical

2ND - 6 Lower Veins

3RD - 5 DESTRUCTION

EXAMPLE: Fulguration venous lesion | CMS Ex: Fulguration polyp

DESTRUCTION: Physical eradication of all or a portion of a body part by the direct use of energy, force, or a destructive agent.

EXPLANATION: None of the body part is physically taken out

Body Part – 4TH		Approach – 5TH	Device – 6TH	Qualifier – 7TH
0 Inferior Vena Cava	H Hypogastric Vein, Right	0 Open	Z No device	Z No qualifier
1 Splenic Vein	J Hypogastric Vein, Left	3 Percutaneous		
2 Gastric Vein	M Femoral Vein, Right	4 Percutaneous endoscopic		
3 Esophageal Vein	N Femoral Vein, Left			
4 Hepatic Vein	P Greater Saphenous Vein, Right			
5 Superior Mesenteric Vein	Q Greater Saphenous Vein, Left			
6 Inferior Mesenteric Vein				
7 Colic Vein	R Lesser Saphenous Vein, Right			
8 Portal Vein				
9 Renal Vein, Right	S Lesser Saphenous Vein, Left			
B Renal Vein, Left				
C Common Iliac Vein, Right	T Foot Vein, Right			
D Common Iliac Vein, Left	V Foot Vein, Left			
F External Iliac Vein, Right				
G External Iliac Vein, Left				
Y Lower Vein		0 Open	Z No device	C Hemorrhoidal Plexus
		3 Percutaneous		Z No qualifier
		4 Percutaneous endoscopic		

TUBULAR GROUP: Bypass, Dilation, Occlusion, Restriction
Root Operations that alter the diameter/route of a tubular body part.

1ST - 0 Medical and Surgical

2ND - 6 Lower Veins

3RD - 7 DILATION

EXAMPLE: Balloon dilation hepatic vein | CMS Ex: Transluminal angioplasty

DILATION: Expanding an orifice or the lumen of a tubular body part.

EXPLANATION: By force (stretching) or cutting ...

Body Part – 4TH		Approach – 5TH	Device – 6TH	Qualifier – 7TH
0 Inferior Vena Cava	H Hypogastric Vein, Right	0 Open	D Intraluminal device	Z No qualifier
1 Splenic Vein	J Hypogastric Vein, Left	3 Percutaneous	Z No device	
2 Gastric Vein	M Femoral Vein, Right	4 Percutaneous endoscopic		
3 Esophageal Vein	N Femoral Vein, Left			
4 Hepatic Vein	P Greater Saphenous Vein, Right			
5 Superior Mesenteric Vein	Q Greater Saphenous Vein, Left			
6 Inferior Mesenteric Vein				
7 Colic Vein	R Lesser Saphenous Vein, Right			
8 Portal Vein				
9 Renal Vein, Right	S Lesser Saphenous Vein, Left			
B Renal Vein, Left				
C Common Iliac Vein, Right	T Foot Vein, Right			
D Common Iliac Vein, Left	V Foot Vein, Left			
F External Iliac Vein, Right	Y Lower Vein			
G External Iliac Vein, Left				

DRAINAGE GROUP: Drainage, Extirpation, (Fragmentation)
Root Operations that take out solids/fluids/gases from a body part.

1ST - 0 Medical and Surgical	EXAMPLE: Phlebotomy iliac vein	CMS Ex: Thoracentesis

2ND - **6** Lower Veins

3RD - **9 DRAINAGE**

DRAINAGE: Taking or letting out fluids and/or gases from a body part.

EXPLANATION: Qualifier "X Diagnostic" indicates biopsy ...

Body Part – 4TH		Approach – 5TH	Device – 6TH	Qualifier – 7TH
0 Inferior Vena Cava 1 Splenic Vein 2 Gastric Vein 3 Esophageal Vein 4 Hepatic Vein 5 Superior Mesenteric Vein 6 Inferior Mesenteric Vein 7 Colic Vein 8 Portal Vein 9 Renal Vein, Right B Renal Vein, Left C Common Iliac Vein, Right D Common Iliac Vein, Left F External Iliac Vein, Right G External Iliac Vein, Left	H Hypogastric Vein, Right J Hypogastric Vein, Left M Femoral Vein, Right N Femoral Vein, Left P Greater Saphenous Vein, Right Q Greater Saphenous Vein, Left R Lesser Saphenous Vein, Right S Lesser Saphenous Vein, Left T Foot Vein, Right V Foot Vein, Left Y Lower Vein	0 Open 3 Percutaneous 4 Percutaneous endoscopic	0 Drainage device	Z No qualifier
0 Inferior Vena Cava 1 Splenic Vein 2 Gastric Vein 3 Esophageal Vein 4 Hepatic Vein 5 Superior Mesenteric Vein 6 Inferior Mesenteric Vein 7 Colic Vein 8 Portal Vein 9 Renal Vein, Right B Renal Vein, Left C Common Iliac Vein, Right D Common Iliac Vein, Left F External Iliac Vein, Right G External Iliac Vein, Left	H Hypogastric Vein, Right J Hypogastric Vein, Left M Femoral Vein, Right N Femoral Vein, Left P Greater Saphenous Vein, Right Q Greater Saphenous Vein, Left R Lesser Saphenous Vein, Right S Lesser Saphenous Vein, Left T Foot Vein, Right V Foot Vein, Left Y Lower Vein	0 Open 3 Percutaneous 4 Percutaneous endoscopic	Z No device	X Diagnostic Z No qualifier

LOWER VEINS 069

EXCISION GROUP: Excision, (Resection), Destruction, Extraction, (Detachment)
Root Operations that take out some or all of a body part.

1ST - **0** Medical and Surgical

2ND - **6** Lower Veins

3RD - **B EXCISION**

EXAMPLE: Harvest saphenous vein

CMS Ex: Liver biopsy

EXCISION: Cutting out or off, without replacement, a portion of a body part.

EXPLANATION: Qualifier "X Diagnostic" indicates biopsy ...

Body Part – 4TH		Approach – 5TH	Device – 6TH	Qualifier – 7TH
0 Inferior Vena Cava	H Hypogastric Vein, Right	0 Open	Z No device	X Diagnostic
1 Splenic Vein	J Hypogastric Vein, Left	3 Percutaneous		Z No qualifier
2 Gastric Vein	M Femoral Vein, Right	4 Percutaneous		
3 Esophageal Vein	N Femoral Vein, Left	endoscopic		
4 Hepatic Vein	P Greater Saphenous			
5 Superior Mesenteric Vein	Vein, Right			
6 Inferior Mesenteric Vein	Q Greater Saphenous			
7 Colic Vein	Vein, Left			
8 Portal Vein	R Lesser Saphenous			
9 Renal Vein, Right	Vein, Right			
B Renal Vein, Left	S Lesser Saphenous			
C Common Iliac Vein, Right	Vein, Left			
D Common Iliac Vein, Left	T Foot Vein, Right			
F External Iliac Vein, Right	V Foot Vein, Left			
G External Iliac Vein, Left				
Y Lower Vein		0 Open	Z No device	C Hemorrhoidal
		3 Percutaneous		Plexus
		4 Percutaneous		X Diagnostic
		endoscopic		Z No qualifier

LOWER VEINS

0
6
B

DRAINAGE GROUP: Drainage, Extirpation, (Fragmentation)
Root Operations that take out solids/fluids/gases from a body part.

1ST - **0** Medical and Surgical

2ND - **6** Lower Veins

3RD - **C EXTIRPATION**

EXAMPLE: Mechanical thrombectomy | CMS Ex: Choledocholithotomy

EXTIRPATION: Taking or cutting out solid matter from a body part.

EXPLANATION: Abnormal byproduct or foreign body ...

Body Part – 4TH	Approach – 5TH	Device – 6TH	Qualifier – 7TH
0 Inferior Vena Cava	0 Open	Z No device	Z No qualifier
1 Splenic Vein	3 Percutaneous		
2 Gastric Vein	4 Percutaneous		
3 Esophageal Vein	endoscopic		
4 Hepatic Vein			
5 Superior Mesenteric Vein			
6 Inferior Mesenteric Vein			
7 Colic Vein			
8 Portal Vein			
9 Renal Vein, Right			
B Renal Vein, Left			
C Common Iliac Vein, Right			
D Common Iliac Vein, Left			
F External Iliac Vein, Right			
G External Iliac Vein, Left			
H Hypogastric Vein, Right			
J Hypogastric Vein, Left			
M Femoral Vein, Right			
N Femoral Vein, Left			
P Greater Saphenous Vein, Right			
Q Greater Saphenous Vein, Left			
R Lesser Saphenous Vein, Right			
S Lesser Saphenous Vein, Left			
T Foot Vein, Right			
V Foot Vein, Left			
Y Lower Vein			

EXCISION GROUP: Excision, (Resection), Destruction, Extraction, (Detachment)
Root Operations that take out some or all of a body part.

1ST - **0** Medical and Surgical

2ND - **6** Lower Veins

3RD - **D EXTRACTION**

EXAMPLE: Vein ligation and stripping | CMS Ex: D&C

EXTRACTION: Pulling or stripping out or off all or a portion of a body part by the use of force.

EXPLANATION: None for this Body System

Body Part – 4TH	Approach – 5TH	Device – 6TH	Qualifier – 7TH
M Femoral Vein, Right	0 Open	Z No device	Z No qualifier
N Femoral Vein, Left	3 Percutaneous		
P Greater Saphenous Vein, Right	4 Percutaneous		
Q Greater Saphenous Vein, Left	endoscopic		
R Lesser Saphenous Vein, Right			
S Lesser Saphenous Vein, Left			
T Foot Vein, Right			
V Foot Vein, Left			
Y Lower Vein			

DEVICE GROUP: (Change), Insertion, Removal, Replacement, Revision, Supplement
Root Operations that always involve a device.

1ST - 0 Medical and Surgical

2ND - 6 Lower Veins

3RD - H INSERTION

EXAMPLE: Insertion IVC filter	CMS Ex: Insertion central venous catheter

INSERTION: Putting in a nonbiological appliance that monitors, assists, performs, or prevents a physiological function but does not physically take the place of a body part.

EXPLANATION: None

Body Part – 4TH		Approach – 5TH	Device – 6TH	Qualifier – 7TH
0	Inferior Vena Cava	0 Open 3 Percutaneous	3 Infusion device	T Via Umbilical Vein Z No qualifier
0	Inferior Vena Cava	0 Open 3 Percutaneous	D Intraluminal device	Z No qualifier
0	Inferior Vena Cava	4 Percutaneous endoscopic	3 Infusion device D Intraluminal device	Z No qualifier
1 Splenic Vein 2 Gastric Vein 3 Esophageal Vein 4 Hepatic Vein 5 Superior Mesenteric Vein 6 Inferior Mesenteric Vein 7 Colic Vein 8 Portal Vein 9 Renal Vein, Right B Renal Vein, Left C Common Iliac Vein, Right D Common Iliac Vein, Left F External Iliac Vein, Right G External Iliac Vein, Left	H Hypogastric Vein, Right J Hypogastric Vein, Left M Femoral Vein, Right N Femoral Vein, Left P Greater Saphenous Vein, Right Q Greater Saphenous Vein, Left R Lesser Saphenous Vein, Right S Lesser Saphenous Vein, Left T Foot Vein, Right V Foot Vein, Left	0 Open 3 Percutaneous 4 Percutaneous endoscopic	3 Infusion device D Intraluminal device	Z No qualifier
Y	Lower Vein	0 Open 3 Percutaneous 4 Percutaneous endoscopic	2 Monitoring device 3 Infusion device D Intraluminal device	Z No qualifier

EXAMINATION GROUP: Inspection, (Map)
Root Operations involving examination only.

1ST - 0 Medical and Surgical

2ND - 6 Lower Veins

3RD - J INSPECTION

EXAMPLE: Open iliac vein examination	CMS Ex: Colonoscopy

INSPECTION: Visually and/or manually exploring a body part.

EXPLANATION: Direct or instrumental visualization ...

Body Part – 4TH	Approach – 5TH	Device – 6TH	Qualifier – 7TH
Y Lower Vein	0 Open 3 Percutaneous 4 Percutaneous endoscopic X External	Z No device	Z No qualifier

© 2016 Channel Publishing, Ltd.

TUBULAR GROUP: Bypass, Dilation, Occlusion, Restriction
Root Operations that alter the diameter/route of a tubular body part.

1ST - 0 Medical and Surgical	EXAMPLE: Ligation esophageal varices CMS Ex: Fallopian tube ligation
2ND - 6 Lower Veins	OCCLUSION: Completely closing an orifice or lumen of a tubular body part.
3RD - L OCCLUSION	EXPLANATION: Natural or artificially created orifice …

Body Part – 4TH	Approach – 5TH	Device – 6TH	Qualifier – 7TH
0 Inferior Vena Cava 1 Splenic Vein 2 Gastric Vein 3 Esophageal Vein 4 Hepatic Vein 5 Superior Mesenteric Vein 6 Inferior Mesenteric Vein 7 Colic Vein 8 Portal Vein 9 Renal Vein, Right B Renal Vein, Left C Common Iliac Vein, Right D Common Iliac Vein, Left F External Iliac Vein, Right G External Iliac Vein, Left H Hypogastric Vein, Right J Hypogastric Vein, Left M Femoral Vein, Right N Femoral Vein, Left P Greater Saphenous Vein, Right Q Greater Saphenous Vein, Left R Lesser Saphenous Vein, Right S Lesser Saphenous Vein, Left T Foot Vein, Right V Foot Vein, Left	0 Open 3 Percutaneous 4 Percutaneous endoscopic	C Extraluminal device D Intraluminal device Z No device	Z No qualifier
Y Lower Vein	0 Open 3 Percutaneous 4 Percutaneous endoscopic	C Extraluminal device D Intraluminal device Z No device	C Hemorrhoidal Plexus Z No qualifier

DIVISION GROUP: (Division), Release
Root Operations involving cutting or separation only.

1ST - 0 Medical and Surgical	EXAMPLE: Adhesiolysis hepatic vein CMS Ex: Carpal tunnel release
2ND - 6 Lower Veins	RELEASE: Freeing a body part from an abnormal physical constraint by cutting or by the use of force.
3RD - N RELEASE	EXPLANATION: None of the body part is taken out …

Body Part – 4TH	Approach – 5TH	Device – 6TH	Qualifier – 7TH
0 Inferior Vena Cava 1 Splenic Vein 2 Gastric Vein 3 Esophageal Vein 4 Hepatic Vein 5 Superior Mesenteric Vein 6 Inferior Mesenteric Vein 7 Colic Vein 8 Portal Vein 9 Renal Vein, Right B Renal Vein, Left C Common Iliac Vein, Right D Common Iliac Vein, Left F External Iliac Vein, Right G External Iliac Vein, Left H Hypogastric Vein, Right J Hypogastric Vein, Left M Femoral Vein, Right N Femoral Vein, Left P Greater Saphenous Vein, Right Q Greater Saphenous Vein, Left R Lesser Saphenous Vein, Right S Lesser Saphenous Vein, Left T Foot Vein, Right V Foot Vein, Left Y Lower Vein	0 Open 3 Percutaneous 4 Percutaneous endoscopic	Z No device	Z No qualifier

---

DEVICE GROUP: (Change), **Insertion, Removal, Replacement, Revision, Supplement**
Root Operations that always involve a device.

1ST - **0** Medical and Surgical	EXAMPLE: Removal IVC filter CMS Ex: Chest tube removal
2ND - **6** Lower Veins	**REMOVAL:** Taking out or off a device from a body part.
3RD - **P REMOVAL**	EXPLANATION: Removal device without reinsertion ...

Body Part – 4TH	Approach – 5TH	Device – 6TH	Qualifier – 7TH
Y Lower Vein	0 Open 3 Percutaneous 4 Percutaneous endoscopic	0 Drainage device 2 Monitoring device 3 Infusion device 7 Autologous tissue substitute C Extraluminal device D Intraluminal device J Synthetic substitute K Nonautologous tissue substitute	Z No qualifier
Y Lower Vein	X External	0 Drainage device 2 Monitoring device 3 Infusion device D Intraluminal device	Z No qualifier

---

OTHER REPAIRS GROUP: (Control), **Repair**
Root Operations that define other repairs.

1ST - **0** Medical and Surgical	EXAMPLE: Suture varicose vein CMS Ex: Suture laceration
2ND - **6** Lower Veins	**REPAIR:** Restoring, to the extent possible, a body part to its normal anatomic structure and function.
3RD - **Q REPAIR**	EXPLANATION: Only when no other root operation applies ...

Body Part – 4TH	Approach – 5TH	Device – 6TH	Qualifier – 7TH
0 Inferior Vena Cava 1 Splenic Vein 2 Gastric Vein 3 Esophageal Vein 4 Hepatic Vein 5 Superior Mesenteric Vein 6 Inferior Mesenteric Vein 7 Colic Vein 8 Portal Vein 9 Renal Vein, Right B Renal Vein, Left C Common Iliac Vein, Right D Common Iliac Vein, Left F External Iliac Vein, Right G External Iliac Vein, Left	H Hypogastric Vein, Right J Hypogastric Vein, Left M Femoral Vein, Right N Femoral Vein, Left P Greater Saphenous Vein, Right Q Greater Saphenous Vein, Left R Lesser Saphenous Vein, Right S Lesser Saphenous Vein, Left T Foot Vein, Right V Foot Vein, Left Y Lower Vein 0 Open 3 Percutaneous 4 Percutaneous endoscopic	Z No device	Z No qualifier

DEVICE GROUP: (Change), Insertion, Removal, Replacement, Revision, Supplement
Root Operations that always involve a device.

1ST - **0** Medical and Surgical	EXAMPLE: Portal vein reconstruction graft CMS Ex: Total hip
2ND - **6** Lower Veins	**REPLACEMENT:** Putting in or on a biological or synthetic material that physically takes the place and/or function of all or a portion of a body part.
3RD - **R REPLACEMENT**	EXPLANATION: Includes taking out body part, or eradication...

Body Part – 4TH	Approach – 5TH	Device – 6TH	Qualifier – 7TH
0 Inferior Vena Cava H Hypogastric Vein, Right 1 Splenic Vein J Hypogastric Vein, Left 2 Gastric Vein M Femoral Vein, Right 3 Esophageal Vein N Femoral Vein, Left 4 Hepatic Vein P Greater Saphenous 5 Superior Mesenteric Vein Vein, Right 6 Inferior Mesenteric Vein Q Greater Saphenous 7 Colic Vein Vein, Left 8 Portal Vein R Lesser Saphenous 9 Renal Vein, Right Vein, Right B Renal Vein, Left S Lesser Saphenous C Common Iliac Vein, Right Vein, Left D Common Iliac Vein, Left T Foot Vein, Right F External Iliac Vein, Right V Foot Vein, Left G External Iliac Vein, Left Y Lower Vein	0 Open 4 Percutaneous endoscopic	7 Autologous tissue substitute J Synthetic substitute K Nonautologous tissue substitute	Z No qualifier

MOVE GROUP: (Reattachment), Reposition, (Transfer), (Transplantation)
Root Operations that put in/put back or move some/all of a body part.

1ST - **0** Medical and Surgical	EXAMPLE: Relocate hypogastric vein CMS Ex: Fracture reduction
2ND - **6** Lower Veins	**REPOSITION:** Moving to its normal location, or other suitable location, all or a portion of a body part.
3RD - **S REPOSITION**	EXPLANATION: May or may not be cut to be moved ...

Body Part – 4TH	Approach – 5TH	Device – 6TH	Qualifier – 7TH
0 Inferior Vena Cava H Hypogastric Vein, Right 1 Splenic Vein J Hypogastric Vein, Left 2 Gastric Vein M Femoral Vein, Right 3 Esophageal Vein N Femoral Vein, Left 4 Hepatic Vein P Greater Saphenous 5 Superior Mesenteric Vein Vein, Right 6 Inferior Mesenteric Vein Q Greater Saphenous 7 Colic Vein Vein, Left 8 Portal Vein R Lesser Saphenous 9 Renal Vein, Right Vein, Right B Renal Vein, Left S Lesser Saphenous C Common Iliac Vein, Right Vein, Left D Common Iliac Vein, Left T Foot Vein, Right F External Iliac Vein, Right V Foot Vein, Left G External Iliac Vein, Left Y Lower Vein	0 Open 3 Percutaneous 4 Percutaneous endoscopic	Z No device	Z No qualifier

LOWER VEINS   0 6 R

DEVICE GROUP: (Change), Insertion, Removal, Replacement, Revision, Supplement
Root Operations that always involve a device.

1ST - **0** Medical and Surgical

2ND - **6** Lower Veins

3RD - **U SUPPLEMENT**

EXAMPLE: Patch graft venoplasty | CMS Ex: Hernia repair with mesh

SUPPLEMENT: Putting in or on biological or synthetic material that physically reinforces and/or augments the function of a portion of a body part.

EXPLANATION: Biological material from same individual ...

Body Part – 4TH		Approach – 5TH	Device – 6TH	Qualifier – 7TH
0 Inferior Vena Cava	H Hypogastric Vein, Right	0 Open	7 Autologous tissue substitute	Z No qualifier
1 Splenic Vein	J Hypogastric Vein, Left	3 Percutaneous	J Synthetic substitute	
2 Gastric Vein	M Femoral Vein, Right	4 Percutaneous endoscopic	K Nonautologous tissue substitute	
3 Esophageal Vein	N Femoral Vein, Left			
4 Hepatic Vein	P Greater Saphenous Vein, Right			
5 Superior Mesenteric Vein	Q Greater Saphenous Vein, Left			
6 Inferior Mesenteric Vein	R Lesser Saphenous Vein, Right			
7 Colic Vein	S Lesser Saphenous Vein, Left			
8 Portal Vein	T Foot Vein, Right			
9 Renal Vein, Right	V Foot Vein, Left			
B Renal Vein, Left	Y Lower Vein			
C Common Iliac Vein, Right				
D Common Iliac Vein, Left				
F External Iliac Vein, Right				
G External Iliac Vein, Left				

TUBULAR GROUP: Bypass, Dilation, Occlusion, Restriction
Root Operations that alter the diameter/route of a tubular body part.

1ST - **0** Medical and Surgical

2ND - **6** Lower Veins

3RD - **V RESTRICTION**

EXAMPLE: Restrictive venous stent | CMS Ex: Cervical cerclage

RESTRICTION: Partially closing an orifice or the lumen of a tubular body part.

EXPLANATION: Natural or artificially created orifice ...

Body Part – 4TH		Approach – 5TH	Device – 6TH	Qualifier – 7TH
0 Inferior Vena Cava	H Hypogastric Vein, Right	0 Open	C Extraluminal device	Z No qualifier
1 Splenic Vein	J Hypogastric Vein, Left	3 Percutaneous	D Intraluminal device	
2 Gastric Vein	M Femoral Vein, Right	4 Percutaneous endoscopic	Z No device	
3 Esophageal Vein	N Femoral Vein, Left			
4 Hepatic Vein	P Greater Saphenous Vein, Right			
5 Superior Mesenteric Vein	Q Greater Saphenous Vein, Left			
6 Inferior Mesenteric Vein	R Lesser Saphenous Vein, Right			
7 Colic Vein	S Lesser Saphenous Vein, Left			
8 Portal Vein	T Foot Vein, Right			
9 Renal Vein, Right	V Foot Vein, Left			
B Renal Vein, Left	Y Lower Vein			
C Common Iliac Vein, Right				
D Common Iliac Vein, Left				
F External Iliac Vein, Right				
G External Iliac Vein, Left				

DEVICE GROUP: (Change), Insertion, Removal, Replacement, Revision, Supplement			
Root Operations that always involve a device.			

1ST - 0 Medical and Surgical

2ND - 6 Lower Veins

3RD - W REVISION

EXAMPLE: Reposition IVC filter   CMS Ex: Adjustment pacemaker lead

REVISION: Correcting, to the extent possible, a portion of a malfunctioning device or the position of a displaced device.

EXPLANATION: May replace components of a device ...

Body Part – 4TH	Approach – 5TH	Device – 6TH	Qualifier – 7TH
Y Lower Vein	0 Open 3 Percutaneous 4 Percutaneous endoscopic X External	0 Drainage device 2 Monitoring device 3 Infusion device 7 Autologous tissue substitute C Extraluminal device D Intraluminal device J Synthetic substitute K Nonautologous tissue substitute	Z No qualifier

Educational Annotations | 7 – Lymphatic and Hemic Systems

Body System Specific Educational Annotations for the Lymphatic and Hemic Systems include:

- Anatomy and Physiology Review
- Anatomical Illustrations
- Definitions of Common Procedures
- AHA Coding Clinic® Reference Notations
- Body Part Key Listings
- Device Key Listings
- Device Aggregation Table Listings
- Coding Notes

Anatomy and Physiology Review of Lymphatic and Hemic Systems

BODY PART VALUES – 7 - LYMPHATIC AND HEMIC SYSTEMS

Bone Marrow – ANATOMY – The soft tissue on the inside of bones that is comprised of red and yellow bone marrow tissue. PHYSIOLOGY – Red bone marrow produces red blood cells, platelets, and most white blood cells. Yellow bone marrow has a minor role in cell production and consists primarily of fat cells.

Cisterna Chyli – ANATOMY – The cisterna chyli is a sac-like structure formed by the junction of the lumbar, intestinal, and descending intercostal lymphatic trunks that empties into the thoracic duct. PHYSIOLOGY – The cisterna chyli collects the lymph from the lower body and chyle from the intestines.

Lymphatic – ANATOMY – The general term for structures and tissues of the lymphatic system. The lymphatic system is part of the circulatory system and its major components include: Thymus, spleen, bone marrow, cisterna chyli, thoracic duct, lymph vessels, lymph nodes, and lymph node chains. PHYSIOLOGY – The lymphatic system serves multiple functions including: Immune system defense, draining the interstitial fluid, removing waste products and cellular debris, and maintaining the balance of body fluids.

Spleen – ANATOMY – The spleen is a gland-like organ, located in the upper abdomen behind the stomach and at the tail of the pancreas, and is about 5 inches (13 cm) in length. The spleen contains both white pulp and red pulp. PHYSIOLOGY – The spleen functions as both a large lymph node (white pulp) that filters the blood and produces lymphocytes and monocytes, and as a red blood cell reservoir (red pulp) and disintegrator of worn-out red blood cells. It also plays a role in producing antibodies. Although important, the spleen is not essential to life.

Thoracic Duct – ANATOMY – The largest of the lymphatic vessels extending from the middle lumbar region to the base of the neck. PHYSIOLOGY – The thoracic duct collects most of the body's the lymphatic fluid from the chest down and drains it into the left subclavian vein.

Thymus – ANATOMY – The thymus is the small, flat bi-lobed organ lying behind the sternum, and is composed of lymphoid material. PHYSIOLOGY – The thymus functions substantially during childhood by producing lymphocytes and aids in the development of the individual's immunity.

Anatomical Illustrations of Lymphatic and Hemic Systems

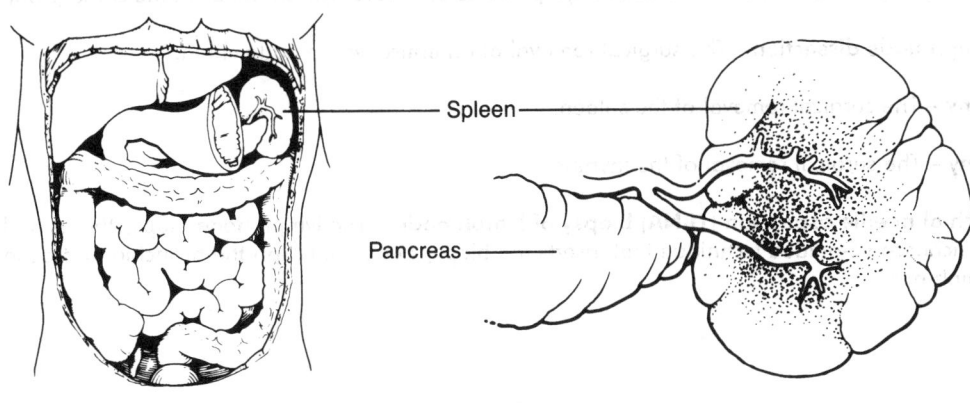

Spleen

Pancreas

SPLEEN

Continued on next page

LYMPHATIC & HEMIC 07

Educational Annotations | 7 – Lymphatic and Hemic Systems

Anatomical Illustrations of Lymphatic and Hemic Systems

Continued from previous page

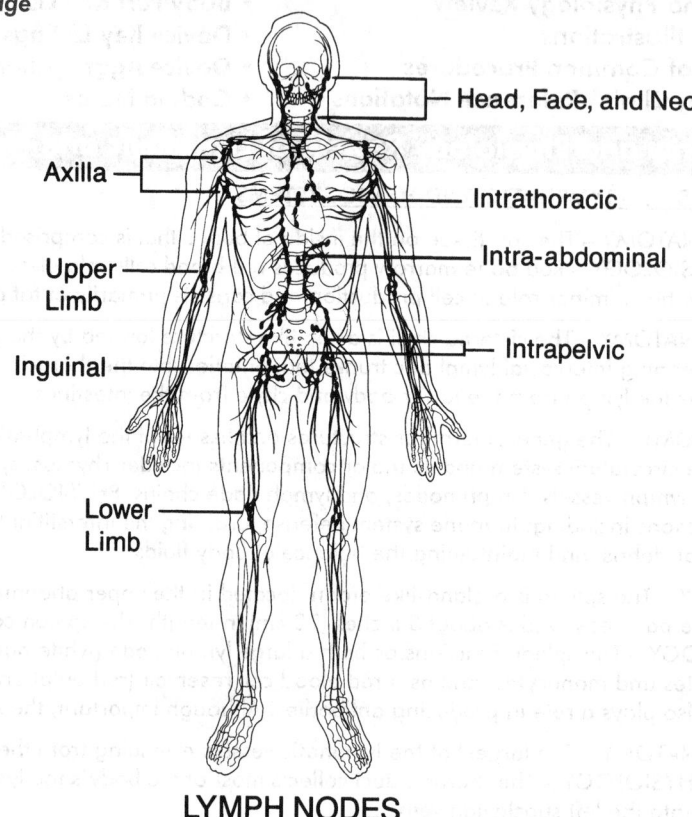

LYMPH NODES

Definitions of Common Procedures of Lymphatic and Hemic Systems

Bone marrow biopsy – The removal of living bone marrow tissue for microscopic examination using a special needle that extracts a core (cylindrical sample) of tissue.

Lymphadenectomy – The surgical removal of a lymph node or several lymph nodes in the same group.

Radical lymph node dissection – The surgical removal of an entire lymph node chain.

Splenectomy – The surgical removal of the spleen.

Thymectomy – The surgical removal of the thymus.

Transbronchial needle aspiration (TBNA) biopsy of lymph node – The lymph node biopsy that is performed using a bronchoscopic-guided technique that inserts the biopsy needle through the bronchial or tracheal wall and into the lymph node.

Educational Annotations | 7 – Lymphatic and Hemic Systems

AHA Coding Clinic® Reference Notations of Lymphatic and Hemic Systems

ROOT OPERATION SPECIFIC - 7 - LYMPHATIC AND HEMIC SYSTEMS
CHANGE - 2
DESTRUCTION - 5
DRAINAGE - 9
EXCISION - B
  Removal of some paratracheal lymph nodes..AHA 14:3Q:p10
  Transbronchial endoscopic needle aspiration biopsy of right lung
    lymph nodes ....AHA 14:1Q:p20
  Transbronchial endoscopic lymph node aspiration biopsy
    (*see also* AHA 13:4Q:p111)..AHA 14:1Q:p26
EXTIRPATION - C
EXTRACTION - D
  Bone marrow biopsy ....AHA 13:4Q:p111
INSERTION - H
INSPECTION - J
OCCLUSION - L
RELEASE - N
REMOVAL - P
REPAIR - Q
REPOSITION - S
RESECTION - T
  Infratemporal fossa malignancy with lymph node level resection................AHA 16:2Q:p12
  Radical resection of level I lymph nodes, bilateral ....AHA 14:3Q:p9
  Resection of lymph node levels..AHA 16:1Q:p30
  Resection of thymus ....AHA 14:3Q:p16
SUPPLEMENT - U
RESTRICTION - V
REVISION - W
TRANSPLANTATION - Y

Body Part Key Listings of Lymphatic and Hemic Systems

See also Body Part Key in Appendix C
Accessory spleen ....*use* Spleen
Anterior (pectoral) lymph node ....*use* Lymphatic, Axillary, Left/Right
Apical (subclavicular) lymph node ....*use* Lymphatic, Axillary, Left/Right
Brachial (lateral) lymph node............................*use* Lymphatic, Axillary, Left/Right
Buccinator lymph node ....*use* Lymphatic, Head
Celiac lymph node ....*use* Lymphatic, Aortic
Central axillary lymph node............................*use* Lymphatic, Axillary, Left/Right
Cervical lymph node ....*use* Lymphatic, Neck, Left/Right
Common iliac (subaortic) lymph node ....*use* Lymphatic, Pelvis
Cubital lymph node ....*use* Lymphatic, Upper Extremity, Left/Right
Deltopectoral (infraclavicular) lymph node ......*use* Lymphatic, Upper Extremity, Left/Right
Epitrochlear lymph node ....*use* Lymphatic, Upper Extremity, Left/Right
Femoral lymph node ....*use* Lymphatic, Lower Extremity, Left/Right
Gastric lymph node ....*use* Lymphatic, Aortic
Gluteal lymph node ....*use* Lymphatic, Pelvis
Hepatic lymph node...*use* Lymphatic, Aortic
Iliac lymph node ....*use* Lymphatic, Pelvis
Continued on next page

Educational Annotations | 7 – Lymphatic and Hemic Systems

Body Part Key Listings of Lymphatic and Hemic Systems

Continued from previous page

Inferior epigastric lymph node	*use* Lymphatic, Pelvis
Inferior mesenteric lymph node	*use* Lymphatic, Mesenteric
Infraauricular lymph node	*use* Lymphatic, Head
Infraclavicular (deltopectoral) lymph node	*use* Lymphatic, Upper Extremity, Left/Right
Infraparotid lymph node	*use* Lymphatic, Head
Intercostal lymph node	*use* Lymphatic, Thorax
Intestinal lymphatic trunk	*use* Cisterna Chyli
Jugular lymph node	*use* Lymphatic, Neck, Left/Right
Lateral (brachial) lymph node	*use* Lymphatic, Axillary, Left/Right
Left jugular trunk	*use* Thoracic Duct
Left subclavian trunk	*use* Thoracic Duct
Lumbar lymph node	*use* Lymphatic, Aortic
Lumbar lymphatic trunk	*use* Cisterna Chyli
Mastoid (postauricular) lymph node	*use* Lymphatic, Neck, Left/Right
Mediastinal lymph node	*use* Lymphatic, Thorax
Obturator lymph node	*use* Lymphatic, Pelvis
Occipital lymph node	*use* Lymphatic, Neck, Left/Right
Pancreaticosplenic lymph node	*use* Lymphatic, Aortic
Paraaortic lymph node	*use* Lymphatic, Aortic
Pararectal lymph node	*use* Lymphatic, Mesenteric
Parasternal lymph node	*use* Lymphatic, Thorax
Paratracheal lymph node	*use* Lymphatic, Thorax
Parotid lymph node	*use* Lymphatic, Head
Pectoral (anterior) lymph node	*use* Lymphatic, Axillary, Left/Right
Popliteal lymph node	*use* Lymphatic, Lower Extremity, Left/Right
Postauricular (mastoid) lymph node	*use* Lymphatic, Neck, Left/Right
Posterior (subscapular) lymph node	*use* Lymphatic, Axillary, Left/Right
Preauricular lymph node	*use* Lymphatic, Head
Retroperitoneal lymph node	*use* Lymphatic, Aortic
Retropharyngeal lymph node	*use* Lymphatic, Neck, Left/Right
Right jugular trunk	*use* Lymphatic, Right Neck
Right lymphatic duct	*use* Lymphatic, Right Neck
Right subclavian trunk	*use* Lymphatic, Right Neck
Sacral lymph node	*use* Lymphatic, Pelvis
Subaortic (common iliac) lymph node	*use* Lymphatic, Pelvis
Subclavicular (apical) lymph node	*use* Lymphatic, Axillary, Left/Right
Submandibular lymph node	*use* Lymphatic, Head
Submaxillary lymph node	*use* Lymphatic, Head
Submental lymph node	*use* Lymphatic, Head
Subparotid lymph node	*use* Lymphatic, Head
Subscapular (posterior) lymph node	*use* Lymphatic, Axillary, Left/Right
Superior mesenteric lymph node	*use* Lymphatic, Mesenteric
Supraclavicular (Virchow's) lymph node	*use* Lymphatic, Neck, Left/Right
Suprahyoid lymph node	*use* Lymphatic, Head
Suprainguinal lymph node	*use* Lymphatic, Pelvis
Supratrochlear lymph node	*use* Lymphatic, Upper Extremity, Left/Right
Thymus gland	*use* Thymus
Tracheobronchial lymph node	*use* Lymphatic, Thorax
Virchow's (supraclavicular) lymph node	*use* Lymphatic, Neck, Left/Right

Educational Annotations | 7 – Lymphatic and Hemic Systems

Device Key Listings of Lymphatic and Hemic Systems

See also Device Key in Appendix D

Autograft ....*use* Autologous Tissue Substitute
Tissue bank graft ....*use* Nonautologous Tissue Substitute

Device Aggregation Table Listings of Lymphatic and Hemic Systems

See also Device Aggregation Table in Appendix E

Specific Device	For Operation	In Body System	General Device
None Listed in Device Aggregation Table for this Body System			

Coding Notes of Lymphatic and Hemic Systems

Body System Specific PCS Reference Manual Exercises

PCS CODE	7 – LYMPHATIC AND HEMIC SYSTEMS EXERCISES
0 7 T 6 0 Z Z	Open left axillary total lymphadenectomy. (Resection is coded for cutting out a chain of lymph nodes.)
0 7 V K 3 D Z	Restriction of thoracic duct with intraluminal stent, percutaneous.

LYMPHATIC & HEMIC 07

Educational Annotations | 7 – Lymphatic and Hemic Systems

NOTES

DEVICE GROUP: Change, Insertion, Removal, (Replacement), Revision, Supplement
Root Operations that always involve a device.

1ST - **0** Medical and Surgical

2ND - **7** Lymphatic and Hemic Systems

3RD - **2 CHANGE**

EXAMPLE: Exchange drain tube | CMS Ex: Changing urinary catheter

CHANGE: Taking out or off a device from a body part and putting back an identical or similar device in or on the same body part without cutting or puncturing the skin or a mucous membrane.

EXPLANATION: ALL Changes use EXTERNAL approach only...

Body Part – 4TH		Approach – 5TH	Device – 6TH	Qualifier – 7TH
K Thoracic Duct	N Lymphatic	X External	0 Drainage device	Z No qualifier
L Cisterna Chyli	P Spleen		Y Other device	
M Thymus	T Bone Marrow			

EXCISION GROUP: Excision, Resection, Destruction, Extraction (Detachment)
Root Operations that take out some or all of a body part.

1ST - **0** Medical and Surgical

2ND - **7** Lymphatic and Hemic Systems

3RD - **5 DESTRUCTION**

EXAMPLE: Radiofrequency node ablation | CMS Ex: Fulguration polyp

DESTRUCTION: Physical eradication of all or a portion of a body part by the direct use of energy, force, or a destructive agent.

EXPLANATION: None of the body part is physically taken out

Body Part – 4TH		Approach – 5TH	Device – 6TH	Qualifier – 7TH
0 Lymphatic, Head	B Lymphatic, Mesenteric	0 Open	Z No device	Z No qualifier
1 Lymphatic, Right Neck	C Lymphatic, Pelvis	3 Percutaneous		
2 Lymphatic, Left Neck	D Lymphatic, Aortic	4 Percutaneous endoscopic		
3 Lymphatic, Right Upper Extremity	F Lymphatic, Right Lower Extremity			
4 Lymphatic, Left Upper Extremity	G Lymphatic, Left Lower Extremity			
5 Lymphatic, Right Axillary	H Lymphatic, Right Inguinal			
6 Lymphatic, Left Axillary	J Lymphatic, Left Inguinal			
7 Lymphatic, Thorax	K Thoracic Duct			
8 Lymphatic, Internal Mammary, Right	L Cisterna Chyli			
9 Lymphatic, Internal Mammary, Left	M Thymus			
	P Spleen			

LYMPHATIC & HEMIC 075

241

DRAINAGE GROUP: Drainage, Extirpation, (Fragmentation)
Root Operations that take out solids/fluids/gases from a body part.

1ST - 0 Medical and Surgical	EXAMPLE: Drainage Cisterna Chyli	CMS Ex: Thoracentesis

2ND - 7 Lymphatic and Hemic Systems

3RD - 9 DRAINAGE

DRAINAGE: Taking or letting out fluids and/or gases from a body part.

EXPLANATION: Qualifier "X Diagnostic" indicates biopsy ...

Body Part – 4TH		Approach – 5TH	Device – 6TH	Qualifier – 7TH
0 Lymphatic, Head 1 Lymphatic, Right Neck 2 Lymphatic, Left Neck 3 Lymphatic, Right Upper Extremity 4 Lymphatic, Left Upper Extremity 5 Lymphatic, Right Axillary 6 Lymphatic, Left Axillary 7 Lymphatic, Thorax 8 Lymphatic, Internal Mammary, Right 9 Lymphatic, Internal Mammary, Left	B Lymphatic, Mesenteric C Lymphatic, Pelvis D Lymphatic, Aortic F Lymphatic, Right Lower Extremity G Lymphatic, Left Lower Extremity H Lymphatic, Right Inguinal J Lymphatic, Left Inguinal K Thoracic Duct L Cisterna Chyli M Thymus P Spleen T Bone Marrow	0 Open 3 Percutaneous 4 Percutaneous endoscopic	0 Drainage device	Z No qualifier
0 Lymphatic, Head 1 Lymphatic, Right Neck 2 Lymphatic, Left Neck 3 Lymphatic, Right Upper Extremity 4 Lymphatic, Left Upper Extremity 5 Lymphatic, Right Axillary 6 Lymphatic, Left Axillary 7 Lymphatic, Thorax 8 Lymphatic, Internal Mammary, Right 9 Lymphatic, Internal Mammary, Left	B Lymphatic, Mesenteric C Lymphatic, Pelvis D Lymphatic, Aortic F Lymphatic, Right Lower Extremity G Lymphatic, Left Lower Extremity H Lymphatic, Right Inguinal J Lymphatic, Left Inguinal K Thoracic Duct L Cisterna Chyli M Thymus P Spleen T Bone Marrow	0 Open 3 Percutaneous 4 Percutaneous endoscopic	Z No device	X Diagnostic Z No qualifier

EXCISION GROUP: Excision, Resection, Destruction, Extraction, (Detachment)
Root Operations that take out some or all of a body part.

| | | EXAMPLE: Removal single lymph node | CMS Ex: Liver biopsy |

1ST - 0 Medical and Surgical

2ND - 7 Lymphatic and Hemic Systems

3RD - B EXCISION

EXCISION: Cutting out or off, without replacement, a portion of a body part.

EXPLANATION: Qualifier "X Diagnostic" indicates biopsy ...

Body Part – 4TH	Approach – 5TH	Device – 6TH	Qualifier – 7TH
0 Lymphatic, Head 1 Lymphatic, Right Neck 2 Lymphatic, Left Neck 3 Lymphatic, Right Upper Extremity 4 Lymphatic, Left Upper Extremity 5 Lymphatic, Right Axillary 6 Lymphatic, Left Axillary 7 Lymphatic, Thorax 8 Lymphatic, Internal Mammary, Right 9 Lymphatic, Internal Mammary, Left B Lymphatic, Mesenteric C Lymphatic, Pelvis D Lymphatic, Aortic F Lymphatic, Right Lower Extremity G Lymphatic, Left Lower Extremity H Lymphatic, Right Inguinal J Lymphatic, Left Inguinal K Thoracic Duct L Cisterna Chyli M Thymus P Spleen	0 Open 3 Percutaneous 4 Percutaneous endoscopic	Z No device	X Diagnostic Z No qualifier

DRAINAGE GROUP: Drainage, Extirpation, (Fragmentation)
Root Operations that take out solids/fluids/gases from a body part.

| | | EXAMPLE: Removal foreign body spleen | CMS Ex: Choledocholithotomy |

1ST - 0 Medical and Surgical

2ND - 7 Lymphatic and Hemic Systems

3RD - C EXTIRPATION

EXTIRPATION: Taking or cutting out solid matter from a body part.

EXPLANATION: Abnormal byproduct or foreign body ...

Body Part – 4TH	Approach – 5TH	Device – 6TH	Qualifier – 7TH
0 Lymphatic, Head 1 Lymphatic, Right Neck 2 Lymphatic, Left Neck 3 Lymphatic, Right Upper Extremity 4 Lymphatic, Left Upper Extremity 5 Lymphatic, Right Axillary 6 Lymphatic, Left Axillary 7 Lymphatic, Thorax 8 Lymphatic, Internal Mammary, Right 9 Lymphatic, Internal Mammary, Left B Lymphatic, Mesenteric C Lymphatic, Pelvis D Lymphatic, Aortic F Lymphatic, Right Lower Extremity G Lymphatic, Left Lower Extremity H Lymphatic, Right Inguinal J Lymphatic, Left Inguinal K Thoracic Duct L Cisterna Chyli M Thymus P Spleen	0 Open 3 Percutaneous 4 Percutaneous endoscopic	Z No device	Z No qualifier

---

EXCISION GROUP: Excision, Resection, Destruction, Extraction, (Detachment)
Root Operations that take out some or all of a body part.

1ST – **0** Medical and Surgical

2ND – **7** Lymphatic and Hemic Systems

3RD – **D EXTRACTION**

EXAMPLE: Bone marrow biopsy | CMS Ex: D&C

__EXTRACTION:__ Pulling or stripping out or off all or a portion of a body part by the use of force.

EXPLANATION: Qualifier "X Diagnostic" indicates biopsy ...

Body Part – 4TH	Approach – 5TH	Device – 6TH	Qualifier – 7TH
Q Bone Marrow, Sternum R Bone Marrow, Iliac S Bone Marrow, Vertebral	0 Open 3 Percutaneous	Z No device	X Diagnostic Z No qualifier

---

DEVICE GROUP: Change, Insertion, Removal, (Replacement), Revision, Supplement
Root Operations that always involve a device.

1ST – **0** Medical and Surgical

2ND – **7** Lymphatic and Hemic Systems

3RD – **H INSERTION**

EXAMPLE: Insertion infusion device | CMS Ex: Central venous catheter

__INSERTION:__ Putting in a nonbiological appliance that monitors, assists, performs, or prevents a physiological function but does not physically take the place of a body part.

EXPLANATION: None

Body Part – 4TH	Approach – 5TH	Device – 6TH	Qualifier – 7TH
K Thoracic Duct L Cisterna Chyli M Thymus N Lymphatic P Spleen	0 Open 3 Percutaneous 4 Percutaneous endoscopic	3 Infusion device	Z No qualifier

---

EXAMINATION GROUP: Inspection, (Map)
Root Operations involving examination only.

1ST – **0** Medical and Surgical

2ND – **7** Lymphatic and Hemic Systems

3RD – **J INSPECTION**

EXAMPLE: Examination of spleen | CMS Ex: Colonoscopy

__INSPECTION:__ Visually and/or manually exploring a body part.

EXPLANATION: Direct or instrumental visualization ...

Body Part – 4TH	Approach – 5TH	Device – 6TH	Qualifier – 7TH
K Thoracic Duct L Cisterna Chyli M Thymus T Bone Marrow	0 Open 3 Percutaneous 4 Percutaneous endoscopic	Z No device	Z No qualifier
N Lymphatic P Spleen	0 Open 3 Percutaneous 4 Percutaneous endoscopic X External	Z No device	Z No qualifier

TUBULAR GROUP: (Bypass), (Dilation), Occlusion, Restriction
Root Operations that alter the diameter/route of a tubular body part.

1ST - **0** Medical and Surgical

2ND - **7** Lymphatic and Hemic Systems

3RD - **L** OCCLUSION

EXAMPLE: Occlusion para-aortic lymph | CMS Ex: Fallopian tube ligation

OCCLUSION: Completely closing an orifice or lumen of a tubular body part.

EXPLANATION: Natural or artificially created orifice ...

Body Part – 4TH		Approach – 5TH	Device – 6TH	Qualifier – 7TH
0 Lymphatic, Head	B Lymphatic, Mesenteric	0 Open	C Extraluminal device	Z No qualifier
1 Lymphatic, Right Neck	C Lymphatic, Pelvis	3 Percutaneous	D Intraluminal device	
2 Lymphatic, Left Neck	D Lymphatic, Aortic	4 Percutaneous endoscopic	Z No device	
3 Lymphatic, Right Upper Extremity	F Lymphatic, Right Lower Extremity			
4 Lymphatic, Left Upper Extremity	G Lymphatic, Left Lower Extremity			
5 Lymphatic, Right Axillary	H Lymphatic, Right Inguinal			
6 Lymphatic, Left Axillary	J Lymphatic, Left Inguinal			
7 Lymphatic, Thorax	K Thoracic Duct			
8 Lymphatic, Internal Mammary, Right	L Cisterna Chyli			
9 Lymphatic, Internal Mammary, Left				

DIVISION GROUP: (Division), Release
Root Operations involving cutting or separation only.

1ST - **0** Medical and Surgical

2ND - **7** Lymphatic and Hemic Systems

3RD - **N** RELEASE

EXAMPLE: Lysis of splenic adhesions | CMS Ex: Carpal tunnel release

RELEASE: Freeing a body part from an abnormal physical constraint by cutting or by the use of force.

EXPLANATION: None of the body part is taken out ...

Body Part – 4TH		Approach – 5TH	Device – 6TH	Qualifier – 7TH
0 Lymphatic, Head	B Lymphatic, Mesenteric	0 Open	Z No device	Z No qualifier
1 Lymphatic, Right Neck	C Lymphatic, Pelvis	3 Percutaneous		
2 Lymphatic, Left Neck	D Lymphatic, Aortic	4 Percutaneous endoscopic		
3 Lymphatic, Right Upper Extremity	F Lymphatic, Right Lower Extremity			
4 Lymphatic, Left Upper Extremity	G Lymphatic, Left Lower Extremity			
5 Lymphatic, Right Axillary	H Lymphatic, Right Inguinal			
6 Lymphatic, Left Axillary	J Lymphatic, Left Inguinal			
7 Lymphatic, Thorax	K Thoracic Duct			
8 Lymphatic, Internal Mammary, Right	L Cisterna Chyli			
9 Lymphatic, Internal Mammary, Left	M Thymus			
	P Spleen			

LYMPHATIC & HEMIC 07N

DEVICE GROUP: Change, Insertion, Removal, (Replacement), Revision, Supplement
Root Operations that always involve a device.

1ST - 0 Medical and Surgical	EXAMPLE: Removal drain tube	CMS Ex: Chest tube removal
2ND - 7 Lymphatic and Hemic Systems	**REMOVAL:** Taking out or off a device from a body part.	
3RD - P REMOVAL	EXPLANATION: Removal device without reinsertion ...	

Body Part – 4TH	Approach – 5TH	Device – 6TH	Qualifier – 7TH
K Thoracic Duct L Cisterna Chyli N Lymphatic	0 Open 3 Percutaneous 4 Percutaneous endoscopic	0 Drainage device 3 Infusion device 7 Autologous tissue substitute C Extraluminal device D Intraluminal device J Synthetic substitute K Nonautologous tissue substitute	Z No qualifier
K Thoracic Duct L Cisterna Chyli N Lymphatic	X External	0 Drainage device 3 Infusion device D Intraluminal device	Z No qualifier
M Thymus P Spleen	0 Open 3 Percutaneous 4 Percutaneous endoscopic X External	0 Drainage device 3 Infusion device	Z No qualifier
T Bone Marrow	0 Open 3 Percutaneous 4 Percutaneous endoscopic X External	0 Drainage device	Z No qualifier

OTHER REPAIRS GROUP: (Control), Repair
Root Operations that define other repairs.

1ST – **0** Medical and Surgical

2ND – **7** Lymphatic and Hemic Systems

3RD – **Q REPAIR**

EXAMPLE: Splenorrhaphy | CMS Ex: Suture laceration

REPAIR: Restoring, to the extent possible, a body part to its normal anatomic structure and function.

EXPLANATION: Only when no other root operation applies ...

Body Part – 4TH		Approach – 5TH	Device – 6TH	Qualifier – 7TH
0 Lymphatic, Head	B Lymphatic, Mesenteric	0 Open	Z No device	Z No qualifier
1 Lymphatic, Right Neck	C Lymphatic, Pelvis	3 Percutaneous		
2 Lymphatic, Left Neck	D Lymphatic, Aortic	4 Percutaneous endoscopic		
3 Lymphatic, Right Upper Extremity	F Lymphatic, Right Lower Extremity			
4 Lymphatic, Left Upper Extremity	G Lymphatic, Left Lower Extremity			
5 Lymphatic, Right Axillary	H Lymphatic, Right Inguinal			
6 Lymphatic, Left Axillary	J Lymphatic, Left Inguinal			
7 Lymphatic, Thorax	K Thoracic Duct			
8 Lymphatic, Internal Mammary, Right	L Cisterna Chyli			
	M Thymus			
9 Lymphatic, Internal Mammary, Left	P Spleen			

MOVE GROUP: (Reattachment), Reposition, (Transfer), Transplantation
Root Operations that put in/put back or move some/all of a body part.

1ST – **0** Medical and Surgical

2ND – **7** Lymphatic and Hemic Systems

3RD – **S REPOSITION**

EXAMPLE: Relocation spleen | CMS Ex: Fracture reduction

REPOSITION: Moving to its normal location, or other suitable location, all or a portion of a body part.

EXPLANATION: May or may not be cut to be moved ...

Body Part – 4TH	Approach – 5TH	Device – 6TH	Qualifier – 7TH
M Thymus	0 Open	Z No device	Z No qualifier
P Spleen			

LYMPHATIC & HEMIC **07S**

EXCISION GROUP: Excision, Resection, Destruction, Extraction, (Detachment)
Root Operations that take out some or all of a body part.

1ST - 0 Medical and Surgical

2ND - 7 Lymphatic and Hemic Systems

3RD - T RESECTION

EXAMPLE: Excision lymph node chain	CMS Ex: Cholecystectomy

RESECTION: Cutting out or off, without replacement, all of a body part.

EXPLANATION: None

Body Part – 4TH		Approach – 5TH	Device – 6TH	Qualifier – 7TH
0 Lymphatic, Head	B Lymphatic, Mesenteric	0 Open	Z No device	Z No qualifier
1 Lymphatic, Right Neck	C Lymphatic, Pelvis	4 Percutaneous		
2 Lymphatic, Left Neck	D Lymphatic, Aortic	endoscopic		
3 Lymphatic, Right Upper Extremity	F Lymphatic, Right Lower Extremity			
4 Lymphatic, Left Upper Extremity	G Lymphatic, Left Lower Extremity			
5 Lymphatic, Right Axillary	H Lymphatic, Right Inguinal			
6 Lymphatic, Left Axillary	J Lymphatic, Left Inguinal			
7 Lymphatic, Thorax	K Thoracic Duct			
8 Lymphatic, Internal Mammary, Right	L Cisterna Chyli			
9 Lymphatic, Internal Mammary, Left	M Thymus			
	P Spleen			

DEVICE GROUP: Change, Insertion, Removal, (Replacement), Revision, Supplement
Root Operations that always involve a device.

1ST - 0 Medical and Surgical

2ND - 7 Lymphatic and Hemic Systems

3RD - U SUPPLEMENT

EXAMPLE: Overlay splenic graft	CMS Ex: Hernia repair with mesh

SUPPLEMENT: Putting in or on biological or synthetic material that physically reinforces and/or augments the function of a portion of a body part.

EXPLANATION: Biological material from same individual ...

Body Part – 4TH		Approach – 5TH	Device – 6TH	Qualifier – 7TH
0 Lymphatic, Head	B Lymphatic, Mesenteric	0 Open	7 Autologous tissue substitute	Z No qualifier
1 Lymphatic, Right Neck	C Lymphatic, Pelvis	4 Percutaneous	J Synthetic substitute	
2 Lymphatic, Left Neck	D Lymphatic, Aortic	endoscopic	K Nonautologous tissue substitute	
3 Lymphatic, Right Upper Extremity	F Lymphatic, Right Lower Extremity			
4 Lymphatic, Left Upper Extremity	G Lymphatic, Left Lower Extremity			
5 Lymphatic, Right Axillary	H Lymphatic, Right Inguinal			
6 Lymphatic, Left Axillary	J Lymphatic, Left Inguinal			
7 Lymphatic, Thorax	K Thoracic Duct			
8 Lymphatic, Internal Mammary, Right	L Cisterna Chyli			
9 Lymphatic, Internal Mammary, Left				

LYMPHATIC & HEMIC 07T

TUBULAR GROUP: (Bypass), (Dilation), **Occlusion, Restriction**
Root Operations that alter the diameter/route of a tubular body part.

1ST - **0** Medical and Surgical	EXAMPLE: Thoracic duct restrictive stent　｜　CMS Ex: Cervical cerclage
2ND - **7** Lymphatic and Hemic Systems	**RESTRICTION:** Partially closing an orifice or the lumen of a tubular body part.
3RD - **V RESTRICTION**	EXPLANATION: Natural or artificially created orifice ...

Body Part – 4TH		Approach – 5TH	Device – 6TH	Qualifier – 7TH
0　Lymphatic, Head	B　Lymphatic, Mesenteric	0　Open	C　Extraluminal device	Z　No qualifier
1　Lymphatic, Right Neck	C　Lymphatic, Pelvis	3　Percutaneous	D　Intraluminal device	
2　Lymphatic, Left Neck	D　Lymphatic, Aortic	4　Percutaneous endoscopic	Z　No device	
3　Lymphatic, Right Upper Extremity	F　Lymphatic, Right Lower Extremity			
4　Lymphatic, Left Upper Extremity	G　Lymphatic, Left Lower Extremity			
5　Lymphatic, Right Axillary	H　Lymphatic, Right Inguinal			
6　Lymphatic, Left Axillary	J　Lymphatic, Left Inguinal			
7　Lymphatic, Thorax	K　Thoracic Duct			
8　Lymphatic, Internal Mammary, Right	L　Cisterna Chyli			
9　Lymphatic, Internal Mammary, Left				

LYMPHATIC & HEMIC 0 7 V

DEVICE GROUP: Change, Insertion, Removal, (Replacement), Revision, Supplement
Root Operations that always involve a device.

1ST - 0 Medical and Surgical	EXAMPLE: Reposition drainage tube	CMS Ex: Adjustment pacemaker lead

2ND - 7 Lymphatic and Hemic Systems

3RD - W REVISION

REVISION: Correcting, to the extent possible, a portion of a malfunctioning device or the position of a displaced device.

EXPLANATION: May replace components of a device ...

Body Part – 4TH	Approach – 5TH	Device – 6TH	Qualifier – 7TH
K Thoracic Duct L Cisterna Chyli N Lymphatic	0 Open 3 Percutaneous 4 Percutaneous endoscopic X External	0 Drainage device 3 Infusion device 7 Autologous tissue substitute C Extraluminal device D Intraluminal device J Synthetic substitute K Nonautologous tissue substitute	Z No qualifier
M Thymus P Spleen	0 Open 3 Percutaneous 4 Percutaneous endoscopic X External	0 Drainage device 3 Infusion device	Z No qualifier
T Bone Marrow	0 Open 3 Percutaneous 4 Percutaneous endoscopic X External	0 Drainage device	Z No qualifier

MOVE GROUP: (Reattachment), Reposition, (Transfer), Transplantation
Root Operations that put in/put back or move some/all of a body part.

1ST - 0 Medical and Surgical	EXAMPLE: Spleen transplant	CMS Ex: Kidney transplant

2ND - 7 Lymphatic and Hemic Systems

3RD - Y TRANSPLANTATION

TRANSPLANTATION: Putting in or on all or a portion of a living body part taken from another individual or animal to physically take the place and/or function of all or a portion of a similar body part.

EXPLANATION: May take over all or part of its function ...

Body Part – 4TH	Approach – 5TH	Device – 6TH	Qualifier – 7TH
M Thymus P Spleen	0 Open	Z No device	0 Allogeneic 1 Syngeneic 2 Zooplastic

Educational Annotations | 8 – Eye

Body System Specific Educational Annotations for the Eye include:

- Anatomy and Physiology Review
- Anatomical Illustrations
- Definitions of Common Procedures
- AHA Coding Clinic® Reference Notations
- Body Part Key Listings
- Device Key Listings
- Device Aggregation Table Listings
- Coding Notes

Anatomy and Physiology Review of Eye

BODY PART VALUES – 8 - EYE

Anterior Chamber – The anterior chamber contains the watery fluid between the iris and cornea.

Choroid – ANATOMY – The choroid is the vascular layer lying between the retina and the sclera that contains the dark brown pigment. PHYSIOLOGY – The choroid functions as a vascular blood supply to most eye structures and absorbs excess light through its dark pigment.

Ciliary Body – The ciliary body consists of smooth muscle with suspensory ligaments which holds the lens in place and adjusts the focus of the lens.

Conjunctiva – ANATOMY – The conjunctiva is the delicate mucous membrane that lines the eyelids and covers the exposed surface of the sclera. PHYSIOLOGY – The conjunctiva is the protective mucous-producing membrane covering the eyelids and exposed portion of the sclera. In addition to providing lubrication, it helps prevent the entry of microorganisms.

Cornea – ANATOMY – The transparent tissue layer that covers the front part of the eye including the iris, pupil, and anterior chamber. PHYSIOLOGY – The cornea refracts and focuses most of the light entering the eye.

Extraocular Muscle – ANATOMY – The extraocular muscles attach the eyeball to the orbit by 6 different muscles. PHYSIOLOGY – The extraocular muscles function to rotate the eyeballs to look at desired objects. Four muscles move the eyeball up, down, right, and left. The other two muscles control the adjustments involved in counteracting head movement while maintaining the target.

Eye – ANATOMY – The eyes are hollow spherical structures about 1 inch (2.5 cm) in diameter, located in and protected by the orbital socket in the skull. PHYSIOLOGY – The eyes are the primary organ of sight, and are directly connected to the brain through the retina and optic nerve.

Eyelid – ANATOMY – The thin folds of skin that cover the eye when muscles draw the eyelids together. PHYSIOLOGY – The eyelids protect the eye from injury and foreign objects and aid in tear flow and distribution.

Iris – ANATOMY – The iris is a muscular diaphragm that controls the dilation of the pupil. PHYSIOLOGY – The iris contracts or dilates, allowing for varying amounts of light to enter the eye and retina.

Lacrimal Duct – ANATOMY – The lacrimal duct is located at the inner lower corner of each eye and connects the lacrimal sac with the nasal cavity. PHYSIOLOGY – The lacrimal duct drains the tears from the eyes into the nasal cavities.

Lacrimal Gland – ANATOMY – The lacrimal glands are almond-shaped glands located in the upper outer corner of each orbit. PHYSIOLOGY – The lacrimal glands produce the tears that function to keep protective fluid on the conjunctiva and cornea.

Lens – ANATOMY – The crystalline lens is a transparent elastic, biconvex structure whose shape is controlled by the action of ciliary muscles. PHYSIOLOGY – The lens and cornea refract light waves to focus them on the retina.

Retina – ANATOMY – The retina is the inner layer of the eye and is continuous with the optic nerve. It contains the visual receptor cells including the rods and cones. PHYSIOLOGY – The rods are responsible for colorless vision, like in dim light, and the cones are responsible for color vision through their light-sensitive pigment sets.

Retinal Vessels – The small arteries and veins that circulate the blood to the retina. The retinal arteries are branches of the ophthalmic artery.

Sclera – ANATOMY – The protective, outer layer of the eye (white of the eye). PHYSIOLOGY – The sclera maintains the shape of the globe and serves as the attachment insertions for the extraocular muscles. Its anterior portion, the cornea, is transparent so that it can refract light entering the eye.

Vitreous – ANATOMY – The clear, gelatinous substance filling the globe of the eye between the lens and retina. PHYSIOLOGY – The thick, gel-like substance maintains the shape of the eye globe.

Educational Annotations | 8 – Eye

Anatomical Illustrations of Eye

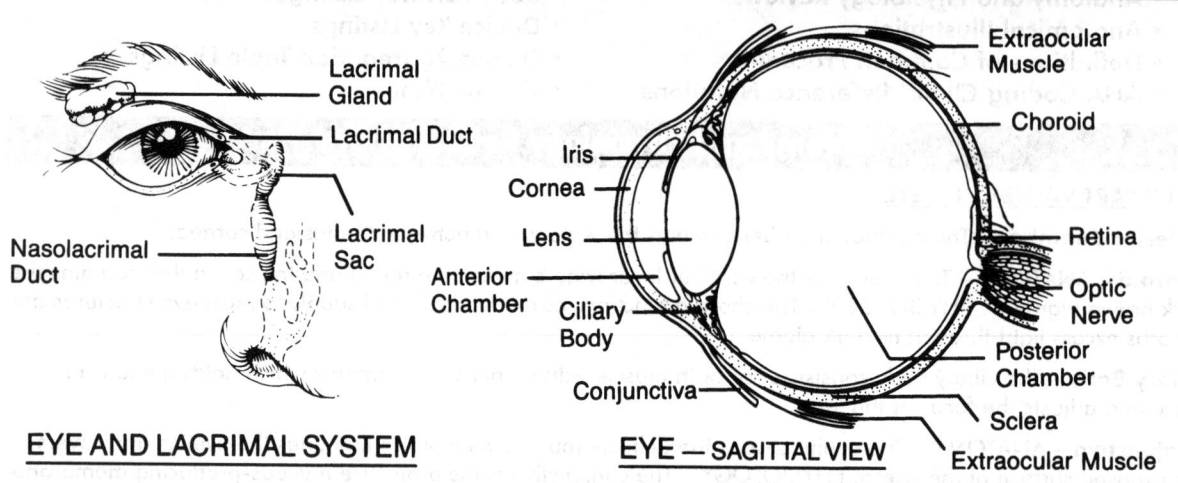

EYE AND LACRIMAL SYSTEM   **EYE — SAGITTAL VIEW**

Definitions of Common Procedures – Body System Specific

Blepharoplasty – The plastic surgical correction of eyelid defects and deformities. It may also be done for cosmetic reasons.

Cataract extraction – The surgical removal of a cloudy lens (normally clear) that is most often immediately replaced with an artificial lens substitute.

Conjunctivoplasty – The surgical procedure to correct a conjunctival defect or conjunctivochalasis.

Corneal transplant – The replacement of the cornea with a donor cornea graft. Also referred to as a keratoplasty.

Dacryocystorhinostomy – The surgical creation of a communicating passage between the lacrimal sac and the nasal cavity to restore the flow of tears.

Enucleation of eyeball – The surgical removal of the entire eyeball (globe) that leaves the eyelids and eye socket structures intact.

Evisceration of eyeball – The surgical removal of the iris, cornea, lens, retina, and vitreous while leaving the sclera, optic nerve, and extraocular eye muscles intact so that an artificial eye prosthesis (integrated orbital implant) moves naturally with the other eye.

Exenteration of eyeball – The surgical removal of all of the contents of the eye socket including the extraocular muscles and often including the eyelids.

Scleral buckling – The surgical placement of synthetic material around the eyeball to create an inward indentation of the sclera from the exterior creating a ridge (or buckle) that corrects the effects of retinal detachment.

Strabismus surgery – The surgical correction of strabismus by repositioning, shortening, or lengthening of one or more of the extraocular eye muscles.

Educational Annotations | 8 – Eye

AHA Coding Clinic® Reference Notations of Eye

ROOT OPERATION SPECIFIC - 8 - EYE
ALTERATION - 0
BYPASS - 1
CHANGE - 2
DESTRUCTION - 5
DILATION - 7
DRAINAGE - 9
    Laser trabeculoplasty ....AHA 16:2Q:p21
EXCISION - B
    Core vitrectomy with gas replacement ....AHA 14:4Q:p35
    Posterior pars plana vitrectomy..AHA 14:4Q:p36
EXTIRPATION - C
EXTRACTION - D
FRAGMENTATION - F
INSERTION - H
INSPECTION - J
    Unsuccessful removal of foreign body of eye ....AHA 15:1Q:p35
OCCLUSION - L
REATTACHMENT - M
RELEASE - N
    Lysis of iris adhesions...AHA 15:2Q:p24
REMOVAL - P
REPAIR - Q
REPLACEMENT - R
    Penetrating keratoplasty with anterior segment reconstruction ....AHA 15:2Q:p24
    Penetrating keratoplasty with viscoelastic filling ....AHA 15:2Q:p25
REPOSITION - S
RESECTION - T
    Radical resection of eyelid and orbital tumor ....AHA 15:2Q:p12
SUPPLEMENT - U
    Amniotic membrane corneal transplantation ....AHA 14:3Q:p31
RESTRICTION - V
REVISION - W
TRANSFER - X

Body Part Key Listings of Eye

See also Body Part Key in Appendix C
Aqueous humour ....*use* Anterior Chamber, Left/Right
Ciliary body ....*use* Eye, Left/Right
Fovea ....*use* Retina, Left/Right
Inferior oblique muscle ....*use* Extraocular Muscle, Left/Right
Inferior rectus muscle........................*use* Extraocular Muscle, Left/Right
Inferior tarsal plate ....*use* Lower Eyelid, Left/Right
Lacrimal canaliculus...........................*use* Lacrimal Duct, Left/Right
Lacrimal punctum ....*use* Lacrimal Duct, Left/Right
Lacrimal sac ....*use* Lacrimal Duct, Left/Right
Lateral canthus..................................*use* Upper Eyelid, Left/Right
Lateral rectus muscle ....*use* Extraocular Muscle, Left/Right
Levator palpebrae superioris muscle ....*use* Upper Eyelid, Left/Right
Macula ....*use* Retina, Left/Right
Medial canthus..................................*use* Lower Eyelid, Left/Right
Medial rectus muscle ....*use* Extraocular Muscle, Left/Right
Continued on next page

Educational Annotations | 8 – Eye

Body Part Key Listings of Eye

Continued from previous page

Nasolacrimal duct	*use* Lacrimal Duct, Left/Right
Optic disc	*use* Retina, Left/Right
Orbicularis oculi muscle	*use* Upper Eyelid, Left/Right
Plica semilunaris	*use* Conjunctiva, Left/Right
Posterior chamber	*use* Eye, Left/Right
Superior oblique muscle	*use* Extraocular Muscle, Left/Right
Superior rectus muscle	*use* Extraocular Muscle, Left/Right
Superior tarsal plate	*use* Upper Eyelid, Left/Right
Vitreous body	*use* Vitreous, Left/Right
Zonule of Zinn	*use* Lens, Left/Right

Device Key Listings of Eye

See also Device Key in Appendix D

Autograft	*use* Autologous Tissue Substitute
Brachytherapy seeds	*use* Radioactive Element
Ex-PRESS™ mini glaucoma shunt	*use* Synthetic Substitute
Implantable Miniature Telescope™ (IMT)	*use* Synthetic Substitute, Intraocular Telescope for Replacement in Eye
Tissue bank graft	*use* Nonautologous Tissue Substitute

Device Aggregation Table Listings of Eye

See also Device Aggregation Table in Appendix E

Specific Device	For Operation	In Body System	General Device	
Epiretinal Visual Prosthesis	All applicable	Eye	J	Synthetic Substitute
Synthetic Substitute, Intraocular Telescope	Replacement	Eye	J	Synthetic Substitute

Coding Notes of Eye

Body System Specific PCS Reference Manual Exercises

PCS CODE	8 – EYE EXERCISES
0 8 5 G 3 Z Z	Laser coagulation of right retinal vessel hemorrhage, percutaneous. (The "Retinal Vessel" body part values are in the "Eye" body system.)
0 8 7 X 7 D Z	Trans-nasal dilation and stent placement in right lacrimal duct.
0 8 C 8 X Z Z	Removal of foreign body, right cornea.
0 8 C X 0 Z Z	Incision and removal of right lacrimal duct stone.
0 8 D J 3 Z Z	Extraction of right intraocular lens without replacement, percutaneous.
0 8 R 8 3 K Z	Penetrating keratoplasty of right cornea with donor matched cornea, percutaneous approach.
0 8 R J 3 J Z	Percutaneous phacoemulsification of right eye cataract with prosthetic lens insertion.
0 8 U 9 X 7 Z	Onlay lamellar keratoplasty of left cornea using autograft, external approach.
0 8 V X 7 D Z	Non-incisional, trans-nasal placement of restrictive stent in right lacrimal duct.

OTHER OBJECTIVES GROUP: Alteration, (Creation), (Fusion)
Root Operations that define other objectives.

1ST - **0** Medical and Surgical

2ND - **8** Eye

3RD - **0 ALTERATION**

EXAMPLE: Cosmetic blepharoplasty | CMS Ex: Face lift

ALTERATION: Modifying the anatomic structure of a body part without affecting the function of the body part.

EXPLANATION: Principal purpose is to improve appearance

Body Part – 4TH	Approach – 5TH	Device – 6TH	Qualifier – 7TH
N Upper Eyelid, Right P Upper Eyelid, Left Q Lower Eyelid, Right R Lower Eyelid, Left	0 Open 3 Percutaneous X External	7 Autologous tissue substitute J Synthetic substitute K Nonautologous tissue substitute Z No device	Z No qualifier

TUBULAR GROUP: Bypass, Dilation, Occlusion, Restriction
Root Operations that alter the diameter/route of a tubular body part.

1ST - **0** Medical and Surgical

2ND - **8** Eye

3RD - **1 BYPASS**

EXAMPLE: Dacryocystorhinostomy | CMS Ex: Coronary artery bypass

BYPASS: Altering the route of passage of the contents of a tubular body part.

EXPLANATION: Rerouting contents to a downstream part ...

Body Part – 4TH	Approach – 5TH	Device – 6TH	Qualifier – 7TH
2 Anterior Chamber, Right 3 Anterior Chamber, Left	3 Percutaneous	J Synthetic substitute K Nonautologous tissue substitute Z No device	4 Sclera
X Lacrimal Duct, Right Y Lacrimal Duct, Left	0 Open 3 Percutaneous	J Synthetic substitute K Nonautologous tissue substitute Z No device	3 Nasal Cavity

DEVICE GROUP: Change, Insertion, Removal, Replacement, Revision, Supplement
Root Operations that always involve a device.

1ST - **0** Medical and Surgical

2ND - **8** Eye

3RD - **2 CHANGE**

EXAMPLE: Exchange drain tube | CMS Ex: Changing urinary catheter

CHANGE: Taking out or off a device from a body part and putting back an identical or similar device in or on the same body part without cutting or puncturing the skin or a mucous membrane.

EXPLANATION: ALL Changes use EXTERNAL approach only...

Body Part – 4TH	Approach – 5TH	Device – 6TH	Qualifier – 7TH
0 Eye, Right 1 Eye, Left	X External	0 Drainage device Y Other device	Z No qualifier

EXCISION GROUP: Excision, Resection, Destruction, Extraction, (Detachment)
Root Operations that take out some or all of a body part.

1ST - 0 Medical and Surgical	EXAMPLE: Cryoablation eyelid lesion	CMS Ex: Fulguration polyp
2ND - 8 Eye	**DESTRUCTION:** Physical eradication of all or a portion of a body part by the direct use of energy, force, or a destructive agent.	
3RD - 5 DESTRUCTION	EXPLANATION: None of the body part is physically taken out	

Body Part – 4TH		Approach – 5TH	Device – 6TH	Qualifier – 7TH
0 Eye, Right 1 Eye, Left 6 Sclera, Right 7 Sclera, Left	8 Cornea, Right 9 Cornea, Left S Conjunctiva, Right T Conjunctiva, Left	X External	Z No device	Z No qualifier
2 Anterior Chamber, Right 3 Anterior Chamber, Left 4 Vitreous, Right 5 Vitreous, Left C Iris, Right D Iris, Left	E Retina, Right F Retina, Left G Retinal Vessel, Right H Retinal Vessel, Left J Lens, Right K Lens, Left	3 Percutaneous	Z No device	Z No qualifier
A Choroid, Right B Choroid, Left L Extraocular Muscle, Right	M Extraocular Muscle, Left V Lacrimal Gland, Right W Lacrimal Gland, Left	0 Open 3 Percutaneous	Z No device	Z No qualifier
N Upper Eyelid, Right P Upper Eyelid, Left Q Lower Eyelid, Right R Lower Eyelid, Left		0 Open 3 Percutaneous X External	Z No device	Z No qualifier
X Lacrimal Duct, Right Y Lacrimal Duct, Left		0 Open 3 Percutaneous 7 Via natural or artificial opening 8 Via natural or artificial opening endoscopic	Z No device	Z No qualifier

TUBULAR GROUP: Bypass, Dilation, Occlusion, Restriction
Root Operations that alter the diameter/route of a tubular body part.

1ST - 0 Medical and Surgical	EXAMPLE: Dilation lacrimal duct	CMS Ex: Transluminal angioplasty
2ND - 8 Eye	**DILATION:** Expanding an orifice or the lumen of a tubular body part.	
3RD - 7 DILATION	EXPLANATION: By force (stretching) or cutting ...	

Body Part – 4TH	Approach – 5TH	Device – 6TH	Qualifier – 7TH
X Lacrimal Duct, Right Y Lacrimal Duct, Left	0 Open 3 Percutaneous 7 Via natural or artificial opening 8 Via natural or artificial opening endoscopic	D Intraluminal device Z No device	Z No qualifier

DRAINAGE GROUP: Drainage, Extirpation, Fragmentation
Root Operations that take out solids/fluids/gases from a body part.

1ST - 0 Medical and Surgical	EXAMPLE: Drainage of lacrimal gland	CMS Ex: Thoracentesis

2ND - 8 Eye

3RD - 9 DRAINAGE

DRAINAGE: Taking or letting out fluids and/or gases from a body part.

EXPLANATION: Qualifier "X Diagnostic" indicates biopsy …

Body Part – 4TH		Approach – 5TH	Device – 6TH	Qualifier – 7TH
0 Eye, Right 1 Eye, Left 6 Sclera, Right 7 Sclera, Left	8 Cornea, Right 9 Cornea, Left S Conjunctiva, Right T Conjunctiva, Left	X External	0 Drainage device	Z No qualifier
0 Eye, Right 1 Eye, Left 6 Sclera, Right 7 Sclera, Left	8 Cornea, Right 9 Cornea, Left S Conjunctiva, Right T Conjunctiva, Left	X External	Z No device	X Diagnostic Z No qualifier
2 Anterior Chamber, Right 3 Anterior Chamber, Left 4 Vitreous, Right 5 Vitreous, Left C Iris, Right D Iris, Left	E Retina, Right F Retina, Left G Retinal Vessel, Right H Retinal Vessel, Left J Lens, Right K Lens, Left	3 Percutaneous	0 Drainage device	Z No qualifier
2 Anterior Chamber, Right 3 Anterior Chamber, Left 4 Vitreous, Right 5 Vitreous, Left C Iris, Right D Iris, Left	E Retina, Right F Retina, Left G Retinal Vessel, Right H Retinal Vessel, Left J Lens, Right K Lens, Left	3 Percutaneous	Z No device	X Diagnostic Z No qualifier
A Choroid, Right B Choroid, Left L Extraocular Muscle, Right	M Extraocular Muscle, Left V Lacrimal Gland, Right W Lacrimal Gland, Left	0 Open 3 Percutaneous	0 Drainage device	Z No qualifier
A Choroid, Right B Choroid, Left L Extraocular Muscle, Right	M Extraocular Muscle, Left V Lacrimal Gland, Right W Lacrimal Gland, Left	0 Open 3 Percutaneous	Z No device	X Diagnostic Z No qualifier
N Upper Eyelid, Right P Upper Eyelid, Left Q Lower Eyelid, Right R Lower Eyelid, Left		0 Open 3 Percutaneous X External	0 Drainage device	Z No qualifier
N Upper Eyelid, Right P Upper Eyelid, Left Q Lower Eyelid, Right R Lower Eyelid, Left		0 Open 3 Percutaneous X External	Z No device	X Diagnostic Z No qualifier
X Lacrimal Duct, Right Y Lacrimal Duct, Left		0 Open 3 Percutaneous 7 Via natural or artificial opening 8 Via natural or artificial opening endoscopic	0 Drainage device	Z No qualifier
X Lacrimal Duct, Right Y Lacrimal Duct, Left		0 Open 3 Percutaneous 7 Via natural or artificial opening 8 Via natural or artificial opening endoscopic	Z No device	X Diagnostic Z No qualifier

EYE 089

EXCISION GROUP: Excision, Resection, Destruction, Extraction, (Detachment)
Root Operations that take out some or all of a body part.

1ST - **0** Medical and Surgical	EXAMPLE: Sclerectomy CMS Ex: Liver biopsy
2ND - **8** Eye	**EXCISION:** Cutting out or off, without replacement, a portion of a body part.
3RD - **B EXCISION**	EXPLANATION: Qualifier "X Diagnostic" indicates biopsy …

Body Part – 4TH		Approach – 5TH	Device – 6TH	Qualifier – 7TH
0 Eye, Right 1 Eye, Left N Upper Eyelid, Right	P Upper Eyelid, Left Q Lower Eyelid, Right R Lower Eyelid, Left	0 Open 3 Percutaneous X External	Z No device	X Diagnostic Z No qualifier
4 Vitreous, Right 5 Vitreous, Left C Iris, Right D Iris, Left	E Retina, Right F Retina, Left J Lens, Right K Lens, Left	3 Percutaneous	Z No device	X Diagnostic Z No qualifier
6 Sclera, Right 7 Sclera, Left 8 Cornea, Right	9 Cornea, Left S Conjunctiva, Right T Conjunctiva, Left	X External	Z No device	X Diagnostic Z No qualifier
A Choroid, Right B Choroid, Left L Extraocular Muscle, Right	M Extraocular Muscle, Left V Lacrimal Gland, Right W Lacrimal Gland, Left	0 Open 3 Percutaneous	Z No device	X Diagnostic Z No qualifier
X Lacrimal Duct, Right Y Lacrimal Duct, Left		0 Open 3 Percutaneous 7 Via natural or artificial opening 8 Via natural or artificial opening endoscopic	Z No device	X Diagnostic Z No qualifier

EYE

0
8
B

DRAINAGE GROUP: Drainage, Extirpation, Fragmentation
Root Operations that take out solids/fluids/gases from a body part.

1ST - **0** Medical and Surgical

2ND - **8** Eye

3RD - **C EXTIRPATION**

EXAMPLE: Magnetic extraction, metal splinter | CMS Ex: Choledocholithotomy

EXTIRPATION: Taking or cutting out solid matter from a body part.

EXPLANATION: Abnormal byproduct or foreign body …

Body Part – 4TH		Approach – 5TH	Device – 6TH	Qualifier – 7TH
0 Eye, Right 1 Eye, Left 6 Sclera, Right 7 Sclera, Left	8 Cornea, Right 9 Cornea, Left S Conjunctiva, Right T Conjunctiva, Left	X External	Z No device	Z No qualifier
2 Anterior Chamber, Right 3 Anterior Chamber, Left 4 Vitreous, Right 5 Vitreous, Left C Iris, Right D Iris, Left	E Retina, Right F Retina, Left G Retinal Vessel, Right H Retinal Vessel, Left J Lens, Right K Lens, Left	3 Percutaneous X External	Z No device	Z No qualifier
A Choroid, Right B Choroid, Left L Extraocular Muscle, Right M Extraocular Muscle, Left N Upper Eyelid, Right	P Upper Eyelid, Left Q Lower Eyelid, Right R Lower Eyelid, Left V Lacrimal Gland, Right W Lacrimal Gland, Left	0 Open 3 Percutaneous X External	Z No device	Z No qualifier
X Lacrimal Duct, Right Y Lacrimal Duct, Left		0 Open 3 Percutaneous 7 Via natural or artificial opening 8 Via natural or artificial opening endoscopic	Z No device	Z No qualifier

EYE

0 8 D

EXCISION GROUP: Excision, Resection, Destruction, Extraction, (Detachment)
Root Operations that take out some or all of a body part.

1ST - **0** Medical and Surgical

2ND - **8** Eye

3RD - **D EXTRACTION**

EXAMPLE: Lens extraction without replacement | CMS Ex: D&C

EXTRACTION: Pulling or stripping out or off all or a portion of a body part by the use of force.

EXPLANATION: Qualifier "X Diagnostic" indicates biopsy …

Body Part – 4TH	Approach – 5TH	Device – 6TH	Qualifier – 7TH
8 Cornea, Right 9 Cornea, Left	X External	Z No device	X Diagnostic Z No qualifier
J Lens, Right K Lens, Left	3 Percutaneous	Z No device	Z No qualifier

---

DRAINAGE GROUP: Drainage, Extirpation, Fragmentation
Root Operations that take out solids/fluids/gases from a body part.

1ST - 0 Medical and Surgical 2ND - 8 Eye 3RD - F FRAGMENTATION	EXAMPLE: Lithotripsy, vitreous	CMS Ex: Extracorporeal shockwave lithotripsy
	FRAGMENTATION: Breaking solid matter in a body part into pieces.	
	EXPLANATION: Pieces are not taken out during procedure ...	

Body Part – 4TH	Approach – 5TH	Device – 6TH	Qualifier – 7TH
4 Vitreous, Right 5 Vitreous, Left	3 Percutaneous X External NC*	Z No device	Z No qualifier

NC* – Non-covered by Medicare. See current Medicare Code Editor for details.

DEVICE GROUP: Change, Insertion, Removal, Replacement, Revision, Supplement
Root Operations that always involve a device.

1ST - 0 Medical and Surgical 2ND - 8 Eye 3RD - H INSERTION	EXAMPLE: Implantation EpiRet	CMS Ex: Insertion central venous catheter
	INSERTION: Putting in a nonbiological appliance that monitors, assists, performs, or prevents a physiological function but does not physically take the place of a body part.	
	EXPLANATION: None	

Body Part – 4TH	Approach – 5TH	Device – 6TH	Qualifier – 7TH
0 Eye, Right 1 Eye, Left	0 Open	5 Epiretinal visual prosthesis	Z No qualifier
0 Eye, Right 1 Eye, Left	3 Percutaneous X External	1 Radioactive element 3 Infusion device	Z No qualifier

---

EXAMINATION GROUP: Inspection, (Map)
Root Operations involving examination only.

1ST - 0 Medical and Surgical 2ND - 8 Eye 3RD - J INSPECTION	EXAMPLE: Eye examination	CMS Ex: Colonoscopy
	INSPECTION: Visually and/or manually exploring a body part.	
	EXPLANATION: Direct or instrumental visualization ...	

Body Part – 4TH	Approach – 5TH	Device – 6TH	Qualifier – 7TH
0 Eye, Right 1 Eye, Left J Lens, Right K Lens, Left	X External	Z No device	Z No qualifier
L Extraocular Muscle, Right M Extraocular Muscle, Left	0 Open X External	Z No device	Z No qualifier

EYE

0 8 F

TUBULAR GROUP: Bypass, Dilation, Occlusion, Restriction
Root Operations that alter the diameter/route of a tubular body part.

1ST - 0 Medical and Surgical
2ND - 8 Eye
3RD - L OCCLUSION

EXAMPLE: Punctal occlusion   **CMS Ex: Fallopian tube ligation**

OCCLUSION: Completely closing an orifice or lumen of a tubular body part.

EXPLANATION: Natural or artificially created orifice ...

Body Part – 4TH	Approach – 5TH	Device – 6TH	Qualifier – 7TH
X Lacrimal Duct, Right Y Lacrimal Duct, Left	0 Open 3 Percutaneous	C Extraluminal device D Intraluminal device Z No device	Z No qualifier
X Lacrimal Duct, Right Y Lacrimal Duct, Left	7 Via natural or artificial opening 8 Via natural or artificial opening endoscopic	D Intraluminal device Z No device	Z No qualifier

MOVE GROUP: Reattachment, Reposition, Transfer, (Transplantation)
Root Operations that put in/put back or move some/all of a body part.

1ST - 0 Medical and Surgical
2ND - 8 Eye
3RD - M REATTACHMENT

EXAMPLE: Reattachment avulsed eyelid   **CMS Ex: Reattachment hand**

REATTACHMENT: Putting back in or on all or a portion of a separated body part to its normal location or other suitable location.

EXPLANATION: With/without reconnection of vessels/nerves...

Body Part – 4TH	Approach – 5TH	Device – 6TH	Qualifier – 7TH
N Upper Eyelid, Right P Upper Eyelid, Left Q Lower Eyelid, Right R Lower Eyelid, Left	X External	Z No device	Z No qualifier

DIVISION GROUP: (Division), Release

Root Operations involving cutting or separation only.

1ST - **0** Medical and Surgical	EXAMPLE: Adhesiolysis lateral rectus	CMS Ex: Carpal tunnel release

2ND - **8** Eye

3RD - **N RELEASE**

RELEASE: Freeing a body part from an abnormal physical constraint by cutting or by the use of force.

EXPLANATION: None of the body part is taken out ...

Body Part – 4TH		Approach – 5TH	Device – 6TH	Qualifier – 7TH
0 Eye, Right	8 Cornea, Right	X External	Z No device	Z No qualifier
1 Eye, Left	9 Cornea, Left			
6 Sclera, Right	S Conjunctiva, Right			
7 Sclera, Left	T Conjunctiva, Left			
2 Anterior Chamber, Right	E Retina, Right	3 Percutaneous	Z No device	Z No qualifier
3 Anterior Chamber, Left	F Retina, Left			
4 Vitreous, Right	G Retinal Vessel, Right			
5 Vitreous, Left	H Retinal Vessel, Left			
C Iris, Right	J Lens, Right			
D Iris, Left	K Lens, Left			
A Choroid, Right	M Extraocular Muscle, Left	0 Open	Z No device	Z No qualifier
B Choroid, Left	V Lacrimal Gland, Right	3 Percutaneous		
L Extraocular Muscle, Right	W Lacrimal Gland, Left			
N Upper Eyelid, Right		0 Open	Z No device	Z No qualifier
P Upper Eyelid, Left		3 Percutaneous		
Q Lower Eyelid, Right		X External		
R Lower Eyelid, Left				
X Lacrimal Duct, Right		0 Open	Z No device	Z No qualifier
Y Lacrimal Duct, Left		3 Percutaneous		
		7 Via natural or artificial opening		
		8 Via natural or artificial opening endoscopic		

EYE

08N

DEVICE GROUP: Change, Insertion, Removal, Replacement, Revision, Supplement
Root Operations that always involve a device.

1ST - **0** Medical and Surgical

2ND - **8** Eye

3RD - **P REMOVAL**

EXAMPLE: Removal eye drain tube | **CMS Ex:** Chest tube removal

REMOVAL: Taking out or off a device from a body part.

EXPLANATION: Removal without reinsertion ...

Body Part – 4TH	Approach – 5TH	Device – 6TH	Qualifier – 7TH
0 Eye, Right 1 Eye, Left	0 Open 3 Percutaneous 7 Via natural or artificial opening 8 Via natural or artificial opening endoscopic X External	0 Drainage device 1 Radioactive element 3 Infusion device 7 Autologous tissue substitute C Extraluminal device D Intraluminal device J Synthetic substitute K Nonautologous tissue substitute	Z No qualifier
J Lens, Right K Lens, Left	3 Percutaneous	J Synthetic substitute	Z No qualifier
L Extraocular Muscle, Right M Extraocular Muscle, Left	0 Open 3 Percutaneous	0 Drainage device 7 Autologous tissue substitute J Synthetic substitute K Nonautologous tissue substitute	Z No qualifier

EYE

0
8
P

OTHER REPAIRS GROUP: (Control), **Repair**
Root Operations that define other repairs.

1ST - **0** Medical and Surgical	EXAMPLE: Iris mattress suture	CMS Ex: Suture laceration
2ND - **8** Eye	**REPAIR:** Restoring, to the extent possible, a body part to its normal anatomic structure and function.	
3RD - **Q REPAIR**	EXPLANATION: Only when no other root operation applies ...	

Body Part – 4TH		Approach – 5TH	Device – 6TH	Qualifier – 7TH
0 Eye, Right 1 Eye, Left 6 Sclera, Right 7 Sclera, Left	8 Cornea, Right NC* 9 Cornea, Left NC* S Conjunctiva, Right T Conjunctiva, Left	X External	Z No device	Z No qualifier
2 Anterior Chamber, Right 3 Anterior Chamber, Left 4 Vitreous, Right 5 Vitreous, Left C Iris, Right D Iris, Left	E Retina, Right F Retina, Left G Retinal Vessel, Right H Retinal Vessel, Left J Lens, Right K Lens, Left	3 Percutaneous	Z No device	Z No qualifier
A Choroid, Right B Choroid, Left L Extraocular Muscle, Right	M Extraocular Muscle, Left V Lacrimal Gland, Right W Lacrimal Gland, Left	0 Open 3 Percutaneous	Z No device	Z No qualifier
N Upper Eyelid, Right P Upper Eyelid, Left Q Lower Eyelid, Right R Lower Eyelid, Left		0 Open 3 Percutaneous X External	Z No device	Z No qualifier
X Lacrimal Duct, Right Y Lacrimal Duct, Left		0 Open 3 Percutaneous 7 Via natural or artificial opening 8 Via natural or artificial opening endoscopic	Z No device	Z No qualifier

NC* – Non-covered by Medicare. See current Medicare Code Editor for details.

DEVICE GROUP: Change, Insertion, Removal, Replacement, Revision, Supplement
Root Operations that always involve a device.

1ST - 0 Medical and Surgical			
2ND - 8 Eye			
3RD - R REPLACEMENT			

EXAMPLE: Extraction lens with prosthetic insertion | CMS Ex: Total hip

REPLACEMENT: Putting in or on a biological or synthetic material that physically takes the place and/or function of all or a portion of a body part.

EXPLANATION: Includes taking out body part, or eradication...

Body Part – 4TH	Approach – 5TH	Device – 6TH	Qualifier – 7TH
0 Eye, Right 1 Eye, Left A Choroid, Right B Choroid, Left	0 Open 3 Percutaneous	7 Autologous tissue substitute J Synthetic substitute K Nonautologous tissue substitute	Z No qualifier
4 Vitreous, Right 5 Vitreous, Left C Iris, Right D Iris, Left G Retinal Vessel, Right H Retinal Vessel, Left	3 Percutaneous	7 Autologous tissue substitute J Synthetic substitute K Nonautologous tissue substitute	Z No qualifier
6 Sclera, Right 7 Sclera, Left S Conjunctiva, Right T Conjunctiva, Left	X External	7 Autologous tissue substitute J Synthetic substitute K Nonautologous tissue substitute	Z No qualifier
8 Cornea, Right 9 Cornea, Left	3 Percutaneous X External	7 Autologous tissue substitute J Synthetic substitute K Nonautologous tissue substitute	Z No qualifier
J Lens, Right K Lens, Left	3 Percutaneous	0 Synthetic substitute, intraocular telescope 7 Autologous tissue substitute J Synthetic substitute K Nonautologous tissue substitute	Z No qualifier
N Upper Eyelid, Right P Upper Eyelid, Left Q Lower Eyelid, Right R Lower Eyelid, Left	0 Open 3 Percutaneous X External	7 Autologous tissue substitute J Synthetic substitute K Nonautologous tissue substitute	Z No qualifier
X Lacrimal Duct, Right Y Lacrimal Duct, Left	0 Open 3 Percutaneous 7 Via natural or artificial opening 8 Via natural or artificial opening endoscopic	7 Autologous tissue substitute J Synthetic substitute K Nonautologous tissue substitute	Z No qualifier

EYE   0 8 R

MOVE GROUP: Reattachment, Reposition, Transfer, (Transplantation)
Root Operations that put in/put back or move some/all of a body part.

1ST - **0** Medical and Surgical

2ND - **8** Eye

3RD - **S REPOSITION**

EXAMPLE: Relocation eye muscle (strabismus) | CMS Ex: FX reduction

REPOSITION: Moving to its normal location, or other suitable location, all or a portion of a body part.

EXPLANATION: May or may not be cut to be moved ...

Body Part – 4TH	Approach – 5TH	Device – 6TH	Qualifier – 7TH
C Iris, Right H Retinal Vessel, Left D Iris, Left J Lens, Right G Retinal Vessel, Right K Lens, Left	3 Percutaneous	Z No device	Z No qualifier
L Extraocular Muscle, Right M Extraocular Muscle, Left V Lacrimal Gland, Right W Lacrimal Gland, Left	0 Open 3 Percutaneous	Z No device	Z No qualifier
N Upper Eyelid, Right P Upper Eyelid, Left Q Lower Eyelid, Right R Lower Eyelid, Left	0 Open 3 Percutaneous X External	Z No device	Z No qualifier
X Lacrimal Duct, Right Y Lacrimal Duct, Left	0 Open 3 Percutaneous 7 Via natural or artificial opening 8 Via natural or artificial opening endoscopic	Z No device	Z No qualifier

E Y E

0 8 S

EXCISION GROUP: Excision, Resection, Destruction, Extraction, (Detachment)
Root Operations that take out some or all of a body part.

1ST - 0 Medical and Surgical	**EXAMPLE:** Enucleation eyeball **CMS Ex:** Cholecystectomy
2ND - 8 Eye	**RESECTION:** Cutting out or off, without replacement, all of a body part.
3RD - T RESECTION	**EXPLANATION:** None

Body Part – 4TH		Approach – 5TH	Device – 6TH	Qualifier – 7TH
0 Eye, Right 1 Eye, Left	8 Cornea, Right 9 Cornea, Left	X External	Z No device	Z No qualifier
4 Vitreous, Right 5 Vitreous, Left C Iris, Right	D Iris, Left J Lens, Right K Lens, Left	3 Percutaneous	Z No device	Z No qualifier
L Extraocular Muscle, Right M Extraocular Muscle, Left V Lacrimal Gland, Right W Lacrimal Gland, Left		0 Open 3 Percutaneous	Z No device	Z No qualifier
N Upper Eyelid, Right P Upper Eyelid, Left Q Lower Eyelid, Right R Lower Eyelid, Left		0 Open X External	Z No device	Z No qualifier
X Lacrimal Duct, Right Y Lacrimal Duct, Left		0 Open 3 Percutaneous 7 Via natural or artificial opening 8 Via natural or artificial opening endoscopic	Z No device	Z No qualifier

E Y E

0 8 T

DEVICE GROUP: Change, Insertion, Removal, Replacement, Revision, Supplement
Root Operations that always involve a device.

1ST - **0** Medical and Surgical	EXAMPLE: Scleral buckle with implant — CMS Ex: Hernia repair with mesh
2ND - **8** Eye	**SUPPLEMENT:** Putting in or on biological or synthetic material that physically reinforces and/or augments the function of a portion of a body part.
3RD - **U SUPPLEMENT**	EXPLANATION: Biological material from same individual …

Body Part – 4TH		Approach – 5TH	Device – 6TH	Qualifier – 7TH
0 Eye, Right 1 Eye, Left C Iris, Right D Iris, Left E Retina, Right F Retina, Left	G Retinal Vessel, Right H Retinal Vessel, Left L Extraocular Muscle, Right M Extraocular Muscle, Left	0 Open 3 Percutaneous	7 Autologous tissue substitute J Synthetic substitute K Nonautologous tissue substitute	Z No qualifier
8 Cornea, Right NC* 9 Cornea, Left NC* N Upper Eyelid, Right P Upper Eyelid, Left Q Lower Eyelid, Right R Lower Eyelid, Left		0 Open 3 Percutaneous X External	7 Autologous tissue substitute J Synthetic substitute K Nonautologous tissue substitute	Z No qualifier
X Lacrimal Duct, Right Y Lacrimal Duct, Left		0 Open 3 Percutaneous 7 Via natural or artificial opening 8 Via natural or artificial opening endoscopic	7 Autologous tissue substitute J Synthetic substitute K Nonautologous tissue substitute	Z No qualifier

NC* – Some procedures are considered non-covered by Medicare. See current Medicare Code Editor for details.

TUBULAR GROUP: Bypass, Dilation, Occlusion, Restriction
Root Operations that alter the diameter/route of a tubular body part.

1ST - **0** Medical and Surgical	EXAMPLE: Lacrimal duct restrictive stent — CMS Ex: Cervical cerclage
2ND - **8** Eye	**RESTRICTION:** Partially closing an orifice or the lumen of a tubular body part.
3RD - **V RESTRICTION**	EXPLANATION: Natural or artificially created orifice …

Body Part – 4TH	Approach – 5TH	Device – 6TH	Qualifier – 7TH
X Lacrimal Duct, Right Y Lacrimal Duct, Left	0 Open 3 Percutaneous	C Extraluminal device D Intraluminal device Z No device	Z No qualifier
X Lacrimal Duct, Right Y Lacrimal Duct, Left	7 Via natural or artificial opening 8 Via natural or artificial opening endoscopic	D Intraluminal device Z No device	Z No qualifier

DEVICE GROUP: Change, Insertion, Removal, Replacement, Revision, Supplement
Root Operations that always involve a device.

1ST - 0 Medical and Surgical	EXAMPLE: Reposition prosthetic lens | CMS Ex: Adjustment pacemaker lead
2ND - 8 Eye	**REVISION:** Correcting, to the extent possible, a portion of a malfunctioning device or the position of a displaced device.
3RD - W REVISION	EXPLANATION: May replace components of a device ...

Body Part – 4TH	Approach – 5TH	Device – 6TH	Qualifier – 7TH
0 Eye, Right 1 Eye, Left	0 Open 3 Percutaneous 7 Via natural or artificial opening 8 Via natural or artificial opening endoscopic X External	0 Drainage device 3 Infusion device 7 Autologous tissue substitute C Extraluminal device D Intraluminal device J Synthetic substitute K Nonautologous tissue substitute	Z No qualifier
J Lens, Right K Lens, Left	3 Percutaneous X External	J Synthetic substitute	Z No qualifier
L Extraocular Muscle, Right M Extraocular Muscle, Left	0 Open 3 Percutaneous	0 Drainage device 7 Autologous tissue substitute J Synthetic substitute K Nonautologous tissue substitute	Z No qualifier

MOVE GROUP: Reattachment, Reposition, Transfer, (Transplantation)
Root Operations that put in/put back or move some/all of a body part.

1ST - 0 Medical and Surgical	EXAMPLE: Transfer medial rectus muscle | CMS Ex: Tendon transfer
2ND - 8 Eye	**TRANSFER:** Moving, without taking out, all or a portion of a body part to another location to take over the function of all or a portion of a body part.
3RD - X TRANSFER	EXPLANATION: The body part remains connected ...

Body Part – 4TH	Approach – 5TH	Device – 6TH	Qualifier – 7TH
L Extraocular Muscle, Right M Extraocular Muscle, Left	0 Open 3 Percutaneous	Z No device	Z No qualifier

NOTES

Educational Annotations | 9 – Ear, Nose, Sinus

Body System Specific Educational Annotations for the Ear, Nose, Sinus include:

- Anatomy and Physiology Review
- Anatomical Illustrations
- Definitions of Common Procedures
- AHA Coding Clinic® Reference Notations
- Body Part Key Listings
- Device Key Listings
- Device Aggregation Table Listings
- Coding Notes

Anatomy and Physiology Review of Ear, Nose, Sinus

BODY PART VALUES – 9 - EAR, NOSE, SINUS

Accessory Sinus – A paranasal sinus that is not identified as one of the four paired nasal sinuses (maxillary, frontal, ethmoid, and sphenoid).

Auditory Ossicle – ANATOMY – The three small bones of the middle ear (malleus, incus, and stapes). PHYSIOLOGY – These bones transfer the sound waves from the tympanic membrane to the oval window of the inner ear while modulating and amplifying the sound.

Ear – ANATOMY – The organ of hearing comprised of the external ear (auricle or pinna), middle ear (malleus, incus, and stapes bones), and inner ear (cochlea). PHYSIOLOGY – The external ear collects the sound, the middle ear transfers and amplifies the sound to the inner ear, and the inner ear converts it into neural impulses.

Ethmoid Sinus – The one of four paired, air-filled paranasal sinuses located within the ethmoid bone cavities that lies between the nose and the eyes.

Eustachian Tube – ANATOMY – The Eustachian (auditory) tube connects the middle ear with the nasopharynx. PHYSIOLOGY – The tube allows for proper equalization of atmospheric pressure between the atmosphere and the middle ear, and for mucous drainage from the middle ear.

External Auditory Canal – That cylindrical portion of the external ear that focuses the sound waves onto the tympanic membrane.

External Ear – ANATOMY – The visible outer portion of the ear (auricle or pinna) that includes the ear canal and outer tympanic membrane (ear drum). PHYSIOLOGY – The external ear collects the sound onto the tympanic membrane.

Frontal Sinus – The one of four paired, air-filled paranasal sinuses located above the eye in the frontal bone.

Inner Ear – ANATOMY – The fluid-filled (endolymph) inner ear is that portion behind the middle ear and comprised of the cochlea and the semicircular canals. PHYSIOLOGY – The sound waves travel through the endolymph of the cochlea stimulating millions of hairs that in turn send neural signals through the vestibulo-cochlear nerve to the brain where the brain interprets it as sound. The semicircular canals allow the individual to sense physical balance and motion.

Mastoid Sinus – The numerous, small air-filled cavities within the mastoid process of the temporal bone.

Maxillary Sinus – The largest of the one of four paired, air-filled paranasal sinuses located under the eye in the maxillary bone.

Middle Ear – ANATOMY – The middle ear is the air-filled space behind the tympanic membrane of the external ear that connects the inner ear, mastoid cells, and Eustachian tube. PHYSIOLOGY – The middle ear transfers, modulates, and amplifies the sound to the inner ear.

Nasal Septum – The bone and cartilage that divides the left and right nasal cavities and airways.

Nasal Turbinate – ANATOMY – The cartilage-like mucosal tissue grooves that divide the nasal airways into passages. PHYSIOLOGY – The turbinates assist in directing and smoothing the airflow through the nasal airways. They also sense heat and cold and help regulate the temperature and humidity of the inhaled air.

Nasopharynx – The upper portion of the pharynx from the base of skull and the nasal cavities to the top of the soft palate and the oral portion of the pharynx.

Nose – ANATOMY – The organ of sense of smell in the middle of the face and skull with the external portion extending out from the face. PHYSIOLOGY – The nose contains the organs and tissues (olfactory epithelium) that collect scent molecules and transmit impulses to the brain. The nose also warms, filters, and humidifies the air inhaled into the lungs.

Continued on next page

Educational Annotations | 9 – Ear, Nose, Sinus

Anatomy and Physiology Review of Ear, Nose, Sinus

<u>BODY PART VALUES – 9 - EAR, NOSE, SINUS</u>
Continued from previous page

Sinus – ANATOMY – The group of four paired, air-filled mucous-membrane-lined skull bone cavities (maxillary, frontal, ethmoid, and sphenoid) that are linked to the nasal airways and the mastoid and accessory sinus bone cavities. PHYSIOLOGY – The sinuses function to warm and humidify the inhaled air, filter airborne pathogens, increase the resonance of the voice, lighten the weight of the skull, and provide a role in immunological response.

Sphenoid Sinus – The one of four paired, air-filled paranasal sinuses in the sphenoid bone and located behind the eye and nose.

Tympanic Membrane – ANATOMY – The membrane at the innermost portion of the ear canal that separates the external ear from the middle ear. PHYSIOLOGY – Transmits sound waves to the middle ear bones, and serves as a barrier to organisms and microorganisms.

Anatomical Illustrations of Ear, Nose, Sinus

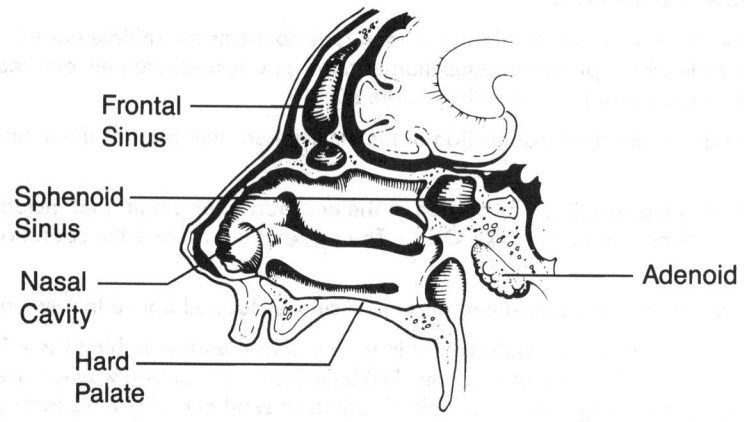

Frontal Sinus
Sphenoid Sinus
Nasal Cavity
Hard Palate
Adenoid

NASOPHARYNX

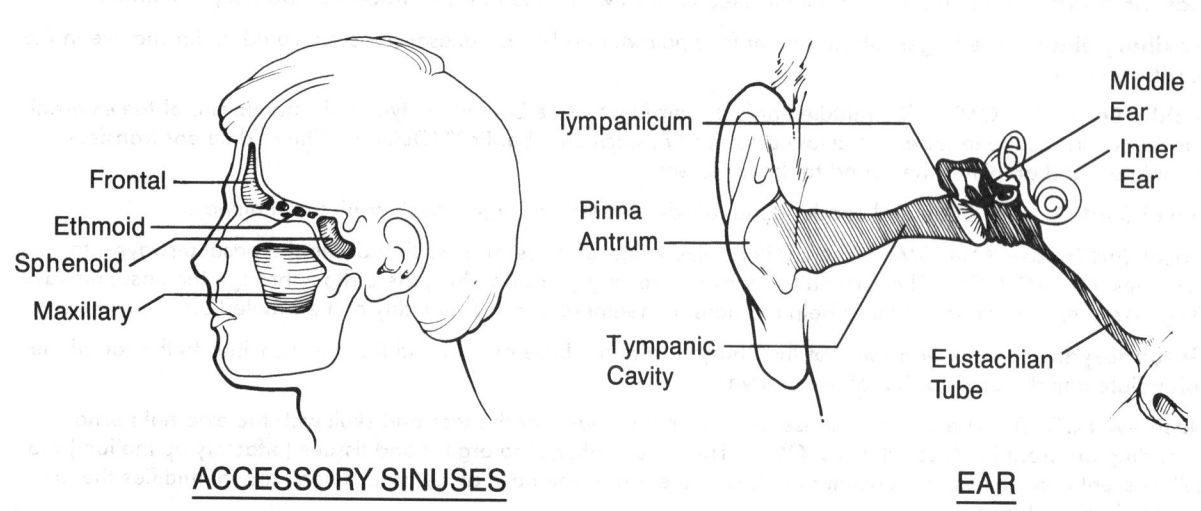

Frontal
Ethmoid
Sphenoid
Maxillary

ACCESSORY SINUSES

Tympanicum
Pinna
Antrum
Tympanic Cavity
Middle Ear
Inner Ear
Eustachian Tube

EAR

Educational Annotations | 9 – Ear, Nose, Sinus

Definitions of Common Procedures of Ear, Nose, Sinus

Cochlear implant – The surgical implantation of a small, complex electronic hearing device (microphone, speech processor, transmitter, and electrical array) that can help to provide a sense of sound to individuals that are profoundly deaf. It is implanted behind the ear and connected to the auditory nerve.

Mastoidectomy – The surgical procedure to remove diseased mastoid air cells (chronic mastoiditis, cholesteatoma). A radical mastoidectomy also involves removing portions of the middle ear and tympanic membrane.

Rhinoplasty – The surgical repair of nasal defects or cosmetic reconstruction of the exterior shape of the nose.

Septoplasty – The surgical correction of a nasal septum defect (deviated nasal septum).

Sinusectomy – The surgical excision of paranasal sinus tissue to remove diseased or excessive tissue and/or to create a larger sinus cavity and promote more efficient drainage.

Sinusotomy (antrostomy) – The surgical incision/excision of paranasal sinus tissue to increase the drainage passage opening.

Stapedectomy/stapedotomy – The surgical correction of a dysfunctional stapes (middle ear) bone by implanting a small, movable prosthesis to allow the transfer of sound vibrations from the tympanic membrane to the middle ear and then on to the inner ear.

Turbinectomy – The surgical procedure to remove the turbinate bones of the nasal cavity that are causing nasal cavity obstruction.

AHA Coding Clinic® Reference Notations of Ear, Nose, Sinus

<u>ROOT OPERATION - 9 - EAR, NOSE, SINUS</u>
ALTERATION - 0
BYPASS - 1
CHANGE - 2
DESTRUCTION - 5
DILATION - 7
DIVISION - 8
DRAINAGE - 9
EXCISION - B
EXTIRPATION - C
EXTRACTION - D
INSERTION - H
INSPECTION - J
REATTACHMENT - M
RELEASE - N
REMOVAL - P
REPAIR - Q
    Endoscopic balloon sinuplasty (dilation) ....AHA 13:4Q:p114
    Epistaxis control using sutures ....AHA 14:4Q:p20
    Fat graft to seal sphenoid sinus and sella ....AHA 14:3Q:p22
REPLACEMENT - R
REPOSITION - S
RESECTION - T
SUPPLEMENT - U
REVISION - W

Educational Annotations | 9 – Ear, Nose, Sinus

Body Part Key Listings of Ear, Nose, Sinus

See also Body Part Key in Appendix C

Antihelix	*use* External Ear, Bilateral/Left/Right
Antitragus	*use* External Ear, Bilateral/Left/Right
Antrum of Highmore	*use* Maxillary Sinus, Left/Right
Auditory tube	*use* Eustachian Tube, Left/Right
Auricle	*use* External Ear, Bilateral/Left/Right
Bony labyrinth	*use* Inner Ear, Left/Right
Bony vestibule	*use* Inner Ear, Left/Right
Choana	*use* Nasopharynx
Cochlea	*use* Inner Ear, Left/Right
Columella	*use* Nose
Earlobe	*use* External Ear, Bilateral/Left/Right
Ethmoidal air cell	*use* Ethmoid Sinus, Left/Right
External auditory meatus	*use* External Auditory Canal, Left/Right
External naris	*use* Nose
Fossa of Rosenmuller	*use* Nasopharynx
Greater alar cartilage	*use* Nose
Helix	*use* External Ear, Bilateral/Left/Right
Incus	*use* Auditory Ossicle, Left/Right
Inferior turbinate	*use* Nasal Turbinate
Internal naris	*use* Nose
Lateral nasal cartilage	*use* Nose
Lesser alar cartilage	*use* Nose
Malleus	*use* Auditory Ossicle, Left/Right
Mastoid air cells	*use* Mastoid Sinus, Left/Right
Middle turbinate	*use* Nasal Turbinate
Nasal cavity	*use* Nose
Nasal concha	*use* Nasal Turbinate
Nostril	*use* Nose
Oval window	*use* Middle Ear, Left/Right
Pars flaccida	*use* Tympanic Membrane, Left/Right
Pharyngeal recess	*use* Nasopharynx
Pharyngotympanic tube	*use* Eustachian Tube, Left/Right
Pinna	*use* External Ear, Bilateral/Left/Right
Quadrangular cartilage	*use* Nasal Septum
Rhinopharynx	*use* Nasopharynx
Round window	*use* Inner Ear, Left/Right
Semicircular canal	*use* Inner Ear, Left/Right
Septal cartilage	*use* Nasal Septum
Stapes	*use* Auditory Ossicle, Left/Right
Superior turbinate	*use* Nasal Turbinate
Tragus	*use* External Ear, Bilateral/Left/Right
Tympanic cavity	*use* Middle Ear, Left/Right
Vomer bone	*use* Nasal Septum

EAR NOSE SINUS 09

Educational Annotations | 9 – Ear, Nose, Sinus

Device Key Listings of Ear, Nose, Sinus

See also Device Key in Appendix D

Autograft ....*use* Autologous Tissue Substitute
Bone anchored hearing device ....*use* Hearing Device, Bone Conduction for Insertion in Ear, Nose, Sinus
Cochlear implant (CI), multiple channel (electrode)*use* Hearing Device, Multiple Channel Cochlear Prosthesis for Insertion in Ear, Nose, Sinus
Cochlear implant (CI), single channel (electrode) ..*use* Hearing Device, Single Channel Cochlear Prosthesis for Insertion in Ear, Nose, Sinus
Esteem® implantable hearing system.......................*use* Hearing Device in Ear, Nose, Sinus
Nasopharyngeal airway (NPA) ....*use* Intraluminal Device, Airway in Ear, Nose, Sinus
Tissue bank graft ....*use* Nonautologous Tissue Substitute

Device Aggregation Table Listings of Ear, Nose, Sinus

See also Device Aggregation Table in Appendix E

Specific Device	For Operation	In Body System	General Device	
Hearing Device, Bone Conduction	Insertion	Ear, Nose, Sinus	S	Hearing Device
Hearing Device, Multiple Channel Cochlear Prosthesis	Insertion	Ear, Nose, Sinus	S	Hearing Device
Hearing Device, Single Channel Cochlear Prosthesis	Insertion	Ear, Nose, Sinus	S	Hearing Device
Intraluminal Device, Airway	All applicable	Ear, Nose, Sinus	D	Intraluminal Device

Coding Notes of Ear, Nose, Sinus

Body System Specific PCS Reference Manual Exercises

PCS CODE	9 – EAR, NOSE, SINUS EXERCISES
0 9 0 K 0 7 Z	Cosmetic rhinoplasty with septal reduction and tip elevation using local tissue graft, open.
0 9 5 K X Z Z	Cautery of nosebleed.
0 9 9 V 4 Z Z	Endoscopic drainage of left ethmoid sinus.
0 9 C K X Z Z	Forceps removal of foreign body in right nostril. (Nostril is coded to the "Nose" body part value.)
0 9 D 7 7 Z Z	Removal of tattered right ear drum fragments with tweezers.
0 9 H E 0 6 Z	Open insertion of multiple channel cochlear implant, left ear.
0 9 M 0 X Z Z	Reattachment of severed right ear.
0 9 T Q 4 Z Z	Endoscopic bilateral total maxillary sinusectomy.
0 9 T R 4 Z Z	

Educational Annotations | 9 – Ear, Nose, Sinus

NOTES

OTHER OBJECTIVES GROUP: Alteration, (Creation), (Fusion)
Root Operations that define other objectives.

1ST - 0 Medical and Surgical	EXAMPLE: Cosmetic rhinoplasty		CMS Ex: Face lift
2ND - 9 Ear, Nose, Sinus	ALTERATION: Modifying the anatomic structure of a body part without affecting the function of the body part.		
3RD - 0 ALTERATION	EXPLANATION: Principal purpose is to improve appearance		

Body Part – 4TH	Approach – 5TH	Device – 6TH	Qualifier – 7TH
0 External Ear, Right	0 Open	7 Autologous tissue substitute	Z No qualifier
1 External Ear, Left	3 Percutaneous	J Synthetic substitute	
2 External Ear, Bilateral	4 Percutaneous endoscopic	K Nonautologous tissue substitute	
K Nose	X External	Z No device	

TUBULAR GROUP: Bypass, Dilation, (Occlusion), (Restriction)
Root Operations that alter the diameter/route of a tubular body part.

1ST - 0 Medical and Surgical	EXAMPLE: Endolymphatic bypass		CMS Ex: Coronary artery bypass
2ND - 9 Ear, Nose, Sinus	BYPASS: Altering the route of passage of the contents of a tubular body part.		
3RD - 1 BYPASS	EXPLANATION: Rerouting contents to a downstream part ...		

Body Part – 4TH	Approach – 5TH	Device – 6TH	Qualifier – 7TH
D Inner Ear, Right	0 Open	7 Autologous tissue substitute	0 Endolymphatic
E Inner Ear, Left		J Synthetic substitute	
		K Nonautologous tissue substitute	
		Z No device	

DEVICE GROUP: Change, Insertion, Removal, Replacement, Revision, Supplement
Root Operations that always involve a device.

1ST - 0 Medical and Surgical	EXAMPLE: Exchange drain tube		CMS Ex: Changing urinary catheter
2ND - 9 Ear, Nose, Sinus	CHANGE: Taking out or off a device from a body part and putting back an identical or similar device in or on the same body part without cutting or puncturing the skin or a mucous membrane.		
3RD - 2 CHANGE	EXPLANATION: ALL Changes use EXTERNAL approach only...		

Body Part – 4TH	Approach – 5TH	Device – 6TH	Qualifier – 7TH
H Ear, Right	X External	0 Drainage device	Z No qualifier
J Ear, Left		Y Other device	
K Nose			
Y Sinus			

EAR NOSE SINUS 0 9 2

EXCISION GROUP: Excision, Resection, Destruction, Extraction, (Detachment)
Root Operations that take out some or all of a body part.

1ST - **0** Medical and Surgical	**EXAMPLE:** Cautery epistaxis	**CMS Ex:** Fulguration polyp
2ND - **9** Ear, Nose, Sinus	**DESTRUCTION:** Physical eradication of all or a portion of a body part by the direct use of energy, force, or a destructive agent.	
3RD - **5 DESTRUCTION**	**EXPLANATION:** None of the body part is physically taken out	

Body Part – 4TH	Approach – 5TH	Device – 6TH	Qualifier – 7TH
0 External Ear, Right 1 External Ear, Left K Nose	0 Open 3 Percutaneous 4 Percutaneous endoscopic X External	Z No device	Z No qualifier
3 External Auditory Canal, Right 4 External Auditory Canal, Left	0 Open 3 Percutaneous 4 Percutaneous endoscopic 7 Via natural or artificial opening 8 Via natural or artificial opening endoscopic X External	Z No device	Z No qualifier
5 Middle Ear, Right A Auditory Ossicle, Left 6 Middle Ear, Left D Inner Ear, Right 9 Auditory Ossicle, Right E Inner Ear, Left	0 Open	Z No device	Z No qualifier
7 Tympanic Membrane, Right 8 Tympanic Membrane, Left F Eustachian Tube, Right G Eustachian Tube, Left L Nasal Turbinate N Nasopharynx	0 Open 3 Percutaneous 4 Percutaneous endoscopic 7 Via natural or artificial opening 8 Via natural or artificial opening endoscopic	Z No device	Z No qualifier
B Mastoid Sinus, Right S Frontal Sinus, Right C Mastoid Sinus, Left T Frontal Sinus, Left M Nasal Septum U Ethmoid Sinus, Right P Accessory Sinus V Ethmoid Sinus, Left Q Maxillary Sinus, Right W Sphenoid Sinus, Right R Maxillary Sinus, Left X Sphenoid Sinus, Left	0 Open 3 Percutaneous 4 Percutaneous endoscopic	Z No device	Z No qualifier

TUBULAR GROUP: Bypass, Dilation, (Occlusion), (Restriction)
Root Operations that alter the diameter/route of a tubular body part.

1ST - 0 Medical and Surgical	EXAMPLE: Balloon dilation Eustachian	CMS Ex: Transluminal angioplasty
2ND - 9 Ear, Nose, Sinus	**DILATION:** Expanding an orifice or the lumen of a tubular body part.	
3RD - 7 DILATION	EXPLANATION: By force (stretching) or cutting ...	

Body Part – 4TH	Approach – 5TH	Device – 6TH	Qualifier – 7TH
F Eustachian Tube, Right G Eustachian Tube, Left	0 Open 7 Via natural or artificial opening 8 Via natural or artificial opening endoscopic	D Intraluminal device Z No device	Z No qualifier
F Eustachian Tube, Right G Eustachian Tube, Left	3 Percutaneous 4 Percutaneous endoscopic	Z No device	Z No qualifier

DIVISION GROUP: Division, Release
Root Operations involving cutting or separation only.

1ST - 0 Medical and Surgical	EXAMPLE: Division nasal turbinate	CMS Ex: Osteotomy
2ND - 9 Ear, Nose, Sinus	**DIVISION:** Cutting into a body part without draining fluids and/or gases from the body part in order to separate or transect a body part.	
3RD - 8 DIVISION	EXPLANATION: Separated into two or more portions ...	

Body Part – 4TH	Approach – 5TH	Device – 6TH	Qualifier – 7TH
L Nasal Turbinate	0 Open 3 Percutaneous 4 Percutaneous endoscopic 7 Via natural or artificial opening 8 Via natural or artificial opening endoscopic	Z No device	Z No qualifier

DRAINAGE GROUP: Drainage, Extirpation, (Fragmentation)
Root Operations that take out solids/fluids/gases from a body part.

| 1ST - 0 Medical and Surgical | | EXAMPLE: Sinusotomy for drainage | | CMS Ex: Thoracentesis |

2ND - 9 Ear, Nose, Sinus

3RD - 9 DRAINAGE

DRAINAGE: Taking or letting out fluids and/or gases from a body part.

EXPLANATION: Qualifier "X Diagnostic" indicates biopsy ...

Body Part – 4TH	Approach – 5TH	Device – 6TH	Qualifier – 7TH
0 External Ear, Right 1 External Ear, Left K Nose	0 Open 3 Percutaneous 4 Percutaneous endoscopic X External	0 Drainage device	Z No qualifier
0 External Ear, Right 1 External Ear, Left K Nose	0 Open 3 Percutaneous 4 Percutaneous endoscopic X External	Z No device	X Diagnostic Z No qualifier
3 External Auditory Canal, Right 4 External Auditory Canal, Left	0 Open 3 Percutaneous 4 Percutaneous endoscopic 7 Via natural or artificial opening 8 Via natural or artificial opening endoscopic X External	0 Drainage device	Z No qualifier
3 External Auditory Canal, Right 4 External Auditory Canal, Left	0 Open 3 Percutaneous 4 Percutaneous endoscopic 7 Via natural or artificial opening 8 Via natural or artificial opening endoscopic X External	Z No device	X Diagnostic Z No qualifier
5 Middle Ear, Right A Auditory Ossicle, Left 6 Middle Ear, Left D Inner Ear, Right 9 Auditory Ossicle, Right E Inner Ear, Left	0 Open	0 Drainage device	Z No qualifier
5 Middle Ear, Right A Auditory Ossicle, Left 6 Middle Ear, Left D Inner Ear, Right 9 Auditory Ossicle, Right E Inner Ear, Left	0 Open	Z No device	X Diagnostic Z No qualifier

continued ⇨

EAR NOSE SINUS 099

0 9 9 DRAINAGE – continued

Body Part – 4TH	Approach – 5TH	Device – 6TH	Qualifier – 7TH
7 Tympanic Membrane, Right 8 Tympanic Membrane, Left F Eustachian Tube, Right G Eustachian Tube, Left L Nasal Turbinate N Nasopharynx	0 Open 3 Percutaneous 4 Percutaneous endoscopic 7 Via natural or artificial opening 8 Via natural or artificial opening endoscopic	0 Drainage device	Z No qualifier
7 Tympanic Membrane, Right 8 Tympanic Membrane, Left F Eustachian Tube, Right G Eustachian Tube, Left L Nasal Turbinate N Nasopharynx	0 Open 3 Percutaneous 4 Percutaneous endoscopic 7 Via natural or artificial opening 8 Via natural or artificial opening endoscopic	Z No device	X Diagnostic Z No qualifier
B Mastoid Sinus, Right S Frontal Sinus, Right C Mastoid Sinus, Left T Frontal Sinus, Left M Nasal Septum U Ethmoid Sinus, Right P Accessory Sinus V Ethmoid Sinus, Left Q Maxillary Sinus, Right W Sphenoid Sinus, Right R Maxillary Sinus, Left X Sphenoid Sinus, Left	0 Open 3 Percutaneous 4 Percutaneous endoscopic	0 Drainage device	Z No qualifier
B Mastoid Sinus, Right S Frontal Sinus, Right C Mastoid Sinus, Left T Frontal Sinus, Left M Nasal Septum U Ethmoid Sinus, Right P Accessory Sinus V Ethmoid Sinus, Left Q Maxillary Sinus, Right W Sphenoid Sinus, Right R Maxillary Sinus, Left X Sphenoid Sinus, Left	0 Open 3 Percutaneous 4 Percutaneous endoscopic	Z No device	X Diagnostic Z No qualifier

EXCISION GROUP: Excision, Resection, Destruction, Extraction, (Detachment)
Root Operations that take out some or all of a body part.

1ST - 0 Medical and Surgical	EXAMPLE: Excision lesion nose	CMS Ex: Liver biopsy

2ND - 9 Ear, Nose, Sinus

3RD - B EXCISION

EXCISION: Cutting out or off, without replacement, a portion of a body part.

EXPLANATION: Qualifier "X Diagnostic" indicates biopsy ...

Body Part – 4TH	Approach – 5TH	Device – 6TH	Qualifier – 7TH
0 External Ear, Right 1 External Ear, Left K Nose	0 Open 3 Percutaneous 4 Percutaneous endoscopic X External	Z No device	X Diagnostic Z No qualifier
3 External Auditory Canal, Right 4 External Auditory Canal, Left	0 Open 3 Percutaneous 4 Percutaneous endoscopic 7 Via natural or artificial opening 8 Via natural or artificial opening endoscopic X External	Z No device	X Diagnostic Z No qualifier
5 Middle Ear, Right A Auditory Ossicle, Left 6 Middle Ear, Left D Inner Ear, Right 9 Auditory Ossicle, Right E Inner Ear, Left	0 Open	Z No device	X Diagnostic Z No qualifier
7 Tympanic Membrane, Right 8 Tympanic Membrane, Left F Eustachian Tube, Right G Eustachian Tube, Left L Nasal Turbinate N Nasopharynx	0 Open 3 Percutaneous 4 Percutaneous endoscopic 7 Via natural or artificial opening 8 Via natural or artificial opening endoscopic	Z No device	X Diagnostic Z No qualifier
B Mastoid Sinus, Right S Frontal Sinus, Right C Mastoid Sinus, Left T Frontal Sinus, Left M Nasal Septum U Ethmoid Sinus, Right P Accessory Sinus V Ethmoid Sinus, Left Q Maxillary Sinus, Right W Sphenoid Sinus, Right R Maxillary Sinus, Left X Sphenoid Sinus, Left	0 Open 3 Percutaneous 4 Percutaneous endoscopic	Z No device	X Diagnostic Z No qualifier

DRAINAGE GROUP: Drainage, Extirpation, (Fragmentation)
Root Operations that take out solids/fluids/gases from a body part.

1ST - 0 Medical and Surgical

2ND - 9 Ear, Nose, Sinus

3RD - C EXTIRPATION

EXAMPLE: Removal foreign body nose | CMS Ex: Choledocholithotomy

EXTIRPATION: Taking or cutting out solid matter from a body part.

EXPLANATION: Abnormal byproduct or foreign body ...

Body Part – 4TH	Approach – 5TH	Device – 6TH	Qualifier – 7TH
0 External Ear, Right 1 External Ear, Left K Nose	0 Open 3 Percutaneous 4 Percutaneous endoscopic X External	Z No device	Z No qualifier
3 External Auditory Canal, Right 4 External Auditory Canal, Left	0 Open 3 Percutaneous 4 Percutaneous endoscopic 7 Via natural or artificial opening 8 Via natural or artificial opening endoscopic X External	Z No device	Z No qualifier
5 Middle Ear, Right A Auditory Ossicle, Left 6 Middle Ear, Left D Inner Ear, Right 9 Auditory Ossicle, Right E Inner Ear, Left	0 Open	Z No device	Z No qualifier
7 Tympanic Membrane, Right 8 Tympanic Membrane, Left F Eustachian Tube, Right G Eustachian Tube, Left L Nasal Turbinate N Nasopharynx	0 Open 3 Percutaneous 4 Percutaneous endoscopic 7 Via natural or artificial opening 8 Via natural or artificial opening endoscopic	Z No device	Z No qualifier
B Mastoid Sinus, Right S Frontal Sinus, Right C Mastoid Sinus, Left T Frontal Sinus, Left M Nasal Septum U Ethmoid Sinus, Right P Accessory Sinus V Ethmoid Sinus, Left Q Maxillary Sinus, Right W Sphenoid Sinus, Right R Maxillary Sinus, Left X Sphenoid Sinus, Left	0 Open 3 Percutaneous 4 Percutaneous endoscopic	Z No device	Z No qualifier

EAR NOSE SINUS 0 9 C

EXCISION GROUP: Excision, Resection, Destruction, Extraction, (Detachment)
Root Operations that take out some or all of a body part.

1ST – 0 Medical and Surgical

2ND – 9 Ear, Nose, Sinus

3RD – D EXTRACTION

EXAMPLE: Removal sinus lining membrane | CMS Ex: D&C

EXTRACTION: Pulling or stripping out or off all or a portion of a body part by the use of force.

EXPLANATION: None for this Body System

Body Part – 4TH	Approach – 5TH	Device – 6TH	Qualifier – 7TH
7 Tympanic Membrane, Right 8 Tympanic Membrane, Left L Nasal Turbinate	0 Open 3 Percutaneous 4 Percutaneous endoscopic 7 Via natural or artificial opening 8 Via natural or artificial opening endoscopic	Z No device	Z No qualifier
9 Auditory Ossicle, Right A Auditory Ossicle, Left	0 Open	Z No device	Z No qualifier
B Mastoid Sinus, Right S Frontal Sinus, Right C Mastoid Sinus, Left T Frontal Sinus, Left M Nasal Septum U Ethmoid Sinus, Right P Accessory Sinus V Ethmoid Sinus, Left Q Maxillary Sinus, Right W Sphenoid Sinus, Right R Maxillary Sinus, Left X Sphenoid Sinus, Left	0 Open 3 Percutaneous 4 Percutaneous endoscopic	Z No device	Z No qualifier

EAR NOSE SINUS 09D

DEVICE GROUP: Change, Insertion, Removal, Replacement, Revision, Supplement
Root Operations that always involve a device.

1ST - 0 Medical and Surgical	EXAMPLE: Cochlear implant	CMS Ex: Insertion central venous catheter

2ND - 9 Ear, Nose, Sinus

3RD - H INSERTION

INSERTION: Putting in a nonbiological appliance that monitors, assists, performs, or prevents a physiological function but does not physically take the place of a body part.

EXPLANATION: None

Body Part – 4TH	Approach – 5TH	Device – 6TH	Qualifier – 7TH
D Inner Ear, Right E Inner Ear, Left	0 Open 3 Percutaneous 4 Percutaneous endoscopic	4 Hearing device, bone conduction 5 Hearing device, single channel cochlear prosthesis 6 Hearing device, multiple channel cochlear prosthesis S Hearing device	Z No qualifier
N Nasopharynx	7 Via natural or artificial opening 8 Via natural or artificial opening endoscopic	B Intraluminal device, airway	Z No qualifier

---

EXAMINATION GROUP: Inspection, (Map)
Root Operations involving examination only.

1ST - **0** Medical and Surgical

2ND - **9** Ear, Nose, Sinus

3RD - **J** INSPECTION

EXAMPLE: Sinus endoscopy

CMS Ex: Colonoscopy

INSPECTION: Visually and/or manually exploring a body part.

EXPLANATION: Direct or instrumental visualization ...

Body Part – 4TH	Approach – 5TH	Device – 6TH	Qualifier – 7TH
7 Tympanic Membrane, Right 8 Tympanic Membrane, Left H Ear, Right J Ear, Left	0 Open 3 Percutaneous 4 Percutaneous endoscopic 7 Via natural or artificial opening 8 Via natural or artificial opening endoscopic X External	Z No device	Z No qualifier
D Inner Ear, Right E Inner Ear, Left K Nose Y Sinus	0 Open 3 Percutaneous 4 Percutaneous endoscopic X External	Z No device	Z No qualifier

---

MOVE GROUP: Reattachment, Reposition, (Transfer), (Transplantation)
Root Operations that put in/put back or move some/all of a body part.

1ST - **0** Medical and Surgical

2ND - **9** Ear, Nose, Sinus

3RD - **M** REATTACHMENT

EXAMPLE: Reattachment severed ear

CMS Ex: Reattachment hand

REATTACHMENT: Putting back in or on all or a portion of a separated body part to its normal location or other suitable location.

EXPLANATION: With/without reconnection of vessels/nerves...

Body Part – 4TH	Approach – 5TH	Device – 6TH	Qualifier – 7TH
0 External Ear, Right 1 External Ear, Left K Nose	X External	Z No device	Z No qualifier

DIVISION GROUP: Division, Release
Root Operations involving cutting or separation only.

1ST - 0 Medical and Surgical

2ND - 9 Ear, Nose, Sinus

3RD - N RELEASE

EXAMPLE: Adhesiolysis middle ear | CMS Ex: Carpal tunnel release

RELEASE: Freeing a body part from an abnormal physical constraint by cutting or by the use of force.

EXPLANATION: None of the body part is taken out ...

Body Part – 4TH	Approach – 5TH	Device – 6TH	Qualifier – 7TH
0 External Ear, Right 1 External Ear, Left K Nose	0 Open 3 Percutaneous 4 Percutaneous endoscopic X External	Z No device	Z No qualifier
3 External Auditory Canal, Right 4 External Auditory Canal, Left	0 Open 3 Percutaneous 4 Percutaneous endoscopic 7 Via natural or artificial opening 8 Via natural or artificial opening endoscopic X External	Z No device	Z No qualifier
5 Middle Ear, Right A Auditory Ossicle, Left 6 Middle Ear, Left D Inner Ear, Right 9 Auditory Ossicle, Right E Inner Ear, Left	0 Open	Z No device	Z No qualifier
7 Tympanic Membrane, Right 8 Tympanic Membrane, Left F Eustachian Tube, Right G Eustachian Tube, Left L Nasal Turbinate N Nasopharynx	0 Open 3 Percutaneous 4 Percutaneous endoscopic 7 Via natural or artificial opening 8 Via natural or artificial opening endoscopic	Z No device	Z No qualifier
B Mastoid Sinus, Right S Frontal Sinus, Right C Mastoid Sinus, Left T Frontal Sinus, Left M Nasal Septum U Ethmoid Sinus, Right P Accessory Sinus V Ethmoid Sinus, Left Q Maxillary Sinus, Right W Sphenoid Sinus, Right R Maxillary Sinus, Left X Sphenoid Sinus, Left	0 Open 3 Percutaneous 4 Percutaneous endoscopic	Z No device	Z No qualifier

DEVICE GROUP: Change, Insertion, Removal, Replacement, Revision, Supplement
Root Operations that always involve a device.

1ST - **0** Medical and Surgical

2ND - **9** Ear, Nose, Sinus

3RD - **P REMOVAL**

EXAMPLE: Removal drain tube

CMS Ex: Chest tube removal

REMOVAL: Taking out or off a device from a body part.

EXPLANATION: Removal device without reinsertion ...

Body Part – 4TH	Approach – 5TH	Device – 6TH	Qualifier – 7TH
7 Tympanic Membrane, Right 8 Tympanic Membrane, Left	0 Open 7 Via natural or artificial opening 8 Via natural or artificial opening endoscopic X External	0 Drainage device	Z No qualifier
D Inner Ear, Right E Inner Ear, Left	0 Open 7 Via natural or artificial opening 8 Via natural or artificial opening endoscopic	S Hearing device	Z No qualifier
H Ear, Right J Ear, Left K Nose	0 Open 3 Percutaneous 4 Percutaneous endoscopic 7 Via natural or artificial opening 8 Via natural or artificial opening endoscopic X External	0 Drainage device 7 Autologous tissue substitute D Intraluminal device J Synthetic substitute K Nonautologous tissue substitute	Z No qualifier
Y Sinus	0 Open 3 Percutaneous 4 Percutaneous endoscopic X External	0 Drainage device	Z No qualifier

OTHER REPAIRS GROUP: (Control), Repair
Root Operations that define other repairs.

1ST - 0 Medical and Surgical

2ND - 9 Ear, Nose, Sinus

3RD - Q REPAIR

EXAMPLE: Epistaxis control using sutures | CMS Ex: Suture laceration

REPAIR: Restoring, to the extent possible, a body part to its normal anatomic structure and function.

EXPLANATION: Only when no other root operation applies ...

Body Part – 4TH	Approach – 5TH	Device – 6TH	Qualifier – 7TH
0 External Ear, Right 1 External Ear, Left 2 External Ear, Bilateral K Nose	0 Open 3 Percutaneous 4 Percutaneous endoscopic X External	Z No device	Z No qualifier
3 External Auditory Canal, Right 4 External Auditory Canal, Left F Eustachian Tube, Right G Eustachian Tube, Left	0 Open 3 Percutaneous 4 Percutaneous endoscopic 7 Via natural or artificial opening 8 Via natural or artificial opening endoscopic X External	Z No device	Z No qualifier
5 Middle Ear, Right A Auditory Ossicle, Left 6 Middle Ear, Left D Inner Ear, Right 9 Auditory Ossicle, Right E Inner Ear, Left	0 Open	Z No device	Z No qualifier
7 Tympanic Membrane, Right 8 Tympanic Membrane, Left L Nasal Turbinate N Nasopharynx	0 Open 3 Percutaneous 4 Percutaneous endoscopic 7 Via natural or artificial opening 8 Via natural or artificial opening endoscopic	Z No device	Z No qualifier
B Mastoid Sinus, Right S Frontal Sinus, Right C Mastoid Sinus, Left T Frontal Sinus, Left M Nasal Septum U Ethmoid Sinus, Right P Accessory Sinus V Ethmoid Sinus, Left Q Maxillary Sinus, Right W Sphenoid Sinus, Right R Maxillary Sinus, Left X Sphenoid Sinus, Left	0 Open 3 Percutaneous 4 Percutaneous endoscopic	Z No device	Z No qualifier

EAR NOSE SINUS 0 9 Q

DEVICE GROUP: Change, Insertion, Removal, Replacement, Revision, Supplement
Root Operations that always involve a device.

1ST - **0** Medical and Surgical 2ND - **9** Ear, Nose, Sinus 3RD - **R REPLACEMENT**	EXAMPLE: External ear reconstruction CMS Ex: Total hip **REPLACEMENT:** Putting in or on a biological or synthetic material that physically takes the place and/or function of all or a portion of a body part. EXPLANATION: Includes taking out body part, or eradication...

Body Part – 4TH	Approach – 5TH	Device – 6TH	Qualifier – 7TH
0 External Ear, Right 1 External Ear, Left 2 External Ear, Bilateral K Nose	0 Open X External	7 Autologous tissue substitute J Synthetic substitute K Nonautologous tissue substitute	Z No qualifier
5 Middle Ear, Right A Auditory Ossicle, Left 6 Middle Ear, Left D Inner Ear, Right 9 Auditory Ossicle, Right E Inner Ear, Left	0 Open	7 Autologous tissue substitute J Synthetic substitute K Nonautologous tissue substitute	Z No qualifier
7 Tympanic Membrane, Right 8 Tympanic Membrane, Left N Nasopharynx	0 Open 7 Via natural or artificial opening 8 Via natural or artificial opening endoscopic	7 Autologous tissue substitute J Synthetic substitute K Nonautologous tissue substitute	Z No qualifier
L Nasal Turbinate	0 Open 3 Percutaneous 4 Percutaneous endoscopic 7 Via natural or artificial opening 8 Via natural or artificial opening endoscopic	7 Autologous tissue substitute J Synthetic substitute K Nonautologous tissue substitute	Z No qualifier
M Nasal Septum	0 Open 3 Percutaneous 4 Percutaneous endoscopic	7 Autologous tissue substitute J Synthetic substitute K Nonautologous tissue substitute	Z No qualifier

EAR NOSE SINUS 09R

MOVE GROUP: Reattachment, Reposition, (Transfer), (Transplantation)
Root Operations that put in/put back or move some/all of a body part.

1ST - 0 Medical and Surgical
2ND - 9 Ear, Nose, Sinus
3RD - S REPOSITION

EXAMPLE: Deviated septum septoplasty | CMS Ex: Fracture reduction

REPOSITION: Moving to its normal location, or other suitable location, all or a portion of a body part.

EXPLANATION: May or may not be cut to be moved ...

Body Part – 4TH	Approach – 5TH	Device – 6TH	Qualifier – 7TH
0 External Ear, Right 1 External Ear, Left 2 External Ear, Bilateral K Nose	0 Open 4 Percutaneous endoscopic X External	Z No device	Z No qualifier
7 Tympanic Membrane, Right 8 Tympanic Membrane, Left F Eustachian Tube, Right G Eustachian Tube, Left L Nasal Turbinate	0 Open 4 Percutaneous endoscopic 7 Via natural or artificial opening 8 Via natural or artificial opening endoscopic	Z No device	Z No qualifier
9 Auditory Ossicle, Right A Auditory Ossicle, Left M Nasal Septum	0 Open 4 Percutaneous endoscopic	Z No device	Z No qualifier

EAR NOSE SINUS 09S

EXCISION GROUP: Excision, Resection, Destruction, Extraction, (Detachment)
Root Operations that take out some or all of a body part.

1ST - 0 Medical and Surgical	EXAMPLE: Total maxillary sinusectomy	CMS Ex: Cholecystectomy

2ND - 9 Ear, Nose, Sinus

3RD - T RESECTION

RESECTION: Cutting out or off, without replacement, all of a body part.

EXPLANATION: None

Body Part – 4TH	Approach – 5TH	Device – 6TH	Qualifier – 7TH
0 External Ear, Right 1 External Ear, Left K Nose	0 Open 4 Percutaneous endoscopic X External	Z No device	Z No qualifier
5 Middle Ear, Right A Auditory Ossicle, Left 6 Middle Ear, Left D Inner Ear, Right 9 Auditory Ossicle, Right E Inner Ear, Left	0 Open	Z No device	Z No qualifier
7 Tympanic Membrane, Right 8 Tympanic Membrane, Left F Eustachian Tube, Right G Eustachian Tube, Left L Nasal Turbinate N Nasopharynx	0 Open 4 Percutaneous endoscopic 7 Via natural or artificial opening 8 Via natural or artificial opening endoscopic	Z No device	Z No qualifier
B Mastoid Sinus, Right S Frontal Sinus, Right C Mastoid Sinus, Left T Frontal Sinus, Left M Nasal Septum U Ethmoid Sinus, Right P Accessory Sinus V Ethmoid Sinus, Left Q Maxillary Sinus, Right W Sphenoid Sinus, Right R Maxillary Sinus, Left X Sphenoid Sinus, Left	0 Open 4 Percutaneous endoscopic	Z No device	Z No qualifier

DEVICE GROUP: Change, Insertion, Removal, Replacement, Revision, Supplement			
Root Operations that always involve a device.			

1ST - 0 Medical and Surgical

2ND - 9 Ear, Nose, Sinus

3RD - U SUPPLEMENT

EXAMPLE: Overlay graft myringoplasty | **CMS Ex:** Hernia repair with mesh

SUPPLEMENT: Putting in or on biological or synthetic material that physically reinforces and/or augments the function of a portion of a body part.

EXPLANATION: Biological material from same individual ...

Body Part – 4TH	Approach – 5TH	Device – 6TH	Qualifier – 7TH
0 External Ear, Right 1 External Ear, Left 2 External Ear, Bilateral K Nose	0 Open X External	7 Autologous tissue substitute J Synthetic substitute K Nonautologous tissue substitute	Z No qualifier
5 Middle Ear, Right　A Auditory Ossicle, Left 6 Middle Ear, Left　D Inner Ear, Right 9 Auditory Ossicle, Right　E Inner Ear, Left	0 Open	7 Autologous tissue substitute J Synthetic substitute K Nonautologous tissue substitute	Z No qualifier
7 Tympanic Membrane, Right 8 Tympanic Membrane, Left N Nasopharynx	0 Open 7 Via natural or artificial opening 8 Via natural or artificial opening endoscopic	7 Autologous tissue substitute J Synthetic substitute K Nonautologous tissue substitute	Z No qualifier
L Nasal Turbinate	0 Open 3 Percutaneous 4 Percutaneous endoscopic 7 Via natural or artificial opening 8 Via natural or artificial opening endoscopic	7 Autologous tissue substitute J Synthetic substitute K Nonautologous tissue substitute	Z No qualifier
M Nasal Septum	0 Open 3 Percutaneous 4 Percutaneous endoscopic	7 Autologous tissue substitute J Synthetic substitute K Nonautologous tissue substitute	Z No qualifier

EAR NOSE SINUS 09U

DEVICE GROUP: Change, Insertion, Removal, Replacement, Revision, Supplement
Root Operations that always involve a device.

| 1ST - 0 Medical and Surgical |
| 2ND - 9 Ear, Nose, Sinus |
| 3RD - W REVISION |

EXAMPLE: Reposition cochlear implant | CMS Ex: Adjustment pacemaker lead

REVISION: Correcting, to the extent possible, a portion of a malfunctioning device or the position of a displaced device.

EXPLANATION: May replace components of a device ...

Body Part – 4TH	Approach – 5TH	Device – 6TH	Qualifier – 7TH
7 Tympanic Membrane, Right 8 Tympanic Membrane, Left 9 Auditory Ossicle, Right A Auditory Ossicle, Left	0 Open 7 Via natural or artificial opening 8 Via natural or artificial opening endoscopic	7 Autologous tissue substitute J Synthetic substitute K Nonautologous tissue substitute	Z No qualifier
D Inner Ear, Right E Inner Ear, Left	0 Open 7 Via natural or artificial opening 8 Via natural or artificial opening endoscopic	S Hearing device	Z No qualifier
H Ear, Right J Ear, Left K Nose	0 Open 3 Percutaneous 4 Percutaneous endoscopic 7 Via natural or artificial opening 8 Via natural or artificial opening endoscopic X External	0 Drainage device 7 Autologous tissue substitute D Intraluminal device J Synthetic substitute K Nonautologous tissue substitute	Z No qualifier
Y Sinus	0 Open 3 Percutaneous 4 Percutaneous endoscopic X External	0 Drainage device	Z No qualifier

Educational Annotations | B – Respiratory System

Body System Specific Educational Annotations for the Respiratory System include:

- **Anatomy and Physiology Review**
- **Anatomical Illustrations**
- **Definitions of Common Procedures**
- **AHA Coding Clinic® Reference Notations**
- **Body Part Key Listings**
- **Device Key Listings**
- **Device Aggregation Table Listings**
- **Coding Notes**

Anatomy and Physiology Review of Respiratory System

BODY PART VALUES – B - RESPIRATORY SYSTEM

Carina – ANATOMY – The carina is a ridge of cartilaginous tissue within the trachea at the tracheal bifurcation at the lower end of the trachea. PHYSIOLOGY – The sensitive mucous membrane of the carina is responsible for triggering a cough reflex.

Diaphragm – ANATOMY – The diaphragm is dome-shaped sheet of skeletal muscle between the thoracic and abdominal cavities. PHYSIOLOGY – The diaphragm is the primary muscle in respiration and when it contracts, air is drawn into the lungs.

Lingula Bronchus – The secondary bronchi serving a lung lingula.

Lower Lobe Bronchus – The secondary bronchi serving a lower lung lobe (left or right).

Lower Lobe Lung – The lower lung lobes are soft, spongy, cone-shaped organs of respiration (left or right).

Lung – ANATOMY – The lungs are soft, spongy, cone-shaped organs located in the thoracic cavity. The right and left lungs are separated medially by the heart and the mediastinum, and they are enclosed by the diaphragm and the thoracic cage. The right lung is divided into 3 lobes called the upper (superior), middle, and lower (inferior). The left lung is divided into 2 lobes, the upper and lower. The lobes are subdivided into lobules which are composed of bronchioles, alveolar sacs, alveoli, nerves, and associated blood and lymphatic vessels. The alveoli are thin-walled, microscopic air sacs that open only on the side communicating with the inhaled air. PHYSIOLOGY – The lungs are organs that perform pulmonary ventilation. The alveoli are the microscopic structures responsible for the exchange of oxygen into the blood and carbon dioxide out of the body. Inspiration (inhalation) and expiration (exhalation) are complex central nervous system functions. Two groups of nerve cell bodies in the medulla of the brain compose the inspiratory center and the expiratory center. These two centers act reciprocally; that is, when one is stimulated and discharging, the other is inhibited. Both centers discharge nerve impulses to the intercostal muscles. When the inspiration center discharges nerve impulses, the diaphragm moves down and the external intercostal muscles contract, causing inflation. Inflation of the lungs causes stimulation of stretch receptors, which send impulses to the medulla, which in turn stimulates the expiratory center. Two other respiratory centers are contained in the pons which modify and control the medullary centers' activities, and are called the apneustic center and the pneumotaxic center. In addition to the above centers, there is also a chemical reaction which helps to control pulmonary ventilation. The carbon dioxide level in the blood is directly measured by the medulla, and respiration is adjusted accordingly. A decrease in the oxygen level, sensed by nerve endings in the common carotid artery and the aortic arch, will also stimulate a respiratory adjustment, but it does not play a noticeable difference in pulmonary ventilation.

Lung Lingula – The downward projection of the upper lobe of the left lung.

Main Bronchus – ANATOMY – The bronchial tree consists of branched airways leading from the trachea to the microscopic air sacs. The two main branches, the right and left bronchi, subdivide into secondary or lobar bronchi, which in turn branch into finer tubes down to the bronchioles. PHYSIOLOGY – The trachea and bronchi allow for the rapid transport of air to and from the lung tissue.

Middle Lobe Bronchus – The secondary bronchi serving a middle lung lobe (right).

Middle Lobe Lung – The middle lung lobe is the soft, spongy, cone-shaped organ of respiration (right).

Pleura – ANATOMY – The pleura are closed, double-layered serous membranous sacs surrounding the lungs. The parietal pleura is the layer which lines the thoracic walls opposite to the visceral pleura. The visceral pleura is the layer which adheres to the lungs and together with the parietal, forms the pleural cavity. PHYSIOLOGY – The pleura functions to prevent friction of the lungs against the thoracic wall during respiration. There is a small amount of serous fluid in the pleural cavity which lubricates the facing membranes.

Continued on next page

Educational Annotations | B – Respiratory System

Anatomy and Physiology Review of Respiratory System

BODY PART VALUES – B - RESPIRATORY SYSTEM
Continued from previous page

Trachea – ANATOMY – The trachea is a cylindrical tube about 1 inch (2.5 cm) in diameter. It extends downward from the larynx in front of the esophagus and into the thoracic cavity, where it splits into the right and left main bronchi. PHYSIOLOGY – The trachea and bronchi allow for the rapid transport of air to and from the lung tissue.

Tracheobronchial Tree – The trachea, main bronchi, secondary (lobar) bronchi, and bronchioles.

Upper Lobe Bronchus – The secondary bronchi serving a lower lung lobe (left or right).

Upper Lobe Lung – The upper lung lobes are soft, spongy, cone-shaped organs of respiration (left or right).

Anatomical Illustrations of Respiratory System

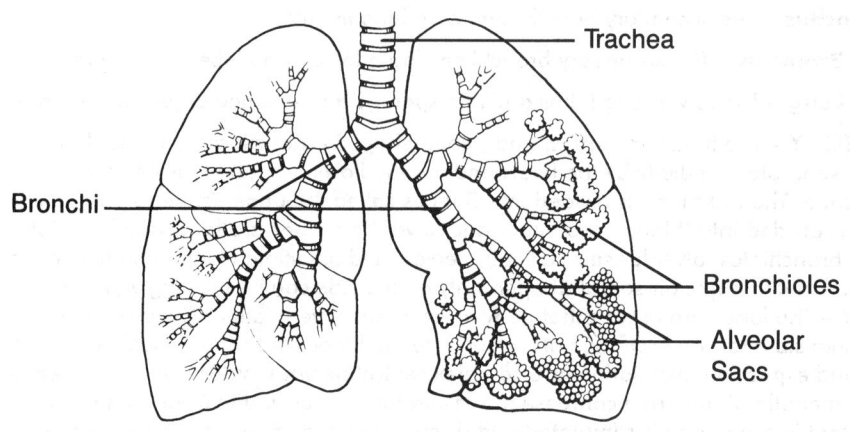

LUNGS — ANTERIOR (CUT-AWAY) VIEW

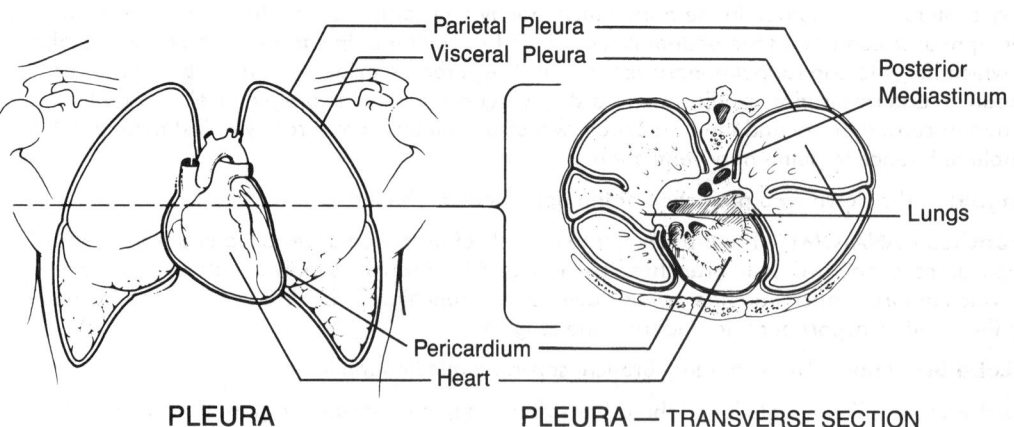

PLEURA

PLEURA — TRANSVERSE SECTION

Educational Annotations | B – Respiratory System

Definitions of Common Procedures of Respiratory System

Bronchoscopy – The use of a flexible bronchoscope to visualize and perform procedures on the bronchi and lungs.

Endobronchial valve insertion – The bronchoscopic placement of one-way bronchial airflow valves that prevent air from entering the designated lobe segments while allowing trapped air and secretions to flow out. The valves are used primarily to treat emphysema by not allowing that segment to inflate and thus allowing other healthier segments to inflate and exhale more easily and efficiently.

Endotracheal intubation – The placement of a flexible, plastic breathing tube into the trachea through the oral cavity and occasionally through the nose.

Lobectomy of lung – The surgical removal of an entire lobe of a lung.

Lung transplant – The surgical replacement of a diseased lung by implantation of a donor lung.

Pleurodesis – The medical procedure to eliminate the pleural cavity space by instilling a substance (chemical, talc, etc.) through a chest tube that adheres the visceral and parietal pleura together.

Tracheostomy – The creation of a surgical opening in the front of neck and into the trachea with the placement of a tube through the opening and into the trachea to maintain the patency of the new airway for breathing and secretion removal.

AHA Coding Clinic® Reference Notations of Respiratory System

ROOT OPERATION SPECIFIC - B - RESPIRATORY SYSTEM
BYPASS - 1
CHANGE - 2
DESTRUCTION - 5
    Photodynamic therapy of diaphragm and pleura ....AHA 16:2Q:p17
DILATION - 7
DRAINAGE - 9
    Bronchoalveolar lavage ....AHA 16:1Q:p26,27
EXCISION - B
    Bronchial brush biopsies ....AHA 16:1Q:p26,27
    Endoscopic transbronchial needle aspiration biopsy of right lung ....AHA 14:1Q:p20
    Cricotracheal resection ....AHA 15:1Q:p15
EXTIRPATION - C
EXTRACTION - D
FRAGMENTATION - F
INSERTION - H
    Endotracheal intubation ....AHA 14:4Q:p3
INSPECTION - J
    Bronchoscopic placement of fiducial marker ....AHA 14:1Q:p20
    Endoscopic viewing of talc placement in pleural cavity ....AHA 15:2Q:p31
OCCLUSION - L
REATTACHMENT - M
RELEASE - N
    Release of tracheal vascular ring ....AHA 15:3Q:p15
REMOVAL - P
REPAIR - Q
    Diaphragm hiatal hernia repair ....AHA 16:2Q:p22
    Repair of midline diaphragm (paraesophageal) hernia ....AHA 14:3Q:p28
REPOSITION - S
RESECTION - T

Continued on next page

R E S P I R A T O R Y

0 B

Educational Annotations | B – Respiratory System

AHA Coding Clinic® Reference Notations of Respiratory System

Continued from previous page
SUPPLEMENT - U
  Omental flap repair of bronchopleural fistula ....AHA 15:1Q:p28
RESTRICTION - V
REVISION - W
TRANSPLANTATION - Y

Body Part Key Listings of Respiratory System

See also Body Part Key in Appendix C
Bronchus intermedius ....*use* Main Bronchus, Right
Cricoid cartilage..*use* Trachea
Intermediate bronchus.....................................*use* Main Bronchus, Right

Device Key Listings of Respiratory System

See also Device Key in Appendix D
Autograft ....*use* Autologous Tissue Substitute
Brachytherapy seeds ....*use* Radioactive Element
Endotracheal tube (cuffed) (double-lumen) ....*use* Intraluminal Device, Endotracheal Airway in Respiratory System
Phrenic nerve stimulator lead ....*use* Diaphragmatic Pacemaker Lead in Respiratory System
Spiration IBV™ Valve System ....*use* Intraluminal Device, Endobronchial Valve in Respiratory System
Tissue bank graft ....*use* Nonautologous Tissue Substitute
Tracheostomy tube...*use* Tracheostomy Device in Respiratory System

Device Aggregation Table Listings of Respiratory System

See also Device Aggregation Table in Appendix E

Specific Device	For Operation	In Body System	General Device	
Intraluminal Device, Endobronchial Valve	All applicable	Respiratory System	D	Intraluminal Device
Intraluminal Device, Endotracheal Airway	All applicable	Respiratory System	D	Intraluminal Device

Coding Notes of Respiratory System

Body System Relevant Coding Guidelines

Branches of body parts
  B4.2
    Where a specific branch of a body part does not have its own body part value in PCS, the body part is typically coded to the closest proximal branch that has a specific body part value. In the cardiovascular body systems, if a general body part is available in the correct root operation table, and coding to a proximal branch would require assigning a code in a different body system, the procedure is coded using the general body part value.
    Examples: A procedure performed on the mandibular branch of the trigeminal nerve is coded to the trigeminal nerve body part value.
    Occlusion of the bronchial artery is coded to the body part value Upper Artery in the body system Upper Arteries, and not to the body part value Thoracic Aorta, Descending in the body system Heart and Great Vessels.

Body System Specific PCS Reference Manual Exercises

PCS CODE	B – RESPIRATORY SYSTEM EXERCISES
0 B 1 1 3 F 4	Tracheostomy formation with tracheostomy tube placement, percutaneous.
0 B 2 1 X F Z	Tracheostomy tube exchange.
0 B 5 P 4 Z Z	Thoracoscopy with mechanical abrasion and application of talc for pleurodesis.
0 B 7 1 8 Z Z	Tracheoscopy with intraluminal dilation of tracheal stenosis.
0 B H 0 8 1 Z	Bronchoscopy with insertion of brachytherapy seeds, right main bronchus.
0 B P 1 X D Z	Extubation, endotracheal tube.
0 B Y K 0 Z 0	Right lung transplant, open, using organ donor match.

TUBULAR GROUP: Bypass, Dilation, Occlusion, Restriction
Root Operations that alter the diameter/route of a tubular body part.

1ST - 0 Medical and Surgical

2ND - B Respiratory System

3RD - 1 BYPASS

EXAMPLE: Tracheostomy tube placement | CMS Ex: Coronary artery bypass

BYPASS: Altering the route of passage of the contents of a tubular body part.

EXPLANATION: Rerouting contents to a downstream part ...

Body Part – 4TH	Approach – 5TH	Device – 6TH	Qualifier – 7TH
1 Trachea	0 Open	D Intraluminal device	6 Esophagus
1 Trachea	0 Open	F Tracheostomy device Z No device	4 Cutaneous
1 Trachea	3 Percutaneous 4 Percutaneous endoscopic	F Tracheostomy device Z No device	4 Cutaneous

DEVICE GROUP: Change, Insertion, Removal, (Replacement), Revision, Supplement
Root Operations that always involve a device.

1ST - 0 Medical and Surgical

2ND - B Respiratory System

3RD - 2 CHANGE

EXAMPLE: Exchange trachea tube | CMS Ex: Changing urinary catheter

CHANGE: Taking out or off a device from a body part and putting back an identical or similar device in or on the same body part without cutting or puncturing the skin or a mucous membrane.

EXPLANATION: ALL Changes use EXTERNAL approach only...

Body Part – 4TH	Approach – 5TH	Device – 6TH	Qualifier – 7TH
0 Tracheobronchial Tree Q Pleura K Lung, Right T Diaphragm L Lung, Left	X External	0 Drainage device Y Other device	Z No qualifier
1 Trachea	X External	0 Drainage device E Intraluminial device, endotracheal airway F Tracheostomy device Y Other device	Z No qualifier

RESPIRATORY

0 B 2

EXCISION GROUP: Excision, Resection, Destruction, Extraction, (Detachment)
Root Operations that take out some or all of a body part.

1ST - **0** Medical and Surgical	**EXAMPLE:** Pleurodesis with talc **CMS Ex:** Fulguration polyp
2ND - **B** Respiratory System	**DESTRUCTION:** Physical eradication of all or a portion of a body part by the direct use of energy, force, or a destructive agent.
3RD - **5 DESTRUCTION**	**EXPLANATION:** None of the body part is physically taken out

Body Part – 4TH	Approach – 5TH	Device – 6TH	Qualifier – 7TH

1 Trachea 9 Lingula Bronchus
2 Carina B Lower Lobe Bronchus, Left
3 Main Bronchus, Right C Upper Lung Lobe, Right
4 Upper Lobe Bronchus, Right D Middle Lung Lobe, Right
5 Middle Lobe Bronchus, Right F Lower Lung Lobe, Right
  G Upper Lung Lobe, Left
6 Lower Lobe Bronchus, Right H Lung Lingula
7 Main Bronchus, Left J Lower Lung Lobe, Left
  K Lung, Right
8 Upper Lobe Bronchus, Left L Lung, Left
  M Lungs, Bilateral
	0 Open
	3 Percutaneous
	4 Percutaneous endoscopic
	7 Via natural or artificial opening
	8 Via natural or artificial opening endoscopic
		Z No device	Z No qualifier

N Pleura, Right P Pleura, Left R Diaphragm, Right S Diaphragm, Left	0 Open 3 Percutaneous 4 Percutaneous endoscopic	Z No device	Z No qualifier

---

TUBULAR GROUP: Bypass, Dilation, Occlusion, Restriction
Root Operations that alter the diameter/route of a tubular body part.

1ST - **0** Medical and Surgical	**EXAMPLE:** Dilation tracheal stenosis **CMS Ex:** Transluminal angioplasty
2ND - **B** Respiratory System	**DILATION:** Expanding an orifice or the lumen of a tubular body part.
3RD - **7 DILATION**	**EXPLANATION:** By force (stretching) or cutting ...

Body Part – 4TH	Approach – 5TH	Device – 6TH	Qualifier – 7TH
1 Trachea 2 Carina 3 Main Bronchus, Right 4 Upper Lobe Bronchus, Right 5 Middle Lobe Bronchus, Right 6 Lower Lobe Bronchus, Right 7 Main Bronchus, Left 8 Upper Lobe Bronchus, Left 9 Lingula Bronchus B Lower Lobe Bronchus, Left	0 Open 3 Percutaneous 4 Percutaneous endoscopic 7 Via natural or artificial opening 8 Via natural or artificial opening endoscopic	D Intraluminal device Z No device	Z No qualifier

DRAINAGE GROUP: Drainage, Extirpation, Fragmentation
Root Operations that take out solids/fluids/gases from a body part.

1ST - **0** Medical and Surgical

2ND - **B** Respiratory System

3RD - **9 DRAINAGE**

EXAMPLE: Needle aspiration lung abscess | CMS Ex: Thoracentesis

DRAINAGE: Taking or letting out fluids and/or gases from a body part.

EXPLANATION: Qualifier "X Diagnostic" indicates biopsy ...

Body Part – 4TH		Approach – 5TH	Device – 6TH	Qualifier – 7TH
1 Trachea 2 Carina 3 Main Bronchus, Right 4 Upper Lobe Bronchus, Right 5 Middle Lobe Bronchus, Right 6 Lower Lobe Bronchus, Right 7 Main Bronchus, Left 8 Upper Lobe Bronchus, Left	9 Lingula Bronchus B Lower Lobe Bronchus, Left C Upper Lung Lobe, Right D Middle Lung Lobe, Right F Lower Lung Lobe, Right G Upper Lung Lobe, Left H Lung Lingula J Lower Lung Lobe, Left K Lung, Right L Lung, Left M Lungs, Bilateral	0 Open 3 Percutaneous 4 Percutaneous endoscopic 7 Via natural or artificial opening 8 Via natural or artificial opening endoscopic	0 Drainage device	Z No qualifier
1 Trachea 2 Carina 3 Main Bronchus, Right 4 Upper Lobe Bronchus, Right 5 Middle Lobe Bronchus, Right 6 Lower Lobe Bronchus, Right 7 Main Bronchus, Left 8 Upper Lobe Bronchus, Left	9 Lingula Bronchus B Lower Lobe Bronchus, Left C Upper Lung Lobe, Right D Middle Lung Lobe, Right F Lower Lung Lobe, Right G Upper Lung Lobe, Left H Lung Lingula J Lower Lung Lobe, Left K Lung, Right L Lung, Left M Lungs, Bilateral	0 Open 3 Percutaneous 4 Percutaneous endoscopic 7 Via natural or artificial opening 8 Via natural or artificial opening endoscopic	Z No device	X Diagnostic Z No qualifier
N Pleura, Right P Pleura, Left R Diaphragm, Right S Diaphragm, Left		0 Open 3 Percutaneous 4 Percutaneous endoscopic	0 Drainage device	Z No qualifier
N Pleura, Right P Pleura, Left R Diaphragm, Right S Diaphragm, Left		0 Open 3 Percutaneous 4 Percutaneous endoscopic	Z No device	X Diagnostic Z No qualifier

RESPIRATORY 0 B 9

EXCISION GROUP: Excision, Resection, Destruction, Extraction, (Detachment)
Root Operations that take out some or all of a body part.

1ST - 0 Medical and Surgical	EXAMPLE: Endoscopic biopsy of lung	CMS Ex: Liver biopsy
2ND - B Respiratory System	**EXCISION:** Cutting out or off, without replacement, a portion of a body part.	
3RD - B EXCISION	EXPLANATION: Qualifier "X Diagnostic" indicates biopsy ...	

Body Part – 4TH		Approach – 5TH	Device – 6TH	Qualifier – 7TH
1 Trachea	9 Lingula Bronchus	0 Open	Z No device	X Diagnostic
2 Carina	B Lower Lobe Bronchus, Left	3 Percutaneous		Z No qualifier
3 Main Bronchus, Right	C Upper Lung Lobe, Right	4 Percutaneous endoscopic		
4 Upper Lobe Bronchus, Right	D Middle Lung Lobe, Right	7 Via natural or artificial opening		
5 Middle Lobe Bronchus, Right	F Lower Lung Lobe, Right	8 Via natural or artificial opening endoscopic		
	G Upper Lung Lobe, Left			
	H Lung Lingula			
6 Lower Lobe Bronchus, Right	J Lower Lung Lobe, Left			
	K Lung, Right			
7 Main Bronchus, Left	L Lung, Left			
8 Upper Lobe Bronchus, Left	M Lungs, Bilateral			
N Pleura, Right		0 Open	Z No device	X Diagnostic
P Pleura, Left		3 Percutaneous		Z No qualifier
R Diaphragm, Right		4 Percutaneous endoscopic		
S Diaphragm, Left				

DRAINAGE GROUP: Drainage, Extirpation, Fragmentation
Root Operations that take out solids/fluids/gases from a body part.

1ST - 0 Medical and Surgical	EXAMPLE: Removal bronchial foreign body	CMS Ex: Choledocholithotomy
2ND - B Respiratory System	**EXTIRPATION:** Taking or cutting out solid matter from a body part.	
3RD - C EXTIRPATION	EXPLANATION: Abnormal byproduct or foreign body ...	

Body Part – 4TH		Approach – 5TH	Device – 6TH	Qualifier – 7TH
1 Trachea	9 Lingula Bronchus	0 Open	Z No device	Z No qualifier
2 Carina	B Lower Lobe Bronchus, Left	3 Percutaneous		
3 Main Bronchus, Right	C Upper Lung Lobe, Right	4 Percutaneous endoscopic		
4 Upper Lobe Bronchus, Right	D Middle Lung Lobe, Right	7 Via natural or artificial opening		
5 Middle Lobe Bronchus, Right	F Lower Lung Lobe, Right	8 Via natural or artificial opening endoscopic		
	G Upper Lung Lobe, Left			
	H Lung Lingula			
6 Lower Lobe Bronchus, Right	J Lower Lung Lobe, Left			
	K Lung, Right			
7 Main Bronchus, Left	L Lung, Left			
8 Upper Lobe Bronchus, Left	M Lungs, Bilateral			
N Pleura, Right		0 Open	Z No device	Z No qualifier
P Pleura, Left		3 Percutaneous		
R Diaphragm, Right		4 Percutaneous endoscopic		
S Diaphragm, Left				

© 2016 Channel Publishing, Ltd.

EXCISION GROUP: Excision, Resection, Destruction, Extraction, (Detachment)
Root Operations that take out some or all of a body part.

1ST – 0 Medical and Surgical	EXAMPLE: Pleural extraction	CMS Ex: D&C
2ND – B Respiratory System		
3RD – D EXTRACTION	**EXTRACTION:** Pulling or stripping out or off all or a portion of a body part by the use of force.	
	EXPLANATION: Qualifier "X Diagnostic" indicates biopsy ...	

Body Part – 4TH	Approach – 5TH	Device – 6TH	Qualifier – 7TH
N Pleura, Right P Pleura, Left	0 Open 3 Percutaneous 4 Percutaneous endoscopic	Z No device	X Diagnostic Z No qualifier

---

DRAINAGE GROUP: Drainage, Extirpation, Fragmentation
Root Operations that take out solids/fluids/gases from a body part.

1ST – 0 Medical and Surgical	EXAMPLE: Lithotripsy broncholithiasis	CMS Ex: ESWL
2ND – B Respiratory System		
3RD – F FRAGMENTATION	**FRAGMENTATION:** Breaking solid matter in a body part into pieces.	
	EXPLANATION: Pieces are not taken out during procedure ...	

Body Part – 4TH	Approach – 5TH	Device – 6TH	Qualifier – 7TH
1 Trachea 2 Carina 3 Main Bronchus, Right 4 Upper Lobe Bronchus, Right 5 Middle Lobe Bronchus, Right 6 Lower Lobe Bronchus, Right 7 Main Bronchus, Left 8 Upper Lobe Bronchus, Left 9 Lingula Bronchus B Lower Lobe Bronchus, Left	0 Open 3 Percutaneous 4 Percutaneous endoscopic 7 Via natural or artificial opening 8 Via natural or artificial opening endoscopic X External NC*	Z No device	Z No qualifier

NC* – Non-covered by Medicare. See current Medicare Code Editor for details.

RESPIRATORY   0 B F

DEVICE GROUP: Change, Insertion, Removal, (Replacement), Revision, Supplement
Root Operations that always involve a device.

1ST - 0 Medical and Surgical

2ND - B Respiratory System

3RD - H INSERTION

EXAMPLE: Endotracheal intubation   CMS Ex: Central venous catheter

INSERTION: Putting in a nonbiological appliance that monitors, assists, performs, or prevents a physiological function but does not physically take the place of a body part.

EXPLANATION: None

Body Part – 4TH	Approach – 5TH	Device – 6TH	Qualifier – 7TH
0 Tracheobronchial Tree	0 Open 3 Percutaneous 4 Percutaneous endoscopic 7 Via natural or artificial opening 8 Via natural or artificial opening endoscopic	1 Radioactive element 2 Monitoring device 3 Infusion device D Intraluminal device	Z No qualifier
1 Trachea	0 Open	2 Monitoring device D Intraluminal device	Z No qualifier
1 Trachea	3 Percutaneous	D Intraluminal device E Intraluminal device, endotracheal airway	Z No qualifier
1 Trachea	4 Percutaneous endoscopic	D Intraluminal device	Z No qualifier
1 Trachea	7 Via natural or artificial opening 8 Via natural or artificial opening endoscopic	2 Monitoring device D Intraluminal device E Intraluminal device, endotracheal airway	Z No qualifier
3 Main Bronchus, Right 4 Upper Lobe Bronchus, Right 5 Middle Lobe Bronchus, Right 6 Lower Lobe Bronchus, Right 7 Main Bronchus, Left 8 Upper Lobe Bronchus, Left 9 Lingula Bronchus B Lower Lobe Bronchus, Left	0 Open 3 Percutaneous 4 Percutaneous endoscopic 7 Via natural or artificial opening 8 Via natural or artificial opening endoscopic	G Intraluminal device, endobronchial valve	Z No qualifier
K Lung, Right L Lung, Left	0 Open 3 Percutaneous 4 Percutaneous endoscopic 7 Via natural or artificial opening 8 Via natural or artificial opening endoscopic	1 Radioactive element 2 Monitoring device 3 Infusion device	Z No qualifier
R Diaphragm, Right S Diaphragm, Left	0 Open 3 Percutaneous 4 Percutaneous endoscopic	2 Monitoring device M Diaphragmatic pacemaker lead	Z No qualifier

---

EXAMINATION GROUP: Inspection, (Map)
Root Operations involving examination only.

1ST – 0 Medical and Surgical	EXAMPLE: Diagnostic bronchoscopy	CMS Ex: Colonoscopy
2ND – B Respiratory System	**INSPECTION:** Visually and/or manually exploring a body part.	
3RD – J INSPECTION	EXPLANATION: Direct or instrumental visualization …	

Body Part – 4TH	Approach – 5TH	Device – 6TH	Qualifier – 7TH
0 Tracheobronchial Tree 1 Trachea K Lung, Right L Lung, Left Q Pleura T Diaphragm	0 Open 3 Percutaneous 4 Percutaneous endoscopic 7 Via natural or artificial opening 8 Via natural or artificial opening endoscopic X External	Z No device	Z No qualifier

---

TUBULAR GROUP: Bypass, Dilation, Occlusion, Restriction
Root Operations that alter the diameter/route of a tubular body part.

1ST – 0 Medical and Surgical	EXAMPLE: Suture closure bronchus	CMS Ex: Fallopian tube ligation
2ND – B Respiratory System	**OCCLUSION:** Completely closing an orifice or lumen of a tubular body part.	
3RD – L OCCLUSION	EXPLANATION: Natural or artificially created orifice …	

Body Part – 4TH	Approach – 5TH	Device – 6TH	Qualifier – 7TH
1 Trachea 2 Carina 3 Main Bronchus, Right 4 Upper Lobe Bronchus, Right 5 Middle Lobe Bronchus, Right 6 Lower Lobe Bronchus, Right 7 Main Bronchus, Left 8 Upper Lobe Bronchus, Left 9 Lingula Bronchus B Lower Lobe Bronchus, Left	0 Open 3 Percutaneous 4 Percutaneous endoscopic	C Extraluminal device D Intraluminal device Z No device	Z No qualifier
1 Trachea 2 Carina 3 Main Bronchus, Right 4 Upper Lobe Bronchus, Right 5 Middle Lobe Bronchus, Right 6 Lower Lobe Bronchus, Right 7 Main Bronchus, Left 8 Upper Lobe Bronchus, Left 9 Lingula Bronchus B Lower Lobe Bronchus, Left	7 Via natural or artificial opening 8 Via natural or artificial opening endoscopic	D Intraluminal device Z No device	Z No qualifier

RESPIRATORY 0 B L

MOVE GROUP: Reattachment, Reposition, (Transfer), Transplantation
Root Operations that put in/put back or move some/all of a body part.

1ST – O Medical and Surgical	EXAMPLE: Reattachment ruptured diaphragm	CMS Ex: Reattach hand
2ND – B Respiratory System	**REATTACHMENT:** Putting back in or on all or a portion of a separated body part to its normal location or other suitable location.	
3RD – M REATTACHMENT	EXPLANATION: With/without reconnection of vessels/nerves…	

Body Part – 4TH		Approach – 5TH	Device – 6TH	Qualifier – 7TH
1 Trachea	B Lower Lobe Bronchus, Left	0 Open	Z No device	Z No qualifier
2 Carina	C Upper Lung Lobe, Right			
3 Main Bronchus, Right	D Middle Lung Lobe, Right			
4 Upper Lobe Bronchus, Right	F Lower Lung Lobe, Right			
5 Middle Lobe Bronchus, Right	G Upper Lung Lobe, Left			
	H Lung Lingula			
6 Lower Lobe Bronchus, Right	J Lower Lung Lobe, Left			
7 Main Bronchus, Left	K Lung, Right			
8 Upper Lobe Bronchus, Left	L Lung, Left			
	R Diaphragm, Right			
9 Lingula Bronchus	S Diaphragm, Left			

DIVISION GROUP: (Division), Release
Root Operations involving cutting or separation only.

1ST – O Medical and Surgical	EXAMPLE: Lysis adhesions lung	CMS Ex: Carpal tunnel release
2ND – B Respiratory System	**RELEASE:** Freeing a body part from an abnormal physical constraint by cutting or by the use of force.	
3RD – N RELEASE	EXPLANATION: None of the body part is taken out …	

Body Part – 4TH		Approach – 5TH	Device – 6TH	Qualifier – 7TH
1 Trachea	9 Lingula Bronchus	0 Open	Z No device	Z No qualifier
2 Carina	B Lower Lobe Bronchus, Left	3 Percutaneous		
3 Main Bronchus, Right	C Upper Lung Lobe, Right	4 Percutaneous endoscopic		
4 Upper Lobe Bronchus, Right	D Middle Lung Lobe, Right	7 Via natural or artificial opening		
5 Middle Lobe Bronchus, Right	F Lower Lung Lobe, Right	8 Via natural or artificial opening endoscopic		
	G Upper Lung Lobe, Left			
	H Lung Lingula			
6 Lower Lobe Bronchus, Right	J Lower Lung Lobe, Left			
	K Lung, Right			
7 Main Bronchus, Left	L Lung, Left			
8 Upper Lobe Bronchus, Left	M Lungs, Bilateral			
N Pleura, Right		0 Open	Z No device	Z No qualifier
P Pleura, Left		3 Percutaneous		
R Diaphragm, Right		4 Percutaneous endoscopic		
S Diaphragm, Left				

DEVICE GROUP: Change, Insertion, Removal, (Replacement), Revision, Supplement
Root Operations that always involve a device.

1ST - 0 Medical and Surgical

2ND - B Respiratory System

3RD - P REMOVAL

EXAMPLE: Removal tracheostomy tube | CMS Ex: Chest tube removal

REMOVAL: Taking out or off a device from a body part.

EXPLANATION: Removal device without reinsertion ...

Body Part – 4TH	Approach – 5TH	Device – 6TH	Qualifier – 7TH
0 Tracheobronchial Tree	0 Open 3 Percutaneous 4 Percutaneous endoscopic 7 Via natural or artificial opening 8 Via natural or artificial opening endoscopic	0 Drainage device 1 Radioactive element 2 Monitoring device 3 Infusion device 7 Autologous tissue substitute C Extraluminal device D Intraluminal device J Synthetic substitute K Nonautologous tissue substitute	Z No qualifier
0 Tracheobronchial Tree	X External	0 Drainage device 1 Radioactive element 2 Monitoring device 3 Infusion device D Intraluminal device	Z No qualifier
1 Trachea	0 Open 3 Percutaneous 4 Percutaneous endoscopic 7 Via natural or artificial opening 8 Via natural or artificial opening endoscopic	0 Drainage device 2 Monitoring device 7 Autologous tissue substitute C Extraluminal device D Intraluminal device F Tracheostomy device J Synthetic substitute K Nonautologous tissue substitute	Z No qualifier
1 Trachea	X External	0 Drainage device 2 Monitoring device D Intraluminal device F Tracheostomy device	Z No qualifier

RESPIRATORY 0 B P

continued ⇨

0   B   P   REMOVAL – continued

Body Part – 4TH	Approach – 5TH	Device – 6TH	Qualifier – 7TH
K Lung, Right L Lung, Left	0 Open 3 Percutaneous 4 Percutaneous endoscopic 7 Via natural or artificial opening 8 Via natural or artificial opening endoscopic X External	0 Drainage device 1 Radioactive element 2 Monitoring device 3 Infusion device	Z No qualifier
Q Pleura	0 Open 3 Percutaneous 4 Percutaneous endoscopic 7 Via natural or artificial opening 8 Via natural or artificial opening endoscopic X External	0 Drainage device 1 Radioactive element 2 Monitoring device	Z No qualifier
T Diaphragm	0 Open 3 Percutaneous 4 Percutaneous endoscopic 7 Via natural or artificial opening 8 Via natural or artificial opening endoscopic	0 Drainage device 2 Monitoring device 7 Autologous tissue substitute J Synthetic substitute K Nonautologous tissue substitute M Diaphragmatic pacemaker lead	Z No qualifier
T Diaphragm	X External	0 Drainage device 2 Monitoring device M Diaphragmatic pacemaker lead	Z No qualifier

OTHER REPAIRS GROUP: (Control), Repair
Root Operations that define other repairs.

1ST - **0** Medical and Surgical	EXAMPLE: Repair diaphragmatic hernia	CMS Ex: Suture laceration
2ND - **B** Respiratory System	**REPAIR:** Restoring, to the extent possible, a body part to its normal anatomic structure and function.	
3RD - **Q REPAIR**	EXPLANATION: Only when no other root operation applies ...	

Body Part – 4TH		Approach – 5TH	Device – 6TH	Qualifier – 7TH
1 Trachea 2 Carina 3 Main Bronchus, Right 4 Upper Lobe Bronchus, Right 5 Middle Lobe Bronchus, Right 6 Lower Lobe Bronchus, Right 7 Main Bronchus, Left 8 Upper Lobe Bronchus, Left	9 Lingula Bronchus B Lower Lobe Bronchus, Left C Upper Lung Lobe, Right D Middle Lung Lobe, Right F Lower Lung Lobe, Right G Upper Lung Lobe, Left H Lung Lingula J Lower Lung Lobe, Left K Lung, Right L Lung, Left M Lungs, Bilateral	0 Open 3 Percutaneous 4 Percutaneous endoscopic 7 Via natural or artificial opening 8 Via natural or artificial opening endoscopic	Z No device	Z No qualifier
N Pleura, Right P Pleura, Left R Diaphragm, Right S Diaphragm, Left		0 Open 3 Percutaneous 4 Percutaneous endoscopic	Z No device	Z No qualifier

MOVE GROUP: Reattachment, Reposition, (Transfer), Transplantation
Root Operations that put in/put back or move some/all of a body part.

1ST - **0** Medical and Surgical	EXAMPLE: Tracheal relocation	CMS Ex: Fracture reduction
2ND - **B** Respiratory System	**REPOSITION:** Moving to its normal location, or other suitable location, all or a portion of a body part.	
3RD - **S REPOSITION**	EXPLANATION: May or may not be cut to be moved ...	

Body Part – 4TH		Approach – 5TH	Device – 6TH	Qualifier – 7TH
1 Trachea 2 Carina 3 Main Bronchus, Right 4 Upper Lobe Bronchus, Right 5 Middle Lobe Bronchus, Right 6 Lower Lobe Bronchus, Right 7 Main Bronchus, Left 8 Upper Lobe Bronchus, Left 9 Lingula Bronchus	B Lower Lobe Bronchus, Left C Upper Lung Lobe, Right D Middle Lung Lobe, Right F Lower Lung Lobe, Right G Upper Lung Lobe, Left H Lung Lingula J Lower Lung Lobe, Left K Lung, Right L Lung, Left R Diaphragm, Right S Diaphragm, Left	0 Open	Z No device	Z No qualifier

RESPIRATORY **0 B S**

EXCISION GROUP: Excision, Resection, Destruction, Extraction, (Detachment)
Root Operations that take out some or all of a body part.

1ST - O Medical and Surgical	EXAMPLE: Lobectomy		CMS Ex: Cholecystectomy

1ST - O Medical and Surgical

2ND - B Respiratory System

3RD - T RESECTION

EXAMPLE: Lobectomy   CMS Ex: Cholecystectomy

RESECTION: Cutting out or off, without replacement, all of a body part.

EXPLANATION: None

Body Part – 4TH		Approach – 5TH	Device – 6TH	Qualifier – 7TH
1 Trachea	B Lower Lobe Bronchus, Left	0 Open	Z No device	Z No qualifier
2 Carina	C Upper Lung Lobe, Right	4 Percutaneous endoscopic		
3 Main Bronchus, Right	D Middle Lung Lobe, Right			
4 Upper Lobe Bronchus, Right	F Lower Lung Lobe, Right			
5 Middle Lobe Bronchus, Right	G Upper Lung Lobe, Left			
6 Lower Lobe Bronchus, Right	H Lung Lingula			
7 Main Bronchus, Left	J Lower Lung Lobe, Left			
8 Upper Lobe Bronchus, Left	K Lung, Right			
9 Lingula Bronchus	L Lung, Left			
	M Lungs, Bilateral			
	R Diaphragm, Right			
	S Diaphragm, Left			

DEVICE GROUP: Change, Insertion, Removal, (Replacement), Revision, Supplement
Root Operations that always involve a device.

1ST - O Medical and Surgical

2ND - B Respiratory System

3RD - U SUPPLEMENT

EXAMPLE: Graft repair diaphragm defect   CMS Ex: Hernia repair with mesh

SUPPLEMENT: Putting in or on biological or synthetic material that physically reinforces and/or augments the function of a portion of a body part.

EXPLANATION: Biological material from same individual ...

Body Part – 4TH	Approach – 5TH	Device – 6TH	Qualifier – 7TH
1 Trachea	0 Open	7 Autologous tissue substitute	Z No qualifier
2 Carina	4 Percutaneous endoscopic	J Synthetic substitute	
3 Main Bronchus, Right		K Nonautologous tissue substitute	
4 Upper Lobe Bronchus, Right			
5 Middle Lobe Bronchus, Right			
6 Lower Lobe Bronchus, Right			
7 Main Bronchus, Left			
8 Upper Lobe Bronchus, Left			
9 Lingula Bronchus			
B Lower Lobe Bronchus, Left			
R Diaphragm, Right			
S Diaphragm, Left			

RESPIRATORY   0 B T

TUBULAR GROUP: Bypass, Dilation, Occlusion, Restriction
Root Operations that alter the diameter/route of a tubular body part.

1ST - **0** Medical and Surgical	EXAMPLE: Bronchial restrictive stent CMS Ex: Cervical cerclage
2ND - **B** Respiratory System	**RESTRICTION:** Partially closing an orifice or the lumen of a tubular body part.
3RD - **V RESTRICTION**	EXPLANATION: Natural or artificially created orifice ...

Body Part – 4TH	Approach – 5TH	Device – 6TH	Qualifier – 7TH
1 Trachea 2 Carina 3 Main Bronchus, Right 4 Upper Lobe Bronchus, Right 5 Middle Lobe Bronchus, Right 6 Lower Lobe Bronchus, Right 7 Main Bronchus, Left 8 Upper Lobe Bronchus, Left 9 Lingula Bronchus B Lower Lobe Bronchus, Left	0 Open 3 Percutaneous 4 Percutaneous endoscopic	C Extraluminal device D Intraluminal device Z No device	Z No qualifier
1 Trachea 2 Carina 3 Main Bronchus, Right 4 Upper Lobe Bronchus, Right 5 Middle Lobe Bronchus, Right 6 Lower Lobe Bronchus, Right 7 Main Bronchus, Left 8 Upper Lobe Bronchus, Left 9 Lingula Bronchus B Lower Lobe Bronchus, Left	7 Via natural or artificial opening 8 Via natural or artificial opening endoscopic	D Intraluminal device Z No device	Z No qualifier

R E S P I R A T O R Y

0 B V

DEVICE GROUP: Change, Insertion, Removal, (Replacement), Revision, Supplement
Root Operations that always involve a device.

1ST - 0 Medical and Surgical	EXAMPLE: Reposition diaphragm lead	CMS Ex: Adjustment pacemaker lead
2ND - B Respiratory System	REVISION: Correcting, to the extent possible, a portion of a malfunctioning device or the position of a displaced device.	
3RD - W REVISION	EXPLANATION: May replace components of a device ...	

Body Part – 4TH	Approach – 5TH	Device – 6TH	Qualifier – 7TH
0 Tracheobronchial Tree	0 Open 3 Percutaneous 4 Percutaneous endoscopic 7 Via natural or artificial opening 8 Via natural or artificial opening endoscopic X External	0 Drainage device 2 Monitoring device 3 Infusion device 7 Autologous tissue substitute C Extraluminal device D Intraluminal device J Synthetic substitute K Nonautologous tissue substitute	Z No qualifier
1 Trachea	0 Open 3 Percutaneous 4 Percutaneous endoscopic 7 Via natural or artificial opening 8 Via natural or artificial opening endoscopic X External	0 Drainage device 2 Monitoring device 7 Autologous tissue substitute C Extraluminal device D Intraluminal device F Tracheostomy device J Synthetic substitute K Nonautologous tissue substitute	Z No qualifier
K Lung, Right L Lung, Left	0 Open 3 Percutaneous 4 Percutaneous endoscopic 7 Via natural or artificial opening 8 Via natural or artificial opening endoscopic X External	0 Drainage device 2 Monitoring device 3 Infusion device	Z No qualifier
Q Pleura	0 Open 3 Percutaneous 4 Percutaneous endoscopic 7 Via natural or artificial opening 8 Via natural or artificial opening endoscopic X External	0 Drainage device 2 Monitoring device	Z No qualifier
T Diaphragm	0 Open 3 Percutaneous 4 Percutaneous endoscopic 7 Via natural or artificial opening 8 Via natural or artificial opening endoscopic X External	0 Drainage device 2 Monitoring device 7 Autologous tissue substitute J Synthetic substitute K Nonautologous tissue substitute M Diaphragmatic pacemaker lead	Z No qualifier

<table>
<tr><td colspan="4"> <u>MOVE GROUP:</u> Reattachment, Reposition, (Transfer), Transplantation
Root Operations that put in/put back or move some/all of a body part. </td></tr>
</table>

1ST - 0 Medical and Surgical	EXAMPLE: Lung transplant		CMS Ex: Kidney transplant
2ND - B Respiratory System	<u>TRANSPLANTATION:</u> Putting in or on all or a portion of a living body part taken from another individual or animal to physically take the place and/or function of all or a portion of a similar body part.		
3RD - Y TRANSPLANTATION	EXPLANATION: May take over all or part of its function ...		

Body Part – 4TH	Approach – 5TH	Device – 6TH	Qualifier – 7TH
C Upper Lung Lobe, Right LC* D Middle Lung Lobe, Right LC* F Lower Lung Lobe, Right LC* G Upper Lung Lobe, Left LC* H Lung Lingula LC* J Lower Lung Lobe, Left LC* K Lung, Right LC* L Lung, Left LC* M Lungs, Bilateral LC*	0 Open	Z No device	0 Allogeneic 1 Syngeneic 2 Zooplastic

LC* – Some procedures are considered limited coverage by Medicare. See current Medicare Code Editor for details.

RESPIRATORY 0 B Y

NOTES

Educational Annotations | C – Mouth and Throat

Body System Specific Educational Annotations for the Mouth and Throat include:

- Anatomy and Physiology Review
- Anatomical Illustrations
- Definitions of Common Procedures
- AHA Coding Clinic® Reference Notations
- Body Part Key Listings
- Device Key Listings
- Device Aggregation Table Listings
- Coding Notes

Anatomy and Physiology Review of Mouth and Throat

BODY PART VALUES – C - MOUTH AND THROAT

Adenoids – ANATOMY – The adenoids (nasopharyngeal tonsils) are masses of lymphatic tissue located behind the nasal cavity and on roof of the nasopharynx. PHYSIOLOGY – The adenoids help in the prevention of bacteria entering the body.

Buccal Mucosa – The mucous membrane lining of the mouth and inside of cheeks.

Epiglottis – ANATOMY – The epiglottis is a mucous-membrane-covered flap of elastic cartilage tissue that is attached to the entrance of the larynx. PHYSIOLOGY – The epiglottis prevents food from going into the trachea and channels it into the esophagus.

Gingiva – ANATOMY – The gingiva (gums) are fibrous and mucous membrane tissue that surround the roots of erupted teeth and the crowns of unerupted teeth, and cover the alveolar process of the maxilla and mandible. PHYSIOLOGY – The gingiva (gums) function to help protect and support the roots of the teeth.

Hard Palate – The hard palate is the superior wall of the oral cavity formed by the palatine processes of the maxilla that separates the oral cavity from the nasal cavity.

Larynx – ANATOMY – The larynx is the musculocartilaginous structure, lined with mucous membrane located between the root of the tongue and the trachea. The glottis is the slit-like opening of the larynx formed by the true vocal cords. The supraglottis is that portion of the larynx situated above the glottis. There are nine laryngeal cartilages, three paired and three single. PHYSIOLOGY – The larynx functions to guard the entrance of the trachea from food and liquids, to control the expulsion of air, and to produce sound. The glottis produces sound, controls pitch, and when closed prevents food from entering the trachea. The supraglottis is an area of the larynx which helps to prevent food and liquid from entering the trachea. The laryngeal cartilages frame and support the larynx and its muscles.

Lip – ANATOMY – The soft tissue opening of the mouth comprised of skin, connective tissue, and muscle. PHYSIOLOGY – The lips contain sensitive nerve endings that provide sensory information about food. The lips secure the closure of the mouth during chewing and swallowing. They also are involved in sound production and facial expression.

Minor Salivary Gland – Any of the large number of small salivary glands in the oral mucosa of the mouth.

Parotid Duct – The tube (Stenson's ducts) beginning in the parotid gland and emptying into the oral cavity.

Parotid Gland – The two parotid glands lie above the mouth, and below and in front of the ears, with ducts (Stenson's ducts) that run down through the cheeks and empty into the roof of the mouth opposite of the second molar.

Pharynx – ANATOMY – The portion of the throat comprised of the oropharynx and the laryngopharynx. PHYSIOLOGY – The pharynx serves as a passageway for food and air.

Salivary Gland – ANATOMY – There are three pairs of major salivary glands; the parotids, the submandibular, and the sublingual glands. Both sympathetic and parasympathetic nerves stimulate the major salivary glands. PHYSIOLOGY – The major salivary glands function to secrete saliva which moistens food particles, help to bind them together, and begin digestion of carbohydrates. Saliva also dissolves various food chemicals so they can be tasted. There are two types of secretory cells. Serous cells produce a watery fluid which contain a digestive enzyme called amylase. Mucous cells produce a thick stringy liquid that bind food together and act as a lubricant during swallowing. Sympathetic nerves stimulate the glands to secrete a small quantity of saliva to keep the mouth moist. Parasympathetic nerves stimulate the glands reflexly when the person sees, smells, or even thinks about pleasant food.

Soft Palate – ANATOMY – The soft palate is the muscular extension of the hard palate in the superior-posterior oral cavity. PHYSIOLOGY – The soft palate contracts to allow swallowing and prevents food from entering the nasal cavity.

Continued on next page

Educational Annotations | C – Mouth and Throat

Anatomy and Physiology Review of Mouth and Throat

BODY PART VALUES – C - MOUTH AND THROAT

Continued from previous page

Subligual Gland – The two sublingual glands lie beneath the tongue, with ducts opening near the frenulum of the tongue.

Submaxillary Gland – The two submaxillary (submandibular) glands lie in the floor of the mouth on the inside surface of the mandible, with ducts (Wharton's ducts) opening beneath the tongue, and with other ducts opening near the frenulum of the tongue.

Teeth – ANATOMY – The teeth consist of the bony substance dentine, which surround the soft inner pulp that contain blood vessels and nerves and are embedded in rows in the upper (maxilla) and lower (mandible) jaw bones. PHYSIOLOGY – The teeth function primarily to chew food into smaller parts in preparation for swallowing and digestion.

Tongue – ANATOMY – The tongue is the movable, muscular organ on the floor of the mouth. The lingual tonsils are a mass of lymphoid tissue at the root, and the frenulum is the mucous membrane fold which attaches the undersurface of the tongue to the floor of the mouth. PHYSIOLOGY – The tongue functions primarily as the organ of sense of taste, as well as aiding in the chewing and swallowing of food, and the articulation of sound. The lingual tonsils aid in the elimination of bacteria entering the oral cavity. The frenulum somewhat restricts the movement of the tongue.

Tonsils – ANATOMY – The tonsils (palatine tonsils) are masses of lymphatic tissue located on either side of the tongue in the posterior oral cavity. The tonsillar fossa is the depression in which the tonsils are located. The tonsillar pillars are the mucous membrane folds attached to the soft palate. PHYSIOLOGY – The tonsils function to help fight off bacteria by releasing bacteria-consuming phagocytes.

Uvula – The uvula is the cone-shaped projection of the soft palate.

Vocal Cord – ANATOMY – The vocal cords are folds of mucous membranes located within the larynx. PHYSIOLOGY – The vocal cords are primarily responsible for voice production. Sound is produced by the vibration of the folds as air is exhaled from the lungs.

Anatomical Illustrations of Mouth and Throat

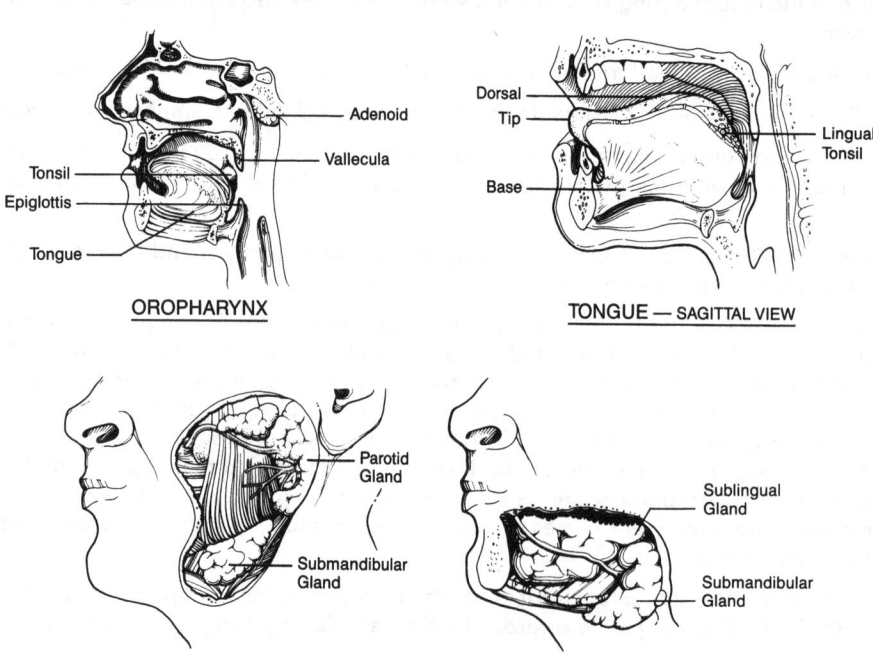

OROPHARYNX

TONGUE — SAGITTAL VIEW

MAJOR SALIVARY GLANDS

Continued on next page

Educational Annotations | C – Mouth and Throat

Anatomical Illustrations of Mouth and Throat

Continued from previous page

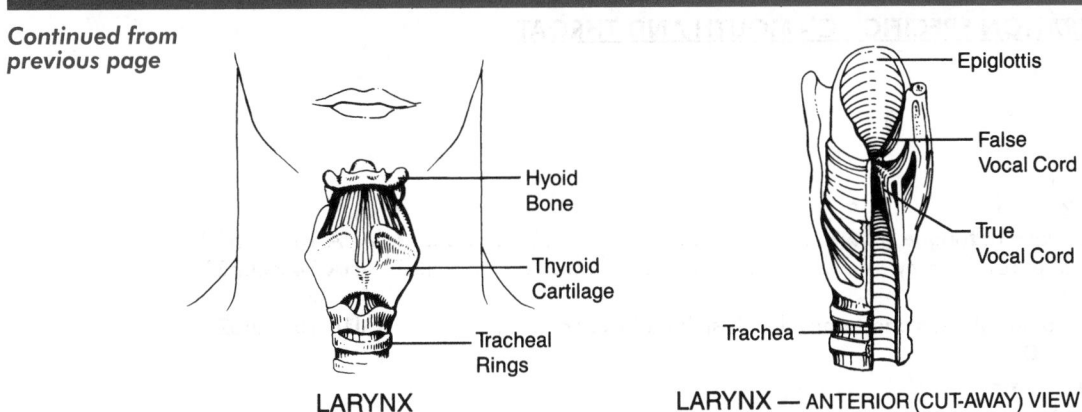

LARYNX

LARYNX — ANTERIOR (CUT-AWAY) VIEW

Definitions of Common Procedures of Mouth and Throat

Ablation of vocal cord lesion – The destruction of a vocal cord lesion using a tissue destroying technique (laser, radiofrequency heat, etc.).

Cleft palate repair – The reconstructing surgical repair of a cleft palate (defect in the roof of the mouth) by excising and moving tissue from the palate and other oral tissues and closing in layers while realigning the palatal muscles.

Glossectomy – The excision of all or a portion of the tongue.

Laser-assisted uvuloplasty – The use of repeated laser treatments to destroy and modify the uvula tissue in order to reduce or eliminate snoring.

Sialoadenectomy – The excision of a salivary gland.

Sialolithotomy – The incision of a salivary gland to remove a stone from the gland or its duct.

Tonsillectomy – The excision of the tonsils performed by a direct approach (external).

Total laryngectomy – The surgical removal of all of the larynx and usually with the insertion of an artificial voice box prosthesis.

Uvulopalatopharyngoplasty – The reconstructing surgical repair of the back of the oral cavity by removing the tonsils, and reshaping the uvula, pharynx, and soft palate to correct obstructive sleep apnea.

MOUTH & THROAT 0 C

Educational Annotations | C – Mouth and Throat

AHA Coding Clinic® Reference Notations of Mouth and Throat

ROOT OPERATION SPECIFIC - C - MOUTH AND THROAT

ALTERATION - 0
CHANGE - 2
DESTRUCTION - 5
DILATION - 7
DRAINAGE - 9
EXCISION - B
    Biopsy of base of tongue ....AHA 16:2Q:p19
    Superficial parotidectomy..AHA 14:3Q:p21
EXTIRPATION - C
    Submandibular gland stone removal with sialoendoscope ....AHA 16:2Q:p20
EXTRACTION - D
FRAGMENTATION - F
INSERTION - H
INSPECTION - J
OCCLUSION - L
REATTACHMENT - M
RELEASE - N
REMOVAL - P
REPAIR - Q
REPLACEMENT - R
    Intraoral graft using Oasis® acellular matrix ....AHA 14:2Q:p5,6
    Wide local excision of soft palate with placement of a maxillary
        surgical obturator ....AHA 14:3Q:p25
REPOSITION - S
RESECTION - T
    Extraction of impacted teeth ....AHA 14:3Q:p23
    Infratemporal fossa malignancy with parotidectomy ....AHA 16:2Q:p12
SUPPLEMENT - U
RESTRICTION - V
REVISION - W
TRANSFER - X

Body Part Key Listings of Mouth and Throat

See also Body Part Key in Appendix C
Anterior lingual gland ....*use* Minor Salivary Gland
Aryepiglottic fold ....*use* Larynx
Arytenoid cartilage ....*use* Larynx
Base of tongue ....*use* Pharynx
Buccal gland ....*use* Buccal Mucosa
Corniculate cartilage ....*use* Larynx
Cuneiform cartilage ....*use* Larynx
False vocal cord ....*use* Larynx
Frenulum labii inferioris................................*use* Lower Lip
Frenulum labii superioris ....*use* Upper Lip
Frenulum linguae................................*use* Tongue
Glossoepiglottic fold ....*use* Epiglottis
Glottis................................*use* Larynx
Hypopharynx ....*use* Pharynx
Continued on next page

Educational Annotations | C – Mouth and Throat

Body Part Key Listings of Mouth and Throat

Continued from previous page

Labial gland ....*use* Upper Lip, Lower Lip
Laryngopharynx ....*use* Pharynx
Lingual tonsil ....*use* Tongue
Molar gland ....*use* Buccal Mucosa
Oropharynx ....*use* Pharynx
Palatine gland ....*use* Buccal Mucosa
Palatine tonsil..*use* Tonsils
Palatine uvula ....*use* Uvula
Pharyngeal tonsil ....*use* Adenoids
Piriform recess (sinus) ....*use* Pharynx
Rima glottidis ....*use* Larynx
Stensen's duct..*use* Parotid Duct, Left/Right
Submandibular gland ....*use* Submaxillary Gland, Left/Right
Thyroid cartilage ....*use* Larynx
Tongue, base of   ....*use* Pharynx
Ventricular fold ....*use* Larynx
Vermilion border ....*use* Upper Lip, Lower Lip
Vocal fold ....*use* Vocal Cord, Left/Right

Device Key Listings of Mouth and Throat

See also Device Key in Appendix D

Autograft ....*use* Autologous Tissue Substitute
Brachytherapy seeds ....*use* Radioactive Element
Guedel airway ....*use* Intraluminal Device, Airway in Mouth and Throat
Oropharyngeal airway (OPA) ....*use* Intraluminal Device, Airway in Mouth and Throat
Tissue bank graft ....*use* Nonautologous Tissue Substitute

Device Aggregation Table Listings of Mouth and Throat

See also Device Aggregation Table in Appendix E

Specific Device	For Operation	In Body System	General Device
Intraluminal Device, Airway	All applicable	Mouth and Throat	D Intraluminal Device

MOUTH & THROAT 0 C

Educational Annotations | C – Mouth and Throat

Coding Notes of Mouth and Throat

Body System Specific PCS Reference Manual Exercises

PCS CODE	C – MOUTH AND THROAT EXERCISES
0 C 5 T 3 Z Z	Percutaneous radiofrequency ablation of right vocal cord lesion.
0 C B 1 X Z Z	Excision of basal cell carcinoma of lower lip.
0 C D W X Z 2	Forceps total mouth extraction, upper and lower teeth.
0 C D X X Z 2	
0 C J S 8 Z Z	Diagnostic laryngoscopy.
0 C M X X Z 1	Closed replantation of three avulsed teeth, lower jaw.
0 C N 7 X Z Z	Frenulotomy for treatment of tongue-tie syndrome. (The frenulum is coded to the body part value Tongue.)

OTHER OBJECTIVES GROUP: Alteration, (Creation), (Fusion)
Root Operations that define other objectives.

1ST – 0 Medical and Surgical	EXAMPLE: Cosmetic lip augmentation		CMS Ex: Face lift
2ND – C Mouth and Throat	**ALTERATION:** Modifying the anatomic structure of a body part without affecting the function of the body part.		
3RD – 0 **ALTERATION**			
	EXPLANATION: Principal purpose is to improve appearance		

Body Part – 4TH	Approach – 5TH	Device – 6TH	Qualifier – 7TH
0 Upper Lip 1 Lower Lip	X External	7 Autologous tissue substitute J Synthetic substitute K Nonautologous tissue substitute Z No device	Z No qualifier

---

DEVICE GROUP: Change, Insertion, Removal, Replacement, Revision, Supplement
Root Operations that always involve a device.

1ST – 0 Medical and Surgical	EXAMPLE: Exchange drain tube	CMS Ex: Changing urinary catheter
2ND – C Mouth and Throat	**CHANGE:** Taking out or off a device from a body part and putting back an identical or similar device in or on the same body part without cutting or puncturing the skin or a mucous membrane.	
3RD – 2 **CHANGE**		
	EXPLANATION: ALL Changes use EXTERNAL approach only...	

Body Part – 4TH	Approach – 5TH	Device – 6TH	Qualifier – 7TH
A Salivary Gland S Larynx Y Mouth and Throat	X External	0 Drainage device Y Other device	Z No qualifier

MOUTH & THROAT 0 C 2

EXCISION GROUP: Excision, Resection, Destruction, Extraction, (Detachment)
Root Operations that take out some or all of a body part.

1ST - 0 Medical and Surgical	EXAMPLE: Ablation vocal cord lesion	CMS Ex: Fulguration polyp
2ND - C Mouth and Throat	**DESTRUCTION:** Physical eradication of all or a portion of a body part by the direct use of energy, force, or a destructive agent.	
3RD - 5 DESTRUCTION	EXPLANATION: None of the body part is physically taken out	

Body Part – 4TH	Approach – 5TH	Device – 6TH	Qualifier – 7TH
0 Upper Lip 5 Upper Gingiva 1 Lower Lip 6 Lower Gingiva 2 Hard Palate 7 Tongue 3 Soft Palate N Uvula 4 Buccal Mucosa P Tonsils Q Adenoids	0 Open 3 Percutaneous X External	Z No device	Z No qualifier
8 Parotid Gland, Right D Sublingual Gland, Right 9 Parotid Gland, Left F Sublingual Gland, Left B Parotid Duct, Right G Submaxillary Gland, Right C Parotid Duct, Left H Submaxillary Gland, Left J Minor Salivary Gland	0 Open 3 Percutaneous	Z No device	Z No qualifier
M Pharynx R Epiglottis S Larynx T Vocal Cord, Right V Vocal Cord, Left	0 Open 3 Percutaneous 4 Percutaneous endoscopic 7 Via natural or artificial opening 8 Via natural or artificial opening endoscopic	Z No device	Z No qualifier
W Upper Tooth X Lower Tooth	0 Open X External	Z No device	0 Single 1 Multiple 2 All

© 2016 Channel Publishing, Ltd.

TUBULAR GROUP: (Bypass), **Dilation, Occlusion, Restriction**
Root Operations that alter the diameter/route of a tubular body part.

1ST - 0 Medical and Surgical	EXAMPLE: Dilation laryngeal stenosis CMS Ex: Transluminal angioplasty
2ND - C Mouth and Throat	**DILATION:** Expanding an orifice or the lumen of a tubular body part.
3RD - 7 DILATION	EXPLANATION: By force (stretching) or cutting ...

Body Part – 4TH	Approach – 5TH	Device – 6TH	Qualifier – 7TH
B Parotid Duct, Right C Parotid Duct, Left	0 Open 3 Percutaneous 7 Via natural or artificial opening	D Intraluminal device Z No device	Z No qualifier
M Pharynx	7 Via natural or artificial opening 8 Via natural or artificial opening endoscopic	D Intraluminal device Z No device	Z No qualifier
S Larynx	0 Open 3 Percutaneous 4 Percutaneous endoscopic 7 Via natural or artificial opening 8 Via natural or artificial opening endoscopic	D Intraluminal device Z No device	Z No qualifier

MOUTH & THROAT
0 C 7

DRAINAGE GROUP: Drainage, Extirpation, Fragmentation
Root Operations that take out solids/fluids/gases from a body part.

1ST – **0** Medical and Surgical	EXAMPLE: I&D parotid gland abscess	CMS Ex: Thoracentesis
2ND – **C** Mouth and Throat	**DRAINAGE:** Taking or letting out fluids and/or gases from a body part.	
3RD – **9 DRAINAGE**	EXPLANATION: Qualifier "X Diagnostic" indicates biopsy …	

Body Part – 4TH	Approach – 5TH	Device – 6TH	Qualifier – 7TH
0 Upper Lip 5 Upper Gingiva 1 Lower Lip 6 Lower Gingiva 2 Hard Palate 7 Tongue 3 Soft Palate N Uvula 4 Buccal Mucosa P Tonsils Q Adenoids	0 Open 3 Percutaneous X External	0 Drainage device	Z No qualifier
0 Upper Lip 5 Upper Gingiva 1 Lower Lip 6 Lower Gingiva 2 Hard Palate 7 Tongue 3 Soft Palate N Uvula 4 Buccal Mucosa P Tonsils Q Adenoids	0 Open 3 Percutaneous X External	Z No device	X Diagnostic Z No qualifier
8 Parotid Gland, Right D Sublingual Gland, Right 9 Parotid Gland, Left F Sublingual Gland, Left B Parotid Duct, Right G Submaxillary Gland, Right C Parotid Duct, Left H Submaxillary Gland, Left J Minor Salivary Gland	0 Open 3 Percutaneous	0 Drainage device	Z No qualifier
8 Parotid Gland, Right D Sublingual Gland, Right 9 Parotid Gland, Left F Sublingual Gland, Left B Parotid Duct, Right G Submaxillary Gland, Right C Parotid Duct, Left H Submaxillary Gland, Left J Minor Salivary Gland	0 Open 3 Percutaneous	Z No device	X Diagnostic Z No qualifier
M Pharynx R Epiglottis S Larynx T Vocal Cord, Right V Vocal Cord, Left	0 Open 3 Percutaneous 4 Percutaneous endoscopic 7 Via natural or artificial opening 8 Via natural or artificial opening endoscopic	0 Drainage device	Z No qualifier
M Pharynx R Epiglottis S Larynx T Vocal Cord, Right V Vocal Cord, Left	0 Open 3 Percutaneous 4 Percutaneous endoscopic 7 Via natural or artificial opening 8 Via natural or artificial opening endoscopic	Z No device	X Diagnostic Z No qualifier
W Upper Tooth X Lower Tooth	0 Open X External	0 Drainage device Z No device	0 Single 1 Multiple 2 All

MOUTH & THROAT 0 C 9

EXCISION GROUP: Excision, Resection, Destruction, Extraction, (Detachment)
Root Operations that take out some or all of a body part.

1ST - 0 Medical and Surgical

2ND - C Mouth and Throat

3RD - B EXCISION

EXAMPLE: Excision lesion lip | **CMS Ex:** Liver biopsy

EXCISION: Cutting out or off, without replacement, a portion of a body part.

EXPLANATION: Qualifier "X Diagnostic" indicates biopsy ...

Body Part – 4TH		Approach – 5TH	Device – 6TH	Qualifier – 7TH
0 Upper Lip 1 Lower Lip 2 Hard Palate 3 Soft Palate 4 Buccal Mucosa	5 Upper Gingiva 6 Lower Gingiva 7 Tongue N Uvula P Tonsils Q Adenoids	0 Open 3 Percutaneous X External	Z No device	X Diagnostic Z No qualifier
8 Parotid Gland, Right 9 Parotid Gland, Left B Parotid Duct, Right C Parotid Duct, Left	D Sublingual Gland, Right F Sublingual Gland, Left G Submaxillary Gland, Right H Submaxillary Gland, Left J Minor Salivary Gland	0 Open 3 Percutaneous	Z No device	X Diagnostic Z No qualifier
M Pharynx R Epiglottis S Larynx T Vocal Cord, Right V Vocal Cord, Left		0 Open 3 Percutaneous 4 Percutaneous endoscopic 7 Via natural or artificial opening 8 Via natural or artificial opening endoscopic	Z No device	X Diagnostic Z No qualifier
W Upper Tooth X Lower Tooth		0 Open X External	Z No device	0 Single 1 Multiple 2 All

MOUTH & THROAT

0 C B

DRAINAGE GROUP: Drainage, Extirpation, Fragmentation
Root Operations that take out solids/fluids/gases from a body part.

1ST – **0** Medical and Surgical	EXAMPLE: Sialolithotomy		CMS Ex: Choledocholithotomy
2ND – **C** Mouth and Throat	**EXTIRPATION:** Taking or cutting out solid matter from a body part.		
3RD – **C EXTIRPATION**	EXPLANATION: Abnormal byproduct or foreign body ...		

Body Part – 4TH		Approach – 5TH	Device – 6TH	Qualifier – 7TH
0 Upper Lip 1 Lower Lip 2 Hard Palate 3 Soft Palate 4 Buccal Mucosa	5 Upper Gingiva 6 Lower Gingiva 7 Tongue N Uvula P Tonsils Q Adenoids	0 Open 3 Percutaneous X External	Z No device	Z No qualifier
8 Parotid Gland, Right 9 Parotid Gland, Left B Parotid Duct, Right C Parotid Duct, Left	D Sublingual Gland, Right F Sublingual Gland, Left G Submaxillary Gland, Right H Submaxillary Gland, Left J Minor Salivary Gland	0 Open 3 Percutaneous	Z No device	Z No qualifier
M Pharynx R Epiglottis S Larynx T Vocal Cord, Right V Vocal Cord, Left		0 Open 3 Percutaneous 4 Percutaneous endoscopic 7 Via natural or artificial opening 8 Via natural or artificial opening endoscopic	Z No device	Z No qualifier
W Upper Tooth X Lower Tooth		0 Open X External	Z No device	0 Single 1 Multiple 2 All

EXCISION GROUP: Excision, Resection, Destruction, Extraction, (Detachment)
Root Operations that take out some or all of a body part.

1ST – **0** Medical and Surgical	EXAMPLE: Tooth extraction		CMS Ex: D&C
2ND – **C** Mouth and Throat	**EXTRACTION:** Pulling or stripping out or off all or a portion of a body part by the use of force.		
3RD – **D EXTRACTION**	EXPLANATION: None for this Body System		

Body Part – 4TH	Approach – 5TH	Device – 6TH	Qualifier – 7TH
T Vocal Cord, Right V Vocal Cord, Left	0 Open 3 Percutaneous 4 Percutaneous endoscopic 7 Via natural or artificial opening 8 Via natural or artificial opening endoscopic	Z No device	Z No qualifier
W Upper Tooth X Lower Tooth	X External	Z No device	0 Single 1 Multiple 2 All

DRAINAGE GROUP: Drainage, Extirpation, Fragmentation
Root Operations that take out solids/fluids/gases from a body part.

1ST - **0** Medical and Surgical

2ND - **C** Mouth and Throat

3RD - **F FRAGMENTATION**

EXAMPLE: Lithotripsy parotid stone | CMS Ex: Extracorporeal shockwave lithotripsy

FRAGMENTATION: Breaking solid matter in a body part into pieces.

EXPLANATION: Pieces are not taken out during procedure ...

Body Part – 4TH	Approach – 5TH	Device – 6TH	Qualifier – 7TH
B Parotid Duct, Right C Parotid Duct, Left	0 Open 3 Percutaneous 7 Via natural or artificial opening X External NC*	Z No device	Z No qualifier

NC* – Non-covered by Medicare. See current Medicare Code Editor for details.

DEVICE GROUP: Change, Insertion, Removal, Replacement, Revision, Supplement
Root Operations that always involve a device.

1ST - **0** Medical and Surgical

2ND - **C** Mouth and Throat

3RD - **H INSERTION**

EXAMPLE: Insertion oral airway | CMS Ex: Central venous catheter

INSERTION: Putting in a nonbiological appliance that monitors, assists, performs, or prevents a physiological function but does not physically take the place of a body part.

EXPLANATION: None

Body Part – 4TH	Approach – 5TH	Device – 6TH	Qualifier – 7TH
7 Tongue	0 Open 3 Percutaneous X External	1 Radioactive element	Z No qualifier

Y Mouth and Throat	7 Via natural or
	   artificial opening
	8 Via natural or
	   artificial opening
	   endoscopic
		B Intraluminal
		   device, airway
			Z No qualifier

EXAMINATION GROUP: Inspection, (Map)
Root Operations involving examination only.

1ST – 0 Medical and Surgical	EXAMPLE: Diagnostic laryngoscopy	CMS Ex: Colonoscopy
2ND – C Mouth and Throat	**INSPECTION:** Visually and/or manually exploring a body part.	
3RD – J INSPECTION	EXPLANATION: Direct or instrumental visualization ...	

Body Part – 4TH	Approach – 5TH	Device – 6TH	Qualifier – 7TH
A Salivary Gland	0 Open 3 Percutaneous X External	Z No device	Z No qualifier
S Larynx Y Mouth and Throat	0 Open 3 Percutaneous 4 Percutaneous endoscopic 7 Via natural or artificial opening 8 Via natural or artificial opening endoscopic X External	Z No device	Z No qualifier

TUBULAR GROUP: (Bypass), Dilation, Occlusion, Restriction
Root Operations that alter the diameter/route of a tubular body part.

1ST – 0 Medical and Surgical	EXAMPLE: Ligation Stensen's duct	CMS Ex: Fallopian tube ligation
2ND – C Mouth and Throat	**OCCLUSION:** Completely closing an orifice or lumen of a tubular body part.	
3RD – L OCCLUSION	EXPLANATION: Natural or artificially created orifice ...	

Body Part – 4TH	Approach – 5TH	Device – 6TH	Qualifier – 7TH
B Parotid Duct, Right C Parotid Duct, Left	0 Open 3 Percutaneous 4 Percutaneous endoscopic	C Extraluminal device D Intraluminal device Z No device	Z No qualifier
B Parotid Duct, Right C Parotid Duct, Left	7 Via natural or artificial opening 8 Via natural or artificial opening endoscopic	D Intraluminal device Z No device	Z No qualifier

---

MOVE GROUP: Reattachment, Reposition, Transfer, (Transplantation)
Root Operations that put in/put back or move some/all of a body part.

1ST - **0** Medical and Surgical

2ND - **C** Mouth and Throat

3RD - **M REATTACHMENT**

EXAMPLE: Replantation tooth | CMS Ex: Reattachment hand

REATTACHMENT: Putting back in or on all or a portion of a separated body part to its normal location or other suitable location.

EXPLANATION: With/without reconnection of vessels/nerves...

Body Part – 4TH	Approach – 5TH	Device – 6TH	Qualifier – 7TH
0 Upper Lip 1 Lower Lip 3 Soft Palate 7 Tongue N Uvula	0 Open	Z No device	Z No qualifier
W Upper Tooth X Lower Tooth	0 Open X External	Z No device	0 Single 1 Multiple 2 All

---

DIVISION GROUP: (Division), Release
Root Operations involving cutting or separation only.

1ST - **0** Medical and Surgical

2ND - **C** Mouth and Throat

3RD - **N RELEASE**

EXAMPLE: Lysis vocal cord adhesions | CMS Ex: Carpal tunnel release

RELEASE: Freeing a body part from an abnormal physical constraint by cutting or by the use of force.

EXPLANATION: None of the body part is taken out ...

Body Part – 4TH	Approach – 5TH	Device – 6TH	Qualifier – 7TH
0 Upper Lip 5 Upper Gingiva 1 Lower Lip 6 Lower Gingiva 2 Hard Palate 7 Tongue 3 Soft Palate N Uvula 4 Buccal Mucosa P Tonsils Q Adenoids	0 Open 3 Percutaneous X External	Z No device	Z No qualifier
8 Parotid Gland, Right D Sublingual Gland, Right 9 Parotid Gland, Left F Sublingual Gland, Left B Parotid Duct, Right G Submaxillary Gland, Right C Parotid Duct, Left H Submaxillary Gland, Left J Minor Salivary Gland	0 Open 3 Percutaneous	Z No device	Z No qualifier
M Pharynx R Epiglottis S Larynx T Vocal Cord, Right V Vocal Cord, Left	0 Open 3 Percutaneous 4 Percutaneous endoscopic 7 Via natural or artificial opening 8 Via natural or artificial opening endoscopic	Z No device	Z No qualifier
W Upper Tooth X Lower Tooth	0 Open X External	Z No device	0 Single 1 Multiple 2 All

DEVICE GROUP: Change, Insertion, Removal, Replacement, Revision, Supplement
Root Operations that always involve a device.

1ST - **0** Medical and Surgical	EXAMPLE: Removal drain tube	CMS Ex: Chest tube removal
2ND - **C** Mouth and Throat	**REMOVAL:** Taking out or off a device from a body part.	
3RD - **P** REMOVAL	EXPLANATION: Removal device without reinsertion ...	

Body Part – 4TH	Approach – 5TH	Device – 6TH	Qualifier – 7TH
A Salivary Gland	0 Open 3 Percutaneous	0 Drainage device C Extraluminal device	Z No qualifier
S Larynx	0 Open 3 Percutaneous 7 Via natural or artificial opening 8 Via natural or artificial opening endoscopic X External	0 Drainage device 7 Autologous tissue substitute D Intraluminal device J Synthetic substitute K Nonautologous tissue substitute	Z No qualifier
Y Mouth and Throat	0 Open 3 Percutaneous 7 Via natural or artificial opening 8 Via natural or artificial opening endoscopic X External	0 Drainage device 1 Radioactive element 7 Autologous tissue substitute D Intraluminal device J Synthetic substitute K Nonautologous tissue substitute	Z No qualifier

MOUTH & THROAT 0 C P

OTHER REPAIRS GROUP: (Control), Repair
Root Operations that define other repairs.

1ST - 0　Medical and Surgical	EXAMPLE: Cleft palate repair	CMS Ex: Suture laceration
2ND - C　Mouth and Throat	**REPAIR:**　Restoring, to the extent possible, a body part to its normal anatomic structure and function.	
3RD - Q REPAIR	EXPLANATION: Only when no other root operation applies ...	

Body Part – 4TH		Approach – 5TH	Device – 6TH	Qualifier – 7TH
0 Upper Lip 1 Lower Lip 2 Hard Palate 3 Soft Palate 4 Buccal Mucosa	5 Upper Gingiva 6 Lower Gingiva 7 Tongue N Uvula P Tonsils Q Adenoids	0 Open 3 Percutaneous X External	Z No device	Z No qualifier
8 Parotid Gland, Right 9 Parotid Gland, Left B Parotid Duct, Right C Parotid Duct, Left	D Sublingual Gland, Right F Sublingual Gland, Left G Submaxillary Gland, Right H Submaxillary Gland, Left J Minor Salivary Gland	0 Open 3 Percutaneous	Z No device	Z No qualifier
M Pharynx R Epiglottis S Larynx T Vocal Cord, Right V Vocal Cord, Left		0 Open 3 Percutaneous 4 Percutaneous endoscopic 7 Via natural or artificial opening 8 Via natural or artificial opening endoscopic	Z No device	Z No qualifier
W Upper Tooth X Lower Tooth		0 Open X External	Z No device	0 Single 1 Multiple 2 All

MOUTH & THROAT 0 C Q

DEVICE GROUP: Change, Insertion, Removal, Replacement, Revision, Supplement
Root Operations that always involve a device.

| 1ST - 0 Medical and Surgical |
| 2ND - C Mouth and Throat |
| 3RD - R REPLACEMENT |

EXAMPLE: Parotid duct replacement | CMS Ex: Total hip

REPLACEMENT: Putting in or on a biological or synthetic material that physically takes the place and/or function of all or a portion of a body part.

EXPLANATION: Includes taking out body part, or eradication...

Body Part – 4TH	Approach – 5TH	Device – 6TH	Qualifier – 7TH
0 Upper Lip 5 Upper Gingiva 1 Lower Lip 6 Lower Gingiva 2 Hard Palate 7 Tongue 3 Soft Palate N Uvula 4 Buccal Mucosa	0 Open 3 Percutaneous X External	7 Autologous tissue substitute J Synthetic substitute K Nonautologous tissue substitute	Z No qualifier
B Parotid Duct, Right C Parotid Duct, Left	0 Open 3 Percutaneous	7 Autologous tissue substitute J Synthetic substitute K Nonautologous tissue substitute	Z No qualifier
M Pharynx R Epiglottis S Larynx T Vocal Cord, Right V Vocal Cord, Left	0 Open 7 Via natural or artificial opening 8 Via natural or artificial opening endoscopic	7 Autologous tissue substitute J Synthetic substitute K Nonautologous tissue substitute	Z No qualifier
W Upper Tooth X Lower Tooth	0 Open X External	7 Autologous tissue substitute J Synthetic substitute K Nonautologous tissue substitute	0 Single 1 Multiple 2 All

MOUTH & THROAT 0 C R

MOVE GROUP: Reattachment, Reposition, Transfer, (Transplantation)
Root Operations that put in/put back or move some/all of a body part.

1ST - **0** Medical and Surgical

2ND - **C** Mouth and Throat

3RD - **S REPOSITION**

EXAMPLE: Reposition tongue | CMS Ex: Fracture reduction

REPOSITION: Moving to its normal location, or other suitable location, all or a portion of a body part.

EXPLANATION: May or may not be cut to be moved ...

Body Part – 4TH		Approach – 5TH	Device – 6TH	Qualifier – 7TH
0 Upper Lip 1 Lower Lip 2 Hard Palate	3 Soft Palate 7 Tongue N Uvula	0 Open X External	Z No device	Z No qualifier
B Parotid Duct, Right C Parotid Duct, Left		0 Open 3 Percutaneous	Z No device	Z No qualifier
R Epiglottis T Vocal Cord, Right V Vocal Cord, Left		0 Open 7 Via natural or artificial opening 8 Via natural or artificial opening endoscopic	Z No device	Z No qualifier
W Upper Tooth X Lower Tooth		0 Open X External	5 External fixation device Z No device	0 Single 1 Multiple 2 All

MOUTH & THROAT **0 C S**

EXCISION GROUP: Excision, Resection, Destruction, Extraction, (Detachment)
Root Operations that take out some or all of a body part.

1ST – **0** Medical and Surgical	EXAMPLE: Tonsillectomy	CMS Ex: Cholecystectomy
2ND – **C** Mouth and Throat	**RESECTION:** Cutting out or off, without replacement, all of a body part.	
3RD – **T RESECTION**	EXPLANATION: None	

Body Part – 4TH		Approach – 5TH	Device – 6TH	Qualifier – 7TH
0 Upper Lip 1 Lower Lip 2 Hard Palate 3 Soft Palate	7 Tongue N Uvula P Tonsils Q Adenoids	0 Open X External	Z No device	Z No qualifier
8 Parotid Gland, Right 9 Parotid Gland, Left B Parotid Duct, Right C Parotid Duct, Left	D Sublingual Gland, Right F Sublingual Gland, Left G Submaxillary Gland, Right H Submaxillary Gland, Left J Minor Salivary Gland	0 Open	Z No device	Z No qualifier
M Pharynx R Epiglottis S Larynx T Vocal Cord, Right V Vocal Cord, Left		0 Open 4 Percutaneous endoscopic 7 Via natural or artificial opening 8 Via natural or artificial opening endoscopic	Z No device	Z No qualifier
W Upper Tooth X Lower Tooth		0 Open	Z No device	0 Single 1 Multiple 2 All

DEVICE GROUP: Change, Insertion, Removal, Replacement, Revision, Supplement
Root Operations that always involve a device.

1ST – **0** Medical and Surgical	EXAMPLE: Palatoplasty with graft	CMS Ex: Hernia repair with mesh
2ND – **C** Mouth and Throat	**SUPPLEMENT:** Putting in or on biological or synthetic material that physically reinforces and/or augments the function of a portion of a body part.	
3RD – **U SUPPLEMENT**	EXPLANATION: Biological material from same individual …	

Body Part – 4TH		Approach – 5TH	Device – 6TH	Qualifier – 7TH
0 Upper Lip 1 Lower Lip 2 Hard Palate 3 Soft Palate 4 Buccal Mucosa	5 Upper Gingiva 6 Lower Gingiva 7 Tongue N Uvula	0 Open 3 Percutaneous X External	7 Autologous tissue substitute J Synthetic substitute K Nonautologous tissue substitute	Z No qualifier
M Pharynx R Epiglottis S Larynx T Vocal Cord, Right V Vocal Cord, Left		0 Open 7 Via natural or artificial opening 8 Via natural or artificial opening endoscopic	7 Autologous tissue substitute J Synthetic substitute K Nonautologous tissue substitute	Z No qualifier

Mouth & Throat 0 C T

TUBULAR GROUP: (Bypass), Dilation, Occlusion, Restriction
Root Operations that alter the diameter/route of a tubular body part.

1ST - 0 Medical and Surgical

2ND - C Mouth and Throat

3RD - V RESTRICTION

EXAMPLE: Parotid duct restrictive stent | CMS Ex: Cervical cerclage

RESTRICTION: Partially closing an orifice or the lumen of a tubular body part.

EXPLANATION: Natural or artificially created orifice ...

Body Part – 4TH	Approach – 5TH	Device – 6TH	Qualifier – 7TH
B Parotid Duct, Right C Parotid Duct, Left	0 Open 3 Percutaneous	C Extraluminal device D Intraluminal device Z No device	Z No qualifier
B Parotid Duct, Right C Parotid Duct, Left	7 Via natural or artificial opening 8 Via natural or artificial opening endoscopic	D Intraluminal device Z No device	Z No qualifier

DEVICE GROUP: Change, Insertion, Removal, Replacement, Revision, Supplement
Root Operations that always involve a device.

1ST - 0 Medical and Surgical

2ND - C Mouth and Throat

3RD - W REVISION

EXAMPLE: Trimming palatoplasty graft | CMS Ex: Adjustment pacemaker lead

REVISION: Correcting, to the extent possible, a portion of a malfunctioning device or the position of a displaced device.

EXPLANATION: May replace components of a device ...

Body Part – 4TH	Approach – 5TH	Device – 6TH	Qualifier – 7TH
A Salivary Gland	0 Open 3 Percutaneous X External	0 Drainage device C Extraluminal device	Z No qualifier
S Larynx	0 Open 3 Percutaneous 7 Via natural or artificial opening 8 Via natural or artificial opening endoscopic X External	0 Drainage device 7 Autologous tissue substitute D Intraluminal device J Synthetic substitute K Nonautologous tissue substitute	Z No qualifier
Y Mouth and Throat	0 Open 3 Percutaneous 7 Via natural or artificial opening 8 Via natural or artificial opening endoscopic X External	0 Drainage device 1 Radioactive element 7 Autologous tissue substitute D Intraluminal device J Synthetic substitute K Nonautologous tissue substitute	Z No qualifier

MOUTH & THROAT 0 C W

MOVE GROUP: Reattachment, Reposition, Transfer, (Transplantation)
Root Operations that put in/put back or move some/all of a body part.

1ST - **0** Medical and Surgical

2ND - **C** Mouth and Throat

3RD - **X TRANSFER**

EXAMPLE: Gingival pedicle graft   CMS Ex: Tendon transfer

TRANSFER: Moving, without taking out, all or a portion of a body part to another location to take over the function of all or a portion of a body part.

EXPLANATION: The body part remains connected ...

Body Part – 4TH		Approach – 5TH	Device – 6TH	Qualifier – 7TH
0 Upper Lip	5 Upper Gingiva	0 Open	Z No device	Z No qualifier
1 Lower Lip	6 Lower Gingiva	X External		
3 Soft Palate	7 Tongue			
4 Buccal Mucosa				

Educational Annotations | D – Gastrointestinal System

Body System Specific Educational Annotations for the Gastrointestinal System include:

- Anatomy and Physiology Review
- Anatomical Illustrations
- Definitions of Common Procedures
- AHA Coding Clinic® Reference Notations
- Body Part Key Listings
- Device Key Listings
- Device Aggregation Table Listings
- Coding Notes

Anatomy and Physiology Review of Gastrointestinal System

BODY PART VALUES – D - GASTROINTESTINAL SYSTEM

Anal Sphincter – ANATOMY – The anal sphincter is a group of muscles (internal and external) that surrounds the anus. PHYSIOLOGY – Maintains continence by controlling the release of stool from the rectum.

Anus – ANATOMY – The anus is the internal canal from the rectum which ends the alimentary tract at the anal opening. PHYSIOLOGY – The rectum and anus function to eliminate feces from the alimentary tract. A reflex signal is sent when the rectum fills and urgency to defecate is perceived. The external voluntary muscle is voluntarily relaxed to defecate.

Appendix – The appendix is a closed appendage of the colon and projects downward from the cecum.

Ascending Colon – The ascending colon arises from the cecum (the pouch-like structure) and continues upwards where it turns (hepatic flexure) and connects to the transverse colon.

Cecum – ANATOMY – The cecum is an enlarged pouch of the ascending intestine at the junction with the ileum. PHYSIOLOGY – Receives the contents from the small intestine.

Descending Colon – The descending colon extends downward to the rectum, and is called the sigmoid (flexure) colon where it makes an S-shaped curve over the pelvic brim.

Duodenum – The duodenum is the first portion about 10 inches (25 cm) long connected at its proximal end to the stomach.

Esophagogastric Junction – ANATOMY – The lower end of the esophagus at the transition to the stomach identified by the abrupt change from esophageal epithelium to the gastric folds.

Esophagus – ANATOMY – The esophagus, located between the pharynx and stomach, is a collapsible musculomembranous alimentary tract tube about 10 inches (25 cm) long. The esophagus is lined with mucous glands. PHYSIOLOGY – The esophagus is the passageway for food from the mouth to the stomach. The mucous glands moisten and lubricate the inner lining to facilitate the passage of food. Situated just above the stomach opening lie the contracted circular muscles which prevent regurgitation.

Esophagus, Lower – The distal lower one-third of the esophagus (also known as the abdominal esophagus).

Esophagus, Middle – The middle one-third of the esophagus (also known as the thoracic esophagus).

Esophagus, Upper – The proximal upper one-third of the esophagus (also known as the cervical esophagus).

Greater Omentum – The double layer of the peritoneum that extends from the greater curvature of the stomach to the transverse colon.

Ileocecal Valve – ANATOMY – The ileocecal valve is the sphincter muscle valve that separates the small intestine and the large intestine. PHYSIOLOGY – The ileocecal valve prevents contents from the large intestine from backflowing into the small intestine.

Ileum – The ileum is the distal portion of the small intestine which connects with the large intestine.

Jejunum – The jejunum is the middle portion of the small intestine, comprising approximately two-fifths of the intestine.

Large Intestine – ANATOMY – The large intestine (colon) is the tubular organ of the alimentary tract between the small intestine and the rectum, and is about 5 feet (1.5 m) long. The colon has four main segments: Ascending, transverse, descending, and sigmoid. The rectosigmoid junction is that portion of the alimentary tract between the distal end of the sigmoid colon and the proximal end of the rectum. PHYSIOLOGY – The large intestine (colon) functions to absorb water and electrolytes, and to move by peristalsis nonabsorbed substances to the rectum for defecation. Many bacteria normally inhabit the colon and serve to further break down substances for colonic absorption.

Large Intestine, Left – In general, the descending colon and part of the transverse colon.

Continued on next page

Educational Annotations | D – Gastrointestinal System

Anatomy and Physiology Review of Gastrointestinal System

BODY PART VALUES – D - GASTROINTESTINAL SYSTEM

Continued from previous page

Large Intestine, Right – In general, the ascending colon and part of the transverse colon.

Lesser Omentum – The double layer of the peritoneum that extends from the liver to lesser curvature of the stomach.

Lower Intestinal Tract – The gastrointestinal tract from the jejunum down to and including the rectum and anus (see Coding Guideline B4.8).

Mesentery – The mesentery is a fold of membranous tissue that arises from the posterior wall of the peritoneal cavity and attaches the intestine to the abdominal wall and holds it in place.

Omentum – The double layer of the peritoneum that encompasses most of the organs in the abdominal cavity.

Peritoneum – ANATOMY – The peritoneum is the serous membrane (visceral and parietal) which contains most of the abdominal contents, and where doubled upon itself forms supporting structures called ligaments. PHYSIOLOGY – The peritoneum encapsules and protects the abdominal visceral organs allowing them to move slightly without damaging function.

Rectum – ANATOMY – The rectum is the musculomembranous portion of the alimentary tract between the colon and anus, approximately 5 inches (13 cm) long. The rectosigmoid junction is that portion of the alimentary tract between the distal end of the sigmoid colon and the proximal end of the rectum. PHYSIOLOGY – The rectum and anus function to eliminate feces from the alimentary tract. A reflex signal is sent when the rectum fills and urgency to defecate is perceived. The external voluntary muscle is voluntarily relaxed to defecate.

Sigmoid Colon – The descending colon extends downward to the rectum, and is called the sigmoid (flexure) colon where it makes an S-shaped curve over the pelvic brim.

Small Intestine – ANATOMY – The small intestine is the tubular organ of the alimentary tract between the stomach and large intestine and is about 16 to 20 feet (5 to 6 m) long, and has 3 parts: Duodenum, jejunum, and ileum. Both the jejunum and ileum are suspended from the posterior abdominal wall by the mesentery. PHYSIOLOGY – The small intestine functions to absorb the nutrients produced through digestion. The food is passed through the small intestine by the contraction (peristalsis) of its circular smooth muscle layer. The duodenum releases several enzymes and mixes the pancreatic and bile juices with food from the stomach. The jejunum and ileum continue mixing and absorbing until the remaining substances pass into the large intestine.

Stomach – ANATOMY – The stomach, located in the upper abdomen, is a pouch-like organ of the alimentary tract connecting with the esophagus in the proximal (upper) portion and the duodenum in the distal (lower) portion and is about 10 to 12 inches (25 to 30 cm) long. The cardia lies at the opening of the esophagus at the fundus of the stomach. The fundus is the upper ballooned area of the stomach. The body is the main part of the stomach and is located between the fundus and the pyloric antrum and the duodenum. When empty, the mucous membrane on the interior surface forms longitudinal folds (rugae). There are three mucosal glands which secrete digestive juices and mucous. These are the gastric glands, which are located throughout the body of the stomach; the cardiac glands, which are found near the esophageal opening; and the pyloric glands, which are located in the pyloric (distal) region. The vagus nerve stimulates the gastric glands. There are three layers of smooth muscle and a serosal covering of the visceral peritoneum. The stomach has a rich arterial blood supply through the celiac artery. The venous blood is drained into the hepatic portal system. PHYSIOLOGY – The stomach functions to receive food from the esophagus, mixes it with the gastric juice, initiates the digestion of proteins with pepsin, carries on a limited amount of absorption, and moves food into the small intestine by peristaltic muscle action. The gastric glands produce mucous, digestive enzymes (pepsin), hydrochloric acid, and an intrinsic factor, forming the gastric juice. The mucous is thought to help prevent the pepsin and hydrochloric acid from digesting the stomach surface. The stomach may absorb small quantities of water, glucose, certain salts, and alcohol. The parasympathetic vagus nerve stimulates the gastric glands to secrete large amounts of gastric juice, which in turn releases gastrin, a hormone that causes the gastric glands to increase their secretory activity.

Stomach, Pylorus – The pylorus is the lower section of the stomach that connects to the duodenum and allows emptying of the contents into the small intestine.

Transverse Colon – The transverse colon extends horizontally and turns (splenic flexure) downward connecting to the descending colon.

Upper Intestinal Tract – The gastrointestinal tract from the esophagus down to and including the duodenum (see Coding Guideline B4.8).

Educational Annotations | D – Gastrointestinal System

Anatomical Illustrations of Gastrointestinal System

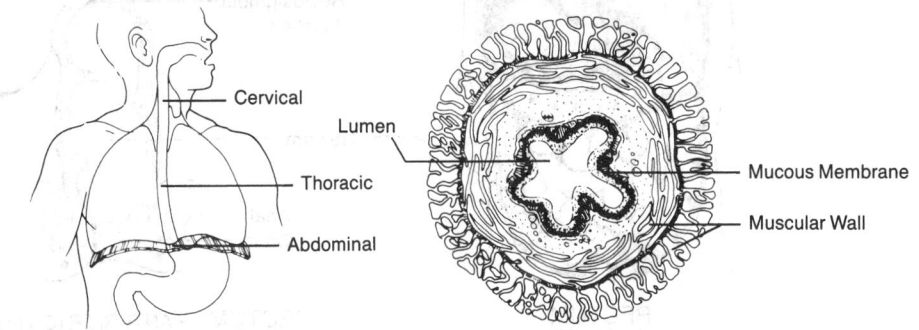

ESOPHAGUS — ANTERIOR VIEW   ESOPHAGUS — SECTION

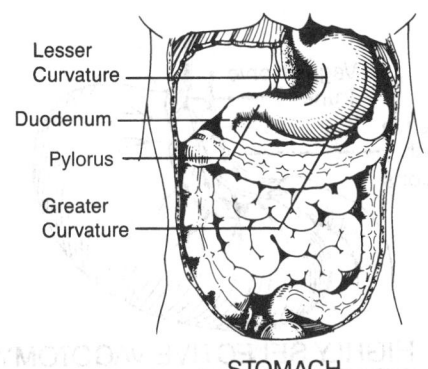
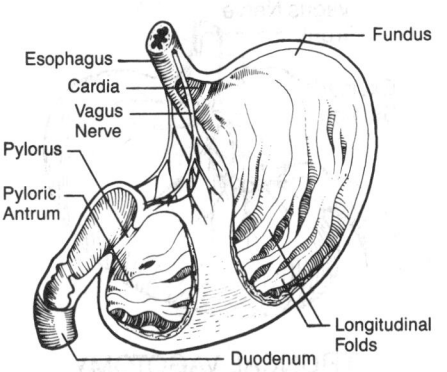

STOMACH   STOMACH — ANTERIOR (CUT-AWAY) VIEW

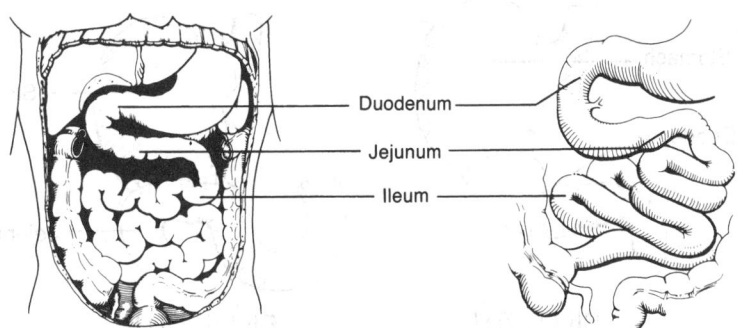

SMALL INTESTINE

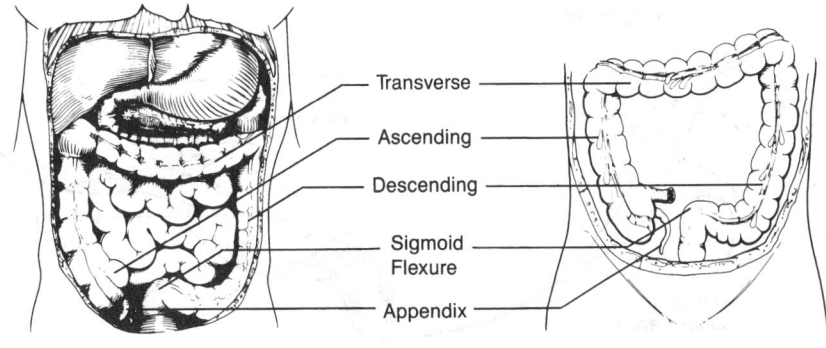

LARGE INTESTINE (COLON)

Continued on next page

Educational Annotations | D – Gastrointestinal System

Continued from previous page

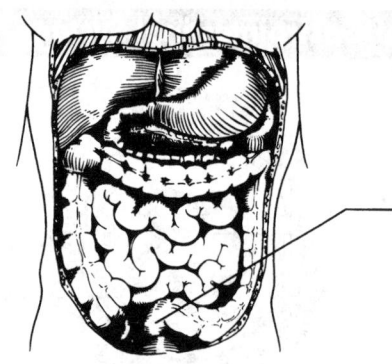

RECTUM

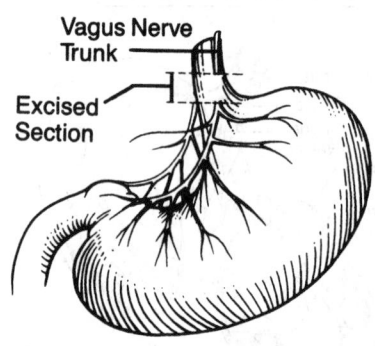

RECTUM — ANTERIOR (CUT-AWAY) VIEW

TRUNCAL VAGOTOMY

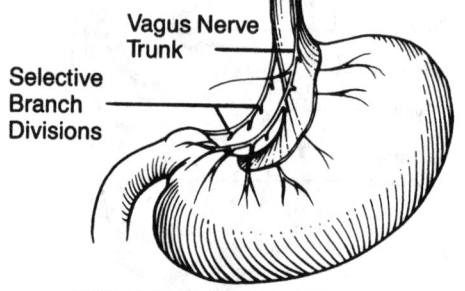

HIGHLY SELECTIVE VAGOTOMY

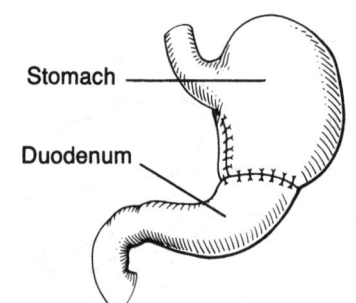

BILLROTH I

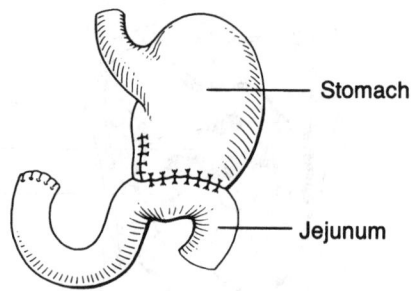

BILLROTH II

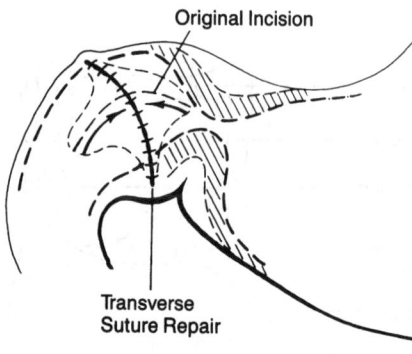

PYLOROPLASTY

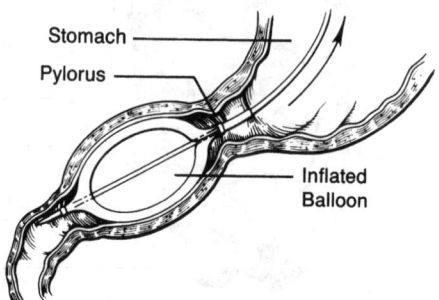

BALLOON DILATATION OF PYLORUS

Continued on next page

GASTROINTESTINAL 0 D

Educational Annotations | D – Gastrointestinal System

Continued from previous page

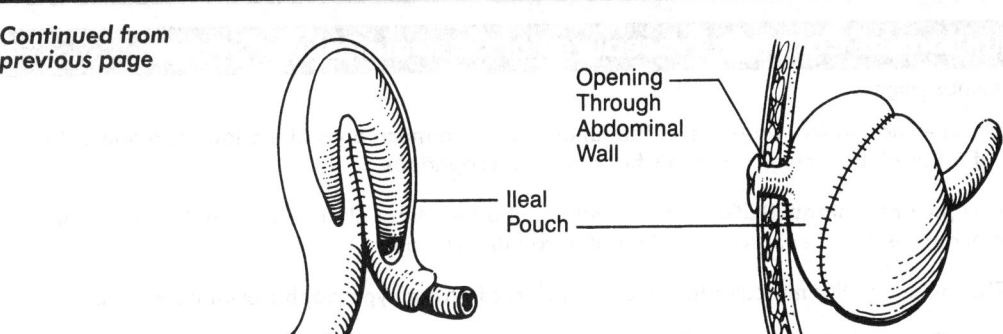

Opening Through Abdominal Wall

Ileal Pouch

Stage I   Stage II

CONTINENT ILEOSTOMY

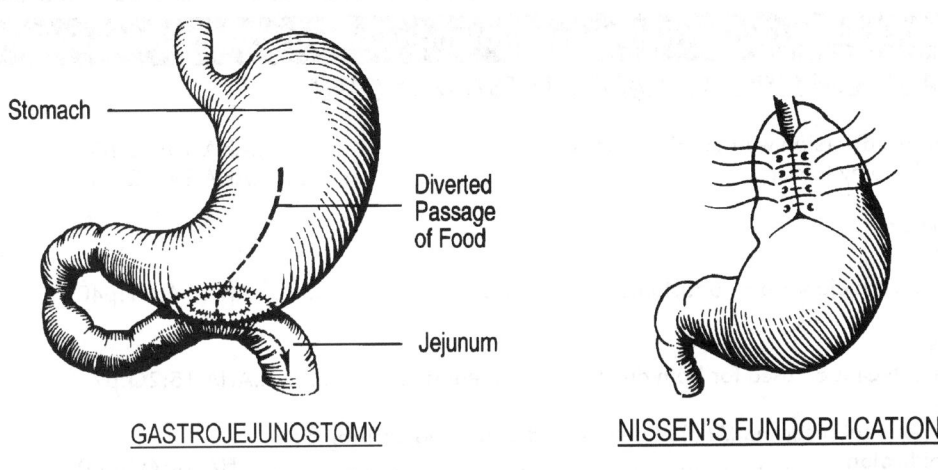

Stomach

Diverted Passage of Food

Jejunum

GASTROJEJUNOSTOMY   NISSEN'S FUNDOPLICATION

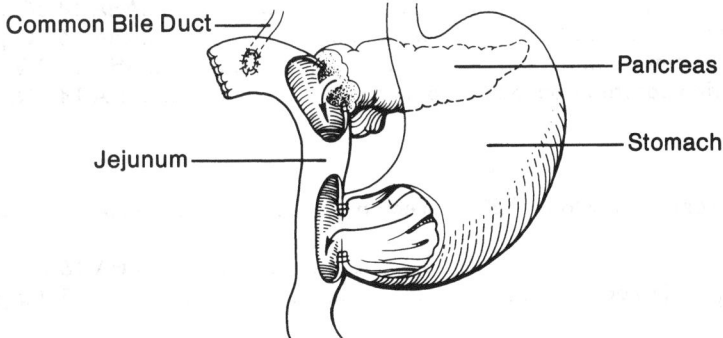

Common Bile Duct

Pancreas

Stomach

Jejunum

WHIPPLE PROCEDURE

GASTROINTESTINAL 0 D

Definitions of Common Procedures of Gastrointestinal System

Anal sphincterotomy – The incision of the anal sphincter muscle to prevent spasms and intentionally weaken the muscle during healing.

Colostomy – The creation of an artificial opening of the colon through the abdominal wall.

Gastrojejunostomy – The surgical creation of an anastomosis between the stomach and the jejunum (the second portion of the small intestine) to bypass and relieve gastric outlet obstruction.

Continued on next page

Educational Annotations | D – Gastrointestinal System

Definitions of Common Procedures of Gastrointestinal System

Continued from previous page

Nissen's fundoplication – The surgical wrapping of the fundus of the stomach around the lower portion of the esophagus to prevent reflux of the stomach contents back into the esophagus.

Percutaneous endoscopic gastrostomy (PEG) – The placement of a tube through an abdominal wall incision from inside the stomach by using an endoscope and a pull-through technique.

Pyloromyotomy – The incision in the muscular layers of the pylorus to treat hypertrophic pyloric stenosis.

Right hemicolectomy – The surgical removal of the cecum, ascending colon, and hepatic flexure portion of the tranverse colon, and usually end-to-end anastomosis between the small intestine and the transverse colon.

Vertical sleeve gastrectomy – The surgical excision of a large portion of the stomach along a vertical line of the stomach to reduce the stomach volume and limit the amount of food that can be consumed at one time.

AHA Coding Clinic® Reference Notations of Gastrointestinal System

<u>ROOT OPERATION SPECIFIC - D - GASTROINTESTINAL SYSTEM</u>

BYPASS - 1
   Biliopancreatic diversion with duodenal switch ....AHA 16:2Q:p31
   Sigmoid colostomy to skin ....AHA 14:4Q:p41
CHANGE - 2
DESTRUCTION - 5
DILATION - 7
   Dilation of gastrojejunostomy anastomosis ....AHA 14:4Q:p40
DIVISION - 8
DRAINAGE - 9
   Nasogastric (NG) tube used for both drainage and feeding ....AHA 15:2Q:p2
EXCISION - B
   Abdominoperineal resection (APR) of rectum and anus, and excision of
      sigmoid colon ....AHA 14:4Q:p40
   Esophageal brush biopsy ....AHA 16:1Q:p24
   Ileostomy takedown ....AHA 14:3Q:p28
   Perineal proctectomy ....AHA 16:1Q:p22
   Vertical sleeve gastrectomy ....AHA 16:2Q:p31
   Whipple pyloric sparing pancreaticoduodenectomy....................................AHA 14:3Q:p32
EXTIRPATION - C
FRAGMENTATION - F
INSERTION - H
   Percutaneous endoscopic gastrostomy (PEG) placement ....AHA 13:4Q:p117
INSPECTION - J
   Capsule endoscopy ....AHA 16:2Q:p20
   EGD with epinephrine injection ....AHA 15:3Q:p24
OCCLUSION - L
REATTACHMENT - M
RELEASE - N
   Lysis of adhesions, integral or code separately ....AHA 14:1Q:p3
   Release of esophageal vascular ring..AHA 15:3Q:p15,16
REMOVAL - P
REPAIR - Q
   Clips to control bleeding duodenal ulcer ....AHA 14:4Q:p20
   Repair of third and fourth degree perineal lacerations ....AHA 16:1Q:p6-8
REPLACEMENT - R
REPOSITION - S

Continued on next page

Educational Annotations | D – Gastrointestinal System

AHA Coding Clinic® Reference Notations of Gastrointestinal System

Continued from previous page

RESECTION - T

Abdominoperineal resection (APR) of rectum and anus, and excision of
sigmoid colon ....AHA 14:4Q:p40
Colectomy, right..AHA 14:3Q:p6
Colectomy with side-to-side anastomosis ....AHA 14:4Q:p42
Ileocecectomy ....AHA 14:3Q:p6

SUPPLEMENT - U

RESTRICTION - V

Nissen fundoplication ....AHA 14:3Q:p28
....AHA 16:2Q:p22

REVISION - W

TRANSFER - X

Collis gastroplasty ....AHA 16:2Q:p22

TRANSPLANTATION - Y

Body Part Key Listings of Gastrointestinal System

See also Body Part Key in Appendix C

Abdominal esophagus ....*use* Esophagus, Lower
Anal orifice ....*use* Anus
Anorectal junction ....*use* Rectum
Cardia ....*use* Esophagogastric Junction
Cardioesophageal junction ....*use* Esophagogastric Junction
Cervical esophagus ....*use* Esophagus, Upper
Duodenojejunal flexure ....*use* Jejunum
Epiploic foramen ....*use* Peritoneum
External anal sphincter ....*use* Anal Sphincter
Gastrocolic ligament ....*use* Greater Omentum
Gastrocolic omentum ....*use* Greater Omentum
Gastroesophageal (GE) junction .....*use* Esophagogastric Junction
Gastrohepatic omentum ....*use* Lesser Omentum
Gastrophrenic ligament ....*use* Greater Omentum
Gastrosplenic ligament ....*use* Greater Omentum
Hepatic flexure................................*use* Ascending Colon
Hepatogastric ligament ....*use* Lesser Omentum
Internal anal sphincter....................*use* Anal Sphincter
Mesoappendix ....*use* Mesentery
Mesocolon ....*use* Mesentery
Pyloric antrum ....*use* Stomach, Pylorus
Pyloric canal.....................................*use* Stomach, Pylorus
Pyloric sphincter.............................*use* Stomach, Pylorus
Rectosigmoid junction ....*use* Sigmoid Colon
Sigmoid flexure ....*use* Sigmoid Colon
Splenic flexure ....*use* Transverse Colon
Thoracic esophagus ....*use* Esophagus, Middle
Vermiform appendix ....*use* Appendix

Device Key Listings of Gastrointestinal System

See also Device Key in Appendix D

Artificial anal sphincter (AAS) ....*use* Artificial Sphincter in Gastrointestinal System
Artificial bowel sphincter (neosphincter) ....*use* Artificial Sphincter in Gastrointestinal System
Autograft ....*use* Autologous Tissue Substitute
Brachytherapy seeds ....*use* Radioactive Element

Continued on next page

Educational Annotations | D – Gastrointestinal System

Device Key Listings of Gastrointestinal System

Continued from previous page

Colonic Z-Stent®..*use* Intraluminal Device

Cook Biodesign® Fistula Plug(s) ....*use* Nonautologous Tissue Substitute

Esophageal obturator airway (EOA) ....*use* Intraluminal Device, Airway in Gastrointestinal System

Gastric electrical stimulation (GES) lead ....*use* Stimulator Lead in Gastrointestinal System

Gastric pacemaker lead ....*use* Stimulator Lead in Gastrointestinal System

LAP-BAND® adjustable gastric banding system ......*use* Extraluminal Device

Percutaneous endoscopic gastrojejunostomy (PEG/J) tube...*use* Feeding Device in Gastrointestinal System

Percutaneous endoscopic gastrostomy (PEG) tube..*use* Feeding Device in Gastrointestinal System

REALIZE® Adjustable Gastric Band ....*use* Extraluminal Device

Tissue bank graft ....*use* Nonautologous Tissue Substitute

Ultraflex™ Precision Colonic Stent System...............*use* Intraluminal Device

Device Aggregation Table Listings of Gastrointestinal System

See also Device Aggregation Table in Appendix E

Specific Device	For Operation	In Body System	General Device
Intraluminal Device, Airway	All applicable	Gastrointestinal System	D Intraluminal Device

Coding Notes of Gastrointestinal System

Body System Relevant Coding Guidelines

Upper and lower intestinal tract

B4.8

In the Gastrointestinal body system, the general body part values Upper Intestinal Tract and Lower Intestinal Tract are provided as an option for the root operations Change, Inspection, Removal and Revision. Upper Intestinal Tract includes the portion of the gastrointestinal tract from the esophagus down to and including the duodenum, and Lower Intestinal Tract includes the portion of the gastrointestinal tract from the jejunum down to and including the rectum and anus.

Example: In the root operation Change table, change of a device in the jejunum is coded using the body part Lower Intestinal Tract.

Body System Specific PCS Reference Manual Exercises

PCS CODE	D – GASTROINTESTINAL SYSTEM EXERCISES
0 D 1 6 0 Z A	Open gastric bypass with Roux-en-Y limb to jejunum.
0 D 1 L 0 Z 4	Colostomy formation, open, transverse colon to abdominal wall.
0 D 7 1 7 Z Z	Dilation of upper esophageal stricture, direct visualization, with Bougie sound.
0 D 8 4 8 Z Z	EGD with esophagotomy of esophagogastric junction.
0 D 9 Q X Z Z	Incision and drainage of external anal abscess.
0 D B 6 4 Z 3	Laparoscopic vertical sleeve gastrectomy.
0 D B 6 8 Z X	EGD with gastric biopsy.
0 D B N 8 Z Z	Sigmoidoscopy with sigmoid polypectomy.
0 D C 6 8 Z Z	Esophagogastroscopy with removal of bezoar from stomach.
0 D C V 4 Z Z	Laparoscopy with excision of old suture from mesentery.
0 D J 0 8 Z Z	EGD (esophagogastroduodenoscopy).
0 D J D 7 Z Z	Digital rectal exam.
0 D J D 8 Z Z	Colonoscopy, discontinued at sigmoid colon.
0 D N W 4 Z Z	Laparoscopy with lysis of peritoneal adhesions.
0 D P 6 X 0 Z	Removal of nasogastric drainage tube for decompression.
0 D P 6 X U Z	Non-incisional PEG tube removal.
0 D Q 9 0 Z Z	Laparotomy with suture repair of blunt force duodenal laceration.
0 D S 6 4 Z Z	Laparoscopy with gastropexy for malrotation.
0 D T H 0 Z Z	Open resection of cecum.
0 D Y E 0 Z 0	Transplant of large intestine, organ donor match.

TUBULAR GROUP: Bypass, Dilation, Occlusion, Restriction
Root Operations that alter the diameter/route of a tubular body part.

1ST - 0 Medical and Surgical	**EXAMPLE:** Colostomy formation	CMS Ex: Coronary artery bypass
2ND - D Gastrointestinal System	**BYPASS:** Altering the route of passage of the contents of a tubular body part.	
3RD - 1 BYPASS	**EXPLANATION:** Rerouting contents to a downstream part ...	

Body Part – 4TH	Approach – 5TH	Device – 6TH	Qualifier – 7TH
1 Esophagus, Upper 2 Esophagus, Middle 3 Esophagus, Lower 5 Esophagus	0 Open 4 Percutaneous endoscopic 8 Via natural or artificial opening endoscopic	7 Autologous tissue substitute J Synthetic substitute K Nonautologous tissue substitute Z No device	4 Cutaneous 6 Stomach 9 Duodenum A Jejunum B Ileum
1 Esophagus, Upper 2 Esophagus, Middle 3 Esophagus, Lower 5 Esophagus	3 Percutaneous	J Synthetic substitute	4 Cutaneous
6 Stomach 9 Duodenum	0 Open 4 Percutaneous endoscopic 8 Via natural or artificial opening endoscopic	7 Autologous tissue substitute J Synthetic substitute K Nonautologous tissue substitute Z No device	4 Cutaneous 9 Duodenum A Jejunum B Ileum L Transverse Colon
6 Stomach 9 Duodenum	3 Percutaneous	J Synthetic substitute	4 Cutaneous
A Jejunum	0 Open 4 Percutaneous endoscopic 8 Via natural or artificial opening endoscopic	7 Autologous tissue substitute J Synthetic substitute K Nonautologous tissue substitute Z No device	4 Cutaneous A Jejunum B Ileum H Cecum K Ascending Colon L Transverse Colon M Descending Colon N Sigmoid Colon P Rectum Q Anus
A Jejunum	3 Percutaneous	J Synthetic substitute	4 Cutaneous

GASTROINTESTINAL 0 D 1

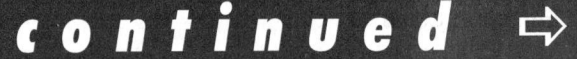

continued ⇨

0	D	1	BYPASS – *continued*

GASTROINTESTINAL 0 D 1

Body Part – 4TH	Approach – 5TH	Device – 6TH	Qualifier – 7TH
B Ileum	0 Open 4 Percutaneous endoscopic 8 Via natural or artificial opening endoscopic	7 Autologous tissue substitute J Synthetic substitute K Nonautologous tissue substitute Z No device	4 Cutaneous B Ileum H Cecum K Ascending Colon L Transverse Colon M Descending Colon N Sigmoid Colon P Rectum Q Anus
B Ileum	3 Percutaneous	J Synthetic substitute	4 Cutaneous
H Cecum	0 Open 4 Percutaneous endoscopic 8 Via natural or artificial opening endoscopic	7 Autologous tissue substitute J Synthetic substitute K Nonautologous tissue substitute Z No device	4 Cutaneous H Cecum K Ascending Colon L Transverse Colon M Descending Colon N Sigmoid Colon P Rectum
H Cecum	3 Percutaneous	J Synthetic substitute	4 Cutaneous
K Ascending Colon	0 Open 4 Percutaneous endoscopic 8 Via natural or artificial opening endoscopic	7 Autologous tissue substitute J Synthetic substitute K Nonautologous tissue substitute Z No device	4 Cutaneous K Ascending Colon L Transverse Colon M Descending Colon N Sigmoid Colon P Rectum
K Ascending Colon	3 Percutaneous	J Synthetic substitute	4 Cutaneous
L Transverse Colon	0 Open 4 Percutaneous endoscopic 8 Via natural or artificial opening endoscopic	7 Autologous tissue substitute J Synthetic substitute K Nonautologous tissue substitute Z No device	4 Cutaneous L Transverse Colon M Descending Colon N Sigmoid Colon P Rectum
L Transverse Colon	3 Percutaneous	J Synthetic substitute	4 Cutaneous

continued ⇨

0   D   1   BYPASS – *continued*

Body Part – 4TH	Approach – 5TH	Device – 6TH	Qualifier – 7TH
M Descending Colon	0 Open 4 Percutaneous endoscopic 8 Via natural or artificial opening endoscopic	7 Autologous tissue substitute J Synthetic substitute K Nonautologous tissue substitute Z No device	4 Cutaneous M Descending Colon N Sigmoid Colon P Rectum
M Descending Colon	3 Percutaneous	J Synthetic substitute	4 Cutaneous
N Sigmoid Colon	0 Open 4 Percutaneous endoscopic 8 Via natural or artificial opening endoscopic	7 Autologous tissue substitute J Synthetic substitute K Nonautologous tissue substitute Z No device	4 Cutaneous N Sigmoid Colon P Rectum
N Sigmoid Colon	3 Percutaneous	J Synthetic substitute	4 Cutaneous

GASTROINTESTINAL 0 D 1

DEVICE GROUP: Change, Insertion, Removal, Replacement, Revision, Supplement
Root Operations that always involve a device.

1ST – **0** Medical and Surgical	EXAMPLE: Exchange feeding tube	CMS Ex: Changing urinary catheter
2ND – **D** Gastrointestinal System	**CHANGE:** Taking out or off a device from a body part and putting back an identical or similar device in or on the same body part without cutting or puncturing the skin or a mucous membrane.	
3RD – **2 CHANGE**	EXPLANATION: ALL Changes use EXTERNAL approach only...	

Body Part – 4TH	Approach – 5TH	Device – 6TH	Qualifier – 7TH
0 Upper Intestinal Tract D Lower Intestinal Tract	X External	0 Drainage device U Feeding device Y Other device	Z No qualifier
U Omentum V Mesentery W Peritoneum	X External	0 Drainage device Y Other device	Z No qualifier

---

EXCISION GROUP: Excision, Resection, Destruction, (Extraction), (Detachment)
Root Operations that take out some or all of a body part.

1ST – **0** Medical and Surgical	EXAMPLE: Ablation esophageal polyp	CMS Ex: Fulguration polyp
2ND – **D** Gastrointestinal System	**DESTRUCTION:** Physical eradication of all or a portion of a body part by the direct use of energy, force, or a destructive agent.	
3RD – **5 DESTRUCTION**	EXPLANATION: None of the body part is physically taken out	

Body Part – 4TH		Approach – 5TH	Device – 6TH	Qualifier – 7TH
1 Esophagus, Upper 2 Esophagus, Middle 3 Esophagus, Lower 4 Esophagogastric Junction 5 Esophagus 6 Stomach 7 Stomach, Pylorus 8 Small Intestine 9 Duodenum A Jejunum B Ileum	C Ileocecal Valve E Large Intestine F Large Intestine, Right G Large Intestine, Left H Cecum J Appendix K Ascending Colon L Transverse Colon M Descending Colon N Sigmoid Colon P Rectum	0 Open 3 Percutaneous 4 Percutaneous endoscopic 7 Via natural or artificial opening 8 Via natural or artificial opening endoscopic	Z No device	Z No qualifier
Q Anus		0 Open 3 Percutaneous 4 Percutaneous endoscopic 7 Via natural or artificial opening 8 Via natural or artificial opening endoscopic X External	Z No device	Z No qualifier
R Anal Sphincter S Greater Omentum T Lesser Omentum V Mesentery W Peritoneum		0 Open 3 Percutaneous 4 Percutaneous endoscopic	Z No device	Z No qualifier

TUBULAR GROUP: Bypass, Dilation, Occlusion, Restriction
Root Operations that alter the diameter/route of a tubular body part.

1ST – 0 Medical and Surgical	EXAMPLE: Dilation rectal stricture	CMS Ex: Transluminal angioplasty
2ND – D Gastrointestinal System	**DILATION:** Expanding an orifice or the lumen of a tubular body part.	
3RD – 7 DILATION	EXPLANATION: By force (stretching) or cutting ...	

Body Part – 4TH		Approach – 5TH	Device – 6TH	Qualifier – 7TH
1 Esophagus, Upper	C Ileocecal Valve	0 Open	D Intraluminal device	Z No qualifier
2 Esophagus, Middle	E Large Intestine	3 Percutaneous	Z No device	
3 Esophagus, Lower	F Large Intestine, Right	4 Percutaneous endoscopic		
4 Esophagogastric Junction	G Large Intestine, Left	7 Via natural or artificial opening		
5 Esophagus	H Cecum	8 Via natural or artificial opening endoscopic		
6 Stomach	K Ascending Colon			
7 Stomach, Pylorus	L Transverse Colon			
8 Small Intestine	M Descending Colon			
9 Duodenum	N Sigmoid Colon			
A Jejunum	P Rectum			
B Ileum	Q Anus			

DIVISION GROUP: Division, Release
Root Operations involving cutting or separation only.

1ST – 0 Medical and Surgical	EXAMPLE: Pyloromyotomy	CMS Ex: Osteotomy
2ND – D Gastrointestinal System	**DIVISION:** Cutting into a body part without draining fluids and/or gases from the body part in order to separate or transect a body part.	
3RD – 8 DIVISION	EXPLANATION: Separated into two or more portions ...	

Body Part – 4TH	Approach – 5TH	Device – 6TH	Qualifier – 7TH
4 Esophagogastric Junction	0 Open	Z No device	Z No qualifier
7 Stomach, Pylorus	3 Percutaneous		
	4 Percutaneous endoscopic		
	7 Via natural or artificial opening		
	8 Via natural or artificial opening endoscopic		
R Anal Sphincter	0 Open	Z No device	Z No qualifier
	3 Percutaneous		

GASTROINTESTINAL 0 D 8

0 D 9

DRAINAGE GROUP: Drainage, Extirpation, Fragmentation
Root Operations that take out solids/fluids/gases from a body part.

1ST - 0 Medical and Surgical	EXAMPLE: I&D perianal abscess	CMS Ex: Thoracentesis

2ND - D Gastrointestinal System	**DRAINAGE:** Taking or letting out fluids and/or gases from a body part.

3RD - 9 DRAINAGE

EXPLANATION: Qualifier "X Diagnostic" indicates biopsy ...

Body Part – 4TH		Approach – 5TH	Device – 6TH	Qualifier – 7TH
1 Esophagus, Upper 2 Esophagus, Middle 3 Esophagus, Lower 4 Esophagogastric Junction 5 Esophagus 6 Stomach 7 Stomach, Pylorus 8 Small Intestine 9 Duodenum A Jejunum B Ileum	C Ileocecal Valve E Large Intestine F Large Intestine, Right G Large Intestine, Left H Cecum J Appendix K Ascending Colon L Transverse Colon M Descending Colon N Sigmoid Colon P Rectum	0 Open 3 Percutaneous 4 Percutaneous endoscopic 7 Via natural or artificial opening 8 Via natural or artificial opening endoscopic	0 Drainage device	Z No qualifier
1 Esophagus, Upper 2 Esophagus, Middle 3 Esophagus, Lower 4 Esophagogastric Junction 5 Esophagus 6 Stomach 7 Stomach, Pylorus 8 Small Intestine 9 Duodenum A Jejunum B Ileum	C Ileocecal Valve E Large Intestine F Large Intestine, Right G Large Intestine, Left H Cecum J Appendix K Ascending Colon L Transverse Colon M Descending Colon N Sigmoid Colon P Rectum	0 Open 3 Percutaneous 4 Percutaneous endoscopic 7 Via natural or artificial opening 8 Via natural or artificial opening endoscopic	Z No device	X Diagnostic Z No qualifier
Q Anus		0 Open 3 Percutaneous 4 Percutaneous endoscopic 7 Via natural or artificial opening 8 Via natural or artificial opening endoscopic X External	0 Drainage device	Z No qualifier
Q Anus		0 Open 3 Percutaneous 4 Percutaneous endoscopic 7 Via natural or artificial opening 8 Via natural or artificial opening endoscopic X External	Z No device	X Diagnostic Z No qualifier

GASTROINTESTINAL 0 D 9

continued ⇨

0 D 9		DRAINAGE – *continued*		
Body Part – 4TH		**Approach – 5TH**	**Device – 6TH**	**Qualifier – 7TH**
R Anal Sphincter S Greater Omentum T Lesser Omentum V Mesentery W Peritoneum		0 Open 3 Percutaneous 4 Percutaneous endoscopic	0 Drainage device	Z No qualifier
R Anal Sphincter S Greater Omentum T Lesser Omentum V Mesentery W Peritoneum		0 Open 3 Percutaneous 4 Percutaneous endoscopic	Z No device	X Diagnostic Z No qualifier

GASTROINTESTINAL 0 D 9

EXCISION GROUP: Excision, Resection, Destruction, (Extraction), (Detachment)
Root Operations that take out some or all of a body part.

1ST - 0 Medical and Surgical	**EXAMPLE:** Vertical sleeve gastrectomy · **CMS Ex:** Liver biopsy
2ND - D Gastrointestinal System	**EXCISION:** Cutting out or off, without replacement, a portion of a body part.
3RD - B EXCISION	**EXPLANATION:** Qualifier "X Diagnostic" indicates biopsy ...

Body Part – 4TH	Approach – 5TH	Device – 6TH	Qualifier – 7TH
1 Esophagus, Upper C Ileocecal Valve 2 Esophagus, Middle E Large Intestine 3 Esophagus, Lower F Large Intestine, Right 4 Esophagogastric Junction G Large Intestine, Left 5 Esophagus H Cecum 7 Stomach, Pylorus J Appendix 8 Small Intestine K Ascending Colon 9 Duodenum L Transverse Colon A Jejunum M Descending Colon B Ileum N Sigmoid Colon P Rectum	0 Open 3 Percutaneous 4 Percutaneous endoscopic 7 Via natural or artificial opening 8 Via natural or artificial opening endoscopic	Z No device	X Diagnostic Z No qualifier
6 Stomach	0 Open 3 Percutaneous 4 Percutaneous endoscopic 7 Via natural or artificial opening 8 Via natural or artificial opening endoscopic	Z No device	3 Vertical X Diagnostic Z No qualifier
Q Anus	0 Open 3 Percutaneous 4 Percutaneous endoscopic 7 Via natural or artificial opening 8 Via natural or artificial opening endoscopic X External	Z No device	X Diagnostic Z No qualifier
R Anal Sphincter S Greater Omentum T Lesser Omentum V Mesentery W Peritoneum	0 Open 3 Percutaneous 4 Percutaneous endoscopic	Z No device	X Diagnostic Z No qualifier

GASTROINTESTINAL 0 D B

DRAINAGE GROUP: Drainage, Extirpation, Fragmentation
Root Operations that take out solids/fluids/gases from a body part.

1ST - **0** Medical and Surgical

2ND - **D** Gastrointestinal System

3RD - **C** EXTIRPATION

EXAMPLE: Removal gastric bezoar | CMS Ex: Choledocholithotomy

EXTIRPATION: Taking or cutting out solid matter from a body part.

EXPLANATION: Abnormal byproduct or foreign body …

Body Part – 4TH	Approach – 5TH	Device – 6TH	Qualifier – 7TH
1 Esophagus, Upper C Ileocecal Valve 2 Esophagus, Middle E Large Intestine 3 Esophagus, Lower F Large Intestine, Right 4 Esophagogastric Junction G Large Intestine, Left 5 Esophagus H Cecum 6 Stomach J Appendix 7 Stomach, Pylorus K Ascending Colon 8 Small Intestine L Transverse Colon 9 Duodenum M Descending Colon A Jejunum N Sigmoid Colon B Ileum P Rectum	0 Open 3 Percutaneous 4 Percutaneous endoscopic 7 Via natural or artificial opening 8 Via natural or artificial opening endoscopic	Z No device	Z No qualifier
Q Anus	0 Open 3 Percutaneous 4 Percutaneous endoscopic 7 Via natural or artificial opening 8 Via natural or artificial opening endoscopic X External	Z No device	Z No qualifier
R Anal Sphincter S Greater Omentum T Lesser Omentum V Mesentery W Peritoneum	0 Open 3 Percutaneous 4 Percutaneous endoscopic	Z No device	Z No qualifier

---

DRAINAGE GROUP: Drainage, Extirpation, Fragmentation
Root Operations that take out solids/fluids/gases from a body part.

1ST - **0** Medical and Surgical

2ND - **D** Gastrointestinal System

3RD - **F** FRAGMENTATION

EXAMPLE: Breaking apart gastric bezoar | CMS Ex: Shockwave lithotripsy

FRAGMENTATION: Breaking solid matter in a body part into pieces.

EXPLANATION: Pieces are not taken out during procedure …

Body Part – 4TH	Approach – 5TH	Device – 6TH	Qualifier – 7TH
5 Esophagus H Cecum 6 Stomach J Appendix 8 Small Intestine K Ascending Colon 9 Duodenum L Transverse Colon A Jejunum M Descending Colon B Ileum N Sigmoid Colon E Large Intestine P Rectum F Large Intestine, Right Q Anus G Large Intestine, Left	0 Open 3 Percutaneous 4 Percutaneous endoscopic 7 Via natural or artificial opening 8 Via natural or artificial opening endoscopic X External NC*	Z No device	Z No qualifier

NC* – Non-covered by Medicare. See current Medicare Code Editor for details.

GASTROINTESTINAL 0 D F

GASTROINTESTINAL 0 D H

DEVICE GROUP: Change, Insertion, Removal, Replacement, Revision, Supplement
Root Operations that always involve a device.

1ST – **0** Medical and Surgical	**EXAMPLE:** Placement artificial anal sphincter CMS Ex: CVP catheter
2ND – **D** Gastrointestinal System	**INSERTION:** Putting in a nonbiological appliance that monitors, assists, performs, or prevents a physiological function but does not physically take the place of a body part.
3RD – **H** INSERTION	**EXPLANATION:** None

Body Part – 4TH	Approach – 5TH	Device – 6TH	Qualifier – 7TH
5 Esophagus	0 Open 3 Percutaneous 4 Percutaneous endoscopic	1 Radioactive element 2 Monitoring device 3 Infusion device D Intraluminal device U Feeding device	Z No qualifier
5 Esophagus	7 Via natural or artificial opening 8 Via natural or artificial opening endoscopic	1 Radioactive element 2 Monitoring device 3 Infusion device B Intraluminal device, airway D Intraluminal device U Feeding device	Z No qualifier
6 Stomach	0 Open 3 Percutaneous 4 Percutaneous endoscopic	2 Monitoring device 3 Infusion device D Intraluminal device M Stimulator lead U Feeding device	Z No qualifier
6 Stomach	7 Via natural or artificial opening 8 Via natural or artificial opening endoscopic	2 Monitoring device 3 Infusion device D Intraluminal device U Feeding device	Z No qualifier
8 Small Intestine 9 Duodenum A Jejunum B Ileum	0 Open 3 Percutaneous 4 Percutaneous endoscopic 7 Via natural or artificial opening 8 Via natural or artificial opening endoscopic	2 Monitoring device 3 Infusion device D Intraluminal device U Feeding device	Z No qualifier

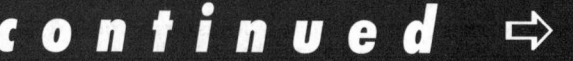

continued ⇨

0   D   H   INSERTION – *continued*

Body Part – 4TH	Approach – 5TH	Device – 6TH	Qualifier – 7TH
E Large Intestine	0 Open 3 Percutaneous 4 Percutaneous endoscopic 7 Via natural or artificial opening 8 Via natural or artificial opening endoscopic	D Intraluminal device	Z No qualifier
P Rectum	0 Open 3 Percutaneous 4 Percutaneous endoscopic 7 Via natural or artificial opening 8 Via natural or artificial opening endoscopic	1 Radioactive element D Intraluminal device	Z No qualifier
Q Anus	0 Open 3 Percutaneous 4 Percutaneous endoscopic	D Intraluminal device L Artificial sphincter	Z No qualifier
Q Anus	7 Via natural or artificial opening 8 Via natural or artificial opening endoscopic	D Intraluminal device	Z No qualifier
R Anal Sphincter	0 Open 3 Percutaneous 4 Percutaneous endoscopic	M Stimulator lead	Z No qualifier

GASTROINTESTINAL 0 D H

EXAMINATION GROUP: Inspection, (Map)
Root Operations involving examination only.

1ST - **0** Medical and Surgical	**EXAMPLE:** Esophagogastroduodenoscopy **CMS Ex:** Colonoscopy
2ND - **D** Gastrointestinal System	**INSPECTION:** Visually and/or manually exploring a body part.
3RD - **J INSPECTION**	**EXPLANATION:** Direct or instrumental visualization ...

Body Part – 4TH	Approach – 5TH	Device – 6TH	Qualifier – 7TH
0 Upper Intestinal Tract 6 Stomach D Lower Intestinal Tract	0 Open 3 Percutaneous 4 Percutaneous endoscopic 7 Via natural or artificial opening 8 Via natural or artificial opening endoscopic X External	Z No device	Z No qualifier
U Omentum V Mesentery W Peritoneum	0 Open 3 Percutaneous 4 Percutaneous endoscopic X External	Z No device	Z No qualifier

TUBULAR GROUP: Bypass, Dilation, Occlusion, Restriction
Root Operations that alter the diameter/route of a tubular body part.

1ST - 0 Medical and Surgical

2ND - D Gastrointestinal System

3RD - L OCCLUSION

EXAMPLE: Closure of rectal stump | CMS Ex: Fallopian tube ligation

OCCLUSION: Completely closing an orifice or lumen of a tubular body part.

EXPLANATION: Natural or artificially created orifice ...

Body Part – 4TH		Approach – 5TH	Device – 6TH	Qualifier – 7TH
1 Esophagus, Upper C Ileocecal Valve 2 Esophagus, Middle E Large Intestine 3 Esophagus, Lower F Large Intestine, Right 4 Esophagogastric Junction G Large Intestine, Left 5 Esophagus H Cecum 6 Stomach K Ascending Colon 7 Stomach, Pylorus L Transverse Colon 8 Small Intestine M Descending Colon 9 Duodenum N Sigmoid Colon A Jejunum P Rectum B Ileum		0 Open 3 Percutaneous 4 Percutaneous endoscopic	C Extraluminal device D Intraluminal device Z No device	Z No qualifier
1 Esophagus, Upper C Ileocecal Valve 2 Esophagus, Middle E Large Intestine 3 Esophagus, Lower F Large Intestine, Right 4 Esophagogastric Junction G Large Intestine, Left 5 Esophagus H Cecum 6 Stomach K Ascending Colon 7 Stomach, Pylorus L Transverse Colon 8 Small Intestine M Descending Colon 9 Duodenum N Sigmoid Colon A Jejunum P Rectum B Ileum		7 Via natural or artificial opening 8 Via natural or artificial opening endoscopic	D Intraluminal device Z No device	Z No qualifier
Q Anus		0 Open 3 Percutaneous 4 Percutaneous endoscopic X External	C Extraluminal device D Intraluminal device Z No device	Z No qualifier
Q Anus		7 Via natural or artificial opening 8 Via natural or artificial opening endoscopic	D Intraluminal device Z No device	Z No qualifier

GASTROINTESTINAL 0 D L

357

MOVE GROUP: Reattachment, Reposition, Transfer, Transplantation
Root Operations that put in/put back or move some/all of a body part.

1ST - **0** Medical and Surgical

2ND - **D** Gastrointestinal System

3RD - **M REATTACHMENT**

EXAMPLE: Reattachment of avulsed esophagus | CMS Ex: Reattach hand

REATTACHMENT: Putting back in or on all or a portion of a separated body part to its normal location or other suitable location.

EXPLANATION: With/without reconnection of vessels/nerves...

Body Part – 4TH		Approach – 5TH	Device – 6TH	Qualifier – 7TH
5 Esophagus	G Large Intestine, Left	0 Open	Z No device	Z No qualifier
6 Stomach	H Cecum	4 Percutaneous endoscopic		
8 Small Intestine	K Ascending Colon			
9 Duodenum	L Transverse Colon			
A Jejunum	M Descending Colon			
B Ileum	N Sigmoid Colon			
E Large Intestine	P Rectum			
F Large Intestine, Right				

DIVISION GROUP: Division, Release
Root Operations involving cutting or separation only.

1ST - **0** Medical and Surgical

2ND - **D** Gastrointestinal System

3RD - **N RELEASE**

EXAMPLE: Adhesiolysis colon | CMS Ex: Carpal tunnel release

RELEASE: Freeing a body part from an abnormal physical constraint by cutting or by the use of force.

EXPLANATION: None of the body part is taken out ...

Body Part – 4TH	Approach – 5TH	Device – 6TH	Qualifier – 7TH
1 Esophagus, Upper 2 Esophagus, Middle 3 Esophagus, Lower 4 Esophagogastric Junction 5 Esophagus 6 Stomach 7 Stomach, Pylorus 8 Small Intestine 9 Duodenum A Jejunum B Ileum C Ileocecal Valve E Large Intestine F Large Intestine, Right G Large Intestine, Left H Cecum J Appendix K Ascending Colon L Transverse Colon M Descending Colon N Sigmoid Colon P Rectum	0 Open 3 Percutaneous 4 Percutaneous endoscopic 7 Via natural or artificial opening 8 Via natural or artificial opening endoscopic	Z No device	Z No qualifier
Q Anus	0 Open 3 Percutaneous 4 Percutaneous endoscopic 7 Via natural or artificial opening 8 Via natural or artificial opening endoscopic X External	Z No device	Z No qualifier
R Anal Sphincter S Greater Omentum T Lesser Omentum V Mesentery W Peritoneum	0 Open 3 Percutaneous 4 Percutaneous endoscopic	Z No device	Z No qualifier

GASTROINTESTINAL 0 D N

DEVICE GROUP: Change, Insertion, Removal, Replacement, Revision, Supplement
Root Operations that always involve a device.

1ST - 0 Medical and Surgical	EXAMPLE: Removal artificial sphincter	CMS Ex: Chest tube removal

2ND - **D** Gastrointestinal System

3RD - **P REMOVAL**

REMOVAL: Taking out or off a device from a body part.

EXPLANATION: Removal device without reinsertion ...

Body Part – 4TH	Approach – 5TH	Device – 6TH	Qualifier – 7TH
0 Upper Intestinal Tract D Lower Intestinal Tract	0 Open 3 Percutaneous 4 Percutaneous endoscopic 7 Via natural or artificial opening 8 Via natural or artificial opening endoscopic	0 Drainage device 2 Monitoring device 3 Infusion device 7 Autologous tissue substitute C Extraluminal device D Intraluminal device J Synthetic substitute K Nonautologous tissue substitute U Feeding device	Z No qualifier
0 Upper Intestinal Tract D Lower Intestinal Tract	X External	0 Drainage device 2 Monitoring device 3 Infusion device D Intraluminal device U Feeding device	Z No qualifier
5 Esophagus	0 Open 3 Percutaneous 4 Percutaneous endoscopic	1 Radioactive element 2 Monitoring device 3 Infusion device U Feeding device	Z No qualifier
5 Esophagus	7 Via natural or artificial opening 8 Via natural or artificial opening endoscopic	1 Radioactive element D Intraluminal device	Z No qualifier
5 Esophagus	X External	1 Radioactive element 2 Monitoring device 3 Infusion device D Intraluminal device U Feeding device	Z No qualifier

c o n t i n u e d ⇨

GASTROINTESTINAL 0 D P

0   D   P   REMOVAL – continued

Body Part – 4TH	Approach – 5TH	Device – 6TH	Qualifier – 7TH
6 Stomach	0 Open 3 Percutaneous 4 Percutaneous endoscopic	0 Drainage device 2 Monitoring device 3 Infusion device 7 Autologous tissue substitute C Extraluminal device D Intraluminal device J Synthetic substitute K Nonautologous tissue substitute M Stimulator lead U Feeding device	Z No qualifier
6 Stomach	7 Via natural or artificial opening 8 Via natural or artificial opening endoscopic	0 Drainage device 2 Monitoring device 3 Infusion device 7 Autologous tissue substitute C Extraluminal device D Intraluminal device J Synthetic substitute K Nonautologous tissue substitute U Feeding device	Z No qualifier
6 Stomach	X External	0 Drainage device 2 Monitoring device 3 Infusion device D Intraluminal device U Feeding device	Z No qualifier
P Rectum	0 Open 3 Percutaneous 4 Percutaneous endoscopic 7 Via natural or artificial opening 8 Via natural or artificial opening endoscopic X External	1 Radioactive element	Z No qualifier
Q Anus	0 Open 3 Percutaneous 4 Percutaneous endoscopic 7 Via natural or artificial opening 8 Via natural or artificial opening endoscopic	L Artificial sphincter	Z No qualifier
R Anal Sphincter	0 Open 3 Percutaneous 4 Percutaneous endoscopic	M Stimulator lead	Z No qualifier
U Omentum V Mesentery W Peritoneum	0 Open 3 Percutaneous 4 Percutaneous endoscopic	0 Drainage device 1 Radioactive element 7 Autologous tissue substitute J Synthetic substitute K Nonautologous tissue substitute	Z No qualifier

GASTROINTESTINAL 0 D P

OTHER REPAIRS GROUP: (Control), **Repair**
Root Operations that define other repairs.

1ST - **0** Medical and Surgical	EXAMPLE: Suture duodenal laceration	CMS Ex: Suture laceration
2ND - **D** Gastrointestinal System	**REPAIR:** Restoring, to the extent possible, a body part to its normal anatomic structure and function.	
3RD - **Q REPAIR**	EXPLANATION: Only when no other root operation applies …	

Body Part – 4TH	Approach – 5TH	Device – 6TH	Qualifier – 7TH
1 Esophagus, Upper C Ileocecal Valve 2 Esophagus, Middle E Large Intestine 3 Esophagus, Lower F Large Intestine, Right 4 Esophagogastric Junction G Large Intestine, Left 5 Esophagus H Cecum 6 Stomach J Appendix 7 Stomach, Pylorus K Ascending Colon 8 Small Intestine L Transverse Colon 9 Duodenum M Descending Colon A Jejunum N Sigmoid Colon B Ileum P Rectum	0 Open 3 Percutaneous 4 Percutaneous endoscopic 7 Via natural or artificial opening 8 Via natural or artificial opening endoscopic	Z No device	Z No qualifier
Q Anus	0 Open 3 Percutaneous 4 Percutaneous endoscopic 7 Via natural or artificial opening 8 Via natural or artificial opening endoscopic X External	Z No device	Z No qualifier
R Anal Sphincter S Greater Omentum T Lesser Omentum V Mesentery W Peritoneum	0 Open 3 Percutaneous 4 Percutaneous endoscopic	Z No device	Z No qualifier

DEVICE GROUP: Change, Insertion, Removal, Replacement, Revision, Supplement
Root Operations that always involve a device.

1ST - **0** Medical and Surgical

2ND - **D** Gastrointestinal System

3RD - **R REPLACEMENT**

EXAMPLE: Esophageal segment replacement | CMS Ex: Total hip

REPLACEMENT: Putting in or on a biological or synthetic material that physically takes the place and/or function of all or a portion of a body part.

EXPLANATION: Includes taking out body part, or eradication...

Body Part – 4TH	Approach – 5TH	Device – 6TH	Qualifier – 7TH
5 Esophagus	0 Open 4 Percutaneous endoscopic 7 Via natural or artificial opening 8 Via natural or artificial opening endoscopic	7 Autologous tissue substitute J Synthetic substitute K Nonautologous tissue substitute	Z No qualifier
R Anal Sphincter S Greater Omentum T Lesser Omentum V Mesentery W Peritoneum	0 Open 4 Percutaneous endoscopic	7 Autologous tissue substitute J Synthetic substitute K Nonautologous tissue substitute	Z No qualifier

MOVE GROUP: Reattachment, Reposition, Transfer, Transplantation
Root Operations that put in/put back or move some/all of a body part.

1ST - **0** Medical and Surgical

2ND - **D** Gastrointestinal System

3RD - **S REPOSITION**

EXAMPLE: Gastropexy for malrotation | CMS Ex: Fracture reduction

REPOSITION: Moving to its normal location, or other suitable location, all or a portion of a body part.

EXPLANATION: May or may not be cut to be moved ...

Body Part – 4TH	Approach – 5TH	Device – 6TH	Qualifier – 7TH
5 Esophagus 6 Stomach 9 Duodenum A Jejunum B Ileum H Cecum K Ascending Colon L Transverse Colon M Descending Colon N Sigmoid Colon P Rectum Q Anus	0 Open 4 Percutaneous endoscopic 7 Via natural or artificial opening 8 Via natural or artificial opening endoscopic X External	Z No device	Z No qualifier

GASTROINTESTINAL 0 D S

EXCISION GROUP: Excision, Resection, Destruction, (Extraction), (Detachment)
Root Operations that take out some or all of a body part.

1ST - O Medical and Surgical	EXAMPLE: Sigmoid colectomy	CMS Ex: Cholecystectomy
2ND - D Gastrointestinal System	RESECTION: Cutting out or off, without replacement, all of a body part.	
3RD - T RESECTION		
	EXPLANATION: None	

Body Part – 4TH		Approach – 5TH	Device – 6TH	Qualifier – 7TH
1 Esophagus, Upper 2 Esophagus, Middle 3 Esophagus, Lower 4 Esophagogastric Junction 5 Esophagus 6 Stomach 7 Stomach, Pylorus 8 Small Intestine 9 Duodenum A Jejunum B Ileum	C Ileocecal Valve E Large Intestine F Large Intestine, Right G Large Intestine, Left H Cecum J Appendix K Ascending Colon L Transverse Colon M Descending Colon N Sigmoid Colon P Rectum Q Anus	0 Open 4 Percutaneous endoscopic 7 Via natural or artificial opening 8 Via natural or artificial opening endoscopic	Z No device	Z No qualifier
R Anal Sphincter S Greater Omentum T Lesser Omentum		0 Open 4 Percutaneous endoscopic	Z No device	Z No qualifier

DEVICE GROUP: Change, Insertion, Removal, Replacement, Revision, Supplement	
Root Operations that always involve a device.	

1ST - 0 Medical and Surgical	EXAMPLE: Parastomal hernia repair with graft	CMS Ex: Hernia mesh

2ND - D Gastrointestinal System

3RD - U SUPPLEMENT

SUPPLEMENT: Putting in or on biological or synthetic material that physically reinforces and/or augments the function of a portion of a body part.

EXPLANATION: Biological material from same individual ...

Body Part – 4TH	Approach – 5TH	Device – 6TH	Qualifier – 7TH
1 Esophagus, Upper 2 Esophagus, Middle 3 Esophagus, Lower 4 Esophagogastric Junction 5 Esophagus 6 Stomach 7 Stomach, Pylorus 8 Small Intestine 9 Duodenum A Jejunum B Ileum C Ileocecal Valve E Large Intestine F Large Intestine, Right G Large Intestine, Left H Cecum K Ascending Colon L Transverse Colon M Descending Colon N Sigmoid Colon P Rectum	0 Open 4 Percutaneous endoscopic 7 Via natural or artificial opening 8 Via natural or artificial opening endoscopic	7 Autologous tissue substitute J Synthetic substitute K Nonautologous tissue substitute	Z No qualifier
Q Anus	0 Open 4 Percutaneous endoscopic 7 Via natural or artificial opening 8 Via natural or artificial opening endoscopic X External	7 Autologous tissue substitute J Synthetic substitute K Nonautologous tissue substitute	Z No qualifier
R Anal Sphincter S Greater Omentum T Lesser Omentum V Mesentery W Peritoneum	0 Open 4 Percutaneous endoscopic	7 Autologous tissue substitute J Synthetic substitute K Nonautologous tissue substitute	Z No qualifier

GASTROINTESTINAL 0 D U

TUBULAR GROUP: Bypass, Dilation, Occlusion, Restriction
Root Operations that alter the diameter/route of a tubular body part.

1ST – **0** Medical and Surgical

2ND – **D** Gastrointestinal System

3RD – **V RESTRICTION**

EXAMPLE: Nissen fundoplication

CMS Ex: Cervical cerclage

RESTRICTION: Partially closing an orifice or the lumen of a tubular body part.

EXPLANATION: Natural or artificially created orifice ...

Body Part – 4TH	Approach – 5TH	Device – 6TH	Qualifier – 7TH
1 Esophagus, Upper C Ileocecal Valve 2 Esophagus, Middle E Large Intestine 3 Esophagus, Lower F Large Intestine, Right 4 Esophagogastric Junction G Large Intestine, Left 5 Esophagus H Cecum 6 Stomach K Ascending Colon 7 Stomach, Pylorus L Transverse Colon 8 Small Intestine M Descending Colon 9 Duodenum N Sigmoid Colon A Jejunum P Rectum B Ileum	0 Open 3 Percutaneous 4 Percutaneous endoscopic	C Extraluminal device D Intraluminal device Z No device	Z No qualifier
1 Esophagus, Upper C Ileocecal Valve 2 Esophagus, Middle E Large Intestine 3 Esophagus, Lower F Large Intestine, Right 4 Esophagogastric Junction G Large Intestine, Left 5 Esophagus H Cecum 6 Stomach NC* K Ascending Colon 7 Stomach, Pylorus L Transverse Colon 8 Small Intestine M Descending Colon 9 Duodenum N Sigmoid Colon A Jejunum P Rectum B Ileum	7 Via natural or artificial opening 8 Via natural or artificial opening endoscopic	D Intraluminal device Z No device	Z No qualifier
Q Anus	0 Open 3 Percutaneous 4 Percutaneous endoscopic X External	C Extraluminal device D Intraluminal device Z No device	Z No qualifier
Q Anus	7 Via natural or artificial opening 8 Via natural or artificial opening endoscopic	D Intraluminal device Z No device	Z No qualifier

NC* – Some procedures are considered non-covered by Medicare. See current Medicare Code Editor for details.

DEVICE GROUP: Change, Insertion, Removal, Replacement, Revision, Supplement
Root Operations that always involve a device.

1ST - 0 Medical and Surgical	EXAMPLE: Reposition artificial anal sphincter	CMS Ex: Adjustment lead

2ND - D Gastrointestinal System

3RD - W REVISION

REVISION: Correcting, to the extent possible, a portion of a malfunctioning device or the position of a displaced device.

EXPLANATION: May replace components of a device …

Body Part – 4TH	Approach – 5TH	Device – 6TH	Qualifier – 7TH
0 Upper Intestinal Tract D Lower Intestinal Tract	0 Open 3 Percutaneous 4 Percutaneous endoscopic 7 Via natural or artificial opening 8 Via natural or artificial opening endoscopic X External	0 Drainage device 2 Monitoring device 3 Infusion device 7 Autologous tissue substitute C Extraluminal device D Intraluminal device J Synthetic substitute K Nonautologous tissue substitute U Feeding device	Z No qualifier
5 Esophagus	7 Via natural or artificial opening 8 Via natural or artificial opening endoscopic X External	D Intraluminal device	Z No qualifier
6 Stomach	0 Open 3 Percutaneous 4 Percutaneous endoscopic	0 Drainage device 2 Monitoring device 3 Infusion device 7 Autologous tissue substitute C Extraluminal device D Intraluminal device J Synthetic substitute K Nonautologous tissue substitute M Stimulator lead U Feeding device	Z No qualifier
6 Stomach	7 Via natural or artificial opening 8 Via natural or artificial opening endoscopic X External	0 Drainage device 2 Monitoring device 3 Infusion device 7 Autologous tissue substitute C Extraluminal device D Intraluminal device J Synthetic substitute K Nonautologous tissue substitute U Feeding device	Z No qualifier
8 Small Intestine E Large Intestine	0 Open 4 Percutaneous endoscopic 7 Via natural or artificial opening 8 Via natural or artificial opening endoscopic	7 Autologous tissue substitute J Synthetic substitute K Nonautologous tissue substitute	Z No qualifier
Q Anus	0 Open 3 Percutaneous 4 Percutaneous endoscopic 7 Via natural or artificial opening 8 Via natural or artificial opening endoscopic	L Artificial sphincter	Z No qualifier

GASTROINTESTINAL 0 D W

continued ⇨

0 D W REVISION – continued

Body Part – 4TH	Approach – 5TH	Device – 6TH	Qualifier – 7TH
R Anal Sphincter	0 Open 3 Percutaneous 4 Percutaneous endoscopic	M Stimulator lead	Z No qualifier
U Omentum V Mesentery W Peritoneum	0 Open 3 Percutaneous 4 Percutaneous endoscopic	0 Drainage device 7 Autologous tissue substitute J Synthetic substitute K Nonautologous tissue substitute	Z No qualifier

---

MOVE GROUP: Reattachment, Reposition, Transfer, Transplantation
Root Operations that put in/put back or move some/all of a body part.

1ST - **0** Medical and Surgical

2ND - **D** Gastrointestinal System

3RD - **X** TRANSFER

EXAMPLE: Colon-interposition esophagus | CMS Ex: Tendon transfer

TRANSFER: Moving, without taking out, all or a portion of a body part to another location to take over the function of all or a portion of a body part.

EXPLANATION: The body part remains connected ...

Body Part – 4TH	Approach – 5TH	Device – 6TH	Qualifier – 7TH
6 Stomach 8 Small Intestine E Large Intestine	0 Open 4 Percutaneous endoscopic	Z No device	5 Esophagus

---

MOVE GROUP: Reattachment, Reposition, Transfer, Transplantation
Root Operations that put in/put back or move some/all of a body part.

1ST - **0** Medical and Surgical

2ND - **D** Gastrointestinal System

3RD - **Y** TRANSPLANTATION

EXAMPLE: Esophagus transplant | CMS Ex: Kidney transplant

TRANSPLANTATION: Putting in or on all or a portion of a living body part taken from another individual or animal to physically take the place and/or function of all or a portion of a similar body part.

EXPLANATION: May take over all or part of its function ...

Body Part – 4TH	Approach – 5TH	Device – 6TH	Qualifier – 7TH
5 Esophagus 6 Stomach 8 Small Intestine LC* E Large Intestine LC*	0 Open	Z No device	0 Allogeneic 1 Syngeneic 2 Zooplastic

LC* – Some procedures are considered limited coverage by Medicare. See current Medicare Code Editor for details.

GASTROINTESTINAL 0 D W

Educational Annotations | F – Hepatobiliary System and Pancreas

Body System Specific Educational Annotations for the Hepatobiliary System and Pancreas include:

- Anatomy and Physiology Review
- Anatomical Illustrations
- Definitions of Common Procedures
- AHA Coding Clinic® Reference Notations
- Body Part Key Listings
- Device Key Listings
- Device Aggregation Table Listings
- Coding Notes

Anatomy and Physiology Review of Hepatobiliary System and Pancreas

BODY PART VALUES – F - HEPATOBILIARY SYSTEM AND PANCREAS

Ampulla of Vater – The common bile duct merges with the pancreatic duct in the dilated area known as the ampulla of Vater.

Common Bile Duct – ANATOMY – The common bile duct is formed by the merger of the cystic duct from the gallbladder and the common hepatic duct. PHYSIOLOGY – The cystic duct, hepatic duct, and common bile duct convey the bile into the duodenum.

Cystic Duct – ANATOMY – The cystic duct is the tubular drain of the gallbladder which merges with the hepatic duct to form the common bile duct. PHYSIOLOGY – The cystic duct, hepatic duct, and common bile duct convey the bile into the duodenum.

Gallbladder – ANATOMY – The gallbladder is the musculomembranous, pear-shaped bile reservoir located on the undersurface of the liver. PHYSIOLOGY – The gallbladder functions to store and concentrate the bile and release the bile on demand to the small intestine for the digestion of fats.

Hepatic Duct – ANATOMY – The common hepatic duct is formed by the merger of the right and left hepatic ducts that drain the smaller intrahepatic ducts. PHYSIOLOGY – The cystic duct, hepatic duct, and common bile duct convey the bile into the duodenum.

Hepatobiliary Duct – The ducts of the hepatobiliary system including the cystic duct, hepatic ducts, and common bile duct.

Liver – ANATOMY – The liver is the largest organ in the body, weighing about 3 pounds (1 kg) in the adult. Located in the upper right quadrant of the abdominal cavity, its superior surface lies under the dome of the diaphragm. There are 4 lobes of the liver; the left, right (the right lobe has two smaller lobes, the caudate and quadrate). The common bile duct is formed by the joining of the hepatic duct, which carries bile from the liver, and the cystic duct, which carries bile from the gallbladder. The common duct then carries the bile into the duodenum through an opening on the duodenal papilla. The hepatic artery furnishes arterial blood for the nourishment of the liver cells. The portal vein carries blood containing products of digestion from the intestinal tract into the liver. Internally, the liver lobules are the functional units of liver substance. Bile is secreted by the liver cells into tiny canals, or canaliculi, and then emptied into a bile duct. PHYSIOLOGY – One of the regulatory functions of the liver is controlling the blood sugar level. The liver is able to both absorb excess sugar and dispense it into the blood. The liver also stores and secretes other essential nutrients. It chemically processes these materials and detoxifies many substances that could be harmful if allowed to accumulate in the body. Its bile salts are necessary for the absorption of vitamin K from the gastrointestinal tract, which in turn are needed for the production of prothrombin. Another important liver function is producing bile. A brownish-yellow fluid, it is secreted continuously by the liver in amounts averaging about 20 fluid ounces (600 ml) per day. Bile contains the bile salts which are very important in the digestion of fat.

Liver, Left Lobe – One of the two common lobes of the liver.

Liver, Right Lobe – One of the two common lobes of the liver.

Continued on next page

HEPATOBILIARY 0 F

Educational Annotations | F – Hepatobiliary System and Pancreas

Anatomy and Physiology Review of Hepatobiliary System and Pancreas

BODY PART VALUES – F - HEPATOBILIARY SYSTEM AND PANCREAS
Continued from previous page

Pancreas – ANATOMY – The pancreas is a slender organ about 6 to 9 inches (15 to 23 cm) long lying horizontally and located in the abdomen behind and under the stomach. The pancreas is divided into 3 areas: The head, lying in the curve formed by the duodenum; the body, the main portion lying between the head and tail; and the tail, the most lateral portion blunting up against the spleen. The cells that produce pancreatic juice are called pancreatic acinar cells, and they make up the bulk of the pancreas. These cells are clustered around tiny tubes which drain into the pancreatic duct (duct of Wirsung). This duct connects with the duodenum at the same place where the bile ducts join the duodenum. The second type of pancreatic cells are arranged in groups closely associated with blood vessels and are called islets of Langerhans. The pancreas arterial blood is supplied via the common hepatic artery, the gastroduodenal artery, the pancreatico-duodenal arches, the splenic artery, and also from the superior mesenteric artery. PHYSIOLOGY – The pancreas functions as both an exocrine gland, producing pancreatic juice, and as an endocrine gland, producing the hormones insulin and glucagen. The pancreatic juice contains enzymes capable of digesting carbohydrates, fats, proteins, and nucleic acids, and is produced by the pancreatic acinar cells. This juice is drained into the duodenum. The pancreatic hormones which are produced by the islets of Langerhans cells regulate blood glucose level.

Pancreatic Duct – The pancreatic duct connects with the duodenum at the dilated area known as the ampulla of Vater.

Pancreatic Duct, Accessory – The presence of an additional pancreatic duct that connects directly with the duodenum.

Anatomical Illustrations of Hepatobiliary System and Pancreas

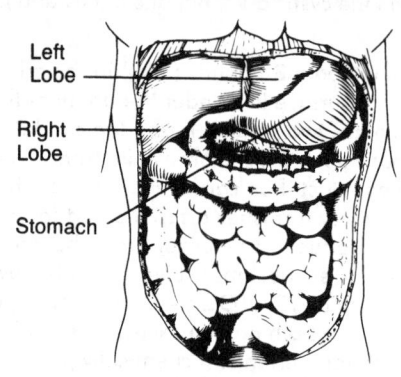

LIVER — ANTERIOR VIEW

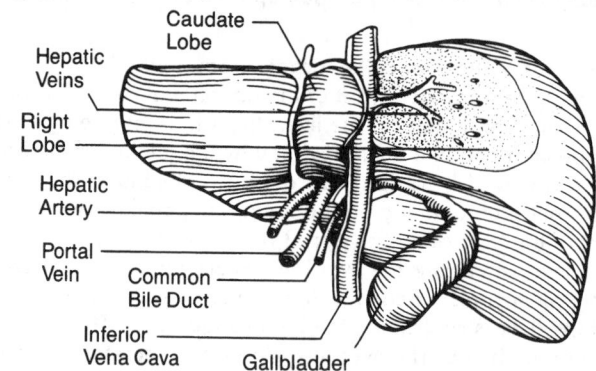

LIVER — POSTERIOR VIEW

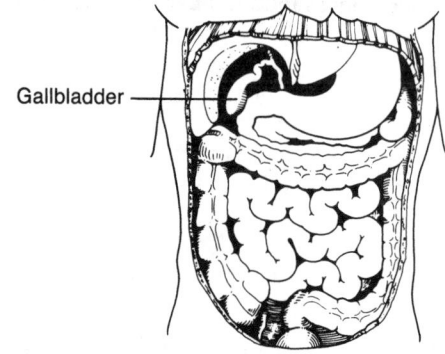

GALLBLADDER

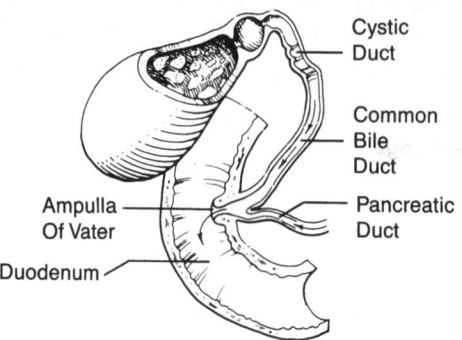

GALLBLADDER — ANTERIOR (CUT-AWAY) VIEW

Continued on next page

Educational Annotations | F – Hepatobiliary System and Pancreas

Anatomical Illustrations of Hepatobiliary System and Pancreas

Continued from previous page

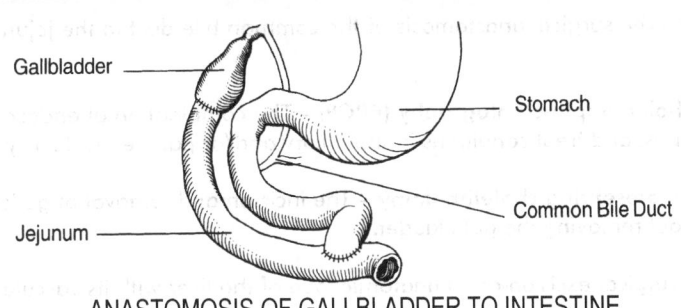

ANASTOMOSIS OF GALLBLADDER TO INTESTINE

AHA Coding Clinic® Reference Notations of Hepatobiliary System and Pancreas

ROOT OPERATION SPECIFIC - F - HEPATOBILIARY SYSTEM AND PANCREAS

BYPASS - 1

CHANGE - 2

DESTRUCTION - 5

DILATION - 7
Dilation of common bile duct ....AHA 14:3Q:p15

DIVISION - 8

DRAINAGE - 9
ERCP with pseudocyst drainage ....AHA 14:3Q:p15
Placement of external-internal biliary drainage catheter ....AHA 15:1Q:p32

EXCISION - B
Brush biopsy of pancreatic and common bile ducts ....AHA 16:1Q:p25
Needle biopsy of common hepatic duct ....AHA 16:1Q:p23
Whipple pyloric sparing pancreaticoduodenectomy..................................AHA 14:3Q:p32

EXTIRPATION - C

FRAGMENTATION - F

INSERTION - H

INSPECTION - J

OCCLUSION - L

REATTACHMENT - M

RELEASE - N

REMOVAL - P

REPAIR - Q

REPLACEMENT - R

REPOSITION - S

RESECTION - T
Resection of liver to capture "domino liver transplant" ....AHA 12:4Q:p99

SUPPLEMENT - U

RESTRICTION - V

REVISION - W

TRANSPLANTATION - Y
"Domino liver transplant"..AHA 12:4Q:p99
Orthotopic liver allotransplant ....AHA 14:3Q:p13

HEPATOBILIARY 0 F

Educational Annotations | F – Hepatobiliary System and Pancreas

Definitions of Common Procedures of Hepatobiliary System and Pancreas

Choledochojejunostomy – The surgical anastomosis of the common bile duct to the jejunum to relieve biliary obstruction symptoms.

Endoscopic retrograde cholangiopancreatography (ERCP) – The combination of endoscopic and fluoroscopy to visualize, obtain radiographs, and treat conditions in the biliary and/or pancreatic duct systems.

Laparoscopic gallbladder-preserving cholelithotomy – The incision and removal of gallstones that is performed laparoscopically and without removing the gallbladder.

Lobectomy of liver – The surgical excision of an anatomic lobe of the liver with its vascular connections.

Wedge resection of liver – The surgical excision of less than a whole anatomic liver segment or parts of two anatomic segments.

Whipple procedure (pancreatoduodenectomy) – The surgical excision of the head of the pancreas that usually includes a duodenectomy, cholecystectomy, and a portion of the stomach including the pylorus, with anastomosis of the common bile duct, pancreas, and stomach to the jejunum. A pyloric-sparing version keeps the stomach and pylorus intact.

Body Part Key Listings of Hepatobiliary System and Pancreas

See also Body Part Key in Appendix C
Duct of Santorini ....*use* Pancreatic Duct, Accessory
Duct of Wirsung ....*use* Pancreatic Duct
Duodenal ampulla ....*use* Ampulla of Vater
Hepatopancreatic ampulla ....*use* Ampulla of Vater
Quadrate lobe ....*use* Liver

Device Key Listings of Hepatobiliary System and Pancreas

See also Device Key in Appendix D
Autograft ....*use* Autologous Tissue Substitute
Brachytherapy seeds ....*use* Radioactive Element
Stent, intraluminal (cardiovascular)
   (gastrointestinal) (hepatobiliary) (urinary) ......*use* Intraluminal Device
Tissue bank graft ....*use* Nonautologous Tissue Substitute

Device Aggregation Table Listings of Hepatobiliary System and Pancreas

See also Device Aggregation Table in Appendix E

Specific Device	For Operation	In Body System	General Device
None Listed in Device Aggregation Table for this Body System			

Educational Annotations | F – Hepatobiliary System and Pancreas

Coding Notes of Hepatobiliary System and Pancreas

Body System Specific PCS Reference Manual Exercises

PCS CODE	F – HEPATOBILIARY SYSTEM AND PANCREAS EXERCISES
0 F 7 9 8 Z Z	ERCP with balloon dilation of common bile duct.
0 F 9 1 0 0 Z	Laparotomy with drain placement for liver abscess, right lobe.
0 F B 2 0 Z Z	Laparotomy with wedge resection of left lateral segment of liver.
0 F B G 0 Z Z	Open excision of tail of pancreas.
0 F F 9 8 Z Z	Endoscopic Retrograde Cholangiopancreatography (ERCP) with lithotripsy of common bile duct stone. (ERCP is performed through the mouth to the biliary system via the duodenum, so the approach value is Via Natural or Artificial Opening Endoscopic.)
0 F J 0 0 Z Z	Laparotomy with palpation of liver.
0 F P G 0 0 Z	Laparotomy with removal of pancreatic drain.
0 F T 4 4 Z Z	Laparoscopic cholecystectomy.
0 F Y 0 0 Z 0	Liver transplant with donor matched liver.
0 F Y G 0 Z 0	Left kidney/pancreas organ bank transplant.
0 T Y 1 0 Z 0	

HEPATOBILIARY

0 F

Educational Annotations | F – Hepatobiliary System and Pancreas

NOTES

TUBULAR GROUP: Bypass, Dilation, Occlusion, Restriction
Root Operations that alter the diameter/route of a tubular body part.

1ST – 0 Medical and Surgical

2ND – F Hepatobiliary System and Pancreas

3RD – 1 BYPASS

EXAMPLE: Choledochojejunostomy | CMS Ex: Coronary artery bypass

BYPASS: Altering the route of passage of the contents of a tubular body part.

EXPLANATION: Rerouting contents to a downstream part …

Body Part – 4TH	Approach – 5TH	Device – 6TH	Qualifier – 7TH
4 Gallbladder 5 Hepatic Duct, Right 6 Hepatic Duct, Left 8 Cystic Duct 9 Common Bile Duct	0 Open 4 Percutaneous endoscopic	D Intraluminal device Z No device	3 Duodenum 4 Stomach 5 Hepatic Duct, Right 6 Hepatic Duct, Left 7 Hepatic Duct, Caudate 8 Cystic Duct 9 Common Bile Duct B Small Intestine
D Pancreatic Duct F Pancreatic Duct, Accessory G Pancreas	0 Open 4 Percutaneous endoscopic	D Intraluminal device Z No device	3 Duodenum B Small Intestine C Large Intestine

DEVICE GROUP: Change, Insertion, Removal, Replacement, Revision, Supplement
Root Operations that always involve a device.

1ST – 0 Medical and Surgical

2ND – F Hepatobiliary System and Pancreas

3RD – 2 CHANGE

EXAMPLE: Exchange drain tube | CMS Ex: Changing urinary catheter

CHANGE: Taking out or off a device from a body part and putting back an identical or similar device in or on the same body part without cutting or puncturing the skin or a mucous membrane.

EXPLANATION: ALL Changes use EXTERNAL approach only…

Body Part – 4TH		Approach – 5TH	Device – 6TH	Qualifier – 7TH
0 Liver 4 Gallbladder B Hepatobiliary Duct	D Pancreatic Duct G Pancreas	X External	0 Drainage device Y Other device	Z No qualifier

HEPATOBILIARY 0 F 2

EXCISION GROUP: Excision, Resection, Destruction, (Extraction), (Detachment)
Root Operations that take out some or all of a body part.

1ST - 0 Medical and Surgical	EXAMPLE: RF ablation liver lesion	CMS Ex: Fulguration polyp
2ND - F Hepatobiliary System and Pancreas 3RD - 5 DESTRUCTION	**DESTRUCTION:** Physical eradication of all or a portion of a body part by the direct use of energy, force, or a destructive agent.	
	EXPLANATION: None of the body part is physically taken out	

Body Part – 4TH	Approach – 5TH	Device – 6TH	Qualifier – 7TH
0 Liver 1 Liver, Right Lobe 2 Liver, Left Lobe 4 Gallbladder G Pancreas	0 Open 3 Percutaneous 4 Percutaneous endoscopic	Z No device	Z No qualifier
5 Hepatic Duct, Right 6 Hepatic Duct, Left 8 Cystic Duct 9 Common Bile Duct C Ampulla of Vater D Pancreatic Duct F Pancreatic Duct, Accessory	0 Open 3 Percutaneous 4 Percutaneous endoscopic 7 Via natural or artificial opening 8 Via natural or artificial opening endoscopic	Z No device	Z No qualifier

---

TUBULAR GROUP: Bypass, Dilation, Occlusion, Restriction
Root Operations that alter the diameter/route of a tubular body part.

1ST - 0 Medical and Surgical	EXAMPLE: ERCP dilation pancreatic duct	CMS Ex: Transluminal angioplasty
2ND - F Hepatobiliary System and Pancreas 3RD - 7 DILATION	**DILATION:** Expanding an orifice or the lumen of a tubular body part.	
	EXPLANATION: By force (stretching) or cutting ...	

Body Part – 4TH	Approach – 5TH	Device – 6TH	Qualifier – 7TH
5 Hepatic Duct, Right 6 Hepatic Duct, Left 8 Cystic Duct 9 Common Bile Duct C Ampulla of Vater D Pancreatic Duct F Pancreatic Duct, Accessory	0 Open 3 Percutaneous 4 Percutaneous endoscopic 7 Via natural or artificial opening 8 Via natural or artificial opening endoscopic	D Intraluminal device Z No device	Z No qualifier

DIVISION GROUP: Division, Release
Root Operations involving cutting or separation only.

	EXAMPLE: Pancreatotomy	CMS Ex: Osteotomy
1ST – **0** Medical and Surgical	**DIVISION:** Cutting into a body part without draining fluids and/or gases from the body part in order to separate or transect a body part.	
2ND – **F** Hepatobiliary System and Pancreas		
3RD – **8 DIVISION**	EXPLANATION: Separated into two or more portions …	

Body Part – 4TH	Approach – 5TH	Device – 6TH	Qualifier – 7TH
G Pancreas	0 Open 3 Percutaneous 4 Percutaneous endoscopic	Z No device	Z No qualifier

DRAINAGE GROUP: Drainage, Extirpation, Fragmentation
Root Operations that take out solids/fluids/gases from a body part.

	EXAMPLE: ERCP pseudocyst drainage	CMS Ex: Thoracentesis
1ST – **0** Medical and Surgical	**DRAINAGE:** Taking or letting out fluids and/or gases from a body part.	
2ND – **F** Hepatobiliary System and Pancreas		
3RD – **9 DRAINAGE**	EXPLANATION: Qualifier "X Diagnostic" indicates biopsy …	

Body Part – 4TH	Approach – 5TH	Device – 6TH	Qualifier – 7TH
0 Liver 1 Liver, Right Lobe 2 Liver, Left Lobe 4 Gallbladder G Pancreas	0 Open 3 Percutaneous 4 Percutaneous endoscopic	0 Drainage device	Z No qualifier
0 Liver 1 Liver, Right Lobe 2 Liver, Left Lobe 4 Gallbladder G Pancreas	0 Open 3 Percutaneous 4 Percutaneous endoscopic	Z No device	X Diagnostic Z No qualifier
5 Hepatic Duct, Right 6 Hepatic Duct, Left 8 Cystic Duct 9 Common Bile Duct C Ampulla of Vater D Pancreatic Duct F Pancreatic Duct, Accessory	0 Open 3 Percutaneous 4 Percutaneous endoscopic 7 Via natural or artificial opening 8 Via natural or artificial opening endoscopic	0 Drainage device	Z No qualifier
5 Hepatic Duct, Right 6 Hepatic Duct, Left 8 Cystic Duct 9 Common Bile Duct C Ampulla of Vater D Pancreatic Duct F Pancreatic Duct, Accessory	0 Open 3 Percutaneous 4 Percutaneous endoscopic 7 Via natural or artificial opening 8 Via natural or artificial opening endoscopic	Z No device	X Diagnostic Z No qualifier

HEPATOBILIARY **0 F 9**

EXCISION GROUP: Excision, Resection, Destruction, (Extraction), (Detachment)
Root Operations that take out some or all of a body part.

1ST - 0 Medical and Surgical	EXAMPLE: Wedge resection liver		CMS Ex: Liver biopsy
2ND - F Hepatobiliary System and Pancreas 3RD - B EXCISION	**EXCISION:** Cutting out or off, without replacement, a portion of a body part.		
	EXPLANATION: Qualifier "X Diagnostic" indicates biopsy …		

Body Part – 4TH	Approach – 5TH	Device – 6TH	Qualifier – 7TH
0 Liver 1 Liver, Right Lobe 2 Liver, Left Lobe 4 Gallbladder G Pancreas	0 Open 3 Percutaneous 4 Percutaneous endoscopic	Z No device	X Diagnostic Z No qualifier
5 Hepatic Duct, Right 6 Hepatic Duct, Left 8 Cystic Duct 9 Common Bile Duct C Ampulla of Vater D Pancreatic Duct F Pancreatic Duct, Accessory	0 Open 3 Percutaneous 4 Percutaneous endoscopic 7 Via natural or artificial opening 8 Via natural or artificial opening endoscopic	Z No device	X Diagnostic Z No qualifier

DRAINAGE GROUP: Drainage, Extirpation, Fragmentation
Root Operations that take out solids/fluids/gases from a body part.

1ST - 0 Medical and Surgical	EXAMPLE: Cholelithotomy		CMS Ex: Choledocholithotomy
2ND - F Hepatobiliary System and Pancreas 3RD - C EXTIRPATION	**EXTIRPATION:** Taking or cutting out solid matter from a body part.		
	EXPLANATION: Abnormal byproduct or foreign body …		

Body Part – 4TH	Approach – 5TH	Device – 6TH	Qualifier – 7TH
0 Liver 1 Liver, Right Lobe 2 Liver, Left Lobe 4 Gallbladder G Pancreas	0 Open 3 Percutaneous 4 Percutaneous endoscopic	Z No device	Z No qualifier
5 Hepatic Duct, Right 6 Hepatic Duct, Left 8 Cystic Duct 9 Common Bile Duct C Ampulla of Vater D Pancreatic Duct F Pancreatic Duct, Accessory	0 Open 3 Percutaneous 4 Percutaneous endoscopic 7 Via natural or artificial opening 8 Via natural or artificial opening endoscopic	Z No device	Z No qualifier

DRAINAGE GROUP: Drainage, Extirpation, Fragmentation
Root Operations that take out solids/fluids/gases from a body part.

1ST - **0** Medical and Surgical

2ND - **F** Hepatobiliary System and Pancreas

3RD - **F FRAGMENTATION**

EXAMPLE: Lithotripsy gallstones | CMS Ex: Extracorporeal shockwave lithotripsy

FRAGMENTATION: Breaking solid matter in a body part into pieces.

EXPLANATION: Pieces are not taken out during procedure ...

Body Part – 4TH	Approach – 5TH	Device – 6TH	Qualifier – 7TH
4 Gallbladder	0 Open	Z No device	Z No qualifier
5 Hepatic Duct, Right	3 Percutaneous		
6 Hepatic Duct, Left	4 Percutaneous		
8 Cystic Duct	endoscopic		
9 Common Bile Duct	7 Via natural or		
C Ampulla of Vater	artificial opening		
D Pancreatic Duct	8 Via natural or		
F Pancreatic Duct, Accessory	artificial opening		
	endoscopic		
	X External NC*		

NC* – Non-covered by Medicare. See current Medicare Code Editor for details.

DEVICE GROUP: Change, Insertion, Removal, Replacement, Revision, Supplement
Root Operations that always involve a device.

1ST - **0** Medical and Surgical

2ND - **F** Hepatobiliary System and Pancreas

3RD - **H INSERTION**

EXAMPLE: Insertion infusion pump pancreas | CMS Ex: CVP catheter

INSERTION: Putting in a nonbiological appliance that monitors, assists, performs, or prevents a physiological function but does not physically take the place of a body part.

EXPLANATION: None

Body Part – 4TH	Approach – 5TH	Device – 6TH	Qualifier – 7TH
0 Liver	0 Open	2 Monitoring device	Z No qualifier
1 Liver, Right Lobe	3 Percutaneous	3 Infusion device	
2 Liver, Left Lobe	4 Percutaneous		
4 Gallbladder	endoscopic		
G Pancreas			
B Hepatobiliary Duct	0 Open	1 Radioactive element	Z No qualifier
D Pancreatic Duct	3 Percutaneous	2 Monitoring device	
	4 Percutaneous	3 Infusion device	
	endoscopic	D Intraluminal device	
	7 Via natural or		
	artificial opening		
	8 Via natural or		
	artificial opening		
	endoscopic		

HEPATOBILIARY 0 F H

EXAMINATION GROUP: Inspection, (Map)
Root Operations involving examination only.

1ST - 0 Medical and Surgical	EXAMPLE: Exploration of common bile duct	CMS Ex: Colonoscopy
2ND - F Hepatobiliary System and Pancreas	**INSPECTION:** Visually and/or manually exploring a body part.	
3RD - J INSPECTION	EXPLANATION: Direct or instrumental visualization ...	

Body Part – 4TH	Approach – 5TH	Device – 6TH	Qualifier – 7TH
0 Liver 4 Gallbladder G Pancreas	0 Open 3 Percutaneous 4 Percutaneous endoscopic X External	Z No device	Z No qualifier
B Hepatobiliary Duct D Pancreatic Duct	0 Open 3 Percutaneous 4 Percutaneous endoscopic 7 Via natural or artificial opening 8 Via natural or artificial opening endoscopic	Z No device	Z No qualifier

---

TUBULAR GROUP: Bypass, Dilation, Occlusion, Restriction
Root Operations that alter the diameter/route of a tubular body part.

1ST - 0 Medical and Surgical	EXAMPLE: Clipping accessory pancreatic duct	CMS Ex: Tubal ligation
2ND - F Hepatobiliary System and Pancreas	**OCCLUSION:** Completely closing an orifice or lumen of a tubular body part.	
3RD - L OCCLUSION	EXPLANATION: Natural or artificially created orifice ...	

Body Part – 4TH	Approach – 5TH	Device – 6TH	Qualifier – 7TH
5 Hepatic Duct, Right 6 Hepatic Duct, Left 8 Cystic Duct 9 Common Bile Duct C Ampulla of Vater D Pancreatic Duct F Pancreatic Duct, Accessory	0 Open 3 Percutaneous 4 Percutaneous endoscopic	C Extraluminal device D Intraluminal device Z No device	Z No qualifier
5 Hepatic Duct, Right 6 Hepatic Duct, Left 8 Cystic Duct 9 Common Bile Duct C Ampulla of Vater D Pancreatic Duct F Pancreatic Duct, Accessory	7 Via natural or artificial opening 8 Via natural or artificial opening endoscopic	D Intraluminal device Z No device	Z No qualifier

HEPATOBILIARY 0 F J

MOVE GROUP: Reattachment, Reposition, (Transfer), Transplantation
Root Operations that put in/put back or move some/all of a body part.

1ST - 0   Medical and Surgical

2ND - F   Hepatobiliary System and Pancreas

3RD - M   REATTACHMENT

EXAMPLE: Reattachment avulsed pancreas | CMS Ex: Reattachment hand

REATTACHMENT: Putting back in or on all or a portion of a separated body part to its normal location or other suitable location.

EXPLANATION: With/without reconnection of vessels/nerves...

Body Part – 4TH	Approach – 5TH	Device – 6TH	Qualifier – 7TH
0 Liver 1 Liver, Right Lobe 2 Liver, Left Lobe 4 Gallbladder 5 Hepatic Duct, Right 6 Hepatic Duct, Left 8 Cystic Duct 9 Common Bile Duct C Ampulla of Vater D Pancreatic Duct F Pancreatic Duct, Accessory G Pancreas	0 Open 4 Percutaneous endoscopic	Z No device	Z No qualifier

DIVISION GROUP: Division, Release
Root Operations involving cutting or separation only.

1ST - 0   Medical and Surgical

2ND - F   Hepatobiliary System and Pancreas

3RD - N   RELEASE

EXAMPLE: Lysis adhesions gallbladder | CMS Ex: Carpal tunnel release

RELEASE: Freeing a body part from an abnormal physical constraint by cutting or by the use of force.

EXPLANATION: None of the body part is taken out ...

Body Part – 4TH	Approach – 5TH	Device – 6TH	Qualifier – 7TH
0 Liver 1 Liver, Right Lobe 2 Liver, Left Lobe 4 Gallbladder G Pancreas	0 Open 3 Percutaneous 4 Percutaneous endoscopic	Z No device	Z No qualifier
5 Hepatic Duct, Right 6 Hepatic Duct, Left 8 Cystic Duct 9 Common Bile Duct C Ampulla of Vater D Pancreatic Duct F Pancreatic Duct, Accessory	0 Open 3 Percutaneous 4 Percutaneous endoscopic 7 Via natural or artificial opening 8 Via natural or artificial opening endoscopic	Z No device	Z No qualifier

HEPATOBILIARY   0 F N

DEVICE GROUP: Change, Insertion, Removal, Replacement, Revision, Supplement
Root Operations that always involve a device.

1ST - O Medical and Surgical	EXAMPLE: Removal drain tube · CMS Ex: Chest tube removal
2ND - F Hepatobiliary System and Pancreas	**REMOVAL:** Taking out or off a device from a body part.
3RD - P REMOVAL	EXPLANATION: Removal device without reinsertion ...

Body Part – 4TH	Approach – 5TH	Device – 6TH	Qualifier – 7TH
0 Liver	0 Open 3 Percutaneous 4 Percutaneous endoscopic X External	0 Drainage device 2 Monitoring device 3 Infusion device	Z No qualifier
4 Gallbladder G Pancreas	0 Open 3 Percutaneous 4 Percutaneous endoscopic X External	0 Drainage device 2 Monitoring device 3 Infusion device D Intraluminal device	Z No qualifier
B Hepatobiliary Duct D Pancreatic Duct	0 Open 3 Percutaneous 4 Percutaneous endoscopic 7 Via natural or artificial opening 8 Via natural or artificial opening endoscopic	0 Drainage device 1 Radioactive element 2 Monitoring device 3 Infusion device 7 Autologous tissue substitute C Extraluminal device D Intraluminal device J Synthetic substitute K Nonautologous tissue substitute	Z No qualifier
B Hepatobiliary Duct D Pancreatic Duct	X External	0 Drainage device 1 Radioactive element 2 Monitoring device 3 Infusion device D Intraluminal device	Z No qualifier

---

OTHER REPAIRS GROUP: (Control), **Repair**
Root Operations that define other repairs.

1ST - 0 Medical and Surgical	EXAMPLE: Repair liver laceration		CMS Ex: Suture laceration
2ND - F Hepatobiliary System and Pancreas	**REPAIR:**	Restoring, to the extent possible, a body part to its normal anatomic structure and function.	
3RD - Q REPAIR	EXPLANATION: Only when no other root operation applies ...		

Body Part – 4TH	Approach – 5TH	Device – 6TH	Qualifier – 7TH
0 Liver 1 Liver, Right Lobe 2 Liver, Left Lobe 4 Gallbladder G Pancreas	0 Open 3 Percutaneous 4 Percutaneous endoscopic	Z No device	Z No qualifier
5 Hepatic Duct, Right 6 Hepatic Duct, Left 8 Cystic Duct 9 Common Bile Duct C Ampulla of Vater D Pancreatic Duct F Pancreatic Duct, Accessory	0 Open 3 Percutaneous 4 Percutaneous endoscopic 7 Via natural or artificial opening 8 Via natural or artificial opening endoscopic	Z No device	Z No qualifier

---

DEVICE GROUP: Change, Insertion, Removal, Replacement, Revision, Supplement
Root Operations that always involve a device.

1ST - 0 Medical and Surgical	EXAMPLE: Hepatic duct replacement		CMS Ex: Total hip
2ND - F Hepatobiliary System and Pancreas	**REPLACEMENT:** Putting in or on a biological or synthetic material that physically takes the place and/or function of all or a portion of a body part.		
3RD - R REPLACEMENT	EXPLANATION: Includes taking out body part, or eradication...		

Body Part – 4TH	Approach – 5TH	Device – 6TH	Qualifier – 7TH
5 Hepatic Duct, Right 6 Hepatic Duct, Left 8 Cystic Duct 9 Common Bile Duct C Ampulla of Vater D Pancreatic Duct F Pancreatic Duct, Accessory	0 Open 4 Percutaneous endoscopic	7 Autologous tissue substitute J Synthetic substitute K Nonautologous tissue substitute	Z No qualifier

HEPATOBILIARY

0 F R

MOVE GROUP: Reattachment, Reposition, (Transfer), Transplantation
Root Operations that put in/put back or move some/all of a body part.

1ST - **0** Medical and Surgical	**EXAMPLE:** Relocation cystic duct **CMS Ex:** Fracture reduction
2ND - **F** Hepatobiliary System and Pancreas	**REPOSITION:** Moving to its normal location, or other suitable location, all or a portion of a body part.
3RD - **S** REPOSITION	**EXPLANATION:** May or may not be cut to be moved ...

Body Part – 4TH		Approach – 5TH	Device – 6TH	Qualifier – 7TH
0 Liver	9 Common Bile Duct	0 Open	Z No device	Z No qualifier
4 Gallbladder	C Ampulla of Vater	4 Percutaneous endoscopic		
5 Hepatic Duct, Right	D Pancreatic Duct			
6 Hepatic Duct, Left	F Pancreatic Duct, Accessory			
8 Cystic Duct	G Pancreas			

EXCISION GROUP: Excision, Resection, Destruction, (Extraction), (Detachment)
Root Operations that take out some or all of a body part.

1ST - **0** Medical and Surgical	**EXAMPLE:** Liver lobectomy **CMS Ex:** Cholecystectomy
2ND - **F** Hepatobiliary System and Pancreas	**RESECTION:** Cutting out or off, without replacement, all of a body part.
3RD - **T** RESECTION	**EXPLANATION:** None

Body Part – 4TH	Approach – 5TH	Device – 6TH	Qualifier – 7TH
0 Liver 1 Liver, Right Lobe 2 Liver, Left Lobe 4 Gallbladder G Pancreas	0 Open 4 Percutaneous endoscopic	Z No device	Z No qualifier
5 Hepatic Duct, Right 6 Hepatic Duct, Left 8 Cystic Duct 9 Common Bile Duct C Ampulla of Vater D Pancreatic Duct F Pancreatic Duct, Accessory	0 Open 4 Percutaneous endoscopic 7 Via natural or artificial opening 8 Via natural or artificial opening endoscopic	Z No device	Z No qualifier

Hepatobiliary 0 F S

DEVICE GROUP: Change, Insertion, Removal, Replacement, Revision, Supplement
Root Operations that always involve a device.

1ST - **0** Medical and Surgical

2ND - **F** Hepatobiliary System and Pancreas

3RD - **U SUPPLEMENT**

EXAMPLE: Tissue graft ductal repair | CMS Ex: Hernia repair with mesh

SUPPLEMENT: Putting in or on biological or synthetic material that physically reinforces and/or augments the function of a portion of a body part.

EXPLANATION: Biological material from same individual ...

Body Part – 4TH	Approach – 5TH	Device – 6TH	Qualifier – 7TH
5 Hepatic Duct, Right 6 Hepatic Duct, Left 8 Cystic Duct 9 Common Bile Duct C Ampulla of Vater D Pancreatic Duct F Pancreatic Duct, Accessory	0 Open 3 Percutaneous 4 Percutaneous endoscopic	7 Autologous tissue substitute J Synthetic substitute K Nonautologous tissue substitute	Z No qualifier

TUBULAR GROUP: Bypass, Dilation, Occlusion, Restriction
Root Operations that alter the diameter/route of a tubular body part.

1ST - **0** Medical and Surgical

2ND - **F** Hepatobiliary System and Pancreas

3RD - **V RESTRICTION**

EXAMPLE: Restrictive ductal stent | CMS Ex: Cervical cerclage

RESTRICTION: Partially closing an orifice or the lumen of a tubular body part.

EXPLANATION: Natural or artificially created orifice ...

Body Part – 4TH	Approach – 5TH	Device – 6TH	Qualifier – 7TH
5 Hepatic Duct, Right 6 Hepatic Duct, Left 8 Cystic Duct 9 Common Bile Duct C Ampulla of Vater D Pancreatic Duct F Pancreatic Duct, Accessory	0 Open 3 Percutaneous 4 Percutaneous endoscopic	C Extraluminal device D Intraluminal device Z No device	Z No qualifier
5 Hepatic Duct, Right 6 Hepatic Duct, Left 8 Cystic Duct 9 Common Bile Duct C Ampulla of Vater D Pancreatic Duct F Pancreatic Duct, Accessory	7 Via natural or artificial opening 8 Via natural or artificial opening endoscopic	D Intraluminal device Z No device	Z No qualifier

HEPATOBILIARY 0 F V

DEVICE GROUP: Change, Insertion, Removal, Replacement, Revision, Supplement
Root Operations that always involve a device.

1ST - 0 Medical and Surgical	EXAMPLE: Reposition drainage tube	CMS Ex: Adjustment pacemaker lead

2ND - F Hepatobiliary System and Pancreas

3RD - W REVISION

REVISION: Correcting, to the extent possible, a portion of a malfunctioning device or the position of a displaced device.

EXPLANATION: May replace components of a device ...

Body Part – 4TH	Approach – 5TH	Device – 6TH	Qualifier – 7TH
0 Liver	0 Open 3 Percutaneous 4 Percutaneous endoscopic X External	0 Drainage device 2 Monitoring device 3 Infusion device	Z No qualifier
4 Gallbladder G Pancreas	0 Open 3 Percutaneous 4 Percutaneous endoscopic X External	0 Drainage device 2 Monitoring device 3 Infusion device D Intraluminal device	Z No qualifier
B Hepatobiliary Duct D Pancreatic Duct	0 Open 3 Percutaneous 4 Percutaneous endoscopic 7 Via natural or artificial opening 8 Via natural or artificial opening endoscopic X External	0 Drainage device 2 Monitoring device 3 Infusion device 7 Autologous tissue substitute C Extraluminal device D Intraluminal device J Synthetic substitute K Nonautologous tissue substitute	Z No qualifier

MOVE GROUP: Reattachment, Reposition, (Transfer), Transplantation
Root Operations that put in/put back or move some/all of a body part.

1ST - 0 Medical and Surgical	EXAMPLE: Liver transplant	CMS Ex: Kidney transplant

2ND - F Hepatobiliary System and Pancreas

3RD - Y TRANSPLANTATION

TRANSPLANTATION: Putting in or on all or a portion of a living body part taken from another individual or animal to physically take the place and/or function of all or a portion of a similar body part.

EXPLANATION: May take over all or part of its function ...

Body Part – 4TH	Approach – 5TH	Device – 6TH	Qualifier – 7TH
0 Liver G Pancreas NC*	0 Open	Z No device	0 Allogeneic 1 Syngeneic 2 Zooplastic NC*

NC* – Some procedures are considered non-covered by Medicare. See current Medicare Code Editor for details.

Educational Annotations | G – Endocrine System

Body System Specific Educational Annotations for the Endocrine System include:

- Anatomy and Physiology Review
- Anatomical Illustrations
- Definitions of Common Procedures
- AHA Coding Clinic® Reference Notations
- Body Part Key Listings
- Device Key Listings
- Device Aggregation Table Listings
- Coding Notes

Anatomy and Physiology Review of Endocrine System

BODY PART VALUES – G - ENDOCRINE SYSTEM

Adrenal Gland – ANATOMY – The adrenal gland is the highly vascular, pyramid-shaped endocrine gland that sits upon the top of each kidney. PHYSIOLOGY – The adrenal gland produces several important hormones, among them: Adrenalin, noradrenalin, aldosterone, cortisol, and some sex hormones.

Aortic Body – ANATOMY – The aortic body is the small neurovascular structure located at the aortic arch. PHYSIOLOGY – The aortic body monitors and regulates the reflex respiration and blood pressure.

Carotid Body – ANATOMY – The carotid bodies are small neurovascular structures at the carotid bifurcation. PHYSIOLOGY – The carotid bodies function as a blood oxygen, carbon dioxide, and Ph sensor.

Coccygeal Glomus – The coccygeal glomus is a very small (2.5mm), oval mass exocrine gland tissue located beneath the coccyx tip.

Endocrine Gland – A gland that secretes hormones.

Glomus Jugulare – A mass of neuroendocrine cells in the jugular foramen area of the temporal bone near the middle and inner ear.

Para-aortic Body – ANATOMY – The para-aortic body is the small mass of chromaffin tissue located alongside the abdominal aorta. PHYSIOLOGY – The para-aortic body produces catecholamines.

Paraganglion Extremity – Groups of extra-adrenal neuroendocrine cells usually found in the peripheral nervous system that produce adrenaline.

Parathyroid Gland – ANATOMY – The parathyroid glands are 4 small glands, 2 on the posterior surface of the thyroid lobes. PHYSIOLOGY – The parathyroid gland secretes one hormone, the parathyroid hormone which causes an increase in the blood calcium level and a decrease in the blood phosphate level.

Pineal Gland – ANATOMY – The pineal gland is the small endocrine gland located below the posterior base of the corpus callosum, and attached to the upper portion of the thalamus. PHYSIOLOGY – The pineal gland produces the hormone melatonin.

Pituitary Gland – ANATOMY – The pituitary gland is the small endocrine gland with two lobes located in the sella turcica of the sphenoid bone at the base of the cerebrum, and is about 0.4 inches (1 cm) in diameter. PHYSIOLOGY – The pituitary gland functions as the central endocrine gland by producing hormones which stimulate many of the other endocrine glands, and has two lobes. The anterior lobe (adenohypophysis) produces the growth hormone (prolactin), thyroid-stimulating hormone, follicle-stimulating and luteinizing hormones, and adrenocorticotropic hormone. The posterior lobe (neurohypophysis) secretes the antidiuretic hormone and oxytocin.

Thyroid Gland – ANATOMY – The thyroid gland is the bi-lobed endocrine gland of the front of the neck and is connected by a narrow isthmus. PHYSIOLOGY – The thyroid gland produces the hormones thyroxine and triiodothyronine that help to regulate the metabolic rate of the body.

Thyroid Gland Isthmus – The narrow, middle portion connecting the two thyroid lobes.

ENDOCRINE

0 G

Educational Annotations | G – Endocrine System

Anatomical Illustrations of Endocrine System

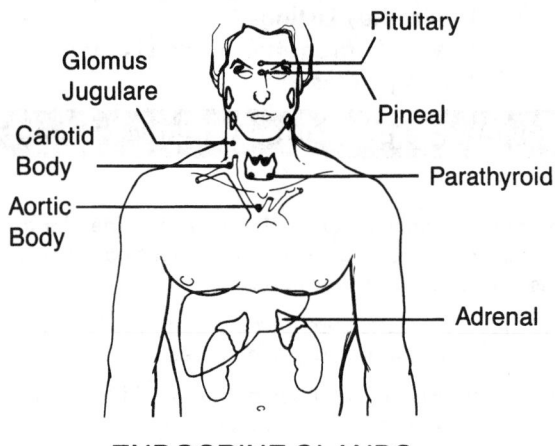

ENDOCRINE GLANDS

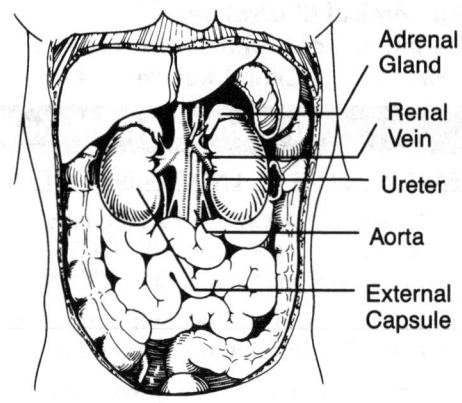

KIDNEY — ANTERIOR VIEW

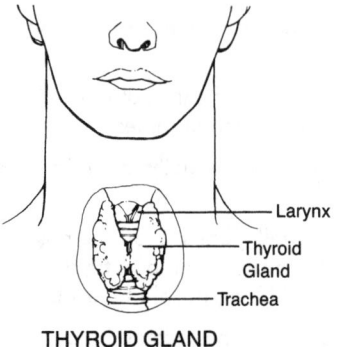

THYROID GLAND

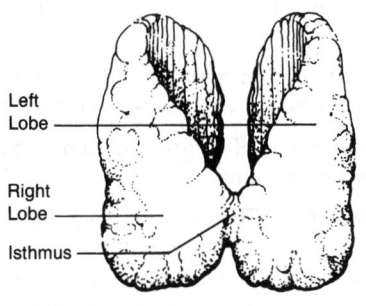

THYROID GLAND — ANTERIOR (DETAIL) VIEW

Definitions of Common Procedures of Endocrine System

Adrenalectomy – The surgical removal of one or both of the adrenal glands.

Hypophysectomy – The surgical removal of the pituitary gland (hypophysis).

Thyroid lobectomy – The surgical removal of one of the two lobes of the thyroid.

Total thyroidectomy – The surgical removal of both lobes and the isthmus of the thyroid.

Educational Annotations | G – Endocrine System

AHA Coding Clinic® Reference Notations of Endocrine System

ROOT OPERATION SPECIFIC - G - ENDOCRINE SYSTEM
CHANGE - 2
DESTRUCTION - 5
DIVISION - 8
DRAINAGE - 9
EXCISION - B
    Removal of pituitary tumor ....AHA 14:3Q:p22
EXTIRPATION - C
INSERTION - H
INSPECTION - J
REATTACHMENT - M
RELEASE - N
REMOVAL - P
REPAIR - Q
REPOSITION - S
RESECTION - T
REVISION - W

Body Part Key Listings of Endocrine System

See also Body Part Key in Appendix C
Adenohypophysis..*use* Pituitary Gland
Carotid glomus ....*use* Carotid Body, Bilateral/Left/Right
Coccygeal body ....*use* Coccygeal Glomus
Hypophysis...*use* Pituitary Gland
Jugular body ....*use* Glomus Jugulare
Neurohypophysis ....*use* Pituitary Gland
Suprarenal gland ....*use* Adrenal Gland, Bilateral/Left/Right

Device Key Listings of Endocrine System

See also Device Key in Appendix D
Autograft ....*use* Autologous Tissue Substitute
Tissue bank graft ....*use* Nonautologous Tissue Substitute

Device Aggregation Table Listings of Endocrine System

See also Device Aggregation Table in Appendix E

Specific Device	For Operation	In Body System	General Device
None Listed in Device Aggregation Table for this Body System			

ENDOCRINE

0 G

Educational Annotations | G – Endocrine System

Coding Notes of Endocrine System

<u>**Body System Specific PCS Reference Manual Exercises**</u>

<u>**PCS CODE**</u>   <u>**G – ENDOCRINE SYSTEM EXERCISES**</u>

0 G T 0 0 Z Z   Total excision of pituitary gland, open.

DEVICE GROUP: Change, Insertion, Removal, (Replacement), Revision, (Supplement)
Root Operations that always involve a device.

1ST - 0 Medical and Surgical

2ND - G Endocrine System

3RD - 2 CHANGE

EXAMPLE: Exchange drain tube | CMS Ex: Changing urinary catheter

CHANGE: Taking out or off a device from a body part and putting back an identical or similar device in or on the same body part without cutting or puncturing the skin or a mucous membrane.

EXPLANATION: ALL Changes use EXTERNAL approach only...

Body Part – 4TH	Approach – 5TH	Device – 6TH	Qualifier – 7TH
0 Pituitary Gland 1 Pineal Body 5 Adrenal Gland K Thyroid Gland R Parathyroid Gland S Endocrine Gland	X External	0 Drainage device Y Other device	Z No qualifier

EXCISION GROUP: Excision, Resection, Destruction, (Extraction), (Detachment)
Root Operations that take out some or all of a body part.

1ST - 0 Medical and Surgical

2ND - G Endocrine System

3RD - 5 DESTRUCTION

EXAMPLE: Radiofrequency ablation | CMS Ex: Fulguration polyp

DESTRUCTION: Physical eradication of all or a portion of a body part by the direct use of energy, force, or a destructive agent.

EXPLANATION: None of the body part is physically taken out

Body Part – 4TH	Approach – 5TH	Device – 6TH	Qualifier – 7TH
0 Pituitary Gland 1 Pineal Body 2 Adrenal Gland, Left 3 Adrenal Gland, Right 4 Adrenal Glands, Bilateral 6 Carotid Body, Left 7 Carotid Body, Right 8 Carotid Bodies, Bilateral 9 Para-aortic Body B Coccygeal Glomus C Glomus Jugulare D Aortic Body F Paraganglion Extremity G Thyroid Gland Lobe, Left H Thyroid Gland Lobe, Right K Thyroid Gland L Superior Parathyroid Gland, Right M Superior Parathyroid Gland, Left N Inferior Parathyroid Gland, Right P Inferior Parathyroid Gland, Left Q Parathyroid Glands, Multiple R Parathyroid Gland	0 Open 3 Percutaneous 4 Percutaneous endoscopic	Z No device	Z No qualifier

ENDOCRINE

0 G 5

DIVISION GROUP: Division, Release
Root Operations involving cutting or separation only.

1ST - **0** Medical and Surgical	EXAMPLE: Transection thyroid isthmus	CMS Ex: Osteotomy
2ND - **G** Endocrine System	**DIVISION:** Cutting into a body part without draining fluids and/or gases from the body part in order to separate or transect a body part.	
3RD - **8 DIVISION**	EXPLANATION: Separated into two or more portions ...	

Body Part – 4TH	Approach – 5TH	Device – 6TH	Qualifier – 7TH
0 Pituitary Gland J Thyroid Gland Isthmus	0 Open 3 Percutaneous 4 Percutaneous endoscopic	Z No device	Z No qualifier

---

DRAINAGE GROUP: Drainage, Extirpation, (Fragmentation)
Root Operations that take out solids/fluids/gases from a body part.

1ST - **0** Medical and Surgical	EXAMPLE: Needle aspiration adrenal abscess	CMS Ex: Thoracentesis
2ND - **G** Endocrine System	**DRAINAGE:** Taking or letting out fluids and/or gases from a body part.	
3RD - **9 DRAINAGE**	EXPLANATION: Qualifier "X Diagnostic" indicates biopsy ...	

Body Part – 4TH	Approach – 5TH	Device – 6TH	Qualifier – 7TH
0 Pituitary Gland G Thyroid Gland Lobe, Left 1 Pineal Body H Thyroid Gland Lobe, Right 2 Adrenal Gland, Left K Thyroid Gland 3 Adrenal Gland, Right L Superior Parathyroid 4 Adrenal Glands, Bilateral Gland, Right 6 Carotid Body, Left M Superior Parathyroid 7 Carotid Body, Right Gland, Left 8 Carotid Bodies, Bilateral N Inferior Parathyroid 9 Para-aortic Body Gland, Right B Coccygeal Glomus P Inferior Parathyroid C Glomus Jugulare Gland, Left D Aortic Body Q Parathyroid Glands, F Paraganglion Extremity Multiple R Parathyroid Gland	0 Open 3 Percutaneous 4 Percutaneous endoscopic	0 Drainage device	Z No qualifier
0 Pituitary Gland G Thyroid Gland Lobe, Left 1 Pineal Body H Thyroid Gland Lobe, Right 2 Adrenal Gland, Left K Thyroid Gland 3 Adrenal Gland, Right L Superior Parathyroid 4 Adrenal Glands, Bilateral Gland, Right 6 Carotid Body, Left M Superior Parathyroid 7 Carotid Body, Right Gland, Left 8 Carotid Bodies, Bilateral N Inferior Parathyroid 9 Para-aortic Body Gland, Right B Coccygeal Glomus P Inferior Parathyroid C Glomus Jugulare Gland, Left D Aortic Body Q Parathyroid Glands, F Paraganglion Extremity Multiple R Parathyroid Gland	0 Open 3 Percutaneous 4 Percutaneous endoscopic	Z No device	X Diagnostic Z No qualifier

EXCISION GROUP: Excision, Resection, Destruction, (Extraction), (Detachment)
Root Operations that take out some or all of a body part.

1ST - **0** Medical and Surgical

2ND - **G** Endocrine System

3RD - **B EXCISION**

EXAMPLE: Needle biopsy parathyroid gland | CMS Ex: Liver biopsy

EXCISION: Cutting out or off, without replacement, a portion of a body part.

EXPLANATION: Qualifier "X Diagnostic" indicates biopsy ...

Body Part – 4TH		Approach – 5TH	Device – 6TH	Qualifier – 7TH
0 Pituitary Gland	G Thyroid Gland Lobe, Left	0 Open	Z No device	X Diagnostic
1 Pineal Body	H Thyroid Gland Lobe, Right	3 Percutaneous		Z No qualifier
2 Adrenal Gland, Left	L Superior Parathyroid Gland, Right	4 Percutaneous endoscopic		
3 Adrenal Gland, Right	M Superior Parathyroid Gland, Left			
4 Adrenal Glands, Bilateral	N Inferior Parathyroid Gland, Right			
6 Carotid Body, Left	P Inferior Parathyroid Gland, Left			
7 Carotid Body, Right	Q Parathyroid Glands, Multiple			
8 Carotid Bodies, Bilateral	R Parathyroid Gland			
9 Para-aortic Body				
B Coccygeal Glomus				
C Glomus Jugulare				
D Aortic Body				
F Paraganglion Extremity				

DRAINAGE GROUP: Drainage, Extirpation, (Fragmentation)
Root Operations that take out solids/fluids/gases from a body part.

1ST - **0** Medical and Surgical

2ND - **G** Endocrine System

3RD - **C EXTIRPATION**

EXAMPLE: Removal foreign body | CMS Ex: Choledocholithotomy

EXTIRPATION: Taking or cutting out solid matter from a body part.

EXPLANATION: Abnormal byproduct or foreign body ...

Body Part – 4TH		Approach – 5TH	Device – 6TH	Qualifier – 7TH
0 Pituitary Gland	G Thyroid Gland Lobe, Left	0 Open	Z No device	Z No qualifier
1 Pineal Body	H Thyroid Gland Lobe, Right	3 Percutaneous		
2 Adrenal Gland, Left	K Thyroid Gland	4 Percutaneous endoscopic		
3 Adrenal Gland, Right	L Superior Parathyroid Gland, Right			
4 Adrenal Glands, Bilateral	M Superior Parathyroid Gland, Left			
6 Carotid Body, Left	N Inferior Parathyroid Gland, Right			
7 Carotid Body, Right	P Inferior Parathyroid Gland, Left			
8 Carotid Bodies, Bilateral	Q Parathyroid Glands, Multiple			
9 Para-aortic Body	R Parathyroid Gland			
B Coccygeal Glomus				
C Glomus Jugulare				
D Aortic Body				
F Paraganglion Extremity				

ENDOCRINE **0 G C**

DEVICE GROUP: Change, Insertion, Removal, (Replacement), Revision, (Supplement)
Root Operations that always involve a device.

1ST - 0 Medical and Surgical

2ND - G Endocrine System

3RD - H INSERTION

EXAMPLE: Insertion infusion device | CMS Ex: Insertion CV catheter

INSERTION: Putting in a nonbiological appliance that monitors, assists, performs, or prevents a physiological function but does not physically take the place of a body part.

EXPLANATION: None

Body Part – 4TH	Approach – 5TH	Device – 6TH	Qualifier – 7TH
S Endocrine Gland	0 Open 3 Percutaneous 4 Percutaneous endoscopic	2 Monitoring device 3 Infusion device	Z No qualifier

EXAMINATION GROUP: Inspection, (Map)
Root Operations involving examination only.

1ST - 0 Medical and Surgical

2ND - G Endocrine System

3RD - J INSPECTION

EXAMPLE: Examination adrenal gland | CMS Ex: Colonoscopy

INSPECTION: Visually and/or manually exploring a body part.

EXPLANATION: Direct or instrumental visualization ...

Body Part – 4TH	Approach – 5TH	Device – 6TH	Qualifier – 7TH
0 Pituitary Gland K Thyroid Gland 1 Pineal Body R Parathyroid Gland 5 Adrenal Gland S Endocrine Gland	0 Open 3 Percutaneous 4 Percutaneous endoscopic	Z No device	Z No qualifier

MOVE GROUP: Reattachment, Reposition, (Transfer), (Transplantation)
Root Operations that put in/put back or move some/all of a body part.

1ST - 0 Medical and Surgical

2ND - G Endocrine System

3RD - M REATTACHMENT

EXAMPLE: Reattachment thyroid | CMS Ex: Reattachment hand

REATTACHMENT: Putting back in or on all or a portion of a separated body part to its normal location or other suitable location.

EXPLANATION: With/without reconnection of vessels/nerves...

Body Part – 4TH	Approach – 5TH	Device – 6TH	Qualifier – 7TH
2 Adrenal Gland, Left 3 Adrenal Gland, Right G Thyroid Gland Lobe, Left H Thyroid Gland Lobe, Right L Superior Parathyroid Gland, Right M Superior Parathyroid Gland, Left N Inferior Parathyroid Gland, Right P Inferior Parathyroid Gland, Left Q Parathyroid Glands, Multiple R Parathyroid Gland	0 Open 4 Percutaneous endoscopic	Z No device	Z No qualifier

ENDOCRINE   0 G H

DIVISION GROUP: Division, Release
Root Operations involving cutting or separation only.

1ST - 0 Medical and Surgical

2ND - G Endocrine System

3RD - N RELEASE

EXAMPLE: Adhesiolysis adrenal gland | CMS Ex: Carpal tunnel release

RELEASE: Freeing a body part from an abnormal physical constraint by cutting or by the use of force.

EXPLANATION: None of the body part is taken out ...

Body Part – 4TH		Approach – 5TH	Device – 6TH	Qualifier – 7TH
0 Pituitary Gland	G Thyroid Gland Lobe, Left	0 Open	Z No device	Z No qualifier
1 Pineal Body	H Thyroid Gland Lobe, Right	3 Percutaneous		
2 Adrenal Gland, Left	K Thyroid Gland	4 Percutaneous endoscopic		
3 Adrenal Gland, Right	L Superior Parathyroid Gland, Right			
4 Adrenal Glands, Bilateral	M Superior Parathyroid Gland, Left			
6 Carotid Body, Left				
7 Carotid Body, Right	N Inferior Parathyroid Gland, Right			
8 Carotid Bodies, Bilateral				
9 Para-aortic Body	P Inferior Parathyroid Gland, Left			
B Coccygeal Glomus				
C Glomus Jugulare	Q Parathyroid Glands, Multiple			
D Aortic Body				
F Paraganglion Extremity	R Parathyroid Gland			

DEVICE GROUP: Change, Insertion, Removal, (Replacement), Revision, (Supplement)
Root Operations that always involve a device.

1ST - 0 Medical and Surgical

2ND - G Endocrine System

3RD - P REMOVAL

EXAMPLE: Removal drain tube | CMS Ex: Chest tube removal

REMOVAL: Taking out or off a device from a body part.

EXPLANATION: Removal device without reinsertion ...

Body Part – 4TH	Approach – 5TH	Device – 6TH	Qualifier – 7TH
0 Pituitary Gland	0 Open	0 Drainage device	Z No qualifier
1 Pineal Body	3 Percutaneous		
5 Adrenal Gland	4 Percutaneous endoscopic		
K Thyroid Gland	X External		
R Parathyroid Gland			
S Endocrine Gland	0 Open	0 Drainage device	Z No qualifier
	3 Percutaneous	2 Monitoring device	
	4 Percutaneous endoscopic	3 Infusion device	
	X External		

OTHER REPAIRS GROUP: (Control), Repair
Root Operations that define other repairs.

1ST – 0 Medical and Surgical
2ND – G Endocrine System
3RD – Q REPAIR

EXAMPLE: Suture thyroid laceration | CMS Ex: Suture laceration

REPAIR: Restoring, to the extent possible, a body part to its normal anatomic structure and function.

EXPLANATION: Only when no other root operation applies …

Body Part – 4TH	Approach – 5TH	Device – 6TH	Qualifier – 7TH
0 Pituitary Gland 1 Pineal Body 2 Adrenal Gland, Left 3 Adrenal Gland, Right 4 Adrenal Glands, Bilateral 6 Carotid Body, Left 7 Carotid Body, Right 8 Carotid Bodies, Bilateral 9 Para-aortic Body B Coccygeal Glomus C Glomus Jugulare D Aortic Body F Paraganglion Extremity G Thyroid Gland Lobe, Left H Thyroid Gland Lobe, Right J Thyroid Gland Isthmus K Thyroid Gland L Superior Parathyroid Gland, Right M Superior Parathyroid Gland, Left N Inferior Parathyroid Gland, Right P Inferior Parathyroid Gland, Left Q Parathyroid Glands, Multiple R Parathyroid Gland	0 Open 3 Percutaneous 4 Percutaneous endoscopic	Z No device	Z No qualifier

MOVE GROUP: Reattachment, Reposition, (Transfer), (Transplantation)
Root Operations that put in/put back or move some/all of a body part.

1ST – 0 Medical and Surgical
2ND – G Endocrine System
3RD – S REPOSITION

EXAMPLE: Relocation parathyroid glands | CMS Ex: Fracture reduction

REPOSITION: Moving to its normal location, or other suitable location, all or a portion of a body part.

EXPLANATION: May or may not be cut to be moved …

Body Part – 4TH	Approach – 5TH	Device – 6TH	Qualifier – 7TH
2 Adrenal Gland, Left 3 Adrenal Gland, Right G Thyroid Gland Lobe, Left H Thyroid Gland Lobe, Right L Superior Parathyroid Gland, Right M Superior Parathyroid Gland, Left N Inferior Parathyroid Gland, Right P Inferior Parathyroid Gland, Left Q Parathyroid Glands, Multiple R Parathyroid Gland	0 Open 4 Percutaneous endoscopic	Z No device	Z No qualifier

EXCISION GROUP: Excision, Resection, Destruction, (Extraction), (Detachment)
Root Operations that take out some or all of a body part.

1ST – **0** Medical and Surgical

2ND – **G** Endocrine System

3RD – **T RESECTION**

EXAMPLE: Thyroid lobectomy		CMS Ex: Cholecystectomy
RESECTION: Cutting out or off, without replacement, all of a body part.		
EXPLANATION: None		

Body Part – 4TH		Approach – 5TH	Device – 6TH	Qualifier – 7TH
0 Pituitary Gland 1 Pineal Body 2 Adrenal Gland, Left 3 Adrenal Gland, Right 4 Adrenal Glands, Bilateral 6 Carotid Body, Left 7 Carotid Body, Right 8 Carotid Bodies, Bilateral 9 Para-aortic Body B Coccygeal Glomus C Glomus Jugulare D Aortic Body F Paraganglion Extremity	G Thyroid Gland Lobe, Left H Thyroid Gland Lobe, Right K Thyroid Gland L Superior Parathyroid Gland, Right M Superior Parathyroid Gland, Left N Inferior Parathyroid Gland, Right P Inferior Parathyroid Gland, Left Q Parathyroid Glands, Multiple R Parathyroid Gland	0 Open 4 Percutaneous endoscopic	Z No device	Z No qualifier

DEVICE GROUP: Change, Insertion, Removal, (Replacement), Revision, (Supplement)
Root Operations that always involve a device.

1ST – **0** Medical and Surgical

2ND – **G** Endocrine System

3RD – **W REVISION**

EXAMPLE: Reposition drainage tube		CMS Ex: Adjustment pacemaker lead
REVISION: Correcting, to the extent possible, a portion of a malfunctioning device or the position of a displaced device.		
EXPLANATION: May replace components of a device ...		

Body Part – 4TH	Approach – 5TH	Device – 6TH	Qualifier – 7TH
0 Pituitary Gland 1 Pineal Body 5 Adrenal Gland K Thyroid Gland R Parathyroid Gland	0 Open 3 Percutaneous 4 Percutaneous endoscopic X External	0 Drainage device	Z No qualifier
S Endocrine Gland	0 Open 3 Percutaneous 4 Percutaneous endoscopic X External	0 Drainage device 2 Monitoring device 3 Infusion device	Z No qualifier

ENDOCRINE

0 G W

NOTES

Educational Annotations | H – Skin and Breast

Body System Specific Educational Annotations for the Skin and Breast include:

- Anatomy and Physiology Review
- Anatomical Illustrations
- Definitions of Common Procedures
- AHA Coding Clinic® Reference Notations
- Body Part Key Listings
- Device Key Listings
- Device Aggregation Table Listings
- Coding Notes

Anatomy and Physiology Review of Skin and Breast

BODY PART VALUES – H - SKIN AND BREAST

Breast, Female – ANATOMY – The female breast is the modified cutaneous glandular cone-shaped prominence overlying the pectoral muscles on the anterior chest, and contains the milk-producing mammary glands. PHYSIOLOGY – The female breast functions to secrete nourishing milk for the newborn. During pregnancy, hormones increase the size of the mammary glands, and following delivery, the pituitary gland secretes prolactin, which stimulates the mammary glands to produce milk. The mammary ducts convey the milk to the nipple.

Breast, Male – ANATOMY – The male breast is the modified cutaneous glandular structure overlying the pectoral muscles of the anterior chest. PHYSIOLOGY – The male breast fails to develop due to the lack of ovarian hormones.

Finger Nail – ANATOMY – The tough keratin covering of the top and end of the fingers. PHYSIOLOGY – The nail functions to protect the end of the finger.

Hair – ANATOMY – Hair is a threadlike structure that grows from follicles found in the dermis and is made of protein. PHYSIOLOGY – Hair serves multiple functions depending on location, including: Sensory transmission, heat retention, skin protection, and protection from particles and organisms.

Nipple – ANATOMY – The nipple is the pigmented projection of the breast and contains the ends of the mammary ducts. The areola is the circular pigmented area around the nipple.

Skin – ANATOMY – The skin is the outer covering of the body, consisting of the epidermis and dermis, that rests upon the subcutaneous tissue. The epidermis is the outermost layer of the skin which develops keratin, a tough, fibrous waterproof protein, and lacks blood vessels. The dermis is the tough, elastic vascular connective tissue layer of the skin which contains the sebaceous and sweat glands. PHYSIOLOGY – The skin functions to protect the body from invading microorganisms, limits the loss of water from deep tissues, assists homeostasis, aids in the regulation of body temperature, acts as the sense organ for the cutaneous senses, and is a source of vitamin D when it is exposed to light.

Supernumerary Breast – The presence of an additional breast (accessory breast) that may or may not have an associated areola and nipple.

Toe Nail – ANATOMY – The tough keratin covering of the top and end of the toes. PHYSIOLOGY – The nail functions to protect the end of the toe.

Anatomical Illustrations of Skin and Breast

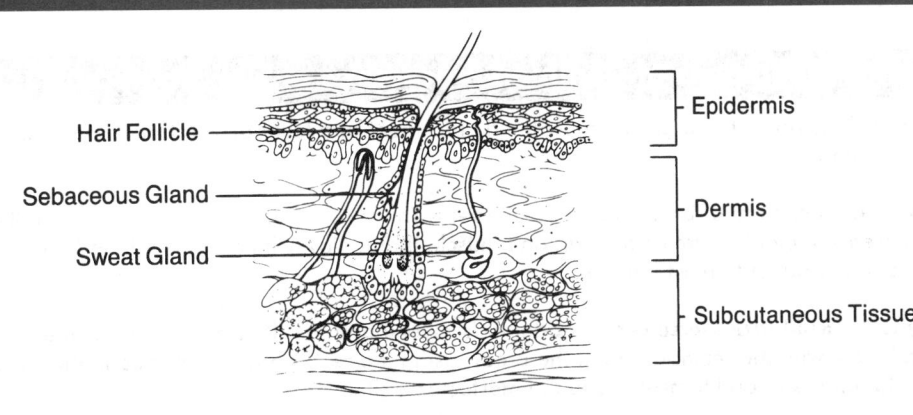

Hair Follicle —
Sebaceous Gland —
Sweat Gland —
Epidermis
Dermis
Subcutaneous Tissue

<u>SKIN</u>

Continued on next page

Educational Annotations | H – Skin and Breast

Anatomical Illustrations of Skin and Breast

Continued from previous page

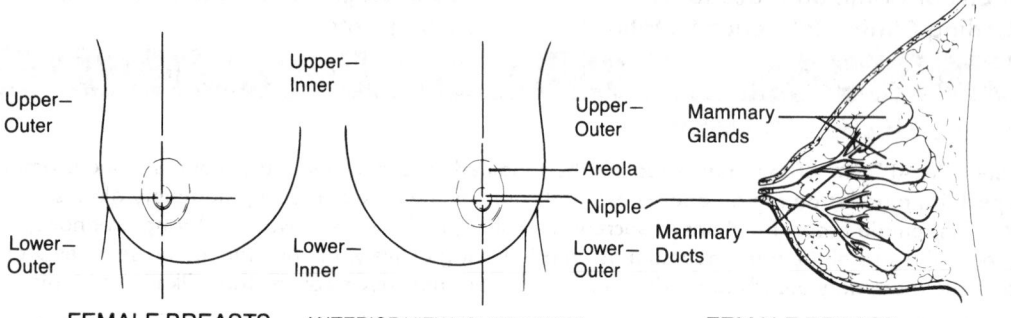

FEMALE BREASTS — ANTERIOR VIEW (QUADRANTS)

FEMALE BREAST — SAGITTAL VIEW

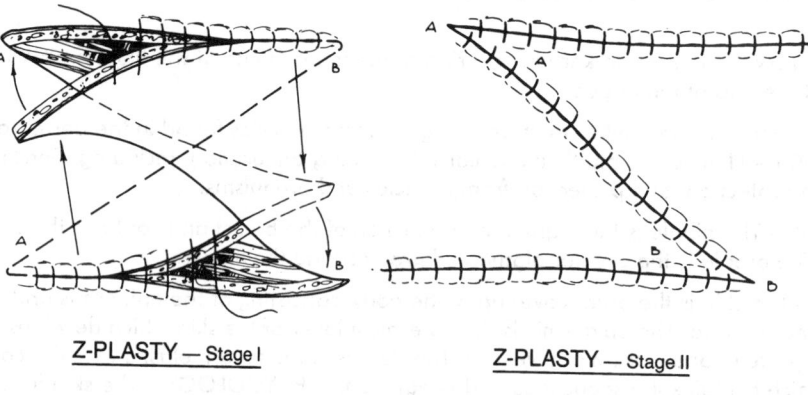

Z-PLASTY — Stage I

Z-PLASTY — Stage II

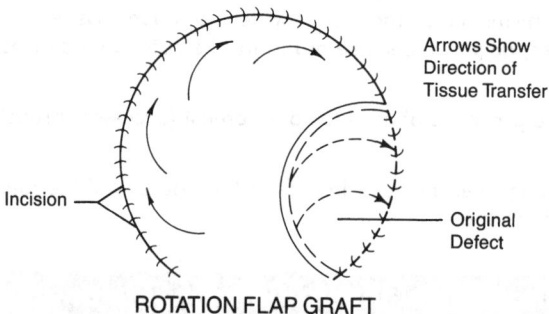

ROTATION FLAP GRAFT

Definitions of Common Procedures of Skin and Breast

Full-thickness skin graft – The surgical removal and placement of a layer of skin that includes the epidermis and entire thickness of the dermis.

Mastectomy with placement of breast tissue expander – The surgical removal of a breast with the placement of an inflatable breast implant to stretch the skin and muscle that is slowly inflated over time (2 to 3 months) to make room for a permanent breast implant.

Mastectomy with TRAM (transverse rectus abdominis myocutaneous) flap breast replacement – The surgical removal of a breast with the replacement of the breast using the rectus abdominis muscle that is raised (including the overlying fat and skin) and transferred to the mastectomy site.

Split-thickness skin graft – The surgical removal and placement of a layer of skin that includes the epidermis and part of the dermis.

Educational Annotations | H – Skin and Breast

AHA Coding Clinic® Reference Notations of Skin and Breast

ROOT OPERATION SPECIFIC - H - SKIN AND BREAST

ALTERATION - 0

CHANGE - 2

DESTRUCTION - 5

DIVISION - 8

DRAINAGE - 9

EXCISION - B
    Excisional debridement ....AHA 15:3Q:p3-8

EXTIRPATION - C

EXTRACTION - D
    Non-excisional debridement ....AHA 15:3Q:p3-8

INSERTION - H
    Bilateral breast tissue expanders ....AHA 14:2Q:p12
    Breast tissue expander using acellular dermal matrix ....AHA 13:4Q:p107

INSPECTION - J

REATTACHMENT - M

RELEASE - N

REMOVAL - P
    Removal of bilateral nonviable TRAM flap.......................................AHA 16:2Q:p27

REPAIR - Q
    Delayed closure of wound using skin clips ....AHA 14:4Q:p31
    Repair of first degree perineal laceration ....AHA 16:1Q:p6-8

REPLACEMENT - R
    Application of TheraSkin®..AHA 14:3Q:p14
    Biologically derived skin substitutes ....AHA 14:2Q:p5

REPOSITION - S

RESECTION - T
    Skin-sparing mastectomy ....AHA 14:4Q:p34

SUPPLEMENT - U

REVISION - W

TRANSFER - X

Body Part Key Listings of Skin and Breast

See also Body Part Key in Appendix C

Areola ....*use* Nipple, Left/Right

Dermis ....*use* Skin

Epidermis ....*use* Skin

Mammary duct ....*use* Breast, Bilateral/Left/Right

Mammary gland ....*use* Breast, Bilateral/Left/Right

Nail bed, Nail plate ....*use* Finger Nail, Toe Nail

Sebaceous gland ....*use* Skin

Sweat gland ....*use* Skin

SKIN & BREAST 0 H

Educational Annotations | H – Skin and Breast

Device Key Listings of Skin and Breast

See also Device Key in Appendix D

Acellular Hydrated Dermis...*use* Nonautologous Tissue Substitute
Autograft ....*use* Autologous Tissue Substitute
Blood glucose monitoring system ....*use* Monitoring Device
Brachytherapy seeds ....*use* Radioactive Element
Continuous Glucose Monitoring (CGM) device........*use* Monitoring Device
Cultured epidermal cell autograft ....*use* Autologous Tissue Substitute
Epicel® cultured epidermal autograft ....*use* Autologous Tissue Substitute
Implantable glucose monitoring device....................*use* Monitoring Device
Tissue bank graft ....*use* Nonautologous Tissue Substitute
Tissue expander (inflatable) (injectable) ....*use* Tissue Expander in Skin and Breast

Device Aggregation Table Listings of Skin and Breast

See also Device Aggregation Table in Appendix E

Specific Device	For Operation	In Body System	General Device
None Listed in Device Aggregation Table for this Body System			

Coding Notes of Skin and Breast

Body System Relevant Coding Guidelines

Skin, subcutaneous tissue and fascia overlying a joint

B4.6

If a procedure is performed on the skin, subcutaneous tissue or fascia overlying a joint, the procedure is coded to the following body part:
- Shoulder is coded to Upper Arm
- Elbow is coded to Lower Arm
- Wrist is coded to Lower Arm
- Hip is coded to Upper Leg
- Knee is coded to Lower Leg
- Ankle is coded to Foot

Body System Specific PCS Reference Manual Exercises

PCS CODE	H – SKIN AND BREAST EXERCISES
0 H 0 V 0 J Z	Bilateral breast augmentation with silicone implants, open.
0 H 5 G X Z Z	Cryotherapy of wart on left hand.
0 H B 2 X Z Z	Excision of malignant melanoma from skin of right ear.
0 H C G X Z Z	Foreign body removal, skin of left thumb. (There is no specific value for thumb skin, so the procedure is coded to the hand.)
0 H D M X Z Z	Non-excisional debridement of skin ulcer, right foot.
0 H D Q X Z Z	Removal of left thumbnail. (No separate body part value is given for thumbnail, so this is coded to Fingernail.)
0 H M 0 X Z Z	Replantation of avulsed scalp.
0 H N D X Z Z	Incision of scar contracture, right elbow. (The skin of the elbow region is coded to the lower arm.)
0 H R D X 7 3	Full-thickness skin graft to right lower arm, autograft (graft harvest not coded for this exercise example).
0 H R V 0 7 6	Bilateral mastectomy with free TRAM flap reconstruction.
0 H R V 0 J Z	Bilateral mastectomy with concomitant saline breast implants, open.

Continued on next page

Educational Annotations | H – Skin and Breast

Continued from previous page

0 H T T 0 Z Z	Right total mastectomy, open.
0 H X 0 X Z Z	Right scalp advancement flap to right temple.
0 H X 6 X Z Z	Skin transfer flap closure of complex open wound, left lower back.

S K I N & B R E A S T

0 H

Educational Annotations | H – Skin and Breast

NOTES

OTHER OBJECTIVES GROUP: Alteration, (Creation), (Fusion)
Root Operations that define other objectives.

1ST - **0** Medical and Surgical

2ND - **H** Skin and Breast

3RD - **0 ALTERATION**

EXAMPLE: Breast augmentation with implants | CMS Ex: Face lift

ALTERATION: Modifying the anatomic structure of a body part without affecting the function of the body part.

EXPLANATION: Principal purpose is to improve appearance

Body Part – 4TH	Approach – 5TH	Device – 6TH	Qualifier – 7TH
T Breast, Right U Breast, Left V Breast, Bilateral	0 Open 3 Percutaneous X External	7 Autologous tissue substitute J Synthetic substitute K Nonautologous tissue substitute Z No device	Z No qualifier

DEVICE GROUP: Change, Insertion, Removal, Replacement, Revision, Supplement
Root Operations that always involve a device.

1ST - **0** Medical and Surgical

2ND - **H** Skin and Breast

3RD - **2 CHANGE**

EXAMPLE: Exchange drain tube | CMS Ex: Changing urinary catheter

CHANGE: Taking out or off a device from a body part and putting back an identical or similar device in or on the same body part without cutting or puncturing the skin or a mucous membrane.

EXPLANATION: ALL Changes use EXTERNAL approach only ...

Body Part – 4TH	Approach – 5TH	Device – 6TH	Qualifier – 7TH
P Skin T Breast, Right U Breast, Left	X External	0 Drainage device Y Other device	Z No qualifier

SKIN & BREAST 0 H 2

EXCISION GROUP: Excision, Resection, Destruction, Extraction, (Detachment)
Root Operations that take out some or all of a body part.

1ST - 0 Medical and Surgical	EXAMPLE: Cryoablation skin lesion	CMS Ex: Fulguration polyp

2ND - H Skin and Breast

3RD - 5 DESTRUCTION

DESTRUCTION: Physical eradication of all or a portion of a body part by the direct use of energy, force, or a destructive agent.

EXPLANATION: None of the body part is physically taken out

Body Part – 4TH		Approach – 5TH	Device – 6TH	Qualifier – 7TH
0 Skin, Scalp 1 Skin, Face 2 Skin, Right Ear 3 Skin, Left Ear 4 Skin, Neck 5 Skin, Chest 6 Skin, Back 7 Skin, Abdomen 8 Skin, Buttock 9 Skin, Perineum A Skin, Genitalia	B Skin, Right Upper Arm C Skin, Left Upper Arm D Skin, Right Lower Arm E Skin, Left Lower Arm F Skin, Right Hand G Skin, Left Hand H Skin, Right Upper Leg J Skin, Left Upper Leg K Skin, Right Lower Leg L Skin, Left Lower Leg M Skin, Right Foot N Skin, Left Foot	X External	Z No device	D Multiple Z No qualifier
Q Finger Nail R Toe Nail		X External	Z No device	Z No qualifier
T Breast, Right U Breast, Left V Breast, Bilateral W Nipple, Right X Nipple, Left		0 Open 3 Percutaneous 7 Via natural or artificial opening 8 Via natural or artificial opening endoscopic X External	Z No device	Z No qualifier

---

DIVISION GROUP: Division, Release
Root Operations involving cutting or separation only.

1ST - 0 Medical and Surgical	EXAMPLE: Division skin	CMS Ex: Osteotomy

2ND - H Skin and Breast

3RD - 8 DIVISION

DIVISION: Cutting into a body part without draining fluids and/or gases from the body part in order to separate or transect a body part.

EXPLANATION: Separated into two or more portions ...

Body Part – 4TH		Approach – 5TH	Device – 6TH	Qualifier – 7TH
0 Skin, Scalp 1 Skin, Face 2 Skin, Right Ear 3 Skin, Left Ear 4 Skin, Neck 5 Skin, Chest 6 Skin, Back 7 Skin, Abdomen 8 Skin, Buttock 9 Skin, Perineum A Skin, Genitalia	B Skin, Right Upper Arm C Skin, Left Upper Arm D Skin, Right Lower Arm E Skin, Left Lower Arm F Skin, Right Hand G Skin, Left Hand H Skin, Right Upper Leg J Skin, Left Upper Leg K Skin, Right Lower Leg L Skin, Left Lower Leg M Skin, Right Foot N Skin, Left Foot	X External	Z No device	Z No qualifier

DRAINAGE GROUP: Drainage, Extirpation, (Fragmentation)
Root Operations that take out solids/fluids/gases from a body part.

	EXAMPLE: Incision and drainage boil	CMS Ex: Thoracentesis

1ST - 0 Medical and Surgical

2ND - H Skin and Breast

3RD - 9 DRAINAGE

DRAINAGE: Taking or letting out fluids and/or gases from a body part.

EXPLANATION: Qualifier "X Diagnostic" indicates biopsy ...

Body Part – 4TH		Approach – 5TH	Device – 6TH	Qualifier – 7TH
0 Skin, Scalp 1 Skin, Face 2 Skin, Right Ear 3 Skin, Left Ear 4 Skin, Neck 5 Skin, Chest 6 Skin, Back 7 Skin, Abdomen 8 Skin, Buttock 9 Skin, Perineum A Skin, Genitalia B Skin, Right Upper Arm C Skin, Left Upper Arm	D Skin, Right Lower Arm E Skin, Left Lower Arm F Skin, Right Hand G Skin, Left Hand H Skin, Right Upper Leg J Skin, Left Upper Leg K Skin, Right Lower Leg L Skin, Left Lower Leg M Skin, Right Foot N Skin, Left Foot Q Finger Nail R Toe Nail	X External	0 Drainage device	Z No qualifier
0 Skin, Scalp 1 Skin, Face 2 Skin, Right Ear 3 Skin, Left Ear 4 Skin, Neck 5 Skin, Chest 6 Skin, Back 7 Skin, Abdomen 8 Skin, Buttock 9 Skin, Perineum A Skin, Genitalia B Skin, Right Upper Arm C Skin, Left Upper Arm	D Skin, Right Lower Arm E Skin, Left Lower Arm F Skin, Right Hand G Skin, Left Hand H Skin, Right Upper Leg J Skin, Left Upper Leg K Skin, Right Lower Leg L Skin, Left Lower Leg M Skin, Right Foot N Skin, Left Foot Q Finger Nail R Toe Nail	X External	Z No device	X Diagnostic Z No qualifier
T Breast, Right U Breast, Left V Breast, Bilateral W Nipple, Right X Nipple, Left		0 Open 3 Percutaneous 7 Via natural or artificial opening 8 Via natural or artificial opening endoscopic X External	0 Drainage device	Z No qualifier
T Breast, Right U Breast, Left V Breast, Bilateral W Nipple, Right X Nipple, Left		0 Open 3 Percutaneous 7 Via natural or artificial opening 8 Via natural or artificial opening endoscopic X External	Z No device	X Diagnostic Z No qualifier

SKIN & BREAST 0 H 9

EXCISION GROUP: Excision, Resection, Destruction, Extraction, (Detachment)
Root Operations that take out some or all of a body part.

1ST - 0 Medical and Surgical	EXAMPLE: Partial mastectomy	CMS Ex: Liver biopsy

2ND - **H** Skin and Breast

3RD - **B EXCISION**

EXCISION: Cutting out or off, without replacement, a portion of a body part.

EXPLANATION: Qualifier "X Diagnostic" indicates biopsy ...

Body Part – 4TH		Approach – 5TH	Device – 6TH	Qualifier – 7TH
0 Skin, Scalp	D Skin, Right Lower Arm	X External	Z No device	X Diagnostic
1 Skin, Face	E Skin, Left Lower Arm			Z No qualifier
2 Skin, Right Ear	F Skin, Right Hand			
3 Skin, Left Ear	G Skin, Left Hand			
4 Skin, Neck	H Skin, Right Upper Leg			
5 Skin, Chest	J Skin, Left Upper Leg			
6 Skin, Back	K Skin, Right Lower Leg			
7 Skin, Abdomen	L Skin, Left Lower Leg			
8 Skin, Buttock	M Skin, Right Foot			
9 Skin, Perineum	N Skin, Left Foot			
A Skin, Genitalia	Q Finger Nail			
B Skin, Right Upper Arm	R Toe Nail			
C Skin, Left Upper Arm				
T Breast, Right		0 Open	Z No device	X Diagnostic
U Breast, Left		3 Percutaneous		Z No qualifier
V Breast, Bilateral		7 Via natural or artificial opening		
W Nipple, Right		8 Via natural or artificial opening endoscopic		
X Nipple, Left		X External		
Y Supernumerary Breast				

DRAINAGE GROUP: Drainage, Extirpation, (Fragmentation)
Root Operations that take out solids/fluids/gases from a body part.

1ST - **0** Medical and Surgical

2ND - **H** Skin and Breast

3RD - **C EXTIRPATION**

EXAMPLE: Removal splinter skin	CMS Ex: Choledocholithotomy

EXTIRPATION: Taking or cutting out solid matter from a body part.

EXPLANATION: Abnormal byproduct or foreign body ...

Body Part – 4TH		Approach – 5TH	Device – 6TH	Qualifier – 7TH
0 Skin, Scalp 1 Skin, Face 2 Skin, Right Ear 3 Skin, Left Ear 4 Skin, Neck 5 Skin, Chest 6 Skin, Back 7 Skin, Abdomen 8 Skin, Buttock 9 Skin, Perineum A Skin, Genitalia B Skin, Right Upper Arm C Skin, Left Upper Arm	D Skin, Right Lower Arm E Skin, Left Lower Arm F Skin, Right Hand G Skin, Left Hand H Skin, Right Upper Leg J Skin, Left Upper Leg K Skin, Right Lower Leg L Skin, Left Lower Leg M Skin, Right Foot N Skin, Left Foot Q Finger Nail R Toe Nail	X External	Z No device	Z No qualifier
T Breast, Right U Breast, Left V Breast, Bilateral W Nipple, Right X Nipple, Left		0 Open 3 Percutaneous 7 Via natural or artificial opening 8 Via natural or artificial opening endoscopic X External	Z No device	Z No qualifier

EXCISION GROUP: Excision, Resection, Destruction, Extraction, (Detachment)
Root Operations that take out some or all of a body part.

1ST - **0** Medical and Surgical

2ND - **H** Skin and Breast

3RD - **D EXTRACTION**

EXAMPLE: Non-excisional debridement skin	CMS Ex: D&C

EXTRACTION: Pulling or stripping out or off all or a portion of a body part by the use of force.

EXPLANATION: None for this Body System

Body Part – 4TH		Approach – 5TH	Device – 6TH	Qualifier – 7TH
0 Skin, Scalp 1 Skin, Face 2 Skin, Right Ear 3 Skin, Left Ear 4 Skin, Neck 5 Skin, Chest 6 Skin, Back 7 Skin, Abdomen 8 Skin, Buttock 9 Skin, Perineum A Skin, Genitalia B Skin, Right Upper Arm C Skin, Left Upper Arm	D Skin, Right Lower Arm E Skin, Left Lower Arm F Skin, Right Hand G Skin, Left Hand H Skin, Right Upper Leg J Skin, Left Upper Leg K Skin, Right Lower Leg L Skin, Left Lower Leg M Skin, Right Foot N Skin, Left Foot Q Finger Nail R Toe Nail S Hair	X External	Z No device	Z No qualifier

SKIN & BREAST 0 H D

DEVICE GROUP: Change, Insertion, Removal, Replacement, Revision, Supplement
Root Operations that always involve a device.

1ST – **O** Medical and Surgical

2ND – **H** Skin and Breast

3RD – **H INSERTION**

EXAMPLE: Insertion breast tissue expander | CMS Ex: Venous catheter

INSERTION: Putting in a nonbiological appliance that monitors, assists, performs, or prevents a physiological function but does not physically take the place of a body part.

EXPLANATION: None

Body Part – 4TH	Approach – 5TH	Device – 6TH	Qualifier – 7TH
T Breast, Right U Breast, Left V Breast, Bilateral W Nipple, Right X Nipple, Left	0 Open 3 Percutaneous 7 Via natural or artificial opening 8 Via natural or artificial opening endoscopic	1 Radioactive element N Tissue expander	Z No qualifier
T Breast, Right U Breast, Left V Breast, Bilateral W Nipple, Right X Nipple, Left	X External	1 Radioactive element	Z No qualifier

EXAMINATION GROUP: Inspection, (Map)
Root Operations involving examination only.

1ST – **O** Medical and Surgical

2ND – **H** Skin and Breast

3RD – **J INSPECTION**

EXAMPLE: Breast exam | CMS Ex: Colonoscopy

INSPECTION: Visually and/or manually exploring a body part.

EXPLANATION: Direct or instrumental visualization ...

Body Part – 4TH	Approach – 5TH	Device – 6TH	Qualifier – 7TH
P Skin Q Finger Nail R Toe Nail	X External	Z No device	Z No qualifier
T Breast, Right U Breast, Left	0 Open 3 Percutaneous 7 Via natural or artificial opening 8 Via natural or artificial opening endoscopic X External	Z No device	Z No qualifier

Skin & Breast OHH

MOVE GROUP: Reattachment, Reposition, Transfer, (Transplantation)
Root Operations that put in/put back or move some/all of a body part.

1ST - 0 Medical and Surgical	EXAMPLE: Replantation avulsed scalp	CMS Ex: Reattachment hand
2ND - H Skin and Breast	**REATTACHMENT:** Putting back in or on all or a portion of a separated body part to its normal location or other suitable location.	
3RD - M REATTACHMENT	EXPLANATION: With/without reconnection of vessels/nerves…	

Body Part – 4TH		Approach – 5TH	Device – 6TH	Qualifier – 7TH
0 Skin, Scalp	F Skin, Right Hand	X External	Z No device	Z No qualifier
1 Skin, Face	G Skin, Left Hand			
2 Skin, Right Ear	H Skin, Right Upper Leg			
3 Skin, Left Ear	J Skin, Left Upper Leg			
4 Skin, Neck	K Skin, Right Lower Leg			
5 Skin, Chest	L Skin, Left Lower Leg			
6 Skin, Back	M Skin, Right Foot			
7 Skin, Abdomen	N Skin, Left Foot			
8 Skin, Buttock	T Breast, Right			
9 Skin, Perineum	U Breast, Left			
A Skin, Genitalia	V Breast, Bilateral			
B Skin, Right Upper Arm	W Nipple, Right			
C Skin, Left Upper Arm	X Nipple, Left			
D Skin, Right Lower Arm				
E Skin, Left Lower Arm				

DIVISION GROUP: Division, Release
Root Operations involving cutting or separation only.

1ST - 0 Medical and Surgical	EXAMPLE: Incision scar contracture	CMS Ex: Carpal tunnel release
2ND - H Skin and Breast	**RELEASE:** Freeing a body part from an abnormal physical constraint by cutting or by the use of force.	
3RD - N RELEASE	EXPLANATION: None of the body part is taken out …	

Body Part – 4TH		Approach – 5TH	Device – 6TH	Qualifier – 7TH
0 Skin, Scalp	D Skin, Right Lower Arm	X External	Z No device	Z No qualifier
1 Skin, Face	E Skin, Left Lower Arm			
2 Skin, Right Ear	F Skin, Right Hand			
3 Skin, Left Ear	G Skin, Left Hand			
4 Skin, Neck	H Skin, Right Upper Leg			
5 Skin, Chest	J Skin, Left Upper Leg			
6 Skin, Back	K Skin, Right Lower Leg			
7 Skin, Abdomen	L Skin, Left Lower Leg			
8 Skin, Buttock	M Skin, Right Foot			
9 Skin, Perineum	N Skin, Left Foot			
A Skin, Genitalia	Q Finger Nail			
B Skin, Right Upper Arm	R Toe Nail			
C Skin, Left Upper Arm				
T Breast, Right		0 Open	Z No device	Z No qualifier
U Breast, Left		3 Percutaneous		
V Breast, Bilateral		7 Via natural or artificial opening		
W Nipple, Right		8 Via natural or artificial opening endoscopic		
X Nipple, Left		X External		

DEVICE GROUP: Change, Insertion, Removal, Replacement, Revision, Supplement
Root Operations that always involve a device.

1ST – 0 Medical and Surgical	**EXAMPLE:** Removal tissue expander	**CMS Ex:** Chest tube removal
2ND – H Skin and Breast	**REMOVAL:** Taking out or off a device from a body part.	
3RD – P REMOVAL	**EXPLANATION:** Removal device without reinsertion ...	

Body Part – 4TH	Approach – 5TH	Device – 6TH	Qualifier – 7TH
P Skin Q Finger Nail R Toe Nail	X External	0 Drainage device 7 Autologous tissue substitute J Synthetic substitute K Nonautologous tissue substitute	Z No qualifier
S Hair	X External	7 Autologous tissue substitute J Synthetic substitute K Nonautologous tissue substitute	Z No qualifier
T Breast, Right U Breast, Left	0 Open 3 Percutaneous 7 Via natural or artificial opening 8 Via natural or artificial opening endoscopic	0 Drainage device 1 Radioactive element 7 Autologous tissue substitute J Synthetic substitute K Nonautologous tissue substitute N Tissue expander	Z No qualifier
T Breast, Right U Breast, Left	X External	0 Drainage device 1 Radioactive element 7 Autologous tissue substitute J Synthetic substitute K Nonautologous tissue substitute	Z No qualifier

SKIN & BREAST 0 H P

OTHER REPAIRS GROUP: (Control), Repair
Root Operations that define other repairs.

1ST - 0 Medical and Surgical

2ND - H Skin and Breast

3RD - Q REPAIR

EXAMPLE: Repair first degree perineum laceration | CMS Ex: Suture

REPAIR: Restoring, to the extent possible, a body part to its normal anatomic structure and function.

EXPLANATION: Only when no other root operation applies ...

Body Part – 4TH		Approach – 5TH	Device – 6TH	Qualifier – 7TH
0 Skin, Scalp	D Skin, Right Lower Arm	X External	Z No device	Z No qualifier
1 Skin, Face	E Skin, Left Lower Arm			
2 Skin, Right Ear	F Skin, Right Hand			
3 Skin, Left Ear	G Skin, Left Hand			
4 Skin, Neck	H Skin, Right Upper Leg			
5 Skin, Chest	J Skin, Left Upper Leg			
6 Skin, Back	K Skin, Right Lower Leg			
7 Skin, Abdomen	L Skin, Left Lower Leg			
8 Skin, Buttock	M Skin, Right Foot			
9 Skin, Perineum	N Skin, Left Foot			
A Skin, Genitalia	Q Finger Nail			
B Skin, Right Upper Arm	R Toe Nail			
C Skin, Left Upper Arm				
T Breast, Right		0 Open	Z No device	Z No qualifier
U Breast, Left		3 Percutaneous		
V Breast, Bilateral		7 Via natural or artificial opening		
W Nipple, Right		8 Via natural or artificial opening endoscopic		
X Nipple, Left		X External		
Y Supernumerary Breast				

SKIN & BREAST

0 H Q

DEVICE GROUP: Change, Insertion, Removal, Replacement, Revision, Supplement
Root Operations that always involve a device.

1ST - 0 Medical and Surgical	
2ND - H Skin and Breast	
3RD - R REPLACEMENT	

EXAMPLE: Mastectomy with implant | CMS Ex: Total hip

REPLACEMENT: Putting in or on a biological or synthetic material that physically takes the place and/or function of all or a portion of a body part.

EXPLANATION: Includes taking out body part, or eradication...

Body Part – 4TH		Approach – 5TH	Device – 6TH	Qualifier – 7TH
0 Skin, Scalp 1 Skin, Face 2 Skin, Right Ear 3 Skin, Left Ear 4 Skin, Neck 5 Skin, Chest 6 Skin, Back 7 Skin, Abdomen 8 Skin, Buttock 9 Skin, Perineum A Skin, Genitalia	B Skin, Right Upper Arm C Skin, Left Upper Arm D Skin, Right Lower Arm E Skin, Left Lower Arm F Skin, Right Hand G Skin, Left Hand H Skin, Right Upper Leg J Skin, Left Upper Leg K Skin, Right Lower Leg L Skin, Left Lower Leg M Skin, Right Foot N Skin, Left Foot	X External	7 Autologous tissue substitute K Nonautologous tissue substitute	3 Full thickness 4 Partial thickness
0 Skin, Scalp 1 Skin, Face 2 Skin, Right Ear 3 Skin, Left Ear 4 Skin, Neck 5 Skin, Chest 6 Skin, Back 7 Skin, Abdomen 8 Skin, Buttock 9 Skin, Perineum A Skin, Genitalia	B Skin, Right Upper Arm C Skin, Left Upper Arm D Skin, Right Lower Arm E Skin, Left Lower Arm F Skin, Right Hand G Skin, Left Hand H Skin, Right Upper Leg J Skin, Left Upper Leg K Skin, Right Lower Leg L Skin, Left Lower Leg M Skin, Right Foot N Skin, Left Foot	X External	J Synthetic substitute	3 Full thickness 4 Partial thickness Z No qualifier
Q Finger Nail R Toe Nail S Hair		X External	7 Autologous tissue substitute J Synthetic substitute K Nonautologous tissue substitute	Z No qualifier

c o n t i n u e d ⇨

0　H　R　REPLACEMENT – *continued*

Body Part – 4TH	Approach – 5TH	Device – 6TH	Qualifier – 7TH
T　Breast, Right U　Breast, Left V　Breast, Bilateral	0　Open	7　Autologous 　　tissue substitute	5　Latissimus Dorsi Myocutaneous Flap 6　Transverse Rectus Abdominis Myocutaneous Flap 7　Deep Inferior Epigastric Artery Perforator Flap 8　Superficial Inferior Epigastric Artery Flap 9　Gluteal Artery Perforator Flap Z　No qualifier
T　Breast, Right U　Breast, Left V　Breast, Bilateral	0　Open	J　Synthetic substitute K　Nonautologous tissue substitute	Z　No qualifier
T　Breast, Right U　Breast, Left V　Breast, Bilateral	3　Percutaneous X　External	7　Autologous tissue substitute J　Synthetic substitute K　Nonautologous tissue substitute	Z　No qualifier
W　Nipple, Right X　Nipple, Left	0　Open 3　Percutaneous X　External	7　Autologous tissue substitute J　Synthetic substitute K　Nonautologous tissue substitute	Z　No qualifier

SKIN & BREAST 0 H S

MOVE GROUP: Reattachment, Reposition, Transfer, (Transplantation)
Root Operations that put in/put back or move some/all of a body part.

1ST – 0 Medical and Surgical

2ND – H Skin and Breast

3RD – S REPOSITION

EXAMPLE: Reposition nipple location　　|　CMS Ex: Fracture reduction

REPOSITION: Moving to its normal location, or other suitable location, all or a portion of a body part.

EXPLANATION: May or may not be cut to be moved ...

Body Part – 4TH	Approach – 5TH	Device – 6TH	Qualifier – 7TH
S　Hair W　Nipple, Right X　Nipple, Left	X　External	Z　No device	Z　No qualifier
T　Breast, Right U　Breast, Left V　Breast, Bilateral	0　Open	Z　No device	Z　No qualifier

---

EXCISION GROUP: Excision, Resection, Destruction, Extraction, (Detachment)
Root Operations that take out some or all of a body part.

1ST - O Medical and Surgical 2ND - H Skin and Breast 3RD - T RESECTION	EXAMPLE: Skin-sparing total mastectomy	CMS Ex: Cholecystectomy
	RESECTION: Cutting out or off, without replacement, all of a body part.	
	EXPLANATION: None	

Body Part – 4TH	Approach – 5TH	Device – 6TH	Qualifier – 7TH
Q Finger Nail R Toe Nail W Nipple, Right X Nipple, Left	X External	Z No device	Z No qualifier
T Breast, Right U Breast, Left V Breast, Bilateral Y Supernumerary Breast	0 Open	Z No device	Z No qualifier

---

DEVICE GROUP: Change, Insertion, Removal, Replacement, Revision, Supplement
Root Operations that always involve a device.

1ST - O Medical and Surgical 2ND - H Skin and Breast 3RD - U SUPPLEMENT	EXAMPLE: Repair inverted nipple with graft	CMS Ex: Hernia mesh
	SUPPLEMENT: Putting in or on biological or synthetic material that physically reinforces and/or augments the function of a portion of a body part.	
	EXPLANATION: Biological material from same individual ...	

Body Part – 4TH	Approach – 5TH	Device – 6TH	Qualifier – 7TH
T Breast, Right U Breast, Left V Breast, Bilateral W Nipple, Right X Nipple, Left	0 Open 3 Percutaneous 7 Via natural or artificial opening 8 Via natural or artificial opening endoscopic X External	7 Autologous tissue substitute J Synthetic substitute K Nonautologous tissue substitute	Z No qualifier

DEVICE GROUP: Change, Insertion, Removal, Replacement, Revision, Supplement
Root Operations that always involve a device.

1ST - 0 Medical and Surgical	EXAMPLE: Reposition tissue expander	CMS Ex: Adjustment pacemaker lead

2ND - H Skin and Breast

3RD - W REVISION

REVISION: Correcting, to the extent possible, a portion of a malfunctioning device or the position of a displaced device.

EXPLANATION: May replace components of a device …

Body Part – 4TH	Approach – 5TH	Device – 6TH	Qualifier – 7TH
P Skin Q Finger Nail R Toe Nail	X External	0 Drainage device 7 Autologous tissue substitute J Synthetic substitute K Nonautologous tissue substitute	Z No qualifier
S Hair	X External	7 Autologous tissue substitute J Synthetic substitute K Nonautologous tissue substitute	Z No qualifier
T Breast, Right U Breast, Left	0 Open 3 Percutaneous 7 Via natural or artificial opening 8 Via natural or artificial opening endoscopic	0 Drainage device 7 Autologous tissue substitute J Synthetic substitute K Nonautologous tissue substitute N Tissue expander	Z No qualifier
T Breast, Right U Breast, Left	X External	0 Drainage device 7 Autologous tissue substitute J Synthetic substitute K Nonautologous tissue substitute	Z No qualifier

SKIN & BREAST 0 H W

MOVE GROUP: Reattachment, Reposition, Transfer, (Transplantation)
Root Operations that put in/put back or move some/all of a body part.

1ST - **0** Medical and Surgical	**EXAMPLE:** Scalp advancement flap **CMS Ex:** Tendon transfer
2ND - **H** Skin and Breast	**TRANSFER:** Moving, without taking out, all or a portion of a body part to another location to take over the function of all or a portion of a body part.
3RD - **X TRANSFER**	**EXPLANATION:** The body part remains connected ...

Body Part – 4TH		Approach – 5TH	Device – 6TH	Qualifier – 7TH
0 Skin, Scalp	B Skin, Right Upper Arm	X External	Z No device	Z No qualifier
1 Skin, Face	C Skin, Left Upper Arm			
2 Skin, Right Ear	D Skin, Right Lower Arm			
3 Skin, Left Ear	E Skin, Left Lower Arm			
4 Skin, Neck	F Skin, Right Hand			
5 Skin, Chest	G Skin, Left Hand			
6 Skin, Back	H Skin, Right Upper Leg			
7 Skin, Abdomen	J Skin, Left Upper Leg			
8 Skin, Buttock	K Skin, Right Lower Leg			
9 Skin, Perineum	L Skin, Left Lower Leg			
A Skin, Genitalia	M Skin, Right Foot			
	N Skin, Left Foot			

SKIN & BREAST

0 H X

Educational Annotations | J – Subcutaneous Tissue and Fascia

Body System Specific Educational Annotations for the Subcutaneous Tissue and Fascia include:

- **Anatomy and Physiology Review**
- **Anatomical Illustrations**
- **Definitions of Common Procedures**
- **AHA Coding Clinic® Reference Notations**
- **Body Part Key Listings**
- **Device Key Listings**
- **Device Aggregation Table Listings**
- **Coding Notes**

Anatomy and Physiology Review of Subcutaneous Tissue and Fascia

BODY PART VALUES – J - SUBCUTANEOUS TISSUE AND FASCIA

Fascia – ANATOMY – The sheets or bands of dense connective tissue located beneath the skin between muscles, organs, and other structures. PHYSIOLOGY – The fascia is strong but flexible and functions to separate, protect, and reduce friction of muscule movement on the organs, blood vessels, nerves, muscles, and other structures within the body.

Subcutaneous Tissue – ANATOMY – The innermost layer of the three layers of the skin (also known as the hypodermis) and comprised of fibous tissue, adipose tissue, elastic fibers, connective tissue, and hair follicle roots. PHYSIOLOGY – The subcutaneous tissue is responsible for regulating body temperature, plays a role in pigmentation, and protects the inner organs and bones.

Anatomical Illustrations of Subcutaneous Tissue and Fascia

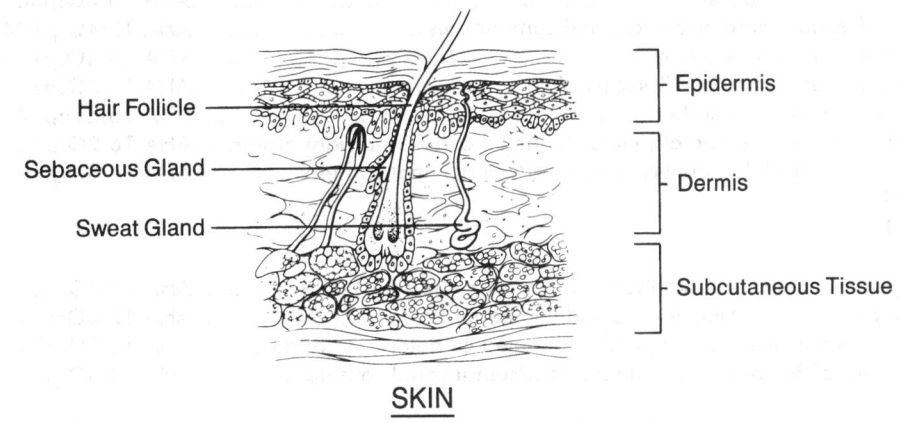

SKIN

Definitions of Common Procedures of Subcutaneous Tissue and Fascia

Free fascia graft – The implantation of fascia to fill a defect using an allograft or donor tissue.

Insertion of pacemaker generator – The surgical placement of a pacemaker generator just under the skin in the subcutaneous tissue.

Liposuction – The surgical removal of excess fat deposits using a hollow cannula that is connected to a strong suction pump.

Pedicle fascia graft – The transfer of fascia to fill a defect without dissecting the graft tissue free from its vascular and nervous supply.

Educational Annotations | J – Subcutaneous Tissue and Fascia

AHA Coding Clinic® Reference Notations of Subcutaneous Tissue and Fascia

ROOT OPERATION SPECIFIC - J - SUBCUTANEOUS TISSUE AND FASCIA

ALTERATION - 0

CHANGE - 2

DESTRUCTION - 5

DIVISION - 8

DRAINAGE - 9

Drainage of subcutaneous abscesses ....AHA 15:3Q:p23

EXCISION - B

Excision of abdominal subcutaneous fat during hernia repair ....AHA 14:4Q:p38

Excision of inclusion cyst of perineum ....AHA 13:4Q:p119

Excisional repair of perineal fistula ....AHA 15:1Q:p29

Graft excision, forearm free flap...AHA 15:2Q:p13

Harvesting of fat graft from abdomen ....AHA 14:3Q:p22

EXTIRPATION - C

EXTRACTION - D

Non-excisional debridement ....AHA 15:3Q:p3-8

Non-excisional debridement using Pulsavac ....AHA 15:1Q:p23

INSERTION - H

Exchange of tunneled hemodialysis catheter with chest port ....AHA 15:4Q:p31

Insertion of infusion pump in chest pocket ....AHA 15:4Q:p14

Insertion of tunneled hemodialysis catheter into superior vena cava

   with port chest pocket ....AHA 15:4Q:p30

Insertion of various cardiac devices and components ....AHA 12:4Q:p104

Insertion of venous access port...AHA 13:4Q:p116

   Official Clarification of 13:4Q:p116 ....AHA 15:2Q:p34

Peritoneal port-a-cath insertion ....AHA 16:2Q:p14

Removal with new insertion of jugular tunneled catheter in right atrium ....AHA 16:2Q:p15

Replacement of Baclofen medication pump/spinal canal catheter ....AHA 14:3Q:p19

INSPECTION - J

RELEASE - N

REMOVAL - P

Exchange of tunneled hemodialysis catheter with chest port ....AHA 15:4Q:p31

Removal of various cardiac devices and components ....AHA 12:4Q:p104

Removal with new insertion of jugular tunneled catheter in right atrium ....AHA 16:2Q:p15

Replacement of Baclofen medication pump/spinal canal catheter ....AHA 14:3Q:p19

REPAIR - Q

Posterior colporrhaphy/rectocele repair ....AHA 14:4Q:p44

REPLACEMENT - R

Reconstruction of orbital defect using forearm free flap..........................AHA 15:2Q:p13

SUPPLEMENT - U

REVISION - W

Externalization of peritoneal dialysis catheter ....AHA 15:4Q:p33

Retunneling and reconnection of VP shunt in periauricular subcutaneous

   tissue ....AHA 15:2Q:p9

Revision of various cardiac devices and components ....AHA 12:4Q:p104

TRANSFER - X

Reverse sural fasciocutaneous pedicle flap ....AHA 14:3Q:p18

Body Part Key Listings of Subcutaneous Tissue and Fascia

See also Body Part Key in Appendix C

Antebrachial fascia ....*use* Subcutaneous Tissue and Fascia, Lower Arm, Left/Right

Axillary fascia..*use* Subcutaneous Tissue and Fascia, Upper Arm, Left/Right

Bicipital aponeurosis ....*use* Subcutaneous Tissue and Fascia, Lower Arm, Left/Right

Continued on next page

© 2016 Channel Publishing, Ltd.

Educational Annotations | J – Subcutaneous Tissue and Fascia

Body Part Key Listings of Subcutaneous Tissue and Fascia

Continued from previous page

Crural fascia	*use* Subcutaneous Tissue and Fascia, Upper Leg, Left/Right
Deep cervical fascia	*use* Subcutaneous Tissue and Fascia, Anterior Neck
Deltoid fascia	*use* Subcutaneous Tissue and Fascia, Upper Arm, Left/Right
External oblique aponeurosis	*use* Subcutaneous Tissue and Fascia, Trunk
Fascia lata	*use* Subcutaneous Tissue and Fascia, Upper Leg, Left/Right
Galea aponeurotica	*use* Subcutaneous Tissue and Fascia, Scalp
Iliac fascia	*use* Subcutaneous Tissue and Fascia, Upper Leg, Left/Right
Iliotibial tract (band)	*use* Subcutaneous Tissue and Fascia, Upper Leg, Left/Right
Infraspinatus fascia	*use* Subcutaneous Tissue and Fascia, Upper Arm, Left/Right
Masseteric fascia	*use* Subcutaneous Tissue and Fascia, Face
Orbital fascia	*use* Subcutaneous Tissue and Fascia, Face
Palmar fascia (aponeurosis)	*use* Subcutaneous Tissue and Fascia, Hand, Left/Right
Pectoral fascia	*use* Subcutaneous Tissue and Fascia, Chest
Plantar fascia (aponeurosis)	*use* Subcutaneous Tissue and Fascia, Foot, Left/Right
Pretracheal fascia	*use* Subcutaneous Tissue and Fascia, Anterior Neck
Prevertebral fascia	*use* Subcutaneous Tissue and Fascia, Posterior Neck
Subscapular aponeurosis	*use* Subcutaneous Tissue and Fascia, Upper Arm, Left/Right
Supraspinatus fascia	*use* Subcutaneous Tissue and Fascia, Upper Arm, Left/Right
Transversalis fascia	*use* Subcutaneous Tissue and Fascia, Trunk

Device Key Listings of Subcutaneous Tissue and Fascia

See also Device Key in Appendix D

Activa PC neurostimulator	*use* Stimulator Generator, Multiple Array for Insertion in Subcutaneous Tissue and Fascia
Activa RC neurostimulator	*use* Stimulator Generator, Multiple Array Rechargeable for Insertion in Subcutaneous Tissue and Fascia
Activa SC neurostimulator	*use* Stimulator Generator, Single Array for Insertion in Subcutaneous Tissue and Fascia
Advisa (MRI)	*use* Pacemaker, Dual Chamber for Insertion in Subcutaneous Tissue and Fascia
Autograft	*use* Autologous Tissue Substitute
Baroreflex Activation Therapy® (BAT®)	*use* Stimulator Generator in Subcutaneous Tissue and Fascia
Brachytherapy seeds	*use* Radioactive Element
COGNIS® CRT-D	*use* Cardiac Resynchronization Defibrillator Pulse Generator for Insertion in Subcutaneous Tissue and Fascia
Concerto II CRT-D	*use* Cardiac Resynchronization Defibrillator Pulse Generator for Insertion in Subcutaneous Tissue and Fascia
Consulta CRT-D	*use* Cardiac Resynchronization Defibrillator Pulse Generator for Insertion in Subcutaneous Tissue and Fascia
Consulta CRT-P	*use* Cardiac Resynchronization Pacemaker Pulse Generator for Insertion in Subcutaneous Tissue and Fascia
CONTAK RENEWAL® 3 RF (HE) CRT-D	*use* Cardiac Resynchronization Defibrillator Pulse Generator for Insertion in Subcutaneous Tissue and Fascia
Cook Biodesign® Fistula Plug(s)	*use* Nonautologous Tissue Substitute
Cook Biodesign® Hernia Graft(s)	*use* Nonautologous Tissue Substitute
Cook Biodesign® Layered Graft(s)	*use* Nonautologous Tissue Substitute
Cook Zenapro™ Layered Graft(s)	*use* Nonautologous Tissue Substitute
Diaphragmatic pacemaker generator	*use* Stimulator Generator in Subcutaneous Tissue and Fascia

Continued on next page

Educational Annotations | J – Subcutaneous Tissue and Fascia

Device Key Listings of Subcutaneous Tissue and Fascia

Continued from previous page

EnRhythm	*use* Pacemaker, Dual Chamber for Insertion in Subcutaneous Tissue and Fascia
Enterra gastric neurostimulator	*use* Stimulator Generator, Multiple Array for Insertion in Subcutaneous Tissue and Fascia
Evera (XT) (S) (DR/VR)	*use* Defibrillator Generator for Insertion in Subcutaneous Tissue and Fascia
Implantable cardioverter-defibrillator (ICD)	*use* Defibrillator Generator for Insertion in Subcutaneous Tissue and Fascia
Implantable drug infusion pump (anti-spasmodic) (chemotherapy) (pain)	*use* Infusion Device, Pump in Subcutaneous Tissue and Fascia
Implantable hemodynamic monitor (IHM)	*use* Monitoring Device, Hemodynamic for Insertion in Subcutaneous Tissue and Fascia
Implantable hemodynamic monitoring system (IHMS)	*use* Monitoring Device, Hemodynamic for Insertion in Subcutaneous Tissue and Fascia
Implanted (venous) (access) port	*use* Vascular Access Device, Reservoir in Subcutaneous Tissue and Fascia
Injection reservoir, port	*use* Vascular Access Device, Reservoir in Subcutaneous Tissue and Fascia
Injection reservoir, pump	*use* Infusion Device, Pump in Subcutaneous Tissue and Fascia
InterStim® Therapy neurostimulator	*use* Stimulator Generator, Single Array for Insertion in Subcutaneous Tissue and Fascia
Itrel (3) (4) neurostimulator	*use* Stimulator Generator, Single Array for Insertion in Subcutaneous Tissue and Fascia
Kappa	*use* Pacemaker, Dual Chamber for Insertion in Subcutaneous Tissue and Fascia
LIVIAN™ CRT-D	*use* Cardiac Resynchronization Defibrillator Pulse Generator for Insertion in Subcutaneous Tissue and Fascia
Loop recorder, implantable	*use* Monitoring Device
Mark IV Breathing Pacemaker System	*use* Stimulator Generator in Subcutaneous Tissue and Fascia
Maximo II DR (VR)	*use* Defibrillator Generator for Insertion in Subcutaneous Tissue and Fascia
Maximo II DR CRT-D	*use* Cardiac Resynchronization Defibrillator Pulse Generator for Insertion in Subcutaneous Tissue and Fascia
Neurostimulator generator, multiple channel	*use* Stimulator Generator, Multiple Array for Insertion in Subcutaneous Tissue and Fascia
Neurostimulator generator, multiple channel rechargeable	*use* Stimulator Generator, Multiple Array Rechargeable for Insertion in Subcutaneous Tissue and Fascia
Neurostimulator generator, single channel	*use* Stimulator Generator, Single Array for Insertion in Subcutaneous Tissue and Fascia
Neurostimulator generator, single channel rechargeable	*use* Stimulator Generator, Single Array Rechargeable for Insertion in Subcutaneous Tissue and Fascia
Optimizer™ III implantable pulse generator	*use* Contractility Modulation Device for Insertion in Subcutaneous Tissue and Fascia
Ovatio™ CRT-D	*use* Cardiac Resynchronization Defibrillator Pulse Generator for Insertion in Subcutaneous Tissue and Fascia
Phrenic nerve stimulator generator	*use* Stimulator Generator in Subcutaneous Tissue and Fascia

Continued on next page

Educational Annotations | J – Subcutaneous Tissue and Fascia

Device Key Listings of Subcutaneous Tissue and Fascia

Continued from previous page

PrimeAdvanced neurostimulator (SureScan) (MRI Safe) ....*use* Stimulator Generator, Multiple Array for Insertion in Subcutaneous Tissue and Fascia

Protecta XT CRT-D ....*use* Cardiac Resynchronization Defibrillator Pulse Generator for Insertion in Subcutaneous Tissue and Fascia

Protecta XT DR (XT VR) ....*use* Defibrillator Generator for Insertion in Subcutaneous Tissue and Fascia

Pump reservoir ....*use* Infusion Device, Pump in Subcutaneous Tissue and Fascia

RestoreAdvanced neurostimulator (SureScan) (MRI Safe) ....*use* Stimulator Generator, Multiple Array Rechargeable for Insertion in Subcutaneous Tissue and Fascia

RestoreSensor neurostimulator (SureScan) (MRI Safe) ....*use* Stimulator Generator, Multiple Array Rechargeable for Insertion in Subcutaneous Tissue and Fascia

RestoreUltra neurostimulator (SureScan) (MRI Safe) ....*use* Stimulator Generator, Multiple Array Rechargeable for Insertion in Subcutaneous Tissue and Fascia

Reveal (DX) (XT) ....*use* Monitoring Device

Revo MRI™ SureScan® pacemaker ....*use* Pacemaker, Dual Chamber for Insertion in Subcutaneous Tissue and Fascia

Rheos® System device ....*use* Stimulator Generator in Subcutaneous Tissue and Fascia

Secura (DR) (VR) ....*use* Defibrillator Generator for Insertion in Subcutaneous Tissue and Fascia

Single lead pacemaker (atrium) (ventricle) ....*use* Pacemaker, Single Chamber for Insertion in Subcutaneous Tissue and Fascia

Single lead rate responsive pacemaker (atrium) (ventricle) ....*use* Pacemaker, Single Chamber Rate Responsive for Insertion in Subcutaneous Tissue and Fascia

Stratos LV ....*use* Cardiac Resynchronization Pacemaker Pulse Generator for Insertion in Subcutaneous Tissue and Fascia

Subcutaneous injection reservoir, port ....*use* Vascular Access Device, Reservoir in Subcutaneous Tissue and Fascia

Subcutaneous injection reservoir, pump ....*use* Infusion Device, Pump in Subcutaneous Tissue and Fascia

Subdermal progesterone implant ....*use* Contraceptive Device in Subcutaneous Tissue and Fascia

Synchra CRT-P ....*use* Cardiac Resynchronization Pacemaker Pulse Generator for Insertion in Subcutaneous Tissue and Fascia

SynchroMed pump ....*use* Infusion Device, Pump in Subcutaneous Tissue and Fascia

Tissue bank graft ....*use* Nonautologous Tissue Substitute

Tissue expander (inflatable) (injectable) ....*use* Tissue Expander in Subcutaneous Tissue and Fascia

Tunneled central venous catheter ....*use* Vascular Access Device in Subcutaneous Tissue and Fascia

Two lead pacemaker ....*use* Pacemaker, Dual Chamber for Insertion in Subcutaneous Tissue and Fascia

Vectra® Vascular Access Graft ....*use* Vascular Access Device in Subcutaneous Tissue and Fascia

Versa ....*use* Pacemaker, Dual Chamber for Insertion in Subcutaneous Tissue and Fascia

Virtuoso (II) (DR) (VR) ....*use* Defibrillator Generator for Insertion in Subcutaneous Tissue and Fascia

Viva (XT) (S) ....*use* Cardiac Resynchronization Defibrillator Pulse Generator for Insertion in Subcutaneous Tissue and Fascia

Educational Annotations | J – Subcutaneous Tissue and Fascia

Device Aggregation Table Listings of Subcutaneous Tissue and Fascia

See also Device Aggregation Table in Appendix E

Specific Device	For Operation	In Body System		General Device
Cardiac Resynchronization Defibrillator Pulse Generator	Insertion	Subcutaneous Tissue and Fascia	P	Cardiac Rhythm Related Device
Cardiac Resynchronization Pacemaker Pulse Generator	Insertion	Subcutaneous Tissue and Fascia	P	Cardiac Rhythm Related Device
Contractility Modulation Device	Insertion	Subcutaneous Tissue and Fascia	P	Cardiac Rhythm Related Device
Defibrillator Generator	Insertion	Subcutaneous Tissue and Fascia	P	Cardiac Rhythm Related Device
Monitoring Device, Hemodynamic	Insertion	Subcutaneous Tissue and Fascia	2	Monitoring Device
Pacemaker, Dual Chamber	Insertion	Subcutaneous Tissue and Fascia	P	Cardiac Rhythm Related Device
Pacemaker, Single Chamber	Insertion	Subcutaneous Tissue and Fascia	P	Cardiac Rhythm Related Device
Pacemaker, Single Chamber Rate Responsive	Insertion	Subcutaneous Tissue and Fascia	P	Cardiac Rhythm Related Device
Stimulator Generator, Multiple Array	Insertion	Subcutaneous Tissue and Fascia	M	Stimulator Generator
Stimulator Generator, Multiple Array Rechargeable	Insertion	Subcutaneous Tissue and Fascia	M	Stimulator Generator
Stimulator Generator, Single Array	Insertion	Subcutaneous Tissue and Fascia	M	Stimulator Generator
Stimulator Generator, Single Array Rechargeable	Insertion	Subcutaneous Tissue and Fascia	M	Stimulator Generator

Coding Notes of Subcutaneous Tissue and Fascia

Body System Relevant Coding Guidelines

Tendons, ligaments, bursae and fascia near a joint

B4.5

Procedures performed on tendons, ligaments, bursae and fascia supporting a joint are coded to the body part in the respective body system that is the focus of the procedure. Procedures performed on joint structures themselves are coded to the body part in the joint body systems.

Examples: Repair of the anterior cruciate ligament of the knee is coded to the knee bursa and ligament body part in the bursae and ligaments body system.

Knee arthroscopy with shaving of articular cartilage is coded to the knee joint body part in the Lower Joints body system.

Skin, subcutaneous tissue and fascia overlying a joint

B4.6

If a procedure is performed on the skin, subcutaneous tissue or fascia overlying a joint, the procedure is coded to the following body part:

- Shoulder is coded to Upper Arm
- Elbow is coded to Lower Arm
- Wrist is coded to Lower Arm
- Hip is coded to Upper Leg
- Knee is coded to Lower Leg
- Ankle is coded to Foot

Body System Specific PCS Reference Manual Exercises

PCS CODE	J – SUBCUTANEOUS TISSUE AND FASCIA EXERCISES
0 J 0 L 3 Z Z 0 J 0 M 3 Z Z	Liposuction of bilateral thighs.
0 J D 8 0 Z Z	Open stripping of abdominal fascia, right side.
0 J D F 3 Z Z	Liposuction for medical purposes, left upper arm. (The Percutaneous approach is inherent in the liposuction technique.)
0 J H 6 0 6 Z	Open placement of dual chamber pacemaker generator in chest wall.
0 J H 8 0 D Z	End-of-life replacement of spinal neurostimulator generator, multiple array, in lower abdomen. (Taking out the old generator is coded separately to the root operation Removal.)
0 J U C 0 J Z	Anterior colporrhaphy with polypropylene mesh reinforcement, open approach.
0 J W T 0 X Z	Revision of totally implantable VAD port placement in chest wall, causing patient discomfort, open.
0 J X 4 3 Z Z	Percutaneous fascia transfer to fill defect, anterior neck.
0 J X M 0 Z C	Fasciocutaneous flap closure of left thigh, open. (The qualifier identifies the body layers in addition to fascia included in the procedure.)

SUBCUTANEOUS 0 J

OTHER OBJECTIVES GROUP: Alteration, (Creation), (Fusion)
Root Operations that define other objectives.

1ST - **0** Medical and Surgical

2ND - **J** Subcutaneous Tissue and Fascia

3RD - **0 ALTERATION**

EXAMPLE: Liposuction thighs | CMS Ex: Face lift

ALTERATION: Modifying the anatomic structure of a body part without affecting the function of the body part.

EXPLANATION: Principal purpose is to improve appearance

Body Part – 4TH	Approach – 5TH	Device – 6TH	Qualifier – 7TH
1 Subcutaneous Tissue and Fascia, Face	0 Open	Z No device	Z No qualifier
4 Subcutaneous Tissue and Fascia, Anterior Neck	3 Percutaneous		
5 Subcutaneous Tissue and Fascia, Posterior Neck			
6 Subcutaneous Tissue and Fascia, Chest			
7 Subcutaneous Tissue and Fascia, Back			
8 Subcutaneous Tissue and Fascia, Abdomen			
9 Subcutaneous Tissue and Fascia, Buttock			
D Subcutaneous Tissue and Fascia, Right Upper Arm			
F Subcutaneous Tissue and Fascia, Left Upper Arm			
G Subcutaneous Tissue and Fascia, Right Lower Arm			
H Subcutaneous Tissue and Fascia, Left Lower Arm			
L Subcutaneous Tissue and Fascia, Right Upper Leg			
M Subcutaneous Tissue and Fascia, Left Upper Leg			
N Subcutaneous Tissue and Fascia, Right Lower Leg			
P Subcutaneous Tissue and Fascia, Left Lower Leg			

DEVICE GROUP: Change, Insertion, Removal, Replacement, Revision, Supplement
Root Operations that always involve a device.

1ST - **0** Medical and Surgical

2ND - **J** Subcutaneous Tissue and Fascia

3RD - **2 CHANGE**

EXAMPLE: Exchange drain tube | CMS Ex: Changing urinary catheter

CHANGE: Taking out or off a device from a body part and putting back an identical or similar device in or on the same body part without cutting or puncturing the skin or a mucous membrane.

EXPLANATION: ALL Changes use EXTERNAL approach only ...

Body Part – 4TH	Approach – 5TH	Device – 6TH	Qualifier – 7TH
S Subcutaneous Tissue and Fascia, Head and Neck	X External	0 Drainage device	Z No qualifier
T Subcutaneous Tissue and Fascia, Trunk		Y Other device	
V Subcutaneous Tissue and Fascia, Upper Extremity			
W Subcutaneous Tissue and Fascia, Lower Extremity			

SUBCUTANEOUS 0 J 2

EXCISION GROUP: Excision, (Resection), Destruction, Extraction (Detachment)
Root Operations that take out some or all of a body part.

1ST - 0 Medical and Surgical

2ND - J Subcutaneous Tissue and Fascia

3RD - 5 DESTRUCTION

EXAMPLE: Radiofrequency ablation	CMS Ex: Fulguration polyp

DESTRUCTION: Physical eradication of all or a portion of a body part by the direct use of energy, force, or a destructive agent.

EXPLANATION: None of the body part is physically taken out

Body Part – 4TH	Approach – 5TH	Device – 6TH	Qualifier – 7TH
0 Subcutaneous Tissue and Fascia, Scalp	0 Open	Z No device	Z No qualifier
1 Subcutaneous Tissue and Fascia, Face	3 Percutaneous		
4 Subcutaneous Tissue and Fascia, Anterior Neck			
5 Subcutaneous Tissue and Fascia, Posterior Neck			
6 Subcutaneous Tissue and Fascia, Chest			
7 Subcutaneous Tissue and Fascia, Back			
8 Subcutaneous Tissue and Fascia, Abdomen			
9 Subcutaneous Tissue and Fascia, Buttock			
B Subcutaneous Tissue and Fascia, Perineum			
C Subcutaneous Tissue and Fascia, Pelvic Region			
D Subcutaneous Tissue and Fascia, Right Upper Arm			
F Subcutaneous Tissue and Fascia, Left Upper Arm			
G Subcutaneous Tissue and Fascia, Right Lower Arm			
H Subcutaneous Tissue and Fascia, Left Lower Arm			
J Subcutaneous Tissue and Fascia, Right Hand			
K Subcutaneous Tissue and Fascia, Left Hand			
L Subcutaneous Tissue and Fascia, Right Upper Leg			
M Subcutaneous Tissue and Fascia, Left Upper Leg			
N Subcutaneous Tissue and Fascia, Right Lower Leg			
P Subcutaneous Tissue and Fascia, Left Lower Leg			
Q Subcutaneous Tissue and Fascia, Right Foot			
R Subcutaneous Tissue and Fascia, Left Foot			

SUBCUTANEOUS 0 J 5

| **DIVISION GROUP: Division, Release** | | | |
| Root Operations involving cutting or separation only. | | | |

	EXAMPLE: Division plantar fascia		CMS Ex: Osteotomy

1ST - 0 Medical and Surgical

2ND - J Subcutaneous Tissue and Fascia

3RD - 8 DIVISION

DIVISION: Cutting into a body part without draining fluids and/or gases from the body part in order to separate or transect a body part.

EXPLANATION: Separated into two or more portions ...

Body Part – 4TH	Approach – 5TH	Device – 6TH	Qualifier – 7TH
0 Subcutaneous Tissue and Fascia, Scalp	0 Open	Z No device	Z No qualifier
1 Subcutaneous Tissue and Fascia, Face	3 Percutaneous		
4 Subcutaneous Tissue and Fascia, Anterior Neck			
5 Subcutaneous Tissue and Fascia, Posterior Neck			
6 Subcutaneous Tissue and Fascia, Chest			
7 Subcutaneous Tissue and Fascia, Back			
8 Subcutaneous Tissue and Fascia, Abdomen			
9 Subcutaneous Tissue and Fascia, Buttock			
B Subcutaneous Tissue and Fascia, Perineum			
C Subcutaneous Tissue and Fascia, Pelvic Region			
D Subcutaneous Tissue and Fascia, Right Upper Arm			
F Subcutaneous Tissue and Fascia, Left Upper Arm			
G Subcutaneous Tissue and Fascia, Right Lower Arm			
H Subcutaneous Tissue and Fascia, Left Lower Arm			
J Subcutaneous Tissue and Fascia, Right Hand			
K Subcutaneous Tissue and Fascia, Left Hand			
L Subcutaneous Tissue and Fascia, Right Upper Leg			
M Subcutaneous Tissue and Fascia, Left Upper Leg			
N Subcutaneous Tissue and Fascia, Right Lower Leg			
P Subcutaneous Tissue and Fascia, Left Lower Leg			
Q Subcutaneous Tissue and Fascia, Right Foot			
R Subcutaneous Tissue and Fascia, Left Foot			
S Subcutaneous Tissue and Fascia, Head and Neck			
T Subcutaneous Tissue and Fascia, Trunk			
V Subcutaneous Tissue and Fascia, Upper Extremity			
W Subcutaneous Tissue and Fascia, Lower Extremity			

SUBCUTANEOUS

0 J 8

DRAINAGE GROUP: Drainage, Extirpation, (Fragmentation)
Root Operations that take out solids/fluids/gases from a body part.

1ST - **0** Medical and Surgical	EXAMPLE: I&D fascial abscess CMS Ex: Thoracentesis
2ND - **J** Subcutaneous Tissue and Fascia	**DRAINAGE:** Taking or letting out fluids and/or gases from a body part.
3RD - **9 DRAINAGE**	EXPLANATION: Qualifier "X Diagnostic" indicates biopsy ...

Body Part – 4TH	Approach – 5TH	Device – 6TH	Qualifier – 7TH
0 Subcutaneous Tissue and Fascia, Scalp 1 Subcutaneous Tissue and Fascia, Face 4 Subcutaneous Tissue and Fascia, Anterior Neck 5 Subcutaneous Tissue and Fascia, Posterior Neck 6 Subcutaneous Tissue and Fascia, Chest 7 Subcutaneous Tissue and Fascia, Back 8 Subcutaneous Tissue and Fascia, Abdomen 9 Subcutaneous Tissue and Fascia, Buttock B Subcutaneous Tissue and Fascia, Perineum C Subcutaneous Tissue and Fascia, Pelvic Region D Subcutaneous Tissue and Fascia, Right Upper Arm F Subcutaneous Tissue and Fascia, Left Upper Arm G Subcutaneous Tissue and Fascia, Right Lower Arm H Subcutaneous Tissue and Fascia, Left Lower Arm J Subcutaneous Tissue and Fascia, Right Hand K Subcutaneous Tissue and Fascia, Left Hand L Subcutaneous Tissue and Fascia, Right Upper Leg M Subcutaneous Tissue and Fascia, Left Upper Leg N Subcutaneous Tissue and Fascia, Right Lower Leg P Subcutaneous Tissue and Fascia, Left Lower Leg Q Subcutaneous Tissue and Fascia, Right Foot R Subcutaneous Tissue and Fascia, Left Foot	0 Open 3 Percutaneous	0 Drainage device	Z No qualifier
0 Subcutaneous Tissue and Fascia, Scalp 1 Subcutaneous Tissue and Fascia, Face 4 Subcutaneous Tissue and Fascia, Anterior Neck 5 Subcutaneous Tissue and Fascia, Posterior Neck 6 Subcutaneous Tissue and Fascia, Chest 7 Subcutaneous Tissue and Fascia, Back 8 Subcutaneous Tissue and Fascia, Abdomen 9 Subcutaneous Tissue and Fascia, Buttock B Subcutaneous Tissue and Fascia, Perineum C Subcutaneous Tissue and Fascia, Pelvic Region D Subcutaneous Tissue and Fascia, Right Upper Arm F Subcutaneous Tissue and Fascia, Left Upper Arm G Subcutaneous Tissue and Fascia, Right Lower Arm H Subcutaneous Tissue and Fascia, Left Lower Arm J Subcutaneous Tissue and Fascia, Right Hand K Subcutaneous Tissue and Fascia, Left Hand L Subcutaneous Tissue and Fascia, Right Upper Leg M Subcutaneous Tissue and Fascia, Left Upper Leg N Subcutaneous Tissue and Fascia, Right Lower Leg P Subcutaneous Tissue and Fascia, Left Lower Leg Q Subcutaneous Tissue and Fascia, Right Foot R Subcutaneous Tissue and Fascia, Left Foot	0 Open 3 Percutaneous	Z No device	X Diagnostic Z No qualifier

SUBCUTANEOUS 0 J 9

EXCISION GROUP: Excision, (Resection), Destruction, Extraction (Detachment)
Root Operations that take out some or all of a body part.

1ST - 0 Medical and Surgical	EXAMPLE: Harvesting fat for graft CMS Ex: Liver biopsy
2ND - J Subcutaneous Tissue and Fascia	**EXCISION:** Cutting out or off, without replacement, a portion of a body part.
3RD - B EXCISION	EXPLANATION: Qualifier "X Diagnostic" indicates biopsy ...

Body Part – 4TH	Approach – 5TH	Device – 6TH	Qualifier – 7TH
0 Subcutaneous Tissue and Fascia, Scalp	0 Open	Z No device	X Diagnostic
1 Subcutaneous Tissue and Fascia, Face	3 Percutaneous		Z No qualifier
4 Subcutaneous Tissue and Fascia, Anterior Neck			
5 Subcutaneous Tissue and Fascia, Posterior Neck			
6 Subcutaneous Tissue and Fascia, Chest			
7 Subcutaneous Tissue and Fascia, Back			
8 Subcutaneous Tissue and Fascia, Abdomen			
9 Subcutaneous Tissue and Fascia, Buttock			
B Subcutaneous Tissue and Fascia, Perineum			
C Subcutaneous Tissue and Fascia, Pelvic Region			
D Subcutaneous Tissue and Fascia, Right Upper Arm			
F Subcutaneous Tissue and Fascia, Left Upper Arm			
G Subcutaneous Tissue and Fascia, Right Lower Arm			
H Subcutaneous Tissue and Fascia, Left Lower Arm			
J Subcutaneous Tissue and Fascia, Right Hand			
K Subcutaneous Tissue and Fascia, Left Hand			
L Subcutaneous Tissue and Fascia, Right Upper Leg			
M Subcutaneous Tissue and Fascia, Left Upper Leg			
N Subcutaneous Tissue and Fascia, Right Lower Leg			
P Subcutaneous Tissue and Fascia, Left Lower Leg			
Q Subcutaneous Tissue and Fascia, Right Foot			
R Subcutaneous Tissue and Fascia, Left Foot			

SUBCUTANEOUS

0
J
B

0JC

DRAINAGE GROUP: Drainage, Extirpation, (Fragmentation)
Root Operations that take out solids/fluids/gases from a body part.

1ST - 0 Medical and Surgical	**EXAMPLE:** Removal foreign body **CMS Ex:** Choledocholithotomy
2ND - J Subcutaneous Tissue and Fascia	**EXTIRPATION:** Taking or cutting out solid matter from a body part.
3RD - C EXTIRPATION	**EXPLANATION:** Abnormal byproduct or foreign body ...

Body Part – 4TH	Approach – 5TH	Device – 6TH	Qualifier – 7TH
0 Subcutaneous Tissue and Fascia, Scalp	0 Open	Z No device	Z No qualifier
1 Subcutaneous Tissue and Fascia, Face	3 Percutaneous		
4 Subcutaneous Tissue and Fascia, Anterior Neck			
5 Subcutaneous Tissue and Fascia, Posterior Neck			
6 Subcutaneous Tissue and Fascia, Chest			
7 Subcutaneous Tissue and Fascia, Back			
8 Subcutaneous Tissue and Fascia, Abdomen			
9 Subcutaneous Tissue and Fascia, Buttock			
B Subcutaneous Tissue and Fascia, Perineum			
C Subcutaneous Tissue and Fascia, Pelvic Region			
D Subcutaneous Tissue and Fascia, Right Upper Arm			
F Subcutaneous Tissue and Fascia, Left Upper Arm			
G Subcutaneous Tissue and Fascia, Right Lower Arm			
H Subcutaneous Tissue and Fascia, Left Lower Arm			
J Subcutaneous Tissue and Fascia, Right Hand			
K Subcutaneous Tissue and Fascia, Left Hand			
L Subcutaneous Tissue and Fascia, Right Upper Leg			
M Subcutaneous Tissue and Fascia, Left Upper Leg			
N Subcutaneous Tissue and Fascia, Right Lower Leg			
P Subcutaneous Tissue and Fascia, Left Lower Leg			
Q Subcutaneous Tissue and Fascia, Right Foot			
R Subcutaneous Tissue and Fascia, Left Foot			

SUBCUTANEOUS 0JC

EXCISION GROUP: Excision, (Resection), Destruction, Extraction (Detachment)
Root Operations that take out some or all of a body part.

1ST - **0** Medical and Surgical

2ND - **J** Subcutaneous Tissue and Fascia

3RD - **D EXTRACTION**

EXAMPLE: Non-excisional debridement | CMS Ex: D&C

EXTRACTION: Pulling or stripping out or off all or a portion of a body part by the use of force.

EXPLANATION: None for this Body System

Body Part – 4TH	Approach – 5TH	Device – 6TH	Qualifier – 7TH
0 Subcutaneous Tissue and Fascia, Scalp	0 Open	Z No device	Z No qualifier
1 Subcutaneous Tissue and Fascia, Face	3 Percutaneous		
4 Subcutaneous Tissue and Fascia, Anterior Neck			
5 Subcutaneous Tissue and Fascia, Posterior Neck			
6 Subcutaneous Tissue and Fascia, Chest			
7 Subcutaneous Tissue and Fascia, Back			
8 Subcutaneous Tissue and Fascia, Abdomen			
9 Subcutaneous Tissue and Fascia, Buttock			
B Subcutaneous Tissue and Fascia, Perineum			
C Subcutaneous Tissue and Fascia, Pelvic Region			
D Subcutaneous Tissue and Fascia, Right Upper Arm			
F Subcutaneous Tissue and Fascia, Left Upper Arm			
G Subcutaneous Tissue and Fascia, Right Lower Arm			
H Subcutaneous Tissue and Fascia, Left Lower Arm			
J Subcutaneous Tissue and Fascia, Right Hand			
K Subcutaneous Tissue and Fascia, Left Hand			
L Subcutaneous Tissue and Fascia, Right Upper Leg			
M Subcutaneous Tissue and Fascia, Left Upper Leg			
N Subcutaneous Tissue and Fascia, Right Lower Leg			
P Subcutaneous Tissue and Fascia, Left Lower Leg			
Q Subcutaneous Tissue and Fascia, Right Foot			
R Subcutaneous Tissue and Fascia, Left Foot			

SUBCUTANEOUS 0 J D

DEVICE GROUP: Change, Insertion, Removal, Replacement, Revision, Supplement
Root Operations that always involve a device.

1ST - **0** Medical and Surgical	EXAMPLE: Placement pacemaker generator	CMS Ex: CVP catheter
2ND - **J** Subcutaneous Tissue and Fascia	**INSERTION:** Putting in a nonbiological appliance that monitors, assists, performs, or prevents a physiological function but does not physically take the place of a body part.	
3RD - **H INSERTION**	EXPLANATION: None	

Body Part – 4TH	Approach – 5TH	Device – 6TH	Qualifier – 7TH
0 Subcutaneous Tissue and Fascia, Scalp 1 Subcutaneous Tissue and Fascia, Face 4 Subcutaneous Tissue and Fascia, Anterior Neck 5 Subcutaneous Tissue and Fascia, Posterior Neck 9 Subcutaneous Tissue and Fascia, Buttock B Subcutaneous Tissue and Fascia, Perineum C Subcutaneous Tissue and Fascia, Pelvic Region J Subcutaneous Tissue and Fascia, Right Hand K Subcutaneous Tissue and Fascia, Left Hand Q Subcutaneous Tissue and Fascia, Right Foot R Subcutaneous Tissue and Fascia, Left Foot	0 Open 3 Percutaneous	N Tissue Expander	Z No qualifier
6 Subcutaneous Tissue and Fascia, Chest 8 Subcutaneous Tissue and Fascia, Abdomen	0 Open 3 Percutaneous	0 Monitoring device, hemodynamic 2 Monitoring device 4 Pacemaker, single chamber 5 Pacemaker, single chamber rate responsive 6 Pacemaker, dual chamber 7 Cardiac resynchronization pacemaker pulse generator 8 Defibrillator generator 9 Cardiac resynchronization defibrillator pulse generator A Contractility modulation device B Stimulator generator, single array C Stimulator generator, single array rechargeable D Stimulator generator, multiple array E Stimulator generator, multiple array rechargeable H Contraceptive device M Stimulator generator NC* N Tissue expander P Cardiac rhythm related device V Infusion device, pump W Vascular access device, reservoir X Vascular access device	Z No qualifier

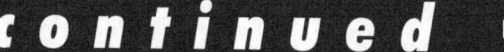

0 J H   INSERTION – continued

Body Part – 4TH	Approach – 5TH	Device – 6TH	Qualifier – 7TH
7 Subcutaneous Tissue and Fascia, Back	0 Open 3 Percutaneous	B Stimulator generator, single array C Stimulator generator, single array rechargeable D Stimulator generator, multiple array E Stimulator generator, multiple array rechargeable M Stimulator generator NC* N Tissue expander V Infusion device, pump	Z No qualifier
D Subcutaneous Tissue and Fascia, Right Upper Arm F Subcutaneous Tissue and Fascia, Left Upper Arm G Subcutaneous Tissue and Fascia, Right Lower Arm H Subcutaneous Tissue and Fascia, Left Lower Arm L Subcutaneous Tissue and Fascia, Right Upper Leg M Subcutaneous Tissue and Fascia, Left Upper Leg N Subcutaneous Tissue and Fascia, Right Lower Leg P Subcutaneous Tissue and Fascia, Left Lower Leg	0 Open 3 Percutaneous	H Contraceptive device N Tissue expander V Infusion device, pump W Vascular access device, reservoir X Vascular access device	Z No qualifier
S Subcutaneous Tissue and Fascia, Head and Neck V Subcutaneous Tissue and Fascia, Upper Extremity W Subcutaneous Tissue and Fascia, Lower Extremity	0 Open 3 Percutaneous	1 Radioactive element 3 Infusion device	Z No qualifier
T Subcutaneous Tissue and Fascia, Trunk	0 Open 3 Percutaneous	1 Radioactive element 3 Infusion device V Infusion device, pump	Z No qualifier

NC* – Some procedures are considered non-covered by Medicare. See current Medicare Code Editor for details.

SUBCUTANEOUS 0 J J

EXAMINATION GROUP: Inspection, (Map)
Root Operations involving examination only.

1ST - 0 Medical and Surgical
2ND - J Subcutaneous Tissue and Fascia
3RD - J INSPECTION

EXAMPLE: Exploration abdominal fascia   CMS Ex: Colonoscopy

INSPECTION: Visually and/or manually exploring a body part.

EXPLANATION: Direct or instrumental visualization ...

Body Part – 4TH	Approach – 5TH	Device – 6TH	Qualifier – 7TH
S Subcutaneous Tissue and Fascia, Head and Neck T Subcutaneous Tissue and Fascia, Trunk V Subcutaneous Tissue and Fascia, Upper Extremity W Subcutaneous Tissue and Fascia, Lower Extremity	0 Open 3 Percutaneous X External	Z No device	Z No qualifier

DIVISION GROUP: Division, Release
Root Operations involving cutting or separation only.

1ST - 0 Medical and Surgical	EXAMPLE: Lysis fascial adhesions	CMS Ex: Carpal tunnel release
2ND - J Subcutaneous Tissue and Fascia	**RELEASE:**	Freeing a body part from an abnormal physical constraint by cutting or by the use of force.
3RD - N RELEASE		

EXPLANATION: None of the body part is taken out ...

Body Part – 4TH	Approach – 5TH	Device – 6TH	Qualifier – 7TH
0 Subcutaneous Tissue and Fascia, Scalp	0 Open	Z No device	Z No qualifier
1 Subcutaneous Tissue and Fascia, Face	3 Percutaneous		
4 Subcutaneous Tissue and Fascia, Anterior Neck	X External		
5 Subcutaneous Tissue and Fascia, Posterior Neck			
6 Subcutaneous Tissue and Fascia, Chest			
7 Subcutaneous Tissue and Fascia, Back			
8 Subcutaneous Tissue and Fascia, Abdomen			
9 Subcutaneous Tissue and Fascia, Buttock			
B Subcutaneous Tissue and Fascia, Perineum			
C Subcutaneous Tissue and Fascia, Pelvic Region			
D Subcutaneous Tissue and Fascia, Right Upper Arm			
F Subcutaneous Tissue and Fascia, Left Upper Arm			
G Subcutaneous Tissue and Fascia, Right Lower Arm			
H Subcutaneous Tissue and Fascia, Left Lower Arm			
J Subcutaneous Tissue and Fascia, Right Hand			
K Subcutaneous Tissue and Fascia, Left Hand			
L Subcutaneous Tissue and Fascia, Right Upper Leg			
M Subcutaneous Tissue and Fascia, Left Upper Leg			
N Subcutaneous Tissue and Fascia, Right Lower Leg			
P Subcutaneous Tissue and Fascia, Left Lower Leg			
Q Subcutaneous Tissue and Fascia, Right Foot			
R Subcutaneous Tissue and Fascia, Left Foot			

DEVICE GROUP: Change, Insertion, Removal, Replacement, Revision, Supplement
Root Operations that always involve a device.

1ST - **0** Medical and Surgical	EXAMPLE: Removal VAD reservoir	CMS Ex: Chest tube removal
2ND - **J** Subcutaneous Tissue and Fascia	**REMOVAL:** Taking out or off a device from a body part.	
3RD - **P REMOVAL**	EXPLANATION: Removal device without reinsertion ...	

Body Part – 4TH	Approach – 5TH	Device – 6TH	Qualifier – 7TH
S Subcutaneous Tissue and Fascia, Head and Neck	0 Open 3 Percutaneous	0 Drainage device 1 Radioactive element 3 Infusion device 7 Autologous tissue substitute J Synthetic substitute K Nonautologous tissue substitute N Tissue expander	Z No qualifier
S Subcutaneous Tissue and Fascia, Head and Neck	X External	0 Drainage device 1 Radioactive element 3 Infusion device	Z No qualifier
T Subcutaneous Tissue and Fascia, Trunk	0 Open 3 Percutaneous	0 Drainage device 1 Radioactive element 2 Monitoring device 3 Infusion device 7 Autologous tissue substitute H Contraceptive device J Synthetic substitute K Nonautologous tissue substitute M Stimulator generator N Tissue expander P Cardiac rhythm related device V Infusion device, pump W Vascular access device, reservoir X Vascular access device	Z No qualifier
T Subcutaneous Tissue and Fascia, Trunk	X External	0 Drainage device 1 Radioactive element 2 Monitoring device 3 Infusion device H Contraceptive device V Infusion device, pump X Vascular access device	Z No qualifier

SUBCUTANEOUS 0 J P

continued ⇨

0 J P REMOVAL – continued

Body Part – 4TH	Approach – 5TH	Device – 6TH	Qualifier – 7TH
V Subcutaneous Tissue and Fascia, Upper Extremity W Subcutaneous Tissue and Fascia, Lower Extremity	0 Open 3 Percuta-neous	0 Drainage device 1 Radioactive element 2 Monitoring device 3 Infusion device 7 Autologous tissue substitute H Contraceptive device J Synthetic substitute K Nonautologous tissue substitute N Tissue expander V Infusion device, pump W Vascular access device, reservoir X Vascular access device	Z No qualifier
V Subcutaneous Tissue and Fascia, Upper Extremity W Subcutaneous Tissue and Fascia, Lower Extremity	X External	0 Drainage device 1 Radioactive element 3 Infusion device H Contraceptive device V Infusion device, pump X Vascular access device	Z No qualifier

---

OTHER REPAIRS GROUP: (Control), Repair
Root Operations that define other repairs.

1ST - **0** Medical and Surgical

2ND - **J** Subcutaneous Tissue and Fascia

3RD - **Q REPAIR**

EXAMPLE: Rectocele repair with sutures | CMS Ex: Suture laceration

REPAIR: Restoring, to the extent possible, a body part to its normal anatomic structure and function.

EXPLANATION: Only when no other root operation applies ...

Body Part – 4TH	Approach – 5TH	Device – 6TH	Qualifier – 7TH
0 Subcutaneous Tissue and Fascia, Scalp 1 Subcutaneous Tissue and Fascia, Face 4 Subcutaneous Tissue and Fascia, Anterior Neck 5 Subcutaneous Tissue and Fascia, Posterior Neck 6 Subcutaneous Tissue and Fascia, Chest 7 Subcutaneous Tissue and Fascia, Back 8 Subcutaneous Tissue and Fascia, Abdomen 9 Subcutaneous Tissue and Fascia, Buttock B Subcutaneous Tissue and Fascia, Perineum C Subcutaneous Tissue and Fascia, Pelvic Region D Subcutaneous Tissue and Fascia, Right Upper Arm F Subcutaneous Tissue and Fascia, Left Upper Arm G Subcutaneous Tissue and Fascia, Right Lower Arm H Subcutaneous Tissue and Fascia, Left Lower Arm J Subcutaneous Tissue and Fascia, Right Hand K Subcutaneous Tissue and Fascia, Left Hand L Subcutaneous Tissue and Fascia, Right Upper Leg M Subcutaneous Tissue and Fascia, Left Upper Leg N Subcutaneous Tissue and Fascia, Right Lower Leg P Subcutaneous Tissue and Fascia, Left Lower Leg Q Subcutaneous Tissue and Fascia, Right Foot R Subcutaneous Tissue and Fascia, Left Foot	0 Open 3 Percutaneous	Z No device	Z No qualifier

DEVICE GROUP: Change, Insertion, Removal, Replacement, Revision, Supplement
Root Operations that always involve a device.

1ST - 0 Medical and Surgical	EXAMPLE: Free fascia lata graft	CMS Ex: Total hip

1ST - 0 Medical and Surgical

2ND - J Subcutaneous Tissue and Fascia

3RD - R REPLACEMENT

REPLACEMENT: Putting in or on a biological or synthetic material that physically takes the place and/or function of all or a portion of a body part.

EXPLANATION: Includes taking out body part, or eradication...

Body Part – 4TH	Approach – 5TH	Device – 6TH	Qualifier – 7TH
0 Subcutaneous Tissue and Fascia, Scalp	0 Open	7 Autologous tissue substitute	Z No qualifier
1 Subcutaneous Tissue and Fascia, Face	3 Percutaneous	J Synthetic substitute	
4 Subcutaneous Tissue and Fascia, Anterior Neck		K Nonautologous tissue substitute	
5 Subcutaneous Tissue and Fascia, Posterior Neck			
6 Subcutaneous Tissue and Fascia, Chest			
7 Subcutaneous Tissue and Fascia, Back			
8 Subcutaneous Tissue and Fascia, Abdomen			
9 Subcutaneous Tissue and Fascia, Buttock			
B Subcutaneous Tissue and Fascia, Perineum			
C Subcutaneous Tissue and Fascia, Pelvic Region			
D Subcutaneous Tissue and Fascia, Right Upper Arm			
F Subcutaneous Tissue and Fascia, Left Upper Arm			
G Subcutaneous Tissue and Fascia, Right Lower Arm			
H Subcutaneous Tissue and Fascia, Left Lower Arm			
J Subcutaneous Tissue and Fascia, Right Hand			
K Subcutaneous Tissue and Fascia, Left Hand			
L Subcutaneous Tissue and Fascia, Right Upper Leg			
M Subcutaneous Tissue and Fascia, Left Upper Leg			
N Subcutaneous Tissue and Fascia, Right Lower Leg			
P Subcutaneous Tissue and Fascia, Left Lower Leg			
Q Subcutaneous Tissue and Fascia, Right Foot			
R Subcutaneous Tissue and Fascia, Left Foot			

SUBCUTANEOUS 0 J R

DEVICE GROUP: Change, Insertion, Removal, Replacement, Revision, Supplement			
Root Operations that always involve a device.			

1ST - 0 Medical and Surgical

2ND - J Subcutaneous Tissue and Fascia

3RD - U SUPPLEMENT

EXAMPLE: Rectocele repair with mesh | CMS Ex: Hernia repair with mesh

SUPPLEMENT: Putting in or on biological or synthetic material that physically reinforces and/or augments the function of a portion of a body part.

EXPLANATION: Biological material from same individual ...

Body Part – 4TH	Approach – 5TH	Device – 6TH	Qualifier – 7TH
0 Subcutaneous Tissue and Fascia, Scalp	0 Open	7 Autologous tissue substitute	Z No qualifier
1 Subcutaneous Tissue and Fascia, Face	3 Percutaneous	J Synthetic substitute	
4 Subcutaneous Tissue and Fascia, Anterior Neck		K Nonautologous tissue substitute	
5 Subcutaneous Tissue and Fascia, Posterior Neck			
6 Subcutaneous Tissue and Fascia, Chest			
7 Subcutaneous Tissue and Fascia, Back			
8 Subcutaneous Tissue and Fascia, Abdomen			
9 Subcutaneous Tissue and Fascia, Buttock			
B Subcutaneous Tissue and Fascia, Perineum			
C Subcutaneous Tissue and Fascia, Pelvic Region			
D Subcutaneous Tissue and Fascia, Right Upper Arm			
F Subcutaneous Tissue and Fascia, Left Upper Arm			
G Subcutaneous Tissue and Fascia, Right Lower Arm			
H Subcutaneous Tissue and Fascia, Left Lower Arm			
J Subcutaneous Tissue and Fascia, Right Hand			
K Subcutaneous Tissue and Fascia, Left Hand			
L Subcutaneous Tissue and Fascia, Right Upper Leg			
M Subcutaneous Tissue and Fascia, Left Upper Leg			
N Subcutaneous Tissue and Fascia, Right Lower Leg			
P Subcutaneous Tissue and Fascia, Left Lower Leg			
Q Subcutaneous Tissue and Fascia, Right Foot			
R Subcutaneous Tissue and Fascia, Left Foot			

DEVICE GROUP: Change, Insertion, Removal, Replacement, Revision, Supplement
Root Operations that always involve a device.

1ST - 0 Medical and Surgical	EXAMPLE: Reposition stimulator generator CMS Ex: Adjustment lead
2ND - J Subcutaneous Tissue and Fascia	**REVISION:** Correcting, to the extent possible, a portion of a malfunctioning device or the position of a displaced device.
3RD - W REVISION	EXPLANATION: May replace components of a device ...

Body Part – 4TH	Approach – 5TH	Device – 6TH	Qualifier – 7TH
S Subcutaneous Tissue and Fascia, Head and Neck	0 Open 3 Percutaneous X External	0 Drainage device 3 Infusion device 7 Autologous tissue substitute J Synthetic substitute K Nonautologous tissue substitute N Tissue expander	Z No qualifier
T Subcutaneous Tissue and Fascia, Trunk	0 Open 3 Percutaneous X External	0 Drainage device 2 Monitoring device 3 Infusion device 7 Autologous tissue substitute H Contraceptive device J Synthetic substitute K Nonautologous tissue substitute M Stimulator generator N Tissue expander P Cardiac rhythm related device V Infusion device, pump W Vascular access device, reservoir X Vascular access device	Z No qualifier
V Subcutaneous Tissue and Fascia, Upper Extremity W Subcutaneous Tissue and Fascia, Lower Extremity	0 Open 3 Percutaneous X External	0 Drainage device 3 Infusion device 7 Autologous tissue substitute H Contraceptive device J Synthetic substitute K Nonautologous tissue substitute N Tissue expander V Infusion device, pump W Vascular access device, reservoir X Vascular access device	Z No qualifier

SUBCUTANEOUS 0 J W

MOVE GROUP: (Reattachment), (Reposition), **Transfer,** (Transplantation)
Root Operations that put in/put back or move some/all of a body part.

1ST - **0** Medical and Surgical

2ND - **J** Subcutaneous Tissue and Fascia

3RD - **X TRANSFER**

EXAMPLE: Fasciocutaneous pedicle flap | CMS Ex: Tendon transfer

TRANSFER: Moving, without taking out, all or a portion of a body part to another location to take over the function of all or a portion of a body part.

EXPLANATION: The body part remains connected ...

Body Part – 4TH	Approach – 5TH	Device – 6TH	Qualifier – 7TH
0 Subcutaneous Tissue and Fascia, Scalp	0 Open	Z No device	B Skin and Subcutaneous Tissue
1 Subcutaneous Tissue and Fascia, Face	3 Percutaneous		C Skin, Subcutaneous Tissue and Fascia
4 Subcutaneous Tissue and Fascia, Anterior Neck			Z No qualifier
5 Subcutaneous Tissue and Fascia, Posterior Neck			
6 Subcutaneous Tissue and Fascia, Chest			
7 Subcutaneous Tissue and Fascia, Back			
8 Subcutaneous Tissue and Fascia, Abdomen			
9 Subcutaneous Tissue and Fascia, Buttock			
B Subcutaneous Tissue and Fascia, Perineum			
C Subcutaneous Tissue and Fascia, Pelvic Region			
D Subcutaneous Tissue and Fascia, Right Upper Arm			
F Subcutaneous Tissue and Fascia, Left Upper Arm			
G Subcutaneous Tissue and Fascia, Right Lower Arm			
H Subcutaneous Tissue and Fascia, Left Lower Arm			
J Subcutaneous Tissue and Fascia, Right Hand			
K Subcutaneous Tissue and Fascia, Left Hand			
L Subcutaneous Tissue and Fascia, Right Upper Leg			
M Subcutaneous Tissue and Fascia, Left Upper Leg			
N Subcutaneous Tissue and Fascia, Right Lower Leg			
P Subcutaneous Tissue and Fascia, Left Lower Leg			
Q Subcutaneous Tissue and Fascia, Right Foot			
R Subcutaneous Tissue and Fascia, Left Foot			

Educational Annotations | K – Muscles

Body System Specific Educational Annotations for the Muscles include:
- Anatomy and Physiology Review
- Anatomical Illustrations
- Definitions of Common Procedures
- AHA Coding Clinic® Reference Notations
- Body Part Key Listings
- Device Key Listings
- Device Aggregation Table Listings
- Coding Notes

Anatomy and Physiology Review of Muscles

BODY PART VALUES – K - MUSCLES

Lower Muscle – The muscles located below the diaphragm (see Coding Guideline B2.1b).

Muscle – ANATOMY – Muscles are groups of skeletal muscle tissue, blood vessels, and nerves that are attached to the skeletal bones. Cardiac and smooth muscle tissue is also found in the heart and other organs. PHYSIOLOGY – The muscles contract to allow the movement of the human body.

Upper Muscle – The muscles located above the diaphragm (see Coding Guideline B2.1b).

Anatomical Illustrations of Muscles

None for the Muscles Body System

Definitions of Common Procedures of Muscles

Muscle transfer – The surgical detachment of the distal end of a muscle and subsequent connection to another nearby site while maintaining its vascular and nervous supply.

Muscle transplant – The surgical removal of a muscle with transplantation to a different site and, through microsurgery, connected to blood vessels and a nerve.

TRAM (transverse rectus abdominis myocutaneous) flap breast reconstruction – The post-mastectomy reconstruction of the breast using the transverse rectus abdominis muscle that is raised (including the overlying fat and skin) and transferred to the mastectomy site.

AHA Coding Clinic® Reference Notations of Muscles

ROOT OPERATION SPECIFIC - K - MUSCLES
CHANGE - 2
DESTRUCTION - 5
DIVISION - 8
DRAINAGE - 9
EXCISION - B
EXTIRPATION - C
INSERTION - H
INSPECTION - J
REATTACHMENT - M
RELEASE - N
   Biceps tenotomy...AHA 15:2Q:p22
   Repair of incisional hernia with component release and mesh....................AHA 14:4Q:p39
REMOVAL - P
REPAIR - Q
   Repair of second degree perineal laceration ....AHA 14:4Q:p43
   ....AHA 16:1Q:p6-8
   Repair of second degree perineal laceration including muscle....................AHA 13:4Q:p120
   Repair perineum muscle...AHA 16:2Q:p34
REPOSITION - S
RESECTION - T
   Infratemporal fossa malignancy with neck muscle......................................AHA 16:2Q:p12
   Resection of perineum muscle ....AHA 15:1Q:p38

Continued on next page

MUSCLES

0 K

Educational Annotations | K – Muscles

AHA Coding Clinic® Reference Notations of Muscles

Continued from previous page
SUPPLEMENT - U
REVISION - W
TRANSFER - X

Cleft lip repair, Millard technique	AHA 15:3Q:p33
Ipsilateral pedicle transverse abdominomyocutaneous (TRAM) flap breast reconstruction	AHA 14:2Q:p10
Pedicle latissimus myocutaneous flap breast reconstruction	AHA 14:2Q:p12
Perineal myocutaneous flap closure of abdominoperineal resection	AHA 14:4Q:p41
Posterior pharyngeal flap to the soft palate	AHA 15:2Q:p26

Body Part Key Listings of Muscles

See also Body Part Key in Appendix C

Abductor hallucis muscle	*use* Foot Muscle, Left/Right
Adductor brevis muscle	*use* Upper Leg Muscle, Left/Right
Adductor hallucis muscle	*use* Foot Muscle, Left/Right
Adductor longus muscle	*use* Upper Leg Muscle, Left/Right
Adductor magnus muscle	*use* Upper Leg Muscle, Left/Right
Anatomical snuffbox	*use* Lower Arm and Wrist Muscle, Left/Right
Anterior vertebral muscle	*use* Neck Muscle, Left/Right
Arytenoid muscle	*use* Neck Muscle, Left/Right
Auricularis muscle	*use* Head Muscle
Biceps brachii muscle	*use* Upper Arm Muscle, Left/Right
Biceps femoris muscle	*use* Upper Leg Muscle, Left/Right
Brachialis muscle	*use* Upper Arm Muscle, Left/Right
Brachioradialis muscle	*use* Lower Arm and Wrist Muscle, Left/Right
Buccinator muscle	*use* Facial Muscle
Bulbospongiosus muscle	*use* Perineum Muscle
Chondroglossus muscle	*use* Tongue, Palate, Pharynx Muscle
Coccygeus muscle	*use* Trunk Muscle, Left/Right
Coracobrachialis muscle	*use* Upper Arm Muscle, Left/Right
Corrugator supercilii muscle	*use* Facial Muscle
Cremaster muscle	*use* Perineum Muscle
Cricothyroid muscle	*use* Neck Muscle, Left/Right
Deep transverse perineal muscle	*use* Perineum Muscle
Deltoid muscle	*use* Shoulder Muscle, Left/Right
Depressor anguli oris muscle	*use* Facial Muscle
Depressor labii inferioris muscle	*use* Facial Muscle
Depressor septi nasi muscle	*use* Facial Muscle
Depressor supercilii muscle	*use* Facial Muscle
Erector spinae muscle	*use* Trunk Muscle, Left/Right
Extensor carpi radialis muscle	*use* Lower Arm and Wrist Muscle, Left/Right
Extensor carpi ulnaris muscle	*use* Lower Arm and Wrist Muscle, Left/Right
Extensor digitorum brevis muscle	*use* Foot Muscle, Left/Right
Extensor digitorum longus muscle	*use* Lower Leg Muscle, Left/Right
Extensor hallucis brevis muscle	*use* Foot Muscle, Left/Right
Extensor hallucis longus muscle	*use* Lower Leg Muscle, Left/Right
External oblique muscle	*use* Abdomen Muscle, Left/Right

Continued on next page

Educational Annotations | K – Muscles

Body Part Key Listings of Muscles

Continued from previous page

Fibularis brevis muscle..............................*use* Lower Leg Muscle, Left/Right	
Fibularis longus muscle ....*use* Lower Leg Muscle, Left/Right	
Flexor carpi radialis muscle ....*use* Lower Arm and Wrist Muscle, Left/Right	
Flexor carpi ulnaris muscle ....*use* Lower Arm and Wrist Muscle, Left/Right	
Flexor digitorum brevis muscle ....*use* Foot Muscle, Left/Right	
Flexor digitorum longus muscle ....*use* Lower Leg Muscle, Left/Right	
Flexor hallucis brevis muscle ....*use* Foot Muscle, Left/Right	
Flexor hallucis longus muscle.........................*use* Lower Leg Muscle, Left/Right	
Flexor pollicis longus muscle ....*use* Lower Arm and Wrist Muscle, Left/Right	
Gastrocnemius muscle ....*use* Lower Leg Muscle, Left/Right	
Gemellus muscle ....*use* Hip Muscle, Left/Right	
Genioglossus muscle ....*use* Tongue, Palate, Pharynx Muscle	
Gluteus maximus muscle ....*use* Hip Muscle, Left/Right	
Gluteus medius muscle ....*use* Hip Muscle, Left/Right	
Gluteus minimus muscle ....*use* Hip Muscle, Left/Right	
Gracilis muscle............................*use* Upper Leg Muscle, Left/Right	
Hyoglossus muscle............................*use* Tongue, Palate, Pharynx Muscle	
Hypothenar muscle ....*use* Hand Muscle, Left/Right	
Iliacus muscle............................*use* Hip Muscle, Left/Right	
Inferior longitudinal muscle............................*use* Tongue, Palate, Pharynx Muscle	
Infrahyoid muscle ....*use* Neck Muscle, Left/Right	
Infraspinatus muscle ....*use* Shoulder Muscle, Left/Right	
Intercostal muscle ....*use* Thorax Muscle, Left/Right	
Internal oblique muscle ....*use* Abdomen Muscle, Left/Right	
Interspinalis muscle ....*use* Trunk Muscle, Left/Right	
Intertransversarius muscle ....*use* Trunk Muscle, Left/Right	
Ischiocavernosus muscle ....*use* Perineum Muscle	
Latissimus dorsi muscle ....*use* Trunk Muscle, Left/Right	
Levator anguli oris muscle ....*use* Facial Muscle	
Levator ani muscle............................*use* Perineum Muscle	
Levator labii superioris alaeque nasi muscle ....*use* Facial Muscle	
Levator labii superioris muscle ....*use* Facial Muscle	
Levator scapulae muscle ....*use* Neck Muscle, Left/Right	
Levator veli palatini muscle ....*use* Tongue, Palate, Pharynx Muscle	
Levatores costarum muscle ....*use* Thorax Muscle, Left/Right	
Masseter muscle............................*use* Head Muscle	
Mentalis muscle ....*use* Facial Muscle	
Nasalis muscle............................*use* Facial Muscle	
Obturator muscle............................*use* Hip Muscle, Left/Right	
Occipitofrontalis muscle............................*use* Facial Muscle	
Orbicularis oris muscle ....*use* Facial Muscle	
Palatoglossal muscle ....*use* Tongue, Palate, Pharynx Muscle	
Palatopharyngeal muscle............................*use* Tongue, Palate, Pharynx Muscle	
Palmar interosseous muscle............................*use* Hand Muscle, Left/Right	
Palmaris longus muscle ....*use* Lower Arm and Wrist Muscle, Left/Right	
Pectineus muscle ....*use* Upper Leg Muscle, Left/Right	
Pectoralis major muscle ....*use* Thorax Muscle, Left/Right	
Pectoralis minor muscle ....*use* Thorax Muscle, Left/Right	

Continued on next page

Educational Annotations | K – Muscles

Body Part Key Listings of Muscles

Continued from previous page

Peroneus brevis muscle ....*use* Lower Leg Muscle, Left/Right
Peroneus longus muscle....................................*use* Lower Leg Muscle, Left/Right
Pharyngeal constrictor muscle ....*use* Tongue, Palate, Pharynx Muscle
Piriformis muscle ....*use* Hip Muscle, Left/Right
Platysma muscle...*use* Neck Muscle, Left/Right
Popliteus muscle...*use* Lower Leg Muscle, Left/Right
Procerus muscle ....*use* Facial Muscle
Pronator quadratus muscle ....*use* Lower Arm and Wrist Muscle, Left/Right
Pronator teres muscle ....*use* Lower Arm and Wrist Muscle, Left/Right
Psoas muscle ....*use* Hip Muscle, Left/Right
Pterygoid muscle ....*use* Head Muscle
Pyramidalis muscle ....*use* Abdomen Muscle, Left/Right
Quadratus femoris muscle...............................*use* Hip Muscle, Left/Right
Quadratus lumborum muscle ....*use* Trunk Muscle, Left/Right
Quadratus plantae muscle...............................*use* Foot Muscle, Left/Right
Quadriceps (femoris) ....*use* Upper Leg Muscle, Left/Right
Rectus abdominis muscle ....*use* Abdomen Muscle, Left/Right
Rectus femoris muscle ....*use* Upper Leg Muscle, Left/Right
Rhomboid major muscle ....*use* Trunk Muscle, Left/Right
Rhomboid minor muscle ....*use* Trunk Muscle, Left/Right
Risorius muscle ....*use* Facial Muscle
Salpingopharyngeus muscle ....*use* Tongue, Palate, Pharynx Muscle
Sartorius muscle..*use* Upper Leg Muscle, Left/Right
Scalene muscle...*use* Neck Muscle, Left/Right
Semimembranosus muscle ....*use* Upper Leg Muscle, Left/Right
Semitendinosus muscle ....*use* Upper Leg Muscle, Left/Right
Serratus anterior muscle ....*use* Thorax Muscle, Left/Right
Serratus posterior muscle ....*use* Trunk Muscle, Left/Right
Soleus muscle ....*use* Lower Leg Muscle, Left/Right
Splenius capitis muscle ....*use* Head Muscle
Splenius cervicis muscle..................................*use* Neck Muscle, Left/Right
Sternocleidomastoid muscle............................*use* Neck Muscle, Left/Right
Styloglossus muscle ....*use* Tongue, Palate, Pharynx Muscle
Stylopharyngeus muscle ....*use* Tongue, Palate, Pharynx Muscle
Subclavius muscle ....*use* Thorax Muscle, Left/Right
Subcostal muscle ....*use* Thorax Muscle, Left/Right
Subscapularis muscle......................................*use* Shoulder Muscle, Left/Right
Superficial transverse perineal muscle.............*use* Perineum Muscle
Superior longitudinal muscle ....*use* Tongue, Palate, Pharynx Muscle
Suprahyoid muscle...*use* Neck Muscle, Left/Right
Supraspinatus muscle ....*use* Shoulder Muscle, Left/Right
Temporalis muscle ....*use* Head Muscle
Temporoparietalis muscle ....*use* Head Muscle
Tensor fasciae latae muscle ....*use* Hip Muscle, Left/Right
Tensor veli palatini muscle...............................*use* Tongue, Palate, Pharynx Muscle
Teres major muscle ....*use* Shoulder Muscle, Left/Right
Teres minor muscle ....*use* Shoulder Muscle, Left/Right

Continued on next page

Educational Annotations | K – Muscles

Body Part Key Listings of Muscles

Continued from previous page

Thenar muscle ....*use* Hand Muscle, Left/Right
Thyroarytenoid muscle.......................................*use* Neck Muscle, Left/Right
Tibialis anterior muscle ....*use* Lower Leg Muscle, Left/Right
Tibialis posterior muscle ....*use* Lower Leg Muscle, Left/Right
Transverse thoracis muscle ....*use* Thorax Muscle, Left/Right
Transversospinalis muscle ....*use* Trunk Muscle, Left/Right
Transversus abdominis muscle.....................*use* Abdomen Muscle, Left/Right
Trapezius muscle ....*use* Trunk Muscle, Left/Right
Triceps brachii muscle ....*use* Upper Arm Muscle, Left/Right
Vastus intermedius muscle...............................*use* Upper Leg Muscle, Left/Right
Vastus lateralis muscle.....................................*use* Upper Leg Muscle, Left/Right
Vastus medialis muscle ....*use* Upper Leg Muscle, Left/Right
Zygomaticus muscle...*use* Facial Muscle

Device Key Listings of Muscles

See also Device Key in Appendix D

Autograft ....*use* Autologous Tissue Substitute
Electrical muscle stimulation (EMS) lead ....*use* Stimulator Lead in Muscles
Electronic muscle stimulator lead ....*use* Stimulator Lead in Muscles
Neuromuscular electrical stimulation (NEMS) lead *use* Stimulator Lead in Muscles
Tissue bank graft ....*use* Nonautologous Tissue Substitute

Device Aggregation Table Listings of Muscles

See also Device Aggregation Table in Appendix E

Specific Device	For Operation	In Body System	General Device
None Listed in Device Aggregation Table for this Body System			

Coding Notes of Muscles

Body System Relevant Coding Guidelines

General Guidelines

B2.1b

Where the general body part values "upper" and "lower" are provided as an option in the Upper Arteries, Lower Arteries, Upper Veins, Lower Veins, Muscles and Tendons body systems, "upper" and "lower" specifies body parts located above or below the diaphragm respectively.

Example: Vein body parts above the diaphragm are found in the Upper Veins body system; vein body parts below the diaphragm are found in the Lower Veins body system.

Body System Specific PCS Reference Manual Exercises

PCS CODE	K – MUSCLES EXERCISES
0KBS3ZX	Percutaneous biopsy of right gastrocnemius muscle.
0KMT0ZZ	Reattachment of traumatic left gastrocnemius avulsion, open.
0KXK0Z6	Bilateral TRAM pedicle flap reconstruction status post mastectomy, muscle only, open. (The
0KXL0Z6	transverse rectus abdominus muscle (TRAM) flap is coded for each flap developed.)

Educational Annotations | K – Muscles

NOTES

DEVICE GROUP: Change, Insertion, Removal, (Replacement), Revision, Supplement
Root Operations that always involve a device.

1ST - 0 Medical and Surgical	EXAMPLE: Exchange drain tube	CMS Ex: Changing urinary catheter
2ND - K Muscles 3RD - 2 CHANGE	**CHANGE:** Taking out or off a device from a body part and putting back an identical or similar device in or on the same body part without cutting or puncturing the skin or a mucous membrane.	
	EXPLANATION: ALL Changes use EXTERNAL approach only ...	

Body Part – 4TH	Approach – 5TH	Device – 6TH	Qualifier – 7TH
X Upper Muscle Y Lower Muscle	X External	0 Drainage device Y Other device	Z No qualifier

EXCISION GROUP: Excision, Resection, Destruction, (Extraction), (Detachment)
Root Operations that take out some or all of a body part.

1ST - 0 Medical and Surgical	EXAMPLE: Radiofrequency ablation	CMS Ex: Fulguration polyp
2ND - K Muscles 3RD - 5 DESTRUCTION	**DESTRUCTION:** Physical eradication of all or a portion of a body part by the direct use of energy, force, or a destructive agent.	
	EXPLANATION: None of the body part is physically taken out	

Body Part – 4TH	Approach – 5TH	Device – 6TH	Qualifier – 7TH
0 Head Muscle 1 Facial Muscle 2 Neck Muscle, Right 3 Neck Muscle, Left 4 Tongue, Palate, Pharynx Muscle 5 Shoulder Muscle, Right 6 Shoulder Muscle, Left 7 Upper Arm Muscle, Right 8 Upper Arm Muscle, Left 9 Lower Arm and Wrist Muscle, Right B Lower Arm and Wrist Muscle, Left C Hand Muscle, Right D Hand Muscle, Left F Trunk Muscle, Right G Trunk Muscle, Left H Thorax Muscle, Right J Thorax Muscle, Left K Abdomen Muscle, Right L Abdomen Muscle, Left M Perineum Muscle N Hip Muscle, Right P Hip Muscle, Left Q Upper Leg Muscle, Right R Upper Leg Muscle, Left S Lower Leg Muscle, Right T Lower Leg Muscle, Left V Foot Muscle, Right W Foot Muscle, Left	0 Open 3 Percutaneous 4 Percutaneous endoscopic	Z No device	Z No qualifier

MUSCLES 0 K 5

DIVISION GROUP: Division, Release
Root Operations involving cutting or separation only.

1ST - **0** Medical and Surgical	EXAMPLE: Myotomy hand muscle	CMS Ex: Osteotomy
2ND - **K** Muscles	**DIVISION:** Cutting into a body part without draining fluids and/or gases from the body part in order to separate or transect a body part.	
3RD - **8 DIVISION**	EXPLANATION: Separated into two or more portions ...	

Body Part – 4TH		Approach – 5TH	Device – 6TH	Qualifier – 7TH
0 Head Muscle	C Hand Muscle, Right	0 Open	Z No device	Z No qualifier
1 Facial Muscle	D Hand Muscle, Left	3 Percutaneous		
2 Neck Muscle, Right	F Trunk Muscle, Right	4 Percutaneous endoscopic		
3 Neck Muscle, Left	G Trunk Muscle, Left			
4 Tongue, Palate, Pharynx Muscle	H Thorax Muscle, Right			
	J Thorax Muscle, Left			
5 Shoulder Muscle, Right	K Abdomen Muscle, Right			
6 Shoulder Muscle, Left	L Abdomen Muscle, Left			
7 Upper Arm Muscle, Right	M Perineum Muscle			
8 Upper Arm Muscle, Left	N Hip Muscle, Right			
9 Lower Arm and Wrist Muscle, Right	P Hip Muscle, Left			
	Q Upper Leg Muscle, Right			
B Lower Arm and Wrist Muscle, Left	R Upper Leg Muscle, Left			
	S Lower Leg Muscle, Right			
	T Lower Leg Muscle, Left			
	V Foot Muscle, Right			
	W Foot Muscle, Left			

DRAINAGE GROUP: Drainage, Extirpation, (Fragmentation)		

Root Operations that take out solids/fluids/gases from a body part.

1ST - 0 Medical and Surgical

2ND - K Muscles

3RD - 9 DRAINAGE

EXAMPLE: Aspiration psoas muscle abscess   CMS Ex: Thoracentesis

DRAINAGE: Taking or letting out fluids and/or gases from a body part.

EXPLANATION: Qualifier "X Diagnostic" indicates biopsy ...

Body Part – 4TH		Approach – 5TH	Device – 6TH	Qualifier – 7TH
0 Head Muscle	C Hand Muscle, Right	0 Open	0 Drainage device	Z No qualifier
1 Facial Muscle	D Hand Muscle, Left	3 Percutaneous		
2 Neck Muscle, Right	F Trunk Muscle, Right	4 Percutaneous endoscopic		
3 Neck Muscle, Left	G Trunk Muscle, Left			
4 Tongue, Palate, Pharynx Muscle	H Thorax Muscle, Right			
	J Thorax Muscle, Left			
5 Shoulder Muscle, Right	K Abdomen Muscle, Right			
6 Shoulder Muscle, Left	L Abdomen Muscle, Left			
7 Upper Arm Muscle, Right	M Perineum Muscle			
8 Upper Arm Muscle, Left	N Hip Muscle, Right			
9 Lower Arm and Wrist Muscle, Right	P Hip Muscle, Left			
	Q Upper Leg Muscle, Right			
B Lower Arm and Wrist Muscle, Left	R Upper Leg Muscle, Left			
	S Lower Leg Muscle, Right			
	T Lower Leg Muscle, Left			
	V Foot Muscle, Right			
	W Foot Muscle, Left			
0 Head Muscle	C Hand Muscle, Right	0 Open	Z No device	X Diagnostic
1 Facial Muscle	D Hand Muscle, Left	3 Percutaneous		Z No qualifier
2 Neck Muscle, Right	F Trunk Muscle, Right	4 Percutaneous endoscopic		
3 Neck Muscle, Left	G Trunk Muscle, Left			
4 Tongue, Palate, Pharynx Muscle	H Thorax Muscle, Right			
	J Thorax Muscle, Left			
5 Shoulder Muscle, Right	K Abdomen Muscle, Right			
6 Shoulder Muscle, Left	L Abdomen Muscle, Left			
7 Upper Arm Muscle, Right	M Perineum Muscle			
8 Upper Arm Muscle, Left	N Hip Muscle, Right			
9 Lower Arm and Wrist Muscle, Right	P Hip Muscle, Left			
	Q Upper Leg Muscle, Right			
B Lower Arm and Wrist Muscle, Left	R Upper Leg Muscle, Left			
	S Lower Leg Muscle, Right			
	T Lower Leg Muscle, Left			
	V Foot Muscle, Right			
	W Foot Muscle, Left			

MUSCLES 0 K 9

EXCISION GROUP: Excision, Resection, Destruction, (Extraction), (Detachment)
Root Operations that take out some or all of a body part.

1ST - 0 Medical and Surgical

2ND - K Muscles

3RD - B EXCISION

EXAMPLE: Muscle biopsy   CMS Ex: Liver biopsy

EXCISION: Cutting out or off, without replacement, a portion of a body part.

EXPLANATION: Qualifier "X Diagnostic" indicates biopsy …

Body Part – 4TH		Approach – 5TH	Device – 6TH	Qualifier – 7TH
0 Head Muscle	C Hand Muscle, Right	0 Open	Z No device	X Diagnostic
1 Facial Muscle	D Hand Muscle, Left	3 Percutaneous		Z No qualifier
2 Neck Muscle, Right	F Trunk Muscle, Right	4 Percutaneous endoscopic		
3 Neck Muscle, Left	G Trunk Muscle, Left			
4 Tongue, Palate, Pharynx Muscle	H Thorax Muscle, Right			
	J Thorax Muscle, Left			
5 Shoulder Muscle, Right	K Abdomen Muscle, Right			
6 Shoulder Muscle, Left	L Abdomen Muscle, Left			
7 Upper Arm Muscle, Right	M Perineum Muscle			
8 Upper Arm Muscle, Left	N Hip Muscle, Right			
9 Lower Arm and Wrist Muscle, Right	P Hip Muscle, Left			
B Lower Arm and Wrist Muscle, Left	Q Upper Leg Muscle, Right			
	R Upper Leg Muscle, Left			
	S Lower Leg Muscle, Right			
	T Lower Leg Muscle, Left			
	V Foot Muscle, Right			
	W Foot Muscle, Left			

DRAINAGE GROUP: Drainage, Extirpation, (Fragmentation)
Root Operations that take out solids/fluids/gases from a body part.

1ST - 0 Medical and Surgical

2ND - K Muscles

3RD - C EXTIRPATION

EXAMPLE: Removal foreign body   CMS Ex: Choledocholithotomy

EXTIRPATION: Taking or cutting out solid matter from a body part.

EXPLANATION: Abnormal byproduct or foreign body …

Body Part – 4TH		Approach – 5TH	Device – 6TH	Qualifier – 7TH
0 Head Muscle	C Hand Muscle, Right	0 Open	Z No device	Z No qualifier
1 Facial Muscle	D Hand Muscle, Left	3 Percutaneous		
2 Neck Muscle, Right	F Trunk Muscle, Right	4 Percutaneous endoscopic		
3 Neck Muscle, Left	G Trunk Muscle, Left			
4 Tongue, Palate, Pharynx Muscle	H Thorax Muscle, Right			
	J Thorax Muscle, Left			
5 Shoulder Muscle, Right	K Abdomen Muscle, Right			
6 Shoulder Muscle, Left	L Abdomen Muscle, Left			
7 Upper Arm Muscle, Right	M Perineum Muscle			
8 Upper Arm Muscle, Left	N Hip Muscle, Right			
9 Lower Arm and Wrist Muscle, Right	P Hip Muscle, Left			
B Lower Arm and Wrist Muscle, Left	Q Upper Leg Muscle, Right			
	R Upper Leg Muscle, Left			
	S Lower Leg Muscle, Right			
	T Lower Leg Muscle, Left			
	V Foot Muscle, Right			
	W Foot Muscle, Left			

MUSCLES

0KB

© 2016 Channel Publishing, Ltd.

DEVICE GROUP: Change, Insertion, Removal, (Replacement), Revision, Supplement
Root Operations that always involve a device.

1ST - **0** Medical and Surgical

2ND - **K** Muscles

3RD - **H INSERTION**

EXAMPLE: Insertion stimulator lead	CMS Ex: Central venous catheter

INSERTION: Putting in a nonbiological appliance that monitors, assists, performs, or prevents a physiological function but does not physically take the place of a body part.

EXPLANATION: None

Body Part – 4TH	Approach – 5TH	Device – 6TH	Qualifier – 7TH
X Upper Muscle Y Lower Muscle	0 Open 3 Percutaneous 4 Percutaneous endoscopic	M Stimulator lead	Z No qualifier

EXAMINATION GROUP: Inspection, (Map)
Root Operations involving examination only.

1ST - **0** Medical and Surgical

2ND - **K** Muscles

3RD - **J INSPECTION**

EXAMPLE: Examination pelvic floor muscle	CMS Ex: Colonoscopy

INSPECTION: Visually and/or manually exploring a body part.

EXPLANATION: Direct or instrumental visualization ...

Body Part – 4TH	Approach – 5TH	Device – 6TH	Qualifier – 7TH
X Upper Muscle Y Lower Muscle	0 Open 3 Percutaneous 4 Percutaneous endoscopic X External	Z No device	Z No qualifier

MUSCLES

0 K J

MOVE GROUP: Reattachment, Reposition, Transfer, (Transplantation)
Root Operations that put in/put back or move some/all of a body part.

1ST - **0** Medical and Surgical	**EXAMPLE:** Reattachment arm muscle	**CMS Ex:** Reattachment hand
2ND - **K** Muscles	**REATTACHMENT:** Putting back in or on all or a portion of a separated body part to its normal location or other suitable location.	
3RD - **M REATTACHMENT**	**EXPLANATION:** With/without reconnection of vessels/nerves...	

Body Part – 4TH		Approach – 5TH	Device – 6TH	Qualifier – 7TH
0 Head Muscle	C Hand Muscle, Right	0 Open	Z No device	Z No qualifier
1 Facial Muscle	D Hand Muscle, Left	4 Percutaneous endoscopic		
2 Neck Muscle, Right	F Trunk Muscle, Right			
3 Neck Muscle, Left	G Trunk Muscle, Left			
4 Tongue, Palate, Pharynx Muscle	H Thorax Muscle, Right			
	J Thorax Muscle, Left			
5 Shoulder Muscle, Right	K Abdomen Muscle, Right			
6 Shoulder Muscle, Left	L Abdomen Muscle, Left			
7 Upper Arm Muscle, Right	M Perineum Muscle			
8 Upper Arm Muscle, Left	N Hip Muscle, Right			
9 Lower Arm and Wrist Muscle, Right	P Hip Muscle, Left			
	Q Upper Leg Muscle, Right			
B Lower Arm and Wrist Muscle, Left	R Upper Leg Muscle, Left			
	S Lower Leg Muscle, Right			
	T Lower Leg Muscle, Left			
	V Foot Muscle, Right			
	W Foot Muscle, Left			

DIVISION GROUP: Division, Release
Root Operations involving cutting or separation only.

1ST - **0** Medical and Surgical	**EXAMPLE:** Component muscle separation	**CMS Ex:** Carpal tunnel release
2ND - **K** Muscles	**RELEASE:** Freeing a body part from an abnormal physical constraint by cutting or by the use of force.	
3RD - **N RELEASE**	**EXPLANATION:** None of the body part is taken out ...	

Body Part – 4TH		Approach – 5TH	Device – 6TH	Qualifier – 7TH
0 Head Muscle	C Hand Muscle, Right	0 Open	Z No device	Z No qualifier
1 Facial Muscle	D Hand Muscle, Left	3 Percutaneous		
2 Neck Muscle, Right	F Trunk Muscle, Right	4 Percutaneous endoscopic		
3 Neck Muscle, Left	G Trunk Muscle, Left	X External		
4 Tongue, Palate, Pharynx Muscle	H Thorax Muscle, Right			
	J Thorax Muscle, Left			
5 Shoulder Muscle, Right	K Abdomen Muscle, Right			
6 Shoulder Muscle, Left	L Abdomen Muscle, Left			
7 Upper Arm Muscle, Right	M Perineum Muscle			
8 Upper Arm Muscle, Left	N Hip Muscle, Right			
9 Lower Arm and Wrist Muscle, Right	P Hip Muscle, Left			
	Q Upper Leg Muscle, Right			
B Lower Arm and Wrist Muscle, Left	R Upper Leg Muscle, Left			
	S Lower Leg Muscle, Right			
	T Lower Leg Muscle, Left			
	V Foot Muscle, Right			
	W Foot Muscle, Left			

DEVICE GROUP: Change, Insertion, Removal, (Replacement), Revision, Supplement
Root Operations that always involve a device.

1ST - **0** Medical and Surgical

2ND - **K** Muscles

3RD - **P REMOVAL**

EXAMPLE: Removal stimulator lead | CMS Ex: Chest tube removal

REMOVAL: Taking out or off a device from a body part.

EXPLANATION: Removal device without reinsertion ...

Body Part – 4TH	Approach – 5TH	Device – 6TH	Qualifier – 7TH
X Upper Muscle Y Lower Muscle	0 Open 3 Percutaneous 4 Percutaneous endoscopic	0 Drainage device 7 Autologous tissue substitute J Synthetic substitute K Nonautologous tissue substitute M Stimulator lead	Z No qualifier
X Upper Muscle Y Lower Muscle	X External	0 Drainage device M Stimulator lead	Z No qualifier

OTHER REPAIRS GROUP: (Control), Repair
Root Operations that define other repairs.

1ST - **0** Medical and Surgical

2ND - **K** Muscles

3RD - **Q REPAIR**

EXAMPLE: Repair second degree perineum muscle | CMS Ex: Suture

REPAIR: Restoring, to the extent possible, a body part to its normal anatomic structure and function.

EXPLANATION: Only when no other root operation applies ...

Body Part – 4TH	Approach – 5TH	Device – 6TH	Qualifier – 7TH
0 Head Muscle 1 Facial Muscle 2 Neck Muscle, Right 3 Neck Muscle, Left 4 Tongue, Palate, Pharynx Muscle 5 Shoulder Muscle, Right 6 Shoulder Muscle, Left 7 Upper Arm Muscle, Right 8 Upper Arm Muscle, Left 9 Lower Arm and Wrist Muscle, Right B Lower Arm and Wrist Muscle, Left C Hand Muscle, Right D Hand Muscle, Left F Trunk Muscle, Right G Trunk Muscle, Left H Thorax Muscle, Right J Thorax Muscle, Left K Abdomen Muscle, Right L Abdomen Muscle, Left M Perineum Muscle N Hip Muscle, Right P Hip Muscle, Left Q Upper Leg Muscle, Right R Upper Leg Muscle, Left S Lower Leg Muscle, Right T Lower Leg Muscle, Left V Foot Muscle, Right W Foot Muscle, Left	0 Open 3 Percutaneous 4 Percutaneous endoscopic	Z No device	Z No qualifier

---

MOVE GROUP: Reattachment, Reposition, Transfer, (Transplantation)
Root Operations that put in/put back or move some/all of a body part.

1ST - 0 Medical and Surgical

2ND - K Muscles

3RD - S REPOSITION

EXAMPLE: Relocation shoulder muscle | CMS Ex: Fracture reduction

REPOSITION: Moving to its normal location, or other suitable location, all or a portion of a body part.

EXPLANATION: May or may not be cut to be moved ...

Body Part – 4TH		Approach – 5TH	Device – 6TH	Qualifier – 7TH
0 Head Muscle	C Hand Muscle, Right	0 Open	Z No device	Z No qualifier
1 Facial Muscle	D Hand Muscle, Left	4 Percutaneous endoscopic		
2 Neck Muscle, Right	F Trunk Muscle, Right			
3 Neck Muscle, Left	G Trunk Muscle, Left			
4 Tongue, Palate, Pharynx Muscle	H Thorax Muscle, Right			
	J Thorax Muscle, Left			
5 Shoulder Muscle, Right	K Abdomen Muscle, Right			
6 Shoulder Muscle, Left	L Abdomen Muscle, Left			
7 Upper Arm Muscle, Right	M Perineum Muscle			
8 Upper Arm Muscle, Left	N Hip Muscle, Right			
9 Lower Arm and Wrist Muscle, Right	P Hip Muscle, Left			
	Q Upper Leg Muscle, Right			
B Lower Arm and Wrist Muscle, Left	R Upper Leg Muscle, Left			
	S Lower Leg Muscle, Right			
	T Lower Leg Muscle, Left			
	V Foot Muscle, Right			
	W Foot Muscle, Left			

EXCISION GROUP: Excision, Resection, Destruction, (Extraction), (Detachment)
Root Operations that take out some or all of a body part.

1ST - 0 Medical and Surgical

2ND - K Muscles

3RD - T RESECTION

EXAMPLE: Resection perineum muscle | CMS Ex: Cholecystectomy

RESECTION: Cutting out or off, without replacement, all of a body part.

EXPLANATION: None

Body Part – 4TH		Approach – 5TH	Device – 6TH	Qualifier – 7TH
0 Head Muscle	C Hand Muscle, Right	0 Open	Z No device	Z No qualifier
1 Facial Muscle	D Hand Muscle, Left	4 Percutaneous endoscopic		
2 Neck Muscle, Right	F Trunk Muscle, Right			
3 Neck Muscle, Left	G Trunk Muscle, Left			
4 Tongue, Palate, Pharynx Muscle	H Thorax Muscle, Right			
	J Thorax Muscle, Left			
5 Shoulder Muscle, Right	K Abdomen Muscle, Right			
6 Shoulder Muscle, Left	L Abdomen Muscle, Left			
7 Upper Arm Muscle, Right	M Perineum Muscle			
8 Upper Arm Muscle, Left	N Hip Muscle, Right			
9 Lower Arm and Wrist Muscle, Right	P Hip Muscle, Left			
	Q Upper Leg Muscle, Right			
B Lower Arm and Wrist Muscle, Left	R Upper Leg Muscle, Left			
	S Lower Leg Muscle, Right			
	T Lower Leg Muscle, Left			
	V Foot Muscle, Right			
	W Foot Muscle, Left			

DEVICE GROUP: Change, Insertion, Removal, (Replacement), Revision, Supplement
Root Operations that always involve a device.

1ST - 0 Medical and Surgical

2ND - K Muscles

3RD - U SUPPLEMENT

EXAMPLE: Gracilis muscle graft to face | CMS Ex: Hernia repair with mesh

SUPPLEMENT: Putting in or on biological or synthetic material that physically reinforces and/or augments the function of a portion of a body part.

EXPLANATION: Biological material from same individual ...

Body Part – 4TH		Approach – 5TH	Device – 6TH	Qualifier – 7TH
0 Head Muscle	C Hand Muscle, Right	0 Open	7 Autologous tissue substitute	Z No qualifier
1 Facial Muscle	D Hand Muscle, Left	4 Percutaneous endoscopic	J Synthetic substitute	
2 Neck Muscle, Right	F Trunk Muscle, Right		K Nonautologous tissue substitute	
3 Neck Muscle, Left	G Trunk Muscle, Left			
4 Tongue, Palate, Pharynx Muscle	H Thorax Muscle, Right			
	J Thorax Muscle, Left			
5 Shoulder Muscle, Right	K Abdomen Muscle, Right			
6 Shoulder Muscle, Left	L Abdomen Muscle, Left			
7 Upper Arm Muscle, Right	M Perineum Muscle			
8 Upper Arm Muscle, Left	N Hip Muscle, Right			
9 Lower Arm and Wrist Muscle, Right	P Hip Muscle, Left			
B Lower Arm and Wrist Muscle, Left	Q Upper Leg Muscle, Right			
	R Upper Leg Muscle, Left			
	S Lower Leg Muscle, Right			
	T Lower Leg Muscle, Left			
	V Foot Muscle, Right			
	W Foot Muscle, Left			

DEVICE GROUP: Change, Insertion, Removal, (Replacement), Revision, Supplement
Root Operations that always involve a device.

1ST - 0 Medical and Surgical

2ND - K Muscles

3RD - W REVISION

EXAMPLE: Reposition stimulator lead | CMS Ex: Adjustment pacemaker lead

REVISION: Correcting, to the extent possible, a portion of a malfunctioning device or the position of a displaced device.

EXPLANATION: May replace components of a device ...

Body Part – 4TH	Approach – 5TH	Device – 6TH	Qualifier – 7TH
X Upper Muscle	0 Open	0 Drainage device	Z No qualifier
Y Lower Muscle	3 Percutaneous	7 Autologous tissue substitute	
	4 Percutaneous endoscopic	J Synthetic substitute	
	X External	K Nonautologous tissue substitute	
		M Stimulator lead	

M U S C L E S

0 K W

MOVE GROUP: Reattachment, Reposition, Transfer, (Transplantation)
Root Operations that put in/put back or move some/all of a body part.

| 1ST - 0 Medical and Surgical | EXAMPLE: TRAM flap breast reconstruction | CMS Ex: Tendon transfer |

1ST - 0 Medical and Surgical

2ND - K Muscles

3RD - X TRANSFER

EXAMPLE: TRAM flap breast reconstruction | CMS Ex: Tendon transfer

TRANSFER: Moving, without taking out, all or a portion of a body part to another location to take over the function of all or a portion of a body part.

EXPLANATION: The body part remains connected ...

Body Part – 4TH		Approach – 5TH	Device – 6TH	Qualifier – 7TH
0 Head Muscle 1 Facial Muscle 2 Neck Muscle, Right 3 Neck Muscle, Left 4 Tongue, Palate, Pharynx Muscle 5 Shoulder Muscle, Right 6 Shoulder Muscle, Left 7 Upper Arm Muscle, Right 8 Upper Arm Muscle, Left 9 Lower Arm and Wrist Muscle, Right B Lower Arm and Wrist Muscle, Left	C Hand Muscle, Right D Hand Muscle, Left F Trunk Muscle, Right G Trunk Muscle, Left H Thorax Muscle, Right J Thorax Muscle, Left M Perineum Muscle N Hip Muscle, Right P Hip Muscle, Left Q Upper Leg Muscle, Right R Upper Leg Muscle, Left S Lower Leg Muscle, Right T Lower Leg Muscle, Left V Foot Muscle, Right W Foot Muscle, Left	0 Open 4 Percutaneous endoscopic	Z No device	0 Skin 1 Subcutaneous Tissue 2 Skin and Subcutaneous Tissue Z No qualifier
K Abdomen Muscle, Right L Abdomen Muscle, Left		0 Open 4 Percutaneous endoscopic	Z No device	0 Skin 1 Subcutaneous Tissue 2 Skin and Subcutaneous Tissue 6 Transverse Rectus Abdominis Myocutaneous Flap Z No qualifier

MUSCLES 0KX

Educational Annotations | L – Tendons

Body System Specific Educational Annotations for the Tendons include:

- Anatomy and Physiology Review
- Anatomical Illustrations
- Definitions of Common Procedures
- AHA Coding Clinic® Reference Notations
- Body Part Key Listings
- Device Key Listings
- Device Aggregation Table Listings
- Coding Notes

Anatomy and Physiology Review of Tendons

BODY PART VALUES – L - TENDONS

Lower Tendon – The tendons located below the diaphragm (see Coding Guideline B2.1b).

Tendon – ANATOMY – A tendon is a strong, yet somewhat flexible cord or band of fibrous connective tissue that most often connects muscle to bone. PHYSIOLOGY – Tendons and muscles work together to move the bones.

Upper Tendon – The tendons located above the diaphragm (see Coding Guideline B2.1b).

Anatomical Illustrations of Tendons

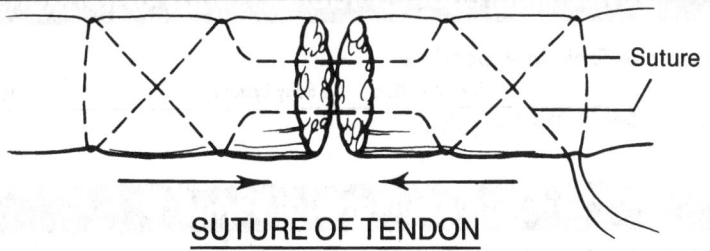

Suture

SUTURE OF TENDON

Definitions of Common Procedures of Tendons

Bridle procedure tendon transfer – The surgical transfer of the distal ends of the posterior tibial, peroneus longus, and the anterior tibialis tendons in a "bridle" configuration to correct the condition of foot drop.

Free tendon graft – The surgical placement of a section of tendon (from another part of the body or donor) to repair a damaged tendon.

AHA Coding Clinic® Reference Notations of Tendons

ROOT OPERATION SPECIFIC - L - TENDONS
CHANGE - 2
DESTRUCTION - 5
DIVISION - 8
DRAINAGE - 9
EXCISION - B
    Excision of tendon for graft ....AHA 15:3Q:p26
    Excisional debridement of nonhealing wound that included tendon...........AHA 14:3Q:p18
    Excisional debridement of ulceration that included tendon ....AHA 14:3Q:p14
EXTIRPATION - C
INSPECTION - H
REATTACHMENT - M
RELEASE - N
REMOVAL - P
REPAIR - Q
    Arthroscopic rotator cuff suture repair ....AHA 13:3Q:p20
REPLACEMENT - R
REPOSITION - S
    Repair by reposition of torn biceps muscle ....AHA 15:3Q:p14
RESECTION - T
SUPPLEMENT - U
    Patellar tendon augmentation with allograft ....AHA 15:2Q:p11
REVISION - W
TRANSFER - X

Educational Annotations | L – Tendons

Body Part Key Listings of Tendons

See also Body Part Key in Appendix C

Achilles tendon ....*use* Lower Leg Tendon, Left/Right

Patellar tendon...*use* Knee Tendon, Left/Right

Device Key Listings of Tendons

See also Device Key in Appendix D

Autograft ....*use* Autologous Tissue Substitute

Tissue bank graft ....*use* Nonautologous Tissue Substitute

Device Aggregation Table Listings of Tendons

See also Device Aggregation Table in Appendix E

Specific Device	For Operation	In Body System	General Device
None Listed in Device Aggregation Table for this Body System			

Coding Notes of Tendons

Body System Relevant Coding Guidelines

General Guidelines
B2.1b

Where the general body part values "upper" and "lower" are provided as an option in the Upper Arteries, Lower Arteries, Upper Veins, Lower Veins, Muscles and Tendons body systems, "upper" and "lower" specifies body parts located above or below the diaphragm respectively.

Example: Vein body parts above the diaphragm are found in the Upper Veins body system; vein body parts below the diaphragm are found in the Lower Veins body system.

Tendons, ligaments, bursae and fascia near a joint
B4.5

Procedures performed on tendons, ligaments, bursae and fascia supporting a joint are coded to the body part in the respective body system that is the focus of the procedure. Procedures performed on joint structures themselves are coded to the body part in the joint body systems.

Examples: Repair of the anterior cruciate ligament of the knee is coded to the knee bursa and ligament body part in the bursae and ligaments body system.

Knee arthroscopy with shaving of articular cartilage is coded to the knee joint body part in the Lower Joints body system.

Body System Specific PCS Reference Manual Exercises

PCS CODE	L – TENDONS EXERCISES
0 L 8 V 3 Z Z	Division of right foot tendon, percutaneous.
0 L B N 0 Z Z	Open excision of lesion from right Achilles tendon.
0 L N P 3 Z Z	Percutaneous left Achilles tendon release.
0 L Q 3 0 Z Z	Suture repair of right biceps tendon laceration, open.
0 L R S 0 K Z	Tenonectomy with graft to right ankle using cadaver graft, open.
0 L U 2 0 7 Z	Tendon graft to strengthen injured left shoulder using autograft, open (do not code graft harvest for this exercise).
0 L X 7 0 Z Z	Right hand open palmaris longus tendon transfer.
0 L X P 4 Z Z	Endoscopic left leg flexor hallucis longus tendon transfer.

DEVICE GROUP: Change, (Insertion), Removal, Replacement, Revision, Supplement
Root Operations that always involve a device.

1ST - 0 Medical and Surgical

2ND - L Tendons

3RD - 2 CHANGE

EXAMPLE: Exchange drain tube	CMS Ex: Changing urinary catheter

CHANGE: Taking out or off a device from a body part and putting back an identical or similar device in or on the same body part without cutting or puncturing the skin or a mucous membrane.

EXPLANATION: ALL Changes use EXTERNAL approach only ...

Body Part – 4TH	Approach – 5TH	Device – 6TH	Qualifier – 7TH
X Upper Tendon Y Lower Tendon	X External	0 Drainage device Y Other device	Z No qualifier

EXCISION GROUP: Excision, Resection, Destruction, (Extraction), (Detachment)
Root Operations that take out some or all of a body part.

1ST - 0 Medical and Surgical

2ND - L Tendons

3RD - 5 DESTRUCTION

EXAMPLE: Radiofrequency ablation	CMS Ex: Fulguration polyp

DESTRUCTION: Physical eradication of all or a portion of a body part by the direct use of energy, force, or a destructive agent.

EXPLANATION: None of the body part is physically taken out

Body Part – 4TH	Approach – 5TH	Device – 6TH	Qualifier – 7TH

0 Head and Neck Tendon   F Abdomen Tendon, Right
1 Shoulder Tendon, Right   G Abdomen Tendon, Left
2 Shoulder Tendon, Left   H Perineum Tendon
3 Upper Arm Tendon, Right   J Hip Tendon, Right
4 Upper Arm Tendon, Left   K Hip Tendon, Left
5 Lower Arm and Wrist   L Upper Leg Tendon, Right
   Tendon, Right   M Upper Leg Tendon, Left
6 Lower Arm and Wrist   N Lower Leg Tendon, Right
   Tendon, Left   P Lower Leg Tendon, Left
7 Hand Tendon, Right   Q Knee Tendon, Right
8 Hand Tendon, Left   R Knee Tendon, Left
9 Trunk Tendon, Right   S Ankle Tendon, Right
B Trunk Tendon, Left   T Ankle Tendon, Left
C Thorax Tendon, Right   V Foot Tendon, Right
D Thorax Tendon, Left   W Foot Tendon, Left
	0 Open
	3 Percutaneous
	4 Percutaneous
	   endoscopic
		Z No device	Z No qualifier

TENDONS 0 L 5

DIVISION GROUP: Division, Release
Root Operations involving cutting or separation only.

1ST - 0 Medical and Surgical	EXAMPLE: Division Achilles tendon	CMS Ex: Osteotomy

2ND - L Tendons

3RD - 8 DIVISION

DIVISION: Cutting into a body part without draining fluids and/or gases from the body part in order to separate or transect a body part.

EXPLANATION: Separated into two or more portions ...

Body Part – 4TH	Approach – 5TH	Device – 6TH	Qualifier – 7TH
0 Head and Neck Tendon 1 Shoulder Tendon, Right 2 Shoulder Tendon, Left 3 Upper Arm Tendon, Right 4 Upper Arm Tendon, Left 5 Lower Arm and Wrist Tendon, Right 6 Lower Arm and Wrist Tendon, Left 7 Hand Tendon, Right 8 Hand Tendon, Left 9 Trunk Tendon, Right B Trunk Tendon, Left C Thorax Tendon, Right D Thorax Tendon, Left F Abdomen Tendon, Right G Abdomen Tendon, Left H Perineum Tendon J Hip Tendon, Right K Hip Tendon, Left L Upper Leg Tendon, Right M Upper Leg Tendon, Left N Lower Leg Tendon, Right P Lower Leg Tendon, Left Q Knee Tendon, Right R Knee Tendon, Left S Ankle Tendon, Right T Ankle Tendon, Left V Foot Tendon, Right W Foot Tendon, Left	0 Open 3 Percutaneous 4 Percutaneous endoscopic	Z No device	Z No qualifier

DRAINAGE GROUP: Drainage, Extirpation, (Fragmentation)
Root Operations that take out solids/fluids/gases from a body part.

1ST - **0** Medical and Surgical	EXAMPLE: I&D tendon sheath abscess　　CMS Ex: Thoracentesis
2ND - **L** Tendons	**DRAINAGE:** Taking or letting out fluids and/or gases from a body part.
3RD - **9 DRAINAGE**	EXPLANATION: Qualifier "X Diagnostic" indicates biopsy ...

Body Part – 4TH		Approach – 5TH	Device – 6TH	Qualifier – 7TH
0　Head and Neck Tendon 1　Shoulder Tendon, Right 2　Shoulder Tendon, Left 3　Upper Arm Tendon, Right 4　Upper Arm Tendon, Left 5　Lower Arm and Wrist 　　Tendon, Right 6　Lower Arm and Wrist 　　Tendon, Left 7　Hand Tendon, Right 8　Hand Tendon, Left 9　Trunk Tendon, Right B　Trunk Tendon, Left C　Thorax Tendon, Right D　Thorax Tendon, Left	F　Abdomen Tendon, Right G　Abdomen Tendon, Left H　Perineum Tendon J　Hip Tendon, Right K　Hip Tendon, Left L　Upper Leg Tendon, Right M　Upper Leg Tendon, Left N　Lower Leg Tendon, Right P　Lower Leg Tendon, Left Q　Knee Tendon, Right R　Knee Tendon, Left S　Ankle Tendon, Right T　Ankle Tendon, Left V　Foot Tendon, Right W　Foot Tendon, Left	0　Open 3　Percutaneous 4　Percutaneous 　　endoscopic	0　Drainage device	Z　No qualifier
0　Head and Neck Tendon 1　Shoulder Tendon, Right 2　Shoulder Tendon, Left 3　Upper Arm Tendon, Right 4　Upper Arm Tendon, Left 5　Lower Arm and Wrist 　　Tendon, Right 6　Lower Arm and Wrist 　　Tendon, Left 7　Hand Tendon, Right 8　Hand Tendon, Left 9　Trunk Tendon, Right B　Trunk Tendon, Left C　Thorax Tendon, Right D　Thorax Tendon, Left	F　Abdomen Tendon, Right G　Abdomen Tendon, Left H　Perineum Tendon J　Hip Tendon, Right K　Hip Tendon, Left L　Upper Leg Tendon, Right M　Upper Leg Tendon, Left N　Lower Leg Tendon, Right P　Lower Leg Tendon, Left Q　Knee Tendon, Right R　Knee Tendon, Left S　Ankle Tendon, Right T　Ankle Tendon, Left V　Foot Tendon, Right W　Foot Tendon, Left	0　Open 3　Percutaneous 4　Percutaneous 　　endoscopic	Z　No device	X　Diagnostic Z　No qualifier

TENDONS

0 L 9

EXCISION GROUP: Excision, Resection, Destruction, (Extraction), (Detachment)
Root Operations that take out some or all of a body part.

1ST - 0 Medical and Surgical	EXAMPLE: Ganglionectomy tendon sheath	CMS Ex: Liver biopsy
2ND - L Tendons	**EXCISION:** Cutting out or off, without replacement, a portion of a body part.	
3RD - B EXCISION	EXPLANATION: Qualifier "X Diagnostic" indicates biopsy …	

Body Part – 4TH		Approach – 5TH	Device – 6TH	Qualifier – 7TH
0 Head and Neck Tendon	F Abdomen Tendon, Right	0 Open	Z No device	X Diagnostic
1 Shoulder Tendon, Right	G Abdomen Tendon, Left	3 Percutaneous		Z No qualifier
2 Shoulder Tendon, Left	H Perineum Tendon	4 Percutaneous endoscopic		
3 Upper Arm Tendon, Right	J Hip Tendon, Right			
4 Upper Arm Tendon, Left	K Hip Tendon, Left			
5 Lower Arm and Wrist Tendon, Right	L Upper Leg Tendon, Right			
	M Upper Leg Tendon, Left			
6 Lower Arm and Wrist Tendon, Left	N Lower Leg Tendon, Right			
	P Lower Leg Tendon, Left			
7 Hand Tendon, Right	Q Knee Tendon, Right			
8 Hand Tendon, Left	R Knee Tendon, Left			
9 Trunk Tendon, Right	S Ankle Tendon, Right			
B Trunk Tendon, Left	T Ankle Tendon, Left			
C Thorax Tendon, Right	V Foot Tendon, Right			
D Thorax Tendon, Left	W Foot Tendon, Left			

DRAINAGE GROUP: Drainage, Extirpation, (Fragmentation)
Root Operations that take out solids/fluids/gases from a body part.

1ST - 0 Medical and Surgical	EXAMPLE: Removal calcium tendon deposits	CMS Ex: Choledocholithotomy
2ND - L Tendons	**EXTIRPATION:** Taking or cutting out solid matter from a body part.	
3RD - C EXTIRPATION	EXPLANATION: Abnormal byproduct or foreign body …	

Body Part – 4TH		Approach – 5TH	Device – 6TH	Qualifier – 7TH
0 Head and Neck Tendon	F Abdomen Tendon, Right	0 Open	Z No device	Z No qualifier
1 Shoulder Tendon, Right	G Abdomen Tendon, Left	3 Percutaneous		
2 Shoulder Tendon, Left	H Perineum Tendon	4 Percutaneous endoscopic		
3 Upper Arm Tendon, Right	J Hip Tendon, Right			
4 Upper Arm Tendon, Left	K Hip Tendon, Left			
5 Lower Arm and Wrist Tendon, Right	L Upper Leg Tendon, Right			
	M Upper Leg Tendon, Left			
6 Lower Arm and Wrist Tendon, Left	N Lower Leg Tendon, Right			
	P Lower Leg Tendon, Left			
7 Hand Tendon, Right	Q Knee Tendon, Right			
8 Hand Tendon, Left	R Knee Tendon, Left			
9 Trunk Tendon, Right	S Ankle Tendon, Right			
B Trunk Tendon, Left	T Ankle Tendon, Left			
C Thorax Tendon, Right	V Foot Tendon, Right			
D Thorax Tendon, Left	W Foot Tendon, Left			

TENDONS

0 L B

EXAMINATION GROUP: Inspection, (Map)
Root Operations involving examination only.

1ST - **0** Medical and Surgical	EXAMPLE: Exploration tendon attachments	CMS Ex: Colonoscopy
2ND - **L** Tendons	**INSPECTION:** Visually and/or manually exploring a body part.	
3RD - **J INSPECTION**	EXPLANATION: Direct or instrumental visualization ...	

Body Part – 4TH	Approach – 5TH	Device – 6TH	Qualifier – 7TH
X Upper Tendon Y Lower Tendon	0 Open 3 Percutaneous 4 Percutaneous endoscopic X External	Z No device	Z No qualifier

---

MOVE GROUP: Reattachment, Reposition, Transfer, (Transplantation)
Root Operations that put in/put back or move some/all of a body part.

1ST - **0** Medical and Surgical	EXAMPLE: Re-anchor torn tendon	CMS Ex: Reattachment hand
2ND - **L** Tendons	**REATTACHMENT:** Putting back in or on all or a portion of a separated body part to its normal location or other suitable location.	
3RD - **M REATTACHMENT**	EXPLANATION: With/without reconnection of vessels/nerves...	

Body Part – 4TH	Approach – 5TH	Device – 6TH	Qualifier – 7TH
0 Head and Neck Tendon 1 Shoulder Tendon, Right 2 Shoulder Tendon, Left 3 Upper Arm Tendon, Right 4 Upper Arm Tendon, Left 5 Lower Arm and Wrist Tendon, Right 6 Lower Arm and Wrist Tendon, Left 7 Hand Tendon, Right 8 Hand Tendon, Left 9 Trunk Tendon, Right B Trunk Tendon, Left C Thorax Tendon, Right D Thorax Tendon, Left F Abdomen Tendon, Right G Abdomen Tendon, Left H Perineum Tendon J Hip Tendon, Right K Hip Tendon, Left L Upper Leg Tendon, Right M Upper Leg Tendon, Left N Lower Leg Tendon, Right P Lower Leg Tendon, Left Q Knee Tendon, Right R Knee Tendon, Left S Ankle Tendon, Right T Ankle Tendon, Left V Foot Tendon, Right W Foot Tendon, Left	0 Open 4 Percutaneous endoscopic	Z No device	Z No qualifier

DIVISION GROUP: Division, Release
Root Operations involving cutting or separation only.

1ST - **0** Medical and Surgical

2ND - **L** Tendons

3RD - **N RELEASE**

EXAMPLE: Extensor tenolysis	CMS Ex: Carpal tunnel release

RELEASE: Freeing a body part from an abnormal physical constraint by cutting or by the use of force.

EXPLANATION: None of the body part is taken out ...

Body Part – 4TH	Approach – 5TH	Device – 6TH	Qualifier – 7TH

0 Head and Neck Tendon F Abdomen Tendon, Right
1 Shoulder Tendon, Right G Abdomen Tendon, Left
2 Shoulder Tendon, Left H Perineum Tendon
3 Upper Arm Tendon, Right J Hip Tendon, Right
4 Upper Arm Tendon, Left K Hip Tendon, Left
5 Lower Arm and Wrist Tendon, Right L Upper Leg Tendon, Right
   M Upper Leg Tendon, Left
6 Lower Arm and Wrist Tendon, Left N Lower Leg Tendon, Right
   P Lower Leg Tendon, Left
7 Hand Tendon, Right Q Knee Tendon, Right
8 Hand Tendon, Left R Knee Tendon, Left
9 Trunk Tendon, Right S Ankle Tendon, Right
B Trunk Tendon, Left T Ankle Tendon, Left
C Thorax Tendon, Right V Foot Tendon, Right
D Thorax Tendon, Left W Foot Tendon, Left
	0 Open
	3 Percutaneous
	4 Percutaneous endoscopic
	X External
		Z No device	Z No qualifier

DEVICE GROUP: Change, (Insertion), Removal, Replacement, Revision, Supplement
Root Operations that always involve a device.

1ST - **0** Medical and Surgical

2ND - **L** Tendons

3RD - **P REMOVAL**

EXAMPLE: Removal drain tube	CMS Ex: Chest tube removal

REMOVAL: Taking out or off a device from a body part.

EXPLANATION: Removal device without reinsertion ...

Body Part – 4TH	Approach – 5TH	Device – 6TH	Qualifier – 7TH
X Upper Tendon Y Lower Tendon	0 Open 3 Percutaneous 4 Percutaneous endoscopic	0 Drainage device 7 Autologous tissue substitute J Synthetic substitute K Nonautologous tissue substitute	Z No qualifier
X Upper Tendon Y Lower Tendon	X External	0 Drainage device	Z No qualifier

OTHER REPAIRS GROUP: (Control), Repair
Root Operations that define other repairs.

| 1ST - **0** Medical and Surgical | EXAMPLE: Tenorrhaphy | | CMS Ex: Suture laceration |

| 2ND - **L** Tendons | **REPAIR:** Restoring, to the extent possible, a body part to its normal anatomic structure and function. |

3RD - Q REPAIR

EXPLANATION: Only when no other root operation applies …

Body Part – 4TH		Approach – 5TH	Device – 6TH	Qualifier – 7TH
0 Head and Neck Tendon	F Abdomen Tendon, Right	0 Open	Z No device	Z No qualifier
1 Shoulder Tendon, Right	G Abdomen Tendon, Left	3 Percutaneous		
2 Shoulder Tendon, Left	H Perineum Tendon	4 Percutaneous endoscopic		
3 Upper Arm Tendon, Right	J Hip Tendon, Right			
4 Upper Arm Tendon, Left	K Hip Tendon, Left			
5 Lower Arm and Wrist Tendon, Right	L Upper Leg Tendon, Right			
	M Upper Leg Tendon, Left			
6 Lower Arm and Wrist Tendon, Left	N Lower Leg Tendon, Right			
	P Lower Leg Tendon, Left			
7 Hand Tendon, Right	Q Knee Tendon, Right			
8 Hand Tendon, Left	R Knee Tendon, Left			
9 Trunk Tendon, Right	S Ankle Tendon, Right			
B Trunk Tendon, Left	T Ankle Tendon, Left			
C Thorax Tendon, Right	V Foot Tendon, Right			
D Thorax Tendon, Left	W Foot Tendon, Left			

DEVICE GROUP: Change, (Insertion), Removal, Replacement, Revision, Supplement
Root Operations that always involve a device.

| 1ST - **0** Medical and Surgical | EXAMPLE: Tendon replacement with cadaver graft | CMS Ex: Total hip |

| 2ND - **L** Tendons | **REPLACEMENT:** Putting in or on a biological or synthetic material that physically takes the place and/or function of all or a portion of a body part. |

3RD - R REPLACEMENT

EXPLANATION: Includes taking out body part, or eradication…

Body Part – 4TH		Approach – 5TH	Device – 6TH	Qualifier – 7TH
0 Head and Neck Tendon	F Abdomen Tendon, Right	0 Open	7 Autologous tissue substitute	Z No qualifier
1 Shoulder Tendon, Right	G Abdomen Tendon, Left	4 Percutaneous endoscopic		
2 Shoulder Tendon, Left	H Perineum Tendon		J Synthetic substitute	
3 Upper Arm Tendon, Right	J Hip Tendon, Right			
4 Upper Arm Tendon, Left	K Hip Tendon, Left		K Nonautologous tissue substitute	
5 Lower Arm and Wrist Tendon, Right	L Upper Leg Tendon, Right			
	M Upper Leg Tendon, Left			
6 Lower Arm and Wrist Tendon, Left	N Lower Leg Tendon, Right			
	P Lower Leg Tendon, Left			
7 Hand Tendon, Right	Q Knee Tendon, Right			
8 Hand Tendon, Left	R Knee Tendon, Left			
9 Trunk Tendon, Right	S Ankle Tendon, Right			
B Trunk Tendon, Left	T Ankle Tendon, Left			
C Thorax Tendon, Right	V Foot Tendon, Right			
D Thorax Tendon, Left	W Foot Tendon, Left			

TENDONS

0 L R

MOVE GROUP: Reattachment, Reposition, Transfer, (Transplantation)
Root Operations that put in/put back or move some/all of a body part.

1ST - 0 Medical and Surgical	EXAMPLE: Relocation extensor tendon hand	CMS Ex: Fracture reduction

2ND - L Tendons	**REPOSITION:** Moving to its normal location, or other suitable location, all or a portion of a body part.
3RD - S REPOSITION	

EXPLANATION: May or may not be cut to be moved …

Body Part – 4TH		Approach – 5TH	Device – 6TH	Qualifier – 7TH
0 Head and Neck Tendon	F Abdomen Tendon, Right	0 Open	Z No device	Z No qualifier
1 Shoulder Tendon, Right	G Abdomen Tendon, Left	4 Percutaneous endoscopic		
2 Shoulder Tendon, Left	H Perineum Tendon			
3 Upper Arm Tendon, Right	J Hip Tendon, Right			
4 Upper Arm Tendon, Left	K Hip Tendon, Left			
5 Lower Arm and Wrist Tendon, Right	L Upper Leg Tendon, Right			
	M Upper Leg Tendon, Left			
6 Lower Arm and Wrist Tendon, Left	N Lower Leg Tendon, Right			
	P Lower Leg Tendon, Left			
7 Hand Tendon, Right	Q Knee Tendon, Right			
8 Hand Tendon, Left	R Knee Tendon, Left			
9 Trunk Tendon, Right	S Ankle Tendon, Right			
B Trunk Tendon, Left	T Ankle Tendon, Left			
C Thorax Tendon, Right	V Foot Tendon, Right			
D Thorax Tendon, Left	W Foot Tendon, Left			

EXCISION GROUP: Excision, Resection, Destruction, (Extraction), (Detachment)
Root Operations that take out some or all of a body part.

1ST - 0 Medical and Surgical	EXAMPLE: Resection flexor tendon hand	CMS Ex: Cholecystectomy

2ND - L Tendons	**RESECTION:** Cutting out or off, without replacement, all of a body part.
3RD - T RESECTION	

EXPLANATION: None

Body Part – 4TH		Approach – 5TH	Device – 6TH	Qualifier – 7TH
0 Head and Neck Tendon	F Abdomen Tendon, Right	0 Open	Z No device	Z No qualifier
1 Shoulder Tendon, Right	G Abdomen Tendon, Left	4 Percutaneous endoscopic		
2 Shoulder Tendon, Left	H Perineum Tendon			
3 Upper Arm Tendon, Right	J Hip Tendon, Right			
4 Upper Arm Tendon, Left	K Hip Tendon, Left			
5 Lower Arm and Wrist Tendon, Right	L Upper Leg Tendon, Right			
	M Upper Leg Tendon, Left			
6 Lower Arm and Wrist Tendon, Left	N Lower Leg Tendon, Right			
	P Lower Leg Tendon, Left			
7 Hand Tendon, Right	Q Knee Tendon, Right			
8 Hand Tendon, Left	R Knee Tendon, Left			
9 Trunk Tendon, Right	S Ankle Tendon, Right			
B Trunk Tendon, Left	T Ankle Tendon, Left			
C Thorax Tendon, Right	V Foot Tendon, Right			
D Thorax Tendon, Left	W Foot Tendon, Left			

DEVICE GROUP: Change, (Insertion), Removal, Replacement, Revision, Supplement
Root Operations that always involve a device.

1ST - 0 Medical and Surgical	EXAMPLE: Tenoplasty augmentation graft CMS Ex: Hernia repair mesh
2ND - L Tendons	**SUPPLEMENT:** Putting in or on biological or synthetic material that physically reinforces and/or augments the function of a portion of a body part.
3RD - U SUPPLEMENT	EXPLANATION: Biological material from same individual ...

Body Part – 4TH		Approach – 5TH	Device – 6TH	Qualifier – 7TH
0 Head and Neck Tendon	F Abdomen Tendon, Right	0 Open	7 Autologous tissue substitute	Z No qualifier
1 Shoulder Tendon, Right	G Abdomen Tendon, Left	4 Percutaneous endoscopic	J Synthetic substitute	
2 Shoulder Tendon, Left	H Perineum Tendon		K Nonautologous tissue substitute	
3 Upper Arm Tendon, Right	J Hip Tendon, Right			
4 Upper Arm Tendon, Left	K Hip Tendon, Left			
5 Lower Arm and Wrist Tendon, Right	L Upper Leg Tendon, Right			
	M Upper Leg Tendon, Left			
6 Lower Arm and Wrist Tendon, Left	N Lower Leg Tendon, Right			
	P Lower Leg Tendon, Left			
7 Hand Tendon, Right	Q Knee Tendon, Right			
8 Hand Tendon, Left	R Knee Tendon, Left			
9 Trunk Tendon, Right	S Ankle Tendon, Right			
B Trunk Tendon, Left	T Ankle Tendon, Left			
C Thorax Tendon, Right	V Foot Tendon, Right			
D Thorax Tendon, Left	W Foot Tendon, Left			

DEVICE GROUP: Change, (Insertion), Removal, Replacement, Revision, Supplement
Root Operations that always involve a device.

1ST - 0 Medical and Surgical	EXAMPLE: Reposition drainage tube CMS Ex: Adjustment pacemaker lead
2ND - L Tendons	**REVISION:** Correcting, to the extent possible, a portion of a malfunctioning device or the position of a displaced device.
3RD - W REVISION	EXPLANATION: May replace components of a device ...

Body Part – 4TH	Approach – 5TH	Device – 6TH	Qualifier – 7TH
X Upper Tendon	0 Open	0 Drainage device	Z No qualifier
Y Lower Tendon	3 Percutaneous	7 Autologous tissue substitute	
	4 Percutaneous endoscopic	J Synthetic substitute	
	X External	K Nonautologous tissue substitute	

T E N D O N S

0 L W

MOVE GROUP: Reattachment, Reposition, Transfer, (Transplantation)
Root Operations that put in/put back or move some/all of a body part.

1ST - 0 Medical and Surgical

2ND - L Tendons

3RD - X TRANSFER

EXAMPLE: Pedicled tendon graft | CMS Ex: Tendon transfer

TRANSFER: Moving, without taking out, all or a portion of a body part to another location to take over the function of all or a portion of a body part.

EXPLANATION: The body part remains connected ...

Body Part – 4TH		Approach – 5TH	Device – 6TH	Qualifier – 7TH
0 Head and Neck Tendon	F Abdomen Tendon, Right	0 Open	Z No device	Z No qualifier
1 Shoulder Tendon, Right	G Abdomen Tendon, Left	4 Percutaneous endoscopic		
2 Shoulder Tendon, Left	H Perineum Tendon			
3 Upper Arm Tendon, Right	J Hip Tendon, Right			
4 Upper Arm Tendon, Left	K Hip Tendon, Left			
5 Lower Arm and Wrist Tendon, Right	L Upper Leg Tendon, Right			
	M Upper Leg Tendon, Left			
6 Lower Arm and Wrist Tendon, Left	N Lower Leg Tendon, Right			
	P Lower Leg Tendon, Left			
7 Hand Tendon, Right	Q Knee Tendon, Right			
8 Hand Tendon, Left	R Knee Tendon, Left			
9 Trunk Tendon, Right	S Ankle Tendon, Right			
B Trunk Tendon, Left	T Ankle Tendon, Left			
C Thorax Tendon, Right	V Foot Tendon, Right			
D Thorax Tendon, Left	W Foot Tendon, Left			

TENDONS

0
L
X

© 2016 Channel Publishing, Ltd.

Educational Annotations | M – Bursae and Ligaments

Body System Specific Educational Annotations for the Bursae and Ligaments include:
- Anatomy and Physiology Review
- Anatomical Illustrations
- Definitions of Common Procedures
- AHA Coding Clinic® Reference Notations
- Body Part Key Listings
- Device Key Listings
- Device Aggregation Table Listings
- Coding Notes

Anatomy and Physiology Review of Bursae and Ligaments

BODY PART VALUES – M - BURSAE AND LIGAMENTS

Bursa – ANATOMY – Bursa are small, synovial fluid-filled sacs that lie between bones, tendons, and muscles around joints. PHYSIOLOGY – Bursa function to allow less friction between the bones, tendons, and muscles around joints during movement.

Ligament – ANATOMY – A ligament is a strong band or sheath of connective tissue that connects bones to bones. PHYSIOLOGY – Ligaments hold bones and joints in proper alignment and allow some flexibility.

Lower Bursa and Ligament – The bursa and ligaments located below the diaphragm (see Coding Guideline B2.1b)

Upper Bursa and Ligament – The bursa and ligaments located above the diaphragm (see Coding Guideline B2.1b).

Anatomical Illustrations of Bursae and Ligaments

None for the Bursae and Ligaments Body System

Definitions of Common Procedures of Bursae and Ligaments

Prepatellar bursectomy – The surgical removal of a prepatellar (knee) bursal sac.

Reattach severed ankle ligament – The repair of a torn ankle ligament using sutures to a small hole drilled in the fibula.

Tommy John surgery – The surgical reconstruction of a torn ulnar collateral ligament by using a tendon graft sewn through small drill holes in the medial epicondyle of the humerus and sublime tubercle of the ulna in a figure 8 pattern with any remnants of the original ligament attached to the tendon.

AHA Coding Clinic® Reference Notations of Bursae and Ligaments

ROOT OPERATION SPECIFIC - M - BURSAE AND LIGAMENTS
CHANGE - 2
DESTRUCTION - 5
DIVISION - 7
DRAINAGE - 9
EXCISION - B
EXTIRPATION - C
EXTRACTION - D
INSPECTION - J
REATTACHMENT - M
    Arthroscopic type 2 SLAP repair ....AHA 13:3Q:p20
RELEASE - N
REMOVAL - P
REPAIR - Q
    Cervical interspinous ligamentoplasty......................................AHA 14:3Q:p9
REPOSITION - S
RESECTION - T
SUPPLEMENT - U
REVISION - W
TRANSFER - X

Educational Annotations | M – Bursae and Ligaments

Body Part Key Listings of Bursae and Ligaments

See also Body Part Key in Appendix C

Acromioclavicular ligament	*use* Shoulder Bursa and Ligament,Left/Right
Alar ligament of axis	*use* Head and Neck Bursa and Ligament
Annular ligament	*use* Elbow Bursa and Ligament, Left/Right
Anterior cruciate ligament (ACL)	*use* Knee Bursa and Ligament, Left/Right
Calcaneocuboid ligament	*use* Foot Bursa and Ligament, Left/Right
Calcaneofibular ligament	*use* Ankle Bursa and Ligament, Left/Right
Carpometacarpal ligament	*use* Hand Bursa and Ligament, Left/Right
Cervical interspinous ligament	*use* Head and Neck Bursa and Ligament
Cervical intertransverse ligament	*use* Head and Neck Bursa and Ligament
Cervical ligamentum flavum	*use* Head and Neck Bursa and Ligament
Coracoacromial ligament	*use* Shoulder Bursa and Ligament, Left/Right
Coracoclavicular ligament	*use* Shoulder Bursa and Ligament, Left/Right
Coracohumeral ligament	*use* Shoulder Bursa and Ligament, Left/Right
Costoclavicular ligament	*use* Shoulder Bursa and Ligament, Left/Right
Costotransverse ligament	*use* Thorax Bursa and Ligament, Left/Right
Costoxiphoid ligament	*use* Thorax Bursa and Ligament, Left/Right
Cuneonavicular ligament	*use* Foot Bursa and Ligament, Left/Right
Deltoid ligament	*use* Ankle Bursa and Ligament, Left/Right
Glenohumeral ligament	*use* Shoulder Bursa and Ligament, Left/Right
Iliofemoral ligament	*use* Hip Bursa and Ligament, Left/Right
Iliolumbar ligament	*use* Trunk Bursa and Ligament, Left/Right
Intercarpal ligament	*use* Hand Bursa and Ligament, Left/Right
Interclavicular ligament	*use* Shoulder Bursa and Ligament, Left/Right
Intercuneiform ligament	*use* Foot Bursa and Ligament, Left/Right
Interphalangeal ligament	*use* Hand Bursa and Ligament, Left/Right
	use Foot Bursa and Ligament, Left/Right
Interspinous ligament	*use* Head and Neck Bursa and Ligament
	use Trunk Bursa and Ligament, Left/Right
Intertransverse ligament	*use* Trunk Bursa and Ligament, Left/Right
Ischiofemoral ligament	*use* Hip Bursa and Ligament, Left/Right
Lateral collateral ligament (LCL)	*use* Knee Bursa and Ligament, Left/Right
Lateral temporomandibular ligament	*use* Head and Neck Bursa and Ligament
Ligament of head of fibula	*use* Knee Bursa and Ligament, Left/Right
Ligament of the lateral malleolus	*use* Ankle Bursa and Ligament, Left/Right
Ligamentum flavum	*use* Trunk Bursa and Ligament, Left/Right
Lunotriquetral ligament	*use* Hand Bursa and Ligament, Left/Right
Medial collateral ligament (MCL)	*use* Knee Bursa and Ligament, Left/Right
Metacarpal ligament	*use* Hand Bursa and Ligament, Left/Right
Metacarpophalangeal ligament	*use* Hand Bursa and Ligament, Left/Right
Metatarsal ligament	*use* Foot Bursa and Ligament, Left/Right
Metatarsophalangeal ligament	*use* Foot Bursa and Ligament, Left/Right
Olecranon bursa	*use* Elbow Bursa and Ligament, Left/Right
Palmar ulnocarpal ligament	*use* Wrist Bursa and Ligament, Left/Right
Patellar ligament	*use* Knee Bursa and Ligament, Left/Right
Pisohamate ligament	*use* Hand Bursa and Ligament, Left/Right
Pisometacarpal ligament	*use* Hand Bursa and Ligament, Left/Right
Popliteal ligament	*use* Knee Bursa and Ligament, Left/Right
Posterior cruciate ligament (PCL)	*use* Knee Bursa and Ligament, Left/Right

Continued on next page

BURSAE & LIGAMENTS 0 M

Educational Annotations | M – Bursae and Ligaments

Body Part Key Listings of Bursae and Ligaments

Continued from previous page

Prepatellar bursa .... *use* Knee Bursa and Ligament, Left/Right
Pubic ligament .... *use* Trunk Bursa and Ligament, Left/Right
Pubofemoral ligament .... *use* Hip Bursa and Ligament, Left/Right
Radial collateral carpal ligament .... *use* Wrist Bursa and Ligament, Left/Right
Radial collateral ligament .... *use* Elbow Bursa and Ligament, Left/Right
Radiocarpal ligament .... *use* Wrist Bursa and Ligament, Left/Right
Radioulnar ligament .... *use* Wrist Bursa and Ligament, Left/Right
Sacrococcygeal ligament .... *use* Trunk Bursa and Ligament, Left/Right
Sacroiliac ligament .... *use* Trunk Bursa and Ligament, Left/Right
Sacrospinous ligament....................................... *use* Trunk Bursa and Ligament, Left/Right
Sacrotuberous ligament..................................... *use* Trunk Bursa and Ligament, Left/Right
Scapholunate ligament .... *use* Hand Bursa and Ligament, Left/Right
Scaphotrapezium ligament .... *use* Hand Bursa and Ligament, Left/Right
Sphenomandibular ligament .... *use* Head and Neck Bursa and Ligament
Sternoclavicular ligament .... *use* Shoulder Bursa and Ligament, Left/Right
Sternocostal ligament .... *use* Thorax Bursa and Ligament, Left/Right
Stylomandibular ligament .... *use* Head and Neck Bursa and Ligament
Subacromial bursa.. *use* Shoulder Bursa and Ligament, Left/Right
Subtalar ligament .... *use* Foot Bursa and Ligament, Left/Right
Supraspinous ligament .... *use* Trunk Bursa and Ligament, Left/Right
Talocalcaneal ligament .... *use* Foot Bursa and Ligament, Left/Right
Talocalcaneonavicular ligament......................... *use* Foot Bursa and Ligament, Left/Right
Talofibular ligament... *use* Ankle Bursa and Ligament, Left/Right
Tarsometatarsal ligament .... *use* Foot Bursa and Ligament, Left/Right
Transverse acetabular ligament .... *use* Hip Bursa and Ligament, Left/Right
Transverse humeral ligament............................. *use* Shoulder Bursa and Ligament, Left/Right
Transverse ligament of atlas .... *use* Head and Neck Bursa and Ligament
Transverse scapular ligament .... *use* Shoulder Bursa and Ligament, Left/Right
Trochanteric bursa .... *use* Hip Bursa and Ligament, Left/Right
Ulnar collateral carpal ligament .... *use* Wrist Bursa and Ligament, Left/Right
Ulnar collateral ligament .... *use* Elbow Bursa and Ligament, Left/Right

Device Key Listings of Bursae and Ligaments

See also Device Key in Appendix D
Autograft .... *use* Autologous Tissue Substitute
Tissue bank graft .... *use* Nonautologous Tissue Substitute

Device Aggregation Table Listings of Bursae and Ligaments

See also Device Aggregation Table in Appendix E

Specific Device	For Operation	In Body System	General Device
None Listed in Device Aggregation Table for this Body System			

Educational Annotations | M – Bursae and Ligaments

Coding Notes of Bursae and Ligaments

Body System Relevant Coding Guidelines

General Guidelines

B2.1b

Where the general body part values "upper" and "lower" are provided as an option in the Upper Arteries, Lower Arteries, Upper Veins, Lower Veins, Muscles and Tendons body systems, "upper" and "lower" specifies body parts located above or below the diaphragm respectively.

Example: Vein body parts above the diaphragm are found in the Upper Veins body system; vein body parts below the diaphragm are found in the Lower Veins body system.

Tendons, ligaments, bursae and fascia near a joint

B4.5

Procedures performed on tendons, ligaments, bursae and fascia supporting a joint are coded to the body part in the respective body system that is the focus of the procedure. Procedures performed on joint structures themselves are coded to the body part in the joint body systems.

Examples: Repair of the anterior cruciate ligament of the knee is coded to the knee bursa and ligament body part in the bursae and ligaments body system.

Knee arthroscopy with shaving of articular cartilage is coded to the knee joint body part in the Lower Joints body system.

Body System Specific PCS Reference Manual Exercises

PCS CODE	M – BURSAE AND LIGAMENTS EXERCISES
0 M N 1 4 Z Z	Right shoulder arthroscopy with coracoacromial ligament release.
0 M S P 4 Z Z	Left knee arthroscopy with reposition of anterior cruciate ligament.

DEVICE GROUP: Change, (Insertion), Removal, (Replacement), Revision, Supplement
Root Operations that always involve a device.

	EXAMPLE: Exchange drain tube	CMS Ex: Changing urinary catheter
1ST - **0** Medical and Surgical 2ND - **M** Bursae and Ligaments 3RD - **2 CHANGE**	**CHANGE:** Taking out or off a device from a body part and putting back an identical or similar device in or on the same body part without cutting or puncturing the skin or a mucous membrane.	
	EXPLANATION: ALL Changes use EXTERNAL approach only ...	

Body Part – 4TH	Approach – 5TH	Device – 6TH	Qualifier – 7TH
X Upper Bursa and Ligament Y Lower Bursa and Ligament	X External	0 Drainage device Y Other device	Z No qualifier

---

EXCISION GROUP: Excision, Resection, Destruction, Extraction, (Detachment)
Root Operations that take out some or all of a body part.

	EXAMPLE: Radiofrequency ablation	CMS Ex: Fulguration polyp
1ST - **0** Medical and Surgical 2ND - **M** Bursae and Ligaments 3RD - **5 DESTRUCTION**	**DESTRUCTION:** Physical eradication of all or a portion of a body part by the direct use of energy, force, or a destructive agent.	
	EXPLANATION: None of the body part is physically taken out	

Body Part – 4TH	Approach – 5TH	Device – 6TH	Qualifier – 7TH
0 Head and Neck Bursa and Ligament 1 Shoulder Bursa and Ligament, Right 2 Shoulder Bursa and Ligament, Left 3 Elbow Bursa and Ligament, Right 4 Elbow Bursa and Ligament, Left 5 Wrist Bursa and Ligament, Right 6 Wrist Bursa and Ligament, Left 7 Hand Bursa and Ligament, Right 8 Hand Bursa and Ligament, Left 9 Upper Extremity Bursa and Ligament, Right B Upper Extremity Bursa and Ligament, Left C Trunk Bursa and Ligament, Right D Trunk Bursa and Ligament, Left F Thorax Bursa and Ligament, Right G Thorax Bursa and Ligament, Left H Abdomen Bursa and Ligament, Right J Abdomen Bursa and Ligament, Left K Perineum Bursa and Ligament L Hip Bursa and Ligament, Right M Hip Bursa and Ligament, Left N Knee Bursa and Ligament, Right P Knee Bursa and Ligament, Left Q Ankle Bursa and Ligament, Right R Ankle Bursa and Ligament, Left S Foot Bursa and Ligament, Right T Foot Bursa and Ligament, Left V Lower Extremity Bursa and Ligament, Right W Lower Extremity Bursa and Ligament, Left	0 Open 3 Percutaneous 4 Percutaneous endoscopic	Z No device	Z No qualifier

BURSAE & LIGAMENTS 0 M 5

DIVISION GROUP: Division, Release
Root Operations involving cutting or separation only.

| 1ST - 0 Medical and Surgical |
| 2ND - M Bursae and Ligaments |
| 3RD - 8 DIVISION |

EXAMPLE: Ligament transection   CMS Ex: Osteotomy

DIVISION: Cutting into a body part without draining fluids and/or gases from the body part in order to separate or transect a body part.

EXPLANATION: Separated into two or more portions ...

Body Part – 4TH	Approach – 5TH	Device – 6TH	Qualifier – 7TH
0 Head and Neck Bursa and Ligament	0 Open	Z No device	Z No qualifier
1 Shoulder Bursa and Ligament, Right	3 Percutaneous		
2 Shoulder Bursa and Ligament, Left	4 Percutaneous endoscopic		
3 Elbow Bursa and Ligament, Right			
4 Elbow Bursa and Ligament, Left			
5 Wrist Bursa and Ligament, Right			
6 Wrist Bursa and Ligament, Left			
7 Hand Bursa and Ligament, Right			
8 Hand Bursa and Ligament, Left			
9 Upper Extremity Bursa and Ligament, Right			
B Upper Extremity Bursa and Ligament, Left			
C Trunk Bursa and Ligament, Right			
D Trunk Bursa and Ligament, Left			
F Thorax Bursa and Ligament, Right			
G Thorax Bursa and Ligament, Left			
H Abdomen Bursa and Ligament, Right			
J Abdomen Bursa and Ligament, Left			
K Perineum Bursa and Ligament			
L Hip Bursa and Ligament, Right			
M Hip Bursa and Ligament, Left			
N Knee Bursa and Ligament, Right			
P Knee Bursa and Ligament, Left			
Q Ankle Bursa and Ligament, Right			
R Ankle Bursa and Ligament, Left			
S Foot Bursa and Ligament, Right			
T Foot Bursa and Ligament, Left			
V Lower Extremity Bursa and Ligament, Right			
W Lower Extremity Bursa and Ligament, Left			

DRAINAGE GROUP: Drainage, Extirpation, (Fragmentation)
Root Operations that take out solids/fluids/gases from a body part.

1ST - 0 Medical and Surgical	**EXAMPLE:** Aspiration prepatellar bursa **CMS Ex:** Thoracentesis
2ND - M Bursae and Ligaments	**DRAINAGE:** Taking or letting out fluids and/or gases from a body part.
3RD - 9 DRAINAGE	**EXPLANATION:** Qualifier "X Diagnostic" indicates biopsy ...

Body Part – 4TH	Approach – 5TH	Device – 6TH	Qualifier – 7TH
0 Head and Neck Bursa and Ligament	0 Open	0 Drainage device	Z No qualifier
1 Shoulder Bursa and Ligament, Right	3 Percutaneous		
2 Shoulder Bursa and Ligament, Left	4 Percutaneous endoscopic		
3 Elbow Bursa and Ligament, Right			
4 Elbow Bursa and Ligament, Left			
5 Wrist Bursa and Ligament, Right			
6 Wrist Bursa and Ligament, Left			
7 Hand Bursa and Ligament, Right			
8 Hand Bursa and Ligament, Left			
9 Upper Extremity Bursa and Ligament, Right			
B Upper Extremity Bursa and Ligament, Left			
C Trunk Bursa and Ligament, Right			
D Trunk Bursa and Ligament, Left			
F Thorax Bursa and Ligament, Right			
G Thorax Bursa and Ligament, Left			
H Abdomen Bursa and Ligament, Right			
J Abdomen Bursa and Ligament, Left			
K Perineum Bursa and Ligament			
L Hip Bursa and Ligament, Right			
M Hip Bursa and Ligament, Left			
N Knee Bursa and Ligament, Right			
P Knee Bursa and Ligament, Left			
Q Ankle Bursa and Ligament, Right			
R Ankle Bursa and Ligament, Left			
S Foot Bursa and Ligament, Right			
T Foot Bursa and Ligament, Left			
V Lower Extremity Bursa and Ligament, Right			
W Lower Extremity Bursa and Ligament, Left			

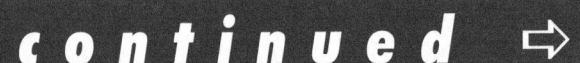

continued ⇨

BURSAE & LIGAMENTS 0 M 9

0 M 9 DRAINAGE – *continued*

Body Part – 4TH	Approach – 5TH	Device – 6TH	Qualifier – 7TH
0 Head and Neck Bursa and Ligament	0 Open	Z No device	X Diagnostic
1 Shoulder Bursa and Ligament, Right	3 Percutaneous		Z No qualifier
2 Shoulder Bursa and Ligament, Left	4 Percutaneous endoscopic		
3 Elbow Bursa and Ligament, Right			
4 Elbow Bursa and Ligament, Left			
5 Wrist Bursa and Ligament, Right			
6 Wrist Bursa and Ligament, Left			
7 Hand Bursa and Ligament, Right			
8 Hand Bursa and Ligament, Left			
9 Upper Extremity Bursa and Ligament, Right			
B Upper Extremity Bursa and Ligament, Left			
C Trunk Bursa and Ligament, Right			
D Trunk Bursa and Ligament, Left			
F Thorax Bursa and Ligament, Right			
G Thorax Bursa and Ligament, Left			
H Abdomen Bursa and Ligament, Right			
J Abdomen Bursa and Ligament, Left			
K Perineum Bursa and Ligament			
L Hip Bursa and Ligament, Right			
M Hip Bursa and Ligament, Left			
N Knee Bursa and Ligament, Right			
P Knee Bursa and Ligament, Left			
Q Ankle Bursa and Ligament, Right			
R Ankle Bursa and Ligament, Left			
S Foot Bursa and Ligament, Right			
T Foot Bursa and Ligament, Left			
V Lower Extremity Bursa and Ligament, Right			
W Lower Extremity Bursa and Ligament, Left			

BURSAE & LIGAMENTS 0 M 9

EXCISION GROUP: Excision, Resection, Destruction, Extraction, (Detachment)
Root Operations that take out some or all of a body part.

1ST - **0** Medical and Surgical	EXAMPLE: Partial bursectomy elbow — CMS Ex: Liver biopsy
2ND - **M** Bursae and Ligaments	**EXCISION:** Cutting out or off, without replacement, a portion of a body part.
3RD - **B EXCISION**	EXPLANATION: Qualifier "X Diagnostic" indicates biopsy ...

Body Part – 4TH	Approach – 5TH	Device – 6TH	Qualifier – 7TH
0 Head and Neck Bursa and Ligament	0 Open	Z No device	X Diagnostic
1 Shoulder Bursa and Ligament, Right	3 Percutaneous		Z No qualifier
2 Shoulder Bursa and Ligament, Left	4 Percutaneous endoscopic		
3 Elbow Bursa and Ligament, Right			
4 Elbow Bursa and Ligament, Left			
5 Wrist Bursa and Ligament, Right			
6 Wrist Bursa and Ligament, Left			
7 Hand Bursa and Ligament, Right			
8 Hand Bursa and Ligament, Left			
9 Upper Extremity Bursa and Ligament, Right			
B Upper Extremity Bursa and Ligament, Left			
C Trunk Bursa and Ligament, Right			
D Trunk Bursa and Ligament, Left			
F Thorax Bursa and Ligament, Right			
G Thorax Bursa and Ligament, Left			
H Abdomen Bursa and Ligament, Right			
J Abdomen Bursa and Ligament, Left			
K Perineum Bursa and Ligament			
L Hip Bursa and Ligament, Right			
M Hip Bursa and Ligament, Left			
N Knee Bursa and Ligament, Right			
P Knee Bursa and Ligament, Left			
Q Ankle Bursa and Ligament, Right			
R Ankle Bursa and Ligament, Left			
S Foot Bursa and Ligament, Right			
T Foot Bursa and Ligament, Left			
V Lower Extremity Bursa and Ligament, Right			
W Lower Extremity Bursa and Ligament, Left			

DRAINAGE GROUP: Drainage, Extirpation, (Fragmentation)
Root Operations that take out solids/fluids/gases from a body part.

1ST – **0** Medical and Surgical	EXAMPLE: Removal calcification CMS Ex: Choledocholithotomy
2ND – **M** Bursae and Ligaments	**EXTIRPATION:** Taking or cutting out solid matter from a body part.
3RD – **C EXTIRPATION**	EXPLANATION: Abnormal byproduct or foreign body …

Body Part – 4TH	Approach – 5TH	Device – 6TH	Qualifier – 7TH
0 Head and Neck Bursa and Ligament	0 Open	Z No device	Z No qualifier
1 Shoulder Bursa and Ligament, Right	3 Percutaneous		
2 Shoulder Bursa and Ligament, Left	4 Percutaneous endoscopic		
3 Elbow Bursa and Ligament, Right			
4 Elbow Bursa and Ligament, Left			
5 Wrist Bursa and Ligament, Right			
6 Wrist Bursa and Ligament, Left			
7 Hand Bursa and Ligament, Right			
8 Hand Bursa and Ligament, Left			
9 Upper Extremity Bursa and Ligament, Right			
B Upper Extremity Bursa and Ligament, Left			
C Trunk Bursa and Ligament, Right			
D Trunk Bursa and Ligament, Left			
F Thorax Bursa and Ligament, Right			
G Thorax Bursa and Ligament, Left			
H Abdomen Bursa and Ligament, Right			
J Abdomen Bursa and Ligament, Left			
K Perineum Bursa and Ligament			
L Hip Bursa and Ligament, Right			
M Hip Bursa and Ligament, Left			
N Knee Bursa and Ligament, Right			
P Knee Bursa and Ligament, Left			
Q Ankle Bursa and Ligament, Right			
R Ankle Bursa and Ligament, Left			
S Foot Bursa and Ligament, Right			
T Foot Bursa and Ligament, Left			
V Lower Extremity Bursa and Ligament, Right			
W Lower Extremity Bursa and Ligament, Left			

BURSAE & LIGAMENTS 0 M C

EXCISION GROUP: Excision, Resection, Destruction, Extraction, (Detachment)
Root Operations that take out some or all of a body part.

1ST - 0 Medical and Surgical	EXAMPLE: Extraction bursal sac		CMS Ex: D&C
2ND - M Bursae and Ligaments	**EXTRACTION:** Pulling or stripping out or off all or a portion of a body part by the use of force.		
3RD - D EXTRACTION	EXPLANATION: None for this Body System		

Body Part – 4TH	Approach – 5TH	Device – 6TH	Qualifier – 7TH
0 Head and Neck Bursa and Ligament 1 Shoulder Bursa and Ligament, Right 2 Shoulder Bursa and Ligament, Left 3 Elbow Bursa and Ligament, Right 4 Elbow Bursa and Ligament, Left 5 Wrist Bursa and Ligament, Right 6 Wrist Bursa and Ligament, Left 7 Hand Bursa and Ligament, Right 8 Hand Bursa and Ligament, Left 9 Upper Extremity Bursa and Ligament, Right B Upper Extremity Bursa and Ligament, Left C Trunk Bursa and Ligament, Right D Trunk Bursa and Ligament, Left F Thorax Bursa and Ligament, Right G Thorax Bursa and Ligament, Left H Abdomen Bursa and Ligament, Right J Abdomen Bursa and Ligament, Left K Perineum Bursa and Ligament L Hip Bursa and Ligament, Right M Hip Bursa and Ligament, Left N Knee Bursa and Ligament, Right P Knee Bursa and Ligament, Left Q Ankle Bursa and Ligament, Right R Ankle Bursa and Ligament, Left S Foot Bursa and Ligament, Right T Foot Bursa and Ligament, Left V Lower Extremity Bursa and Ligament, Right W Lower Extremity Bursa and Ligament, Left	0 Open 3 Percutaneous 4 Percutaneous endoscopic	Z No device	Z No qualifier

EXAMINATION GROUP: Inspection, (Map)
Root Operations involving examination only.

1ST - 0 Medical and Surgical	EXAMPLE: Examination ligament attachments	CMS Ex: Colonoscopy
2ND - M Bursae and Ligaments	**INSPECTION:** Visually and/or manually exploring a body part.	
3RD - J INSPECTION	EXPLANATION: Direct or instrumental visualization ...	

Body Part – 4TH	Approach – 5TH	Device – 6TH	Qualifier – 7TH
X Upper Bursa and Ligament Y Lower Bursa and Ligament	0 Open 3 Percutaneous 4 Percutaneous endoscopic X External	Z No device	Z No qualifier

MOVE GROUP: Reattachment, Reposition, Transfer, (Transplantation)
Root Operations that put in/put back or move some/all of a body part.

1ST - **0** Medical and Surgical

2ND - **M** Bursae and Ligaments

3RD - **M REATTACHMENT**

EXAMPLE: Reattach torn ligament   CMS Ex: Reattachment hand

REATTACHMENT: Putting back in or on all or a portion of a separated body part to its normal location or other suitable location.

EXPLANATION: With/without reconnection of vessels/nerves...

Body Part – 4TH	Approach – 5TH	Device – 6TH	Qualifier – 7TH
0 Head and Neck Bursa and Ligament	0 Open	Z No device	Z No qualifier
1 Shoulder Bursa and Ligament, Right	4 Percutaneous endoscopic		
2 Shoulder Bursa and Ligament, Left			
3 Elbow Bursa and Ligament, Right			
4 Elbow Bursa and Ligament, Left			
5 Wrist Bursa and Ligament, Right			
6 Wrist Bursa and Ligament, Left			
7 Hand Bursa and Ligament, Right			
8 Hand Bursa and Ligament, Left			
9 Upper Extremity Bursa and Ligament, Right			
B Upper Extremity Bursa and Ligament, Left			
C Trunk Bursa and Ligament, Right			
D Trunk Bursa and Ligament, Left			
F Thorax Bursa and Ligament, Right			
G Thorax Bursa and Ligament, Left			
H Abdomen Bursa and Ligament, Right			
J Abdomen Bursa and Ligament, Left			
K Perineum Bursa and Ligament			
L Hip Bursa and Ligament, Right			
M Hip Bursa and Ligament, Left			
N Knee Bursa and Ligament, Right			
P Knee Bursa and Ligament, Left			
Q Ankle Bursa and Ligament, Right			
R Ankle Bursa and Ligament, Left			
S Foot Bursa and Ligament, Right			
T Foot Bursa and Ligament, Left			
V Lower Extremity Bursa and Ligament, Right			
W Lower Extremity Bursa and Ligament, Left			

BURSAE & LIGAMENTS 0 M M

DIVISION GROUP: Division, Release
Root Operations involving cutting or separation only.

1ST - 0 Medical and Surgical	EXAMPLE: Coracoacromial ligament release	CMS Ex: Carpal tunnel
2ND - M Bursae and Ligaments	**RELEASE:** Freeing a body part from an abnormal physical constraint by cutting or by the use of force.	
3RD - N RELEASE	EXPLANATION: None of the body part is taken out ...	

Body Part – 4TH	Approach – 5TH	Device – 6TH	Qualifier – 7TH
0 Head and Neck Bursa and Ligament 1 Shoulder Bursa and Ligament, Right 2 Shoulder Bursa and Ligament, Left 3 Elbow Bursa and Ligament, Right 4 Elbow Bursa and Ligament, Left 5 Wrist Bursa and Ligament, Right 6 Wrist Bursa and Ligament, Left 7 Hand Bursa and Ligament, Right 8 Hand Bursa and Ligament, Left 9 Upper Extremity Bursa and Ligament, Right B Upper Extremity Bursa and Ligament, Left C Trunk Bursa and Ligament, Right D Trunk Bursa and Ligament, Left F Thorax Bursa and Ligament, Right G Thorax Bursa and Ligament, Left H Abdomen Bursa and Ligament, Right J Abdomen Bursa and Ligament, Left K Perineum Bursa and Ligament L Hip Bursa and Ligament, Right M Hip Bursa and Ligament, Left N Knee Bursa and Ligament, Right P Knee Bursa and Ligament, Left Q Ankle Bursa and Ligament, Right R Ankle Bursa and Ligament, Left S Foot Bursa and Ligament, Right T Foot Bursa and Ligament, Left V Lower Extremity Bursa and Ligament, Right W Lower Extremity Bursa and Ligament, Left	0 Open 3 Percutaneous 4 Percutaneous endoscopic X External	Z No device	Z No qualifier

---

DEVICE GROUP: Change, (Insertion), Removal, (Replacement), Revision, Supplement
Root Operations that always involve a device.

1ST - 0 Medical and Surgical	EXAMPLE: Removal drain tube	CMS Ex: Chest tube removal
2ND - M Bursae and Ligaments	**REMOVAL:** Taking out or off a device from a body part.	
3RD - P REMOVAL	EXPLANATION: Removal device without reinsertion ...	

Body Part – 4TH	Approach – 5TH	Device – 6TH	Qualifier – 7TH
X Upper Bursa and Ligament Y Lower Bursa and Ligament	0 Open 3 Percutaneous 4 Percutaneous endoscopic	0 Drainage device 7 Autologous tissue substitute J Synthetic substitute K Nonautologous tissue substitute	Z No qualifier
X Upper Bursa and Ligament Y Lower Bursa and Ligament	X External	0 Drainage device	Z No qualifier

BURSAE & LIGAMENTS 0 M P

OTHER REPAIRS GROUP: (Control), **Repair**
Root Operations that define other repairs.

1ST - 0 Medical and Surgical

2ND - M Bursae and Ligaments

3RD - Q REPAIR

EXAMPLE: Suture torn ligament   CMS Ex: Suture laceration

REPAIR: Restoring, to the extent possible, a body part to its normal anatomic structure and function.

EXPLANATION: Only when no other root operation applies ...

Body Part – 4TH	Approach – 5TH	Device – 6TH	Qualifier – 7TH
0 Head and Neck Bursa and Ligament	0 Open	Z No device	Z No qualifier
1 Shoulder Bursa and Ligament, Right	3 Percutaneous		
2 Shoulder Bursa and Ligament, Left	4 Percutaneous endoscopic		
3 Elbow Bursa and Ligament, Right			
4 Elbow Bursa and Ligament, Left			
5 Wrist Bursa and Ligament, Right			
6 Wrist Bursa and Ligament, Left			
7 Hand Bursa and Ligament, Right			
8 Hand Bursa and Ligament, Left			
9 Upper Extremity Bursa and Ligament, Right			
B Upper Extremity Bursa and Ligament, Left			
C Trunk Bursa and Ligament, Right			
D Trunk Bursa and Ligament, Left			
F Thorax Bursa and Ligament, Right			
G Thorax Bursa and Ligament, Left			
H Abdomen Bursa and Ligament, Right			
J Abdomen Bursa and Ligament, Left			
K Perineum Bursa and Ligament			
L Hip Bursa and Ligament, Right			
M Hip Bursa and Ligament, Left			
N Knee Bursa and Ligament, Right			
P Knee Bursa and Ligament, Left			
Q Ankle Bursa and Ligament, Right			
R Ankle Bursa and Ligament, Left			
S Foot Bursa and Ligament, Right			
T Foot Bursa and Ligament, Left			
V Lower Extremity Bursa and Ligament, Right			
W Lower Extremity Bursa and Ligament, Left			

BURSAE & LIGAMENTS 0 M Q

MOVE GROUP: Reattachment, Reposition, Transfer, (Transplantation)
Root Operations that put in/put back or move some/all of a body part.

1ST - O Medical and Surgical

2ND - M Bursae and Ligaments

3RD - S REPOSITION

EXAMPLE: Reposition ACL ligament	CMS Ex: Fracture reduction

REPOSITION: Moving to its normal location, or other suitable location, all or a portion of a body part.

EXPLANATION: May or may not be cut to be moved ...

Body Part – 4TH	Approach – 5TH	Device – 6TH	Qualifier – 7TH
0 Head and Neck Bursa and Ligament	0 Open	Z No device	Z No qualifier
1 Shoulder Bursa and Ligament, Right	4 Percutaneous endoscopic		
2 Shoulder Bursa and Ligament, Left			
3 Elbow Bursa and Ligament, Right			
4 Elbow Bursa and Ligament, Left			
5 Wrist Bursa and Ligament, Right			
6 Wrist Bursa and Ligament, Left			
7 Hand Bursa and Ligament, Right			
8 Hand Bursa and Ligament, Left			
9 Upper Extremity Bursa and Ligament, Right			
B Upper Extremity Bursa and Ligament, Left			
C Trunk Bursa and Ligament, Right			
D Trunk Bursa and Ligament, Left			
F Thorax Bursa and Ligament, Right			
G Thorax Bursa and Ligament, Left			
H Abdomen Bursa and Ligament, Right			
J Abdomen Bursa and Ligament, Left			
K Perineum Bursa and Ligament			
L Hip Bursa and Ligament, Right			
M Hip Bursa and Ligament, Left			
N Knee Bursa and Ligament, Right			
P Knee Bursa and Ligament, Left			
Q Ankle Bursa and Ligament, Right			
R Ankle Bursa and Ligament, Left			
S Foot Bursa and Ligament, Right			
T Foot Bursa and Ligament, Left			
V Lower Extremity Bursa and Ligament, Right			
W Lower Extremity Bursa and Ligament, Left			

BURSAE & LIGAMENTS **O M S**

EXCISION GROUP: Excision, Resection, Destruction, Extraction, (Detachment)
Root Operations that take out some or all of a body part.

1ST - **0** Medical and Surgical	**EXAMPLE:** Collateral ligament resection **CMS Ex:** Cholecystectomy
2ND - **M** Bursae and Ligaments	**RESECTION:** Cutting out or off, without replacement, all of a body part.
3RD - **T RESECTION**	**EXPLANATION:** None

Body Part – 4TH	Approach – 5TH	Device – 6TH	Qualifier – 7TH
0 Head and Neck Bursa and Ligament	0 Open	Z No device	Z No qualifier
1 Shoulder Bursa and Ligament, Right	4 Percutaneous endoscopic		
2 Shoulder Bursa and Ligament, Left			
3 Elbow Bursa and Ligament, Right			
4 Elbow Bursa and Ligament, Left			
5 Wrist Bursa and Ligament, Right			
6 Wrist Bursa and Ligament, Left			
7 Hand Bursa and Ligament, Right			
8 Hand Bursa and Ligament, Left			
9 Upper Extremity Bursa and Ligament, Right			
B Upper Extremity Bursa and Ligament, Left			
C Trunk Bursa and Ligament, Right			
D Trunk Bursa and Ligament, Left			
F Thorax Bursa and Ligament, Right			
G Thorax Bursa and Ligament, Left			
H Abdomen Bursa and Ligament, Right			
J Abdomen Bursa and Ligament, Left			
K Perineum Bursa and Ligament			
L Hip Bursa and Ligament, Right			
M Hip Bursa and Ligament, Left			
N Knee Bursa and Ligament, Right			
P Knee Bursa and Ligament, Left			
Q Ankle Bursa and Ligament, Right			
R Ankle Bursa and Ligament, Left			
S Foot Bursa and Ligament, Right			
T Foot Bursa and Ligament, Left			
V Lower Extremity Bursa and Ligament, Right			
W Lower Extremity Bursa and Ligament, Left			

DEVICE GROUP: Change, (Insertion), Removal, (Replacement), Revision, Supplement
Root Operations that always involve a device.

1ST - **0** Medical and Surgical

2ND - **M** Bursae and Ligaments

3RD - **U SUPPLEMENT**

EXAMPLE: Augmentation ligamentoplasty | CMS Ex: Hernia repair mesh

SUPPLEMENT: Putting in or on biological or synthetic material that physically reinforces and/or augments the function of a portion of a body part.

EXPLANATION: Biological material from same individual ...

Body Part – 4TH	Approach – 5TH	Device – 6TH	Qualifier – 7TH
0 Head and Neck Bursa and Ligament	0 Open	7 Autologous	Z No qualifier
1 Shoulder Bursa and Ligament, Right	4 Percutaneous	tissue substitute	
2 Shoulder Bursa and Ligament, Left	endoscopic	J Synthetic	
3 Elbow Bursa and Ligament, Right		substitute	
4 Elbow Bursa and Ligament, Left		K Nonautologous	
5 Wrist Bursa and Ligament, Right		tissue substitute	
6 Wrist Bursa and Ligament, Left			
7 Hand Bursa and Ligament, Right			
8 Hand Bursa and Ligament, Left			
9 Upper Extremity Bursa and Ligament, Right			
B Upper Extremity Bursa and Ligament, Left			
C Trunk Bursa and Ligament, Right			
D Trunk Bursa and Ligament, Left			
F Thorax Bursa and Ligament, Right			
G Thorax Bursa and Ligament, Left			
H Abdomen Bursa and Ligament, Right			
J Abdomen Bursa and Ligament, Left			
K Perineum Bursa and Ligament			
L Hip Bursa and Ligament, Right			
M Hip Bursa and Ligament, Left			
N Knee Bursa and Ligament, Right			
P Knee Bursa and Ligament, Left			
Q Ankle Bursa and Ligament, Right			
R Ankle Bursa and Ligament, Left			
S Foot Bursa and Ligament, Right			
T Foot Bursa and Ligament, Left			
V Lower Extremity Bursa and Ligament, Right			
W Lower Extremity Bursa and Ligament, Left			

BURSAE & LIGAMENTS 0 M W

DEVICE GROUP: Change, (Insertion), Removal, (Replacement), Revision, Supplement
Root Operations that always involve a device.

1ST - **0** Medical and Surgical

2ND - **M** Bursae and Ligaments

3RD - **W REVISION**

EXAMPLE: Resuture ligament graft | CMS Ex: Adjustment pacemaker lead

REVISION: Correcting, to the extent possible, a portion of a malfunctioning device or the position of a displaced device.

EXPLANATION: May replace components of a device ...

Body Part – 4TH	Approach – 5TH	Device – 6TH	Qualifier – 7TH
X Upper Bursa and Ligament	0 Open	0 Drainage device	Z No qualifier
Y Lower Bursa and Ligament	3 Percutaneous	7 Autologous	
	4 Percutaneous	tissue substitute	
	endoscopic	J Synthetic	
	X External	substitute	
		K Nonautologous	
		tissue substitute	

MOVE GROUP: Reattachment, Reposition, Transfer, (Transplantation)			
Root Operations that put in/put back or move some/all of a body part.			

1ST - 0 Medical and Surgical

2ND - M Bursae and Ligaments

3RD - X TRANSFER

EXAMPLE: Carpal ligament transfer

CMS Ex: Tendon transfer

TRANSFER: Moving, without taking out, all or a portion of a body part to another location to take over the function of all or a portion of a body part.

EXPLANATION: The body part remains connected ...

Body Part – 4TH	Approach – 5TH	Device – 6TH	Qualifier – 7TH
0 Head and Neck Bursa and Ligament	0 Open	Z No device	Z No qualifier
1 Shoulder Bursa and Ligament, Right	4 Percutaneous		
2 Shoulder Bursa and Ligament, Left	endoscopic		
3 Elbow Bursa and Ligament, Right			
4 Elbow Bursa and Ligament, Left			
5 Wrist Bursa and Ligament, Right			
6 Wrist Bursa and Ligament, Left			
7 Hand Bursa and Ligament, Right			
8 Hand Bursa and Ligament, Left			
9 Upper Extremity Bursa and Ligament, Right			
B Upper Extremity Bursa and Ligament, Left			
C Trunk Bursa and Ligament, Right			
D Trunk Bursa and Ligament, Left			
F Thorax Bursa and Ligament, Right			
G Thorax Bursa and Ligament, Left			
H Abdomen Bursa and Ligament, Right			
J Abdomen Bursa and Ligament, Left			
K Perineum Bursa and Ligament			
L Hip Bursa and Ligament, Right			
M Hip Bursa and Ligament, Left			
N Knee Bursa and Ligament, Right			
P Knee Bursa and Ligament, Left			
Q Ankle Bursa and Ligament, Right			
R Ankle Bursa and Ligament, Left			
S Foot Bursa and Ligament, Right			
T Foot Bursa and Ligament, Left			
V Lower Extremity Bursa and Ligament, Right			
W Lower Extremity Bursa and Ligament, Left			

BURSAE & LIGAMENTS 0 M X

Educational Annotations | N – Head and Facial Bones

Body System Specific Educational Annotations for the Head and Facial Bones include:

- Anatomy and Physiology Review
- Anatomical Illustrations
- Definitions of Common Procedures
- AHA Coding Clinic® Reference Notations
- Body Part Key Listings
- Device Key Listings
- Device Aggregation Table Listings
- Coding Notes

Anatomy and Physiology Review of Head and Facial Bones

BODY PART VALUES – N - HEAD AND FACIAL BONES

Conchae Bone – The 2 small paired bones of the nasal cavity that are attached to the maxilla.

Ethmoid Bone – The single bone located between the orbits that forms the roof of the nasal cavity, part of the floor of the cranial cavity, and part of the orbit.

Facial Bone – Any one of the 14 bones of the facial area below the cranium (2 nasal bones, vomer, 2 conchae, 2 maxilla, mandible, 2 palatine bones, 2 zygomatic bones, 2 lacrimal bones).

Frontal Bone – The single bone in the front of the skull that also forms part of the roof of the nasal cavity and part of the orbit.

Hyoid Bone – The single horseshoe-shaped bone that lies in the front of the neck and just under the chin and aids in tongue movement and swallowing. It is not directly articulated with any other bone and not considered part of the skull.

Lacrimal Bone – The 2 small paired bones that form the medial side of the orbit and the nasolacrimal canal.

Mandible – The single horseshoe-shaped bone forming the lower jaw.

Maxilla – The 2 fused irregularly-shaped bones that form the upper jaw, the roof of the mouth, and a part of the orbit.

Nasal Bone – The 2 small paired bones that form the bridge of the nose.

Occipital Bone – The single bone of the base and back of the skull.

Orbit – The bones (7) which form the orbit (eye socket): Zygomatic, sphenoid, ethmoid, maxilla, lacrimal, palatine, and frontal.

Palatine Bone – The 2 small paired bones at the back of the nasal cavity that form the floor and lateral wall of the nasal cavity, part of the roof of the mouth, and part of the floor of the orbit.

Parietal Bone – The 2 paired bones that form the top and sides of the skull.

Skull – The skull consists of all (22) of the cranial and facial bones. Eight of these bones form the cranium (occipital bone, frontal bone, 2 temporal bones, 2 parietal bones, sphenoid bone, ethmoid bone), and 14 of these bones form the skull below the cranium (2 nasal bones, vomer, 2 conchae, 2 maxilla, mandible, 2 palatine bones, 2 zygomatic bones, 2 lacrimal bones).

Sphenoid Bone – The single winged-shaped bone of the skull floor that forms part of the base of the cranial cavity, sides of the skull, and part of the orbital floor and side.

Temporal Bone – The 2 paired bones that form the lower sides and base of the skull and contain the internal organs and structures of hearing.

Vomer Bone – The single bone of the inferior nasal septum.

Zygomatic Bone – The 2 paired quadrangular bones of the cheeks (also known as the malar bones) that form the cheek prominence and lower-outer part of the orbit.

Educational Annotations | N – Head and Facial Bones

Anatomical Illustrations of Head and Facial Bones

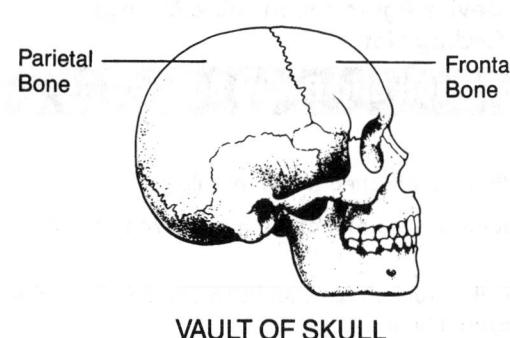

VAULT OF SKULL

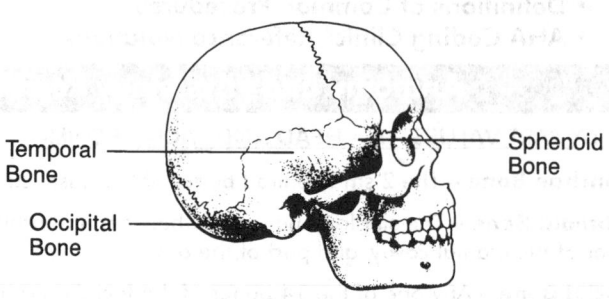

BASE OF SKULL

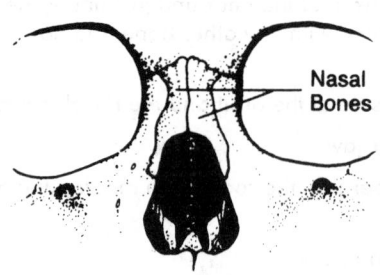

NASAL BONES

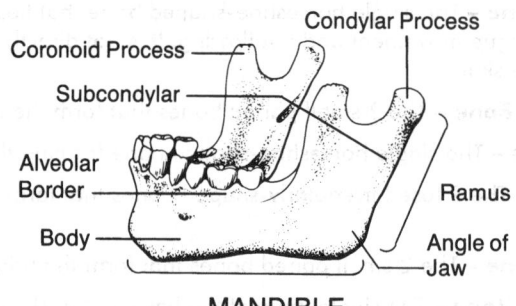

MANDIBLE

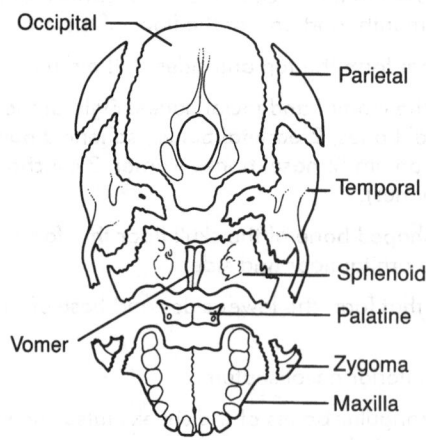

ORBITAL FLOOR AND MALAR BONES

Continued on next page

HEAD & FACIAL BONES 0 N

[2017.PCS]   N – HEAD AND FACIAL BONES   O N

Educational Annotations | N – Head and Facial Bones

Continued from previous page

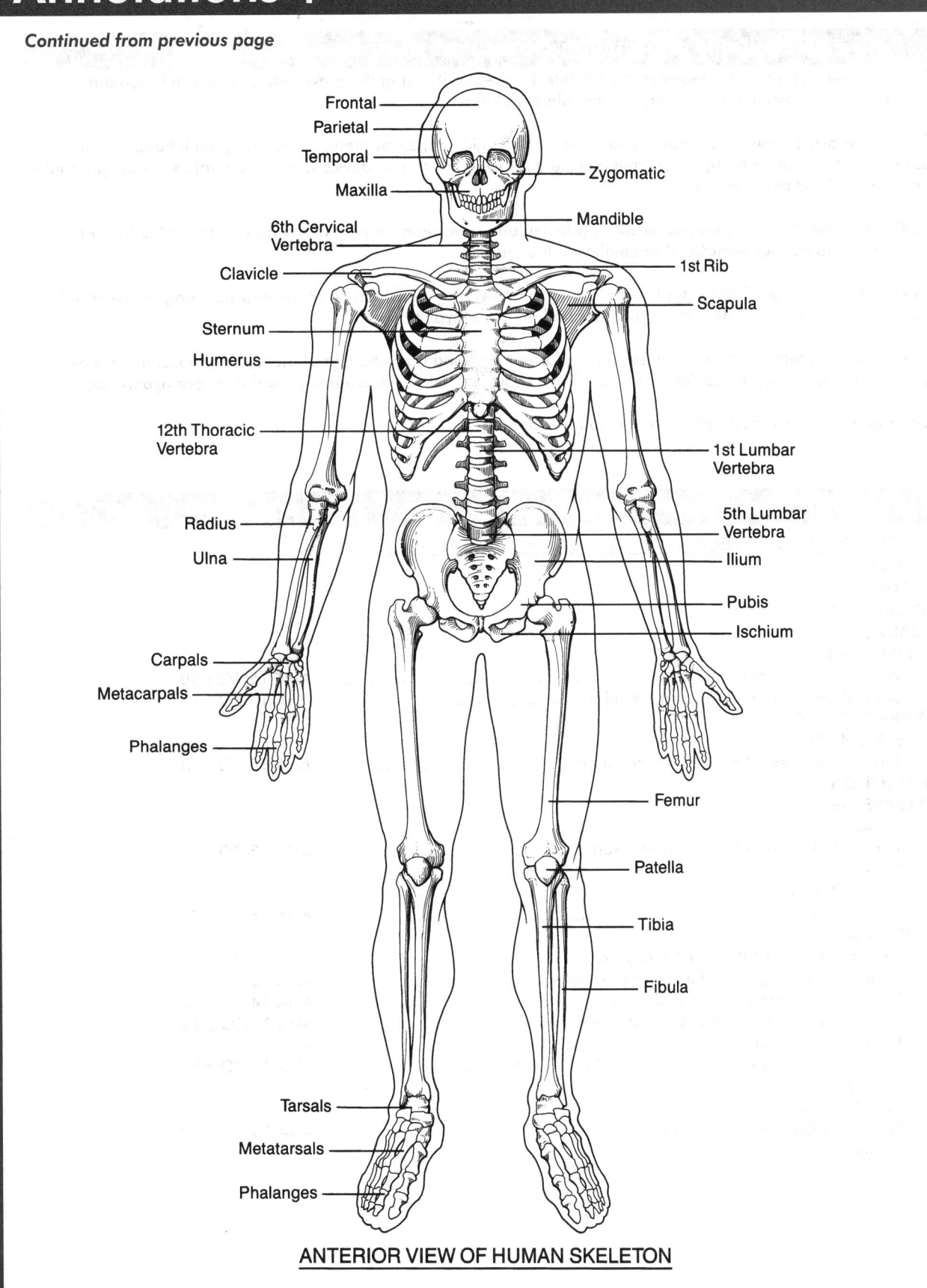

Frontal
Parietal
Temporal
Maxilla
Zygomatic
Mandible
6th Cervical Vertebra
Clavicle
1st Rib
Sternum
Scapula
Humerus
12th Thoracic Vertebra
1st Lumbar Vertebra
Radius
5th Lumbar Vertebra
Ulna
Ilium
Pubis
Ischium
Carpals
Metacarpals
Phalanges
Femur
Patella
Tibia
Fibula
Tarsals
Metatarsals
Phalanges

ANTERIOR VIEW OF HUMAN SKELETON

Educational Annotations | N – Head and Facial Bones

Definitions of Common Procedures of Head and Facial Bones

Cranioplasty – The surgical repair of a skull defect or deformity using the previously excised skull segment, synthetic bone substitute, or synthetic (metal, plastic) plates.

Distraction osteogenesis for craniosynostosis – The surgical repair of prematurely fusing skull bone sutures using osteotomy, bone graft, plates, and an external fixation distractor device to move a portion of skull gradually into a more functional position.

Le Fort I osteotomy – The surgical sectioning (osteotomy) and repositioning of the maxilla along the Le Fort I fracture line to correct dentofacial anomalies of the maxilla.

Le Fort II osteotomy – The surgical sectioning (osteotomy) and repositioning of the maxilla along the Le Fort II fracture line to correct dentofacial anomalies and mid-face hypoplasia.

Le Fort III osteotomy – The surgical sectioning (osteotomy) and repositioning of the maxilla, nose, and cheek bones (zygoma) along the Le Fort III fracture line to correct dentofacial anomalies and mid-face hypoplasia.

Osteotomy – The surgical incision or division of a bone.

AHA Coding Clinic® Reference Notations of Head and Facial Bones

ROOT OPERATION SPECIFIC - N - HEAD AND FACIAL BONES

CHANGE - 2
DESTRUCTION - 5
DIVISION - 8
DRAINAGE - 9
EXCISION - B
    Harvesting of local bone for graft ....AHA 15:1Q:p30
    Radical resection of eyelid and orbital tumor ....AHA 15:2Q:p12
EXTIRPATION - C
INSERTION - H
    Insertion of internal fixation device into skull ....AHA 15:3Q:p13
INSPECTION - J
RELEASE - N
REMOVAL - P
    Removal of internal fixation device from skull ....AHA 15:3Q:p13
REPAIR - Q
REPLACEMENT - R
    Hemi-cranioplasty ....AHA 14:3Q:p7
REPOSITION - S
    Cranial vault reconstruction/reshaping..AHA 15:3Q:p17
    Distraction osteogenesis for craniosynostosis ....AHA 13:3Q:p24
    Le Fort 1 osteotomy ....AHA 14:3Q:p23
    Open reduction internal fixation of frontal bone fracture ....AHA 13:3Q:p25
    Raising of cranium ....AHA 15:3Q:p27
    Removal and placement of skull bone flap in abdominal wall ....AHA 16:2Q:p30
RESECTION - T
SUPPLEMENT - U
    Titanium plates to stabilize bone ....AHA 13:3Q:p 24
REVISION - W

Educational Annotations | N – Head and Facial Bones

Body Part Key Listings of Head and Facial Bones

See also Body Part Key in Appendix C

Alveolar process of mandible ....*use* Mandible, Left/Right
Alveolar process of maxilla ....*use* Maxilla, Left/Right
Bony orbit..*use* Orbit, Left/Right
Condyloid process ....*use* Mandible, Left/Right
Cribriform plate ....*use* Ethmoid Bone, Left/Right
Foramen magnum ....*use* Occipital Bone, Left/Right
Greater wing ....*use* Sphenoid Bone, Left/Right
Lesser wing ....*use* Sphenoid Bone, Left/Right
Mandibular notch...*use* Mandible, Left/Right
Mastoid process ....*use* Temporal Bone, Left/Right
Mental foramen ....*use* Mandible, Left/Right
Optic foramen ....*use* Sphenoid Bone, Left/Right
Orbital portion of ethmoid bone ....*use* Orbit, Left/Right
Orbital portion of frontal bone ....*use* Orbit, Left/Right
Orbital portion of lacrimal bone ....*use* Orbit, Left/Right
Orbital portion of maxilla ....*use* Orbit, Left/Right
Orbital portion of palatine bone ....*use* Orbit, Left/Right
Orbital portion of sphenoid bone ....*use* Orbit, Left/Right
Orbital portion of zygomatic bone...................*use* Orbit, Left/Right
Petrous part of temporal bone ....*use* Temporal Bone, Left/Right
Pterygoid process...*use* Sphenoid Bone, Left/Right
Sella turcica ....*use* Sphenoid Bone, Left/Right
Tympanic part of temporal bone ....*use* Temporal Bone, Left/Right
Vomer of nasal septum ....*use* Nasal Bone
Zygomatic process of frontal bone...................*use* Frontal Bone, Left/Right
Zygomatic process of temporal bone................*use* Temporal Bone, Left/Right

Device Key Listings of Head and Facial Bones

See also Device Key in Appendix D

Autograft ....*use* Autologous Tissue Substitute
Bone anchored hearing device ....*use* Hearing Device in Head and Facial Bones
Bone bank bone graft ....*use* Nonautologous Tissue Substitute
Bone screw (interlocking) (lag) (pedicle) (recessed)*use* Internal Fixation Device in Head and Facial Bones, Upper Bones, Lower Bones
Electrical bone growth stimulator (EBGS) ....*use* Bone Growth Stimulator in Head and Facial Bones, Upper Bones, Lower Bones
External fixator...*use* External Fixation Device in Head and Facial Bones, Upper Bones, Lower Bones, Upper Joints, Lower Joints
Kirschner wire (K-wire) ....*use* Internal Fixation Device in Head and Facial Bones, Upper Bones, Lower Bones, Upper Joints, Lower Joints
Neutralization plate ....*use* Internal Fixation Device in Head and Facial Bones, Upper Bones, Lower Bones
Polymethylmethacrylate (PMMA)...............................*use* Synthetic Substitute
RNS system neurostimulator generator ....*use* Neurostimulator Generator in Head and Facial Bones
Tissue bank graft ....*use* Nonautologous Tissue Substitute
Ultrasonic osteogenic stimulator.............................*use* Bone Growth Stimulator in Head and Facial Bones, Upper Bones, Lower Bones
Ultrasound bone healing system ....*use* Bone Growth Stimulator in Head and Facial Bones, Upper Bones, Lower Bones

Educational Annotations | N – Head and Facial Bones

Device Aggregation Table Listings of Head and Facial Bones

See also Device Aggregation Table in Appendix E

Specific Device	For Operation	In Body System	General Device
None Listed in Device Aggregation Table for this Body System			

Coding Notes of Head and Facial Bones

Body System Relevant Coding Guidelines

Reposition for fracture treatment
B3.15

Reduction of a displaced fracture is coded to the root operation Reposition and the application of a cast or splint in conjunction with the Reposition procedure is not coded separately. Treatment of a nondisplaced fracture is coded to the procedure performed.

Examples: Casting of a nondisplaced fracture is coded to the root operation Immobilization in the Placement section.

Putting a pin in a nondisplaced fracture is coded to the root operation Insertion.

Body System Specific PCS Reference Manual Exercises

<u>PCS CODE</u>   <u>N – HEAD AND FACIAL BONES EXERCISES</u>

None for this Body System

DEVICE GROUP: Change, Insertion, Removal, Replacement, Revision, Supplement
Root Operations that always involve a device.

1ST - **0** Medical and Surgical

2ND - **N** Head and Facial Bones

3RD - **2 CHANGE**

EXAMPLE: Exchange drain tube   CMS Ex: Changing urinary catheter

CHANGE: Taking out or off a device from a body part and putting back an identical or similar device in or on the same body part without cutting or puncturing the skin or a mucous membrane.

EXPLANATION: ALL Changes use EXTERNAL approach only ...

Body Part – 4TH	Approach – 5TH	Device – 6TH	Qualifier – 7TH
0 Skull B Nasal Bone W Facial Bone	X External	0 Drainage device Y Other device	Z No qualifier

EXCISION GROUP: Excision, Resection, Destruction, (Extraction), (Detachment)
Root Operations that take out some or all of a body part.

1ST - **0** Medical and Surgical

2ND - **N** Head and Facial Bones

3RD - **5 DESTRUCTION**

EXAMPLE: Cryoablation bone cyst   CMS Ex: Fulguration polyp

DESTRUCTION: Physical eradication of all or a portion of a body part by the direct use of energy, force, or a destructive agent.

EXPLANATION: None of the body part is physically taken out

Body Part – 4TH		Approach – 5TH	Device – 6TH	Qualifier – 7TH
0 Skull	H Lacrimal Bone, Right	0 Open	Z No device	Z No qualifier
1 Frontal Bone, Right	J Lacrimal Bone, Left	3 Percutaneous		
2 Frontal Bone, Left	K Palatine Bone, Right	4 Percutaneous endoscopic		
3 Parietal Bone, Right	L Palatine Bone, Left			
4 Parietal Bone, Left	M Zygomatic Bone, Right			
5 Temporal Bone, Right	N Zygomatic Bone, Left			
6 Temporal Bone, Left	P Orbit, Right			
7 Occipital Bone, Right	Q Orbit, Left			
8 Occipital Bone, Left	R Maxilla, Right			
B Nasal Bone	S Maxilla, Left			
C Sphenoid Bone, Right	T Mandible, Right			
D Sphenoid Bone, Left	V Mandible, Left			
F Ethmoid Bone, Right	X Hyoid Bone			
G Ethmoid Bone, Left				

HEAD & FACIAL BONES 0 N 5

DIVISION GROUP: Division, Release
Root Operations involving cutting or separation only.

1ST - **0** Medical and Surgical

2ND - **N** Head and Facial Bones

3RD - **8 DIVISION**

EXAMPLE: Mandibular osteotomy | **CMS Ex:** Osteotomy

DIVISION: Cutting into a body part without draining fluids and/or gases from the body part in order to separate or transect a body part.

EXPLANATION: Separated into two or more portions ...

Body Part – 4TH	Approach – 5TH	Device – 6TH	Qualifier – 7TH
0 Skull	0 Open	Z No device	Z No qualifier
1 Frontal Bone, Right	3 Percutaneous		
2 Frontal Bone, Left	4 Percutaneous endoscopic		
3 Parietal Bone, Right			
4 Parietal Bone, Left			
5 Temporal Bone, Right			
6 Temporal Bone, Left			
7 Occipital Bone, Right			
8 Occipital Bone, Left			
B Nasal Bone			
C Sphenoid Bone, Right			
D Sphenoid Bone, Left			
F Ethmoid Bone, Right			
G Ethmoid Bone, Left			
H Lacrimal Bone, Right			
J Lacrimal Bone, Left			
K Palatine Bone, Right			
L Palatine Bone, Left			
M Zygomatic Bone, Right			
N Zygomatic Bone, Left			
P Orbit, Right			
Q Orbit, Left			
R Maxilla, Right			
S Maxilla, Left			
T Mandible, Right			
V Mandible, Left			
X Hyoid Bone			

DRAINAGE GROUP: Drainage, Extirpation, (Fragmentation)
Root Operations that take out solids/fluids/gases from a body part.

1ST - 0 Medical and Surgical	EXAMPLE: Aspiration bone cyst	CMS Ex: Thoracentesis
2ND - N Head and Facial Bones	**DRAINAGE:** Taking or letting out fluids and/or gases from a body part.	
3RD - 9 DRAINAGE	EXPLANATION: Qualifier "X Diagnostic" indicates biopsy ...	

Body Part – 4TH		Approach – 5TH	Device – 6TH	Qualifier – 7TH
0 Skull	H Lacrimal Bone, Right	0 Open	0 Drainage device	Z No qualifier
1 Frontal Bone, Right	J Lacrimal Bone, Left	3 Percutaneous		
2 Frontal Bone, Left	K Palatine Bone, Right	4 Percutaneous endoscopic		
3 Parietal Bone, Right	L Palatine Bone, Left			
4 Parietal Bone, Left	M Zygomatic Bone, Right			
5 Temporal Bone, Right	N Zygomatic Bone, Left			
6 Temporal Bone, Left	P Orbit, Right			
7 Occipital Bone, Right	Q Orbit, Left			
8 Occipital Bone, Left	R Maxilla, Right			
B Nasal Bone	S Maxilla, Left			
C Sphenoid Bone, Right	T Mandible, Right			
D Sphenoid Bone, Left	V Mandible, Left			
F Ethmoid Bone, Right	X Hyoid Bone			
G Ethmoid Bone, Left				
0 Skull	H Lacrimal Bone, Right	0 Open	Z No device	X Diagnostic
1 Frontal Bone, Right	J Lacrimal Bone, Left	3 Percutaneous		Z No qualifier
2 Frontal Bone, Left	K Palatine Bone, Right	4 Percutaneous endoscopic		
3 Parietal Bone, Right	L Palatine Bone, Left			
4 Parietal Bone, Left	M Zygomatic Bone, Right			
5 Temporal Bone, Right	N Zygomatic Bone, Left			
6 Temporal Bone, Left	P Orbit, Right			
7 Occipital Bone, Right	Q Orbit, Left			
8 Occipital Bone, Left	R Maxilla, Right			
B Nasal Bone	S Maxilla, Left			
C Sphenoid Bone, Right	T Mandible, Right			
D Sphenoid Bone, Left	V Mandible, Left			
F Ethmoid Bone, Right	X Hyoid Bone			
G Ethmoid Bone, Left				

HEAD & FACIAL BONES 0 N 9

EXCISION GROUP: Excision, Resection, Destruction, (Extraction), (Detachment)
Root Operations that take out some or all of a body part.

1ST - 0 Medical and Surgical	EXAMPLE: Mandibular sequestrectomy	CMS Ex: Liver biopsy
2ND - N Head and Facial Bones	**EXCISION:** Cutting out or off, without replacement, a portion of a body part.	
3RD - B EXCISION	EXPLANATION: Qualifier "X Diagnostic" indicates biopsy ...	

Body Part – 4TH		Approach – 5TH	Device – 6TH	Qualifier – 7TH
0 Skull	H Lacrimal Bone, Right	0 Open	Z No device	X Diagnostic
1 Frontal Bone, Right	J Lacrimal Bone, Left	3 Percutaneous		Z No qualifier
2 Frontal Bone, Left	K Palatine Bone, Right	4 Percutaneous		
3 Parietal Bone, Right	L Palatine Bone, Left	endoscopic		
4 Parietal Bone, Left	M Zygomatic Bone, Right			
5 Temporal Bone, Right	N Zygomatic Bone, Left			
6 Temporal Bone, Left	P Orbit, Right			
7 Occipital Bone, Right	Q Orbit, Left			
8 Occipital Bone, Left	R Maxilla, Right			
B Nasal Bone	S Maxilla, Left			
C Sphenoid Bone, Right	T Mandible, Right			
D Sphenoid Bone, Left	V Mandible, Left			
F Ethmoid Bone, Right	X Hyoid Bone			
G Ethmoid Bone, Left				

DRAINAGE GROUP: Drainage, Extirpation, (Fragmentation)
Root Operations that take out solids/fluids/gases from a body part.

1ST - 0 Medical and Surgical	EXAMPLE: Removal foreign body	CMS Ex: Choledocholithotomy
2ND - N Head and Facial Bones	**EXTIRPATION:** Taking or cutting out solid matter from a body part.	
3RD - C EXTIRPATION	EXPLANATION: Abnormal byproduct or foreign body ...	

Body Part – 4TH		Approach – 5TH	Device – 6TH	Qualifier – 7TH
1 Frontal Bone, Right	H Lacrimal Bone, Right	0 Open	Z No device	Z No qualifier
2 Frontal Bone, Left	J Lacrimal Bone, Left	3 Percutaneous		
3 Parietal Bone, Right	K Palatine Bone, Right	4 Percutaneous		
4 Parietal Bone, Left	L Palatine Bone, Left	endoscopic		
5 Temporal Bone, Right	M Zygomatic Bone, Right			
6 Temporal Bone, Left	N Zygomatic Bone, Left			
7 Occipital Bone, Right	P Orbit, Right			
8 Occipital Bone, Left	Q Orbit, Left			
B Nasal Bone	R Maxilla, Right			
C Sphenoid Bone, Right	S Maxilla, Left			
D Sphenoid Bone, Left	T Mandible, Right			
F Ethmoid Bone, Right	V Mandible, Left			
G Ethmoid Bone, Left	X Hyoid Bone			

HEAD & FACIAL BONES 0 N B

DEVICE GROUP: Change, Insertion, Removal, Replacement, Revision, Supplement Root Operations that always involve a device.			

EXAMPLE: Bone growth stimulator   CMS Ex: Central venous catheter

1ST - 0 Medical and Surgical

2ND - N Head and Facial Bones

3RD - H INSERTION

INSERTION: Putting in a nonbiological appliance that monitors, assists, performs, or prevents a physiological function but does not physically take the place of a body part.

EXPLANATION: None

Body Part – 4TH	Approach – 5TH	Device – 6TH	Qualifier – 7TH
0 Skull	0 Open	4 Internal fixation device 5 External fixation device M Bone growth stimulator N Neurostimulator generator	Z No qualifier
0 Skull	3 Percutaneous 4 Percutaneous endoscopic	4 Internal fixation device 5 External fixation device M Bone growth stimulator	Z No qualifier
1 Frontal Bone, Right 2 Frontal Bone, Left 3 Parietal Bone, Right 4 Parietal Bone, Left 7 Occipital Bone, Right 8 Occipital Bone, Left C Sphenoid Bone, Right D Sphenoid Bone, Left F Ethmoid Bone, Right G Ethmoid Bone, Left H Lacrimal Bone, Right J Lacrimal Bone, Left K Palatine Bone, Right L Palatine Bone, Left M Zygomatic Bone, Right N Zygomatic Bone, Left P Orbit, Right Q Orbit, Left X Hyoid Bone	0 Open 3 Percutaneous 4 Percutaneous endoscopic	4 Internal fixation device	Z No qualifier
5 Temporal Bone, Right 6 Temporal Bone, Left	0 Open 3 Percutaneous 4 Percutaneous endoscopic	4 Internal fixation device S Hearing device	Z No qualifier
B Nasal Bone	0 Open 3 Percutaneous 4 Percutaneous endoscopic	4 Internal fixation device M Bone growth stimulator	Z No qualifier
R Maxilla, Right S Maxilla, Left T Mandible, Right V Mandible, Left	0 Open 3 Percutaneous 4 Percutaneous endoscopic	4 Internal fixation device 5 External fixation device	Z No qualifier
W Facial Bone	0 Open 3 Percutaneous 4 Percutaneous endoscopic	M Bone growth stimulator	Z No qualifier

HEAD & FACIAL BONES 0 N H

EXAMINATION GROUP: Inspection, (Map)
Root Operations involving examination only.

1ST - **0** Medical and Surgical	EXAMPLE: Examination bone		CMS Ex: Colonoscopy
2ND - **N** Head and Facial Bones	**INSPECTION:** Visually and/or manually exploring a body part.		
3RD - **J** INSPECTION	EXPLANATION: Direct or instrumental visualization ...		

Body Part – 4TH	Approach – 5TH	Device – 6TH	Qualifier – 7TH
0 Skull B Nasal Bone W Facial Bone	0 Open 3 Percutaneous 4 Percutaneous endoscopic X External	Z No device	Z No qualifier

DIVISION GROUP: Division, Release
Root Operations involving cutting or separation only.

1ST - **0** Medical and Surgical	EXAMPLE: Extra-articular bone adhesiolysis		CMS Ex: Carpal tunnel release
2ND - **N** Head and Facial Bones	**RELEASE:** Freeing a body part from an abnormal physical constraint by cutting or by the use of force.		
3RD - **N** RELEASE	EXPLANATION: None of the body part is taken out ...		

Body Part – 4TH		Approach – 5TH	Device – 6TH	Qualifier – 7TH
1 Frontal Bone, Right 2 Frontal Bone, Left 3 Parietal Bone, Right 4 Parietal Bone, Left 5 Temporal Bone, Right 6 Temporal Bone, Left 7 Occipital Bone, Right 8 Occipital Bone, Left B Nasal Bone C Sphenoid Bone, Right D Sphenoid Bone, Left F Ethmoid Bone, Right G Ethmoid Bone, Left	H Lacrimal Bone, Right J Lacrimal Bone, Left K Palatine Bone, Right L Palatine Bone, Left M Zygomatic Bone, Right N Zygomatic Bone, Left P Orbit, Right Q Orbit, Left R Maxilla, Right S Maxilla, Left T Mandible, Right V Mandible, Left X Hyoid Bone	0 Open 3 Percutaneous 4 Percutaneous endoscopic	Z No device	Z No qualifier

DEVICE GROUP: Change, Insertion, Removal, Replacement, Revision, Supplement
Root Operations that always involve a device.

1ST - 0 Medical and Surgical

2ND - N Head and Facial Bones

3RD - P REMOVAL

EXAMPLE: Removal bone growth stimulator | CMS Ex: Chest tube removal

REMOVAL: Taking out or off a device from a body part.

EXPLANATION: Removal device without reinsertion …

Body Part – 4TH	Approach – 5TH	Device – 6TH	Qualifier – 7TH
0 Skull	0 Open	0 Drainage device 4 Internal fixation device 5 External fixation device 7 Autologous tissue substitute J Synthetic substitute K Nonautologous tissue substitute M Bone growth stimulator N Neurostimulator generator S Hearing device	Z No qualifier
0 Skull	3 Percutaneous 4 Percutaneous endoscopic	0 Drainage device 4 Internal fixation device 5 External fixation device 7 Autologous tissue substitute J Synthetic substitute K Nonautologous tissue substitute M Bone growth stimulator S Hearing device	Z No qualifier
0 Skull	X External	0 Drainage device 4 Internal fixation device 5 External fixation device M Bone growth stimulator S Hearing device	Z No qualifier
B Nasal Bone W Facial Bone	0 Open 3 Percutaneous 4 Percutaneous endoscopic	0 Drainage device 4 Internal fixation device 7 Autologous tissue substitute J Synthetic substitute K Nonautologous tissue substitute M Bone growth stimulator	Z No qualifier
B Nasal Bone W Facial Bone	X External	0 Drainage device 4 Internal fixation device M Bone growth stimulator	Z No qualifier

0 N Q

OTHER REPAIRS GROUP: (Control), Repair
Root Operations that define other repairs.

1ST - **0** Medical and Surgical

2ND - **N** Head and Facial Bones

3RD - **Q REPAIR**

EXAMPLE: Orbital osteoplasty | CMS Ex: Suture laceration

REPAIR: Restoring, to the extent possible, a body part to its normal anatomic structure and function.

EXPLANATION: Only when no other root operation applies ...

Body Part – 4TH		Approach – 5TH	Device – 6TH	Qualifier – 7TH
0 Skull	H Lacrimal Bone, Right	0 Open	Z No device	Z No qualifier
1 Frontal Bone, Right	J Lacrimal Bone, Left	3 Percutaneous		
2 Frontal Bone, Left	K Palatine Bone, Right	4 Percutaneous endoscopic		
3 Parietal Bone, Right	L Palatine Bone, Left	X External		
4 Parietal Bone, Left	M Zygomatic Bone, Right			
5 Temporal Bone, Right	N Zygomatic Bone, Left			
6 Temporal Bone, Left	P Orbit, Right			
7 Occipital Bone, Right	Q Orbit, Left			
8 Occipital Bone, Left	R Maxilla, Right			
B Nasal Bone	S Maxilla, Left			
C Sphenoid Bone, Right	T Mandible, Right			
D Sphenoid Bone, Left	V Mandible, Left			
F Ethmoid Bone, Right	X Hyoid Bone			
G Ethmoid Bone, Left				

DEVICE GROUP: Change, Insertion, Removal, Replacement, Revision, Supplement
Root Operations that always involve a device.

1ST - **0** Medical and Surgical

2ND - **N** Head and Facial Bones

3RD - **R REPLACEMENT**

EXAMPLE: Hemi-cranioplasty defect repair | CMS Ex: Total hip

REPLACEMENT: Putting in or on a biological or synthetic material that physically takes the place and/or function of all or a portion of a body part.

EXPLANATION: Includes taking out body part, or eradication...

Body Part – 4TH		Approach – 5TH	Device – 6TH	Qualifier – 7TH
0 Skull	H Lacrimal Bone, Right	0 Open	7 Autologous tissue substitute	Z No qualifier
1 Frontal Bone, Right	J Lacrimal Bone, Left	3 Percutaneous	J Synthetic substitute	
2 Frontal Bone, Left	K Palatine Bone, Right	4 Percutaneous endoscopic	K Nonautologous tissue substitute	
3 Parietal Bone, Right	L Palatine Bone, Left			
4 Parietal Bone, Left	M Zygomatic Bone, Right			
5 Temporal Bone, Right	N Zygomatic Bone, Left			
6 Temporal Bone, Left	P Orbit, Right			
7 Occipital Bone, Right	Q Orbit, Left			
8 Occipital Bone, Left	R Maxilla, Right			
B Nasal Bone	S Maxilla, Left			
C Sphenoid Bone, Right	T Mandible, Right			
D Sphenoid Bone, Left	V Mandible, Left			
F Ethmoid Bone, Right	X Hyoid Bone			
G Ethmoid Bone, Left				

HEAD & FACIAL BONES 0 N Q

MOVE GROUP: (Reattachment), **Reposition**, (Transfer), (Transplantation)
Root Operations that put in/put back or move some/all of a body part.

EXAMPLE: Le Fort 1 maxillary osteotomy	CMS Ex: Fracture reduction

1ST - **0** Medical and Surgical

2ND - **N** Head and Facial Bones

3RD - **S REPOSITION**

REPOSITION: Moving to its normal location, or other suitable location, all or a portion of a body part.

EXPLANATION: May or may not be cut to be moved ...

Body Part – 4TH	Approach – 5TH	Device – 6TH	Qualifier – 7TH
0 Skull R Maxilla, Right S Maxilla, Left T Mandible, Right V Mandible, Left	0 Open 3 Percutaneous 4 Percutaneous endoscopic	4 Internal fixation device 5 External fixation device Z No device	Z No qualifier
0 Skull R Maxilla, Right S Maxilla, Left T Mandible, Right V Mandible, Left	X External	Z No device	Z No qualifier
1 Frontal Bone, Right F Ethmoid Bone, Right 2 Frontal Bone, Left G Ethmoid Bone, Left 3 Parietal Bone, Right H Lacrimal Bone, Right 4 Parietal Bone, Left J Lacrimal Bone, Left 5 Temporal Bone, Right K Palatine Bone, Right 6 Temporal Bone, Left L Palatine Bone, Left 7 Occipital Bone, Right M Zygomatic Bone, Right 8 Occipital Bone, Left N Zygomatic Bone, Left B Nasal Bone P Orbit, Right C Sphenoid Bone, Right Q Orbit, Left D Sphenoid Bone, Left X Hyoid Bone	0 Open 3 Percutaneous 4 Percutaneous endoscopic	4 Internal fixation device Z No device	Z No qualifier
1 Frontal Bone, Right F Ethmoid Bone, Right 2 Frontal Bone, Left G Ethmoid Bone, Left 3 Parietal Bone, Right H Lacrimal Bone, Right 4 Parietal Bone, Left J Lacrimal Bone, Left 5 Temporal Bone, Right K Palatine Bone, Right 6 Temporal Bone, Left L Palatine Bone, Left 7 Occipital Bone, Right M Zygomatic Bone, Right 8 Occipital Bone, Left N Zygomatic Bone, Left B Nasal Bone P Orbit, Right C Sphenoid Bone, Right Q Orbit, Left D Sphenoid Bone, Left X Hyoid Bone	X External	Z No device	Z No qualifier

HEAD & FACIAL BONES **0 N S**

EXCISION GROUP: Excision, Resection, Destruction, (Extraction), (Detachment)
Root Operations that take out some or all of a body part.

1ST - 0 Medical and Surgical	EXAMPLE: Total removal hyoid bone	CMS Ex: Cholecystectomy

2ND - N Head and Facial Bones

3RD - T RESECTION

RESECTION: Cutting out or off, without replacement, all of a body part.

EXPLANATION: None

Body Part – 4TH		Approach – 5TH	Device – 6TH	Qualifier – 7TH
1 Frontal Bone, Right	H Lacrimal Bone, Right	0 Open	Z No device	Z No qualifier
2 Frontal Bone, Left	J Lacrimal Bone, Left			
3 Parietal Bone, Right	K Palatine Bone, Right			
4 Parietal Bone, Left	L Palatine Bone, Left			
5 Temporal Bone, Right	M Zygomatic Bone, Right			
6 Temporal Bone, Left	N Zygomatic Bone, Left			
7 Occipital Bone, Right	P Orbit, Right			
8 Occipital Bone, Left	Q Orbit, Left			
B Nasal Bone	R Maxilla, Right			
C Sphenoid Bone, Right	S Maxilla, Left			
D Sphenoid Bone, Left	T Mandible, Right			
F Ethmoid Bone, Right	V Mandible, Left			
G Ethmoid Bone, Left	X Hyoid Bone			

DEVICE GROUP: Change, Insertion, Removal, Replacement, Revision, Supplement
Root Operations that always involve a device.

1ST - 0 Medical and Surgical	EXAMPLE: Stabilizing plate for defect	CMS Ex: Hernia repair with mesh

2ND - N Head and Facial Bones

3RD - U SUPPLEMENT

SUPPLEMENT: Putting in or on biological or synthetic material that physically reinforces and/or augments the function of a portion of a body part.

EXPLANATION: Biological material from same individual ...

Body Part – 4TH		Approach – 5TH	Device – 6TH	Qualifier – 7TH
0 Skull	H Lacrimal Bone, Right	0 Open	7 Autologous tissue substitute	Z No qualifier
1 Frontal Bone, Right	J Lacrimal Bone, Left	3 Percutaneous	J Synthetic substitute	
2 Frontal Bone, Left	K Palatine Bone, Right	4 Percutaneous endoscopic	K Nonautologous tissue substitute	
3 Parietal Bone, Right	L Palatine Bone, Left			
4 Parietal Bone, Left	M Zygomatic Bone, Right			
5 Temporal Bone, Right	N Zygomatic Bone, Left			
6 Temporal Bone, Left	P Orbit, Right			
7 Occipital Bone, Right	Q Orbit, Left			
8 Occipital Bone, Left	R Maxilla, Right			
B Nasal Bone	S Maxilla, Left			
C Sphenoid Bone, Right	T Mandible, Right			
D Sphenoid Bone, Left	V Mandible, Left			
F Ethmoid Bone, Right	X Hyoid Bone			
G Ethmoid Bone, Left				

DEVICE GROUP: Change, Insertion, Removal, Replacement, Revision, Supplement
Root Operations that always involve a device.

1ST - 0 Medical and Surgical	**EXAMPLE:** Reposition bone stimulator | **CMS Ex:** Adjustment pacemaker lead
2ND - N Head and Facial Bones	**REVISION:** Correcting, to the extent possible, a portion of a malfunctioning device or the position of a displaced device.
3RD - W REVISION	**EXPLANATION:** May replace components of a device ...

Body Part – 4TH	Approach – 5TH	Device – 6TH	Qualifier – 7TH
0 Skull	0 Open	0 Drainage device 4 Internal fixation device 5 External fixation device 7 Autologous tissue substitute J Synthetic substitute K Nonautologous tissue substitute M Bone growth stimulator N Neurostimulator generator S Hearing device	Z No qualifier
0 Skull	3 Percutaneous 4 Percutaneous endoscopic X External	0 Drainage device 4 Internal fixation device 5 External fixation device 7 Autologous tissue substitute J Synthetic substitute K Nonautologous tissue substitute M Bone growth stimulator S Hearing device	Z No qualifier
B Nasal Bone W Facial Bone	0 Open 3 Percutaneous 4 Percutaneous endoscopic X External	0 Drainage device 4 Internal fixation device 7 Autologous tissue substitute J Synthetic substitute K Nonautologous tissue substitute M Bone growth stimulator	Z No qualifier

HEAD & FACIAL BONES 0 N W

NOTES

© 2016 Channel Publishing, Ltd.

Educational Annotations | P – Upper Bones

Body System Specific Educational Annotations for the Upper Bones include:

- Anatomy and Physiology Review
- Anatomical Illustrations
- Definitions of Common Procedures
- AHA Coding Clinic® Reference Notations
- Body Part Key Listings
- Device Key Listings
- Device Aggregation Table Listings
- Coding Notes

Anatomy and Physiology Review of Upper Bones

BODY PART VALUES – P - UPPER BONES

Carpal – The 8 compact bones of the wrist, forming 2 rows of 4 bones each. The proximal row contains the scaphoid, lunate, pisiform, and triquetrum. The distal row contains the trapezium, trapezoid, capitate, and hamate.

Cervical Vertebra – The cervical section of the spinal vertebral column comprised of 7 vertebra, C1-C7.

Clavicle – The paired, straightened S-shaped bones (also known as the collarbones) that connect the sternum with the scapula.

Finger Phalanx – The digital bones of the fingers. Each finger contains three bones: Proximal phalanx, intermediate (middle) phalanx, and distal phalanx.

Glenoid Cavity – The shallow, round depression of the scapula that articulates with the humeral head.

Humeral Head – The upper end of the humerus that is part of the shoulder joint.

Humeral Shaft – The middle, long portion of the humerus.

Humerus – The paired, long bones of the upper arm that articulate at the shoulder and the elbow. The capitulum of the humerus articulates with the head of the radius, and the trochlea of the humerus articulates with the trochlear notch of the ulna.

Metacarpal – One of the 5 cylindrical bones of the palm of the hand connecting the carpals to the phalanges of the hand.

Radius – The paired long bones of the forearms that are further away from the body than the ulnas.

Rib – The 12 paired arched bones of the rib cage that partially enclose and protect the chest cavity.

Scapula – The paired flat, triangular bones located in the upper back behind the shoulder (also called the shoulder blade).

Sternum – The long flat bone (also known as the breast bone) of the chest that connects to the clavicles and most of the ribs.

Thoracic Vertebra – The thoracic section of the spinal vertebral column comprised of 12 vertebra, T1-T12.

Thumb Phalanx – The digital bones of the thumb. The thumb contains two bones: Proximal phalanx and distal phalanx.

Ulna – The paired long bones of the forearms that are closer to the side of the body than the radii.

Upper Bone – Any of the bones designated in the Upper Bones PCS Body System.

Educational Annotations | P – Upper Bones

Anatomical Illustrations of Upper Bones

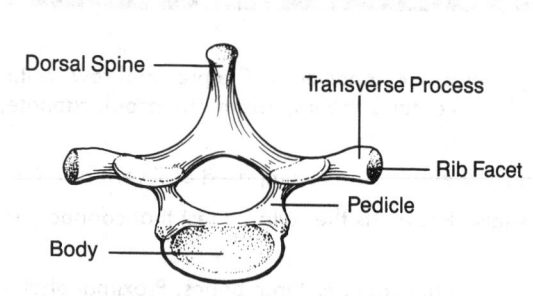

TYPICAL VERTEBRA — SUPERIOR VIEW

Dorsal Spine
Transverse Process
Rib Facet
Pedicle
Body

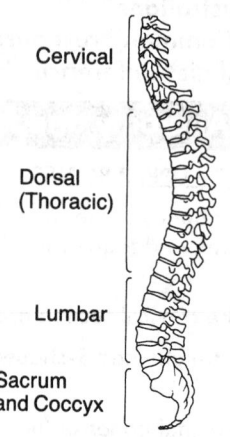

VERTEBRAL COLUMN

Cervical

Dorsal (Thoracic)

Lumbar

Sacrum and Coccyx

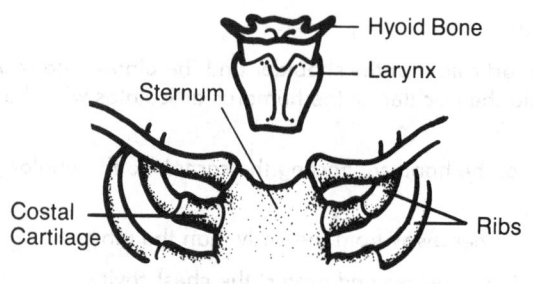

RIBS, STERNUM AND LARYNX

Hyoid Bone
Larynx
Sternum
Costal Cartilage
Ribs

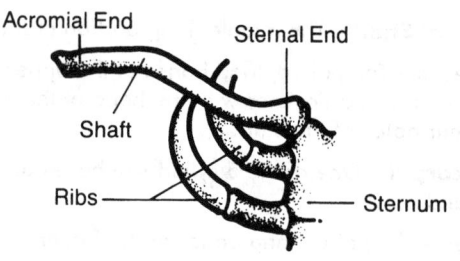

CLAVICLE

Acromial End
Sternal End
Shaft
Ribs
Sternum

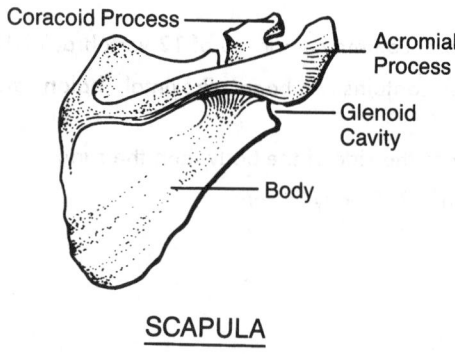

SCAPULA

Coracoid Process
Acromial Process
Glenoid Cavity
Body

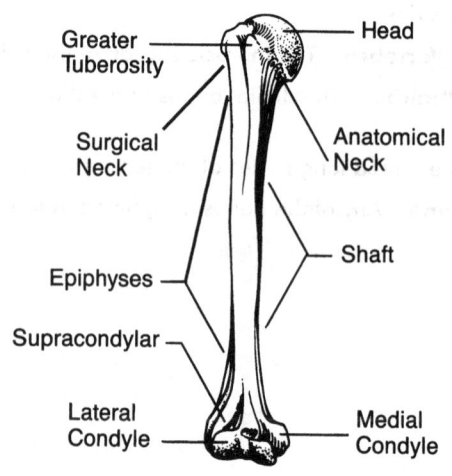

HUMERUS — ANTERIOR VIEW

Greater Tuberosity
Head
Anatomical Neck
Surgical Neck
Shaft
Epiphyses
Supracondylar
Lateral Condyle
Medial Condyle

Educational Annotations | P – Upper Bones

Anatomical Illustrations of Upper Bones

Continued from previous page

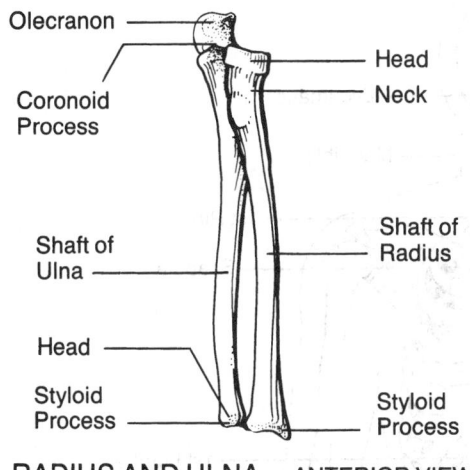

RADIUS AND ULNA — ANTERIOR VIEW

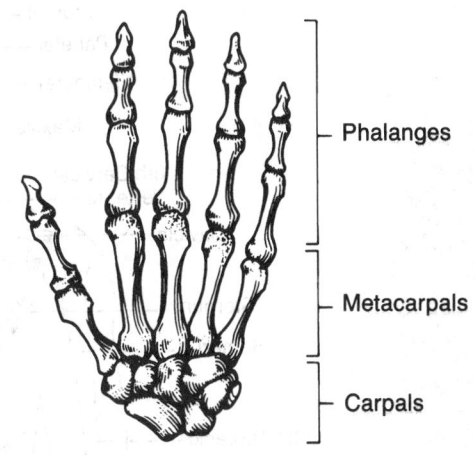

RIGHT HAND — DORSAL VIEW

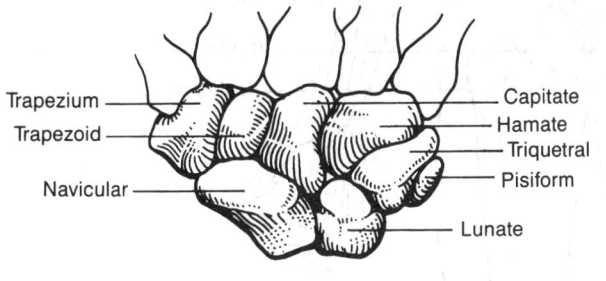

CARPAL BONES — DORSAL VIEW

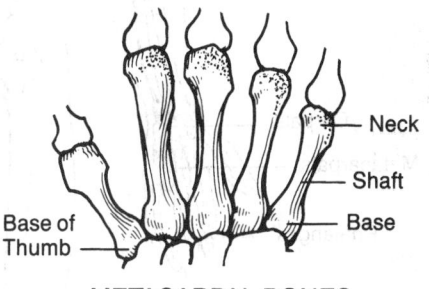

METACARPAL BONES

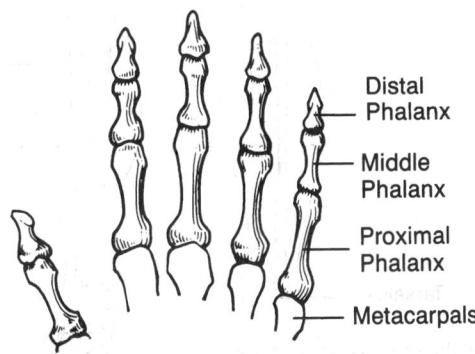

PHALANGES OF HAND

UPPER BONES

0 P

Continued on next page

Educational Annotations | P – Upper Bones

Anatomical Illustrations of Upper Bones

Continued from previous page

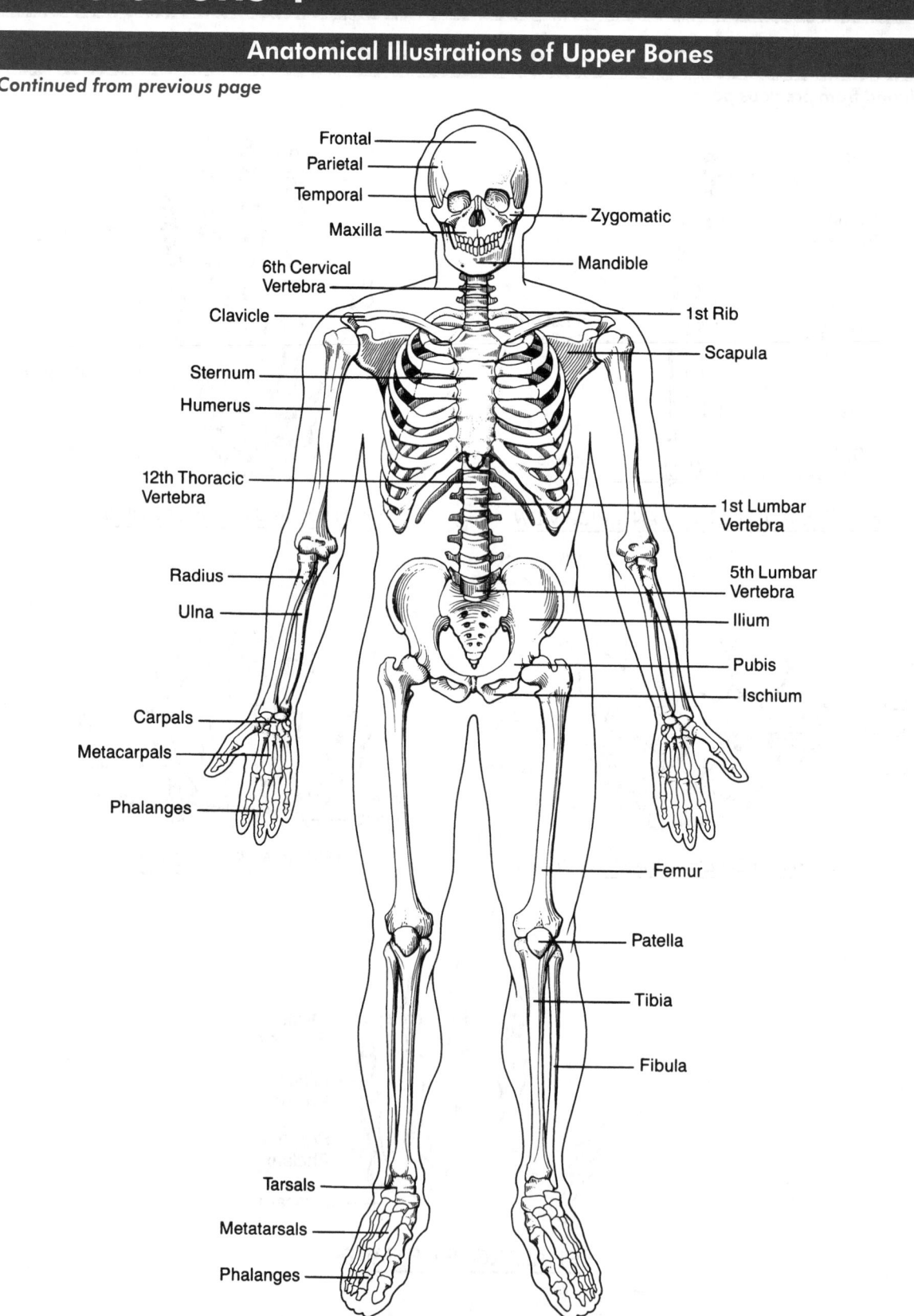

Frontal
Parietal
Temporal
Maxilla
6th Cervical Vertebra
Clavicle
Sternum
Humerus
12th Thoracic Vertebra
Radius
Ulna
Carpals
Metacarpals
Phalanges

Zygomatic
Mandible
1st Rib
Scapula
1st Lumbar Vertebra
5th Lumbar Vertebra
Ilium
Pubis
Ischium
Femur
Patella
Tibia
Fibula

Tarsals
Metatarsals
Phalanges

ANTERIOR VIEW OF HUMAN SKELETON

Continued on next page

© 2016 Channel Publishing, Ltd.

Educational Annotations | P – Upper Bones

Anatomical Illustrations of Upper Bones

Continued from previous page

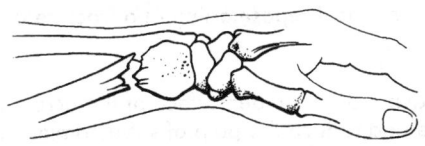

COLLES'

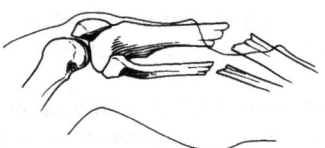

COMPOUND

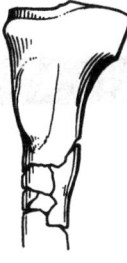

COMMINUTED

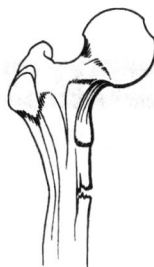

GREENSTICK

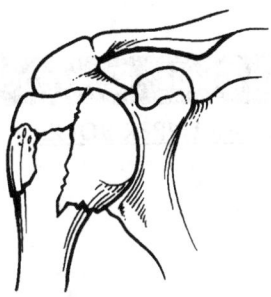

IMPACTED

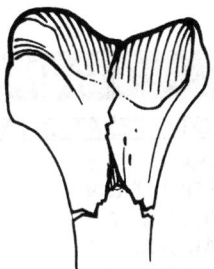

INTERCONDYLAR

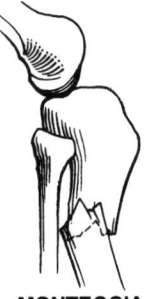

MONTEGGIA

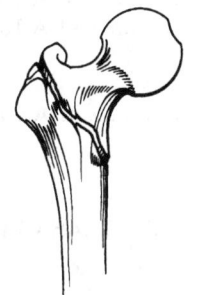

PERTROCHANTERIC

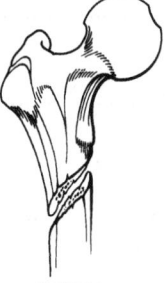

SPIRAL

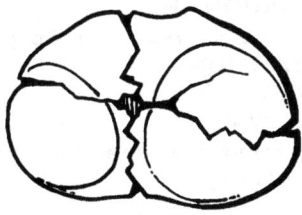

STELLATE

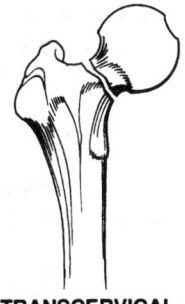

TRANSCERVICAL

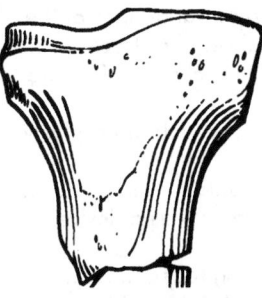

TRANSVERSE

FRACTURE TYPES

Educational Annotations | P – Upper Bones

Definitions of Common Procedures of Upper Bones

Laminectomy – The surgical excision of the lamina of a vertebra, usually to relieve spinal cord compression.

Open reduction, internal fixation of Colles' fracture – The open surgical repositioning of a fracture of the distal radius using internal fixation device(s) (plate, screws, pins).

Subacromial decompression (acromioplasty) – The surgical shaving of the undersurface of the acromial process of the scapula to create more space for the shoulder's soft tissue and reduce the pain of subacromial impingement syndrome.

Total claviculectomy – The surgical removal of the entire clavicle bone.

Vertebroplasty – The surgical injection of bone cement into a fractured vertebra.

AHA Coding Clinic® Reference Notations of Upper Bones

ROOT OPERATION SPECIFIC - P - UPPER BONES

CHANGE - 2
DESTRUCTION - 5
DIVISION - 8
DRAINAGE - 9
EXCISION - B
    Harvesting of local bone for graft ....AHA 15:1Q:p30
    Resection of rib segment ....AHA 12:4Q:p101
    Spinal decompression meaning laminectomy ....AHA 13:4Q:p116
        Official Clarification of 13:4Q:p116 ....AHA 15:2Q:p34
    Subacromial decompression...AHA 13:3Q:p20
EXTIRPATION - C
INSERTION - H
    Insertion/replacement of growing rods.......................................AHA 14:4Q:p28
INSPECTION - J
RELEASE - N
REMOVAL - P
    Removal/replacement of growing rods ....AHA 14:4Q:p28
REPAIR - Q
REPLACEMENT - R
REPOSITION - S
    Elongation derotation flexion cast change ....AHA 16:1Q:p21
    Open reduction internal fixation (ORIF) of forearm bones ....AHA 14:4Q:p32
    Placement of vertical expandable prosthetic titanium rib (VEPTR)..............AHA 14:4Q:p26
    Ravitch procedure (removal of ends of the ribs and reposition of sternum)..AHA 15:4Q:p33
    Reposition of cervical vertebra fracture.......................................AHA 15:2Q:p34
    Reposition of healed distal radius fracture ....AHA 14:3Q:p33
RESECTION - T
    Resection of carpal bone with arthroplasty ....AHA 15:3Q:p26
SUPPLEMENT - U
    Laminoplasty with allograft ....AHA 15:2Q:p20
    Vertebroplasty with cement as a device value ....AHA 14:2Q:p12
REVISION - W
    Lengthening of growing rods ....AHA 14:4Q:p27
    Lengthening of vertical expandable prosthetic titanium rib (VEPTR) ....AHA 14:4Q:p26

UPPER BONES 0 P

Educational Annotations | P – Upper Bones

Body Part Key Listings of Upper Bones

See also Body Part Key in Appendix C

Acromion (process)	*use* Scapula, Left/Right
Capitate bone	*use* Carpal, Left/Right
Coracoid process	*use* Scapula, Left/Right
Distal humerus	*use* Humeral Shaft, Left/Right
Glenoid fossa (of scapula)	*use* Glenoid Cavity, Left/Right
Greater tuberosity	*use* Humeral Head, Left/Right
Hamate bone	*use* Carpal, Left/Right
Humerus, distal	*use* Humeral Shaft, Left/Right
Lateral epicondyle of humerus	*use* Humeral Shaft, Left/Right
Lesser tuberosity	*use* Humeral Head, Left/Right
Lunate bone	*use* Carpal, Left/Right
Manubrium	*use* Sternum
Medial epicondyle of humerus	*use* Humeral Shaft, Left/Right
Neck of humerus (anatomical) (surgical)	*use* Humeral Head, Left/Right
Olecranon process	*use* Ulna, Left/Right
Pisiform bone	*use* Carpal, Left/Right
Radial notch	*use* Ulna, Left/Right
Scaphoid bone	*use* Carpal, Left/Right
Spinous process	*use* Cervical, Thoracic, Lumbar Vertebra
Suprasternal notch	*use* Sternum
Trapezium bone	*use* Carpal, Left/Right
Trapezoid bone	*use* Carpal, Left/Right
Triquetral bone	*use* Carpal, Left/Right
Ulnar notch	*use* Radius, Left/Right
Vertebral arch	*use* Cervical, Thoracic, Lumbar Vertebra
Vertebral foramen	*use* Cervical, Thoracic, Lumbar Vertebra
Vertebral lamina	*use* Cervical, Thoracic, Lumbar Vertebra
Vertebral pedicle	*use* Cervical, Thoracic, Lumbar Vertebra
Xiphoid process	*use* Sternum

Device Key Listings of Upper Bones

See also Device Key in Appendix D

Autograft	*use* Autologous Tissue Substitute
Bone bank bone graft	*use* Nonautologous Tissue Substitute
Bone screw (interlocking) (lag) (pedicle) (recessed)	*use* Internal Fixation Device in Head and Facial Bones, Upper Bones, Lower Bones
Clamp and rod internal fixation system (CRIF)	*use* Internal Fixation Device in Upper Bones, Lower Bones
Delta frame external fixator	*use* External Fixation Device, Hybrid for Insertion in Upper Bones, Lower Bones
	use External Fixation Device, Hybrid for Reposition in Upper Bones, Lower Bones
Electrical bone growth stimulator (EBGS)	*use* Bone Growth Stimulator in Head and Facial Bones, Upper Bones, Lower Bones
External fixator	*use* External Fixation Device in Head and Facial Bones, Upper Bones, Lower Bones, Upper Joints, Lower Joints

Continued on next page

Educational Annotations | P – Upper Bones

Device Key Listings of Upper Bones

Continued from previous page

Ilizarov external fixator ....*use* External Fixation Device, Ring for Insertion in Upper Bones, Lower Bones

....*use* External Fixation Device, Ring for Reposition in Upper Bones, Lower Bones

Ilizarov-Vecklich device..*use* External Fixation Device, Limb Lengthening for Insertion in Upper Bones, Lower Bones

Intramedullary (IM) rod (nail) ....*use* Internal Fixation Device, Intramedullary in Upper Bones, Lower Bones

Intramedullary skeletal kinetic distractor (ISKD) ....*use* Internal Fixation Device, Intramedullary in Upper Bones, Lower Bones

Kirschner wire (K-wire) ....*use* Internal Fixation Device in Head and Facial Bones, Upper Bones, Lower Bones, Upper Joints, Lower Joints

Kuntscher nail..*use* Internal Fixation Device, Intramedullary in Upper Bones, Lower Bones

Neutralization plate ....*use* Internal Fixation Device in Head and Facial Bones, Upper Bones, Lower Bones

Polymethylmethacrylate (PMMA)..............................*use* Synthetic Substitute

Sheffield hybrid external fixator ....*use* External Fixation Device, Hybrid for Insertion in Upper Bones, Lower Bones

....*use* External Fixation Device, Hybrid for Reposition in Upper Bones, Lower Bones

Sheffield ring external fixator ....*use* External Fixation Device, Ring for Insertion in Upper Bones, Lower Bones

....*use* External Fixation Device, Ring for Reposition in Upper Bones, Lower Bones

Tissue bank graft ....*use* Nonautologous Tissue Substitute

Titanium Sternal Fixation System (TSFS) ....*use* Internal Fixation Device, Rigid Plate for Insertion in Upper Bones

....*use* Internal Fixation Device, Rigid Plate for Reposition in Upper Bones

Ultrasonic osteogenic stimulator...............................*use* Bone Growth Stimulator in Head and Facial Bones, Upper Bones, Lower Bones

Ultrasound bone healing system ....*use* Bone Growth Stimulator in Head and Facial Bones, Upper Bones, Lower Bones

Uniplanar external fixator ....*use* External Fixation Device, Monoplanar for Insertion in Upper Bones, Lower Bones

....*use* External Fixation Device, Monoplanar for Reposition in Upper Bones, Lower Bones

Educational Annotations | P – Upper Bones

Device Aggregation Table Listings of Upper Bones

See also Device Aggregation Table in Appendix E

Specific Device	For Operation	In Body System		General Device
External Fixation Device, Hybrid	Insertion	Upper Bones	5	External Fixation Device
External Fixation Device, Hybrid	Reposition	Upper Bones	5	External Fixation Device
External Fixation Device, Limb Lengthening	Insertion	Upper Bones	5	External Fixation Device
External Fixation Device, Monoplanar	Insertion	Upper Bones	5	External Fixation Device
External Fixation Device, Monoplanar	Reposition	Upper Bones	5	External Fixation Device
External Fixation Device, Ring	Insertion	Upper Bones	5	External Fixation Device
External Fixation Device, Ring	Reposition	Upper Bones	5	External Fixation Device
Internal Fixation Device, Intramedullary	All applicable	Upper Bones	4	Internal Fixation Device
Internal Fixation Device, Rigid Plate	Insertion	Upper Bones	4	Internal Fixation Device
Internal Fixation Device, Rigid Plate	Reposition	Upper Bones	4	Internal Fixation Device

Coding Notes of Upper Bones

Body System Relevant Coding Guidelines

Reposition for fracture treatment

B3.15

Reduction of a displaced fracture is coded to the root operation Reposition and the application of a cast or splint in conjunction with the Reposition procedure is not coded separately. Treatment of a nondisplaced fracture is coded to the procedure performed.

Examples: Casting of a nondisplaced fracture is coded to the root operation Immobilization in the Placement section.

Putting a pin in a nondisplaced fracture is coded to the root operation Insertion.

Body System Specific PCS Reference Manual Exercises

PCS CODE	P – UPPER BONES EXERCISES
0 P 8 N 0 Z Z	Open osteotomy of capitate, left hand. (The capitate is one of the carpal bones of the hand.)
0 P P J X 5 Z	Removal of external fixator, left radial fracture.

Educational Annotations | P – Upper Bones

NOTES

DEVICE GROUP: Change, Insertion, Removal, Replacement, Revision, Supplement
Root Operations that always involve a device.

1ST - 0 Medical and Surgical

2ND - P Upper Bones

3RD - 2 CHANGE

EXAMPLE: Exchange drain tube	CMS Ex: Changing urinary catheter

CHANGE: Taking out or off a device from a body part and putting back an identical or similar device in or on the same body part without cutting or puncturing the skin or a mucous membrane.

EXPLANATION: ALL Changes use EXTERNAL approach only …

Body Part – 4TH	Approach – 5TH	Device – 6TH	Qualifier – 7TH
Y Upper Bone	X External	0 Drainage device Y Other device	Z No qualifier

EXCISION GROUP: Excision, Resection, Destruction, (Extraction), (Detachment)
Root Operations that take out some or all of a body part.

1ST - 0 Medical and Surgical

2ND - P Upper Bones

3RD - 5 DESTRUCTION

EXAMPLE: Cryoablation bone cyst	CMS Ex: Fulguration polyp

DESTRUCTION: Physical eradication of all or a portion of a body part by the direct use of energy, force, or a destructive agent.

EXPLANATION: None of the body part is physically taken out

Body Part – 4TH		Approach – 5TH	Device – 6TH	Qualifier – 7TH
0 Sternum	H Radius, Right	0 Open	Z No device	Z No qualifier
1 Rib, Right	J Radius, Left	3 Percutaneous		
2 Rib, Left	K Ulna, Right	4 Percutaneous endoscopic		
3 Cervical Vertebra	L Ulna, Left			
4 Thoracic Vertebra	M Carpal, Right			
5 Scapula, Right	N Carpal, Left			
6 Scapula, Left	P Metacarpal, Right			
7 Glenoid Cavity, Right	Q Metacarpal, Left			
8 Glenoid Cavity, Left	R Thumb Phalanx, Right			
9 Clavicle, Right	S Thumb Phalanx, Left			
B Clavicle, Left	T Finger Phalanx, Right			
C Humeral Head, Right	V Finger Phalanx, Left			
D Humeral Head, Left				
F Humeral Shaft, Right				
G Humeral Shaft, Left				

UPPER BONES 0 P 5

DIVISION GROUP: Division, Release

Root Operations involving cutting or separation only.

1ST - 0 Medical and Surgical	EXAMPLE: Carpal osteotomy	CMS Ex: Osteotomy

2ND - P Upper Bones

3RD - 8 DIVISION

DIVISION: Cutting into a body part without draining fluids and/or gases from the body part in order to separate or transect a body part.

EXPLANATION: Separated into two or more portions ...

Body Part – 4TH		Approach – 5TH	Device – 6TH	Qualifier – 7TH
0 Sternum	H Radius, Right	0 Open	Z No device	Z No qualifier
1 Rib, Right	J Radius, Left	3 Percutaneous		
2 Rib, Left	K Ulna, Right	4 Percutaneous endoscopic		
3 Cervical Vertebra	L Ulna, Left			
4 Thoracic Vertebra	M Carpal, Right			
5 Scapula, Right	N Carpal, Left			
6 Scapula, Left	P Metacarpal, Right			
7 Glenoid Cavity, Right	Q Metacarpal, Left			
8 Glenoid Cavity, Left	R Thumb Phalanx, Right			
9 Clavicle, Right	S Thumb Phalanx, Left			
B Clavicle, Left	T Finger Phalanx, Right			
C Humeral Head, Right	V Finger Phalanx, Left			
D Humeral Head, Left				
F Humeral Shaft, Right				
G Humeral Shaft, Left				

UPPER BONES

0 P 8

DRAINAGE GROUP: Drainage, Extirpation, (Fragmentation)
Root Operations that take out solids/fluids/gases from a body part.

1ST - 0 Medical and Surgical

2ND - P Upper Bones

3RD - 9 DRAINAGE

EXAMPLE: Aspiration bone cyst   CMS Ex: Thoracentesis

<u>DRAINAGE:</u> Taking or letting out fluids and/or gases from a body part.

EXPLANATION: Qualifier "X Diagnostic" indicates biopsy ...

Body Part – 4TH		Approach – 5TH	Device – 6TH	Qualifier – 7TH
0 Sternum 1 Rib, Right 2 Rib, Left 3 Cervical Vertebra 4 Thoracic Vertebra 5 Scapula, Right 6 Scapula, Left 7 Glenoid Cavity, Right 8 Glenoid Cavity, Left 9 Clavicle, Right B Clavicle, Left C Humeral Head, Right D Humeral Head, Left F Humeral Shaft, Right G Humeral Shaft, Left	H Radius, Right J Radius, Left K Ulna, Right L Ulna, Left M Carpal, Right N Carpal, Left P Metacarpal, Right Q Metacarpal, Left R Thumb Phalanx, Right S Thumb Phalanx, Left T Finger Phalanx, Right V Finger Phalanx, Left	0 Open 3 Percutaneous 4 Percutaneous endoscopic	0 Drainage device	Z No qualifier
0 Sternum 1 Rib, Right 2 Rib, Left 3 Cervical Vertebra 4 Thoracic Vertebra 5 Scapula, Right 6 Scapula, Left 7 Glenoid Cavity, Right 8 Glenoid Cavity, Left 9 Clavicle, Right B Clavicle, Left C Humeral Head, Right D Humeral Head, Left F Humeral Shaft, Right G Humeral Shaft, Left	H Radius, Right J Radius, Left K Ulna, Right L Ulna, Left M Carpal, Right N Carpal, Left P Metacarpal, Right Q Metacarpal, Left R Thumb Phalanx, Right S Thumb Phalanx, Left T Finger Phalanx, Right V Finger Phalanx, Left	0 Open 3 Percutaneous 4 Percutaneous endoscopic	Z No device	X Diagnostic Z No qualifier

UPPER BONES 0 P 9

EXCISION GROUP: Excision, Resection, Destruction, (Extraction), (Detachment)
Root Operations that take out some or all of a body part.

1ST - 0	Medical and Surgical
2ND - P	Upper Bones
3RD - B	EXCISION

EXAMPLE: Vertebral laminectomy   **CMS Ex:** Liver biopsy

EXCISION: Cutting out or off, without replacement, a portion of a body part.

EXPLANATION: Qualifier "X Diagnostic" indicates biopsy ...

Body Part – 4TH		Approach – 5TH	Device – 6TH	Qualifier – 7TH
0 Sternum	H Radius, Right	0 Open	Z No device	X Diagnostic
1 Rib, Right	J Radius, Left	3 Percutaneous		Z No qualifier
2 Rib, Left	K Ulna, Right	4 Percutaneous endoscopic		
3 Cervical Vertebra	L Ulna, Left			
4 Thoracic Vertebra	M Carpal, Right			
5 Scapula, Right	N Carpal, Left			
6 Scapula, Left	P Metacarpal, Right			
7 Glenoid Cavity, Right	Q Metacarpal, Left			
8 Glenoid Cavity, Left	R Thumb Phalanx, Right			
9 Clavicle, Right	S Thumb Phalanx, Left			
B Clavicle, Left	T Finger Phalanx, Right			
C Humeral Head, Right	V Finger Phalanx, Left			
D Humeral Head, Left				
F Humeral Shaft, Right				
G Humeral Shaft, Left				

DRAINAGE GROUP: Drainage, Extirpation, (Fragmentation)
Root Operations that take out solids/fluids/gases from a body part.

1ST - 0	Medical and Surgical
2ND - P	Upper Bones
3RD - C	EXTIRPATION

EXAMPLE: Removal foreign body   **CMS Ex:** Choledocholithotomy

EXTIRPATION: Taking or cutting out solid matter from a body part.

EXPLANATION: Abnormal byproduct or foreign body ...

Body Part – 4TH		Approach – 5TH	Device – 6TH	Qualifier – 7TH
0 Sternum	H Radius, Right	0 Open	Z No device	Z No qualifier
1 Rib, Right	J Radius, Left	3 Percutaneous		
2 Rib, Left	K Ulna, Right	4 Percutaneous endoscopic		
3 Cervical Vertebra	L Ulna, Left			
4 Thoracic Vertebra	M Carpal, Right			
5 Scapula, Right	N Carpal, Left			
6 Scapula, Left	P Metacarpal, Right			
7 Glenoid Cavity, Right	Q Metacarpal, Left			
8 Glenoid Cavity, Left	R Thumb Phalanx, Right			
9 Clavicle, Right	S Thumb Phalanx, Left			
B Clavicle, Left	T Finger Phalanx, Right			
C Humeral Head, Right	V Finger Phalanx, Left			
D Humeral Head, Left				
F Humeral Shaft, Right				
G Humeral Shaft, Left				

UPPER BONES

0 P B

DEVICE GROUP: Change, Insertion, Removal, Replacement, Revision, Supplement
Root Operations that always involve a device.

1ST - **0** Medical and Surgical	EXAMPLE: Insertion external fixation pin | CMS Ex: Central venous catheter
2ND - **P** Upper Bones	**INSERTION:** Putting in a nonbiological appliance that monitors, assists, performs, or prevents a physiological function but does not physically take the place of a body part.
3RD - **H INSERTION**	EXPLANATION: None

Body Part – 4TH	Approach – 5TH	Device – 6TH	Qualifier – 7TH
0 Sternum	0 Open 3 Percutaneous 4 Percutaneous endoscopic	0 Internal fixation device, rigid plate 4 Internal fixation device	Z No qualifier
1 Rib, Right 7 Glenoid Cavity, Right 2 Rib, Left 8 Glenoid Cavity, Left 3 Cervical Vertebra 9 Clavicle, Right 4 Thoracic Vertebra B Clavicle, Left 5 Scapula, Right 6 Scapula, Left	0 Open 3 Percutaneous 4 Percutaneous endoscopic	4 Internal fixation device	Z No qualifier
C Humeral Head, Right H Radius, Right D Humeral Head, Left J Radius, Left F Humeral Shaft, Right K Ulna, Right G Humeral Shaft, Left L Ulna, Left	0 Open 3 Percutaneous 4 Percutaneous endoscopic	4 Internal fixation device 5 External fixation device 6 Internal fixation device, intramedullary 8 External fixation device, limb lengthening B External fixation device, monoplanar C External fixation device, ring D External fixation device, hybrid	Z No qualifier
M Carpal, Right R Thumb Phalanx, Right N Carpal, Left S Thumb Phalanx, Left P Metacarpal, Right T Finger Phalanx, Right Q Metacarpal, Left V Finger Phalanx, Left	0 Open 3 Percutaneous 4 Percutaneous endoscopic	4 Internal fixation device 5 External fixation device	Z No qualifier
Y Upper Bone	0 Open 3 Percutaneous 4 Percutaneous endoscopic	M Bone growth stimulator	Z No qualifier

UPPER BONES

0 P H

EXAMINATION GROUP: Inspection, (Map)
Root Operations involving examination only.

1ST - 0 Medical and Surgical	EXAMPLE: Examination bone		CMS Ex: Colonoscopy
2ND - P Upper Bones	**INSPECTION:** Visually and/or manually exploring a body part.		
3RD - J INSPECTION			
	EXPLANATION: Direct or instrumental visualization ...		

Body Part – 4TH	Approach – 5TH	Device – 6TH	Qualifier – 7TH
Y Upper Bone	0 Open 3 Percutaneous 4 Percutaneous endoscopic X External	Z No device	Z No qualifier

DIVISION GROUP: Division, Release
Root Operations involving cutting or separation only.

1ST - 0 Medical and Surgical	EXAMPLE: Extra-articular bone adhesiolysis		CMS Ex: Carpal tunnel release
2ND - P Upper Bones	**RELEASE:** Freeing a body part from an abnormal physical constraint by cutting or by the use of force.		
3RD - N RELEASE			
	EXPLANATION: None of the body part is taken out ...		

Body Part – 4TH		Approach – 5TH	Device – 6TH	Qualifier – 7TH
0 Sternum	H Radius, Right	0 Open	Z No device	Z No qualifier
1 Rib, Right	J Radius, Left	3 Percutaneous		
2 Rib, Left	K Ulna, Right	4 Percutaneous endoscopic		
3 Cervical Vertebra	L Ulna, Left			
4 Thoracic Vertebra	M Carpal, Right			
5 Scapula, Right	N Carpal, Left			
6 Scapula, Left	P Metacarpal, Right			
7 Glenoid Cavity, Right	Q Metacarpal, Left			
8 Glenoid Cavity, Left	R Thumb Phalanx, Right			
9 Clavicle, Right	S Thumb Phalanx, Left			
B Clavicle, Left	T Finger Phalanx, Right			
C Humeral Head, Right	V Finger Phalanx, Left			
D Humeral Head, Left				
F Humeral Shaft, Right				
G Humeral Shaft, Left				

DEVICE GROUP: Change, Insertion, Removal, Replacement, Revision, Supplement
Root Operations that always involve a device.

1ST - **0** Medical and Surgical	**EXAMPLE:** Removal external fixation pin **CMS Ex:** Chest tube removal
2ND - **P** Upper Bones	**REMOVAL:** Taking out or off a device from a body part.
3RD - **P REMOVAL**	**EXPLANATION:** Removal device without reinsertion ...

Body Part – 4TH		Approach – 5TH	Device – 6TH	Qualifier – 7TH
0 Sternum 1 Rib, Right 2 Rib, Left 3 Cervical Vertebra 4 Thoracic Vertebra 5 Scapula, Right 6 Scapula, Left	7 Glenoid Cavity, Right 8 Glenoid Cavity, Left 9 Clavicle, Right B Clavicle, Left	0 Open 3 Percutaneous 4 Percutaneous endoscopic	4 Internal fixation device 7 Autologous tissue substitute J Synthetic substitute K Nonautologous tissue substitute	Z No qualifier
0 Sternum 1 Rib, Right 2 Rib, Left 3 Cervical Vertebra 4 Thoracic Vertebra 5 Scapula, Right 6 Scapula, Left	7 Glenoid Cavity, Right 8 Glenoid Cavity, Left 9 Clavicle, Right B Clavicle, Left	X External	4 Internal fixation device	Z No qualifier
C Humeral Head, Right D Humeral Head, Left F Humeral Shaft, Right G Humeral Shaft, Left H Radius, Right J Radius, Left K Ulna, Right L Ulna, Left	M Carpal, Right N Carpal, Left P Metacarpal, Right Q Metacarpal, Left R Thumb Phalanx, Right S Thumb Phalanx, Left T Finger Phalanx, Right V Finger Phalanx, Left	0 Open 3 Percutaneous 4 Percutaneous endoscopic	4 Internal fixation device 5 External fixation device 7 Autologous tissue substitute J Synthetic substitute K Nonautologous tissue substitute	Z No qualifier
C Humeral Head, Right D Humeral Head, Left F Humeral Shaft, Right G Humeral Shaft, Left H Radius, Right J Radius, Left K Ulna, Right L Ulna, Left	M Carpal, Right N Carpal, Left P Metacarpal, Right Q Metacarpal, Left R Thumb Phalanx, Right S Thumb Phalanx, Left T Finger Phalanx, Right V Finger Phalanx, Left	X External	4 Internal fixation device 5 External fixation device	Z No qualifier
Y Upper Bone		0 Open 3 Percutaneous 4 Percutaneous endoscopic X External	0 Drainage device M Bone growth stimulator	Z No qualifier

UPPER BONES

0 P P

OTHER REPAIRS GROUP: (Control), **Repair**
Root Operations that define other repairs.

1ST - **0**   Medical and Surgical

2ND - **P**   Upper Bones

3RD - **Q REPAIR**

EXAMPLE: Vertebral laminoplasty   CMS Ex: Suture laceration

REPAIR: Restoring, to the extent possible, a body part to its normal anatomic structure and function.

EXPLANATION: Only when no other root operation applies …

Body Part – 4TH		Approach – 5TH	Device – 6TH	Qualifier – 7TH
0 Sternum	H Radius, Right	0 Open	Z No device	Z No qualifier
1 Rib, Right	J Radius, Left	3 Percutaneous		
2 Rib, Left	K Ulna, Right	4 Percutaneous endoscopic		
3 Cervical Vertebra	L Ulna, Left	X External		
4 Thoracic Vertebra	M Carpal, Right			
5 Scapula, Right	N Carpal, Left			
6 Scapula, Left	P Metacarpal, Right			
7 Glenoid Cavity, Right	Q Metacarpal, Left			
8 Glenoid Cavity, Left	R Thumb Phalanx, Right			
9 Clavicle, Right	S Thumb Phalanx, Left			
B Clavicle, Left	T Finger Phalanx, Right			
C Humeral Head, Right	V Finger Phalanx, Left			
D Humeral Head, Left				
F Humeral Shaft, Right				
G Humeral Shaft, Left				

DEVICE GROUP: Change, Insertion, Removal, Replacement, Revision, Supplement
Root Operations that always involve a device.

1ST - **0**   Medical and Surgical

2ND - **P**   Upper Bones

3RD - **R REPLACEMENT**

EXAMPLE: Humeral head replacement   CMS Ex: Total hip

REPLACEMENT: Putting in or on a biological or synthetic material that physically takes the place and/or function of all or a portion of a body part.

EXPLANATION: Includes taking out body part, or eradication…

Body Part – 4TH		Approach – 5TH	Device – 6TH	Qualifier – 7TH
0 Sternum	H Radius, Right	0 Open	7 Autologous tissue substitute	Z No qualifier
1 Rib, Right	J Radius, Left	3 Percutaneous	J Synthetic substitute	
2 Rib, Left	K Ulna, Right	4 Percutaneous endoscopic	K Nonautologous tissue substitute	
3 Cervical Vertebra	L Ulna, Left			
4 Thoracic Vertebra	M Carpal, Right			
5 Scapula, Right	N Carpal, Left			
6 Scapula, Left	P Metacarpal, Right			
7 Glenoid Cavity, Right	Q Metacarpal, Left			
8 Glenoid Cavity, Left	R Thumb Phalanx, Right			
9 Clavicle, Right	S Thumb Phalanx, Left			
B Clavicle, Left	T Finger Phalanx, Right			
C Humeral Head, Right	V Finger Phalanx, Left			
D Humeral Head, Left				
F Humeral Shaft, Right				
G Humeral Shaft, Left				

MOVE GROUP: (Reattachment), **Reposition**, (Transfer), (Transplantation)
Root Operations that put in/put back or move some/all of a body part.

1ST - O Medical and Surgical	**EXAMPLE:** ORIF Colles' fracture **CMS Ex:** Fracture reduction
2ND - P Upper Bones	**REPOSITION:** Moving to its normal location, or other suitable location, all or a portion of a body part.
3RD - S REPOSITION	**EXPLANATION:** May or may not be cut to be moved …

Body Part – 4TH	Approach – 5TH	Device – 6TH	Qualifier – 7TH
0 Sternum	0 Open 3 Percutaneous 4 Percutaneous endoscopic	0 Internal fixation device, rigid plate 4 Internal fixation device Z No device	Z No qualifier
0 Sternum	X External	Z No device	Z No qualifier
1 Rib, Right 6 Scapula, Left 2 Rib, Left 7 Glenoid Cavity, Right 3 Cervical Vertebra 8 Glenoid Cavity, Left 4 Thoracic Vertebra 9 Clavicle, Right 5 Scapula, Right B Clavicle, Left	0 Open 3 Percutaneous 4 Percutaneous endoscopic	4 Internal fixation device Z No device	Z No qualifier
1 Rib, Right 6 Scapula, Left 2 Rib, Left 7 Glenoid Cavity, Right 3 Cervical Vertebra 8 Glenoid Cavity, Left 4 Thoracic Vertebra 9 Clavicle, Right 5 Scapula, Right B Clavicle, Left	X External	Z No device	Z No qualifier
C Humeral Head, Right H Radius, Right D Humeral Head, Left J Radius, Left F Humeral Shaft, Right K Ulna, Right G Humeral Shaft, Left L Ulna, Left	0 Open 3 Percutaneous 4 Percutaneous endoscopic	4 Internal fixation device 5 External fixation device 6 Internal fixation device, intramedullary B External fixation device, monoplanar C External fixation device, ring D External fixation device, hybrid Z No device	Z No qualifier
C Humeral Head, Right H Radius, Right D Humeral Head, Left J Radius, Left F Humeral Shaft, Right K Ulna, Right G Humeral Shaft, Left L Ulna, Left	X External	Z No device	Z No qualifier
M Carpal, Right R Thumb Phalanx, Right N Carpal, Left S Thumb Phalanx, Left P Metacarpal, Right T Finger Phalanx, Right Q Metacarpal, Left V Finger Phalanx, Left	0 Open 3 Percutaneous 4 Percutaneous endoscopic	4 Internal fixation device 5 External fixation device Z No device	Z No qualifier
M Carpal, Right R Thumb Phalanx, Right N Carpal, Left S Thumb Phalanx, Left P Metacarpal, Right T Finger Phalanx, Right Q Metacarpal, Left V Finger Phalanx, Left	X External	Z No device	Z No qualifier

UPPER BONES

O P S

EXCISION GROUP: Excision, Resection, Destruction, (Extraction), (Detachment)
Root Operations that take out some or all of a body part.

1ST - 0 Medical and Surgical	EXAMPLE: Total claviculectomy	CMS Ex: Cholecystectomy
2ND - P Upper Bones	**RESECTION:** Cutting out or off, without replacement, all of a body part.	
3RD - T RESECTION	EXPLANATION: None	

Body Part – 4TH		Approach – 5TH	Device – 6TH	Qualifier – 7TH
0 Sternum	H Radius, Right	0 Open	Z No device	Z No qualifier
1 Rib, Right	J Radius, Left			
2 Rib, Left	K Ulna, Right			
5 Scapula, Right	L Ulna, Left			
6 Scapula, Left	M Carpal, Right			
7 Glenoid Cavity, Right	N Carpal, Left			
8 Glenoid Cavity, Left	P Metacarpal, Right			
9 Clavicle, Right	Q Metacarpal, Left			
B Clavicle, Left	R Thumb Phalanx, Right			
C Humeral Head, Right	S Thumb Phalanx, Left			
D Humeral Head, Left	T Finger Phalanx, Right			
F Humeral Shaft, Right	V Finger Phalanx, Left			
G Humeral Shaft, Left				

DEVICE GROUP: Change, Insertion, Removal, Replacement, Revision, Supplement
Root Operations that always involve a device.

1ST - 0 Medical and Surgical	EXAMPLE: Application bone void filler	CMS Ex: Hernia repair with mesh
2ND - P Upper Bones	**SUPPLEMENT:** Putting in or on biological or synthetic material that physically reinforces and/or augments the function of a portion of a body part.	
3RD - U SUPPLEMENT	EXPLANATION: Biological material from same individual ...	

Body Part – 4TH		Approach – 5TH	Device – 6TH	Qualifier – 7TH
0 Sternum	H Radius, Right	0 Open	7 Autologous tissue substitute	Z No qualifier
1 Rib, Right	J Radius, Left	3 Percutaneous	J Synthetic substitute	
2 Rib, Left	K Ulna, Right	4 Percutaneous endoscopic	K Nonautologous tissue substitute	
3 Cervical Vertebra	L Ulna, Left			
4 Thoracic Vertebra	M Carpal, Right			
5 Scapula, Right	N Carpal, Left			
6 Scapula, Left	P Metacarpal, Right			
7 Glenoid Cavity, Right	Q Metacarpal, Left			
8 Glenoid Cavity, Left	R Thumb Phalanx, Right			
9 Clavicle, Right	S Thumb Phalanx, Left			
B Clavicle, Left	T Finger Phalanx, Right			
C Humeral Head, Right	V Finger Phalanx, Left			
D Humeral Head, Left				
F Humeral Shaft, Right				
G Humeral Shaft, Left				

DEVICE GROUP: Change, Insertion, Removal, Replacement, Revision, Supplement			
Root Operations that always involve a device.			

1ST - 0 Medical and Surgical

2ND - P Upper Bones

3RD - W REVISION

EXAMPLE: Lengthening growing rods | CMS Ex: Adjustment pacemaker lead

REVISION: Correcting, to the extent possible, a portion of a malfunctioning device or the position of a displaced device.

EXPLANATION: May replace components of a device ...

Body Part – 4TH		Approach – 5TH	Device – 6TH	Qualifier – 7TH
0 Sternum 1 Rib, Right 2 Rib, Left 3 Cervical Vertebra 4 Thoracic Vertebra 5 Scapula, Right 6 Scapula, Left	7 Glenoid Cavity, Right 8 Glenoid Cavity, Left 9 Clavicle, Right B Clavicle, Left	0 Open 3 Percutaneous 4 Percutaneous endoscopic X External	4 Internal fixation device 7 Autologous tissue substitute J Synthetic substitute K Nonautologous tissue substitute	Z No qualifier
C Humeral Head, Right D Humeral Head, Left F Humeral Shaft, Right G Humeral Shaft, Left H Radius, Right J Radius, Left K Ulna, Right L Ulna, Left	M Carpal, Right N Carpal, Left P Metacarpal, Right Q Metacarpal, Left R Thumb Phalanx, Right S Thumb Phalanx, Left T Finger Phalanx, Right V Finger Phalanx, Left	0 Open 3 Percutaneous 4 Percutaneous endoscopic X External	4 Internal fixation device 5 External fixation device 7 Autologous tissue substitute J Synthetic substitute K Nonautologous tissue substitute	Z No qualifier
Y Upper Bone		0 Open 3 Percutaneous 4 Percutaneous endoscopic X External	0 Drainage device M Bone growth stimulator	Z No qualifier

UPPER BONES 0 P W

NOTES

Educational Annotations | Q – Lower Bones

Body System Specific Educational Annotations for the Lower Bones include:

- **Anatomy and Physiology Review**
- **Anatomical Illustrations**
- **Definitions of Common Procedures**
- **AHA Coding Clinic® Reference Notations**
- **Body Part Key Listings**
- **Device Key Listings**
- **Device Aggregation Table Listings**
- **Coding Notes**

Anatomy and Physiology Review of Lower Bones

BODY PART VALUES – Q - LOWER BONES

Acetabulum – The round, concave depression in the pelvic bone that articulates with the femoral head forming the hip joint.

Coccyx – The small wedge-shaped bone (also known as the tailbone) at the end of the spinal column.

Femoral Shaft – The middle long portion of the femur.

Femur – The paired long bones (also known as the thigh bone) that articulate at the hip and the knee. It is the longest bone in the body.

Fibula – The paired long slender bones of the lower leg located toward the outside of the lower leg that articulate at the knee and the ankle.

Lower Bone – Any of the bones designated in the Lower Bones PCS Body System.

Lower Femur – The distal end of the femur that articulates with the knee joint.

Lumbar Vertebra – The lumbar section of the spinal vertebral column comprised of 5 vertebra, S1-S5.

Metatarsal – One of the 5 cylindrical bones connecting the tarsals and the phalanges of the foot.

Patella – The paired triangular-shaped bones situated at the front of the knee.

Pelvic Bone – Any of the three bones (ilium, ischium, pubis) that connect with the sacrum to form the pelvic girdle.

Sacrum – The large wedge-shaped vertebra at the lower end of the spine that connects with S5.

Tarsal – The seven bones of the foot (calcaneus, talus, cuboid, navicular, and the medial, intermediate, and lateral cuneiform bones) distal to the tibia and fibula and proximal to the metatarsal bones.

Tibia – The paired long bones of the lower leg (also known as the shin bone) that is the innermost bone of the lower leg supporting and articulating with the knee and with the ankle.

Toe Phalanx – The digital bones of the toes. Each toe contains three bones: Proximal phalanx, intermediate (middle) phalanx, and distal phalanx, except the great toe which only has proximal and distal phalanx bones.

Upper Femur – The proximal end of the femur (head) that articulates with the acetabulum to form the hip joint.

Educational Annotations | Q – Lower Bones

Anatomical Illustrations of Lower Bones

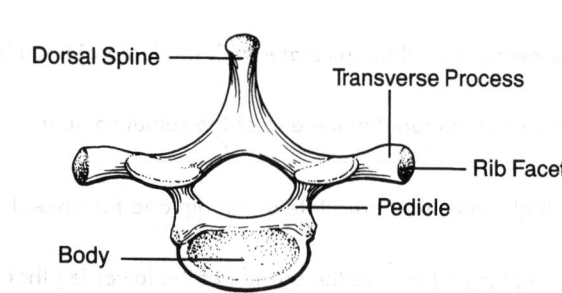

TYPICAL VERTEBRA — SUPERIOR VIEW

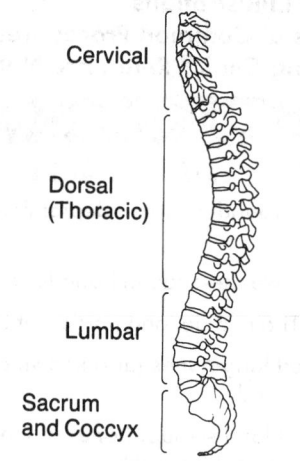

VERTEBRAL COLUMN

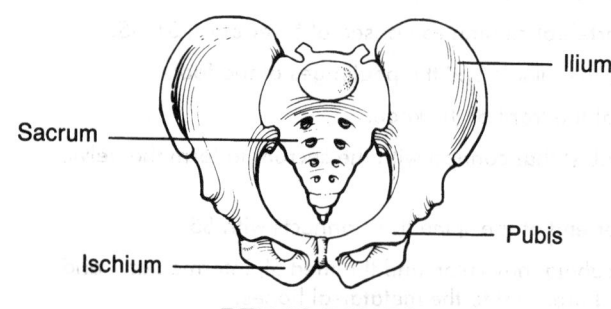

PELVIC BONES

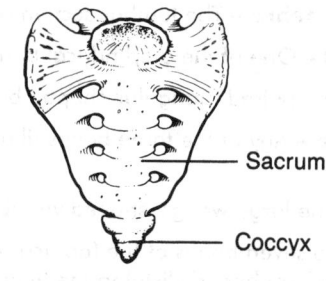

SACRUM AND COCCYX

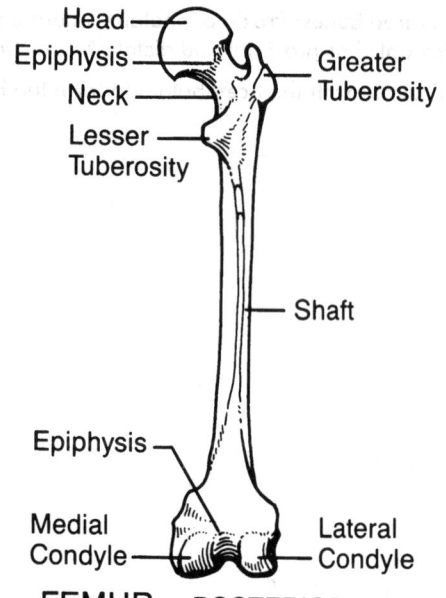

FEMUR — POSTERIOR VIEW

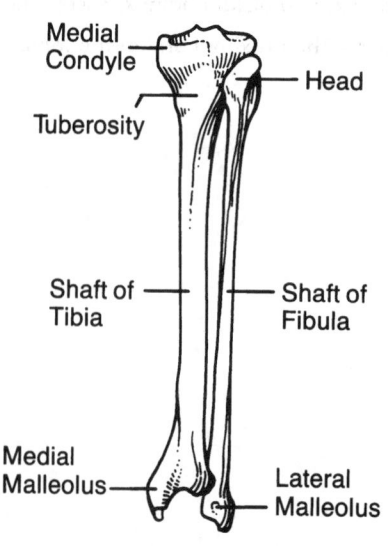

TIBIA AND FIBULA — POSTERIOR VIEW

Continued on next page

Educational Annotations | Q – Lower Bones

Anatomical Illustrations of Lower Bones

Continued from previous page

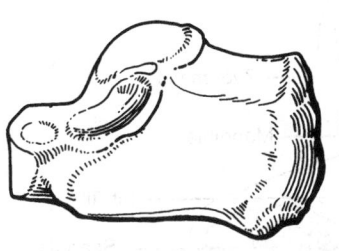

CALCANEUS — MEDIAL VIEW

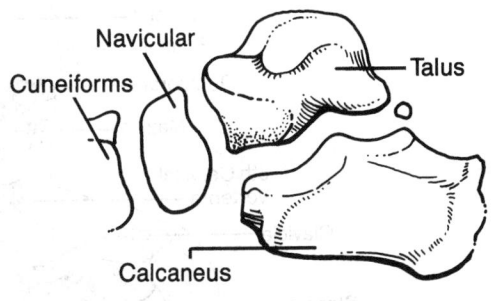

Navicular
Cuneiforms
Talus
Calcaneus

TARSAL BONES

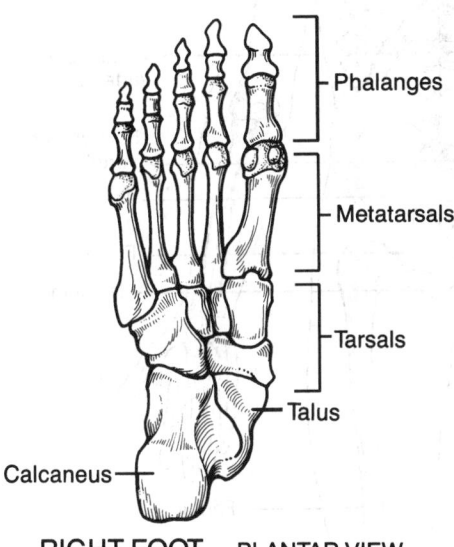

Phalanges
Metatarsals
Tarsals
Talus
Calcaneus

RIGHT FOOT — PLANTAR VIEW

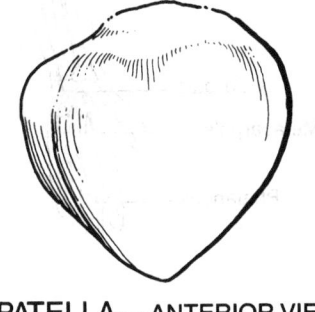

PATELLA — ANTERIOR VIEW

LOWER BONES 0 Q

Continued on next page

Educational Annotations | Q – Lower Bones

Anatomical Illustrations of Lower Bones

Continued from previous page

Continued from previous page

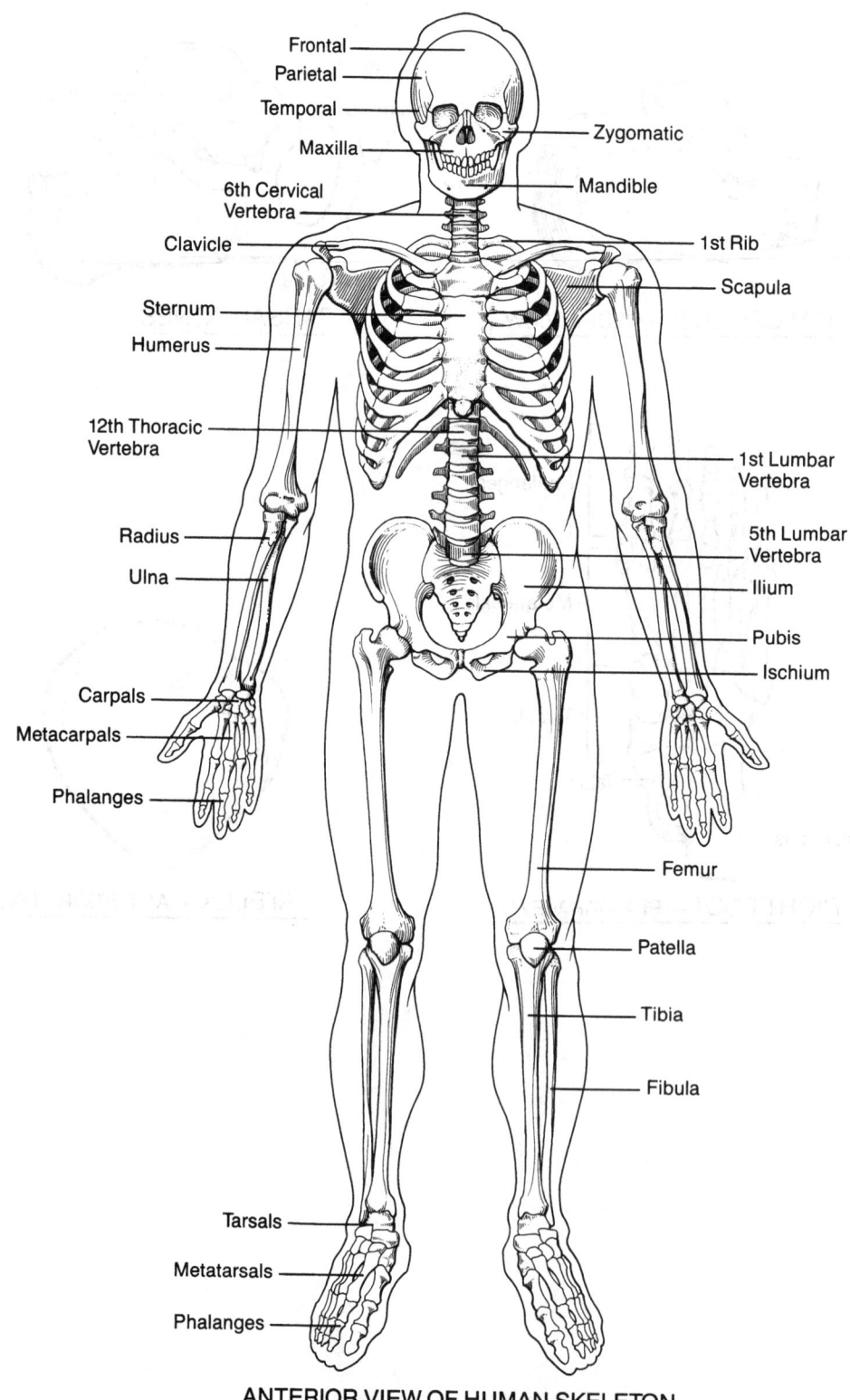

Frontal
Parietal
Temporal
Maxilla
Zygomatic
Mandible
6th Cervical Vertebra
1st Rib
Clavicle
Scapula
Sternum
Humerus
12th Thoracic Vertebra
1st Lumbar Vertebra
5th Lumbar Vertebra
Radius
Ilium
Ulna
Pubis
Ischium
Carpals
Metacarpals
Phalanges
Femur
Patella
Tibia
Fibula
Tarsals
Metatarsals
Phalanges

ANTERIOR VIEW OF HUMAN SKELETON

Continued on next page

LOWER BONES 0 Q

Educational Annotations | Q – Lower Bones

Anatomical Illustrations of Lower Bones

Continued from previous page

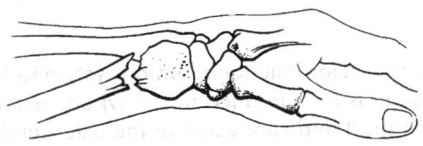

COLLES'

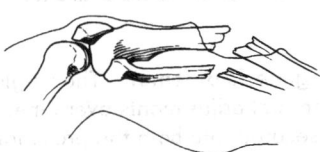

COMPOUND

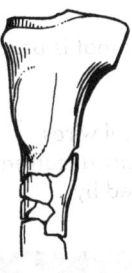

COMMINUTED

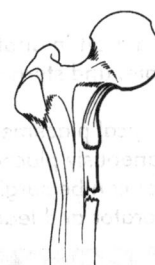

GREENSTICK

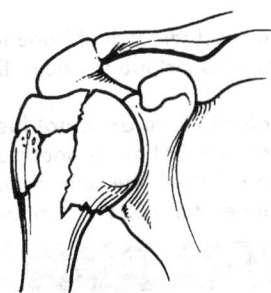

IMPACTED

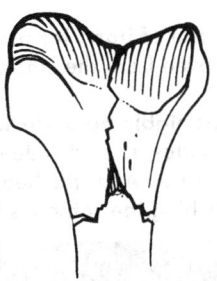

INTERCONDYLAR

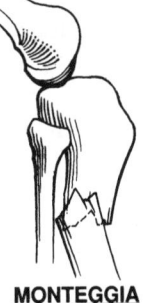

MONTEGGIA

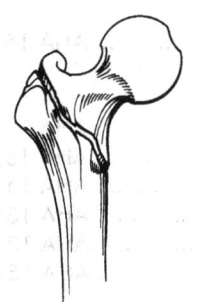

PERTROCHANTERIC

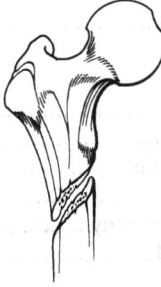

SPIRAL

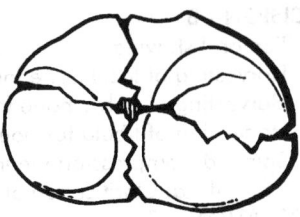

STELLATE

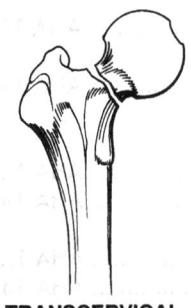

TRANSCERVICAL

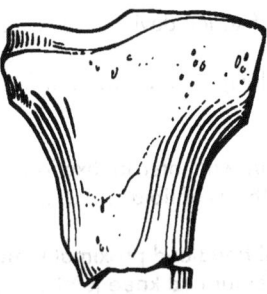

TRANSVERSE

FRACTURE TYPES

LOWER BONES 0 Q

Educational Annotations | Q – Lower Bones

Definitions of Common Procedures of Lower Bones

Bone void filler to iliac crest defect – The surgical placement of a bone void filler (usually synthetic bone material) to fill in a defect in the natural shape of the iliac crest and to enhance the stability and strength of the bone.

Distraction osteogenesis of femur – The surgical placement of a distractor limb lengthening system to lengthen the femur with gradual adjustments over time. The mid-femoral shaft is fractured (corticotomy) and external fixation pins are secured into both the proximal and distal femoral shaft and connected to the external distraction system, allowing new bone to grow and fill the gap.

Femoral head shaving – The surgical grinding down of the femoral head bone that is causing the pain and impaired range of motion (femoroacetabular impingement syndrome). Procedures on the joint tissues often accompany this procedure.

Harvest of bone for graft – The surgical removal of bone to be used as a graft in another location that is usually removed from the iliac crest. Other sites include the tibia, fibula, mandible, and sternum.

Implantable bone growth stimulator in lumbar spinal fusion – The surgical placement of electrical wires (cathodes) to each side of the fusion site that are connected to a subcutaneously placed direct electrical current generator. After the healing is accomplished, the subcutaneous generator can be surgically removed by detaching the cathodes from the generator leads and removing the generator and leads.

AHA Coding Clinic® Reference Notations of Lower Bones

ROOT OPERATION SPECIFIC - Q - LOWER BONES

CHANGE - 2
DESTRUCTION - 5
DIVISION - 8
    Periacetabular osteotomy .... AHA 16:2Q:p31
DRAINAGE - 9
EXCISION - B
    Femoral shaving .... AHA 14:4Q:p25
    Harvesting of local bone for graft .... AHA 15:1Q:p30
    Harvesting of pelvic bone for spinal fusion .... AHA 14:2Q:p6
    Harvesting of fibula for bone graft .... AHA 14:2Q:p6
    Spinal decompression meaning laminectomy .... AHA 13:2Q:p39
       Official Clarification of 13:4Q:p116 .... AHA 15:2Q:p34
EXTIRPATION - C
INSERTION - H
INSPECTION - J
RELEASE - N
REMOVAL - P
    Removal of internal fixation device .... AHA 15:2Q:p6
REPAIR - Q
    Sacrum S1 laminoplasty .... AHA 14:3Q:p24
REPLACEMENT - R
REPOSITION - S
    Realignment of femur with internal fixation .... AHA 14:4Q:p31
    Rotational osteosynthesis of tibia .... AHA 14:4Q:p29
RESECTION - T
    Resection of femoral head and proximal femur .... AHA 15:3Q:p26
    Resection of lower femur and knee joint .... AHA 14:4Q:p29
SUPPLEMENT - U
    Application of bone graft matrix .... AHA 14:4Q:p31
    Bone void filler .... AHA 13:2Q:p35
    Hip replacement with acetabular reconstruction .... AHA 15:3Q:p18
    Vertebroplasty with cement as a device value .... AHA 14:2Q:p12
REVISION - W

Educational Annotations | Q – Lower Bones

Body Part Key Listings of Lower Bones

See also Body Part Key in Appendix C

Body of femur .... *use* Femoral Shaft, Left/Right
Body of fibula .... *use* Fibula, Left/Right
Calcaneus .... *use* Tarsal, Left/Right
Cuboid bone .... *use* Tarsal, Left/Right
Femoral head .... *use* Upper Femur, Left/Right
Greater trochanter .... *use* Upper Femur, Left/Right
Head of fibula .... *use* Fibula, Left/Right
Iliac crest .... *use* Pelvic Bone, Left/Right
Ilium .... *use* Pelvic Bone, Left/Right
Intermediate cuneiform bone .... *use* Tarsal, Left/Right
Ischium .... *use* Pelvic Bone, Left/Right
Lateral condyle of femur .... *use* Lower Femur, Left/Right
Lateral condyle of tibia .... *use* Tibia, Left/Right
Lateral cuneiform bone .... *use* Tarsal, Left/Right
Lateral epicondyle of femur .... *use* Lower Femur, Left/Right
Lateral malleolus .... *use* Fibula, Left/Right
Lesser trochanter .... *use* Upper Femur, Left/Right
Medial condyle of femur .... *use* Lower Femur, Left/Right
Medial condyle of tibia .... *use* Tibia, Left/Right
Medial cuneiform bone .... *use* Tarsal, Left/Right
Medial epicondyle of femur .... *use* Lower Femur, Left/Right
Medial malleolus .... *use* Tibia, Left/Right
Navicular bone .... *use* Tarsal, Left/Right
Neck of femur .... *use* Upper Femur, Left/Right
Pubis .... *use* Pelvic Bone, Left/Right
Spinous process .... *use* Cervical, Thoracic, Lumbar Vertebra
Talus bone .... *use* Tarsal, Left/Right
Vertebral arch .... *use* Cervical, Thoracic, Lumbar Vertebra
Vertebral foramen .... *use* Cervical, Thoracic, Lumbar Vertebra
Vertebral lamina .... *use* Cervical, Thoracic, Lumbar Vertebra
Vertebral pedicle .... *use* Cervical, Thoracic, Lumbar Vertebra

Device Key Listings of Lower Bones

See also Device Key in Appendix D

Autograft .... *use* Autologous Tissue Substitute
Bone bank bone graft .... *use* Nonautologous Tissue Substitute
Bone screw (interlocking) (lag) (pedicle) (recessed) *use* Internal Fixation Device in Head and Facial Bones, Upper Bones, Lower Bones
Clamp and rod internal fixation system (CRIF) .... *use* Internal Fixation Device in Upper Bones, Lower Bones
Delta frame external fixator .... *use* External Fixation Device, Hybrid for Insertion in Upper Bones, Lower Bones
.... *use* External Fixation Device, Hybrid for Reposition in Upper Bones, Lower Bones
Electrical bone growth stimulator (EBGS) .... *use* Bone Growth Stimulator in Head and Facial Bones, Upper Bones, Lower Bones
External fixator .... *use* External Fixation Device in Head and Facial Bones, Upper Bones, Lower Bones, Upper Joints, Lower Joints

Continued on next page

Educational Annotations | Q – Lower Bones

Device Key Listings of Lower Bones

Continued from previous page

Ilizarov external fixator ....*use* External Fixation Device, Ring for Insertion in Upper Bones, Lower Bones

................*use* External Fixation Device, Ring for Reposition in Upper Bones, Lower Bones

Ilizarov-Vecklich device................*use* External Fixation Device, Limb Lengthening for Insertion in Upper Bones, Lower Bones

Intramedullary (IM) rod (nail) ....*use* Internal Fixation Device, Intramedullary in Upper Bones, Lower Bones

Intramedullary skeletal kinetic distractor (ISKD) ....*use* Internal Fixation Device, Intramedullary in Upper Bones, Lower Bones

Kirschner wire (K-wire) ....*use* Internal Fixation Device in Head and Facial Bones, Upper Bones, Lower Bones, Upper Joints, Lower Joints

Kuntscher nail................*use* Internal Fixation Device, Intramedullary in Upper Bones, Lower Bones

Neutralization plate ....*use* Internal Fixation Device in Head and Facial Bones, Upper Bones, Lower Bones

Polymethylmethacrylate (PMMA)................*use* Synthetic Substitute

Sheffield hybrid external fixator ....*use* External Fixation Device, Hybrid for Insertion in Upper Bones, Lower Bones

................*use* External Fixation Device, Hybrid for Reposition in Upper Bones, Lower Bones

Sheffield ring external fixator ....*use* External Fixation Device, Ring for Insertion in Upper Bones, Lower Bones

................*use* External Fixation Device, Ring for Reposition in Upper Bones, Lower Bones

Tissue bank graft ....*use* Nonautologous Tissue Substitute

Ultrasonic osteogenic stimulator................*use* Bone Growth Stimulator in Head and Facial Bones, Upper Bones, Lower Bones

Ultrasound bone healing system ....*use* Bone Growth Stimulator in Head and Facial Bones, Upper Bones, Lower Bones

Uniplanar external fixator ....*use* External Fixation Device, Monoplanar for Insertion in Upper Bones, Lower Bones

................*use* External Fixation Device, Monoplanar for Reposition in Upper Bones, Lower Bones

Device Aggregation Table Listings of Lower Bones

See also Device Aggregation Table in Appendix E

Specific Device	For Operation	In Body System		General Device
External Fixation Device, Hybrid	Insertion	Lower Bones	5	External Fixation Device
External Fixation Device, Hybrid	Reposition	Lower Bones	5	External Fixation Device
External Fixation Device, Limb Lengthening	Insertion	Lower Bones	5	External Fixation Device
External Fixation Device, Monoplanar	Insertion	Lower Bones	5	External Fixation Device
External Fixation Device, Monoplanar	Reposition	Lower Bones	5	External Fixation Device
External Fixation Device, Ring	Insertion	Lower Bones	5	External Fixation Device
External Fixation Device, Ring	Reposition	Lower Bones	5	External Fixation Device
Internal Fixation Device, Intramedullary	All applicable	Lower Bones	4	Internal Fixation Device

Educational Annotations | Q – Lower Bones

Coding Notes of Lower Bones

Body System Relevant Coding Guidelines

Reposition for fracture treatment

B3.15

Reduction of a displaced fracture is coded to the root operation Reposition and the application of a cast or splint in conjunction with the Reposition procedure is not coded separately. Treatment of a nondisplaced fracture is coded to the procedure performed.

Examples: Casting of a nondisplaced fracture is coded to the root operation Immobilization in the Placement section.

Putting a pin in a nondisplaced fracture is coded to the root operation Insertion.

Body System Specific PCS Reference Manual Exercises

PCS CODE	Q – LOWER BONES EXERCISES
0 Q H Y 0 M Z	Open placement of bone growth stimulator, left femoral shaft.
0 Q P N 0 4 Z	Incision with removal of K-wire fixation, right first metatarsal.
0 Q R 7 0 K Z	Excision of necrosed left femoral head with bone bank bone graft to fill the defect, open.
0 Q S 6 3 4 Z	Closed reduction with percutaneous internal fixation of right femoral neck fracture.
0 Q S G 0 Z Z	Open fracture reduction, right tibia.
0 Q W H 0 4 Z	Taking out loose screw and putting larger screw in fracture repair plate, left tibia.

Educational Annotations | Q – Lower Bones

NOTES

DEVICE GROUP: Change, Insertion, Removal, Replacement, Revision, Supplement
Root Operations that always involve a device.

1ST - **0** Medical and Surgical

2ND - **Q** Lower Bones

3RD - **2 CHANGE**

EXAMPLE: Exchange drain tube | CMS Ex: Changing urinary catheter

CHANGE: Taking out or off a device from a body part and putting back an identical or similar device in or on the same body part without cutting or puncturing the skin or a mucous membrane.

EXPLANATION: ALL Changes use EXTERNAL approach only ...

Body Part – 4TH	Approach – 5TH	Device – 6TH	Qualifier – 7TH
Y Lower Bone	X External	0 Drainage device Y Other device	Z No qualifier

EXCISION GROUP: Excision, Resection, Destruction, (Extraction), (Detachment)
Root Operations that take out some or all of a body part.

1ST - **0** Medical and Surgical

2ND - **Q** Lower Bones

3RD - **5 DESTRUCTION**

EXAMPLE: Cryoablation bone cyst | CMS Ex: Fulguration polyp

DESTRUCTION: Physical eradication of all or a portion of a body part by the direct use of energy, force, or a destructive agent.

EXPLANATION: None of the body part is physically taken out

Body Part – 4TH		Approach – 5TH	Device – 6TH	Qualifier – 7TH
0 Lumbar Vertebra	D Patella, Right	0 Open	Z No device	Z No qualifier
1 Sacrum	F Patella, Left	3 Percutaneous		
2 Pelvic Bone, Right	G Tibia, Right	4 Percutaneous endoscopic		
3 Pelvic Bone, Left	H Tibia, Left			
4 Acetabulum, Right	J Fibula, Right			
5 Acetabulum, Left	K Fibula, Left			
6 Upper Femur, Right	L Tarsal, Right			
7 Upper Femur, Left	M Tarsal, Left			
8 Femoral Shaft, Right	N Metatarsal, Right			
9 Femoral Shaft, Left	P Metatarsal, Left			
B Lower Femur, Right	Q Toe Phalanx, Right			
C Lower Femur, Left	R Toe Phalanx, Left			
	S Coccyx			

LOWER BONES 0 Q 5

DIVISION GROUP: Division, Release
Root Operations involving cutting or separation only.

1ST – **0** Medical and Surgical

2ND – **Q** Lower Bones

3RD – **8 DIVISION**

EXAMPLE: Tarsal osteotomy | CMS Ex: Osteotomy

DIVISION: Cutting into a body part without draining fluids and/or gases from the body part in order to separate or transect a body part.

EXPLANATION: Separated into two or more portions ...

Body Part – 4TH		Approach – 5TH	Device – 6TH	Qualifier – 7TH
0 Lumbar Vertebra	D Patella, Right	0 Open	Z No device	Z No qualifier
1 Sacrum	F Patella, Left	3 Percutaneous		
2 Pelvic Bone, Right	G Tibia, Right	4 Percutaneous endoscopic		
3 Pelvic Bone, Left	H Tibia, Left			
4 Acetabulum, Right	J Fibula, Right			
5 Acetabulum, Left	K Fibula, Left			
6 Upper Femur, Right	L Tarsal, Right			
7 Upper Femur, Left	M Tarsal, Left			
8 Femoral Shaft, Right	N Metatarsal, Right			
9 Femoral Shaft, Left	P Metatarsal, Left			
B Lower Femur, Right	Q Toe Phalanx, Right			
C Lower Femur, Left	R Toe Phalanx, Left			
	S Coccyx			

DRAINAGE GROUP: Drainage, Extirpation, (Fragmentation)
Root Operations that take out solids/fluids/gases from a body part.

1ST - 0 Medical and Surgical	**EXAMPLE:** Aspiration bone cyst **CMS Ex:** Thoracentesis
2ND - Q Lower Bones	**DRAINAGE:** Taking or letting out fluids and/or gases from a body part.
3RD - 9 DRAINAGE	**EXPLANATION:** Qualifier "X Diagnostic" indicates biopsy ...

Body Part – 4TH		Approach – 5TH	Device – 6TH	Qualifier – 7TH
0 Lumbar Vertebra 1 Sacrum 2 Pelvic Bone, Right 3 Pelvic Bone, Left 4 Acetabulum, Right 5 Acetabulum, Left 6 Upper Femur, Right 7 Upper Femur, Left 8 Femoral Shaft, Right 9 Femoral Shaft, Left B Lower Femur, Right C Lower Femur, Left	D Patella, Right F Patella, Left G Tibia, Right H Tibia, Left J Fibula, Right K Fibula, Left L Tarsal, Right M Tarsal, Left N Metatarsal, Right P Metatarsal, Left Q Toe Phalanx, Right R Toe Phalanx, Left S Coccyx	0 Open 3 Percutaneous 4 Percutaneous endoscopic	0 Drainage device	Z No qualifier
0 Lumbar Vertebra 1 Sacrum 2 Pelvic Bone, Right 3 Pelvic Bone, Left 4 Acetabulum, Right 5 Acetabulum, Left 6 Upper Femur, Right 7 Upper Femur, Left 8 Femoral Shaft, Right 9 Femoral Shaft, Left B Lower Femur, Right C Lower Femur, Left	D Patella, Right F Patella, Left G Tibia, Right H Tibia, Left J Fibula, Right K Fibula, Left L Tarsal, Right M Tarsal, Left N Metatarsal, Right P Metatarsal, Left Q Toe Phalanx, Right R Toe Phalanx, Left S Coccyx	0 Open 3 Percutaneous 4 Percutaneous endoscopic	Z No device	X Diagnostic Z No qualifier

LOWER BONES 0 Q 9

EXCISION GROUP: Excision, Resection, Destruction, (Extraction), (Detachment)
Root Operations that take out some or all of a body part.

1ST - **0** Medical and Surgical

2ND - **Q** Lower Bones

3RD - **B EXCISION**

EXAMPLE: Harvest bone for graft | CMS Ex: Liver biopsy

EXCISION: Cutting out or off, without replacement, a portion of a body part.

EXPLANATION: Qualifier "X Diagnostic" indicates biopsy …

Body Part – 4TH		Approach – 5TH	Device – 6TH	Qualifier – 7TH
0 Lumbar Vertebra	D Patella, Right	0 Open	Z No device	X Diagnostic
1 Sacrum	F Patella, Left	3 Percutaneous		Z No qualifier
2 Pelvic Bone, Right	G Tibia, Right	4 Percutaneous endoscopic		
3 Pelvic Bone, Left	H Tibia, Left			
4 Acetabulum, Right	J Fibula, Right			
5 Acetabulum, Left	K Fibula, Left			
6 Upper Femur, Right	L Tarsal, Right			
7 Upper Femur, Left	M Tarsal, Left			
8 Femoral Shaft, Right	N Metatarsal, Right			
9 Femoral Shaft, Left	P Metatarsal, Left			
B Lower Femur, Right	Q Toe Phalanx, Right			
C Lower Femur, Left	R Toe Phalanx, Left			
	S Coccyx			

DRAINAGE GROUP: Drainage, Extirpation, (Fragmentation)
Root Operations that take out solids/fluids/gases from a body part.

1ST - **0** Medical and Surgical

2ND - **Q** Lower Bones

3RD - **C EXTIRPATION**

EXAMPLE: Removal foreign body | CMS Ex: Choledocholithotomy

EXTIRPATION: Taking or cutting out solid matter from a body part.

EXPLANATION: Abnormal byproduct or foreign body …

Body Part – 4TH		Approach – 5TH	Device – 6TH	Qualifier – 7TH
0 Lumbar Vertebra	D Patella, Right	0 Open	Z No device	Z No qualifier
1 Sacrum	F Patella, Left	3 Percutaneous		
2 Pelvic Bone, Right	G Tibia, Right	4 Percutaneous endoscopic		
3 Pelvic Bone, Left	H Tibia, Left			
4 Acetabulum, Right	J Fibula, Right			
5 Acetabulum, Left	K Fibula, Left			
6 Upper Femur, Right	L Tarsal, Right			
7 Upper Femur, Left	M Tarsal, Left			
8 Femoral Shaft, Right	N Metatarsal, Right			
9 Femoral Shaft, Left	P Metatarsal, Left			
B Lower Femur, Right	Q Toe Phalanx, Right			
C Lower Femur, Left	R Toe Phalanx, Left			
	S Coccyx			

DEVICE GROUP: Change, Insertion, Removal, Replacement, Revision, Supplement			
Root Operations that always involve a device.			

1ST - **0** Medical and Surgical	EXAMPLE: Insertion growing rods	CMS Ex: Central venous catheter
2ND - **Q** Lower Bones	**INSERTION:** Putting in a nonbiological appliance that monitors, assists, performs, or prevents a physiological function but does not physically take the place of a body part.	
3RD - **H INSERTION**	EXPLANATION: None	

Body Part – 4TH		Approach – 5TH	Device – 6TH	Qualifier – 7TH
0 Lumbar Vertebra 1 Sacrum 2 Pelvic Bone, Right 3 Pelvic Bone, Left 4 Acetabulum, Right 5 Acetabulum, Left D Patella, Right F Patella, Left	L Tarsal, Right M Tarsal, Left N Metatarsal, Right P Metatarsal, Left Q Toe Phalanx, Right R Toe Phalanx, Left S Coccyx	0 Open 3 Percutaneous 4 Percutaneous endoscopic	4 Internal fixation device 5 External fixation device	Z No qualifier
6 Upper Femur, Right 7 Upper Femur, Left 8 Femoral Shaft, Right 9 Femoral Shaft, Left B Lower Femur, Right C Lower Femur, Left G Tibia, Right H Tibia, Left J Fibula, Right K Fibula, Left		0 Open 3 Percutaneous 4 Percutaneous endoscopic	4 Internal fixation device 5 External fixation device 6 Internal fixation device, intramedullary 8 External fixation device, limb lengthening B External fixation device, monoplanar C External fixation device, ring D External fixation device, hybrid	Z No qualifier
Y Lower Bone		0 Open 3 Percutaneous 4 Percutaneous endoscopic	M Bone growth stimulator	Z No qualifier

LOWER BONES

0 Q H

EXAMINATION GROUP: Inspection, (Map)
Root Operations involving examination only.

1ST – **0** Medical and Surgical

2ND – **Q** Lower Bones

3RD – **J** INSPECTION

EXAMPLE: Examination bone   CMS Ex: Colonoscopy

__INSPECTION:__ Visually and/or manually exploring a body part.

EXPLANATION: Direct or instrumental visualization ...

Body Part – 4TH	Approach – 5TH	Device – 6TH	Qualifier – 7TH
Y Lower Bone	0 Open 3 Percutaneous 4 Percutaneous endoscopic X External	Z No device	Z No qualifier

DIVISION GROUP: Division, Release
Root Operations involving cutting or separation only.

1ST – **0** Medical and Surgical

2ND – **Q** Lower Bones

3RD – **N** RELEASE

EXAMPLE: Extra-articular bone adhesiolysis   CMS Ex: Carpal tunnel release

__RELEASE:__ Freeing a body part from an abnormal physical constraint by cutting or by the use of force.

EXPLANATION: None of the body part is taken out ...

Body Part – 4TH		Approach – 5TH	Device – 6TH	Qualifier – 7TH
0 Lumbar Vertebra	D Patella, Right	0 Open	Z No device	Z No qualifier
1 Sacrum	F Patella, Left	3 Percutaneous		
2 Pelvic Bone, Right	G Tibia, Right	4 Percutaneous endoscopic		
3 Pelvic Bone, Left	H Tibia, Left			
4 Acetabulum, Right	J Fibula, Right			
5 Acetabulum, Left	K Fibula, Left			
6 Upper Femur, Right	L Tarsal, Right			
7 Upper Femur, Left	M Tarsal, Left			
8 Femoral Shaft, Right	N Metatarsal, Right			
9 Femoral Shaft, Left	P Metatarsal, Left			
B Lower Femur, Right	Q Toe Phalanx, Right			
C Lower Femur, Left	R Toe Phalanx, Left			
	S Coccyx			

DEVICE GROUP: Change, Insertion, Removal, Replacement, Revision, Supplement
Root Operations that always involve a device.

1ST - 0 Medical and Surgical

2ND - Q Lower Bones

3RD - P REMOVAL

EXAMPLE: Removal growing rods   CMS Ex: Chest tube removal

REMOVAL: Taking out or off a device from a body part.

EXPLANATION: Removal device without reinsertion ...

Body Part – 4TH	Approach – 5TH	Device – 6TH	Qualifier – 7TH
0 Lumbar Vertebra 1 Sacrum 4 Acetabulum, Right 5 Acetabulum, Left S Coccyx	0 Open 3 Percutaneous 4 Percutaneous endoscopic	4 Internal fixation device 7 Autologous tissue substitute J Synthetic substitute K Nonautologous tissue substitute	Z No qualifier
0 Lumbar Vertebra 1 Sacrum 4 Acetabulum, Right 5 Acetabulum, Left S Coccyx	X External	4 Internal fixation device	Z No qualifier
2 Pelvic Bone, Right G Tibia, Right 3 Pelvic Bone, Left H Tibia, Left 6 Upper Femur, Right J Fibula, Right 7 Upper Femur, Left K Fibula, Left 8 Femoral Shaft, Right L Tarsal, Right 9 Femoral Shaft, Left M Tarsal, Left B Lower Femur, Right N Metatarsal, Right C Lower Femur, Left P Metatarsal, Left D Patella, Right Q Toe Phalanx, Right F Patella, Left R Toe Phalanx, Left	0 Open 3 Percutaneous 4 Percutaneous endoscopic	4 Internal fixation device 5 External fixation device 7 Autologous tissue substitute J Synthetic substitute K Nonautologous tissue substitute	Z No qualifier
2 Pelvic Bone, Right G Tibia, Right 3 Pelvic Bone, Left H Tibia, Left 6 Upper Femur, Right J Fibula, Right 7 Upper Femur, Left K Fibula, Left 8 Femoral Shaft, Right L Tarsal, Right 9 Femoral Shaft, Left M Tarsal, Left B Lower Femur, Right N Metatarsal, Right C Lower Femur, Left P Metatarsal, Left D Patella, Right Q Toe Phalanx, Right F Patella, Left R Toe Phalanx, Left	X External	4 Internal fixation device 5 External fixation device	Z No qualifier
Y Lower Bone	0 Open 3 Percutaneous 4 Percutaneous endoscopic X External	0 Drainage device M Bone growth stimulator	Z No qualifier

LOWER BONES

0 Q P

OTHER REPAIRS GROUP: (Control), Repair
Root Operations that define other repairs.

1ST - **0** Medical and Surgical
2ND - **Q** Lower Bones
3RD - **Q REPAIR**

EXAMPLE: Vertebral laminoplasty | CMS Ex: Suture laceration

REPAIR: Restoring, to the extent possible, a body part to its normal anatomic structure and function.

EXPLANATION: Only when no other root operation applies …

Body Part – 4TH		Approach – 5TH	Device – 6TH	Qualifier – 7TH
0 Lumbar Vertebra	D Patella, Right	0 Open	Z No device	Z No qualifier
1 Sacrum	F Patella, Left	3 Percutaneous		
2 Pelvic Bone, Right	G Tibia, Right	4 Percutaneous endoscopic		
3 Pelvic Bone, Left	H Tibia, Left	X External		
4 Acetabulum, Right	J Fibula, Right			
5 Acetabulum, Left	K Fibula, Left			
6 Upper Femur, Right	L Tarsal, Right			
7 Upper Femur, Left	M Tarsal, Left			
8 Femoral Shaft, Right	N Metatarsal, Right			
9 Femoral Shaft, Left	P Metatarsal, Left			
B Lower Femur, Right	Q Toe Phalanx, Right			
C Lower Femur, Left	R Toe Phalanx, Left			
	S Coccyx			

DEVICE GROUP: Change, Insertion, Removal, Replacement, Revision, Supplement
Root Operations that always involve a device.

1ST - **0** Medical and Surgical
2ND - **Q** Lower Bones
3RD - **R REPLACEMENT**

EXAMPLE: Patella replacement | CMS Ex: Total hip

REPLACEMENT: Putting in or on a biological or synthetic material that physically takes the place and/or function of all or a portion of a body part.

EXPLANATION: Includes taking out body part, or eradication…

Body Part – 4TH		Approach – 5TH	Device – 6TH	Qualifier – 7TH
0 Lumbar Vertebra	D Patella, Right	0 Open	7 Autologous tissue substitute	Z No qualifier
1 Sacrum	F Patella, Left	3 Percutaneous	J Synthetic substitute	
2 Pelvic Bone, Right	G Tibia, Right	4 Percutaneous endoscopic	K Nonautologous tissue substitute	
3 Pelvic Bone, Left	H Tibia, Left			
4 Acetabulum, Right	J Fibula, Right			
5 Acetabulum, Left	K Fibula, Left			
6 Upper Femur, Right	L Tarsal, Right			
7 Upper Femur, Left	M Tarsal, Left			
8 Femoral Shaft, Right	N Metatarsal, Right			
9 Femoral Shaft, Left	P Metatarsal, Left			
B Lower Femur, Right	Q Toe Phalanx, Right			
C Lower Femur, Left	R Toe Phalanx, Left			
	S Coccyx			

LOWER BONES   0 Q Q

MOVE GROUP: (Reattachment), **Reposition,** (Transfer), (Transplantation)			
Root Operations that put in/put back or move some/all of a body part.			

1ST - **0** Medical and Surgical	EXAMPLE: Reduction with hybrid device	CMS Ex: Fracture reduction
2ND - **Q** Lower Bones	**REPOSITION:** Moving to its normal location, or other suitable location, all or a portion of a body part.	
3RD - **S REPOSITION**		
	EXPLANATION: May or may not be cut to be moved ...	

Body Part – 4TH		Approach – 5TH	Device – 6TH	Qualifier – 7TH
0 Lumbar Vertebra 1 Sacrum	4 Acetabulum, Right 5 Acetabulum, Left S Coccyx	0 Open 3 Percutaneous 4 Percutaneous endoscopic	4 Internal fixation device Z No device	Z No qualifier
0 Lumbar Vertebra 1 Sacrum	4 Acetabulum, Right 5 Acetabulum, Left S Coccyx	X External	Z No device	Z No qualifier
2 Pelvic Bone, Right 3 Pelvic Bone, Left D Patella, Right F Patella, Left L Tarsal, Right M Tarsal, Left	N Metatarsal, Right P Metatarsal, Left Q Toe Phalanx, Right R Toe Phalanx, Left	0 Open 3 Percutaneous 4 Percutaneous endoscopic	4 Internal fixation device 5 External fixation device Z No device	Z No qualifier
2 Pelvic Bone, Right 3 Pelvic Bone, Left D Patella, Right F Patella, Left L Tarsal, Right M Tarsal, Left	N Metatarsal, Right P Metatarsal, Left Q Toe Phalanx, Right R Toe Phalanx, Left	X External	Z No device	Z No qualifier
6 Upper Femur, Right 7 Upper Femur, Left 8 Femoral Shaft, Right 9 Femoral Shaft, Left B Lower Femur, Right C Lower Femur, Left	G Tibia, Right H Tibia, Left J Fibula, Right K Fibula, Left	0 Open 3 Percutaneous 4 Percutaneous endoscopic	4 Internal fixation device 5 External fixation device 6 Internal fixation device, intramedullary B External fixation device, monoplanar C External fixation device, ring D External fixation device, hybrid Z No device	Z No qualifier
6 Upper Femur, Right 7 Upper Femur, Left 8 Femoral Shaft, Right 9 Femoral Shaft, Left B Lower Femur, Right C Lower Femur, Left	G Tibia, Right H Tibia, Left J Fibula, Right K Fibula, Left	X External	Z No device	Z No qualifier

LOWER BONES

0 Q S

EXCISION GROUP: Excision, Resection, Destruction, (Extraction), (Detachment)
Root Operations that take out some or all of a body part.

1ST - **0** Medical and Surgical	EXAMPLE: Total patellectomy		CMS Ex: Cholecystectomy
2ND - **Q** Lower Bones	**RESECTION:** Cutting out or off, without replacement, all of a body part.		
3RD - **T RESECTION**	EXPLANATION: None		

Body Part – 4TH		Approach – 5TH	Device – 6TH	Qualifier – 7TH
2 Pelvic Bone, Right	G Tibia, Right	0 Open	Z No device	Z No qualifier
3 Pelvic Bone, Left	H Tibia, Left			
4 Acetabulum, Right	J Fibula, Right			
5 Acetabulum, Left	K Fibula, Left			
6 Upper Femur, Right	L Tarsal, Right			
7 Upper Femur, Left	M Tarsal, Left			
8 Femoral Shaft, Right	N Metatarsal, Right			
9 Femoral Shaft, Left	P Metatarsal, Left			
B Lower Femur, Right	Q Toe Phalanx, Right			
C Lower Femur, Left	R Toe Phalanx, Left			
D Patella, Right	S Coccyx			
F Patella, Left				

DEVICE GROUP: Change, Insertion, Removal, Replacement, Revision, Supplement
Root Operations that always involve a device.

1ST - **0** Medical and Surgical	EXAMPLE: Application bone void filler		CMS Ex: Hernia repair with mesh
2ND - **Q** Lower Bones	**SUPPLEMENT:** Putting in or on biological or synthetic material that physically reinforces and/or augments the function of a portion of a body part.		
3RD - **U SUPPLEMENT**	EXPLANATION: Biological material from same individual …		

Body Part – 4TH		Approach – 5TH	Device – 6TH	Qualifier – 7TH
0 Lumbar Vertebra	D Patella, Right	0 Open	7 Autologous tissue substitute	Z No qualifier
1 Sacrum	F Patella, Left	3 Percutaneous	J Synthetic substitute	
2 Pelvic Bone, Right	G Tibia, Right	4 Percutaneous endoscopic	K Nonautologous tissue substitute	
3 Pelvic Bone, Left	H Tibia, Left			
4 Acetabulum, Right	J Fibula, Right			
5 Acetabulum, Left	K Fibula, Left			
6 Upper Femur, Right	L Tarsal, Right			
7 Upper Femur, Left	M Tarsal, Left			
8 Femoral Shaft, Right	N Metatarsal, Right			
9 Femoral Shaft, Left	P Metatarsal, Left			
B Lower Femur, Right	Q Toe Phalanx, Right			
C Lower Femur, Left	R Toe Phalanx, Left			
	S Coccyx			

| DEVICE GROUP: Change, Insertion, Removal, Replacement, Revision, Supplement |
| Root Operations that always involve a device. |

1ST - 0 Medical and Surgical

2ND - Q Lower Bones

3RD - W REVISION

EXAMPLE: Lengthening growing rods | CMS Ex: Adjustment pacemaker lead

REVISION: Correcting, to the extent possible, a portion of a malfunctioning device or the position of a displaced device.

EXPLANATION: May replace components of a device ...

Body Part – 4TH		Approach – 5TH	Device – 6TH	Qualifier – 7TH
0 Lumbar Vertebra 1 Sacrum	4 Acetabulum, Right 5 Acetabulum, Left S Coccyx	0 Open 3 Percutaneous 4 Percutaneous endoscopic X External	4 Internal fixation device 7 Autologous tissue substitute J Synthetic substitute K Nonautologous tissue substitute	Z No qualifier
2 Pelvic Bone, Right 3 Pelvic Bone, Left 6 Upper Femur, Right 7 Upper Femur, Left 8 Femoral Shaft, Right 9 Femoral Shaft, Left B Lower Femur, Right C Lower Femur, Left D Patella, Right F Patella, Left	G Tibia, Right H Tibia, Left J Fibula, Right K Fibula, Left L Tarsal, Right M Tarsal, Left N Metatarsal, Right P Metatarsal, Left Q Toe Phalanx, Right R Toe Phalanx, Left	0 Open 3 Percutaneous 4 Percutaneous endoscopic X External	4 Internal fixation device 5 External fixation device 7 Autologous tissue substitute J Synthetic substitute K Nonautologous tissue substitute	Z No qualifier
Y Lower Bone		0 Open 3 Percutaneous 4 Percutaneous endoscopic X External	0 Drainage device M Bone growth stimulator	Z No qualifier

LOWER BONES 0 Q W

NOTES

Educational Annotations | R – Upper Joints

Body System Specific Educational Annotations for the Upper Joints include:

- **Anatomy and Physiology Review**
- **Anatomical Illustrations**
- **Definitions of Common Procedures**
- **AHA Coding Clinic® Reference Notations**
- **Body Part Key Listings**
- **Device Key Listings**
- **Device Aggregation Table Listings**
- **Coding Notes**

Anatomy and Physiology Review of Upper Joints

BODY PART VALUES – R - UPPER JOINTS

Acromioclavicular Joint – The joint formed between the acromion portion of the scapula and the distal end of the clavicle.

Carpal Joint – A complex collection of joints formed by the interconnection of the 8 carpal bones in the hand.

Cervical Vertebral Disc – The disc-shaped fibrocartilage pad between the cervical spine vertebral bodies comprised of a tough outer portion (annulus fibrosus) and a gel-like inner portion (nucleus pulposus).

Cervical Vertebral Joint – The synovial and cartilaginous joints connecting the vertebra of the cervical spine.

Cervicothoracic Vertebral Disc – The disc-shaped fibrocartilage pad between the C7 vertebral body of the cervical spine and the T1 vertebral body of the thoracic spine comprised of a tough outer portion (annulus fibrosus) and a gel-like inner portion (nucleus pulposus).

Cervicothoracic Vertebral Joint – The synovial and cartilaginous joints connecting the C7 vertebra of the cervical spine and the T1 vertebra of the thoracic spine.

Elbow Joint – A hinge joint between the humerus in the upper arm and the radius and ulna in the forearm.

Finger Phalangeal Joint – Any of 9 hinge joints in the fingers between the proximal and intermediate phalanges (PIP), and the intermediate and distal phalanges (DIP). The thumb has only two phalanges and therefore only one phalangeal joint.

Metacarpocarpal Joint – Any of the 5 joints in the hand that articulate the distal row of carpal bones and the proximal bases of the five metacarpal bones.

Metacarpophalangeal Joint – Any of 5 condyloid joints (except the hinge joint of the thumb) in the hand that articulate the distal heads of the five metacarpal bones and the proximal phalanx of each finger.

Occipital-cervical Joint – The joint formed between the C1 vertebra and the base of the skull (occipital bone).

Shoulder Joint – A multiaxial ball-and-socket joint (also known as the glenohumeral joint) between the head of the humerus and the rounded depression (glenoid fossa) of the scapula.

Sternoclavicular Joint – The joint formed between the upper portion of the sternum and the medial end of the clavicle.

Temporomandibular Joint – The joint formed between the mandible and temporal bone.

Thoracic Vertebral Disc – The disc-shaped fibrocartilage pad between the thoracic spine vertebral bodies comprised of a tough outer portion (annulus fibrosus) and a gel-like inner portion (nucleus pulposus).

Thoracic Vertebral Joint – The synovial and cartilaginous joints connecting the vertebra of the thoracic spine.

Thoracolumbar Vertebral Disc – The disc-shaped fibrocartilage pad between the T12 vertebral body of the thoracic spine and the L1 vertebral body of the lumbar spine comprised of a tough outer portion (annulus fibrosus) and a gel-like inner portion (nucleus pulposus).

Thoracolumbar Vertebral Joint – The synovial and cartilaginous joints connecting the T12 vertebra of the thoracic spine and the L1 vertebra of the lumbar spine.

Upper Joint – Any of the joints designated in the Upper Joints PCS Body System.

Wrist Joint – A pivot joint between the distal radius and the carpus.

UPPER JOINTS

0 R

Educational Annotations | R – Upper Joints

Anatomical Illustrations of Upper Joints

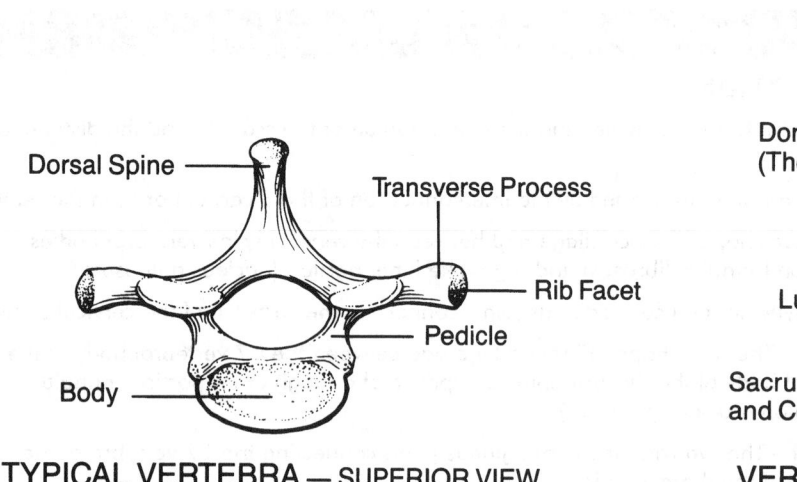

Dorsal Spine

Transverse Process

Rib Facet

Pedicle

Body

TYPICAL VERTEBRA — SUPERIOR VIEW

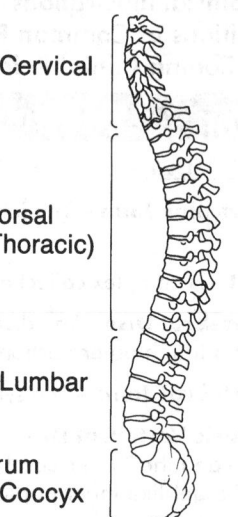

Cervical

Dorsal (Thoracic)

Lumbar

Sacrum and Coccyx

VERTEBRAL COLUMN

Definitions of Common Procedures of Upper Joints

Arthroscopy – The surgical visualization and examination of a joint using an endoscope and often the approach used for joint procedures.

Cervical interbody spinal fusion – The permanent surgical joining of two or more cervical vertebrae together using bone graft placed between the intervertebral space after the disc(s) have been removed and using metal or plastic cage to support the spine while the bone graft hardens.

Cervical spinal fusion – The permanent surgical joining of two or more cervical vertebrae together using a bone graft and immobilization by using plates, rods, screws, and/or wires.

Discectomy – The surgical removal of all (total) or a portion of an intervertebral disc.

Reverse total shoulder arthroplasty – The surgical replacement of the shoulder joint by reversing the cup and head replacement. The cup is placed onto the humerus and the ball is placed in the socket. This procedure is done for patients with severe rotator cuff damage.

Total shoulder arthroplasty – The surgical replacement of the shoulder joint socket (glenoid) cup and humeral head in the normal anatomical configuration.

Type 2 SLAP (superior labral tear from anterior to posterior) repair – The surgical repair of the glenoid labrum of the shoulder joint.

Educational Annotations | R – Upper Joints

AHA Coding Clinic® Reference Notations of Upper Joints

ROOT OPERATION SPECIFIC - R - UPPER JOINTS

CHANGE - 2
DESTRUCTION - 5
DRAINAGE - 9
EXCISION - B
    Spinal fusion with discectomy...AHA 14:2Q:p6
EXTIRPATION - C
FUSION - G
    Components in fusion procedures included in Fusion root operation..........AHA 14:3Q:p30
    Fusion of cervicothoracic vertebral joint with interbody fusion device ....AHA 13:1Q:p29
    ....AHA 14:2Q:p7
    Fusion of multiple vertebral joints ....AHA 13:1Q:p21
INSERTION - H
INSPECTION - J
RELEASE - N
    Release of shoulder joint ....AHA 15:2Q:p23
    Subacromial and rotator cuff decompression ....AHA 15:2Q:p22
REMOVAL - P
REPAIR - Q
    Shoulder thermal capsulorrhaphy..AHA 16:1Q:p30
REPLACEMENT - R
    Replacement of fractured humeral head surface ....AHA 15:3Q:p14
    Reverse total shoulder arthroplasty...AHA 15:1Q:p27
REPOSITION - S
    Manipulation of radioulnar joint dislocation ....AHA 14:4Q:p32
    Reposition of carpal joint ....AHA 14:3Q:p33
    Tongs used to stabilize cervical fracture ....AHA 13:2Q:p39
        Official Correction of 13:2Q:p39..AHA 15:2Q:p34
RESECTION - T
    Spinal fusion with total discectomy ....AHA 14:2Q:p7
SUPPLEMENT - U
    Arthroplasty using tendon graft ....AHA 15:3Q:p26
REVISION - W

Body Part Key Listings of Upper Joints

See also Body Part Key in Appendix C

Atlantoaxial joint ....*use* Cervical Vertebral Joint
Carpometacarpal (CMC) joint ....*use* Metacarpocarpal Joint, Left/Right
Cervical facet joint ....*use* Cervical Vertebral Joint(s)
Cervicothoracic facet joint ....*use* Cervicothoracic Vertebral Joint
Costotransverse joint ....*use* Thoracic Vertebral Joint
Costovertebral joint ....*use* Thoracic Vertebral Joint
Distal humerus, involving joint ....*use* Elbow Joint, Left/Right
Distal radioulnar joint ....*use* Wrist Joint, Left/Right
Glenohumeral joint ....*use* Shoulder Joint, Left/Right
Glenoid ligament (labrum) ....*use* Shoulder Joint, Left/Right
Humeroradial joint ....*use* Elbow Joint, Left/Right
Humeroulnar joint ....*use* Elbow Joint, Left/Right

Continued on next page

Educational Annotations | R – Upper Joints

Body Part Key Listings of Upper Joints

Continued from previous page

Intercarpal joint .... *use* Carpal Joint, Left/Right
Interphalangeal (IP) joint .... *use* Finger Phalangeal Joint, Left/Right
Midcarpal joint.. *use* Carpal Joint, Left/Right
Proximal radioulnar joint .... *use* Elbow Joint, Left/Right
Radiocarpal joint .... *use* Wrist Joint, Left/Right
Thoracic facet joint.. *use* Thoracic Vertebral Joint
Thoracolumbar facet joint .... *use* Thoracolumbar Vertebral Joint

Device Key Listings of Upper Joints

See also Device Key in Appendix D

Autograft .... *use* Autologous Tissue Substitute
BAK/C® Interbody Cervical Fusion System .... *use* Interbody Fusion Device in Upper Joints
BRYAN® Cervical Disc System .... *use* Synthetic Substitute
Delta III Reverse shoulder prosthesis .... *use* Synthetic Substitute, Reverse Ball and Socket for Replacement in Upper Joints
Dynesys® Dynamic Stabilization System .... *use* Spinal Stabilization Device, Pedicle-Based for Insertion in Upper Joints, Lower Joints
External fixator .... *use* External Fixation Device in Head and Facial Bones, Upper Bones, Lower Bones, Upper Joints, Lower Joints
Facet replacement spinal stabilization device.......... *use* Spinal Stabilization Device, Facet Replacement for Insertion in Upper Joints, Lower Joints
Fusion screw (compression) (lag) (locking) .... *use* Internal Fixation Device in Upper Joints, Lower Joints
Interbody fusion (spine) cage .... *use* Interbody Fusion Device in Upper Joints, Lower Joints
Interspinous process spinal stabilization device...... *use* Spinal Stabilization Device, Interspinous Process for Insertion in Upper Joints, Lower Joints
Joint fixation plate .... *use* Internal Fixation Device in Upper Joints, Lower Joints
Joint spacer (antibiotic).. *use* Spacer in Upper Joints, Lower Joints
Kirschner wire (K-wire) .... *use* Internal Fixation Device in Head and Facial Bones, Upper Bones, Lower Bones, Upper Joints, Lower Joints
Pedicle-based dynamic stabilization device .... *use* Spinal Stabilization Device, Pedicle-Based for Insertion in Upper Joints, Lower Joints
Polymethylmethacrylate (PMMA)............................... *use* Synthetic Substitute
PRESTIGE® Cervical Disc .... *use* Synthetic Substitute
Prodisc-C .... *use* Synthetic Substitute
Reverse® Shoulder Prosthesis...................................... *use* Synthetic Substitute, Reverse Ball and Socket for Replacement in Upper Joints
Tissue bank graft .... *use* Nonautologous Tissue Substitute
X-STOP® Spacer .... *use* Spinal Stabilization Device, Interspinous Process for Insertion in Upper Joints, Lower Joints

Device Aggregation Table Listings of Upper Joints

See also Device Aggregation Table in Appendix E

Specific Device	For Operation	In Body System	General Device	
Spinal Stabilization Device, Facet Replacement	Insertion	Upper Joints	4	Internal Fixation Device
Spinal Stabilization Device, Interspinous Process	Insertion	Upper Joints	4	Internal Fixation Device
Spinal Stabilization Device, Pedicle-Based	Insertion	Upper Joints	4	Internal Fixation Device

Educational Annotations | R – Upper Joints

Coding Notes of Upper Joints

Body System Relevant Coding Guidelines

Fusion procedures of the spine

B3.10a

The body part coded for a spinal vertebral joint(s) rendered immobile by a spinal fusion procedure is classified by the level of the spine (e.g. thoracic). There are distinct body part values for a single vertebral joint and for multiple vertebral joints at each spinal level.
Example: Body part values specify Lumbar Vertebral Joint, Lumbar Vertebral Joints, 2 or More and Lumbosacral Vertebral Joint.

B3.10b

If multiple vertebral joints are fused, a separate procedure is coded for each vertebral joint that uses a different device and/or qualifier.
Example: Fusion of lumbar vertebral joint, posterior approach, anterior column and fusion of lumbar vertebral joint, posterior approach, posterior column are coded separately.

B3.10c

Combinations of devices and materials are often used on a vertebral joint to render the joint immobile. When combinations of devices are used on the same vertebral joint, the device value coded for the procedure is as follows:

- If an interbody fusion device is used to render the joint immobile (alone or containing other material like bone graft), the procedure is coded with the device value Interbody Fusion Device
- If bone graft is the only device used to render the joint immobile, the procedure is coded with the device value Nonautologous Tissue Substitute or Autologous Tissue Substitute
- If a mixture of autologous and nonautologous bone graft (with or without biological or synthetic extenders or binders) is used to render the joint immobile, code the procedure with the device value Autologous Tissue Substitute

Examples: Fusion of a vertebral joint using a cage style interbody fusion device containing morsellized bone graft is coded to the device Interbody Fusion Device.

Fusion of a vertebral joint using a bone dowel interbody fusion device made of cadaver bone and packed with a mixture of local morsellized bone and demineralized bone matrix is coded to the device Interbody Fusion Device.

Fusion of a vertebral joint using both autologous bone graft and bone bank bone graft is coded to the device Autologous Tissue Substitute.

Tendons, ligaments, bursae and fascia near a joint

B4.5

Procedures performed on tendons, ligaments, bursae and fascia supporting a joint are coded to the body part in the respective body system that is the focus of the procedure. Procedures performed on joint structures themselves are coded to the body part in the joint body systems.
Examples: Repair of the anterior cruciate ligament of the knee is coded to the knee bursa and ligament body part in the bursae and ligaments body system.
Knee arthroscopy with shaving of articular cartilage is coded to the knee joint body part in the Lower Joints body system.

Body System Specific PCS Reference Manual Exercises

PCS CODE	R – UPPER JOINTS EXERCISES
0 R G P 0 4 Z	Radiocarpal fusion of left hand with internal fixation, open.
0 R G Q 0 K Z	Intercarpal fusion of right hand with bone bank bone graft, open.
0 R J J 4 Z Z	Diagnostic arthroscopy of right shoulder.
0 R N J X Z Z	Manual rupture of right shoulder joint adhesions under general anesthesia.

U P P E R   J O I N T S   0   R

Educational Annotations | R – Upper Joints

NOTES

DEVICE GROUP: Change, Insertion, Removal, Replacement, Revision, Supplement
Root Operations that always involve a device.

1ST - **0** Medical and Surgical

2ND - **R** Upper Joints

3RD - **2 CHANGE**

EXAMPLE: Exchange drain tube | CMS Ex: Changing urinary catheter

CHANGE: Taking out or off a device from a body part and putting back an identical or similar device in or on the same body part without cutting or puncturing the skin or a mucous membrane.

EXPLANATION: ALL Changes use EXTERNAL approach only ...

Body Part – 4TH	Approach – 5TH	Device – 6TH	Qualifier – 7TH
Y Upper Joint	X External	0 Drainage device Y Other device	Z No qualifier

EXCISION GROUP: Excision, Resection, Destruction, (Extraction), (Detachment)
Root Operations that take out some or all of a body part.

1ST - **0** Medical and Surgical

2ND - **R** Upper Joints

3RD - **5 DESTRUCTION**

EXAMPLE: Radiofrequency ablation | CMS Ex: Fulguration polyp

DESTRUCTION: Physical eradication of all or a portion of a body part by the direct use of energy, force, or a destructive agent.

EXPLANATION: None of the body part is physically taken out

Body Part – 4TH	Approach – 5TH	Device – 6TH	Qualifier – 7TH
0 Occipital-cervical Joint 1 Cervical Vertebral Joint 3 Cervical Vertebral Disc 4 Cervicothoracic Vertebral Joint 5 Cervicothoracic Vertebral Disc 6 Thoracic Vertebral Joint 9 Thoracic Vertebral Disc A Thoracolumbar Vertebral Joint B Thoracolumbar Vertebral Disc C Temporomandibular Joint, Right D Temporomandibular Joint, Left E Sternoclavicular Joint, Right F Sternoclavicular Joint, Left G Acromioclavicular Joint, Right H Acromioclavicular Joint, Left J Shoulder Joint, Right K Shoulder Joint, Left L Elbow Joint, Right M Elbow Joint, Left N Wrist Joint, Right P Wrist Joint, Left Q Carpal Joint, Right R Carpal Joint, Left S Metacarpocarpal Joint, Right T Metacarpocarpal Joint, Left U Metacarpophalangeal Joint, Right V Metacarpophalangeal Joint, Left W Finger Phalangeal Joint, Right X Finger Phalangeal Joint, Left	0 Open 3 Percutaneous 4 Percutaneous endoscopic	Z No device	Z No qualifier

DRAINAGE GROUP: Drainage, Extirpation, (Fragmentation)
Root Operations that take out solids/fluids/gases from a body part.

| 1ST - 0 Medical and Surgical | EXAMPLE: Aspiration elbow joint | CMS Ex: Thoracentesis |

1ST - 0 Medical and Surgical

2ND - R Upper Joints

3RD - 9 DRAINAGE

EXAMPLE: Aspiration elbow joint | CMS Ex: Thoracentesis

DRAINAGE: Taking or letting out fluids and/or gases from a body part.

EXPLANATION: Qualifier "X Diagnostic" indicates biopsy …

Body Part – 4TH	Approach – 5TH	Device – 6TH	Qualifier – 7TH
0 Occipital-cervical Joint	0 Open	0 Drainage device	Z No qualifier
1 Cervical Vertebral Joint	3 Percutaneous		
3 Cervical Vertebral Disc	4 Percutaneous endoscopic		
4 Cervicothoracic Vertebral Joint			
5 Cervicothoracic Vertebral Disc			
6 Thoracic Vertebral Joint			
9 Thoracic Vertebral Disc			
A Thoracolumbar Vertebral Joint			
B Thoracolumbar Vertebral Disc			
C Temporomandibular Joint, Right			
D Temporomandibular Joint, Left			
E Sternoclavicular Joint, Right			
F Sternoclavicular Joint, Left			
G Acromioclavicular Joint, Right			
H Acromioclavicular Joint, Left			
J Shoulder Joint, Right			
K Shoulder Joint, Left			
L Elbow Joint, Right			
M Elbow Joint, Left			
N Wrist Joint, Right			
P Wrist Joint, Left			
Q Carpal Joint, Right			
R Carpal Joint, Left			
S Metacarpocarpal Joint, Right			
T Metacarpocarpal Joint, Left			
U Metacarpophalangeal Joint, Right			
V Metacarpophalangeal Joint, Left			
W Finger Phalangeal Joint, Right			
X Finger Phalangeal Joint, Left			

continued ⇨

0 R 9 DRAINAGE – *continued*			
Body Part – 4TH	**Approach – 5TH**	**Device – 6TH**	**Qualifier – 7TH**
0 Occipital-cervical Joint	0 Open	Z No device	X Diagnostic
1 Cervical Vertebral Joint	3 Percutaneous		Z No qualifier
3 Cervical Vertebral Disc	4 Percutaneous		
4 Cervicothoracic Vertebral Joint	endoscopic		
5 Cervicothoracic Vertebral Disc			
6 Thoracic Vertebral Joint			
9 Thoracic Vertebral Disc			
A Thoracolumbar Vertebral Joint			
B Thoracolumbar Vertebral Disc			
C Temporomandibular Joint, Right			
D Temporomandibular Joint, Left			
E Sternoclavicular Joint, Right			
F Sternoclavicular Joint, Left			
G Acromioclavicular Joint, Right			
H Acromioclavicular Joint, Left			
J Shoulder Joint, Right			
K Shoulder Joint, Left			
L Elbow Joint, Right			
M Elbow Joint, Left			
N Wrist Joint, Right			
P Wrist Joint, Left			
Q Carpal Joint, Right			
R Carpal Joint, Left			
S Metacarpocarpal Joint, Right			
T Metacarpocarpal Joint, Left			
U Metacarpophalangeal Joint, Right			
V Metacarpophalangeal Joint, Left			
W Finger Phalangeal Joint, Right			
X Finger Phalangeal Joint, Left			

UPPER JOINTS 0 R 9

EXCISION GROUP: Excision, Resection, Destruction, (Extraction), (Detachment)
Root Operations that take out some or all of a body part.

1ST - **0** Medical and Surgical

2ND - **R** Upper Joints

3RD - **B EXCISION**

EXAMPLE: Partial cervical discectomy   CMS Ex: Liver biopsy

EXCISION: Cutting out or off, without replacement, a portion of a body part.

EXPLANATION: Qualifier "X Diagnostic" indicates biopsy ...

Body Part – 4TH	Approach – 5TH	Device – 6TH	Qualifier – 7TH
0 Occipital-cervical Joint	0 Open	Z No device	X Diagnostic
1 Cervical Vertebral Joint	3 Percutaneous		Z No qualifier
3 Cervical Vertebral Disc	4 Percutaneous		
4 Cervicothoracic Vertebral Joint	endoscopic		
5 Cervicothoracic Vertebral Disc			
6 Thoracic Vertebral Joint			
9 Thoracic Vertebral Disc			
A Thoracolumbar Vertebral Joint			
B Thoracolumbar Vertebral Disc			
C Temporomandibular Joint, Right			
D Temporomandibular Joint, Left			
E Sternoclavicular Joint, Right			
F Sternoclavicular Joint, Left			
G Acromioclavicular Joint, Right			
H Acromioclavicular Joint, Left			
J Shoulder Joint, Right			
K Shoulder Joint, Left			
L Elbow Joint, Right			
M Elbow Joint, Left			
N Wrist Joint, Right			
P Wrist Joint, Left			
Q Carpal Joint, Right			
R Carpal Joint, Left			
S Metacarpocarpal Joint, Right			
T Metacarpocarpal Joint, Left			
U Metacarpophalangeal Joint, Right			
V Metacarpophalangeal Joint, Left			
W Finger Phalangeal Joint, Right			
X Finger Phalangeal Joint, Left			

UPPER JOINTS 0RB

DRAINAGE GROUP: Drainage, Extirpation, (Fragmentation)
Root Operations that take out solids/fluids/gases from a body part.

1ST - **0** Medical and Surgical	EXAMPLE: Removal loose bodies elbow CMS Ex: Choledocholithotomy
2ND - **R** Upper Joints	**EXTIRPATION:** Taking or cutting out solid matter from a body part.
3RD - **C EXTIRPATION**	EXPLANATION: Abnormal byproduct or foreign body ...

Body Part – 4TH	Approach – 5TH	Device – 6TH	Qualifier – 7TH
0 Occipital-cervical Joint	0 Open	Z No device	Z No qualifier
1 Cervical Vertebral Joint	3 Percutaneous		
3 Cervical Vertebral Disc	4 Percutaneous endoscopic		
4 Cervicothoracic Vertebral Joint			
5 Cervicothoracic Vertebral Disc			
6 Thoracic Vertebral Joint			
9 Thoracic Vertebral Disc			
A Thoracolumbar Vertebral Joint			
B Thoracolumbar Vertebral Disc			
C Temporomandibular Joint, Right			
D Temporomandibular Joint, Left			
E Sternoclavicular Joint, Right			
F Sternoclavicular Joint, Left			
G Acromioclavicular Joint, Right			
H Acromioclavicular Joint, Left			
J Shoulder Joint, Right			
K Shoulder Joint, Left			
L Elbow Joint, Right			
M Elbow Joint, Left			
N Wrist Joint, Right			
P Wrist Joint, Left			
Q Carpal Joint, Right			
R Carpal Joint, Left			
S Metacarpocarpal Joint, Right			
T Metacarpocarpal Joint, Left			
U Metacarpophalangeal Joint, Right			
V Metacarpophalangeal Joint, Left			
W Finger Phalangeal Joint, Right			
X Finger Phalangeal Joint, Left			

OTHER OBJECTIVES GROUP: (Alteration), (Creation), **Fusion**

Root Operations that define other objectives.

1ST - **0** Medical and Surgical

2ND - **R** Upper Joints

3RD - **G FUSION**

EXAMPLE: C3-C5 spinal fusion

CMS Ex: Spinal fusion

FUSION: Joining together portions of an articular body part, rendering the articular body part immobile.

EXPLANATION: Use of fixation device, graft, or other means ...

Body Part – 4TH	Approach – 5TH	Device – 6TH	Qualifier – 7TH
0 Occipital-cervical Joint 1 Cervical Vertebral Joint 2 Cervical Vertebral Joints, 2 or more 4 Cervicothoracic Vertebral Joint 6 Thoracic Vertebral Joint 7 Thoracic Vertebral Joints, 2 to 7 8 Thoracic Vertebral Joints, 8 or more A Thoracolumbar Vertebral Joint	0 Open 3 Percutaneous 4 Percutaneous endoscopic	7 Autologous tissue substitute A Interbody fusion device J Synthetic substitute K Nonautologous tissue substitute Z No device	0 Anterior approach, anterior column 1 Posterior approach, posterior column J Posterior approach, anterior column
C Temporomandibular Joint, Right D Temporomandibular Joint, Left E Sternoclavicular Joint, Right F Sternoclavicular Joint, Left G Acromioclavicular Joint, Right H Acromioclavicular Joint, Left J Shoulder Joint, Right K Shoulder Joint, Left	0 Open 3 Percutaneous 4 Percutaneous endoscopic	4 Internal fixation device 7 Autologous tissue substitute J Synthetic substitute K Nonautologous tissue substitute Z No device	Z No qualifier
L Elbow Joint, Right M Elbow Joint, Left N Wrist Joint, Right P Wrist Joint, Left Q Carpal Joint, Right R Carpal Joint, Left S Metacarpocarpal Joint, Right T Metacarpocarpal Joint, Left U Metacarpophalangeal Joint, Right V Metacarpophalangeal Joint, Left W Finger Phalangeal Joint, Right X Finger Phalangeal Joint, Left	0 Open 3 Percutaneous 4 Percutaneous endoscopic	4 Internal fixation device 5 External fixation device 7 Autologous tissue substitute J Synthetic substitute K Nonautologous tissue substitute Z No device	Z No qualifier

DEVICE GROUP: Change, Insertion, Removal, Replacement, Revision, Supplement
Root Operations that always involve a device.

1ST - **0** Medical and Surgical

2ND - **R** Upper Joints

3RD - **H INSERTION**

EXAMPLE: Implantation joint spacer | CMS Ex: Central venous catheter

INSERTION: Putting in a nonbiological appliance that monitors, assists, performs, or prevents a physiological function but does not physically take the place of a body part.

EXPLANATION: None

Body Part – 4TH	Approach – 5TH	Device – 6TH	Qualifier – 7TH
0 Occipital-cervical Joint 1 Cervical Vertebral Joint 4 Cervicothoracic Vertebral Joint 6 Thoracic Vertebral Joint A Thoracolumbar Vertebral Joint	0 Open 3 Percutaneous 4 Percutaneous endoscopic	3 Infusion device 4 Internal fixation device 8 Spacer B Spinal stabilization device, interspinous process C Spinal stabilization device, pedicle-based D Spinal stabilization device, facet replacement	Z No qualifier
3 Cervical Vertebral Disc 5 Cervicothoracic Vertebral Disc 9 Thoracic Vertebral Disc B Thoracolumbar Vertebral Disc	0 Open 3 Percutaneous 4 Percutaneous endoscopic	3 Infusion device	Z No qualifier
C Temporomandibular Joint, Right D Temporomandibular Joint, Left E Sternoclavicular Joint, Right F Sternoclavicular Joint, Left G Acromioclavicular Joint, Right H Acromioclavicular Joint, Left J Shoulder Joint, Right K Shoulder Joint, Left	0 Open 3 Percutaneous 4 Percutaneous endoscopic	3 Infusion device 4 Internal fixation device 8 Spacer	Z No qualifier
L Elbow Joint, Right M Elbow Joint, Left N Wrist Joint, Right P Wrist Joint, Left Q Carpal Joint, Right R Carpal Joint, Left S Metacarpocarpal Joint, Right T Metacarpocarpal Joint, Left U Metacarpophalangeal Joint, Right V Metacarpophalangeal Joint, Left W Finger Phalangeal Joint, Right X Finger Phalangeal Joint, Left	0 Open 3 Percutaneous 4 Percutaneous endoscopic	3 Infusion device 4 Internal fixation device 5 External fixation device 8 Spacer	Z No qualifier

UPPER JOINTS 0 R H

EXAMINATION GROUP: Inspection, (Map)
Root Operations involving examination only.

1ST - 0 Medical and Surgical

2ND - R Upper Joints

3RD - J INSPECTION

EXAMPLE: Diagnostic arthroscopy shoulder | CMS Ex: Colonoscopy

INSPECTION: Visually and/or manually exploring a body part.

EXPLANATION: Direct or instrumental visualization ...

Body Part – 4TH	Approach – 5TH	Device – 6TH	Qualifier – 7TH
0 Occipital-cervical Joint	0 Open	Z No device	Z No qualifier
1 Cervical Vertebral Joint	3 Percutaneous		
3 Cervical Vertebral Disc	4 Percutaneous		
4 Cervicothoracic Vertebral Joint	endoscopic		
5 Cervicothoracic Vertebral Disc	X External		
6 Thoracic Vertebral Joint			
9 Thoracic Vertebral Disc			
A Thoracolumbar Vertebral Joint			
B Thoracolumbar Vertebral Disc			
C Temporomandibular Joint, Right			
D Temporomandibular Joint, Left			
E Sternoclavicular Joint, Right			
F Sternoclavicular Joint, Left			
G Acromioclavicular Joint, Right			
H Acromioclavicular Joint, Left			
J Shoulder Joint, Right			
K Shoulder Joint, Left			
L Elbow Joint, Right			
M Elbow Joint, Left			
N Wrist Joint, Right			
P Wrist Joint, Left			
Q Carpal Joint, Right			
R Carpal Joint, Left			
S Metacarpocarpal Joint, Right			
T Metacarpocarpal Joint, Left			
U Metacarpophalangeal Joint, Right			
V Metacarpophalangeal Joint, Left			
W Finger Phalangeal Joint, Right			
X Finger Phalangeal Joint, Left			

UPPER JOINTS 0RJ

DIVISION GROUP: (Division), Release			
Root Operations involving cutting or separation only.			

1ST - 0 Medical and Surgical

2ND - R Upper Joints

3RD - N RELEASE

EXAMPLE: Manual rupture joint adhesions	CMS Ex: Carpal tunnel release

RELEASE: Freeing a body part from an abnormal physical constraint by cutting or by the use of force.

EXPLANATION: None of the body part is taken out ...

Body Part – 4TH	Approach – 5TH	Device – 6TH	Qualifier – 7TH
0 Occipital-cervical Joint	0 Open	Z No device	Z No qualifier
1 Cervical Vertebral Joint	3 Percutaneous		
3 Cervical Vertebral Disc	4 Percutaneous		
4 Cervicothoracic Vertebral Joint	endoscopic		
5 Cervicothoracic Vertebral Disc	X External		
6 Thoracic Vertebral Joint			
9 Thoracic Vertebral Disc			
A Thoracolumbar Vertebral Joint			
B Thoracolumbar Vertebral Disc			
C Temporomandibular Joint, Right			
D Temporomandibular Joint, Left			
E Sternoclavicular Joint, Right			
F Sternoclavicular Joint, Left			
G Acromioclavicular Joint, Right			
H Acromioclavicular Joint, Left			
J Shoulder Joint, Right			
K Shoulder Joint, Left			
L Elbow Joint, Right			
M Elbow Joint, Left			
N Wrist Joint, Right			
P Wrist Joint, Left			
Q Carpal Joint, Right			
R Carpal Joint, Left			
S Metacarpocarpal Joint, Right			
T Metacarpocarpal Joint, Left			
U Metacarpophalangeal Joint, Right			
V Metacarpophalangeal Joint, Left			
W Finger Phalangeal Joint, Right			
X Finger Phalangeal Joint, Left			

UPPER JOINTS 0 R N

DEVICE GROUP: Change, Insertion, Removal, Replacement, Revision, Supplement
Root Operations that always involve a device.

1ST - 0 Medical and Surgical		
2ND - R Upper Joints		
3RD - P REMOVAL		

EXAMPLE: Removal fixation device	CMS Ex: Chest tube removal

REMOVAL: Taking out or off a device from a body part.

EXPLANATION: Removal device without reinsertion ...

Body Part – 4TH	Approach – 5TH	Device – 6TH	Qualifier – 7TH
0 Occipital-cervical Joint 1 Cervical Vertebral Joint 4 Cervicothoracic Vertebral Joint 6 Thoracic Vertebral Joint A Thoracolumbar Vertebral Joint	0 Open 3 Percutaneous 4 Percutaneous endoscopic	0 Drainage device 3 Infusion device 4 Internal fixation device 7 Autologous tissue substitute 8 Spacer A Interbody fusion device J Synthetic substitute K Nonautologous tissue substitute	Z No qualifier
0 Occipital-cervical Joint 1 Cervical Vertebral Joint 4 Cervicothoracic Vertebral Joint 6 Thoracic Vertebral Joint A Thoracolumbar Vertebral Joint	X External	0 Drainage device 3 Infusion device 4 Internal fixation device	Z No qualifier
3 Cervical Vertebral Disc 5 Cervicothoracic Vertebral Disc 9 Thoracic Vertebral Disc B Thoracolumbar Vertebral Disc	0 Open 3 Percutaneous 4 Percutaneous endoscopic	0 Drainage device 3 Infusion device 7 Autologous tissue substitute J Synthetic substitute K Nonautologous tissue substitute	Z No qualifier
3 Cervical Vertebral Disc 5 Cervicothoracic Vertebral Disc 9 Thoracic Vertebral Disc B Thoracolumbar Vertebral Disc	X External	0 Drainage device 3 Infusion device	Z No qualifier

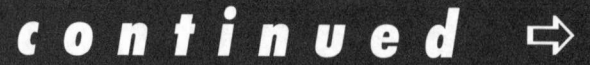
continued ⇨

U P P E R   J O I N T S   0 R P

0 R P REMOVAL – continued

Body Part – 4TH	Approach – 5TH	Device – 6TH	Qualifier – 7TH
C Temporomandibular Joint, Right D Temporomandibular Joint, Left E Sternoclavicular Joint, Right F Sternoclavicular Joint, Left G Acromioclavicular Joint, Right H Acromioclavicular Joint, Left J Shoulder Joint, Right K Shoulder Joint, Left	0 Open 3 Percutaneous 4 Percutaneous endoscopic	0 Drainage device 3 Infusion device 4 Internal fixation device 7 Autologous tissue substitute 8 Spacer J Synthetic substitute K Nonautologous tissue substitute	Z No qualifier
C Temporomandibular Joint, Right D Temporomandibular Joint, Left E Sternoclavicular Joint, Right F Sternoclavicular Joint, Left G Acromioclavicular Joint, Right H Acromioclavicular Joint, Left J Shoulder Joint, Right K Shoulder Joint, Left	X External	0 Drainage device 3 Infusion device 4 Internal fixation device	Z No qualifier
L Elbow Joint, Right M Elbow Joint, Left N Wrist Joint, Right P Wrist Joint, Left Q Carpal Joint, Right R Carpal Joint, Left S Metacarpocarpal Joint, Right T Metacarpocarpal Joint, Left U Metacarpophalangeal Joint, Right V Metacarpophalangeal Joint, Left W Finger Phalangeal Joint, Right X Finger Phalangeal Joint, Left	0 Open 3 Percutaneous 4 Percutaneous endoscopic	0 Drainage device 3 Infusion device 4 Internal fixation device 5 External fixation device 7 Autologous tissue substitute 8 Spacer J Synthetic dubstitute K Nonautologous tissue substitute	Z No qualifier
L Elbow Joint, Right M Elbow Joint, Left N Wrist Joint, Right P Wrist Joint, Left Q Carpal Joint, Right R Carpal Joint, Left S Metacarpocarpal Joint, Right T Metacarpocarpal Joint, Left U Metacarpophalangeal Joint, Right V Metacarpophalangeal Joint, Left W Finger Phalangeal Joint, Right X Finger Phalangeal Joint, Left	X External	0 Drainage device 3 Infusion device 4 Internal fixation device 5 External fixation device	Z No qualifier

UPPER JOINTS 0 R P

OTHER REPAIRS GROUP: (Control), **Repair**
Root Operations that define other repairs.

1ST - 0 Medical and Surgical

2ND - R Upper Joints

3RD - Q REPAIR

EXAMPLE: Suture arthroplasty wrist	CMS Ex: Suture laceration

REPAIR: Restoring, to the extent possible, a body part to its normal anatomic structure and function.

EXPLANATION: Only when no other root operation applies ...

Body Part – 4TH	Approach – 5TH	Device – 6TH	Qualifier – 7TH
0 Occipital-cervical Joint 1 Cervical Vertebral Joint 3 Cervical Vertebral Disc 4 Cervicothoracic Vertebral Joint 5 Cervicothoracic Vertebral Disc 6 Thoracic Vertebral Joint 9 Thoracic Vertebral Disc A Thoracolumbar Vertebral Joint B Thoracolumbar Vertebral Disc C Temporomandibular Joint, Right D Temporomandibular Joint, Left E Sternoclavicular Joint, Right F Sternoclavicular Joint, Left G Acromioclavicular Joint, Right H Acromioclavicular Joint, Left J Shoulder Joint, Right K Shoulder Joint, Left L Elbow Joint, Right M Elbow Joint, Left N Wrist Joint, Right P Wrist Joint, Left Q Carpal Joint, Right R Carpal Joint, Left S Metacarpocarpal Joint, Right T Metacarpocarpal Joint, Left U Metacarpophalangeal Joint, Right V Metacarpophalangeal Joint, Left W Finger Phalangeal Joint, Right X Finger Phalangeal Joint, Left	0 Open 3 Percutaneous 4 Percutaneous endoscopic X External	Z No device	Z No qualifier

UPPER JOINTS 0RQ

1ST - 0 Medical and Surgical			
2ND - R Upper Joints			
3RD - R REPLACEMENT			

DEVICE GROUP: Change, Insertion, Removal, Replacement, Revision, Supplement
Root Operations that always involve a device.

EXAMPLE: Reverse total shoulder arthroplasty   **CMS Ex:** Total hip

REPLACEMENT: Putting in or on a biological or synthetic material that physically takes the place and/or function of all or a portion of a body part.

EXPLANATION: Includes taking out body part, or eradication...

Body Part – 4TH	Approach – 5TH	Device – 6TH	Qualifier – 7TH
0 Occipital-cervical Joint 1 Cervical Vertebral Joint 3 Cervical Vertebral Disc 4 Cervicothoracic Vertebral Joint 5 Cervicothoracic Vertebral Disc 6 Thoracic Vertebral Joint 9 Thoracic Vertebral Disc A Thoracolumbar Vertebral Joint B Thoracolumbar Vertebral Disc C Temporomandibular Joint, Right D Temporomandibular Joint, Left E Sternoclavicular Joint, Right F Sternoclavicular Joint, Left G Acromioclavicular Joint, Right H Acromioclavicular Joint, Left L Elbow Joint, Right M Elbow Joint, Left N Wrist Joint, Right P Wrist Joint, Left Q Carpal Joint, Right R Carpal Joint, Left S Metacarpocarpal Joint, Right T Metacarpocarpal Joint, Left U Metacarpophalangeal Joint, Right V Metacarpophalangeal Joint, Left W Finger Phalangeal Joint, Right X Finger Phalangeal Joint, Left	0 Open	7 Autologous tissue substitute J Synthetic substitute K Nonautologous tissue substitute	Z No qualifier
J Shoulder Joint, Right K Shoulder Joint, Left	0 Open	0 Synthetic substitute, reverse ball and socket 7 Autologous tissue substitute K Nonautologous tissue substitute	Z No qualifier
J Shoulder Joint, Right K Shoulder Joint, Left	0 Open	J Synthetic substitute	6 Humeral Surface 7 Glenoid Surface Z No qualifier

MOVE GROUP: (Reattachment), **Reposition,** (Transfer), (Transplantation)
Root Operations that put in/put back or move some/all of a body part.

1ST - 0 Medical and Surgical	**EXAMPLE:** Closed reduction elbow joint 　 **CMS Ex:** Fracture reduction
2ND - R Upper Joints	**REPOSITION:** Moving to its normal location, or other suitable location, all or a portion of a body part.
3RD - S REPOSITION	**EXPLANATION:** May or may not be cut to be moved ...

Body Part – 4TH	Approach – 5TH	Device – 6TH	Qualifier – 7TH
0 Occipital-cervical Joint 1 Cervical Vertebral Joint 4 Cervicothoracic Vertebral Joint 6 Thoracic Vertebral Joint A Thoracolumbar Vertebral Joint C Temporomandibular Joint, Right D Temporomandibular Joint, Left E Sternoclavicular Joint, Right F Sternoclavicular Joint, Left G Acromioclavicular Joint, Right H Acromioclavicular Joint, Left J Shoulder Joint, Right K Shoulder Joint, Left	0 Open 3 Percutaneous 4 Percutaneous endoscopic X External	4 Internal fixation device Z No device	Z No qualifier
L Elbow Joint, Right M Elbow Joint, Left N Wrist Joint, Right P Wrist Joint, Left Q Carpal Joint, Right R Carpal Joint, Left S Metacarpocarpal Joint, Right T Metacarpocarpal Joint, Left U Metacarpophalangeal Joint, Right V Metacarpophalangeal Joint, Left W Finger Phalangeal Joint, Right X Finger Phalangeal Joint, Left	0 Open 3 Percutaneous 4 Percutaneous endoscopic X External	4 Internal fixation device 5 External fixation device Z No device	Z No qualifier

EXCISION GROUP: Excision, Resection, Destruction, (Extraction), (Detachment)
Root Operations that take out some or all of a body part.

1ST - **0** Medical and Surgical

2ND - **R** Upper Joints

3RD - **T RESECTION**

EXAMPLE: Total cervical discectomy | CMS Ex: Cholecystectomy

RESECTION: Cutting out or off, without replacement, all of a body part.

EXPLANATION: None

Body Part – 4TH	Approach – 5TH	Device – 6TH	Qualifier – 7TH
3 Cervical Vertebral Disc	0 Open	Z No device	Z No qualifier
4 Cervicothoracic Vertebral Joint			
5 Cervicothoracic Vertebral Disc			
9 Thoracic Vertebral Disc			
B Thoracolumbar Vertebral Disc			
C Temporomandibular Joint, Right			
D Temporomandibular Joint, Left			
E Sternoclavicular Joint, Right			
F Sternoclavicular Joint, Left			
G Acromioclavicular Joint, Right			
H Acromioclavicular Joint, Left			
J Shoulder Joint, Right			
K Shoulder Joint, Left			
L Elbow Joint, Right			
M Elbow Joint, Left			
N Wrist Joint, Right			
P Wrist Joint, Left			
Q Carpal Joint, Right			
R Carpal Joint, Left			
S Metacarpocarpal Joint, Right			
T Metacarpocarpal Joint, Left			
U Metacarpophalangeal Joint, Right			
V Metacarpophalangeal Joint, Left			
W Finger Phalangeal Joint, Right			
X Finger Phalangeal Joint, Left			

UPPER JOINTS 0 R T

DEVICE GROUP: Change, Insertion, Removal, Replacement, Revision, Supplement
Root Operations that always involve a device.

1ST - 0 Medical and Surgical

2ND - R Upper Joints

3RD - U SUPPLEMENT

EXAMPLE: Shoulder joint resurfacing	CMS Ex: Hernia repair with mesh

SUPPLEMENT: Putting in or on biological or synthetic material that physically reinforces and/or augments the function of a portion of a body part.

EXPLANATION: Biological material from same individual ...

Body Part – 4TH	Approach – 5TH	Device – 6TH	Qualifier – 7TH
0 Occipital-cervical Joint	0 Open	7 Autologous	Z No qualifier
1 Cervical Vertebral Joint	3 Percutaneous	tissue substitute	
3 Cervical Vertebral Disc	4 Percutaneous	J Synthetic	
4 Cervicothoracic Vertebral Joint	endoscopic	substitute	
5 Cervicothoracic Vertebral Disc		K Nonautologous	
6 Thoracic Vertebral Joint		tissue substitute	
9 Thoracic Vertebral Disc			
A Thoracolumbar Vertebral Joint			
B Thoracolumbar Vertebral Disc			
C Temporomandibular Joint, Right			
D Temporomandibular Joint, Left			
E Sternoclavicular Joint, Right			
F Sternoclavicular Joint, Left			
G Acromioclavicular Joint, Right			
H Acromioclavicular Joint, Left			
J Shoulder Joint, Right			
K Shoulder Joint, Left			
L Elbow Joint, Right			
M Elbow Joint, Left			
N Wrist Joint, Right			
P Wrist Joint, Left			
Q Carpal Joint, Right			
R Carpal Joint, Left			
S Metacarpocarpal Joint, Right			
T Metacarpocarpal Joint, Left			
U Metacarpophalangeal Joint, Right			
V Metacarpophalangeal Joint, Left			
W Finger Phalangeal Joint, Right			
X Finger Phalangeal Joint, Left			

DEVICE GROUP: Change, Insertion, Removal, Replacement, Revision, Supplement
Root Operations that always involve a device.

1ST - 0 Medical and Surgical

2ND - R Upper Joints

3RD - W REVISION

EXAMPLE: Reposition joint spacer | CMS Ex: Adjustment pacemaker lead

REVISION: Correcting, to the extent possible, a portion of a malfunctioning device or the position of a displaced device.

EXPLANATION: May replace components of a device ...

Body Part – 4TH	Approach – 5TH	Device – 6TH	Qualifier – 7TH
0 Occipital-cervical Joint 1 Cervical Vertebral Joint 4 Cervicothoracic Vertebral Joint 6 Thoracic Vertebral Joint A Thoracolumbar Vertebral Joint	0 Open 3 Percutaneous 4 Percutaneous endoscopic X External	0 Drainage device 3 Infusion device 4 Internal fixation device 7 Autologous tissue substitute 8 Spacer A Interbody fusion device J Synthetic substitute K Nonautologous tissue substitute	Z No qualifier
3 Cervical Vertebral Disc 5 Cervicothoracic Vertebral Disc 9 Thoracic Vertebral Disc B Thoracolumbar Vertebral Disc	0 Open 3 Percutaneous 4 Percutaneous endoscopic X External	0 Drainage device 3 Infusion device 7 Autologous tissue substitute J Synthetic substitute K Nonautologous tissue substitute	Z No qualifier
C Temporomandibular Joint, Right D Temporomandibular Joint, Left E Sternoclavicular Joint, Right F Sternoclavicular Joint, Left G Acromioclavicular Joint, Right H Acromioclavicular Joint, Left J Shoulder Joint, Right K Shoulder Joint, Left	0 Open 3 Percutaneous 4 Percutaneous endoscopic X External	0 Drainage device 3 Infusion device 4 Internal fixation device 7 Autologous tissue substitute 8 Spacer J Synthetic substitute K Nonautologous tissue substitute	Z No qualifier
L Elbow Joint, Right M Elbow Joint, Left N Wrist Joint, Right P Wrist Joint, Left Q Carpal Joint, Right R Carpal Joint, Left S Metacarpocarpal Joint, Right T Metacarpocarpal Joint, Left U Metacarpophalangeal Joint, Right V Metacarpophalangeal Joint, Left W Finger Phalangeal Joint, Right X Finger Phalangeal Joint, Left	0 Open 3 Percutaneous 4 Percutaneous endoscopic X External	0 Drainage device 3 Infusion device 4 Internal fixation device 5 External fixation device 7 Autologous tissue substitute 8 Spacer J Synthetic substitute K Nonautologous tissue substitute	Z No qualifier

UPPER JOINTS 0 R W

NOTES

Educational Annotations | S – Lower Joints

Body System Specific Educational Annotations for the Lower Joints include:

- **Anatomy and Physiology Review**
- **Anatomical Illustrations**
- **Definitions of Common Procedures**
- **AHA Coding Clinic® Reference Notations**
- **Body Part Key Listings**
- **Device Key Listings**
- **Device Aggregation Table Listings**
- **Coding Notes**

Anatomy and Physiology Review of Lower Joints

BODY PART VALUES – S - LOWER JOINTS

Ankle Joint – The hinge joint formed between the distal tibia and fibula and the talus.

Coccygeal Joint – The joints formed between the several (3-5) very small bones that make up the coccyx.

Hip Joint – A ball-and-socket joint between the head of the femur and the acetabulum of the pelvis.

Hip Joint, Acetabular Surface – The surface of the acetabulum of the pelvis.

Hip Joint, Femoral Surface – The surface of the femoral head.

Knee Joint – The large hinge joint between the femur and the tibia.

Knee Joint, Femoral Surface – The surface of the femoral condyles.

Knee Joint, Tibial Surface – The surface of the tibial head.

Lower Joint – Any of the joints designated in the Lower Joints PCS Body System.

Lumbar Vertebral Disc – The disc-shaped fibrocartilage pad between the lumbar spine vertebral bodies comprised of a tough outer portion (annulus fibrosus) and a gel-like inner portion (nucleus pulposus).

Lumbar Vertebral Joint – The synovial and cartilaginous joints connecting the vertebra of the lumbar spine.

Lumbosacral Disc – The disc-shaped fibrocartilage pad between the S5 vertebral body of the lumbar spine and the sacrum comprised of a tough outer portion (annulus fibrosus) and a gel-like inner portion (nucleus pulposus).

Lumbosacral Joint – The synovial and cartilaginous joints connecting the S5 vertebra of the thoracic spine and the sacrum.

Metatarsal-Phalangeal Joint – Any of 5 condyloid joints in the foot that articulate the distal heads of the five metatarsal bones and the proximal phalanx of each toe.

Metatarsal-Tarsal Joint – Any of the 5 joints in the foot that articulate the tarsal bones and the proximal bases of the five metatarsal bones.

Sacrococcygeal Joint – The joint formed between the sacrum and coccyx.

Sacroiliac Joint – The strong joint joining the sacrum to the ilium bones that form the rigid pelvis.

Tarsal Joint – A complex collection of joints formed by the interconnection of the 7 tarsal bones in the foot.

Toe Phalangeal Joint – Any of 9 hinge joints in the toes between the proximal and intermediate phalanges (PIP), and the intermediate and distal phalanges (DIP). The great toe has only two phalanges and therefore only one phalangeal joint.

LOWER JOINTS 0 S

Educational Annotations | S – Lower Joints

Anatomical Illustrations of Lower Joints

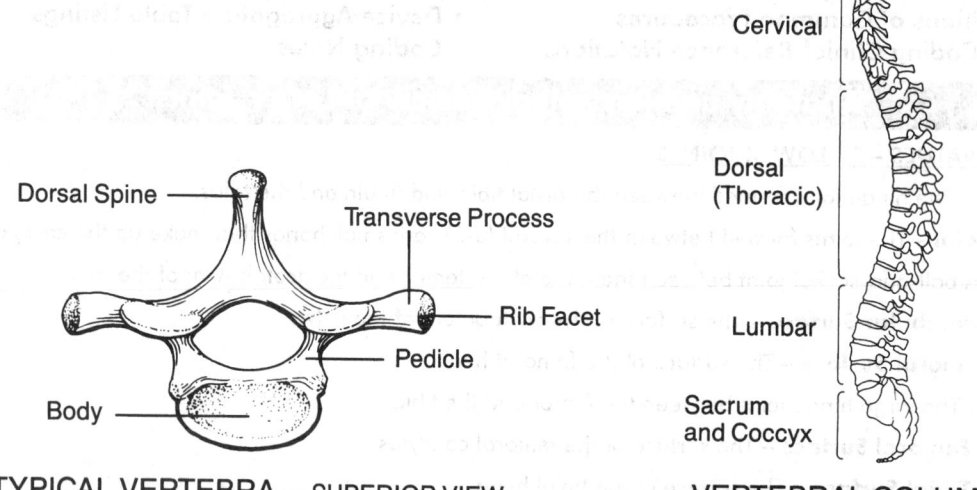

Dorsal Spine
Transverse Process
Rib Facet
Pedicle
Body

TYPICAL VERTEBRA — SUPERIOR VIEW

Cervical

Dorsal (Thoracic)

Lumbar

Sacrum and Coccyx

VERTEBRAL COLUMN

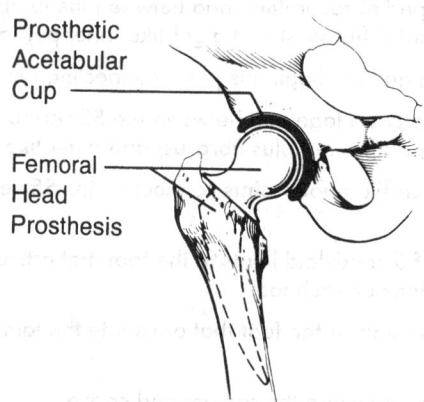

Prosthetic Acetabular Cup

Femoral Head Prosthesis

TOTAL HIP REPLACEMENT

Definitions of Common Procedures of Lower Joints

Arthroscopy – The surgical visualization and examination of a joint using an endoscope and often the approach used for joint procedures.

Discectomy – The surgical removal of all (total) or a portion of an intervertebral disc.

Interspinous process spacer – The surgical placement of a device between the spinous processes of vertebrae to relieve pressure on the spinal nerve roots.

Lumbar interbody spinal fusion – The permanent surgical joining of two or more lumbar vertebrae together using bone graft placed between the intervertebral space after the discs have been removed using metal or plastic cage to support the spine while the bone graft hardens.

Lumbar spinal fusion – The permanent surgical joining of two or more lumbar vertebrae together using a bone graft and immobilization by using plates, rods, screws, and/or wires.

Educational Annotations | S – Lower Joints

AHA Coding Clinic® Reference Notations of Lower Joints

ROOT OPERATION SPECIFIC - S - LOWER JOINTS

CHANGE - 2

DESTRUCTION - 5

DRAINAGE - 9

EXCISION - B
Discectomy with decompressive foraminotomy/laminectomy......................AHA 16:2Q:p16
Menisectomy and abrasion chondroplasty with synovectomy.....................AHA 15:1Q:p34
Spinal fusion with discectomy..AHA 14:2Q:p6

EXTIRPATION - C

FUSION - G
360-degree spinal fusion...AHA 13:3Q:p25
Ankle fusion with bone graft and internal fixation...................................AHA 13:2Q:p39
Components in fusion procedures included in Fusion root operation.........AHA 14:3Q:p30
Fusion of multiple vertebral joints ....AHA 13:1Q:p21
Lumbar spinal fusion at two levels with pelvic bone graft ....AHA 14:2Q:p6
   (see also AHA Correction Notice at 14:3Q:p36)

INSERTION - H

INSPECTION - J

RELEASE - N

REMOVAL - P
Removal of previous total knee replacement components ....AHA 15:2Q:p18
Removal of retained ankle screws...AHA 13:2Q:p39
Removal of synthetic joint components ....AHA 15:2Q:p19

REPAIR - Q
Osteoplasty and labral refixation of hip joint ....AHA 14:4Q:p25

REPLACEMENT - R
Hip replacement with acetabular reconstruction ....AHA 15:3Q:p18
Replacement of femoral surface component ....AHA 15:2Q:p19
Replacement of previous total knee replacement ....AHA 15:2Q:p18

REPOSITION - S
Periacetabular osteotomy...AHA 16:2Q:p31

RESECTION - T
Metatarsophalangeal arthroplasty ....AHA 16:1Q:p20
Resection of lower femur and knee joint...AHA 14:4Q:p29
Spinal fusion with total discectomy...AHA 14:2Q:p7

SUPPLEMENT - U
Placement of new liner...AHA 15:2Q:p19

REVISION - W

Body Part Key Listings of Lower Joints

See also Body Part Key in Appendix C

Acetabulofemoral joint ....*use* Hip Joint, Left/Right

Calcaneocuboid joint ....*use* Tarsal Joint, Left/Right

Cuboideonavicular joint..*use* Tarsal Joint, Left/Right

Cuneonavicular joint ....*use* Tarsal Joint, Left/Right

Femoropatellar joint ....*use* Knee Joint, Left/Right
....*use* Knee Joint, Femoral Surface, Left/Right

Femorotibial joint...*use* Knee Joint, Left/Right
....*use* Knee Joint, Tibial Surface, Left/Right

Continued on next page

Educational Annotations | S – Lower Joints

Body Part Key Listings of Lower Joints

Continued from previous page

Inferior tibiofibular joint	*use* Ankle Joint, Left/Right
Intercuneiform joint	*use* Tarsal Joint, Left/Right
Interphalangeal (IP) joint	*use* Toe Phalangeal Joint, Left/Right
Lateral meniscus	*use* Knee Joint, Left/Right
Lumbar facet joint	*use* Lumbar Vertebral Joint
Lumbosacral facet joint	*use* Lumbosacral Joint
Medial meniscus	*use* Knee Joint, Left/Right
Metatarsophalangeal (MTP) joint	*use* Metatarsal-Phalangeal Joint, Left/Right
Patellofemoral joint	*use* Knee Joint, Left/Right
	use Knee Joint, Femoral Surface, Left/Right
Sacrococcygeal symphysis	*use* Sacrococcygeal Joint
Subtalar (talocalcaneal) joint	*use* Tarsal Joint, Left/Right
Talocalcaneal (subtalar) joint	*use* Tarsal Joint, Left/Right
Talocalcaneonavicular joint	*use* Tarsal Joint, Left/Right
Talocrural joint	*use* Ankle Joint, Left/Right
Tarsometatarsal joint	*use* Metatarsal-Tarsal Joint, Left/Right
Tibiofemoral joint	*use* Knee Joint, Left/Right
	use Knee Joint, Tibial Surface, Left/Right

Device Key Listings of Lower Joints

See also Device Key in Appendix D

Acetabular cup	*use* Liner in Lower Joints
Autograft	*use* Autologous Tissue Substitute
Axial Lumbar Interbody Fusion System	*use* Interbody Fusion Device in Lower Joints
AxiaLIF® System	*use* Interbody Fusion Device in Lower Joints
Ceramic on ceramic bearing surface	*use* Synthetic Substitute, Ceramic for Replacement in Lower Joints
Cobalt/chromium head and polyethylene socket	*use* Synthetic Substitute, Metal on Polyethylene for Replacement in Lower Joints
Cobalt/chromium head and socket	*use* Synthetic Substitute, Ceramic for Replacement in Lower Joints
CONSERVE® PLUS Total Resurfacing Hip System	*use* Resurfacing Device in Lower Joints
Cormet Hip Resurfacing System	*use* Resurfacing Device in Lower Joints
CoRoent® XL	*use* Interbody Fusion Device in Lower Joints
Direct Lateral Interbody Fusion (DLIF) device	*use* Interbody Fusion Device in Lower Joints
Dynesys® Dynamic Stabilization System	*use* Spinal Stabilization Device, Pedicle-Based for Insertion in Upper Joints, Lower Joints
External fixator	*use* External Fixation Device in Head and Facial Bones, Upper Bones, Lower Bones, Upper Joints, Lower Joints
EXtreme Lateral Interbody Fusion (XLIF) device	*use* Interbody Fusion Device in Lower Joints
Facet replacement spinal stabilization device	*use* Spinal Stabilization Device, Facet Replacement for Insertion in Upper Joints, Lower Joints
Fusion screw (compression) (lag) (locking)	*use* Internal Fixation Device in Upper Joints, Lower Joints
Hip (joint) liner	*use* Liner in Lower Joints
Interbody fusion (spine) cage	*use* Interbody Fusion Device in Upper Joints, Lower Joints
Interspinous process spinal stabilization device	*use* Spinal Stabilization Device, Interspinous Process for Insertion in Upper Joints, Lower Joints
Joint fixation plate	*use* Internal Fixation Device in Upper Joints, Lower Joints
Joint liner (insert)	*use* Liner in Lower Joints
Joint spacer (antibiotic)	*use* Spacer in Upper Joints, Lower Joints

Continued on next page

Educational Annotations | S – Lower Joints

Device Key Listings of Lower Joints

Continued from previous page

Kirschner wire (K-wire)	*use* Internal Fixation Device in Head and Facial Bones, Upper Bones, Lower Bones, Upper Joints, Lower Joints
Knee (implant) insert	*use* Liner in Lower Joints
Metal on metal bearing surface	*use* Synthetic Substitute, Metal for Replacement in Lower Joints
Novation® Ceramic AHS® (Articulation Hip System)	*use* Synthetic Substitute, Ceramic for Replacement in Lower Joints
Oxidized zirconium ceramic hip bearing surface	*use* Synthetic Substitute, Ceramic on Polyethylene for Replacement in Lower Joints
Pedicle-based dynamic stabilization device	*use* Spinal Stabilization Device, Pedicle-Based for Insertion in Upper Joints, Lower Joints
Polyethylene socket	*use* Synthetic Substitute, Polyethylene for Replacement in Lower Joints
Polymethylmethacrylate (PMMA)	*use* Synthetic Substitute
Prodisc-L	*use* Synthetic Substitute
Tibial insert	*use* Liner in Lower Joints
Tissue bank graft	*use* Nonautologous Tissue Substitute
X-STOP® Spacer	*use* Spinal Stabilization Device, Interspinous Process for Insertion in Upper Joints, Lower Joints
XLIF® System	*use* Interbody Fusion Device in Lower Joints
Zimmer® NexGen® LPS Mobile Bearing Knee	*use* Synthetic Substitute
Zimmer® NexGen® LPS-Flex Mobile Knee	*use* Synthetic Substitute

Device Aggregation Table Listings of Lower Joints

See also Device Aggregation Table in Appendix E

Specific Device	For Operation	In Body System		General Device
Spinal Stabilization Device, Facet Replacement	Insertion	Lower Joints	4	Internal Fixation Device
Spinal Stabilization Device, Interspinous Process	Insertion	Lower Joints	4	Internal Fixation Device
Spinal Stabilization Device, Pedicle-Based	Insertion	Lower Joints	4	Internal Fixation Device
Synthetic Substitute, Ceramic	Replacement	Lower Joints	J	Synthetic Substitute
Synthetic Substitute, Ceramic on Polyethylene	Replacement	Lower Joints	J	Synthetic Substitute
Synthetic Substitute, Metal	Replacement	Lower Joints	J	Synthetic Substitute
Synthetic Substitute, Metal on Polyethylene	Replacement	Lower Joints	J	Synthetic Substitute
Synthetic Substitute, Polyethylene	Replacement	Lower Joints	J	Synthetic Substitute
Synthetic Substitute, Unicondylar	Replacement	Lower Joints	J	Synthetic Substitute

Coding Notes of Lower Joints

Body System Relevant Coding Guidelines

Fusion procedures of the spine

B3.10a

The body part coded for a spinal vertebral joint(s) rendered immobile by a spinal fusion procedure is classified by the level of the spine (e.g. thoracic). There are distinct body part values for a single vertebral joint and for multiple vertebral joints at each spinal level.

Example: Body part values specify Lumbar Vertebral Joint, Lumbar Vertebral Joints, 2 or More and Lumbosacral Vertebral Joint.

B3.10b

If multiple vertebral joints are fused, a separate procedure is coded for each vertebral joint that uses a different device and/or qualifier.

Example: Fusion of lumbar vertebral joint, posterior approach, anterior column and fusion of lumbar vertebral joint, posterior approach, posterior column are coded separately.

Continued on next page

Educational Annotations | S – Lower Joints

Coding Notes of Lower Joints

Body System Relevant Coding Guidelines

Continued from previous page

B3.10c

Combinations of devices and materials are often used on a vertebral joint to render the joint immobile. When combinations of devices are used on the same vertebral joint, the device value coded for the procedure is as follows:

- If an interbody fusion device is used to render the joint immobile (alone or containing other material like bone graft), the procedure is coded with the device value Interbody Fusion Device
- If bone graft is the only device used to render the joint immobile, the procedure is coded with the device value Nonautologous Tissue Substitute or Autologous Tissue Substitute
- If a mixture of autologous and nonautologous bone graft (with or without biological or synthetic extenders or binders) is used to render the joint immobile, code the procedure with the device value Autologous Tissue Substitute

Examples: Fusion of a vertebral joint using a cage style interbody fusion device containing morsellized bone graft is coded to the device Interbody Fusion Device.

Fusion of a vertebral joint using a bone dowel interbody fusion device made of cadaver bone and packed with a mixture of local morsellized bone and demineralized bone matrix is coded to the device Interbody Fusion Device.

Fusion of a vertebral joint using both autologous bone graft and bone bank bone graft is coded to the device Autologous Tissue Substitute.

Tendons, ligaments, bursae and fascia near a joint

B4.5

Procedures performed on tendons, ligaments, bursae and fascia supporting a joint are coded to the body part in the respective body system that is the focus of the procedure. Procedures performed on joint structures themselves are coded to the body part in the joint body systems.

Examples: Repair of the anterior cruciate ligament of the knee is coded to the knee bursa and ligament body part in the bursae and ligaments body system.

Knee arthroscopy with shaving of articular cartilage is coded to the knee joint body part in the Lower Joints body system.

Body System Specific PCS Reference Manual Exercises

PCS CODE	S – LOWER JOINTS EXERCISES
0 S 2 Y X 0 Z	Exchange of drainage tube from right hip joint.
0 S 9 C 0 0 Z	Right knee arthrotomy with drain placement.
0 S G 1 0 A J	Posterior spinal fusion at L1-L3 level with BAK cage interbody fusion device, open.
0 S G 5 0 7 Z	Sacrococcygeal fusion with bone graft from same operative site, open.
0 S G Q 3 4 Z	Interphalangeal fusion of left great toe, percutaneous pin fixation.
0 S J D 0 Z Z	Exploratory arthrotomy of left knee.
0 S R B 0 3 A	Total left hip replacement using ceramic on ceramic prosthesis, without bone cement.
0 S R C 0 J Z	Total right knee arthroplasty with insertion of total knee prosthesis.
0 S U R 0 B Z	Resurfacing procedure on right femoral head, open approach.
0 S U S 0 9 Z	Exchange of liner in femoral component of previous left hip replacement, open approach. (Taking out the old liner is coded separately to the root operation Removal.)
0 S W 9 0 J Z	Open revision of right hip replacement, with recementing of the prosthesis.

DEVICE GROUP: Change, Insertion, Removal, Replacement, Revision, Supplement
Root Operations that always involve a device.

1ST - **0** Medical and Surgical

2ND - **S** Lower Joints

3RD - **2 CHANGE**

EXAMPLE: Exchange drain tube	CMS Ex: Changing urinary catheter

CHANGE: Taking out or off a device from a body part and putting back an identical or similar device in or on the same body part without cutting or puncturing the skin or a mucous membrane.

EXPLANATION: ALL Changes use EXTERNAL approach only ...

Body Part – 4TH	Approach – 5TH	Device – 6TH	Qualifier – 7TH
Y Lower Joint	X External	0 Drainage device Y Other device	Z No qualifier

EXCISION GROUP: Excision, Resection, Destruction, (Extraction), (Detachment)
Root Operations that take out some or all of a body part.

1ST - **0** Medical and Surgical

2ND - **S** Lower Joints

3RD - **5 DESTRUCTION**

EXAMPLE: Radiofrequency ablation	CMS Ex: Fulguration polyp

DESTRUCTION: Physical eradication of all or a portion of a body part by the direct use of energy, force, or a destructive agent.

EXPLANATION: None of the body part is physically taken out

Body Part – 4TH	Approach – 5TH	Device – 6TH	Qualifier – 7TH
0 Lumbar Vertebral Joints 2 Lumbar Vertebral Disc 3 Lumbosacral Joint 4 Lumbosacral Disc 5 Sacrococcygeal Joint 6 Coccygeal Joint 7 Sacroiliac Joint, Right 8 Sacroiliac Joint, Left 9 Hip Joint, Right B Hip Joint, Left C Knee Joint, Right D Knee Joint, Left F Ankle Joint, Right G Ankle Joint, Left H Tarsal Joint, Right J Tarsal Joint, Left K Metatarsal-Tarsal Joint, Right L Metatarsal-Tarsal Joint, Left M Metatarsal-Phalangeal Joint, Right N Metatarsal-Phalangeal Joint, Left P Toe Phalangeal Joint, Right Q Toe Phalangeal Joint, Left	0 Open 3 Percutaneous 4 Percutaneous endoscopic	Z No device	Z No qualifier

LOWER JOINTS 0 S 5

DRAINAGE GROUP: Drainage, Extirpation, (Fragmentation)
Root Operations that take out solids/fluids/gases from a body part.

1ST - 0 Medical and Surgical	EXAMPLE: Aspiration knee joint	CMS Ex: Thoracentesis
2ND - S Lower Joints	**DRAINAGE:** Taking or letting out fluids and/or gases from a body part.	
3RD - 9 DRAINAGE	EXPLANATION: Qualifier "X Diagnostic" indicates biopsy ...	

Body Part – 4TH		Approach – 5TH	Device – 6TH	Qualifier – 7TH
0 Lumbar Vertebral Joint 2 Lumbar Vertebral Disc 3 Lumbosacral Joint 4 Lumbosacral Disc 5 Sacrococcygeal Joint 6 Coccygeal Joint 7 Sacroiliac Joint, Right 8 Sacroiliac Joint, Left 9 Hip Joint, Right B Hip Joint, Left C Knee Joint, Right D Knee Joint, Left F Ankle Joint, Right G Ankle Joint, Left	H Tarsal Joint, Right J Tarsal Joint, Left K Metatarsal-Tarsal Joint, Right L Metatarsal-Tarsal Joint, Left M Metatarsal-Phalangeal Joint, Right N Metatarsal-Phalangeal Joint, Left P Toe Phalangeal Joint, Right Q Toe Phalangeal Joint, Left	0 Open 3 Percutaneous 4 Percutaneous endoscopic	0 Drainage device	Z No qualifier
0 Lumbar Vertebral Joint 2 Lumbar Vertebral Disc 3 Lumbosacral Joint 4 Lumbosacral Disc 5 Sacrococcygeal Joint 6 Coccygeal Joint 7 Sacroiliac Joint, Right 8 Sacroiliac Joint, Left 9 Hip Joint, Right B Hip Joint, Left C Knee Joint, Right D Knee Joint, Left F Ankle Joint, Right G Ankle Joint, Left	H Tarsal Joint, Right J Tarsal Joint, Left K Metatarsal-Tarsal Joint, Right L Metatarsal-Tarsal Joint, Left M Metatarsal-Phalangeal Joint, Right N Metatarsal-Phalangeal Joint, Left P Toe Phalangeal Joint, Right Q Toe Phalangeal Joint, Left	0 Open 3 Percutaneous 4 Percutaneous endoscopic	Z No device	X Diagnostic Z No qualifier

---

EXCISION GROUP: Excision, Resection, Destruction, (Extraction), (Detachment)
Root Operations that take out some or all of a body part.

1ST - **O** Medical and Surgical	EXAMPLE: Partial medial meniscectomy	CMS Ex: Liver biopsy

2ND - **S** Lower Joints

3RD - **B EXCISION**

EXCISION: Cutting out or off, without replacement, a portion of a body part.

EXPLANATION: Qualifier "X Diagnostic" indicates biopsy ...

Body Part – 4TH		Approach – 5TH	Device – 6TH	Qualifier – 7TH
0 Lumbar Vertebral Joint 2 Lumbar Vertebral Disc 3 Lumbosacral Joint 4 Lumbosacral Disc 5 Sacrococcygeal Joint 6 Coccygeal Joint 7 Sacroiliac Joint, Right 8 Sacroiliac Joint, Left 9 Hip Joint, Right B Hip Joint, Left C Knee Joint, Right D Knee Joint, Left F Ankle Joint, Right G Ankle Joint, Left	H Tarsal Joint, Right J Tarsal Joint, Left K Metatarsal-Tarsal Joint, Right L Metatarsal-Tarsal Joint, Left M Metatarsal-Phalangeal Joint, Right N Metatarsal-Phalangeal Joint, Left P Toe Phalangeal Joint, Right Q Toe Phalangeal Joint, Left	0 Open 3 Percutaneous 4 Percutaneous endoscopic	Z No device	X Diagnostic Z No qualifier

---

DRAINAGE GROUP: Drainage, Extirpation, (Fragmentation)
Root Operations that take out solids/fluids/gases from a body part.

1ST - **O** Medical and Surgical	EXAMPLE: Removal loose bodies knee	CMS Ex: Choledocholithotomy

2ND - **S** Lower Joints

3RD - **C EXTIRPATION**

EXTIRPATION: Taking or cutting out solid matter from a body part.

EXPLANATION: Abnormal byproduct or foreign body ...

Body Part – 4TH		Approach – 5TH	Device – 6TH	Qualifier – 7TH
0 Lumbar Vertebral Joint 2 Lumbar Vertebral Disc 3 Lumbosacral Joint 4 Lumbosacral Disc 5 Sacrococcygeal Joint 6 Coccygeal Joint 7 Sacroiliac Joint, Right 8 Sacroiliac Joint, Left 9 Hip Joint, Right B Hip Joint, Left C Knee Joint, Right D Knee Joint, Left F Ankle Joint, Right G Ankle Joint, Left	H Tarsal Joint, Right J Tarsal Joint, Left K Metatarsal-Tarsal Joint, Right L Metatarsal-Tarsal Joint, Left M Metatarsal-Phalangeal Joint, Right N Metatarsal-Phalangeal Joint, Left P Toe Phalangeal Joint, Right Q Toe Phalangeal Joint, Left	0 Open 3 Percutaneous 4 Percutaneous endoscopic	Z No device	Z No qualifier

OTHER OBJECTIVES GROUP: (Alteration), (Creation), **Fusion**
Root Operations that define other objectives.

1ST - 0	Medical and Surgical
2ND - S	Lower Joints
3RD - G	FUSION

EXAMPLE: Lumbosacral spinal fusion

CMS Ex: Spinal fusion

FUSION: Joining together portions of an articular body part, rendering the articular body part immobile.

EXPLANATION: Use of fixation device, graft, or other means ...

Body Part – 4TH	Approach – 5TH	Device – 6TH	Qualifier – 7TH
0 Lumbar Vertebral Joint 1 Lumbar Vertebral Joints, 2 or more 3 Lumbosacral Joint	0 Open 3 Percutaneous 4 Percutaneous endoscopic	7 Autologous tissue substitute A Interbody fusion device J Synthetic substitute K Nonautologous tissue substitute Z No Device	0 Anterior approach, anterior column 1 Posterior approach, posterior column J Posterior approach, anterior column
5 Sacrococcygeal Joint 6 Coccygeal Joint 7 Sacroiliac Joint, Right 8 Sacroiliac Joint, Left	0 Open 3 Percutaneous 4 Percutaneous endoscopic	4 Internal fixation device 7 Autologous tissue substitute J Synthetic substitute K Nonautologous tissue substitute Z No device	Z No qualifier
9 Hip Joint, Right B Hip Joint, Left C Knee Joint, Right D Knee Joint, Left F Ankle Joint, Right G Ankle Joint, Left H Tarsal Joint, Right J Tarsal Joint, Left K Metatarsal-Tarsal Joint, Right L Metatarsal-Tarsal Joint, Left M Metatarsal-Phalangeal Joint, Right N Metatarsal-Phalangeal Joint, Left P Toe Phalangeal Joint, Right Q Toe Phalangeal Joint, Left	0 Open 3 Percutaneous 4 Percutaneous endoscopic	4 Internal fixation device 5 External fixation device 7 Autologous tissue substitute J Synthetic substitute K Nonautologous tissue substitute Z No device	Z No qualifier

LOWER JOINTS 0 S G

DEVICE GROUP: Change, Insertion, Removal, Replacement, Revision, Supplement
Root Operations that always involve a device.

1ST - **0** Medical and Surgical	EXAMPLE: Implantation joint spacer	CMS Ex: Central venous catheter

2ND - S Lower Joints

3RD - H INSERTION

INSERTION: Putting in a nonbiological appliance that monitors, assists, performs, or prevents a physiological function but does not physically take the place of a body part.

EXPLANATION: None

Body Part – 4TH	Approach – 5TH	Device – 6TH	Qualifier – 7TH
0 Lumbar Vertebral Joint 3 Lumbosacral Joint	0 Open 3 Percutaneous 4 Percutaneous endoscopic	3 Infusion device 4 Internal fixation device 8 Spacer B Spinal stabilization device, interspinous process C Spinal stabilization device, pedicle-based D Spinal stabilization device, facet replacement	Z No qualifier
2 Lumbar Vertebral Disc 4 Lumbosacral Disc	0 Open 3 Percutaneous 4 Percutaneous endoscopic	3 Infusion device 8 Spacer	Z No qualifier
5 Sacrococcygeal Joint 6 Coccygeal Joint 7 Sacroiliac Joint, Right 8 Sacroiliac Joint, Left	0 Open 3 Percutaneous 4 Percutaneous endoscopic	3 Infusion device 4 Internal fixation device 8 Spacer	Z No qualifier
9 Hip Joint, Right B Hip Joint, Left C Knee Joint, Right D Knee Joint, Left F Ankle Joint, Right G Ankle Joint, Left H Tarsal Joint, Right J Tarsal Joint, Left K Metatarsal-Tarsal Joint, Right L Metatarsal-Tarsal Joint, Left M Metatarsal-Phalangeal Joint, Right N Metatarsal-Phalangeal Joint, Left P Toe Phalangeal Joint, Right Q Toe Phalangeal Joint, Left	0 Open 3 Percutaneous 4 Percutaneous endoscopic	3 Infusion device 4 Internal fixation device 5 External fixation device 8 Spacer	Z No qualifier

LOWER JOINTS

0 S H

EXAMINATION GROUP: Inspection, (Map)
Root Operations involving examination only.

1ST – 0 Medical and Surgical	EXAMPLE: Diagnostic arthroscopy knee	CMS Ex: Colonoscopy
2ND – S Lower Joints	**INSPECTION:** Visually and/or manually exploring a body part.	
3RD – J INSPECTION	EXPLANATION: Direct or instrumental visualization ...	

Body Part – 4TH		Approach – 5TH	Device – 6TH	Qualifier – 7TH
0 Lumbar Vertebral Joint	H Tarsal Joint, Right	0 Open	Z No device	Z No qualifier
2 Lumbar Vertebral Disc	J Tarsal Joint, Left	3 Percutaneous		
3 Lumbosacral Joint	K Metatarsal-Tarsal Joint, Right	4 Percutaneous endoscopic		
4 Lumbosacral Disc	L Metatarsal-Tarsal Joint, Left	X External		
5 Sacrococcygeal Joint				
6 Coccygeal Joint	M Metatarsal-Phalangeal Joint, Right			
7 Sacroiliac Joint, Right				
8 Sacroiliac Joint, Left	N Metatarsal-Phalangeal Joint, Left			
9 Hip Joint, Right				
B Hip Joint, Left	P Toe Phalangeal Joint, Right			
C Knee Joint, Right				
D Knee Joint, Left	Q Toe Phalangeal Joint, Left			
F Ankle Joint, Right				
G Ankle Joint, Left				

DIVISION GROUP: (Division), Release
Root Operations involving cutting or separation only.

1ST – 0 Medical and Surgical	EXAMPLE: Manual rupture joint adhesions	CMS Ex: Carpal tunnel release
2ND – S Lower Joints	**RELEASE:** Freeing a body part from an abnormal physical constraint by cutting or by the use of force.	
3RD – N RELEASE	EXPLANATION: None of the body part is taken out ...	

Body Part – 4TH		Approach – 5TH	Device – 6TH	Qualifier – 7TH
0 Lumbar Vertebral Joint	H Tarsal Joint, Right	0 Open	Z No device	Z No qualifier
2 Lumbar Vertebral Disc	J Tarsal Joint, Left	3 Percutaneous		
3 Lumbosacral Joint	K Metatarsal-Tarsal Joint, Right	4 Percutaneous endoscopic		
4 Lumbosacral Disc	L Metatarsal-Tarsal Joint, Left	X External		
5 Sacrococcygeal Joint				
6 Coccygeal Joint	M Metatarsal-Phalangeal Joint, Right			
7 Sacroiliac Joint, Right				
8 Sacroiliac Joint, Left	N Metatarsal-Phalangeal Joint, Left			
9 Hip Joint, Right				
B Hip Joint, Left	P Toe Phalangeal Joint, Right			
C Knee Joint, Right				
D Knee Joint, Left	Q Toe Phalangeal Joint, Left			
F Ankle Joint, Right				
G Ankle Joint, Left				

DEVICE GROUP: Change, Insertion, Removal, Replacement, Revision, Supplement
Root Operations that always involve a device.

1ST - 0 Medical and Surgical	**EXAMPLE:** Removal fixation device **CMS Ex:** Chest tube removal
2ND - S Lower Joints	**REMOVAL:** Taking out or off a device from a body part.
3RD - P REMOVAL	**EXPLANATION:** Removal device without reinsertion ...

Body Part – 4TH	Approach – 5TH	Device – 6TH	Qualifier – 7TH
0 Lumbar Vertebral Joint 3 Lumbosacral Joint	0 Open 3 Percutaneous 4 Percutaneous endoscopic	0 Drainage device 3 Infusion device 4 Internal fixation device 7 Autologous tissue substitute 8 Spacer A Interbody fusion device J Synthetic substitute K Nonautologous tissue substitute	Z No qualifier
0 Lumbar Vertebral Joint 3 Lumbosacral Joint	X External	0 Drainage device 3 Infusion device 4 Internal fixation device	Z No qualifier
2 Lumbar Vertebral Disc 4 Lumbosacral Disc	0 Open 3 Percutaneous 4 Percutaneous endoscopic	0 Drainage device 3 Infusion device 7 Autologous tissue substitute J Synthetic substitute K Nonautologous tissue substitute	Z No qualifier
2 Lumbar Vertebral Disc 4 Lumbosacral Disc	X External	0 Drainage device 3 Infusion device	Z No qualifier
5 Sacrococcygeal Joint 6 Coccygeal Joint 7 Sacroiliac Joint, Right 8 Sacroiliac Joint, Left	0 Open 3 Percutaneous 4 Percutaneous endoscopic	0 Drainage device 3 Infusion device 4 Internal fixation device 7 Autologous tissue substitute 8 Spacer J Synthetic substitute K Nonautologous tissue substitute	Z No qualifier
5 Sacrococcygeal Joint 6 Coccygeal Joint 7 Sacroiliac Joint, Right 8 Sacroiliac Joint, Left	X External	0 Drainage device 3 Infusion device 4 Internal fixation device	Z No qualifier

LOWER JOINTS

0 S P

continued ⇨

0   S   P   REMOVAL – *continued*

Body Part – 4TH	Approach – 5TH	Device – 6TH	Qualifier – 7TH
9 Hip Joint, Right B Hip Joint, Left	0 Open	0 Drainage device 3 Infusion device 4 Internal fixation device 5 External fixation device 7 Autologous tissue substitute 8 Spacer 9 Liner B Resurfacing device J Synthetic substitute K Nonautologous tissue substitute	Z No qualifier
9 Hip Joint, Right B Hip Joint, Left	3 Percutaneous 4 Percutaneous endoscopic	0 Drainage device 3 Infusion device 4 Internal fixation device 5 External fixation device 7 Autologous tissue substitute 8 Spacer J Synthetic substitute K Nonautologous tissue substitute	Z No qualifier
9 Hip Joint, Right B Hip Joint, Left	X External	0 Drainage device 3 Infusion device 4 Internal fixation device 5 External fixation device	Z No qualifier
A Hip Joint, Acetabular Surface, Right E Hip Joint, Acetabular Surface, Left R Hip Joint, Femoral Surface, Right S Hip Joint, Femoral Surface, Left T Knee Joint, Femoral Surface, Right U Knee Joint, Femoral Surface, Left V Knee Joint, Tibial Surface, Right W Knee Joint, Tibial Surface, Left	0 Open 3 Percutaneous 4 Percutaneous endoscopic	J Synthetic substitute	Z No qualifier

c o n t i n u e d ⇨

0 S P REMOVAL – continued

Body Part – 4TH	Approach – 5TH	Device – 6TH	Qualifier – 7TH
C Knee Joint, Right D Knee Joint, Left	0 Open	0 Drainage device 3 Infusion device 4 Internal fixation device 5 External fixation device 7 Autologous tissue substitute 8 Spacer 9 Liner K Nonautologous tissue substitute	Z No qualifier
C Knee Joint, Right D Knee Joint, Left	0 Open	J Synthetic substitute	C Patellar surface Z No qualifier
C Knee Joint, Right D Knee Joint, Left	3 Percutaneous 4 Percutaneous endoscopic	0 Drainage device 3 Infusion device 4 Internal fixation device 5 External fixation device 7 Autologous tissue substitute 8 Spacer K Nonautologous tissue substitute	Z No qualifier
C Knee Joint, Right D Knee Joint, Left	3 Percutaneous 4 Percutaneous endoscopic	J Synthetic Substitute	C Patellar surface Z No qualifier
C Knee Joint, Right D Knee Joint, Left	X External	0 Drainage device 3 Infusion device 4 Internal fixation device 5 External fixation device	Z No qualifier
F Ankle Joint, Right G Ankle Joint, Left H Tarsal Joint, Right J Tarsal Joint, Left K Metatarsal-Tarsal Joint, Right L Metatarsal-Tarsal Joint, Left M Metatarsal-Phalangeal Joint, Right N Metatarsal-Phalangeal Joint, Left P Toe Phalangeal Joint, Right Q Toe Phalangeal Joint, Left	0 Open 3 Percutaneous 4 Percutaneous endoscopic	0 Drainage device 3 Infusion device 4 Internal fixation device 5 External fixation device 7 Autologous tissue substitute 8 Spacer J Synthetic substitute K Nonautologous tissue substitute	Z No qualifier
F Ankle Joint, Right G Ankle Joint, Left H Tarsal Joint, Right J Tarsal Joint, Left K Metatarsal-Tarsal Joint, Right L Metatarsal-Tarsal Joint, Left M Metatarsal-Phalangeal Joint, Right N Metatarsal-Phalangeal Joint, Left P Toe Phalangeal Joint, Right Q Toe Phalangeal Joint, Left	X External	0 Drainage device 3 Infusion device 4 Internal fixation device 5 External fixation device	Z No qualifier

LOWER JOINTS

0 S P

OTHER REPAIRS GROUP: (Control), **Repair**
Root Operations that define other repairs.

1ST - **0** Medical and Surgical	**EXAMPLE:** Suture arthroplasty ankle **CMS Ex:** Suture laceration
2ND - **S** Lower Joints	**REPAIR:** Restoring, to the extent possible, a body part to its normal anatomic structure and function.
3RD - **Q REPAIR**	**EXPLANATION:** Only when no other root operation applies ...

Body Part – 4TH		Approach – 5TH	Device – 6TH	Qualifier – 7TH
0 Lumbar Vertebral Joint	H Tarsal Joint, Right	0 Open	Z No device	Z No qualifier
2 Lumbar Vertebral Disc	J Tarsal Joint, Left	3 Percutaneous		
3 Lumbosacral Joint	K Metatarsal-Tarsal Joint, Right	4 Percutaneous endoscopic		
4 Lumbosacral Disc	L Metatarsal-Tarsal Joint, Left	X External		
5 Sacrococcygeal Joint	M Metatarsal-Phalangeal Joint, Right			
6 Coccygeal Joint				
7 Sacroiliac Joint, Right	N Metatarsal-Phalangeal Joint, Left			
8 Sacroiliac Joint, Left				
9 Hip Joint, Right	P Toe Phalangeal Joint, Right			
B Hip Joint, Left				
C Knee Joint, Right	Q Toe Phalangeal Joint, Left			
D Knee Joint, Left				
F Ankle Joint, Right				
G Ankle Joint, Left				

LOWER JOINTS   0 S Q

DEVICE GROUP: Change, Insertion, Removal, Replacement, Revision, Supplement			
Root Operations that always involve a device.			

1ST - 0 Medical and Surgical

2ND - S Lower Joints

3RD - R REPLACEMENT

EXAMPLE: Total knee replacement — CMS Ex: Total hip

REPLACEMENT: Putting in or on a biological or synthetic material that physically takes the place and/or function of all or a portion of a body part.

EXPLANATION: Includes taking out body part, or eradication...

Body Part – 4TH	Approach – 5TH	Device – 6TH	Qualifier – 7TH
0 Lumbar Vertebral Joint 2 Lumbar Vertebral Disc NC* 3 Lumbosacral Joint 4 Lumbosacral Disc NC* 5 Sacrococcygeal Joint 6 Coccygeal Joint 7 Sacroiliac Joint, Right 8 Sacroiliac Joint, Left H Tarsal Joint, Right J Tarsal Joint, Left K Metatarsal-Tarsal Joint, Right L Metatarsal-Tarsal Joint, Left M Metatarsal-Phalangeal Joint, Right N Metatarsal-Phalangeal Joint, Left P Toe Phalangeal Joint, Right Q Toe Phalangeal Joint, Left	0 Open	7 Autologous tissue substitute J Synthetic substitute K Nonautologous tissue substitute	Z No qualifier
9 Hip Joint, Right B Hip Joint, Left	0 Open	1 Synthetic substitute, metal 2 Synthetic substitute, metal on polyethylene 3 Synthetic substitute, ceramic 4 Synthetic substitute, ceramic on polyethylene J Synthetic substitute	9 Cemented A Uncemented Z No qualifier
9 Hip Joint, Right B Hip Joint, Left	0 Open	7 Autologous tissue substitute K Nonautologous tissue substitute	Z No qualifier

NC* – Some procedures are considered non-covered by Medicare. See current Medicare Code Editor (patient over 60 years with Synthetic substitute) for details.

continued ⇨

0 S R REPLACEMENT – *continued*

LOWER JOINTS   **0 S R**

Body Part – 4TH	Approach – 5TH	Device – 6TH	Qualifier – 7TH
A Hip Joint, Acetabular Surface, Right E Hip Joint, Acetabular Surface, Left	0 Open	0 Synthetic substitute, polyethylene 1 Synthetic substitute, metal 3 Synthetic substitute, ceramic J Synthetic substitute	9 Cemented A Uncemented Z No qualifier
A Hip Joint, Acetabular Surface, Right E Hip Joint, Acetabular Surface, Left	0 Open	7 Autologous tissue substitute K Nonautologous tissue substitute	Z No qualifier
C Knee Joint, Right D Knee Joint, Left	0 Open	7 Autologous tissue substitute K Nonautologous tissue substitute	Z No qualifier
C Knee Joint, Right D Knee Joint, Left	0 Open	J Synthetic substitute L Synthetic substitute, unicondylar	9 Cemented A Uncemented Z No qualifier
F Ankle Joint, Right G Ankle Joint, Left T Knee Joint, Femoral Surface, Right U Knee Joint, Femoral Surface, Left V Knee Joint, Tibial Surface, Right W Knee Joint, Tibial Surface, Left	0 Open	7 Autologous tissue substitute K Nonautologous tissue substitute	Z No qualifier
F Ankle Joint, Right G Ankle Joint, Left T Knee Joint, Femoral Surface, Right U Knee Joint, Femoral Surface, Left V Knee Joint, Tibial Surface, Right W Knee Joint, Tibial Surface, Left	0 Open	J Synthetic substitute	9 Cemented A Uncemented Z No qualifier
R Hip Joint, Femoral Surface, Right S Hip Joint, Femoral Surface, Left	0 Open	1 Synthetic substitute, metal 3 Synthetic substitute, ceramic J Synthetic substitute	9 Cemented A Uncemented Z No qualifier
R Hip Joint, Femoral Surface, Right S Hip Joint, Femoral Surface, Left	0 Open	7 Autologous tissue substitute K Nonautologous tissue substitute	Z No qualifier

MOVE GROUP: (Reattachment), Reposition, (Transfer), (Transplantation)
Root Operations that put in/put back or move some/all of a body part.

1ST - 0 Medical and Surgical 2ND - S Lower Joints 3RD - S REPOSITION	EXAMPLE: Closed reduction hip joint	CMS Ex: Fracture reduction
	REPOSITION: Moving to its normal location, or other suitable location, all or a portion of a body part.	
	EXPLANATION: May or may not be cut to be moved ...	

Body Part – 4TH	Approach – 5TH	Device – 6TH	Qualifier – 7TH
0 Lumbar Vertebral Joint 3 Lumbosacral Joint 5 Sacrococcygeal Joint 6 Coccygeal Joint 7 Sacroiliac Joint, Right 8 Sacroiliac Joint, Left	0 Open 3 Percutaneous 4 Percutaneous endoscopic X External	4 Internal fixation device Z No device	Z No qualifier
9 Hip Joint, Right B Hip Joint, Left C Knee Joint, Right D Knee Joint, Left F Ankle Joint, Right G Ankle Joint, Left H Tarsal Joint, Right J Tarsal Joint, Left K Metatarsal-Tarsal Joint, Right L Metatarsal-Tarsal Joint, Left M Metatarsal-Phalangeal Joint, Right N Metatarsal-Phalangeal Joint, Left P Toe Phalangeal Joint, Right Q Toe Phalangeal Joint, Left	0 Open 3 Percutaneous 4 Percutaneous endoscopic X External	4 Internal fixation device 5 External fixation device Z No device	Z No qualifier

EXCISION GROUP: Excision, Resection, Destruction, (Extraction), (Detachment)
Root Operations that take out some or all of a body part.

1ST - 0 Medical and Surgical 2ND - S Lower Joints 3RD - T RESECTION	EXAMPLE: Total lumbar discectomy	CMS Ex: Cholecystectomy
	RESECTION: Cutting out or off, without replacement, all of a body part.	
	EXPLANATION: None	

Body Part – 4TH	Approach – 5TH	Device – 6TH	Qualifier – 7TH
2 Lumbar Vertebral Disc 4 Lumbosacral Disc 5 Sacrococcygeal Joint 6 Coccygeal Joint 7 Sacroiliac Joint, Right 8 Sacroiliac Joint, Left 9 Hip Joint, Right B Hip Joint, Left C Knee Joint, Right D Knee Joint, Left F Ankle Joint, Right G Ankle Joint, Left H Tarsal Joint, Right J Tarsal Joint, Left K Metatarsal-Tarsal Joint, Right L Metatarsal-Tarsal Joint, Left M Metatarsal-Phalangeal Joint, Right N Metatarsal-Phalangeal Joint, Left P Toe Phalangeal Joint, Right Q Toe Phalangeal Joint, Left	0 Open	Z No device	Z No qualifier

DEVICE GROUP: Change, Insertion, Removal, Replacement, Revision, Supplement
Root Operations that always involve a device.

1ST - **O** Medical and Surgical	**EXAMPLE:** Femoral resurfacing hip joint CMS Ex: Hernia repair with mesh
2ND - **S** Lower Joints	**SUPPLEMENT:** Putting in or on biological or synthetic material that physically reinforces and/or augments the function of a portion of a body part.
3RD - **U SUPPLEMENT**	**EXPLANATION:** Biological material from same individual ...

<table>
<tr><th colspan="2">Body Part – 4TH</th><th>Approach – 5TH</th><th>Device – 6TH</th><th>Qualifier – 7TH</th></tr>
<tr>
<td>0 Lumbar Vertebral Joint
2 Lumbar Vertebral Disc
3 Lumbosacral Joint
4 Lumbosacral Disc
5 Sacrococcygeal Joint
6 Coccygeal Joint
7 Sacroiliac Joint, Right
8 Sacroiliac Joint, Left
F Ankle Joint, Right
G Ankle Joint, Left
H Tarsal Joint, Right
J Tarsal Joint, Left</td>
<td>K Metatarsal-Tarsal Joint, Right
L Metatarsal-Tarsal Joint, Left
M Metatarsal-Phalangeal Joint, Right
N Metatarsal-Phalangeal Joint, Left
P Toe Phalangeal Joint, Right
Q Toe Phalangeal Joint, Left</td>
<td>0 Open
3 Percutaneous
4 Percutaneous endoscopic</td>
<td>7 Autologous tissue substitute
J Synthetic substitute
K Nonautologous tissue substitute</td>
<td>Z No qualifier</td>
</tr>
<tr>
<td colspan="2">9 Hip Joint, Right
B Hip Joint, Left</td>
<td>0 Open</td>
<td>7 Autologous tissue substitute
9 Liner
B Resurfacing device
J Synthetic substitute
K Nonautologous tissue substitute</td>
<td>Z No qualifier</td>
</tr>
<tr>
<td colspan="2">9 Hip Joint, Right
B Hip Joint, Left</td>
<td>3 Percutaneous
4 Percutaneous endoscopic</td>
<td>7 Autologous tissue substitute
J Synthetic substitute
K Nonautologous tissue substitute</td>
<td>Z No qualifier</td>
</tr>
<tr>
<td colspan="2">A Hip Joint, Acetabular Surface, Right
E Hip Joint, Acetabular Surface, Left
R Hip Joint, Femoral Surface, Right
S Hip Joint, Femoral Surface, Left</td>
<td>0 Open</td>
<td>9 Liner
B Resurfacing device</td>
<td>Z No qualifier</td>
</tr>
<tr>
<td colspan="2">C Knee Joint, Right
D Knee Joint, Left</td>
<td>0 Open</td>
<td>7 Autologous tissue substitute
J Synthetic substitute
K Nonautologous tissue substitute</td>
<td>Z No qualifier</td>
</tr>
<tr>
<td colspan="2">C Knee Joint, Right
D Knee Joint, Left</td>
<td>0 Open</td>
<td>9 Liner</td>
<td>C Patellar Surface
Z No qualifier</td>
</tr>
<tr>
<td colspan="2">C Knee Joint, Right
D Knee Joint, Left</td>
<td>3 Percutaneous
4 Percutaneous endoscopic</td>
<td>7 Autologous tissue substitute
J Synthetic substitute
K Nonautologous tissue substitute</td>
<td>Z No qualifier</td>
</tr>
<tr>
<td colspan="2">T Knee Joint, Femoral Surface, Right
U Knee Joint, Femoral Surface, Left
V Knee Joint, Tibial Surface, Right
W Knee Joint, Tibial Surface, Left</td>
<td>0 Open</td>
<td>9 Liner</td>
<td>Z No qualifier</td>
</tr>
</table>

Lower Joints OSU

DEVICE GROUP: Change, Insertion, Removal, Replacement, Revision, Supplement			
Root Operations that always involve a device.			

1ST - 0 Medical and Surgical

2ND - S Lower Joints

3RD - W REVISION

EXAMPLE: Reposition joint spacer | CMS Ex: Adjustment pacemaker lead

REVISION: Correcting, to the extent possible, a portion of a malfunctioning device or the position of a displaced device.

EXPLANATION: May replace components of a device ...

Body Part – 4TH	Approach – 5TH	Device – 6TH	Qualifier – 7TH
0 Lumbar Vertebral Joint 3 Lumbosacral Joint	0 Open 3 Percutaneous 4 Percutaneous endoscopic X External	0 Drainage device 3 Infusion device 4 Internal fixation device 7 Autologous tissue substitute 8 Spacer A Interbody infusion device J Synthetic substitute K Nonautologous tissue substitute	Z No qualifier
2 Lumbar Vertebral Disc 4 Lumbosacral Disc	0 Open 3 Percutaneous 4 Percutaneous endoscopic X External	0 Drainage device 3 Infusion device 7 Autologous tissue substitute J Synthetic substitute K Nonautologous tissue substitute	Z No qualifier
5 Sacrococcygeal Joint 6 Coccygeal Joint 7 Sacroiliac Joint, Right 8 Sacroiliac Joint, Left	0 Open 3 Percutaneous 4 Percutaneous endoscopic X External	0 Drainage device 3 Infusion device 4 Internal fixation device 7 Autologous tissue substitute 8 Spacer J Synthetic substitute K Nonautologous tissue substitute	Z No qualifier
9 Hip Joint, Right B Hip Joint, Left	0 Open	0 Drainage device 3 Infusion device 4 Internal fixation device 5 External fixation device 7 Autologous tissue substitute 8 Spacer 9 Liner B Resurfacing device J Synthetic substitute K Nonautologous tissue substitute	Z No qualifier

continued ⇨

0   S   W   REVISION – *continued*

LOWER JOINTS

0 S W

Body Part – 4TH	Approach – 5TH	Device – 6TH	Qualifier – 7TH
9 Hip Joint, Right B Hip Joint, Left	3 Percutaneous 4 Percutaneous endoscopic X External	0 Drainage device 3 Infusion device 4 Internal fixation device 5 External fixation device 7 Autologous tissue substitute 8 Spacer J Synthetic substitute K Nonautologous tissue substitute	Z No qualifier
A Hip Joint, Acetabular Surface, Right E Hip Joint, Acetabular Surface, Left R Hip Joint, Femoral Surface, Right S Hip Joint, Femoral Surface, Left T Knee Joint, Femoral Surface, Right U Knee Joint, Femoral Surface, Left V Knee Joint, Tibial Surface, Right W Knee Joint, Tibial Surface, Left	0 Open 3 Percutaneous 4 Percutaneous endoscopic X External	J Synthetic substitute	Z No qualifier
C Knee Joint, Right D Knee Joint, Left	0 Open	0 Drainage device 3 Infusion device 4 Internal fixation device 5 External fixation device 7 Autologous tissue substitute 8 Spacer 9 Liner K Nonautologous tissue substitute	Z No qualifier
C Knee Joint, Right D Knee Joint, Left	0 Open	J Synthetic substitute	C Patellar surface Z No qualifier
C Knee Joint, Right D Knee Joint, Left	3 Percutaneous 4 Percutaneous endoscopic X External	0 Drainage device 3 Infusion device 4 Internal fixation device 5 External fixation device 7 Autologous tissue substitute 8 Spacer K Nonautologous tissue substitute	Z No qualifier
C Knee Joint, Right D Knee Joint, Left	3 Percutaneous 4 Percutaneous endoscopic X External	J Synthetic substitute	C Patellar surface Z No qualifier

continued ⇨

© 2016 Channel Publishing, Ltd.

0	**S**	**W**	**REVISION** – *continued*

Body Part – 4TH	Approach – 5TH	Device – 6TH	Qualifier – 7TH
F Ankle Joint, Right G Ankle Joint, Left H Tarsal Joint, Right J Tarsal Joint, Left K Metatarsal-Tarsal Joint, Right L Metatarsal-Tarsal Joint, Left M Metatarsal-Phalangeal Joint, Right N Metatarsal-Phalangeal Joint, Left P Toe Phalangeal Joint, Right Q Toe Phalangeal Joint, Left	0 Open 3 Percutaneous 4 Percutaneous endoscopic X External	0 Drainage device 3 Infusion device 4 Internal fixation device 5 External fixation device 7 Autologous tissue substitute 8 Spacer J Synthetic substitute K Nonautologous tissue substitute	Z No qualifier

NOTES

© 2016 Channel Publishing, Ltd.

Educational Annotations | T – Urinary System

Body System Specific Educational Annotations for the Urinary System include:

- Anatomy and Physiology Review
- Anatomical Illustrations
- Definitions of Common Procedures
- AHA Coding Clinic® Reference Notations
- Body Part Key Listings
- Device Key Listings
- Device Aggregation Table Listings
- Coding Notes

Anatomy and Physiology Review of Urinary System

BODY PART VALUES – T - URINARY SYSTEM

Bladder – ANATOMY – The urinary bladder is a hollow, collapsible musculomembranous organ located within the pelvic cavity behind the symphysis pubis. In the male, it lies against the rectum, and in the female it lies against the vagina and uterus. When filled it may contain 17 fluid ounces (500 ml) of urine and it pushes upward, indenting the abdominal cavity. The trigone area is the floor of the bladder formed by three points, the two ureteral orifices and the urethral orifice. The dome is the expandable superior surface of the bladder. The ureteric orifice is that area surrounding the ureteral openings. The urachus in the adult forms the middle umbilical ligament of the bladder. PHYSIOLOGY – The urinary bladder functions as a reservoir for the urine produced by the kidneys until the individual expels the urine (micturition). Micturition occurs when the bladder becomes distended with urine and stretch receptor nerves signal the micturition center in the sacral spinal cord. Parasympathetic nerve impulses start rhythmically contracting the bladder and the individual senses an urgency to urinate. Following the midbrain decision to urinate, the external urethral sphincter is relaxed, and urination begins as the bladder muscle contracts.

Bladder Neck – The bladder neck is that area surrounding the urethral orifice.

Kidney – ANATOMY – The kidneys are reddish-brown, bean-shaped organs about 4.7 inches (12 cm) long, 2.3 inches (6 cm) wide, and 1.2 inches (3 cm) thick, located on either side of the vertebral column in the retroperitoneal space. The kidneys are supplied with arterial blood from the renal arteries which branch off from the aorta, and are drained by the renal veins which connect with the inferior vena cava. PHYSIOLOGY – The kidneys function to remove metabolic wastes from the blood by transferring them into the urine. They also regulate red blood cell production, blood pressure, calcium absorption, and the pH level of the blood.

Kidney Pelvis – The kidney (renal) pelvis is the funnel-shaped urinary collecting system of the kidney at the upper end of the ureter.

Ureter – The ureter is the musculomembranous tube extending from the renal pelvis to the bladder that transports the urine from the kidney to the bladder using gravity and peristaltic contraction.

Urethra – The urethra is the musculomembranous tube which extends and carries urine from the bladder to the external urethral opening (meatus).

Anatomical Illustrations of Urinary System

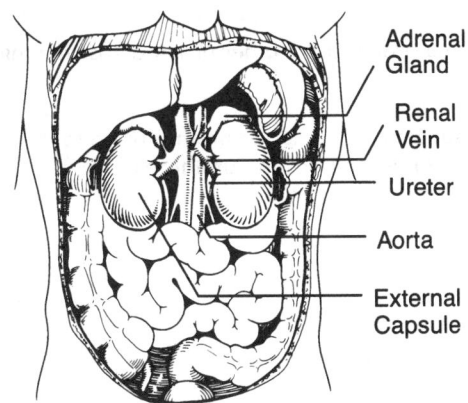

KIDNEY — ANTERIOR VIEW

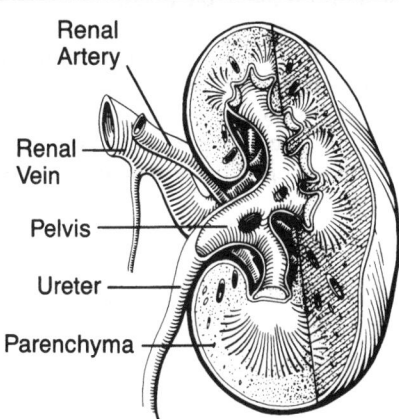

KIDNEY — (CUT AWAY VIEW)

Continued on next page

Educational Annotations | T – Urinary System

Anatomical Illustrations of Urinary System

Continued from previous page

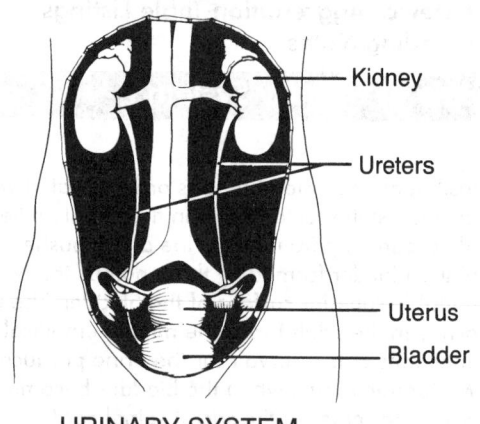

URINARY SYSTEM

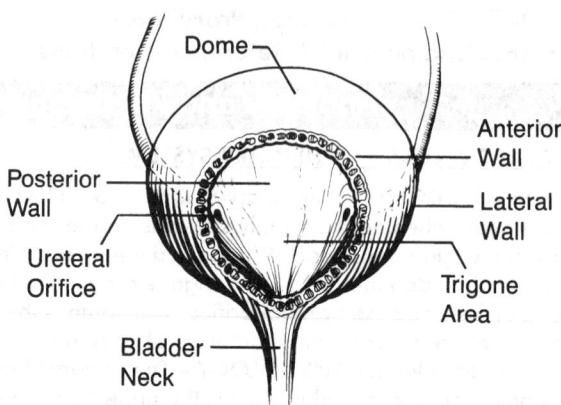

BLADDER — ANTERIOR (CUT-AWAY) VIEW

Definitions of Common Procedures of Urinary System

Bladder neck suspension – The surgical procedure to reposition and support the bladder neck using sutures or a sling of tissue that attaches each end of the sling to pelvic tissue (fascia) or the abdominal wall using stitches.

Cystoscopy – The insertion of an endoscope (cystoscope) through the urethra and into the bladder for visual examination and often to perform procedures on the bladder and urethra.

Extracorporeal shock wave lithotripsy (ESWL) on kidney stone – The breaking apart of kidney stones by using high-energy sound shock waves.

Kidney transplant – The surgical replacement of an end-stage diseased kidney using a donor kidney (living or non-living donor), and sometimes from a genetically identical twin (syngeneic).

Nephrectomy – The surgical removal of a kidney.

Nephropexy – The surgical fixation of a kidney to treat a floating kidney (nephroptosis).

Suprapubic cystostomy – The surgical bypass of the urine from the bladder to outside the body via an implanted catheter placed just above the pubic bone.

Transureteroureterostomy – The surgical anastomosis of one ureter to the other ureter across the midline to bypass distal ureteral obstruction.

Urethroplasty – The surgical repair of a birth defect (hypospadias) or damaged urethra using repositioning, anastomosis, onlay tissue graft, or forming a new urethral channel (Johanson's urethroplasty).

Educational Annotations | T – Urinary System

AHA Coding Clinic® Reference Notations of Urinary System

ROOT OPERATION SPECIFIC - T - URINARY SYSTEM

BYPASS - 1
Rerouting of kinked ileal conduit ....AHA 15:3Q:p34

CHANGE - 2

DESTRUCTION - 5

DILATION - 7
Exchange of ureteral stents ....AHA 16:2Q:p27
Insertion (dilation) of ureteral stent..AHA 15:2Q:p8
Insertion of UroLift® System into prostate ....AHA 13:4Q:p123

DIVISION - 8

DRAINAGE - 9

EXCISION - B
Biopsy of neobladder ....AHA 16:1Q:p19
Excision of Mitrofanoff channel (neo-urethra) polyps ....AHA 15:3Q:p34
Polyp excision in ileal loop (neobladder) ....AHA 14:2Q:p8

EXTIRPATION - C
Extirpation with fragmentation of renal pelvis stone ....AHA 15:2Q:p7
Fragmentation and removal of kidney, ureteral, and bladder stones ....AHA 15:2Q:p8
Ureteroscopic laser lithotripsy with removal of stone fragments.................AHA 13:4Q:p122

EXTRACTION - D

FRAGMENTATION - F
Extracorporeal shock wave lithotripsy (ESWL) on kidney stone ....AHA 13:4Q:p122

INSERTION - H

INSPECTION - J

OCCLUSION - L

REATTACHMENT - M

RELEASE - N

REMOVAL - P
Exchange of ureteral stents ....AHA 16:2Q:p27

REPAIR - Q

REPLACEMENT - R

REPOSITION - S
Pubovaginal sling placement ....AHA 16:1Q:p15

RESECTION - T
Complete nephroureterectomy..AHA 14:3Q:p16

SUPPLEMENT - U

RESTRICTION - V
Deflux injection into bladder at ureteral orifices ....AHA 15:2Q:p11

REVISION - W

TRANSPLANTATION - Y

Body Part Key Listings of Urinary System

See also Body Part Key in Appendix C

Bulbourethral (Cowper's) gland ....*use* Urethra

Cowper's (bulbourethral) gland ....*use* Urethra

External urethral sphincter.............................*use* Urethra

Internal urethral sphincter ....*use* Urethra

Membranous urethra ....*use* Urethra

Penile urethra ....*use* Urethra

Prostatic urethra..*use* Urethra

Continued on next page

U R I N A R Y 0 T

Educational Annotations | T – Urinary System

Body Part Key Listings of Urinary System

Continued from previous page

Renal calyx	*use* Kidney, Bilateral/Left/Right
Renal capsule	*use* Kidney, Bilateral/Left/Right
Renal cortex	*use* Kidney, Bilateral/Left/Right
Renal segment	*use* Kidney, Bilateral/Left/Right
Trigone of bladder	*use* Bladder
Ureteral orifice	*use* Ureter, Bilateral/Left/Right
Ureteropelvic junction (UPJ)	*use* Kidney Pelvis, Left/Right
Ureterovesical orifice	*use* Ureter, Bilateral/Left/Right

Device Key Listings of Urinary System

See also Device Key in Appendix D

AMS 800® Urinary Control System	*use* Artificial Sphincter in Urinary System
Artificial urinary sphincter (AUS)	*use* Artificial Sphincter in Urinary System
Autograft	*use* Autologous Tissue Substitute
Cystostomy tube	*use* Drainage Device
Foley catheter	*use* Drainage Device
Percutaneous nephrostomy catheter	*use* Drainage Device
Sacral nerve modulation (SNM) lead	*use* Stimulator Lead in Urinary System
Sacral neuromodulation lead	*use* Stimulator Lead in Urinary System
Stent, intraluminal (cardiovascular) (gastrointestinal) (hepatobiliary) (urinary)	*use* Intraluminal Device
Tissue bank graft	*use* Nonautologous Tissue Substitute
Urinary incontinence stimulator lead	*use* Stimulator Lead in Urinary System

Device Aggregation Table Listings of Urinary System

See also Device Aggregation Table in Appendix E

Specific Device	For Operation	In Body System	General Device
None Listed in Device Aggregation Table for this Body System			

Coding Notes of Urinary System

Body System Specific PCS Reference Manual Exercises

PCS CODE	T – URINARY SYSTEM EXERCISES
0 T 1 7 0 Z C	Open urinary diversion, left ureter, using ileal conduit to skin.
0 T 2 B X 0 Z	Foley urinary catheter exchange. (This is coded to Drainage Device because urine is being drained.)
0 T 7 7 8 D Z	Cystoscopy with dilation of left ureteral stricture, with stent placement.
0 T 7 C 8 Z Z	Cystoscopy with intraluminal dilation of bladder neck stricture.
0 T 9 B 7 0 Z	Routine Foley catheter placement.
0 T B 0 3 Z X	Percutaneous needle core biopsy of right kidney.
0 T C B 8 Z Z	Transurethral cystoscopy with removal of bladder stone.
0 T F 6 X Z Z	Extracorporeal shock-wave lithotripsy (ESWL), bilateral ureters. (The bilateral ureter body part
0 T F 7 X Z Z	value is not available for the root operation Fragmentation, so the procedures are coded separately.)
0 T F B 8 Z Z	Transurethral cystoscopy with fragmentation of bladder calculus.
0 T J B 8 Z Z	Transurethral diagnostic cystoscopy.
0 T N 6 0 Z Z	Laparotomy with exploration and adhesiolysis of right ureter.
0 T P 9 8 D Z	Cystoscopy with retrieval of left ureteral stent.
0 T T 1 0 Z Z	Explantation of left failed kidney, open.
0 T Y 1 0 Z 0	Left kidney/pancreas organ bank transplant.
0 F Y G 0 Z 0	

TUBULAR GROUP: Bypass, Dilation, Occlusion, Restriction
Root Operations that alter the diameter/route of a tubular body part.

1ST - 0 Medical and Surgical 2ND - T Urinary System 3RD - 1 BYPASS	EXAMPLE: Ileal conduit urinary diversion	CMS Ex: Coronary artery bypass
	BYPASS: Altering the route of passage of the contents of a tubular body part.	
	EXPLANATION: Rerouting contents to a downstream part ...	

Body Part – 4TH	Approach – 5TH	Device – 6TH	Qualifier – 7TH
3 Kidney Pelvis, Right 4 Kidney Pelvis, Left	0 Open 4 Percutaneous endoscopic	7 Autologous tissue substitute J Synthetic substitute K Nonautologous tissue substitute Z No device	3 Kidney Pelvis, Right 4 Kidney Pelvis, Left 6 Ureter, Right 7 Ureter, Left 8 Colon 9 Colocutaneous A Ileum B Bladder C Ileocutaneous D Cutaneous
3 Kidney Pelvis, Right 4 Kidney Pelvis, Left	3 Percutaneous	J Synthetic substitute	D Cutaneous
6 Ureter, Right 7 Ureter, Left 8 Ureters, Bilateral	0 Open 4 Percutaneous endoscopic	7 Autologous tissue substitute J Synthetic substitute K Nonautologous tissue substitute Z No device	6 Ureter, Right 7 Ureter, Left 8 Colon 9 Colocutaneous A Ileum B Bladder C Ileocutaneous D Cutaneous
6 Ureter, Right 7 Ureter, Left 8 Ureters, Bilateral	3 Percutaneous	J Synthetic substitute	D Cutaneous
B Bladder	0 Open 4 Percutaneous endoscopic	7 Autologous tissue substitute J Synthetic substitute K Nonautologous tissue substitute Z No device	9 Colocutaneous C Ileocutaneous D Cutaneous
B Bladder	3 Percutaneous	J Synthetic substitute	D Cutaneous

URINARY

0 T 1

DEVICE GROUP: Change, Insertion, Removal, Replacement, Revision, Supplement
Root Operations that always involve a device.

1ST - 0 Medical and Surgical	EXAMPLE: Exchange Foley catheter	CMS Ex: Changing urinary catheter
2ND - T Urinary System	**CHANGE:** Taking out or off a device from a body part and putting back an identical or similar device in or on the same body part without cutting or puncturing the skin or a mucous membrane.	
3RD - 2 CHANGE	EXPLANATION: ALL Changes use EXTERNAL approach only ...	

Body Part – 4TH	Approach – 5TH	Device – 6TH	Qualifier – 7TH
5 Kidney 9 Ureter B Bladder D Urethra	X External	0 Drainage device Y Other device	Z No qualifier

EXCISION GROUP: Excision, Resection, Destruction, Extraction, (Detachment)
Root Operations that take out some or all of a body part.

1ST - 0 Medical and Surgical	EXAMPLE: Cystoscopic laser ablation	CMS Ex: Fulguration polyp
2ND - T Urinary System	**DESTRUCTION:** Physical eradication of all or a portion of a body part by the direct use of energy, force, or a destructive agent.	
3RD - 5 DESTRUCTION	EXPLANATION: None of the body part is physically taken out	

Body Part – 4TH	Approach – 5TH	Device – 6TH	Qualifier – 7TH
0 Kidney, Right 1 Kidney, Left 3 Kidney Pelvis, Right 4 Kidney Pelvis, Left 6 Ureter, Right 7 Ureter, Left B Bladder C Bladder Neck	0 Open 3 Percutaneous 4 Percutaneous endoscopic 7 Via natural or artificial opening 8 Via natural or artificial opening endoscopic	Z No device	Z No qualifier
D Urethra	0 Open 3 Percutaneous 4 Percutaneous endoscopic 7 Via natural or artificial opening 8 Via natural or artificial opening endoscopic X External	Z No device	Z No qualifier

TUBULAR GROUP: Bypass, Dilation, Occlusion, Restriction
Root Operations that alter the diameter/route of a tubular body part.

1ST - 0 Medical and Surgical

2ND - T Urinary System

3RD - 7 DILATION

EXAMPLE: Urethral dilation   CMS Ex: Transluminal angioplasty

DILATION: Expanding an orifice or the lumen of a tubular body part.

EXPLANATION: By force (stretching) or cutting ...

Body Part – 4TH	Approach – 5TH	Device – 6TH	Qualifier – 7TH
3 Kidney Pelvis, Right 4 Kidney Pelvis, Left 6 Ureter, Right 7 Ureter, Left 8 Ureters, Bilateral B Bladder C Bladder Neck D Urethra	0 Open 3 Percutaneous 4 Percutaneous endoscopic 7 Via natural or artificial opening 8 Via natural or artificial opening endoscopic	D Intraluminal device Z No device	Z No qualifier

DIVISION GROUP: Division, Release
Root Operations involving cutting or separation only.

1ST - 0 Medical and Surgical

2ND - T Urinary System

3RD - 8 DIVISION

EXAMPLE: Division bladder neck   CMS Ex: Osteotomy

DIVISION: Cutting into a body part without draining fluids and/or gases from the body part in order to separate or transect a body part.

EXPLANATION: Separated into two or more portions ...

Body Part – 4TH	Approach – 5TH	Device – 6TH	Qualifier – 7TH
2 Kidneys, Bilateral C Bladder Neck	0 Open 3 Percutaneous 4 Percutaneous endoscopic	Z No device	Z No qualifier

URINARY

0 T 8

DRAINAGE GROUP: Drainage, Extirpation, Fragmentation
Root Operations that take out solids/fluids/gases from a body part.

1ST - 0 Medical and Surgical	EXAMPLE: Foley catheter placement	CMS Ex: Thoracentesis

2ND - T Urinary System

3RD - 9 DRAINAGE

DRAINAGE: Taking or letting out fluids and/or gases from a body part.

EXPLANATION: Qualifier "X Diagnostic" indicates biopsy ...

Body Part – 4TH	Approach – 5TH	Device – 6TH	Qualifier – 7TH
0 Kidney, Right 1 Kidney, Left 3 Kidney Pelvis, Right 4 Kidney Pelvis, Left 6 Ureter, Right 7 Ureter, Left 8 Ureters, Bilateral B Bladder C Bladder Neck	0 Open 3 Percutaneous 4 Percutaneous endoscopic 7 Via natural or artificial opening 8 Via natural or artificial opening endoscopic	0 Drainage device	Z No qualifier
0 Kidney, Right 1 Kidney, Left 3 Kidney Pelvis, Right 4 Kidney Pelvis, Left 6 Ureter, Right 7 Ureter, Left 8 Ureters, Bilateral B Bladder C Bladder Neck	0 Open 3 Percutaneous 4 Percutaneous endoscopic 7 Via natural or artificial opening 8 Via natural or artificial opening endoscopic	Z No device	X Diagnostic Z No qualifier
D Urethra	0 Open 3 Percutaneous 4 Percutaneous endoscopic 7 Via natural or artificial opening 8 Via natural or artificial opening endoscopic X External	0 Drainage device	Z No qualifier
D Urethra	0 Open 3 Percutaneous 4 Percutaneous endoscopic 7 Via natural or artificial opening 8 Via natural or artificial opening endoscopic X External	Z No device	X Diagnostic Z No qualifier

URINARY
0 T 9

EXCISION GROUP: Excision, Resection, Destruction, Extraction, (Detachment)
Root Operations that take out some or all of a body part.

1ST - 0 Medical and Surgical

2ND - T Urinary System

3RD - B EXCISION

EXAMPLE: Needle core biopsy kidney | CMS Ex: Liver biopsy

EXCISION: Cutting out or off, without replacement, a portion of a body part.

EXPLANATION: Qualifier "X Diagnostic" indicates biopsy ...

Body Part – 4TH	Approach – 5TH	Device – 6TH	Qualifier – 7TH
0 Kidney, Right 1 Kidney, Left 3 Kidney Pelvis, Right 4 Kidney Pelvis, Left 6 Ureter, Right 7 Ureter, Left B Bladder C Bladder Neck	0 Open 3 Percutaneous 4 Percutaneous endoscopic 7 Via natural or artificial opening 8 Via natural or artificial opening endoscopic	Z No device	X Diagnostic Z No qualifier
D Urethra	0 Open 3 Percutaneous 4 Percutaneous endoscopic 7 Via natural or artificial opening 8 Via natural or artificial opening endoscopic X External	Z No device	X Diagnostic Z No qualifier

URINARY

0 T B

URINARY

0 T C

DRAINAGE GROUP: Drainage, Extirpation, Fragmentation
Root Operations that take out solids/fluids/gases from a body part.

1ST - **0** Medical and Surgical	EXAMPLE: Removal bladder stone	CMS Ex: Choledocholithotomy
2ND - **T** Urinary System	**EXTIRPATION:** Taking or cutting out solid matter from a body part.	
3RD - **C** EXTIRPATION	EXPLANATION: Abnormal byproduct or foreign body …	

Body Part – 4TH	Approach – 5TH	Device – 6TH	Qualifier – 7TH
0 Kidney, Right 1 Kidney, Left 3 Kidney Pelvis, Right 4 Kidney Pelvis, Left 6 Ureter, Right 7 Ureter, Left B Bladder C Bladder Neck	0 Open 3 Percutaneous 4 Percutaneous endoscopic 7 Via natural or artificial opening 8 Via natural or artificial opening endoscopic	Z No device	Z No qualifier
D Urethra	0 Open 3 Percutaneous 4 Percutaneous endoscopic 7 Via natural or artificial opening 8 Via natural or artificial opening endoscopic X External	Z No device	Z No qualifier

---

EXCISION GROUP: Excision, Resection, Destruction, Extraction, (Detachment)
Root Operations that take out some or all of a body part.

1ST - **0** Medical and Surgical	EXAMPLE: Kidney extraction	CMS Ex: D&C
2ND - **T** Urinary System	**EXTRACTION:** Pulling or stripping out or off all or a portion of a body part by the use of force.	
3RD - **D** EXTRACTION	EXPLANATION: None for this Body System	

Body Part – 4TH	Approach – 5TH	Device – 6TH	Qualifier – 7TH
0 Kidney, Right 1 Kidney, Left	0 Open 3 Percutaneous 4 Percutaneous endoscopic	Z No device	Z No qualifier

DRAINAGE GROUP: Drainage, Extirpation, Fragmentation			
Root Operations that take out solids/fluids/gases from a body part.			

1ST - **0** Medical and Surgical 2ND - **T** Urinary System 3RD - **F FRAGMENTATION**	EXAMPLE: Extracorporeal shockwave lithotripsy	CMS Ex: ESWL
	FRAGMENTATION: Breaking solid matter in a body part into pieces.	
	EXPLANATION: Pieces are not taken out during procedure ...	

Body Part – 4TH	Approach – 5TH	Device – 6TH	Qualifier – 7TH
3　Kidney Pelvis, Right 4　Kidney Pelvis, Left 6　Ureter, Right 7　Ureter, Left B　Bladder C　Bladder Neck D　Urethra NC*	0　Open 3　Percutaneous 4　Percutaneous endoscopic 7　Via natural or artificial opening 8　Via natural or artificial opening endoscopic X　External	Z　No device	Z　No qualifier

NC* – Some procedures are considered non-covered by Medicare. See current Medicare Code Editor for details.

U R I N A R Y

0 T F

DEVICE GROUP: Change, Insertion, Removal, Replacement, Revision, Supplement
Root Operations that always involve a device.

1ST - O Medical and Surgical 2ND - T Urinary System 3RD - H INSERTION	EXAMPLE: Artificial bladder sphincter	CMS Ex: Central venous catheter
	INSERTION: Putting in a nonbiological appliance that monitors, assists, performs, or prevents a physiological function but does not physically take the place of a body part.	
	EXPLANATION: None	

Body Part – 4TH	Approach – 5TH	Device – 6TH	Qualifier – 7TH
5 Kidney	0 Open 3 Percutaneous 4 Percutaneous endoscopic 7 Via natural or artificial opening 8 Via natural or artificial opening endoscopic	2 Monitoring device 3 Infusion device	Z No qualifier
9 Ureter	0 Open 3 Percutaneous 4 Percutaneous endoscopic 7 Via natural or artificial opening 8 Via natural or artificial opening endoscopic	2 Monitoring device 3 Infusion device M Stimulator lead	Z No qualifier
B Bladder	0 Open 3 Percutaneous 4 Percutaneous endoscopic 7 Via natural or artificial opening 8 Via natural or artificial opening endoscopic	2 Monitoring device 3 Infusion device L Artificial sphincter M Stimulator lead NC*	Z No qualifier
C Bladder Neck	0 Open 3 Percutaneous 4 Percutaneous endoscopic 7 Via natural or artificial opening 8 Via natural or artificial opening endoscopic	L Artificial sphincter	Z No qualifier
D Urethra	0 Open 3 Percutaneous 4 Percutaneous endoscopic 7 Via natural or artificial opening 8 Via natural or artificial opening endoscopic X External	2 Monitoring device 3 Infusion device L Artificial sphincter	Z No qualifier

NC* – Non-covered by Medicare. See current Medicare Code Editor for details.

URINARY 0TH

EXAMINATION GROUP: Inspection, (Map)
Root Operations involving examination only.

1ST - **0** Medical and Surgical	EXAMPLE: Ureteroscopy		CMS Ex: Colonoscopy
2ND - **T** Urinary System	**INSPECTION:** Visually and/or manually exploring a body part.		
3RD - **J INSPECTION**			
	EXPLANATION: Direct or instrumental visualization ...		

Body Part – 4TH	Approach – 5TH	Device – 6TH	Qualifier – 7TH
5 Kidney 9 Ureter B Bladder D Urethra	0 Open 3 Percutaneous 4 Percutaneous endoscopic 7 Via natural or artificial opening 8 Via natural or artificial opening endoscopic X External	Z No device	Z No qualifier

TUBULAR GROUP: Bypass, Dilation, Occlusion, Restriction
Root Operations that alter the diameter/route of a tubular body part.

1ST - **0** Medical and Surgical	EXAMPLE: Occlusion kidney pelvis		CMS Ex: Fallopian tube ligation
2ND - **T** Urinary System	**OCCLUSION:** Completely closing an orifice or lumen of a tubular body part.		
3RD - **L OCCLUSION**			
	EXPLANATION: Natural or artificially created orifice ...		

Body Part – 4TH	Approach – 5TH	Device – 6TH	Qualifier – 7TH
3 Kidney Pelvis, Right 4 Kidney Pelvis, Left 6 Ureter, Right 7 Ureter, Left B Bladder C Bladder Neck	0 Open 3 Percutaneous 4 Percutaneous endoscopic	C Extraluminal device D Intraluminal device Z No device	Z No qualifier
3 Kidney Pelvis, Right 4 Kidney Pelvis, Left 6 Ureter, Right 7 Ureter, Left B Bladder C Bladder Neck	7 Via natural or artificial opening 8 Via natural or artificial opening endoscopic	D Intraluminal device Z No device	Z No qualifier
D Urethra	0 Open 3 Percutaneous 4 Percutaneous endoscopic X External	C Extraluminal device D Intraluminal device Z No device	Z No qualifier
D Urethra	7 Via natural or artificial opening 8 Via natural or artificial opening endoscopic	D Intraluminal device Z No device	Z No qualifier

U R I N A R Y

0 T L

MOVE GROUP: Reattachment, Reposition, (Transfer), Transplantation
Root Operations that put in/put back or move some/all of a body part.

1ST - O Medical and Surgical	EXAMPLE: Replantation avulsed kidney	CMS Ex: Reattachment hand
2ND - T Urinary System	**REATTACHMENT:** Putting back in or on all or a portion of a separated body part to its normal location or other suitable location.	
3RD - M REATTACHMENT	EXPLANATION: With/without reconnection of vessels/nerves...	

Body Part – 4TH		Approach – 5TH	Device – 6TH	Qualifier – 7TH
0 Kidney, Right 1 Kidney, Left 2 Kidneys, Bilateral 3 Kidney Pelvis, Right 4 Kidney Pelvis, Left	6 Ureter, Right 7 Ureter, Left 8 Ureters, Bilateral B Bladder C Bladder Neck D Urethra	0 Open 4 Percutaneous endoscopic	Z No device	Z No qualifier

---

DIVISION GROUP: Division, Release
Root Operations involving cutting or separation only.

1ST - O Medical and Surgical	EXAMPLE: Adhesiolysis ureter	CMS Ex: Carpal tunnel release
2ND - T Urinary System	**RELEASE:** Freeing a body part from an abnormal physical constraint by cutting or by the use of force.	
3RD - N RELEASE	EXPLANATION: None of the body part is taken out ...	

Body Part – 4TH	Approach – 5TH	Device – 6TH	Qualifier – 7TH
0 Kidney, Right 1 Kidney, Left 3 Kidney Pelvis, Right 4 Kidney Pelvis, Left 6 Ureter, Right 7 Ureter, Left B Bladder C Bladder Neck	0 Open 3 Percutaneous 4 Percutaneous endoscopic 7 Via natural or artificial opening 8 Via natural or artificial opening endoscopic	Z No device	Z No qualifier
D Urethra	0 Open 3 Percutaneous 4 Percutaneous endoscopic 7 Via natural or artificial opening 8 Via natural or artificial opening endoscopic X External	Z No device	Z No qualifier

URINARY

OTM

DEVICE GROUP: Change, Insertion, Removal, Replacement, Revision, Supplement
Root Operations that always involve a device.

1ST - **0** Medical and Surgical	EXAMPLE: Removal ureteral stent	CMS Ex: Chest tube removal
2ND - **T** Urinary System	**REMOVAL:** Taking out or off a device from a body part.	
3RD - **P REMOVAL**		
	EXPLANATION: Removal device without reinsertion ...	

Body Part – 4TH	Approach – 5TH	Device – 6TH	Qualifier – 7TH
5　Kidney	0　Open 3　Percutaneous 4　Percutaneous endoscopic 7　Via natural or artificial opening 8　Via natural or artificial opening endoscopic	0　Drainage device 2　Monitoring device 3　Infusion device 7　Autologous tissue substitute C　Extraluminal device D　Intraluminal device J　Synthetic substitute K　Nonautologous tissue substitute	Z　No qualifier
5　Kidney	X　External	0　Drainage device 2　Monitoring device 3　Infusion device D　Intraluminal device	Z　No qualifier
9　Ureter	0　Open 3　Percutaneous 4　Percutaneous endoscopic 7　Via natural or artificial opening 8　Via natural or artificial opening endoscopic	0　Drainage device 2　Monitoring device 3　Infusion device 7　Autologous tissue substitute C　Extraluminal device D　Intraluminal device J　Synthetic substitute K　Nonautologous tissue substitute M　Stimulator lead	Z　No qualifier
9　Ureter	X　External	0　Drainage device 2　Monitoring device 3　Infusion device D　Intraluminal device M　Stimulator lead	Z　No qualifier

URINARY

0 T P

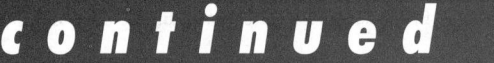

continued ⇨

© 2016 Channel Publishing, Ltd.

0   T   P   REMOVAL – *continued*

Body Part – 4TH	Approach – 5TH	Device – 6TH	Qualifier – 7TH
B Bladder	0 Open 3 Percutaneous 4 Percutaneous endoscopic 7 Via natural or artificial opening 8 Via natural or artificial opening endoscopic	0 Drainage device 2 Monitoring device 3 Infusion device 7 Autologous tissue substitute C Extraluminal device D Intraluminal device J Synthetic substitute K Nonautologous tissue substitute L Artificial sphincter M Stimulator lead NC*	Z No qualifier
B Bladder	X External	0 Drainage device 2 Monitoring device 3 Infusion device D Intraluminal device L Artificial sphincter M Stimulator lead	Z No qualifier
D Urethra	0 Open 3 Percutaneous 4 Percutaneous endoscopic 7 Via natural or artificial opening 8 Via natural or artificial opening endoscopic	0 Drainage device 2 Monitoring device 3 Infusion device 7 Autologous tissue substitute C Extraluminal device D Intraluminal device J Synthetic substitute K Nonautologous tissue substitute L Artificial sphincter	Z No qualifier
D Urethra	X External	0 Drainage device 2 Monitoring device 3 Infusion device D Intraluminal device L Artificial sphincter	Z No qualifier

NC* – Non-covered by Medicare. See current Medicare Code Editor for details.

URINARY

0 T P

© 2016 Channel Publishing, Ltd.

OTHER REPAIRS GROUP: (Control), Repair
Root Operations that define other repairs.

1ST - 0 Medical and Surgical

2ND - T Urinary System

3RD - Q REPAIR

EXAMPLE: Suture lacerated kidney | CMS Ex: Suture laceration

REPAIR: Restoring, to the extent possible, a body part to its normal anatomic structure and function.

EXPLANATION: Only when no other root operation applies ...

Body Part – 4TH	Approach – 5TH	Device – 6TH	Qualifier – 7TH
0 Kidney, Right 1 Kidney, Left 3 Kidney Pelvis, Right 4 Kidney Pelvis, Left 6 Ureter, Right 7 Ureter, Left B Bladder C Bladder Neck	0 Open 3 Percutaneous 4 Percutaneous endoscopic 7 Via natural or artificial opening 8 Via natural or artificial opening endoscopic	Z No device	Z No qualifier
D Urethra	0 Open 3 Percutaneous 4 Percutaneous endoscopic 7 Via natural or artificial opening 8 Via natural or artificial opening endoscopic X External	Z No device	Z No qualifier

---

DEVICE GROUP: Change, Insertion, Removal, Replacement, Revision, Supplement
Root Operations that always involve a device.

1ST - 0 Medical and Surgical

2ND - T Urinary System

3RD - R REPLACEMENT

EXAMPLE: Segmental ureteral replacement | CMS Ex: Total hip

REPLACEMENT: Putting in or on a biological or synthetic material that physically takes the place and/or function of all or a portion of a body part.

EXPLANATION: Includes taking out body part, or eradication...

Body Part – 4TH	Approach – 5TH	Device – 6TH	Qualifier – 7TH
3 Kidney Pelvis, Right 4 Kidney Pelvis, Left 6 Ureter, Right 7 Ureter, Left B Bladder C Bladder Neck	0 Open 4 Percutaneous endoscopic 7 Via natural or artificial opening 8 Via natural or artificial opening endoscopic	7 Autologous tissue substitute J Synthetic substitute K Nonautologous tissue substitute	Z No qualifier
D Urethra	0 Open 4 Percutaneous endoscopic 7 Via natural or artificial opening 8 Via natural or artificial opening endoscopic X External	7 Autologous tissue substitute J Synthetic substitute K Nonautologous tissue substitute	Z No qualifier

URINARY 0 T R

MOVE GROUP: Reattachment, Reposition, (Transfer), Transplantation
Root Operations that put in/put back or move some/all of a body part.

1ST - 0 Medical and Surgical	EXAMPLE: Bladder neck (sling) suspension	CMS Ex: FX reduction

2ND - T Urinary System

3RD - S REPOSITION

REPOSITION: Moving to its normal location, or other suitable location, all or a portion of a body part.

EXPLANATION: May or may not be cut to be moved ...

Body Part – 4TH		Approach – 5TH	Device – 6TH	Qualifier – 7TH
0 Kidney, Right	6 Ureter, Right	0 Open	Z No device	Z No qualifier
1 Kidney, Left	7 Ureter, Left	4 Percutaneous endoscopic		
2 Kidneys, Bilateral	8 Ureters, Bilateral			
3 Kidney Pelvis, Right	B Bladder			
4 Kidney Pelvis, Left	C Bladder Neck			
	D Urethra			

EXCISION GROUP: Excision, Resection, Destruction, Extraction, (Detachment)
Root Operations that take out some or all of a body part.

1ST - 0 Medical and Surgical	EXAMPLE: Nephrectomy	CMS Ex: Cholecystectomy

2ND - T Urinary System

3RD - T RESECTION

RESECTION: Cutting out or off, without replacement, all of a body part.

EXPLANATION: None

Body Part – 4TH	Approach – 5TH	Device – 6TH	Qualifier – 7TH
0 Kidney, Right	0 Open	Z No device	Z No qualifier
1 Kidney, Left	4 Percutaneous endoscopic		
2 Kidneys, Bilateral			
3 Kidney Pelvis, Right	0 Open	Z No device	Z No qualifier
4 Kidney Pelvis, Left	4 Percutaneous endoscopic		
6 Ureter, Right	7 Via natural or artificial opening		
7 Ureter, Left	8 Via natural or artificial opening endoscopic		
B Bladder			
C Bladder Neck			
D Urethra			

URINARY

0 T S

DEVICE GROUP: Change, Insertion, Removal, Replacement, Revision, Supplement
Root Operations that always involve a device.

1ST - 0 Medical and Surgical

2ND - T Urinary System

3RD - U SUPPLEMENT

EXAMPLE: Repair bladder defect with graft | CMS Ex: Hernia repair mesh

SUPPLEMENT: Putting in or on biological or synthetic material that physically reinforces and/or augments the function of a portion of a body part.

EXPLANATION: Biological material from same individual ...

Body Part – 4TH	Approach – 5TH	Device – 6TH	Qualifier – 7TH
3 Kidney Pelvis, Right 4 Kidney Pelvis, Left 6 Ureter, Right 7 Ureter, Left B Bladder C Bladder Neck	0 Open 4 Percutaneous endoscopic 7 Via natural or artificial opening 8 Via natural or artificial opening endoscopic	7 Autologous tissue substitute J Synthetic substitute K Nonautologous tissue substitute	Z No qualifier
D Urethra	0 Open 4 Percutaneous endoscopic 7 Via natural or artificial opening 8 Via natural or artificial opening endoscopic X External	7 Autologous tissue substitute J Synthetic substitute K Nonautologous tissue substitute	Z No qualifier

URINARY

0 T U

TUBULAR GROUP: Bypass, Dilation, Occlusion, Restriction
Root Operations that alter the diameter/route of a tubular body part.

1ST – 0 Medical and Surgical		
2ND – T Urinary System		

3RD – V RESTRICTION

EXAMPLE: Ureteral restrictive stent	CMS Ex: Cervical cerclage

RESTRICTION: Partially closing an orifice or the lumen of a tubular body part.

EXPLANATION: Natural or artificially created orifice ...

Body Part – 4TH	Approach – 5TH	Device – 6TH	Qualifier – 7TH
3 Kidney Pelvis, Right 4 Kidney Pelvis, Left 6 Ureter, Right 7 Ureter, Left B Bladder C Bladder Neck	0 Open 3 Percutaneous 4 Percutaneous endoscopic	C Extraluminal device D Intraluminal device Z No device	Z No qualifier
3 Kidney Pelvis, Right 4 Kidney Pelvis, Left 6 Ureter, Right 7 Ureter, Left B Bladder C Bladder Neck	7 Via natural or artificial opening 8 Via natural or artificial opening endoscopic	D Intraluminal device Z No device	Z No qualifier
D Urethra	0 Open 3 Percutaneous 4 Percutaneous endoscopic	C Extraluminal device D Intraluminal device Z No device	Z No qualifier
D Urethra	7 Via natural or artificial opening 8 Via natural or artificial opening endoscopic	D Intraluminal device Z No device	Z No qualifier
D Urethra	X External	Z No device	Z No qualifier

URINARY

0 T V

	DEVICE GROUP: Change, Insertion, Removal, Replacement, Revision, Supplement		
	Root Operations that always involve a device.		

1ST - 0 Medical and Surgical

2ND - T Urinary System

3RD - W REVISION

EXAMPLE: Reposition stimulator lead | CMS Ex: Adjustment pacemaker lead

REVISION: Correcting, to the extent possible, a portion of a malfunctioning device or the position of a displaced device.

EXPLANATION: May replace components of a device ...

Body Part – 4TH	Approach – 5TH	Device – 6TH	Qualifier – 7TH
5 Kidney	0 Open 3 Percutaneous 4 Percutaneous endoscopic 7 Via natural or artificial opening 8 Via natural or artificial opening endoscopic X External	0 Drainage device 2 Monitoring device 3 Infusion device 7 Autologous tissue substitute C Extraluminal device D Intraluminal device J Synthetic substitute K Nonautologous tissue substitute	Z No qualifier
9 Ureter	0 Open 3 Percutaneous 4 Percutaneous endoscopic 7 Via natural or artificial opening 8 Via natural or artificial opening endoscopic X External	0 Drainage device 2 Monitoring device 3 Infusion device 7 Autologous tissue substitute C Extraluminal device D Intraluminal device J Synthetic substitute K Nonautologous tissue substitute M Stimulator lead	Z No qualifier
B Bladder	0 Open 3 Percutaneous 4 Percutaneous endoscopic 7 Via natural or artificial opening 8 Via natural or artificial opening endoscopic X External	0 Drainage device 2 Monitoring device 3 Infusion device 7 Autologous tissue substitute C Extraluminal device D Intraluminal device J Synthetic substitute K Nonautologous tissue substitute L Artificial sphincter M Stimulator lead	Z No qualifier
D Urethra	0 Open 3 Percutaneous 4 Percutaneous endoscopic 7 Via natural or artificial opening 8 Via natural or artificial opening endoscopic X External	0 Drainage device 2 Monitoring device 3 Infusion device 7 Autologous tissue substitute C Extraluminal device D Intraluminal device J Synthetic substitute K Nonautologous tissue substitute L Artificial sphincter	Z No qualifier

URINARY 0 T W

MOVE GROUP: Reattachment, Reposition, (Transfer), Transplantation
Root Operations that put in/put back or move some/all of a body part.

1ST - 0 Medical and Surgical	EXAMPLE: Kidney transplant	CMS Ex: Kidney transplant
2ND - T Urinary System		
3RD - Y TRANSPLANTATION	**TRANSPLANTATION:** Putting in or on all or a portion of a living body part taken from another individual or animal to physically take the place and/or function of all or a portion of a similar body part.	

EXPLANATION: May take over all or part of its function …

Body Part – 4TH	Approach – 5TH	Device – 6TH	Qualifier – 7TH
0 Kidney, Right LC* 1 Kidney, Left LC*	0 Open	Z No device	0 Allogeneic 1 Syngeneic 2 Zooplastic

LC* – Some procedures are considered limited coverage by Medicare. See current Medicare Code Editor for details.

Educational Annotations | U – Female Reproductive System

Body System Specific Educational Annotations for the Female Reproductive System include:

- Anatomy and Physiology Review
- Anatomical Illustrations
- Definitions of Common Procedures
- AHA Coding Clinic® Reference Notations
- Body Part Key Listings
- Device Key Listings
- Device Aggregation Table Listings
- Coding Notes

Anatomy and Physiology Review of Female Reproductive System

BODY PART VALUES – U - FEMALE REPRODUCTIVE SYSTEM

Cervix – The cervix is the lower portion of the uterus that extends downward into the vagina.

Clitoris – ANATOMY – The highly innervated, sensitive female sex organ that is located above the urethral opening (meatus) and at the junction of the labia minora. PHYSIOLOGY – It is generally accepted as the primary anatomical source of female sexual pleasure.

Cul-de-sac – The deep peritoneal recess between the rectum and back wall of the uterus (also known as the pouch of Douglas and rectouterine pouch).

Endometrium – The mucous membrane interior lining of the uterus that lies upon the thick muscular myometrium of the body.

Fallopian Tube – ANATOMY – The fallopian tubes (also known as oviducts, uterine tubes, and salpinges) are the tubular canals from each side of the uterus to the area immediately next to each ovary (fimbriae). PHYSIOLOGY – The fallopian tubes serve to transport the ova to the uterus.

Hymen – The hymen is a membrane of tissue that surrounds or partially covers the vaginal opening.

Ova – The human reproductive egg(s).

Ovary – ANATOMY – The ovaries are the paired, flat, ovoid female reproductive glands located on each side of the uterus, attached to the broad ligament, and are approximately 1.4 inches (3.5 cm) in length and 0.8 inches (2 cm) in width. PHYSIOLOGY – The ovaries function to produce the human reproductive egg cell (ova, ovum), and to produce hormones. The ovaries secrete estrogen, testosterone, and progesterone.

Uterine Supporting Structure – The ligaments, fibromuscular bands, and connective tissue that support the uterus, ovaries, and fallopian tubes. The broad ligament is the double-layered fold of the peritoneum with the loose connective tissue between its layers, called the parametrium. The round ligaments are the fibromuscular bands attached to the uterus below the fallopian tube orifices and to the pelvic wall.

Uterus – ANATOMY – The uterus is the pear-shaped, hollow, muscular female reproductive organ that is about 2.8 inches (7 cm) in length and up to 2 inches (5 cm) in width, located within the pelvic cavity, and resting slightly above the bladder. The fallopian tubes enter into the upper portion. The cervix is the lower portion that extends downward into the vagina. The isthmus is the narrowed lower end of the body of the uterus. The body is the bulky upper portion with the dome above the fallopian tube orifices (also known as the fundus or corpus uteri). The endometrium is the mucous membrane interior lining lying upon the thick muscular myometrium of the body. The ovarian and uterine arteries supply blood to the uterus. PHYSIOLOGY – The uterus functions to receive the embryo, serve as attachment for the placenta, stretch and enlarge to allow for the fetus to grow, and to rhythmically contract for delivery of the fetus.

Vagina – ANATOMY – The vagina is the elastic, musculomembranous canal extending from the uterus to the vulva, passing in front of the rectum and behind the bladder, attached by loose connective tissue, and is approximately 3-4 inches (7.5-10 cm) in length. PHYSIOLOGY – The vagina functions to receive the penis and ejaculated sperm during intercourse, pass the fetus to birth during delivery, and convey the menstrual discharge out of the body.

Vestibular Gland – The vestibular glands (also known as paraurethral, Bartholin's, and Skene's glands) are small mucous-secreting glands that open on either side of the urethral orifice and vaginal opening.

Vulva – ANATOMY – The vulva is the group of external female genital organs comprising the labia majora, labia minora, clitoris, and vestibular glands. PHYSIOLOGY – The vulva functions to protect the genital organs at the entrance of the vagina, and aid in sexual stimulation and lubrication during intercourse.

FEMALE

0 U

Educational Annotations | U – Female Reproductive System

Anatomical Illustrations of Female Reproductive System

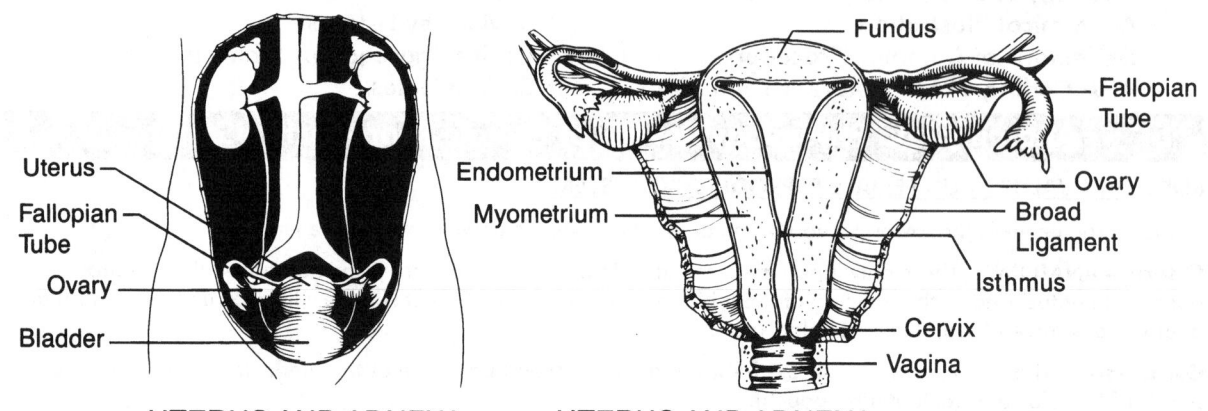

UTERUS AND ADNEXA

Uterus
Fallopian Tube
Ovary
Bladder

UTERUS AND ADNEXA — CUT-AWAY

Fundus
Fallopian Tube
Ovary
Broad Ligament
Isthmus
Cervix
Vagina
Endometrium
Myometrium

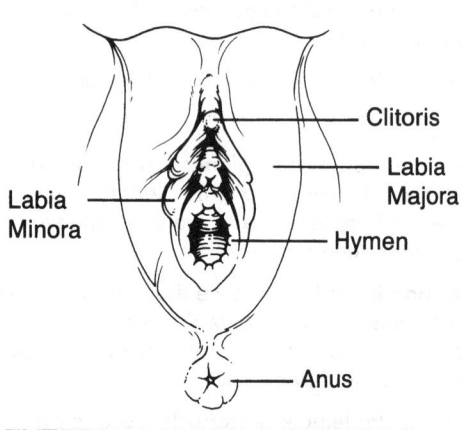
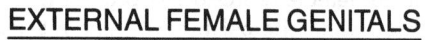

Clitoris
Labia Majora
Hymen
Labia Minora
Anus

EXTERNAL FEMALE GENITALS

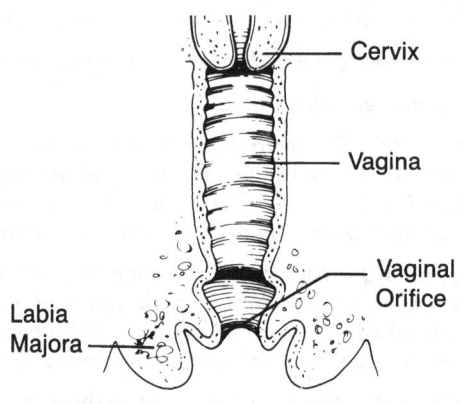

Cervix
Vagina
Vaginal Orifice
Labia Majora

VAGINA — CUT-AWAY VIEW

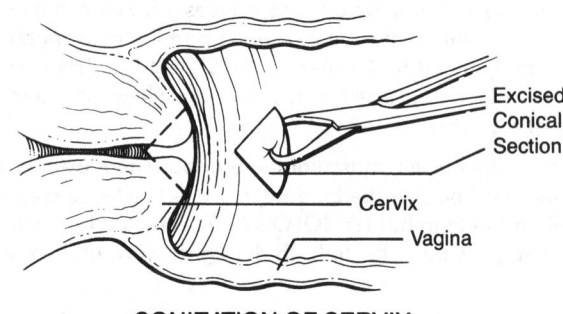

Excised Conical Section
Cervix
Vagina

CONIZATION OF CERVIX

FEMALE

0 U

Educational Annotations | U – Female Reproductive System

Definitions of Common Procedures of Female Reproductive System

Cervical cerclage – The placement of an encircling suture in the cervix to prevent a miscarriage or premature birth.

Hysterectomy – The surgical removal of the uterus (subtotal) and often the cervix (total).

Oophorectomy – The surgical removal of one or both ovaries.

Ovarian cystectomy – The surgical removal of an ovarian cyst leaving the ovary intact.

Salpingectomy – The surgical removal of one or both fallopian tubes.

Vaginoplasty – The plastic surgical restoration of vaginal defects or deformities.

AHA Coding Clinic® Reference Notations of Female Reproductive System

ROOT OPERATION SPECIFIC - U - FEMALE REPRODUCTIVE SYSTEM

BYPASS - 1
CHANGE - 2
DESTRUCTION - 5
DILATION - 7
DIVISION - 8
DRAINAGE - 9
EXCISION - B
  Excision of labia majora skin tags ....AHA 14:3Q:p12
  Partial salpingectomy ....AHA 15:3Q:p31
  Segmental excision of fallopian tubes ....AHA 15:3Q:p31
  Uterine fibroids, multiple ....AHA 14:4Q:p16
EXTIRPATION - C
  Clot evacuation from uterus post delivery ....AHA 13:2Q:p38
  Removal of cervical cerclage ....AHA 15:3Q:p30x2
EXTRACTION - D
FRAGMENTATION - F
INSERTION - H
  IUD insertion during cesarean section ....AHA 13:2Q:p34
INSPECTION - J
  Laparoscopic procedure converted to open ....AHA 15:1Q:p33
OCCLUSION - L
REATTACHMENT - M
RELEASE - N
REMOVAL - P
REPAIR - Q
  Periurethral obstetric laceration repair ....AHA 14:4Q:p18
  Repair of lacerated clitoris ....AHA 13:4Q:p120
REPOSITION - S
  Bimanual retroversion of pregnant uterus ....AHA 16:1Q:p9
RESECTION - T
  Bilateral oophorectomy ....AHA 15:1Q:p33
  Bilateral salpingectomy ....AHA 15:1Q:p33
  Hysterectomy ....AHA 15:1Q:p33
  Removal of cervix ....AHA 15:1Q:p33
  Removal of remaining portion of ovary ....AHA 13:1Q:p24
  Total (open) hysterectomy ....AHA 13:3Q:p28
SUPPLEMENT - U
RESTRICTION - V
  Cervical cerclage ....AHA 15:3Q:p30
REVISION - W
TRANSPLANTATION - Y

Educational Annotations | U – Female Reproductive System

Body Part Key Listings of Female Reproductive System

See also Body Part Key in Appendix C

Bartholin's (greater vestibular) gland	*use* Vestibular Gland
Broad ligament	*use* Uterine Supporting Structure
Fundus uteri	*use* Uterus
Greater vestibular (Bartholin's) gland	*use* Vestibular Gland
Infundibulopelvic ligament	*use* Uterine Supporting Structure
Labia majora	*use* Vulva
Labia minora	*use* Vulva
Myometrium	*use* Uterus
Ovarian ligament	*use* Uterine Supporting Structure
Oviduct	*use* Fallopian Tube, Left/Right
Paraurethral (Skene's) gland	*use* Vestibular Gland
Perimetrium	*use* Uterus
Round ligament of uterus	*use* Uterine Supporting Structure
Salpinx	*use* Fallopian Tube, Left/Right
Skene's (paraurethral) gland	*use* Vestibular Gland
Uterine cornu	*use* Uterus
Uterine tube	*use* Fallopian Tube, Left/Right

Device Key Listings of Female Reproductive System

See also Device Key in Appendix D

Autograft	*use* Autologous Tissue Substitute
Brachytherapy seeds	*use* Radioactive Element
Cook Biodesign® Fistula Plug(s)	*use* Nonautologous Tissue Substitute
Intrauterine device (IUD)	*use* Contraceptive Device in Female Reproductive System
Pessary ring	*use* Intraluminal Device, Pessary in Female Reproductive System
Tissue bank graft	*use* Nonautologous Tissue Substitute
Vaginal pessary	*use* Intraluminal Device, Pessary in Female Reproductive System

Device Aggregation Table Listings of Female Reproductive System

See also Device Aggregation Table in Appendix E

Specific Device	For Operation	In Body System	General Device
Intraluminal Device, Pessary	All applicable	Female Reproductive System	D Intraluminal Device

Educational Annotations | U – Female Reproductive System

Coding Notes of Female Reproductive System

Body System Specific PCS Reference Manual Exercises

PCS CODE	U – FEMALE REPRODUCTIVE SYSTEM EXERCISES
0 U 5 2 4 Z Z	Laparoscopy with destruction of endometriosis, bilateral ovaries.
0 U 7 7 8 Z Z	Hysteroscopy with balloon dilation of bilateral fallopian tubes.
0 U 9 1 4 Z Z	Laparoscopy with left ovarian cystotomy and drainage.
0 U B 1 4 Z Z	Laparoscopy with excision of endometrial implant from left ovary.
0 U C G 7 Z Z	Non-incisional removal of intraluminal foreign body from vagina. (The approach "External" is also a possibility. It is assumed here that since the patient went to the doctor to have the object removed, that it was not in the vaginal orifice.)
0 U D B 8 Z X	Hysteroscopy with D&C, diagnostic.
0 U D N 4 Z Z	Laparoscopy with needle aspiration of ova for in-vitro fertilization.
0 U F 6 8 Z Z	Hysteroscopy with intraluminal lithotripsy of left fallopian tube calcification.
0 U J D 8 Z Z	Colposcopy with diagnostic hysteroscopy.
0 U L 7 4 C Z	Laparoscopy with bilateral occlusion of fallopian tubes using Hulka extraluminal clips.
0 U N 1 4 Z Z	Laparoscopy with freeing of left ovary and fallopian tube.
0 U N 6 4 Z Z	
0 U P H 7 1 Z	Transvaginal removal of brachytherapy seeds.
0 U T 9 F Z Z	Laparoscopic-assisted vaginal hysterectomy, supracervical resection.
0 U V C 7 Z Z	Cervical cerclage using Shirodkar technique.

Educational Annotations | U – Female Reproductive System

NOTES

TUBULAR GROUP: Bypass, Dilation, Occlusion, Restriction
Root Operations that alter the diameter/route of a tubular body part.

1ST - **0** Medical and Surgical

2ND - **U** Female Reproductive System ♀

3RD - **1 BYPASS**

EXAMPLE: Fallopian tube bypass	CMS Ex: Coronary artery bypass

BYPASS: Altering the route of passage of the contents of a tubular body part.

EXPLANATION: Rerouting contents to a downstream part ...

Body Part – 4TH	Approach – 5TH	Device – 6TH	Qualifier – 7TH
5 Fallopian Tube, Right 6 Fallopian Tube, Left	0 Open 4 Percutaneous endoscopic	7 Autologous tissue substitute J Synthetic substitute K Nonautologous tissue substitute Z No device	5 Fallopian Tube, Right 6 Fallopian Tube, Left 9 Uterus

DEVICE GROUP: Change, Insertion, Removal, (Replacement), Revision, Supplement
Root Operations that always involve a device.

1ST - **0** Medical and Surgical

2ND - **U** Female Reproductive System ♀

3RD - **2 CHANGE**

EXAMPLE: Exchange drain tube	CMS Ex: Changing urinary catheter

CHANGE: Taking out or off a device from a body part and putting back an identical or similar device in or on the same body part without cutting or puncturing the skin or a mucous membrane.

EXPLANATION: ALL Changes use EXTERNAL approach only ...

Body Part – 4TH	Approach – 5TH	Device – 6TH	Qualifier – 7TH
3 Ovary 8 Fallopian Tube M Vulva	X External	0 Drainage device Y Other device	Z No qualifier
D Uterus and Cervix	X External	0 Drainage device H Contraceptive device Y Other device	Z No qualifier
H Vagina and Cul-de-sac	X External	0 Drainage device G Intraluminal device, pessary Y Other device	Z No qualifier

FEMALE

0 U 2

EXCISION GROUP: Excision, Resection, Destruction, Extraction, (Detachment)
Root Operations that take out some or all of a body part.

1ST – **0** Medical and Surgical

2ND – **U** Female Reproductive System ♀

3RD – **5 DESTRUCTION**

EXAMPLE: Fulguration endometriosis   CMS Ex: Fulguration polyp

DESTRUCTION: Physical eradication of all or a portion of a body part by the direct use of energy, force, or a destructive agent.

EXPLANATION: None of the body part is physically taken out

Body Part – 4TH	Approach – 5TH	Device – 6TH	Qualifier – 7TH
0 Ovary, Right 1 Ovary, Left 2 Ovaries, Bilateral 4 Uterine Supporting Structure	0 Open 3 Percutaneous 4 Percutaneous endoscopic	Z No device	Z No qualifier
5 Fallopian Tube, Right 6 Fallopian Tube, Left 7 Fallopian Tubes, Bilateral NC* 9 Uterus B Endometrium C Cervix F Cul-de-sac	0 Open 3 Percutaneous 4 Percutaneous endoscopic 7 Via natural or artificial opening 8 Via natural or artificial opening endoscopic	Z No device	Z No qualifier
G Vagina K Hymen	0 Open 3 Percutaneous 4 Percutaneous endoscopic 7 Via natural or artificial opening 8 Via natural or artificial opening endoscopic X External	Z No device	Z No qualifier
J Clitoris L Vestibular Gland M Vulva	0 Open X External	Z No device	Z No qualifier

NC* – Non-covered by Medicare. See current Medicare Code Editor for details.

FEMALE 0 U 5

TUBULAR GROUP: Bypass, Dilation, Occlusion, Restriction
Root Operations that alter the diameter/route of a tubular body part.

1ST – 0 Medical and Surgical

2ND – U Female Reproductive System ♀

3RD – 7 DILATION

EXAMPLE: Dilation fallopian tubes   CMS Ex: Transluminal angioplasty

<u>DILATION:</u> Expanding an orifice or the lumen of a tubular body part.

EXPLANATION: By force (stretching) or cutting ...

Body Part – 4TH	Approach – 5TH	Device – 6TH	Qualifier – 7TH
5 Fallopian Tube, Right 6 Fallopian Tube, Left 7 Fallopian Tubes, Bilateral 9 Uterus C Cervix G Vagina	0 Open 3 Percutaneous 4 Percutaneous endoscopic 7 Via natural or artificial opening 8 Via natural or artificial opening endoscopic	D Intraluminal device Z No device	Z No qualifier
K Hymen	0 Open 3 Percutaneous 4 Percutaneous endoscopic 7 Via natural or artificial opening 8 Via natural or artificial opening endoscopic X External	D Intraluminal device Z No device	Z No qualifier

DIVISION GROUP: Division, Release
Root Operations involving cutting or separation only.

1ST – 0 Medical and Surgical

2ND – U Female Reproductive System ♀

3RD – 8 DIVISION

EXAMPLE: Hymenotomy   CMS Ex: Osteotomy

<u>DIVISION:</u> Cutting into a body part without draining fluids and/or gases from the body part in order to separate or transect a body part.

EXPLANATION: Separated into two or more portions ...

Body Part – 4TH	Approach – 5TH	Device – 6TH	Qualifier – 7TH
0 Ovary, Right 1 Ovary, Left 2 Ovaries, Bilateral 4 Uterine Supporting Structure	0 Open 3 Percutaneous 4 Percutaneous endoscopic	Z No device	Z No qualifier
K Hymen	7 Via natural or artificial opening 8 Via natural or artificial opening endoscopic X External	Z No device	Z No qualifier

DRAINAGE GROUP: Drainage, Extirpation, Fragmentation
Root Operations that take out solids/fluids/gases from a body part.

1ST – 0 Medical and Surgical

2ND – U Female Reproductive System ♀

3RD – 9 DRAINAGE

EXAMPLE: Drainage ovarian cyst   CMS Ex: Thoracentesis

DRAINAGE: Taking or letting out fluids and/or gases from a body part.

EXPLANATION: Qualifier "X Diagnostic" indicates biopsy ...

Body Part – 4TH	Approach – 5TH	Device – 6TH	Qualifier – 7TH
0 Ovary, Right 1 Ovary, Left 2 Ovaries, Bilateral	0 Open 3 Percutaneous 4 Percutaneous endoscopic	0 Drainage device	Z No qualifier
0 Ovary, Right 1 Ovary, Left 2 Ovaries, Bilateral	0 Open 3 Percutaneous 4 Percutaneous endoscopic	Z No device	X Diagnostic Z No qualifier
0 Ovary, Right 1 Ovary, Left 2 Ovaries, Bilateral	X External	Z No device	Z No qualifier
4 Uterine Supporting Structure	0 Open 3 Percutaneous 4 Percutaneous endoscopic	0 Drainage device	Z No qualifier
4 Uterine Supporting Structure	0 Open 3 Percutaneous 4 Percutaneous endoscopic	Z No device	X Diagnostic Z No qualifier
5 Fallopian Tube, Right 6 Fallopian Tube, Left 7 Fallopian Tubes, Bilateral 9 Uterus C Cervix F Cul-de-sac	0 Open 3 Percutaneous 4 Percutaneous endoscopic 7 Via natural or artificial opening 8 Via natural or artificial opening endoscopic	0 Drainage device	Z No qualifier
5 Fallopian Tube, Right 6 Fallopian Tube, Left 7 Fallopian Tubes, Bilateral 9 Uterus C Cervix F Cul-de-sac	0 Open 3 Percutaneous 4 Percutaneous endoscopic 7 Via natural or artificial opening 8 Via natural or artificial opening endoscopic	Z No device	X Diagnostic Z No qualifier

continued ⇨

0 U 9	DRAINAGE – *continued*		
Body Part – 4TH	**Approach – 5TH**	**Device – 6TH**	**Qualifier – 7TH**
G Vagina K Hymen	0 Open 3 Percutaneous 4 Percutaneous endoscopic 7 Via natural or artificial opening 8 Via natural or artificial opening endoscopic X External	0 Drainage device	Z No qualifier
G Vagina K Hymen	0 Open 3 Percutaneous 4 Percutaneous endoscopic 7 Via natural or artificial opening 8 Via natural or artificial opening endoscopic X External	Z No device	X Diagnostic Z No qualifier
J Clitoris L Vestibular Gland M Vulva	0 Open X External	0 Drainage device	Z No qualifier
J Clitoris L Vestibular Gland M Vulva	0 Open X External	Z No device	X Diagnostic Z No qualifier

FEMALE 0 U 9

EXCISION GROUP: Excision, Resection, Destruction, Extraction, (Detachment)
Root Operations that take out some or all of a body part.

1ST - 0 Medical and Surgical	EXAMPLE: Excision uterine fibroids	CMS Ex: Liver biopsy
2ND - U Female Reproductive System ♀	**EXCISION:** Cutting out or off, without replacement, a portion of a body part.	
3RD - B EXCISION	EXPLANATION: Qualifier "X Diagnostic" indicates biopsy ...	

Body Part – 4TH	Approach – 5TH	Device – 6TH	Qualifier – 7TH
0 Ovary, Right 1 Ovary, Left 2 Ovaries, Bilateral 4 Uterine Supporting Structure 5 Fallopian Tube, Right 6 Fallopian Tube, Left 7 Fallopian Tubes, Bilateral 9 Uterus C Cervix F Cul-de-sac	0 Open 3 Percutaneous 4 Percutaneous endoscopic 7 Via natural or artificial opening 8 Via natural or artificial opening endoscopic	Z No device	X Diagnostic Z No qualifier
G Vagina K Hymen	0 Open 3 Percutaneous 4 Percutaneous endoscopic 7 Via natural or artificial opening 8 Via natural or artificial opening endoscopic X External	Z No device	X Diagnostic Z No qualifier
J Clitoris L Vestibular Gland M Vulva	0 Open X External	Z No device	X Diagnostic Z No qualifier

DRAINAGE GROUP: Drainage, Extirpation, Fragmentation
Root Operations that take out solids/fluids/gases from a body part.

1ST - **0** Medical and Surgical

2ND - **U** Female Reproductive System ♀

3RD - **C EXTIRPATION**

EXAMPLE: Clot evacuation post delivery | CMS Ex: Choledocholithotomy

EXTIRPATION: Taking or cutting out solid matter from a body part.

EXPLANATION: Abnormal byproduct or foreign body ...

Body Part – 4TH	Approach – 5TH	Device – 6TH	Qualifier – 7TH
0 Ovary, Right 1 Ovary, Left 2 Ovaries, Bilateral 4 Uterine Supporting Structure	0 Open 3 Percutaneous 4 Percutaneous endoscopic	Z No device	Z No qualifier
5 Fallopian Tube, Right 6 Fallopian Tube, Left 7 Fallopian Tubes, Bilateral 9 Uterus B Endometrium C Cervix F Cul-de-sac	0 Open 3 Percutaneous 4 Percutaneous endoscopic 7 Via natural or artificial opening 8 Via natural or artificial opening endoscopic	Z No device	Z No qualifier
G Vagina K Hymen	0 Open 3 Percutaneous 4 Percutaneous endoscopic 7 Via natural or artificial opening 8 Via natural or artificial opening endoscopic X External	Z No device	Z No qualifier
J Clitoris L Vestibular Gland M Vulva	0 Open X External	Z No device	Z No qualifier

FEMALE

0 U C

© 2016 Channel Publishing, Ltd.

EXCISION GROUP: Excision, Resection, Destruction, Extraction, (Detachment)
Root Operations that take out some or all of a body part.

1ST - **0** Medical and Surgical

2ND - **U** Female Reproductive System ♀

3RD - **D EXTRACTION**

EXAMPLE: Dilation and curettage | CMS Ex: D&C

EXTRACTION: Pulling or stripping out or off all or a portion of a body part by the use of force.

EXPLANATION: Qualifier "X Diagnostic" indicates biopsy ...

Body Part – 4TH	Approach – 5TH	Device – 6TH	Qualifier – 7TH
B Endometrium	7 Via natural or artificial opening 8 Via natural or artificial opening endoscopic	Z No device	X Diagnostic Z No qualifier
N Ova	0 Open 3 Percutaneous 4 Percutaneous endoscopic	Z No device	Z No qualifier

---

DRAINAGE GROUP: Drainage, Extirpation, Fragmentation
Root Operations that take out solids/fluids/gases from a body part.

1ST - **0** Medical and Surgical

2ND - **U** Female Reproductive System ♀

3RD - **F FRAGMENTATION**

EXAMPLE: Lithotripsy fallopian tube calcification | CMS Ex: ESWL

FRAGMENTATION: Breaking solid matter in a body part into pieces.

EXPLANATION: Pieces are not taken out during procedure ...

Body Part – 4TH	Approach – 5TH	Device – 6TH	Qualifier – 7TH
5 Fallopian Tube, Right 6 Fallopian Tube, Left 7 Fallopian Tubes, Bilateral 9 Uterus	0 Open 3 Percutaneous 4 Percutaneous endoscopic 7 Via natural or artificial opening 8 Via natural or artificial opening endoscopic X External NC*	Z No device	Z No qualifier

NC* – Non-covered by Medicare. See current Medicare Code Editor for details.

DEVICE GROUP: Change, Insertion, Removal, (Replacement), Revision, Supplement
Root Operations that always involve a device.

1ST - 0 Medical and Surgical

2ND - U Female Reproductive System ♀

3RD - H INSERTION

EXAMPLE: Insertion of IUD		CMS Ex: Insertion central venous catheter	

INSERTION: Putting in a nonbiological appliance that monitors, assists, performs, or prevents a physiological function but does not physically take the place of a body part.

EXPLANATION: None

Body Part – 4TH	Approach – 5TH	Device – 6TH	Qualifier – 7TH
3 Ovary	0 Open 3 Percutaneous 4 Percutaneous endoscopic	3 Infusion device	Z No qualifier
8 Fallopian Tube D Uterus and Cervix H Vagina and Cul-de-sac	0 Open 3 Percutaneous 4 Percutaneous endoscopic 7 Via natural or artificial opening 8 Via natural or artificial opening endoscopic	3 Infusion device	Z No qualifier
9 Uterus	7 Via natural or artificial opening 8 Via natural or artificial opening endoscopic	H Contraceptive device	Z No qualifier
C Cervix	0 Open 3 Percutaneous 4 Percutaneous endoscopic	1 Radioactive element	Z No qualifier
C Cervix	7 Via natural or artificial opening 8 Via natural or artificial opening endoscopic	1 Radioactive element H Contraceptive device	Z No qualifier
F Cul-de-sac	7 Via natural or artificial opening 8 Via natural or artificial opening endoscopic	G Intraluminal device, pessary	Z No qualifier
G Vagina	0 Open 3 Percutaneous 4 Percutaneous endoscopic X External	1 Radioactive element	Z No qualifier
G Vagina	7 Via natural or artificial opening 8 Via natural or artificial opening endoscopic	1 Radioactive element G Intraluminal device, pessary	Z No qualifier

FEMALE

0 U H

633

EXAMINATION GROUP: Inspection, (Map)

Root Operations involving examination only.

1ST - **0** Medical and Surgical	EXAMPLE: Hysteroscopy			CMS Ex: Colonoscopy
2ND - **U** Female Reproductive System ♀	**INSPECTION:** Visually and/or manually exploring a body part.			
3RD - **J** INSPECTION	EXPLANATION: Direct or instrumental visualization ...			

Body Part – 4TH	Approach – 5TH	Device – 6TH	Qualifier – 7TH
3 Ovary	0 Open 3 Percutaneous 4 Percutaneous endoscopic X External	Z No device	Z No qualifier
8 Fallopian Tube D Uterus and Cervix H Vagina and Cul-de-sac	0 Open 3 Percutaneous 4 Percutaneous endoscopic 7 Via natural or artificial opening 8 Via natural or artificial opening endoscopic X External	Z No device	Z No qualifier
M Vulva	0 Open X External	Z No device	Z No qualifier

TUBULAR GROUP: Bypass, Dilation, Occlusion, Restriction
Root Operations that alter the diameter/route of a tubular body part.

1ST – 0 Medical and Surgical

2ND – U Female Reproductive System ♀

3RD – L OCCLUSION

EXAMPLE: Fallopian tube clipping | CMS Ex: Fallopian tube ligation

OCCLUSION: Completely closing an orifice or lumen of a tubular body part.

EXPLANATION: Natural or artificially created orifice ...

Body Part – 4TH	Approach – 5TH	Device – 6TH	Qualifier – 7TH
5 Fallopian Tube, Right 6 Fallopian Tube, Left 7 Fallopian Tubes, Bilateral NC*	0 Open 3 Percutaneous 4 Percutaneous endoscopic	C Extraluminal device D Intraluminal device Z No device	Z No qualifier
5 Fallopian Tube, Right 6 Fallopian Tube, Left 7 Fallopian Tubes, Bilateral NC*	7 Via natural or artificial opening 8 Via natural or artificial opening endoscopic	D Intraluminal device Z No device	Z No qualifier
F Cul-de-sac G Vagina	7 Via natural or artificial opening 8 Via natural or artificial opening endoscopic	D Intraluminal device Z No device	Z No qualifier

NC* – Non-covered by Medicare. See current Medicare Code Editor for details.

MOVE GROUP: Reattachment, Reposition, (Transfer), Transplantation
Root Operations that put in/put back or move some/all of a body part.

1ST – 0 Medical and Surgical

2ND – U Female Reproductive System ♀

3RD – M REATTACHMENT

EXAMPLE: Reattach avulsed round ligament | CMS Ex: Reattachment hand

REATTACHMENT: Putting back in or on all or a portion of a separated body part to its normal location or other suitable location.

EXPLANATION: With/without reconnection of vessels/nerves...

Body Part – 4TH	Approach – 5TH	Device – 6TH	Qualifier – 7TH
0 Ovary, Right 6 Fallopian Tube, Left 1 Ovary, Left 7 Fallopian Tubes, Bilateral 2 Ovaries, Bilateral 9 Uterus 4 Uterine Supporting C Cervix Structure F Cul-de-sac 5 Fallopian Tube, Right G Vagina	0 Open 4 Percutaneous endoscopic	Z No device	Z No qualifier
J Clitoris M Vulva	X External	Z No device	Z No qualifier
K Hymen	0 Open 4 Percutaneous endoscopic X External	Z No device	Z No qualifier

F E M A L E

0 U M

DIVISION GROUP: Division, Release
Root Operations involving cutting or separation only.

| 1ST - O Medical and Surgical |
| 2ND - U Female Reproductive System ♀ |
| 3RD - N RELEASE |

EXAMPLE: Adhesiolysis ovary and tube | CMS Ex: Carpal tunnel release

RELEASE: Freeing a body part from an abnormal physical constraint by cutting or by the use of force.

EXPLANATION: None of the body part is taken out …

Body Part – 4TH	Approach – 5TH	Device – 6TH	Qualifier – 7TH
0 Ovary, Right 1 Ovary, Left 2 Ovaries, Bilateral 4 Uterine Supporting Structure	0 Open 3 Percutaneous 4 Percutaneous endoscopic	Z No device	Z No qualifier
5 Fallopian Tube, Right 6 Fallopian Tube, Left 7 Fallopian Tubes, Bilateral 9 Uterus C Cervix F Cul-de-sac	0 Open 3 Percutaneous 4 Percutaneous endoscopic 7 Via natural or artificial opening 8 Via natural or artificial opening endoscopic	Z No device	Z No qualifier
G Vagina K Hymen	0 Open 3 Percutaneous 4 Percutaneous endoscopic 7 Via natural or artificial opening 8 Via natural or artificial opening endoscopic X External	Z No device	Z No qualifier
J Clitoris L Vestibular Gland M Vulva	0 Open X External	Z No device	Z No qualifier

FEMALE

O U N

DEVICE GROUP: Change, Insertion, Removal, (Replacement), Revision, Supplement
Root Operations that always involve a device.

1ST - 0 Medical and Surgical

2ND - U Female Reproductive System ♀

3RD - P REMOVAL

EXAMPLE: Removal IUD	CMS Ex: Chest tube removal

REMOVAL: Taking out or off a device from a body part.

EXPLANATION: Removal device without reinsertion ...

Body Part – 4TH	Approach – 5TH	Device – 6TH	Qualifier – 7TH
3 Ovary	0 Open 3 Percutaneous 4 Percutaneous endoscopic X External	0 Drainage device 3 Infusion device	Z No qualifier
8 Fallopian Tube	0 Open 3 Percutaneous 4 Percutaneous endoscopic 7 Via natural or artificial opening 8 Via natural or artificial opening endoscopic	0 Drainage device 3 Infusion device 7 Autologous tissue substitute C Extraluminal device D Intraluminal device J Synthetic substitute K Nonautologous tissue substitute	Z No qualifier
8 Fallopian Tube	X External	0 Drainage device 3 Infusion device D Intraluminal device	Z No qualifier
D Uterus and Cervix	0 Open 3 Percutaneous 4 Percutaneous endoscopic 7 Via natural or artificial opening 8 Via natural or artificial opening endoscopic	0 Drainage device 1 Radioactive element 3 Infusion device 7 Autologous tissue substitute C Extraluminal device D Intraluminal device H Contraceptive device J Synthetic substitute K Nonautologous tissue substitute	Z No qualifier
D Uterus and Cervix	X External	0 Drainage device 3 Infusion device D Intraluminal device H Contraceptive device	Z No qualifier

FEMALE

0 U P

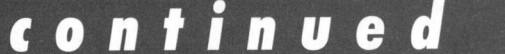

0 U P   REMOVAL – continued

Body Part – 4TH	Approach – 5TH	Device – 6TH	Qualifier – 7TH
H Vagina and Cul-de-sac	0 Open 3 Percutaneous 4 Percutaneous endoscopic 7 Via natural or artificial opening 8 Via natural or artificial opening endoscopic	0 Drainage device 1 Radioactive element 3 Infusion device 7 Autologous tissue substitute D Intraluminal device J Synthetic substitute K Nonautologous tissue substitute	Z No qualifier
H Vagina and Cul-de-sac	X External	0 Drainage device 1 Radioactive element 3 Infusion device D Intraluminal device	Z No qualifier
M Vulva	0 Open	0 Drainage device 7 Autologous tissue substitute J Synthetic substitute K Nonautologous tissue substitute	Z No qualifier
M Vulva	X External	0 Drainage device	Z No qualifier

FEMALE

0 U P

© 2016 Channel Publishing, Ltd.

OTHER REPAIRS GROUP: (Control), Repair
Root Operations that define other repairs.

1ST - 0 Medical and Surgical 2ND - U Female Reproductive System ♀ 3RD - Q REPAIR	EXAMPLE: Repair vulvar laceration		CMS Ex: Suture laceration
	REPAIR: Restoring, to the extent possible, a body part to its normal anatomic structure and function.		
	EXPLANATION: Only when no other root operation applies ...		

Body Part – 4TH	Approach – 5TH	Device – 6TH	Qualifier – 7TH
0 Ovary, Right 1 Ovary, Left 2 Ovaries, Bilateral 4 Uterine Supporting Structure	0 Open 3 Percutaneous 4 Percutaneous endoscopic	Z No device	Z No qualifier
5 Fallopian Tube, Right 6 Fallopian Tube, Left 7 Fallopian Tubes, Bilateral 9 Uterus C Cervix F Cul-de-sac	0 Open 3 Percutaneous 4 Percutaneous endoscopic 7 Via natural or artificial opening 8 Via natural or artificial opening endoscopic	Z No device	Z No qualifier
G Vagina K Hymen	0 Open 3 Percutaneous 4 Percutaneous endoscopic 7 Via natural or artificial opening 8 Via natural or artificial opening endoscopic X External	Z No device	Z No qualifier
J Clitoris L Vestibular Gland M Vulva	0 Open X External	Z No device	Z No qualifier

MOVE GROUP: Reattachment, Reposition, (Transfer), Transplantation
Root Operations that put in/put back or move some/all of a body part.

1ST - 0 Medical and Surgical 2ND - U Female Reproductive System ♀ 3RD - S REPOSITION	EXAMPLE: Relocation fallopian tube		CMS Ex: Fracture reduction
	REPOSITION: Moving to its normal location, or other suitable location, all or a portion of a body part.		
	EXPLANATION: May or may not be cut to be moved ...		

Body Part – 4TH	Approach – 5TH	Device – 6TH	Qualifier – 7TH
0 Ovary, Right 6 Fallopian Tube, Left 1 Ovary, Left 7 Fallopian Tubes, Bilateral 2 Ovaries, Bilateral C Cervix 4 Uterine Supporting F Cul-de-sac Structure 5 Fallopian Tube, Right	0 Open 4 Percutaneous endoscopic	Z No device	Z No qualifier
9 Uterus G Vagina	0 Open 4 Percutaneous endoscopic X External	Z No device	Z No qualifier

FEMALE

0 U S

EXCISION GROUP: Excision, Resection, Destruction, Extraction, (Detachment)
Root Operations that take out some or all of a body part.

1ST – **0** Medical and Surgical

2ND – **U** Female Reproductive System ♀

3RD – **T RESECTION**

EXAMPLE: Bilateral oophorectomy

CMS Ex: Cholecystectomy

RESECTION: Cutting out or off, without replacement, all of a body part.

EXPLANATION: None

Body Part – 4TH	Approach – 5TH	Device – 6TH	Qualifier – 7TH
0 Ovary, Right 1 Ovary, Left 2 Ovaries, Bilateral 5 Fallopian Tube, Right 6 Fallopian Tube, Left 7 Fallopian Tubes, Bilateral 9 Uterus	0 Open 4 Percutaneous endoscopic 7 Via natural or artificial opening 8 Via natural or artificial opening endoscopic F Via natural or artificial opening with percutaneous endoscopic assistance	Z No device	Z No qualifier
4 Uterine Supporting Structure C Cervix F Cul-de-sac G Vagina	0 Open 4 Percutaneous endoscopic 7 Via natural or artificial opening 8 Via natural or artificial opening endoscopic	Z No device	Z No qualifier
J Clitoris L Vestibular Gland M Vulva	0 Open X External	Z No device	Z No qualifier
K Hymen	0 Open 4 Percutaneous endoscopic 7 Via natural or artificial opening 8 Via natural or artificial opening endoscopic X External	Z No device	Z No qualifier

FEMALE

O U T

DEVICE GROUP: Change, Insertion, Removal, (Replacement), Revision, Supplement
Root Operations that always involve a device.

1ST - 0 Medical and Surgical

2ND - U Female Reproductive System ♀

3RD - U SUPPLEMENT

EXAMPLE: Colporrhaphy with mesh | CMS Ex: Hernia repair with mesh

SUPPLEMENT: Putting in or on biological or synthetic material that physically reinforces and/or augments the function of a portion of a body part.

EXPLANATION: Biological material from same individual ...

Body Part – 4TH	Approach – 5TH	Device – 6TH	Qualifier – 7TH
4 Uterine Supporting Structure	0 Open 4 Percutaneous endoscopic	7 Autologous tissue substitute J Synthetic substitute K Nonautologous tissue substitute	Z No qualifier
5 Fallopian Tube, Right 6 Fallopian Tube, Left 7 Fallopian Tubes, Bilateral F Cul-de-sac	0 Open 4 Percutaneous endoscopic 7 Via natural or artificial opening 8 Via natural or artificial opening endoscopic	7 Autologous tissue substitute J Synthetic substitute K Nonautologous tissue substitute	Z No qualifier
G Vagina K Hymen	0 Open 4 Percutaneous endoscopic 7 Via natural or artificial opening 8 Via natural or artificial opening endoscopic X External	7 Autologous tissue substitute J Synthetic substitute K Nonautologous tissue substitute	Z No qualifier
J Clitoris M Vulva	0 Open X External	7 Autologous tissue substitute J Synthetic substitute K Nonautologous tissue substitute	Z No qualifier

FEMALE

0 U U

TUBULAR GROUP: Bypass, Dilation, Occlusion, Restriction			
Root Operations that alter the diameter/route of a tubular body part.			

1ST - 0 Medical and Surgical	EXAMPLE: Cervical cerclage		CMS Ex: Cervical cerclage
2ND - U Female Reproductive System ♀	**RESTRICTION:** Partially closing an orifice or the lumen of a tubular body part.		
3RD - V RESTRICTION	EXPLANATION: Natural or artificially created orifice ...		

Body Part – 4TH	Approach – 5TH	Device – 6TH	Qualifier – 7TH
C Cervix	0 Open 3 Percutaneous 4 Percutaneous endoscopic	C Extraluminal device D Intraluminal device Z No device	Z No qualifier
C Cervix	7 Via natural or artificial opening 8 Via natural or artificial opening endoscopic	D Intraluminal device Z No device	Z No qualifier

FEMALE

0
U
V

© 2016 Channel Publishing, Ltd.

DEVICE GROUP: Change, Insertion, Removal, (Replacement), Revision, Supplement
Root Operations that always involve a device.

1ST – **0** Medical and Surgical	EXAMPLE: Reposition intrauterine device CMS Ex: Adjustment lead
2ND – **U** Female Reproductive System ♀	**REVISION:** Correcting, to the extent possible, a portion of a malfunctioning device or the position of a displaced device.
3RD – **W REVISION**	EXPLANATION: May replace components of a device ...

Body Part – 4TH	Approach – 5TH	Device – 6TH	Qualifier – 7TH
3 Ovary	0 Open 3 Percutaneous 4 Percutaneous endoscopic X External	0 Drainage device 3 Infusion device	Z No qualifier
8 Fallopian Tube	0 Open 3 Percutaneous 4 Percutaneous endoscopic 7 Via natural or artificial opening 8 Via natural or artificial opening endoscopic X External	0 Drainage device 3 Infusion device 7 Autologous tissue substitute C Extraluminal device D Intraluminal device J Synthetic substitute K Nonautologous tissue substitute	Z No qualifier
D Uterus and Cervix	0 Open 3 Percutaneous 4 Percutaneous endoscopic 7 Via natural or artificial opening 8 Via natural or artificial opening endoscopic	0 Drainage device 1 Radioactive element 3 Infusion device 7 Autologous tissue substitute C Extraluminal device D Intraluminal device H Contraceptive device J Synthetic substitute K Nonautologous tissue substitute	Z No qualifier
D Uterus and Cervix	X External	0 Drainage device 3 Infusion device 7 Autologous tissue substitute C Extraluminal device D Intraluminal device H Contraceptive device J Synthetic substitute K Nonautologous tissue substitute	Z No qualifier

FEMALE

0 U W

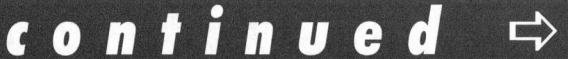

0 U W   REVISION – *continued*

Body Part – 4TH	Approach – 5TH	Device – 6TH	Qualifier – 7TH
H Vagina and Cul-de-sac	0 Open 3 Percutaneous 4 Percutaneous endoscopic 7 Via natural or artificial opening 8 Via natural or artificial opening endoscopic	0 Drainage device 1 Radioactive element 3 Infusion device 7 Autologous tissue substitute D Intraluminal device J Synthetic substitute K Nonautologous tissue substitute	Z No qualifier
H Vagina and Cul-de-sac	X External	0 Drainage device 3 Infusion device 7 Autologous tissue substitute D Intraluminal device J Synthetic substitute K Nonautologous tissue substitute	Z No qualifier
M Vulva	0 Open X External	0 Drainage device 7 Autologous tissue substitute J Synthetic substitute K Nonautologous tissue substitute	Z No qualifier

(Side tab: FEMALE / 0 U W)

MOVE GROUP: Reattachment, Reposition, (Transfer), Transplantation
Root Operations that put in/put back or move some/all of a body part.

1ST – **0** Medical and Surgical

2ND – **U** Female Reproductive System ♀

3RD – **Y** TRANSPLANTATION

EXAMPLE: Ovarian transplant   CMS Ex: Kidney transplant

TRANSPLANTATION: Putting in or on all or a portion of a living body part taken from another individual or animal to physically take the place and/or function of all or a portion of a similar body part.

EXPLANATION: May take over all or part of its function ...

Body Part – 4TH	Approach – 5TH	Device – 6TH	Qualifier – 7TH
0 Ovary, Right 1 Ovary, Left	0 Open	Z No device	0 Allogeneic 1 Syngeneic 2 Zooplastic

Educational Annotations | V – Male Reproductive System

Body System Specific Educational Annotations for the Male Reproductive System include:
- Anatomy and Physiology Review
- Anatomical Illustrations
- Definitions of Common Procedures
- AHA Coding Clinic® Reference Notations
- Body Part Key Listings
- Device Key Listings
- Device Aggregation Table Listings
- Coding Notes

Anatomy and Physiology Review of Male Reproductive System

BODY PART VALUES – V - MALE REPRODUCTIVE SYSTEM

Epididymis – ANATOMY – The epididymis is a tightly coiled, threadlike tube that is about 20 feet (6 m) long. It is connected to ducts within the testis and emerges from the top of the testis, descends along its posterior surface, and then courses upward to become the vas deferens. PHYSIOLOGY – The epididymis functions to store and mature sperm cells, and to transport the sperm from the testicular ducts to the vas deferens.

Penis – ANATOMY – The penis is the cylindrical male sexual organ which contains the urethra and is located at the base of the male perineum. The body (shaft) is composed of 3 columns of erectile tissue, including a pair of dorsally located corpora cavernosa and a single corpus spongiosum below. The corpus spongiosum, through which the urethra extends, is enlarged at its distal end to form a sensitive, cone-shaped glans penis. A loose fold of skin, called the prepuce (foreskin) covers the glans penis, unless removed by circumcision. PHYSIOLOGY – The penis functions as the specialized sexual organ in the male that when erect is inserted into the female vagina for sexual intercourse. It also functions to convey urine and seminal fluid through the urethra to the outside at the urethral opening (meatus). Erection is obtained by sexual excitement, stimulating parasympathetic nerve impulses causing blood engorgement of the corpora cavernosa and corpus spongiosum.

Prepuce – The loose fold of skin (foreskin) that covers the glans penis, unless removed by circumcision.

Prostate – ANATOMY – The walnut-shaped male reproductive organ that surrounds the urethra just below the bladder. PHYSIOLOGY – The prostate secretes a slightly alkaline fluid that constitutes approximately one-third of the volume of the semen. The alkalinity of semen helps neutralize the acidity of the vaginal tract, prolonging the lifespan of sperm.

Scrotum – ANATOMY – The scrotum is a pouch of skin, subcutaneous, and muscular tissue that hangs from the lower abdominal region behind the penis. PHYSIOLOGY – The scrotum protects the testis and spermatic cord by contracting and relaxing the dartos muscle.

Seminal Vesicle – ANATOMY – A pair of tubular male reproductive glands that are located above the prostate and below the bladder. They pass into the prostatic tissue and their excretory ducts open into the vas deferens and form the ejaculatory ducts. PHYSIOLOGY – The seminal vesicles secrete approximately two-thirds of the ejaculated semen volume. The nutrient-rich seminal fluid provides energy for the sperm cells.

Spermatic Cord – ANATOMY – The spermatic cord is a canal of peritoneal tissue about 18 inches (45 cm) long beginning at the testis and ending in the ejaculatory duct, and is externally contained along with the testis in the scrotum. PHYSIOLOGY – The spermatic cord contains and protects the vas deferens, arteries, nerves, and lymphatic vessels.

Testis – ANATOMY – The testes are the male reproductive organs that are ovoid structures in the scrotum, suspended by a spermatic cord, and approximately 2 inches (5 cm) in length and 1.2 inches (3 cm) in diameter. Each testis is enclosed by a tough, white fibrous capsule called the tunica albuginea. PHYSIOLOGY – The testes function to produce sperm cells for human reproduction and secrete male hormones, primarily testosterone.

Tunica Vaginalis – The serous membrane covering of the testes that is comprised of two layers, visceral and parietal.

Vas Deferens – ANATOMY – The vas deferens (ductus deferens) is a muscular tube that begins at the epididymis and ends at the union of the seminal vesicle and forms the ejaculatory duct within the prostatic tissue. PHYSIOLOGY – The vas deferens transports the sperm using peristalsis from the testis/epididymis to the ejaculatory duct.

Educational Annotations | V – Male Reproductive System

Anatomical Illustrations of Male Reproductive System

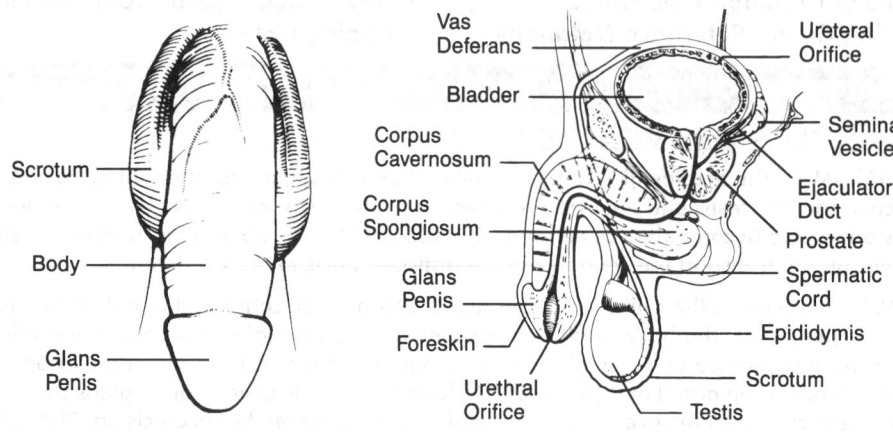

PENIS — FRONTAL VIEW

MALE GENITAL ORGANS — SAGITTAL VIEW

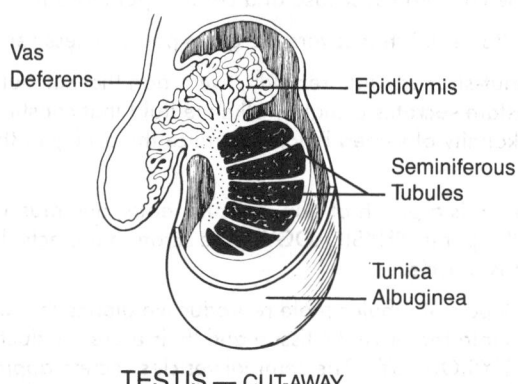

TESTIS — CUT-AWAY

Definitions of Common Procedures of Male Reproductive System

Orchiectomy – The surgical removal of one or both of the testicles.

Orchiopexy – The surgical procedure to move an undescended testicle into the scrotum and secure it in place.

Radical retropubic prostatectomy – The surgical removal of the entire prostate gland and some surrounding tissues that is performed through an open approach between the belly button and pubic bone.

TUNA (transurethral needle ablation of prostate) – The transurethral endoscopic destruction of prostate tissue using radiofrequency (RF) needles that delivers heat to reduce benign prostatic hyperplasia.

TURP (transurethral resection of prostate) – The surgical removal of part or all (total) of the prostate gland through an endoscopic approach.

Vasoepididymostomy – The microsurgical anastomosis of the epididymis to the vas deferens to reverse a vasectomy or to overcome an epididymal obstruction.

Vasovasostomy – The surgical re-anastomosis of the severed vas deferens to reverse a vasectomy.

Educational Annotations | V – Male Reproductive System

AHA Coding Clinic® Reference Notations of Male Reproductive System

<u>ROOT OPERATION SPECIFIC - V - MALE REPRODUCTIVE SYSTEM</u>
BYPASS - 1
CHANGE - 2
DESTRUCTION - 5
DILATION - 7
DRAINAGE - 9
EXCISION - B
    Transurethral resection of ejaculatory ducts ....AHA 16:1Q:p23
EXTIRPATION - C
INSERTION - H
INSPECTION - J
OCCLUSION - L
REATTACHMENT - M
RELEASE - N
REMOVAL - P
    Removal and insertion of penile implant.................................AHA 16:2Q:p28
REPAIR - Q
REPLACEMENT - R
REPOSITION - S
RESECTION - T
    Radical prostatectomy, robotic-assisted, with bilateral resection of
        vas deferens and seminal vesicles ....AHA 14:4Q:p33
SUPPLEMENT - U
    Placement of inflatable penile implant ....AHA 15:3Q:p25
    Removal and insertion of penile implant.................................AHA 16:2Q:p28
REVISION - W

Body Part Key Listings of Male Reproductive System

See also Body Part Key in Appendix C
Corpus cavernosum ....*use* Penis
Corpus spongiosum ....*use* Penis
Ductus deferens ....*use* Vas Deferens, Bilateral/Left/Right
Ejaculatory duct ....*use* Vas Deferens, Bilateral/Left/Right
Foreskin ....*use* Prepuce
Glans penis ....*use* Prepuce

Device Key Listings of Male Reproductive System

See also Device Key in Appendix D
Autograft ....*use* Autologous Tissue Substitute
Brachytherapy seeds ....*use* Radioactive Element
Cook Biodesign® Fistula Plug(s) ....*use* Nonautologous Tissue Substitute
Tissue bank graft ....*use* Nonautologous Tissue Substitute

Device Aggregation Table Listings of Male Reproductive System

See also Device Aggregation Table in Appendix E

Specific Device	For Operation	In Body System	General Device
None Listed in Device Aggregation Table for this Body System

Educational Annotations | V – Male Reproductive System

Coding Notes of Male Reproductive System

Body System Specific PCS Reference Manual Exercises

PCS CODE	V – MALE REPRODUCTIVE SYSTEM EXERCISES
0 V 5 0 8 Z Z	Transurethral endoscopic laser ablation of prostate.
0 V H 0 8 1 Z	Cystoscopy with placement of brachytherapy seeds in prostate gland.
0 V T 0 0 Z Z	Total retropubic prostatectomy, open.

TUBULAR GROUP: Bypass, Dilation, Occlusion, (Restriction)
Root Operations that alter the diameter/route of a tubular body part.

1ST - **0** Medical and Surgical

2ND - **V** Male Reproductive System ♂

3RD - **1 BYPASS**

EXAMPLE: Vasoepididymostomy   CMS Ex: Coronary artery bypass

BYPASS: Altering the route of passage of the contents of a tubular body part.

EXPLANATION: Rerouting contents to a downstream part …

Body Part – 4TH	Approach – 5TH	Device – 6TH	Qualifier – 7TH
N Vas Deferens, Right P Vas Deferens, Left Q Vas Deferens, Bilateral	0 Open 4 Percutaneous endoscopic	7 Autologous tissue substitute J Synthetic substitute K Nonautologous tissue substitute Z No device	J Epididymis, Right K Epididymis, Left N Vas Deferens, Right P Vas Deferens, Left

---

DEVICE GROUP: Change, Insertion, Removal, Replacement, Revision, Supplement
Root Operations that always involve a device.

1ST - **0** Medical and Surgical

2ND - **V** Male Reproductive System ♂

3RD - **2 CHANGE**

EXAMPLE: Exchange drain tube   CMS Ex: Changing urinary catheter

CHANGE: Taking out or off a device from a body part and putting back an identical or similar device in or on the same body part without cutting or puncturing the skin or a mucous membrane.

EXPLANATION: ALL Changes use EXTERNAL approach only …

Body Part – 4TH	Approach – 5TH	Device – 6TH	Qualifier – 7TH
4 Prostate and Seminal Vesicles 8 Scrotum and Tunica Vaginalis D Testis M Epididymis and Spermatic Cord R Vas Deferens S Penis	X External	0 Drainage device Y Other device	Z No qualifier

MALE   0 V 2

EXCISION GROUP: Excision, Resection, Destruction, (Extraction), (Detachment)
Root Operations that take out some or all of a body part.

1ST - **0** Medical and Surgical

2ND - **V** Male Reproductive System ♂

3RD - **5 DESTRUCTION**

EXAMPLE: Needle ablation (TUNA) prostate | CMS Ex: Fulguration polyp

DESTRUCTION: Physical eradication of all or a portion of a body part by the direct use of energy, force, or a destructive agent.

EXPLANATION: None of the body part is physically taken out

Body Part – 4TH	Approach – 5TH	Device – 6TH	Qualifier – 7TH
0 Prostate	0 Open 3 Percutaneous 4 Percutaneous endoscopic 7 Via natural or artificial opening 8 Via natural or artificial opening endoscopic	Z No device	Z No qualifier
1 Seminal Vesicle, Right 2 Seminal Vesicle, Left 3 Seminal Vesicles, Bilateral 6 Tunica Vaginalis, Right 7 Tunica Vaginalis, Left 9 Testis, Right B Testis, Left C Testes, Bilateral F Spermatic Cord, Right G Spermatic Cord, Left H Spermatic Cords, Bilateral J Epididymis, Right K Epididymis, Left L Epididymis, Bilateral N Vas Deferens, Right NC* P Vas Deferens, Left NC* Q Vas Deferens, Bilateral NC*	0 Open 3 Percutaneous 4 Percutaneous endoscopic	Z No device	Z No qualifier
5 Scrotum S Penis T Prepuce	0 Open 3 Percutaneous 4 Percutaneous endoscopic X External	Z No device	Z No qualifier

NC* – Some procedures are considered non-covered by Medicare. See current Medicare Code Editor for details.

TUBULAR GROUP: Bypass, Dilation, Occlusion, (Restriction)
Root Operations that alter the diameter/route of a tubular body part.

1ST - **0** Medical and Surgical

2ND - **V** Male Reproductive System ♂

3RD - **7 DILATION**

EXAMPLE: Dilation vas deferens | CMS Ex: Transluminal angioplasty

DILATION: Expanding an orifice or the lumen of a tubular body part.

EXPLANATION: By force (stretching) or cutting ...

Body Part – 4TH	Approach – 5TH	Device – 6TH	Qualifier – 7TH
N Vas Deferens, Right P Vas Deferens, Left Q Vas Deferens, Bilateral	0 Open 3 Percutaneous 4 Percutaneous endoscopic	D Intraluminal device Z No device	Z No qualifier

MALE

0 V 5

DRAINAGE GROUP: Drainage, Extirpation, (Fragmentation)			
Root Operations that take out solids/fluids/gases from a body part.			

1ST - 0 Medical and Surgical

2ND - V Male Reproductive System ♂

3RD - 9 DRAINAGE

EXAMPLE: Drainage epididymal cyst　　CMS Ex: Thoracentesis

DRAINAGE: Taking or letting out fluids and/or gases from a body part.

EXPLANATION: Qualifier "X Diagnostic" indicates biopsy ...

Body Part – 4TH		Approach – 5TH	Device – 6TH	Qualifier – 7TH
0 Prostate		0 Open 3 Percutaneous 4 Percutaneous endoscopic 7 Via natural or artificial opening 8 Via natural or artificial opening endoscopic	0 Drainage device	Z No qualifier
0 Prostate		0 Open 3 Percutaneous 4 Percutaneous endoscopic 7 Via natural or artificial opening 8 Via natural or artificial opening endoscopic	Z No device	X Diagnostic Z No qualifier
1 Seminal Vesicle, Right 2 Seminal Vesicle, Left 3 Seminal Vesicles, Bilateral 6 Tunica Vaginalis, Right 7 Tunica Vaginalis, Left 9 Testis, Right B Testis, Left C Testes, Bilateral	F Spermatic Cord, Right G Spermatic Cord, Left H Spermatic Cords, Bilateral J Epididymis, Right K Epididymis, Left L Epididymis, Bilateral N Vas Deferens, Right P Vas Deferens, Left Q Vas Deferens, Bilateral	0 Open 3 Percutaneous 4 Percutaneous endoscopic	0 Drainage device	Z No qualifier
1 Seminal Vesicle, Right 2 Seminal Vesicle, Left 3 Seminal Vesicles, Bilateral 6 Tunica Vaginalis, Right 7 Tunica Vaginalis, Left 9 Testis, Right B Testis, Left C Testes, Bilateral	F Spermatic Cord, Right G Spermatic Cord, Left H Spermatic Cords, Bilateral J Epididymis, Right K Epididymis, Left L Epididymis, Bilateral N Vas Deferens, Right P Vas Deferens, Left Q Vas Deferens, Bilateral	0 Open 3 Percutaneous 4 Percutaneous endoscopic	Z No device	X Diagnostic Z No qualifier
5 Scrotum S Penis T Prepuce		0 Open 3 Percutaneous 4 Percutaneous endoscopic X External	0 Drainage device	Z No qualifier
5 Scrotum S Penis T Prepuce		0 Open 3 Percutaneous 4 Percutaneous endoscopic X External	Z No device	X Diagnostic Z No qualifier

MALE

0 V 9

EXCISION GROUP: Excision, Resection, Destruction, (Extraction), (Detachment)
Root Operations that take out some or all of a body part.

1ST - **0** Medical and Surgical

2ND - **V** Male Reproductive System ♂

3RD - **B EXCISION**

EXAMPLE: TURP (non-total) | CMS Ex: Liver biopsy

EXCISION: Cutting out or off, without replacement, a portion of a body part.

EXPLANATION: Qualifier "X Diagnostic" indicates biopsy ...

Body Part – 4TH	Approach – 5TH	Device – 6TH	Qualifier – 7TH
0 Prostate	0 Open 3 Percutaneous 4 Percutaneous endoscopic 7 Via natural or artificial opening 8 Via natural or artificial opening endoscopic	Z No device	X Diagnostic Z No qualifier
1 Seminal Vesicle, Right F Spermatic Cord, Right 2 Seminal Vesicle, Left G Spermatic Cord, Left 3 Seminal Vesicles, Bilateral H Spermatic Cords, Bilateral 6 Tunica Vaginalis, Right J Epididymis, Right 7 Tunica Vaginalis, Left K Epididymis, Left 9 Testis, Right L Epididymis, Bilateral B Testis, Left N Vas Deferens, Right NC* C Testes, Bilateral P Vas Deferens, Left NC* Q Vas Deferens, Bilateral NC*	0 Open 3 Percutaneous 4 Percutaneous endoscopic	Z No device	X Diagnostic Z No qualifier
5 Scrotum S Penis T Prepuce	0 Open 3 Percutaneous 4 Percutaneous endoscopic X External	Z No device	X Diagnostic Z No qualifier

NC* – Some procedures are considered non-covered by Medicare. See current Medicare Code Editor for details.

DRAINAGE GROUP: Drainage, Extirpation, (Fragmentation)
Root Operations that take out solids/fluids/gases from a body part.

1ST - 0 Medical and Surgical	**EXAMPLE:** Removal foreign body **CMS Ex:** Choledocholithotomy
2ND - V Male Reproductive System ♂	**EXTIRPATION:** Taking or cutting out solid matter from a body part.
3RD - C EXTIRPATION	**EXPLANATION:** Abnormal byproduct or foreign body …

Body Part – 4TH	Approach – 5TH	Device – 6TH	Qualifier – 7TH
0 Prostate	0 Open 3 Percutaneous 4 Percutaneous endoscopic 7 Via natural or artificial opening 8 Via natural or artificial opening endoscopic	Z No device	Z No qualifier
1 Seminal Vesicle, Right F Spermatic Cord, Right 2 Seminal Vesicle, Left G Spermatic Cord, Left 3 Seminal Vesicles, Bilateral H Spermatic Cords, Bilateral 6 Tunica Vaginalis, Right J Epididymis, Right 7 Tunica Vaginalis, Left K Epididymis, Left 9 Testis, Right L Epididymis, Bilateral B Testis, Left N Vas Deferens, Right C Testes, Bilateral P Vas Deferens, Left Q Vas Deferens, Bilateral	0 Open 3 Percutaneous 4 Percutaneous endoscopic	Z No device	Z No qualifier
5 Scrotum S Penis T Prepuce	0 Open 3 Percutaneous 4 Percutaneous endoscopic X External	Z No device	Z No qualifier

DEVICE GROUP: Change, Insertion, Removal, Replacement, Revision, Supplement
Root Operations that always involve a device.

1ST - **O** Medical and Surgical

2ND - **V** Male Reproductive System ♂

3RD - **H INSERTION**

EXAMPLE: Insertion radioactive element | CMS Ex: Central venous catheter

INSERTION: Putting in a nonbiological appliance that monitors, assists, performs, or prevents a physiological function but does not physically take the place of a body part.

EXPLANATION: None

Body Part – 4TH	Approach – 5TH	Device – 6TH	Qualifier – 7TH
0 Prostate	0 Open 3 Percutaneous 4 Percutaneous endoscopic 7 Via natural or artificial opening 8 Via natural or artificial opening endoscopic	1 Radioactive element	Z No qualifier
4 Prostate and Seminal Vesicles 8 Scrotum and Tunica Vaginalis D Testis M Epididymis and Spermatic Cord R Vas Deferens	0 Open 3 Percutaneous 4 Percutaneous endoscopic 7 Via natural or artificial opening 8 Via natural or artificial opening endoscopic	3 Infusion device	Z No qualifier
S Penis	0 Open 3 Percutaneous 4 Percutaneous endoscopic X External	3 Infusion device	Z No qualifier

(side tab: MALE — O V H *)*

EXAMINATION GROUP: Inspection (Map)
Root Operations involving examination only.

1ST - **O** Medical and Surgical

2ND - **V** Male Reproductive System ♂

3RD - **J INSPECTION**

EXAMPLE: Prostate exam | CMS Ex: Colonoscopy

INSPECTION: Visually and/or manually exploring a body part.

EXPLANATION: Direct or instrumental visualization ...

Body Part – 4TH	Approach – 5TH	Device – 6TH	Qualifier – 7TH
4 Prostate and Seminal Vesicles 8 Scrotum and Tunica Vaginalis D Testis M Epididymis and Spermatic Cord R Vas Deferens S Penis	0 Open 3 Percutaneous 4 Percutaneous endoscopic X External	Z No device	Z No qualifier

TUBULAR GROUP: Bypass, Dilation, Occlusion, (Restriction)
Root Operations that alter the diameter/route of a tubular body part.

1ST - 0 Medical and Surgical

2ND - V Male Reproductive System ♂

3RD - L OCCLUSION

EXAMPLE: Vasectomy | CMS Ex: Fallopian tube ligation

OCCLUSION: Completely closing an orifice or lumen of a tubular body part.

EXPLANATION: Natural or artificially created orifice ...

Body Part – 4TH	Approach – 5TH	Device – 6TH	Qualifier – 7TH
F Spermatic Cord, Right NC* G Spermatic Cord, Left NC* H Spermatic Cords, Bilateral NC* N Vas Deferens, Right NC* P Vas Deferens, Left NC* Q Vas Deferens, Bilateral NC*	0 Open 3 Percutaneous 4 Percutaneous endoscopic	C Extraluminal device D Intraluminal device Z No device	Z No qualifier

NC* – Some procedures are considered non-covered by Medicare. See current Medicare Code Editor for details.

MOVE GROUP: Reattachment, Reposition, (Transfer), (Transplantation)
Root Operations that put in/put back or move some/all of a body part.

1ST - 0 Medical and Surgical

2ND - V Male Reproductive System ♂

3RD - M REATTACHMENT

EXAMPLE: Penis reattachment | CMS Ex: Reattachment hand

REATTACHMENT: Putting back in or on all or a portion of a separated body part to its normal location or other suitable location.

EXPLANATION: With/without reconnection of vessels/nerves...

Body Part – 4TH	Approach – 5TH	Device – 6TH	Qualifier – 7TH
5 Scrotum S Penis	X External	Z No device	Z No qualifier
6 Tunica Vaginalis, Right F Spermatic Cord, Right 7 Tunica Vaginalis, Left G Spermatic Cord, Left 9 Testis, Right H Spermatic Cords, B Testis, Left Bilateral C Testes, Bilateral	0 Open 4 Percutaneous endoscopic	Z No device	Z No qualifier

DIVISION GROUP: (Division), Release
Root Operations involving cutting or separation only.

1ST - **0** Medical and Surgical

2ND - **V** Male Reproductive System ♂

3RD - **N RELEASE**

EXAMPLE: Adhesiolysis spermatic cord	CMS Ex: Carpal tunnel release

RELEASE: Freeing a body part from an abnormal physical constraint by cutting or by the use of force.

EXPLANATION: None of the body part is taken out ...

Body Part – 4TH	Approach – 5TH	Device – 6TH	Qualifier – 7TH
0 Prostate	0 Open 3 Percutaneous 4 Percutaneous endoscopic 7 Via natural or artificial opening 8 Via natural or artificial opening endoscopic	Z No device	Z No qualifier
1 Seminal Vesicle, Right F Spermatic Cord, Right 2 Seminal Vesicle, Left G Spermatic Cord, Left 3 Seminal Vesicles, Bilateral H Spermatic Cords, Bilateral 6 Tunica Vaginalis, Right J Epididymis, Right 7 Tunica Vaginalis, Left K Epididymis, Left 9 Testis, Right L Epididymis, Bilateral B Testis, Left N Vas Deferens, Right C Testes, Bilateral P Vas Deferens, Left Q Vas Deferens, Bilateral	0 Open 3 Percutaneous 4 Percutaneous endoscopic	Z No device	Z No qualifier
5 Scrotum S Penis T Prepuce	0 Open 3 Percutaneous 4 Percutaneous endoscopic X External	Z No device	Z No qualifier

DEVICE GROUP: Change, Insertion, Removal, Replacement, Revision, Supplement
Root Operations that always involve a device.

1ST - 0 Medical and Surgical

2ND - V Male Reproductive System ♂

3RD - P REMOVAL

EXAMPLE: Removal drain tube

CMS Ex: Chest tube removal

REMOVAL: Taking out or off a device from a body part.

EXPLANATION: Removal device without reinsertion ...

Body Part – 4TH	Approach – 5TH	Device – 6TH	Qualifier – 7TH
4 Prostate and Seminal Vesicles	0 Open 3 Percutaneous 4 Percutaneous endoscopic 7 Via natural or artificial opening 8 Via natural or artificial opening endoscopic	0 Drainage device 1 Radioactive element 3 Infusion device 7 Autologous tissue substitute J Synthetic substitute K Nonautologous tissue substitute	Z No qualifier
4 Prostate and Seminal Vesicles	X External	0 Drainage device 1 Radioactive element 3 Infusion device	Z No qualifier
8 Scrotum and Tunica Vaginalis D Testis S Penis	0 Open 3 Percutaneous 4 Percutaneous endoscopic 7 Via natural or artificial opening 8 Via natural or artificial opening endoscopic	0 Drainage device 3 Infusion device 7 Autologous tissue substitute J Synthetic substitute K Nonautologous tissue substitute	Z No qualifier
8 Scrotum and Tunica Vaginalis D Testis S Penis	X External	0 Drainage device 3 Infusion device	Z No qualifier
M Epididymis and Spermatic Cord	0 Open 3 Percutaneous 4 Percutaneous endoscopic 7 Via natural or artificial opening 8 Via natural or artificial opening endoscopic	0 Drainage device 3 Infusion device 7 Autologous tissue substitute C Extraluminal device J Synthetic substitute K Nonautologous tissue substitute	Z No qualifier
M Epididymis and Spermatic Cord	X External	0 Drainage device 3 Infusion device	Z No qualifier
R Vas Deferens	0 Open 3 Percutaneous 4 Percutaneous endoscopic 7 Via natural or artificial opening 8 Via natural or artificial opening endoscopic	0 Drainage device 3 Infusion device 7 Autologous tissue substitute C Extraluminal device D Intraluminal device J Synthetic substitute K Nonautologous tissue substitute	Z No qualifier
R Vas Deferens	X External	0 Drainage device 3 Infusion device D Intraluminal device	Z No qualifier

OTHER REPAIRS GROUP: (Control), **Repair**
Root Operations that define other repairs.

1ST – 0 Medical and Surgical	EXAMPLE: Repair laceration scrotum	CMS Ex: Suture laceration
2ND – V Male Reproductive System ♂	**REPAIR:** Restoring, to the extent possible, a body part to its normal anatomic structure and function.	
3RD – Q REPAIR	EXPLANATION: Only when no other root operation applies …	

Body Part – 4TH		Approach – 5TH	Device – 6TH	Qualifier – 7TH
0 Prostate		0 Open 3 Percutaneous 4 Percutaneous endoscopic 7 Via natural or artificial opening 8 Via natural or artificial opening endoscopic	Z No device	Z No qualifier
1 Seminal Vesicle, Right 2 Seminal Vesicle, Left 3 Seminal Vesicles, Bilateral 6 Tunica Vaginalis, Right 7 Tunica Vaginalis, Left 9 Testis, Right B Testis, Left C Testes, Bilateral	F Spermatic Cord, Right G Spermatic Cord, Left H Spermatic Cords, Bilateral J Epididymis, Right K Epididymis, Left L Epididymis, Bilateral N Vas Deferens, Right P Vas Deferens, Left Q Vas Deferens, Bilateral	0 Open 3 Percutaneous 4 Percutaneous endoscopic	Z No device	Z No qualifier
5 Scrotum S Penis T Prepuce		0 Open 3 Percutaneous 4 Percutaneous endoscopic X External	Z No device	Z No qualifier

DEVICE GROUP: Change, Insertion, Removal, Replacement, Revision, Supplement
Root Operations that always involve a device.

1ST – 0 Medical and Surgical	EXAMPLE: Testis removal with replacement	CMS Ex: Total hip
2ND – V Male Reproductive System ♂	**REPLACEMENT:** Putting in or on a biological or synthetic material that physically takes the place and/or function of all or a portion of a body part.	
3RD – R REPLACEMENT	EXPLANATION: Includes taking out body part, or eradication…	

Body Part – 4TH	Approach – 5TH	Device – 6TH	Qualifier – 7TH
9 Testis, Right B Testis, Left C Testes, Bilateral	0 Open	J Synthetic substitute	Z No qualifier

MALE

0 V Q

© 2016 Channel Publishing, Ltd.

MOVE GROUP: Reattachment, Reposition, (Transfer), (Transplantation)
Root Operations that put in/put back or move some/all of a body part.

1ST - 0 Medical and Surgical

2ND - V Male Reproductive System ♂

3RD - S REPOSITION

EXAMPLE: Relocation undescended testis	CMS Ex: Fracture reduction

REPOSITION: Moving to its normal location, or other suitable location, all or a portion of a body part.

EXPLANATION: May or may not be cut to be moved ...

Body Part – 4TH		Approach – 5TH	Device – 6TH	Qualifier – 7TH

9 Testis, Right
B Testis, Left
C Testes, Bilateral
	F Spermatic Cord, Right
	G Spermatic Cord, Left
	H Spermatic Cords,
	   Bilateral
		0 Open
		3 Percutaneous
		4 Percutaneous
		   endoscopic
			Z No device	Z No qualifier

EXCISION GROUP: Excision, Resection, Destruction, (Extraction), (Detachment)
Root Operations that take out some or all of a body part.

1ST - 0 Medical and Surgical

2ND - V Male Reproductive System ♂

3RD - T RESECTION

EXAMPLE: Total retropubic prostatectomy	CMS Ex: Cholecystectomy

RESECTION: Cutting out or off, without replacement, all of a body part.

EXPLANATION: None

Body Part – 4TH		Approach – 5TH	Device – 6TH	Qualifier – 7TH

0 Prostate		0 Open
		4 Percutaneous
		   endoscopic
		7 Via natural or
		   artificial opening
		8 Via natural or
		   artificial opening
		   endoscopic
			Z No device	Z No qualifier

1 Seminal Vesicle, Right
2 Seminal Vesicle, Left
3 Seminal Vesicles,
   Bilateral
6 Tunica Vaginalis, Right
7 Tunica Vaginalis, Left
9 Testis, Right
B Testis, Left
C Testes, Bilateral
	F Spermatic Cord, Right
	G Spermatic Cord, Left
	H Spermatic Cords,
	   Bilateral
	J Epididymis, Right
	K Epididymis, Left
	L Epididymis, Bilateral
	N Vas Deferens, Right NC*
	P Vas Deferens, Left NC*
	Q Vas Deferens,
	   Bilateral NC*
		0 Open
		4 Percutaneous
		   endoscopic
			Z No device	Z No qualifier

5 Scrotum S Penis T Prepuce		0 Open 4 Percutaneous endoscopic X External	Z No device	Z No qualifier

NC* – Some procedures are considered non-covered by Medicare. See current Medicare Code Editor for details.

DEVICE GROUP: Change, Insertion, Removal, Replacement, Revision, Supplement
Root Operations that always involve a device.

1ST – **0** Medical and Surgical

2ND – **V** Male Reproductive System ♂

3RD – **U SUPPLEMENT**

EXAMPLE: Tunica vaginalis repair with graft | CMS Ex: Hernia with mesh

SUPPLEMENT: Putting in or on biological or synthetic material that physically reinforces and/or augments the function of a portion of a body part.

EXPLANATION: Biological material from same individual ...

Body Part – 4TH		Approach – 5TH	Device – 6TH	Qualifier – 7TH
1 Seminal Vesicle, Right 2 Seminal Vesicle, Left 3 Seminal Vesicles, Bilateral 6 Tunica Vaginalis, Right 7 Tunica Vaginalis, Left F Spermatic Cord, Right G Spermatic Cord, Left H Spermatic Cords, Bilateral	J Epididymis, Right K Epididymis, Left L Epididymis, Bilateral N Vas Deferens, Right P Vas Deferens, Left Q Vas Deferens, Bilateral	0 Open 4 Percutaneous endoscopic	7 Autologous tissue substitute J Synthetic substitute K Nonautologous tissue substitute	Z No qualifier
5 Scrotum S Penis T Prepuce		0 Open 4 Percutaneous endoscopic X External	7 Autologous tissue substitute J Synthetic substitute K Nonautologous tissue substitute	Z No qualifier
9 Testis, Right B Testis, Left C Testes, Bilateral		0 Open	7 Autologous tissue substitute J Synthetic substitute K Nonautologous tissue substitute	Z No qualifier

MALE

0 V U

DEVICE GROUP: Change, Insertion, Removal, Replacement, Revision, Supplement
Root Operations that always involve a device.

1ST - **0**　Medical and Surgical	EXAMPLE: Reposition drain tube	CMS Ex: Adjustment pacemaker lead
2ND - **V**　Male Reproductive System ♂	**REVISION:**　Correcting, to the extent possible, a portion of a malfunctioning device or the position of a displaced device.	
3RD - **W REVISION**		
	EXPLANATION: May replace components of a device ...	

Body Part – 4TH	Approach – 5TH	Device – 6TH	Qualifier – 7TH
4　Prostate and Seminal Vesicles 8　Scrotum and Tunica Vaginalis D　Testis S　Penis	0　Open 3　Percutaneous 4　Percutaneous endoscopic 7　Via natural or artificial opening 8　Via natural or artificial opening endoscopic X　External	0　Drainage device 3　Infusion device 7　Autologous tissue substitute J　Synthetic substitute K　Nonautologous tissue substitute	Z　No qualifier
M　Epididymis and Spermatic Cord	0　Open 3　Percutaneous 4　Percutaneous endoscopic 7　Via natural or artificial opening 8　Via natural or artificial opening endoscopic X　External	0　Drainage device 3　Infusion device 7　Autologous tissue substitute C　Extraluminal device J　Synthetic substitute K　Nonautologous tissue substitute	Z　No qualifier
R　Vas Deferens	0　Open 3　Percutaneous 4　Percutaneous endoscopic 7　Via natural or artificial opening 8　Via natural or artificial opening endoscopic X　External	0　Drainage device 3　Infusion device 7　Autologous tissue substitute C　Extraluminal device D　Intraluminal device J　Synthetic substitute K　Nonautologous tissue substitute	Z　No qualifier

MALE

0 V W

NOTES

Educational Annotations | W – Anatomical Regions, General

Body System Specific Educational Annotations for the Anatomical Regions, General include:

- Anatomy and Physiology Review
- Anatomical Illustrations
- Definitions of Common Procedures
- AHA Coding Clinic® Reference Notations
- Body Part Key Listings
- Device Key Listings
- Device Aggregation Table Listings
- Coding Notes

Anatomy and Physiology Review of Anatomical Regions, General

BODY PART VALUES – W - ANATOMICAL REGIONS, GENERAL

Coding Guideline B2.1a - Body System, General Guideline – The procedure codes in the general anatomical regions body systems ~~should only~~ can be used when the procedure is performed on an anatomical region rather than a specific body part (e.g., root operations Control and Detachment, Drainage of a body cavity) or on the rare occasion when no information is available to support assignment of a code to a specific body part. **Examples:** Control of postoperative hemorrhage is coded to the root operation Control found in the general anatomical regions body systems.
Chest tube drainage of the pleural cavity is coded to the root operation Drainage found in the general anatomical regions body systems. Suture repair of the abdominal wall is coded to the root operation Repair in the General Anatomical Regions body system.

Abdominal Wall – The multi-tissue-layered covering of the abdominal and pelvic portions of the trunk.

Back – The multi-tissue-layered covering of the back portion of the trunk.

Chest Wall – The multi-tissue-layered covering of the thoracic portion of the trunk.

Cranial Cavity – The space inside the skull.

Face – The multi-tissue-layered covering of the anterior portion of the head.

Gastrointestinal Tract – The alimentary tract from the esophagus to the anus.

Genitourinary Tract – The organs and structures of the urinary and reproductive systems.

Head – The portion of the human body above the neck.

Jaw – The anterior, lower, movable, articulated portion of the head.

Mediastinum – The central portion of the thoracic cavity that lies between the right pleura, left pleura, sternum, and vertebral column and contains the heart, great vessels, esophagus, bronchi, and thymus.

Neck – The portion of the human body above the trunk and below the head.

Oral Cavity and Throat – The space formed by the mouth, pharynx, and larynx.

Pelvic Cavity – The lower abdominal space containing the rectum, bladder, and reproductive organs.

Pericardial Cavity – The thoracic, fluid-filled space formed by the double-walled peritoneal sac that contains the heart.

Perineum, Female – The multi-tissue-layered area between the vulva and the anus.

Perineum, Male – The multi-tissue-layered area between the scrotum and the anus.

Peritoneal Cavity – The abdominal space between the parietal peritoneum and visceral peritoneum.

Pleural Cavity – The thoracic, fluid-filled space between the visceral pleura and parietal pleura.

Respiratory Tract – The organs and structures involved in respiration.

Retroperitoneum – The space behind the peritoneum that borders the deep muscles of the back and contains the kidneys, adrenals, most of the duodenum, ascending and descending colon, and the pancreas.

Anatomical Illustrations of Anatomical Regions, General

None for the Anatomical Regions, General Body System

Educational Annotations | W – Anatomical Regions, General

Definitions of Common Procedures of Anatomical Regions, General

Abdominoplasty (tummy tuck) – The cosmetic plastic surgical procedure to remove excess fat and skin from the abdominal wall area.

Chest tube for pneumothorax – The surgical insertion of a plastic tube through the chest wall and into the pleural space to remove the air of a pneumothorax.

Episiotomy – The surgical incision of the perineum (with subsequent closure) to expand the opening of the vagina and prevent tearing of the perineal tissues during delivery.

Face lift (rhytidectomy) – The cosmetic plastic surgical procedure to remove the visible signs of aging in the face and neck including removing excess skin and fat with resulting tightening of the facial skin. The procedure often includes a cosmetic blepharoplasty of the eyelids.

Paracentesis – The procedural insertion of a needle or catheter through the abdominal wall and into the peritoneal cavity to drain excess fluid.

Pleuroperitoneal shunt – The shunting redirection of excessive pleural fluid by placing a catheter into the pleural space and tunneling it into the peritoneal cavity.

Thoracentesis – The procedural insertion of a needle or catheter through the chest wall and into the pleural space to drain fluid (pleural effusion, empyema, blood, chyle).

AHA Coding Clinic® Reference Notations of Anatomical Regions, General

ROOT OPERATION SPECIFIC - W - ANATOMICAL REGIONS, GENERAL

ALTERATION - 0
Browpexy..AHA 15:1Q:p31
BYPASS - 1
Creation of percutaneous cutaneoperitoneal fistula for peritoneal
   dialysis ....AHA 13:4Q:p126
   Official Correction of 13:4Q:p126 & 127 ....AHA 15:2Q:p36
Creation of percutaneous cutaneoperitoneal fistula
   laparoscopically for peritoneal dialysis...............................AHA 13:4Q:p127
   Official Correction of 13:4Q:p126 & 127 ....AHA 15:2Q:p36
CHANGE - 2
CONTROL - 3
Control of post vaginal delivery bleeding ....AHA 14:4Q:p44
CREATION - 4
DIVISION - 8
DRAINAGE - 9
EXCISION - B
Excision of inclusion cyst of perineum ....AHA 13:4Q:p119
Excision of urachal mass ....AHA 16:1Q:p21
EXTIRPATION - C
FRAGMENTATION - F
INSERTION - H
Peritoneal port-a-cath insertion ....AHA 16:2Q:p14
Placement of peritoneal dialysis device..................................AHA 15:2Q:p36
INSPECTION - J
Ventriculoperitoneal (VP) shunt with laparoscopic assistance ......AHA 13:2Q:p36
REATTACHMENT - M
REMOVAL - P
REPAIR - Q
Abdominoplasty of ventral hernia..AHA 14:4Q:p38
Parastomal hernia repair ....AHA 14:3Q:p28
Continued on next page

Educational Annotations | W – Anatomical Regions, General

AHA Coding Clinic® Reference Notations of Anatomical Regions, General

Continued from previous page
SUPPLEMENT - U
Reconstruction of chest wall using Marlex overlay plate .... AHA 12:4Q:p101
Repair of incisional hernia with component release and mesh .... AHA 14:4Q:p39
REVISION - W
Replacement of disconnected abdominal portion of VP shunt .... AHA 15:2Q:p9

Body Part Key Listings of Anatomical Regions, General

See also Body Part Key in Appendix C
Retroperitoneal space .... *use* Retroperitoneum
Retropubic space .... *use* Pelvic Cavity

Device Key Listings of Anatomical Regions, General

See also Device Key in Appendix D
Autograft .... *use* Autologous Tissue Substitute
Bard® Composix® Kugel® patch .... *use* Synthetic Substitute
Bard® Ventralex™ hernia patch .... *use* Synthetic Substitute
Bard® Composix® (E/X)(LP) mesh .... *use* Synthetic Substitute
Bard® Dulex™ mesh .... *use* Synthetic Substitute
Brachytherapy seeds .... *use* Radioactive Element
Cook Biodesign® Hernia Graft(s) .... *use* Nonautologous Tissue Substitute
Cook Biodesign® Layered Graft(s) .... *use* Nonautologous Tissue Substitute
Cook Zenapro™ Layered Graft(s) .... *use* Nonautologous Tissue Substitute
Flexible Composite Mesh .... *use* Synthetic Substitute
GORE® DUALMESH® .... *use* Synthetic Substitute
Nitinol framed polymer mesh .... *use* Synthetic Substitute
Partially absorbable mesh .... *use* Synthetic Substitute
PHYSIOMESH™ Flexible Composite Mesh .... *use* Synthetic Substitute
Polypropylene mesh .... *use* Synthetic Substitute
PROCEED™ Ventral Patch .... *use* Synthetic Substitute
PROLENE Polypropylene Hernia System (PHS) .... *use* Synthetic Substitute
Rebound HRD® (Hernia Repair Device) .... *use* Synthetic Substitute
Thoracostomy tube .... *use* Drainage Device
Tissue bank graft .... *use* Nonautologous Tissue Substitute
ULTRAPRO Hernia System (UHS) .... *use* Synthetic Substitute
ULTRAPRO Partially Absorbable Lightweight Mesh *use* Synthetic Substitute
ULTRAPRO Plug .... *use* Synthetic Substitute
Ventrio™ Hernia Patch .... *use* Synthetic Substitute

Aggregation Key Listings of Anatomical Regions, General

See also Device Aggregation Table in Appendix E

Specific Device	For Operation	In Body System	General Device
None Listed in Device Aggregation Table for this Body System			

Educational Annotations | W – Anatomical Regions, General

Coding Notes of Anatomical Regions, General

Body System Relevant Coding Guidelines

General Guidelines
B2.1a

The procedure codes in the general anatomical regions body systems ~~should only~~ can be used when the procedure is performed on an anatomical region rather than a specific body part (e.g., root operations Control and Detachment, Drainage of a body cavity) or on the rare occasion when no information is available to support assignment of a code to a specific body part.

Examples: Control of postoperative hemorrhage is coded to the root operation Control found in the general anatomical regions body systems.

Chest tube drainage of the pleural cavity is coded to the root operation Drainage found in the general anatomical regions body systems. Suture repair of the abdominal wall is coded to the root operation Repair in the General Anatomical Regions body system.

Control vs. more definitive root operations
B3.7

The root operation Control is defined as, "Stopping, or attempting to stop, postprocedural or other acute bleeding." If an attempt to stop postprocedural or other acute bleeding is initially unsuccessful, and to stop the bleeding requires performing any of the definitive root operations Bypass, Detachment, Excision, Extraction, Reposition, Replacement, or Resection, then that root operation is coded instead of Control.

Example: Resection of spleen to stop ~~postprocedural~~ bleeding is coded to Resection instead of Control.

Body System Specific PCS Reference Manual Exercises

PCS CODE	W – ANATOMICAL REGIONS, GENERAL EXERCISES
0 W 0 2 0 Z Z	Cosmetic face lift, open, no other information available.
0 W 0 F 0 Z Z	Abdominoplasty (tummy tuck), open.
0 W 1 9 0 J G	Open pleuroperitoneal shunt, right pleural cavity, using synthetic device.
0 W 2 B X 0 Z	Change chest tube for left pneumothorax.
0 W 3 D 0 Z Z	Reopening of thoracotomy site with drainage and control of post-op hemopericardium.
0 W 3 H 0 Z Z	Control of post-operative retroperitoneal bleeding via laparotomy.
0 W 3 R 8 Z Z	Hysteroscopy with cautery of post-hysterectomy oozing and evacuation of clot.
0 W 4 M 0 J 0	Creation of vagina in male patient using synthetic material.
0 W 4 N 0 K 1	Creation of penis in female patient using tissue bank donor graft.
0 W 9 9 3 0 Z	Percutaneous chest tube placement for right pneumothorax.
0 W 9 B 3 Z Z	Thoracentesis of left pleural effusion. (This is drainage of the pleural cavity.)
0 W 9 G 3 Z Z	Percutaneous drainage of ascites. (This is drainage of the cavity and not the peritoneal membrane itself.)
0 W J 9 0 Z Z	Thoracotomy with exploration of right pleural cavity.
0 W Q F 0 Z Z	Closure of abdominal wall stab wound.
0 W Q N 0 Z Z	Perineoplasty with repair of old obstetric laceration, open.
0 W U F 0 J Z	Abdominal wall herniorrhaphy, open, using synthetic mesh.

OTHER OBJECTIVES GROUP: Alteration, Creation, (Fusion)
Root Operations that define other objectives.

1ST - 0 Medical and Surgical

2ND - W Anatomical Regions, General

3RD - 0 ALTERATION

EXAMPLE: Abdominoplasty (tummy tuck) | CMS Ex: Face lift

ALTERATION: Modifying the anatomic structure of a body part without affecting the function of the body part.

EXPLANATION: Principal purpose is to improve appearance

Body Part – 4TH		Approach – 5TH	Device – 6TH	Qualifier – 7TH
0 Head 2 Face 4 Upper Jaw 5 Lower Jaw 6 Neck 8 Chest Wall	F Abdominal Wall K Upper Back L Lower Back M Perineum, Male ♂ N Perineum, Female ♀	0 Open 3 Percutaneous 4 Percutaneous endoscopic	7 Autologous tissue substitute J Synthetic substitute K Nonautologous tissue substitute Z No device	Z No qualifier

TUBULAR GROUP: Bypass, (Dilation), (Occlusion), (Restriction)
Root Operations that alter the diameter/route of a tubular body part.

1ST - 0 Medical and Surgical

2ND - W Anatomical Regions, General

3RD - 1 BYPASS

EXAMPLE: Pleuroperitoneal shunt | CMS Ex: Coronary artery bypass

BYPASS: Altering the route of passage of the contents of a tubular body part.

EXPLANATION: Rerouting contents to a downstream part ...

Body Part – 4TH	Approach – 5TH	Device – 6TH	Qualifier – 7TH
1 Cranial Cavity	0 Open	J Synthetic substitute	9 Pleural Cavity, Right B Pleural Cavity, Left G Peritoneal Cavity J Pelvic Cavity
9 Pleural Cavity, Right B Pleural Cavity, Left G Peritoneal Cavity J Pelvic Cavity	0 Open 4 Percutaneous endoscopic	J Synthetic substitute	4 Cutaneous 9 Pleural Cavity, Right B Pleural Cavity, Left G Peritoneal Cavity J Pelvic Cavity Y Lower Vein
9 Pleural Cavity, Right B Pleural Cavity, Left G Peritoneal Cavity J Pelvic Cavity	3 Percutaneous	J Synthetic substitute	4 Cutaneous

REGIONS GENERAL 0 W 1

DEVICE GROUP: Change, Insertion, Removal, (Replacement), Revision, Supplement
Root Operations that always involve a device.

1ST - 0 Medical and Surgical		EXAMPLE: Exchange chest tube	CMS Ex: Changing urinary catheter

2ND - W Anatomical Regions, General

3RD - 2 CHANGE

EXAMPLE: Exchange chest tube | **CMS Ex:** Changing urinary catheter

CHANGE: Taking out or off a device from a body part and putting back an identical or similar device in or on the same body part without cutting or puncturing the skin or a mucous membrane.

EXPLANATION: ALL Changes use EXTERNAL approach only ...

Body Part – 4TH		Approach – 5TH	Device – 6TH	Qualifier – 7TH
0 Head	D Pericardial Cavity	X External	0 Drainage device	Z No qualifier
1 Cranial Cavity	F Abdominal Wall		Y Other device	
2 Face	G Peritoneal Cavity			
4 Upper Jaw	H Retroperitoneum			
5 Lower Jaw	J Pelvic Cavity			
6 Neck	K Upper Back			
8 Chest Wall	L Lower Back			
9 Pleural Cavity, Right	M Perineum, Male ♂			
B Pleural Cavity, Left	N Perineum, Female ♀			
C Mediastinum				

OTHER REPAIRS GROUP: Control, Repair
Root Operations that define other repairs.

1ST - **0** Medical and Surgical	EXAMPLE: Cautery post-op oozing	CMS Ex: Control post-op hemorrhage

2ND - **W** Anatomical Regions, General

3RD - **3 CONTROL**

<u>CONTROL:</u> Stopping, or attempting to stop, postprocedural or other acute bleeding.

EXPLANATION: Bleeding site coded to an anatomical region...

Body Part – 4TH		Approach – 5TH	Device – 6TH	Qualifier – 7TH
0 Head	D Pericardial Cavity	0 Open	Z No device	Z No qualifier
1 Cranial Cavity	F Abdominal Wall	3 Percutaneous		
2 Face	G Peritoneal Cavity	4 Percutaneous		
4 Upper Jaw	H Retroperitoneum	endoscopic		
5 Lower Jaw	J Pelvic Cavity			
6 Neck	K Upper Back			
8 Chest Wall	L Lower Back			
9 Pleural Cavity, Right	M Perineum, Male ♂			
B Pleural Cavity, Left	N Perineum, Female ♀			
C Mediastinum				
3 Oral Cavity and Throat		0 Open	Z No device	Z No qualifier
		3 Percutaneous		
		4 Percutaneous endoscopic		
		7 Via natural or artificial opening		
		8 Via natural or artificial opening endoscopic		
		X External		
P Gastrointestinal Tract		0 Open	Z No device	Z No qualifier
Q Respiratory Tract		3 Percutaneous		
R Genitourinary Tract		4 Percutaneous endoscopic		
		7 Via natural or artificial opening		
		8 Via natural or artificial opening endoscopic		

REGIONS GENERAL **0 W 3**

OTHER OBJECTIVES GROUP: Alteration, Creation, (Fusion)
Root Operations that define other objectives.

1ST – 0 Medical and Surgical	EXAMPLE: Creation penis in female	CMS Ex: Creation vagina in male

2ND – W Anatomical Regions, General

3RD – 4 CREATION

CREATION: Putting in or on biological or synthetic material to form a new body part that to the extent possible replicates the anatomic structure or function of an absent body part.

EXPLANATION: Gender reassignment, anomaly correction

Body Part – 4TH	Approach – 5TH	Device – 6TH	Qualifier – 7TH
M Perineum, Male ♂ NC*	0 Open	7 Autologous tissue substitute J Synthetic substitute K Nonautologous tissue substitute Z No device	0 Vagina
N Perineum, Female ♀ NC*	0 Open	7 Autologous tissue substitute J Synthetic substitute K Nonautologous tissue substitute Z No device	1 Penis

NC* – Non-covered by Medicare. See current Medicare Code Editor for details.

DIVISION GROUP: Division, (Release)
Root Operations involving cutting or separation only.

1ST – 0 Medical and Surgical	EXAMPLE: Episiotomy	CMS Ex: Osteotomy

2ND – W Anatomical Regions, General

3RD – 8 DIVISION

DIVISION: Cutting into a body part without draining fluids and/or gases from the body part in order to separate or transect a body part.

EXPLANATION: Separated into two or more portions ...

Body Part – 4TH	Approach – 5TH	Device – 6TH	Qualifier – 7TH
N Perineum, Female ♀	X External	Z No device	Z No qualifier

DRAINAGE GROUP: Drainage, Extirpation, Fragmentation
Root Operations that take out solids/fluids/gases from a body part.

1ST - **0** Medical and Surgical

2ND - **W** Anatomical Regions, General

3RD - **9 DRAINAGE**

EXAMPLE: Paracentesis for ascites   CMS Ex: Thoracentesis

DRAINAGE: Taking or letting out fluids and/or gases from a body part.

EXPLANATION: Qualifier "X Diagnostic" indicates biopsy ...

Body Part – 4TH		Approach – 5TH	Device – 6TH	Qualifier – 7TH
0 Head 1 Cranial Cavity 2 Face 3 Oral Cavity and Throat 4 Upper Jaw 5 Lower Jaw 6 Neck 8 Chest Wall 9 Pleural Cavity, Right B Pleural Cavity, Left	C Mediastinum D Pericardial Cavity F Abdominal Wall G Peritoneal Cavity H Retroperitoneum J Pelvic Cavity K Upper Back L Lower Back M Perineum, Male ♂ N Perineum, Female ♀	0 Open 3 Percutaneous 4 Percutaneous endoscopic	0 Drainage device	Z No qualifier
0 Head 1 Cranial Cavity 2 Face 3 Oral Cavity and Throat 4 Upper Jaw 5 Lower Jaw 6 Neck 8 Chest Wall 9 Pleural Cavity, Right B Pleural Cavity, Left	C Mediastinum D Pericardial Cavity F Abdominal Wall G Peritoneal Cavity H Retroperitoneum J Pelvic Cavity K Upper Back L Lower Back M Perineum, Male ♂ N Perineum, Female ♀	0 Open 3 Percutaneous 4 Percutaneous endoscopic	Z No device	X Diagnostic Z No qualifier

REGIONS GENERAL 0 W 9

EXCISION GROUP: Excision, (Resection), (Destruction), (Extraction), (Detachment)
Root Operations that take out some or all of a body part.

1ST - 0 Medical and Surgical	EXAMPLE: Excision perineal inclusion cyst	CMS Ex: Liver biopsy

2ND - **W** Anatomical Regions, General

3RD - **B** EXCISION

EXCISION: Cutting out or off, without replacement, a portion of a body part.

EXPLANATION: Qualifier "X Diagnostic" indicates biopsy ...

Body Part – 4TH		Approach – 5TH	Device – 6TH	Qualifier – 7TH
0 Head 2 Face 4 Upper Jaw 5 Lower Jaw 8 Chest Wall	K Upper Back L Lower Back M Perineum, Male ♂ N Perineum, Female ♀	0 Open 3 Percutaneous 4 Percutaneous endoscopic X External	Z No device	X Diagnostic Z No qualifier
6 Neck F Abdominal Wall		0 Open 3 Percutaneous 4 Percutaneous endoscopic	Z No device	X Diagnostic Z No qualifier
6 Neck F Abdominal Wall		X External	Z No device	2 Stoma X Diagnostic Z No qualifier
C Mediastinum H Retroperitoneum		0 Open 3 Percutaneous 4 Percutaneous endoscopic	Z No device	X Diagnostic Z No qualifier

---

DRAINAGE GROUP: Drainage, Extirpation, Fragmentation
Root Operations that take out solids/fluids/gases from a body part.

1ST - **0** Medical and Surgical	EXAMPLE: Evacuation clot cranial cavity	CMS Ex: Choledocholithotomy
2ND - **W** Anatomical Regions, General	**EXTIRPATION:** Taking or cutting out solid matter from a body part.	
3RD - **C** EXTIRPATION		
	EXPLANATION: Abnormal byproduct or foreign body ...	

Body Part – 4TH	Approach – 5TH	Device – 6TH	Qualifier – 7TH
1 Cranial Cavity C Mediastinum 3 Oral Cavity and Throat D Pericardial Cavity 9 Pleural Cavity, Right G Peritoneal Cavity B Pleural Cavity, Left J Pelvic Cavity	0 Open 3 Percutaneous 4 Percutaneous endoscopic X External	Z No device	Z No qualifier
P Gastrointestinal Tract Q Respiratory Tract R Genitourinary Tract	0 Open 3 Percutaneous 4 Percutaneous endoscopic 7 Via natural or artificial opening 8 Via natural or artificial opening endoscopic X External	Z No device	Z No qualifier

---

DRAINAGE GROUP: Drainage, Extirpation, Fragmentation
Root Operations that take out solids/fluids/gases from a body part.

1ST - **0** Medical and Surgical	EXAMPLE: Lithotripsy pericardial cavity	CMS Ex: EWSL
2ND - **W** Anatomical Regions, General	**FRAGMENTATION:** Breaking solid matter in a body part into pieces.	
3RD - **F** FRAGMENTATION		
	EXPLANATION: Pieces are not taken out during procedure ...	

Body Part – 4TH	Approach – 5TH	Device – 6TH	Qualifier – 7TH
1 Cranial Cavity C Mediastinum 3 Oral Cavity and Throat D Pericardial Cavity 9 Pleural Cavity, Right G Peritoneal Cavity B Pleural Cavity, Left J Pelvic Cavity	0 Open 3 Percutaneous 4 Percutaneous endoscopic X External NC*	Z No device	Z No qualifier
P Gastrointestinal Tract Q Respiratory Tract R Genitourinary Tract	0 Open 3 Percutaneous 4 Percutaneous endoscopic 7 Via natural or artificial opening 8 Via natural or artificial opening endoscopic X External NC*	Z No device	Z No qualifier

NC* – Some procedures are considered non-covered by Medicare. See current Medicare Code Editor for details.

DEVICE GROUP: Change, Insertion, Removal, (Replacement), Revision, Supplement
Root Operations that always involve a device.

1ST - **0** Medical and Surgical

2ND - **W** Anatomical Regions, General

3RD - **H INSERTION**

EXAMPLE: Implantation infusion pump | CMS Ex: Central venous catheter

INSERTION: Putting in a nonbiological appliance that monitors, assists, performs, or prevents a physiological function but does not physically take the place of a body part.

EXPLANATION: None

Body Part – 4TH		Approach – 5TH	Device – 6TH	Qualifier – 7TH
0 Head 1 Cranial Cavity 2 Face 3 Oral Cavity and Throat 4 Upper Jaw 5 Lower Jaw 6 Neck 8 Chest Wall 9 Pleural Cavity, Right B Pleural Cavity, Left	C Mediastinum D Pericardial Cavity F Abdominal Wall G Peritoneal Cavity H Retroperitoneum J Pelvic Cavity K Upper Back L Lower Back M Perineum, Male ♂ N Perineum, Female ♀	0 Open 3 Percutaneous 4 Percutaneous endoscopic	1 Radioactive element 3 Infusion device Y Other device	Z No qualifier
P Gastrointestinal Tract Q Respiratory Tract R Genitourinary Tract		0 Open 3 Percutaneous 4 Percutaneous endoscopic 7 Via natural or artificial opening 8 Via natural or artificial opening endoscopic	1 Radioactive element 3 Infusion device Y Other device	Z No qualifier

EXAMINATION GROUP: Inspection, (Map)
Root Operations involving examination only.

1ST - **0** Medical and Surgical	EXAMPLE: Exploration peritoneal cavity	CMS Ex: Colonoscopy

2ND - **W** Anatomical Regions, General

3RD - **J INSPECTION**

INSPECTION: Visually and/or manually exploring a body part.

EXPLANATION: Direct or instrumental visualization ...

Body Part – 4TH	Approach – 5TH	Device – 6TH	Qualifier – 7TH
0 Head 8 Chest Wall 2 Face F Abdominal Wall 3 Oral Cavity and Throat K Upper Back 4 Upper Jaw L Lower Back 5 Lower Jaw M Perineum, Male ♂ 6 Neck N Perineum, Female ♀	0 Open 3 Percutaneous 4 Percutaneous endoscopic X External	Z No device	Z No qualifier
1 Cranial Cavity D Pericardial Cavity 9 Pleural Cavity, Right G Peritoneal Cavity B Pleural Cavity, Left H Retroperitoneum C Mediastinum J Pelvic Cavity	0 Open 3 Percutaneous 4 Percutaneous endoscopic	Z No device	Z No qualifier
P Gastrointestinal Tract Q Respiratory Tract R Genitourinary Tract	0 Open 3 Percutaneous 4 Percutaneous endoscopic 7 Via natural or artificial opening 8 Via natural or artificial opening endoscopic	Z No device	Z No qualifier

MOVE GROUP: Reattachment, (Reposition), (Transfer), (Transplantation)
Root Operations that put in/put back or move some/all of a body part.

1ST - **0** Medical and Surgical	EXAMPLE: Replantation avulsed perineum	CMS Ex: Reattachment hand

2ND - **W** Anatomical Regions, General

3RD - **M REATTACHMENT**

REATTACHMENT: Putting back in or on all or a portion of a separated body part to its normal location or other suitable location.

EXPLANATION: With/without reconnection of vessels/nerves...

Body Part – 4TH	Approach – 5TH	Device – 6TH	Qualifier – 7TH
2 Face F Abdominal Wall 4 Upper Jaw K Upper Back 5 Lower Jaw L Lower Back 6 Neck M Perineum, Male ♂ 8 Chest Wall N Perineum, Female ♀	0 Open	Z No device	Z No qualifier

DEVICE GROUP: Change, Insertion, Removal, (Replacement), Revision, Supplement		
Root Operations that always involve a device.		

	EXAMPLE: Removal infusion pump	CMS Ex: Chest tube removal
1ST – **0** Medical and Surgical 2ND – **W** Anatomical Regions, General 3RD – **P REMOVAL**	**REMOVAL:** Taking out or off a device from a body part.	
	EXPLANATION: Removal device without reinsertion …	

Body Part – 4TH	Approach – 5TH	Device – 6TH	Qualifier – 7TH
0 Head C Mediastinum 2 Face F Abdominal Wall 4 Upper Jaw K Upper Back 5 Lower Jaw L Lower Back 6 Neck M Perineum, Male ♂ 8 Chest Wall N Perineum, Female ♀	0 Open 3 Percutaneous 4 Percutaneous endoscopic X External	0 Drainage device 1 Radioactive element 3 Infusion device 7 Autologous tissue substitute J Synthetic substitute K Nonautologous tissue substitute Y Other device	Z No qualifier
1 Cranial Cavity 9 Pleural Cavity, Right B Pleural Cavity, Left G Peritoneal Cavity J Pelvic Cavity	0 Open 3 Percutaneous 4 Percutaneous endoscopic	0 Drainage device 1 Radioactive element 3 Infusion device J Synthetic substitute Y Other device	Z No qualifier
1 Cranial Cavity 9 Pleural Cavity, Right B Pleural Cavity, Left G Peritoneal Cavity J Pelvic Cavity	X External	0 Drainage device 1 Radioactive element 3 Infusion device	Z No qualifier
D Pericardial Cavity H Retroperitoneum	0 Open 3 Percutaneous 4 Percutaneous endoscopic	0 Drainage device 1 Radioactive element 3 Infusion device Y Other device	Z No qualifier
D Pericardial Cavity H Retroperitoneum	X External	0 Drainage device 1 Radioactive element 3 Infusion device	Z No qualifier
P Gastrointestinal Tract Q Respiratory Tract R Genitourinary Tract	0 Open 3 Percutaneous 4 Percutaneous endoscopic 7 Via natural or artificial opening 8 Via natural or artificial opening endoscopic X External	1 Radioactive element 3 Infusion device Y Other device	Z No qualifier

OTHER REPAIRS GROUP: Control, Repair
Root Operations that define other repairs.

1ST - **0** Medical and Surgical	EXAMPLE: Parastomal hernia repair	CMS Ex: Suture laceration

2ND - **W** Anatomical Regions, General

3RD - **Q REPAIR**

REPAIR: Restoring, to the extent possible, a body part to its normal anatomic structure and function.

EXPLANATION: Only when no other root operation applies …

Body Part – 4TH		Approach – 5TH	Device – 6TH	Qualifier – 7TH
0 Head 2 Face 4 Upper Jaw 5 Lower Jaw 8 Chest Wall	K Upper Back L Lower Back M Perineum, Male ♂ N Perineum, Female ♀	0 Open 3 Percutaneous 4 Percutaneous endoscopic X External	Z No device	Z No qualifier
6 Neck F Abdominal Wall		0 Open 3 Percutaneous 4 Percutaneous endoscopic	Z No device	Z No qualifier
6 Neck F Abdominal Wall		X External	Z No device	2 Stoma Z No qualifier
C Mediastinum		0 Open 3 Percutaneous 4 Percutaneous endoscopic	Z No device	Z No qualifier

DEVICE GROUP: Change, Insertion, Removal, (Replacement), Revision, Supplement
Root Operations that always involve a device.

1ST - **0** Medical and Surgical	EXAMPLE: Parastomal hernia repair with mesh	CMS Ex: With mesh

2ND - **W** Anatomical Regions, General

3RD - **U SUPPLEMENT**

SUPPLEMENT: Putting in or on biological or synthetic material that physically reinforces and/or augments the function of a portion of a body part.

EXPLANATION: Biological material from same individual …

Body Part – 4TH		Approach – 5TH	Device – 6TH	Qualifier – 7TH
0 Head 2 Face 4 Upper Jaw 5 Lower Jaw 6 Neck 8 Chest Wall	C Mediastinum F Abdominal Wall K Upper Back L Lower Back M Perineum, Male ♂ N Perineum, Female ♀	0 Open 4 Percutaneous endoscopic	7 Autologous tissue substitute J Synthetic substitute K Nonautologous tissue substitute	Z No qualifier

---

DEVICE GROUP: Change, Insertion, Removal, (Replacement), Revision, Supplement
Root Operations that always involve a device.

1ST – 0 Medical and Surgical	EXAMPLE: Reposition infusion pump	CMS Ex: Adjustment pacemaker lead
2ND – W Anatomical Regions, General	**REVISION:** Correcting, to the extent possible, a portion of a malfunctioning device or the position of a displaced device.	
3RD – W REVISION	EXPLANATION: May replace components of a device ...	

Body Part – 4TH	Approach – 5TH	Device – 6TH	Qualifier – 7TH
0 Head C Mediastinum 2 Face F Abdominal Wall 4 Upper Jaw K Upper Back 5 Lower Jaw L Lower Back 6 Neck M Perineum, Male ♂ 8 Chest Wall N Perineum, Female ♀	0 Open 3 Percutaneous 4 Percutaneous endoscopic X External	0 Drainage device 1 Radioactive element 3 Infusion device 7 Autologous tissue substitute J Synthetic substitute K Nonautologous tissue substitute Y Other device	Z No qualifier
1 Cranial Cavity 9 Pleural Cavity, Right B Pleural Cavity, Left G Peritoneal Cavity J Pelvic Cavity	0 Open 3 Percutaneous 4 Percutaneous endoscopic X External	0 Drainage device 1 Radioactive element 3 Infusion device J Synthetic substitute Y Other device	Z No qualifier
D Pericardial Cavity H Retroperitoneum	0 Open 3 Percutaneous 4 Percutaneous endoscopic X External	0 Drainage device 1 Radioactive element 3 Infusion device Y Other device	Z No qualifier
P Gastrointestinal Tract Q Respiratory Tract R Genitourinary Tract	0 Open 3 Percutaneous 4 Percutaneous endoscopic 7 Via natural or artificial opening 8 Via natural or artificial opening endoscopic X External	1 Radioactive element 3 Infusion device Y Other device	Z No qualifier

---

MOVE GROUP: Reattachment, (Reposition), (Transfer), Transplantation
Root Operations that put in/put back or move some/all of a body part.

1ST – 0 Medical and Surgical	EXAMPLE: Face transplant	CMS Ex: Kidney transplant
2ND – W Anatomical Regions, General	**TRANSPLANTATION:** Putting in or on all or a portion of a living body part taken from another individual or animal to physically take the place and/or function of all or a portion of a similar body part.	
3RD – Y TRANSPLANTATION	EXPLANATION: May take over all or part of its function ...	

Body Part – 4TH	Approach – 5TH	Device – 6TH	Qualifier – 7TH
2 Face	0 Open	Z No device	0 Allogeneic 1 Syngeneic

Educational Annotations | X – Anatomical Regions, Upper Extremities

Body System Specific Educational Annotations for the Anatomical Regions, Upper Extremities include:

- Anatomy and Physiology Review
- Anatomical Illustrations
- Definitions of Common Procedures
- AHA Coding Clinic® Reference Notations
- Body Part Key Listings
- Device Key Listings
- Device Aggregation Table Listings
- Coding Notes

Anatomy and Physiology Review of Anatomical Regions, Upper Extremities

BODY PART VALUES – X - ANATOMICAL REGIONS, UPPER EXTREMITIES

Coding Guideline B2.1a - Body System, General Guideline – The procedure codes in the general anatomical regions body systems ~~should only~~ can be used when the procedure is performed on an anatomical region rather than a specific body part (e.g., root operations Control and Detachment, Drainage of a body cavity) or on the rare occasion when no information is available to support assignment of a code to a specific body part. **Example*s*:** Control of postoperative hemorrhage is coded to the root operation Control found in the general anatomical regions body systems.

Chest tube drainage of the pleural cavity is coded to the root operation Drainage found in the general anatomical regions body systems. Suture repair of the abdominal wall is coded to the root operation Repair in the General Anatomical Regions body system.

1st Ray – The first digit of the hand and its associated first metacarpal bone.

2nd Ray – The second digit of the hand and its associated second metacarpal bone.

3rd Ray – The third digit of the hand and its associated third metacarpal bone.

4th Ray – The fourth digit of the hand and its associated fourth metacarpal bone.

5th Ray – The fifth digit of the hand and its associated fifth metacarpal bone.

Axilla – The multi-tissue-layered area at the junction of the arm and trunk on the underside of the shoulder joint.

Elbow Region – The multi-tissue-layered elbow joint area.

Forequarter – The portion of the body including the upper extremity, scapula, and clavicle.

Hand – The portion of the upper extermity distal to the forearm.

Index Finger – The second digit of the hand.

Little Finger – The fifth digit of the hand.

Lower Arm – The portion of the upper extermity distal to the elbow.

Middle Finger – The third digit of the hand.

Ring Finger – The fourth digit of the hand.

Shoulder Region – The multi-tissue-layered shoulder joint area.

Thumb – The first digit of the hand.

Upper Arm – The portion of the upper extermity distal to the shoulder and proximal to the elbow.

Upper Extremity – The entire upper extremity (arm).

Wrist Region – The multi-tissue-layered wrist joint area.

Educational Annotations | X – Anatomical Regions, Upper Extremities

Anatomical Illustrations of Anatomical Regions, Upper Extremities

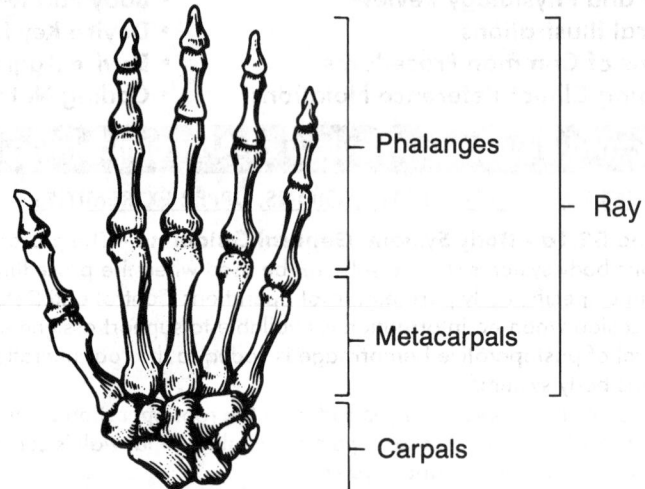

RIGHT HAND — DORSAL VIEW

Definitions of Common Procedures of Anatomical Regions, Upper Extremities

Amputation through elbow – The surgical detachment and removal of the lower arm including the entire radius and ulna that is performed through the elbow joint.

Forequarter amputation – The surgical detachment and removal of the entire arm including part or all of the scapula and clavicle.

Reattachment of severed thumb – The surgical reconnection of a thumb that has been traumatically amputated.

Transfer of index finger to thumb – The surgical dissection and migration of the index finger, including division of the metacarpal index ray bone that is positioned to function as the thumb.

Transplantation of toe to thumb – The surgical detachment of the great toe or second toe and microsurgical connection at the thumb site to function as the thumb.

Educational Annotations | X – Anatomical Regions, Upper Extremities

AHA Coding Clinic® Reference Notations of Anatomical Regions, Upper Extremities

<u>ROOT OPERATION SPECIFIC - X - ANATOMICAL REGIONS, UPPER EXTREMITIES</u>
ALTERATION - 0
CHANGE - 2
CONTROL - 3
    Control of post arterial bypass bleeding ....AHA 15:1Q:p35
DETACHMENT - 6
DRAINAGE - 9
EXCISION - B
INSERTION - H
INSPECTION - J
REATTACHMENT - M
REMOVAL - P
REPAIR - Q
REPLACEMENT - R
SUPPLEMENT - U
REVISION - W
TRANSFER - X

Body Part Key Listings of Anatomical Regions, Upper Extremities

See also Body Part Key in Appendix C
None for the Anatomical Regions, Upper Extremities Body System

Device Key Listings of Anatomical Regions, Upper Extremities

See also Device Key in Appendix D
Autograft ....*use* Autologous Tissue Substitute
Brachytherapy seeds ....*use* Radioactive Element
Tissue bank graft ....*use* Nonautologous Tissue Substitute

Device Aggregation Table Listings of Anatomical Regions, Upper Extremities

See also Device Aggregation Table in Appendix E

Specific Device	For Operation	In Body System	General Device
None Listed in Device Aggregation Table for this Body System			

Educational Annotations | X – Anatomical Regions, Upper Extremities

Coding Notes of Anatomical Regions, Upper Extremities

Body System Relevant Coding Guidelines

General Guidelines

B2.1a

The procedure codes in the general anatomical regions body systems ~~should only~~ can be used when the procedure is performed on an anatomical region rather than a specific body part (e.g., root operations Control and Detachment, Drainage of a body cavity) or on the rare occasion when no information is available to support assignment of a code to a specific body part.

Examples: Control of postoperative hemorrhage is coded to the root operation Control found in the general anatomical regions body systems.

Chest tube drainage of the pleural cavity is coded to the root operation Drainage found in the general anatomical regions body systems. Suture repair of the abdominal wall is coded to the root operation Repair in the General Anatomical Regions body system.

Control vs. more definitive root operations

B3.7

The root operation Control is defined as, "Stopping, or attempting to stop, postprocedural or other acute bleeding." If an attempt to stop postprocedural or other acute bleeding is initially unsuccessful, and to stop the bleeding requires performing any of the definitive root operations Bypass, Detachment, Excision, Extraction, Reposition, Replacement, or Resection, then that root operation is coded instead of Control.

Example: Resection of spleen to stop ~~postprocedural~~ bleeding is coded to Resection instead of Control.

Body System Specific PCS Reference Manual Exercises

PCS CODE	X – ANATOMICAL REGIONS, UPPER EXTREMITIES EXERCISES
0 X 3 F 0 Z Z	Open exploration and ligation of post-op arterial bleeder, left forearm.
0 X 6 0 0 Z Z	Right forequarter amputation. (The Forequarter body part includes amputation along any part of the scapula and clavicle.)
0 X 6 8 0 Z 2	Mid-shaft amputation, right humerus.
0 X 6 B 0 Z Z	Amputation at right elbow level.
0 X 6 J 0 Z 0	Right wrist joint amputation. (Amputation at the wrist joint is actually complete amputation of the hand.)
0 X 6 K 0 Z 8	Fifth ray carpometacarpal joint amputation, left hand. (A "Complete" ray amputation is through the carpometacarpal joint.)
0 X 6 L 0 Z 3	DIP joint amputation of right thumb. (The qualifier "Low" here means through the distal interphalangeal joint.)
0 X M K 0 Z Z	Reattachment of severed left hand.
0 X X P 0 Z M	Transfer left index finger to left thumb position, open.

OTHER OBJECTIVES GROUP: Alteration, (Creation), (Fusion)
Root Operations that define other objectives.

1ST - 0 Medical and Surgical
2ND - X Anatomical Regions, Upper Extremities
3RD - 0 ALTERATION

EXAMPLE: Cosmetic deltoid augmentation | CMS Ex: Face lift

ALTERATION: Modifying the anatomic structure of a body part without affecting the function of the body part.

EXPLANATION: Principal purpose is to improve appearance

Body Part – 4TH		Approach – 5TH	Device – 6TH	Qualifier – 7TH
2 Shoulder Region, Right	B Elbow Region, Right	0 Open	7 Autologous tissue substitute	Z No qualifier
3 Shoulder Region, Left	C Elbow Region, Left	3 Percutaneous	J Synthetic substitute	
4 Axilla, Right	D Lower Arm, Right	4 Percutaneous endoscopic	K Nonautologous tissue substitute	
5 Axilla, Left	F Lower Arm, Left		Z No device	
6 Upper Extremity, Right	G Wrist Region, Right			
7 Upper Extremity, Left	H Wrist Region, Left			
8 Upper Arm, Right				
9 Upper Arm, Left				

DEVICE GROUP: Change, Insertion, Removal, Replacement, Revision, Supplement
Root Operations that always involve a device.

1ST - 0 Medical and Surgical
2ND - X Anatomical Regions, Upper Extremities
3RD - 2 CHANGE

EXAMPLE: Exchange drain tube | CMS Ex: Changing urinary catheter

CHANGE: Taking out or off a device from a body part and putting back an identical or similar device in or on the same body part without cutting or puncturing the skin or a mucous membrane.

EXPLANATION: ALL Changes use EXTERNAL approach only ...

Body Part – 4TH	Approach – 5TH	Device – 6TH	Qualifier – 7TH
6 Upper Extremity, Right	X External	0 Drainage device	Z No qualifier
7 Upper Extremity, Left		Y Other device	

OTHER REPAIRS GROUP: Control, Repair
Root Operations that define other repairs.

1ST - 0 Medical and Surgical
2ND - X Anatomical Regions, Upper Extremities
3RD - 3 CONTROL

EXAMPLE: Ligation post-op bleeder | CMS Ex: Control post-op hemorrhage

CONTROL: Stopping, or attempting to stop, postprocedural or other acute bleeding.

EXPLANATION: Bleeding site coded to an anatomical region...

Body Part – 4TH		Approach – 5TH	Device – 6TH	Qualifier – 7TH
2 Shoulder Region, Right	B Elbow Region, Right	0 Open	Z No device	Z No qualifier
3 Shoulder Region, Left	C Elbow Region, Left	3 Percutaneous		
4 Axilla, Right	D Lower Arm, Right	4 Percutaneous endoscopic		
5 Axilla, Left	F Lower Arm, Left			
6 Upper Extremity, Right	G Wrist Region, Right			
7 Upper Extremity, Left	H Wrist Region, Left			
8 Upper Arm, Right	J Hand, Right			
9 Upper Arm, Left	K Hand, Left			

EXCISION GROUP: Excision, (Resection), (Destruction), (Extraction), **Detachment**
Root Operations that take out some or all of a body part.

1ST - **0** Medical and Surgical	EXAMPLE: Amputation hand CMS Ex: Leg amputation
2ND - **X** Anatomical Regions, Upper Extremities	<u>DETACHMENT:</u> Cutting off all or portion of the upper or lower extremities.
3RD - **6 DETACHMENT**	EXPLANATION: Qualifier specifies amputation level ...

Body Part – 4TH	Approach – 5TH	Device – 6TH	Qualifier – 7TH
0 Forequarter, Right 3 Shoulder Region, Left 1 Forequarter, Left B Elbow Region, Right 2 Shoulder Region, Right C Elbow Region, Left	0 Open	Z No device	Z No qualifier
8 Upper Arm, Right 9 Upper Arm, Left D Lower Arm, Right F Lower Arm, Left	0 Open	Z No device	1 High 2 Mid 3 Low
J Hand, Right K Hand, Left	0 Open	Z No device	0 Complete 4 Complete 1st Ray 5 Complete 2nd Ray 6 Complete 3rd Ray 7 Complete 4th Ray 8 Complete 5th Ray 9 Partial 1st Ray B Partial 2nd Ray C Partial 3rd Ray D Partial 4th Ray F Partial 5th Ray
L Thumb, Right S Ring Finger, Right M Thumb, Left T Ring Finger, Left N Index Finger, Right V Little Finger, Right P Index Finger, Left W Little Finger, Left Q Middle Finger, Right R Middle Finger, Left	0 Open	Z No device	0 Complete 1 High 2 Mid 3 Low

REGIONS UPPER EXT 0 X 6

DRAINAGE GROUP: Drainage, (Extirpation), (Fragmentation)
Root Operations that take out solids/fluids/gases from a body part.

1ST – 0 Medical and Surgical	EXAMPLE: I&D deep wound infection CMS Ex: Thoracentesis
2ND – X Anatomical Regions, Upper Extremities	**DRAINAGE:** Taking or letting out fluids and/or gases from a body part.
3RD – 9 DRAINAGE	EXPLANATION: Qualifier "X Diagnostic" indicates biopsy …

Body Part – 4TH	Approach – 5TH	Device – 6TH	Qualifier – 7TH
2 Shoulder Region, Right B Elbow Region, Right 3 Shoulder Region, Left C Elbow Region, Left 4 Axilla, Right D Lower Arm, Right 5 Axilla, Left F Lower Arm, Left 6 Upper Extremity, Right G Wrist Region, Right 7 Upper Extremity, Left H Wrist Region, Left 8 Upper Arm, Right J Hand, Right 9 Upper Arm, Left K Hand, Left	0 Open 3 Percutaneous 4 Percutaneous endoscopic	0 Drainage device	Z No qualifier
2 Shoulder Region, Right B Elbow Region, Right 3 Shoulder Region, Left C Elbow Region, Left 4 Axilla, Right D Lower Arm, Right 5 Axilla, Left F Lower Arm, Left 6 Upper Extremity, Right G Wrist Region, Right 7 Upper Extremity, Left H Wrist Region, Left 8 Upper Arm, Right J Hand, Right 9 Upper Arm, Left K Hand, Left	0 Open 3 Percutaneous 4 Percutaneous endoscopic	Z No device	X Diagnostic Z No qualifier

---

EXCISION GROUP: Excision, (Resection), (Destruction), (Extraction), **Detachment**
Root Operations that take out some or all of a body part.

1ST – 0 Medical and Surgical	EXAMPLE: Excision tumor axilla region CMS Ex: Liver biopsy
2ND – X Anatomical Regions, Upper Extremities	**EXCISION:** Cutting out or off, without replacement, a portion of a body part.
3RD – B EXCISION	EXPLANATION: Qualifier "X Diagnostic" indicates biopsy …

Body Part – 4TH	Approach – 5TH	Device – 6TH	Qualifier – 7TH
2 Shoulder Region, Right B Elbow Region, Right 3 Shoulder Region, Left C Elbow Region, Left 4 Axilla, Right D Lower Arm, Right 5 Axilla, Left F Lower Arm, Left 6 Upper Extremity, Right G Wrist Region, Right 7 Upper Extremity, Left H Wrist Region, Left 8 Upper Arm, Right J Hand, Right 9 Upper Arm, Left K Hand, Left	0 Open 3 Percutaneous 4 Percutaneous endoscopic	Z No device	X Diagnostic Z No qualifier

REGIONS UPPER EXT 0 X B

DEVICE GROUP: Change, Insertion, Removal, Replacement, Revision, Supplement
Root Operations that always involve a device.

1ST - **0** Medical and Surgical	EXAMPLE: Implant infusion device	CMS Ex: Central venous catheter

2ND - **X** Anatomical Regions, Upper Extremities

3RD - **H INSERTION**

INSERTION: Putting in a nonbiological appliance that monitors, assists, performs, or prevents a physiological function but does not physically take the place of a body part.

EXPLANATION: None

Body Part – 4TH		Approach – 5TH	Device – 6TH	Qualifier – 7TH
2 Shoulder Region, Right	B Elbow Region, Right	0 Open	1 Radioactive element	Z No qualifier
3 Shoulder Region, Left	C Elbow Region, Left	3 Percutaneous	3 Infusion device	
4 Axilla, Right	D Lower Arm, Right	4 Percutaneous endoscopic	Y Other device	
5 Axilla, Left	F Lower Arm, Left			
6 Upper Extremity, Right	G Wrist Region, Right			
7 Upper Extremity, Left	H Wrist Region, Left			
8 Upper Arm, Right	J Hand, Right			
9 Upper Arm, Left	K Hand, Left			

EXAMINATION GROUP: Inspection, (Map)
Root Operations involving examination only.

1ST - **0** Medical and Surgical	EXAMPLE: Exploration axilla region	CMS Ex: Colonoscopy

2ND - **X** Anatomical Regions, Upper Extremities

3RD - **J INSPECTION**

INSPECTION: Visually and/or manually exploring a body part.

EXPLANATION: Direct or instrumental visualization ...

Body Part – 4TH		Approach – 5TH	Device – 6TH	Qualifier – 7TH
2 Shoulder Region, Right	B Elbow Region, Right	0 Open	Z No device	Z No qualifier
3 Shoulder Region, Left	C Elbow Region, Left	3 Percutaneous		
4 Axilla, Right	D Lower Arm, Right	4 Percutaneous endoscopic		
5 Axilla, Left	F Lower Arm, Left	X External		
6 Upper Extremity, Right	G Wrist Region, Right			
7 Upper Extremity, Left	H Wrist Region, Left			
8 Upper Arm, Right	J Hand, Right			
9 Upper Arm, Left	K Hand, Left			

REGIONS UPPER EXT 0 X H

MOVE GROUP: Reattachment, (Reposition), Transfer, (Transplantation)
Root Operations that put in/put back or move some/all of a body part.

1ST – 0 Medical and Surgical
2ND – X Anatomical Regions, Upper Extremities
3RD – M REATTACHMENT

EXAMPLE: Reattachment severed thumb | CMS Ex: Reattachment hand

REATTACHMENT: Putting back in or on all or a portion of a separated body part to its normal location or other suitable location.

EXPLANATION: With/without reconnection of vessels/nerves…

Body Part – 4TH	Approach – 5TH	Device – 6TH	Qualifier – 7TH
0 Forequarter, Right / G Wrist Region, Right	0 Open	Z No device	Z No qualifier
1 Forequarter, Left / H Wrist Region, Left			
2 Shoulder Region, Right / J Hand, Right			
3 Shoulder Region, Left / K Hand, Left			
4 Axilla, Right / L Thumb, Right			
5 Axilla, Left / M Thumb, Left			
6 Upper Extremity, Right / N Index Finger, Right			
7 Upper Extremity, Left / P Index Finger, Left			
8 Upper Arm, Right / Q Middle Finger, Right			
9 Upper Arm, Left / R Middle Finger, Left			
B Elbow Region, Right / S Ring Finger, Right			
C Elbow Region, Left / T Ring Finger, Left			
D Lower Arm, Right / V Little Finger, Right			
F Lower Arm, Left / W Little Finger, Left			

DEVICE GROUP: Change, Insertion, Removal, Replacement, Revision, Supplement
Root Operations that always involve a device.

1ST – 0 Medical and Surgical
2ND – X Anatomical Regions, Upper Extremities
3RD – P REMOVAL

EXAMPLE: Removal drain tube | CMS Ex: Chest tube removal

REMOVAL: Taking out or off a device from a body part.

EXPLANATION: Removal device without reinsertion …

Body Part – 4TH	Approach – 5TH	Device – 6TH	Qualifier – 7TH
6 Upper Extremity, Right	0 Open	0 Drainage device	Z No qualifier
7 Upper Extremity, Left	3 Percutaneous	1 Radioactive element	
	4 Percutaneous endoscopic	3 Infusion device	
	X External	7 Autologous tissue substitute	
		J Synthetic substitute	
		K Nonautologous tissue substitute	
		Y Other device	

REGIONS UPPER EXT 0 X P

0 X Q

MEDICAL AND SURGICAL SECTION – 2017 ICD-10-PCS

OTHER REPAIRS GROUP: Control, Repair

Root Operations that define other repairs.

1ST - 0 Medical and Surgical

2ND - X Anatomical Regions, Upper Extremities

3RD - Q REPAIR

EXAMPLE: Repair lower arm

CMS Ex: Suture laceration

REPAIR: Restoring, to the extent possible, a body part to its normal anatomic structure and function.

EXPLANATION: Only when no other root operation applies …

Body Part – 4TH		Approach – 5TH	Device – 6TH	Qualifier – 7TH
2 Shoulder Region, Right	J Hand, Right	0 Open	Z No device	Z No qualifier
3 Shoulder Region, Left	K Hand, Left	3 Percutaneous		
4 Axilla, Right	L Thumb, Right	4 Percutaneous endoscopic		
5 Axilla, Left	M Thumb, Left	X External		
6 Upper Extremity, Right	N Index Finger, Right			
7 Upper Extremity, Left	P Index Finger, Left			
8 Upper Arm, Right	Q Middle Finger, Right			
9 Upper Arm, Left	R Middle Finger, Left			
B Elbow Region, Right	S Ring Finger, Right			
C Elbow Region, Left	T Ring Finger, Left			
D Lower Arm, Right	V Little Finger, Right			
F Lower Arm, Left	W Little Finger, Left			
G Wrist Region, Right				
H Wrist Region, Left				

DEVICE GROUP: Change, Insertion, Removal, Replacement, Revision, Supplement

Root Operations that always involve a device.

1ST - 0 Medical and Surgical

2ND - X Anatomical Regions, Upper Extremities

3RD - R REPLACEMENT

EXAMPLE: Replacement thumb with toe

CMS Ex: Total hip

REPLACEMENT: Putting in or on a biological or synthetic material that physically takes the place and/or function of all or a portion of a body part.

EXPLANATION: Includes taking out body part, or eradication…

Body Part – 4TH	Approach – 5TH	Device – 6TH	Qualifier – 7TH
L Thumb, Right	0 Open	7 Autologous tissue substitute	N Toe, Right
M Thumb, Left	4 Percutaneous endoscopic		P Toe, Left

REGIONS UPPER EXT 0 X Q

© 2016 Channel Publishing, Ltd.

688

DEVICE GROUP: Change, Insertion, Removal, Replacement, Revision, Supplement
Root Operations that always involve a device.

1ST - **0** Medical and Surgical

2ND - **X** Anatomical Regions, Upper Extremities

3RD - **U SUPPLEMENT**

EXAMPLE: Augmentation graft axilla | CMS Ex: Hernia repair with mesh

SUPPLEMENT: Putting in or on biological or synthetic material that physically reinforces and/or augments the function of a portion of a body part.

EXPLANATION: Biological material from same individual ...

Body Part – 4TH		Approach – 5TH	Device – 6TH	Qualifier – 7TH
2 Shoulder Region, Right	J Hand, Right	0 Open	7 Autologous tissue substitute	Z No qualifier
3 Shoulder Region, Left	K Hand, Left	4 Percutaneous endoscopic	J Synthetic substitute	
4 Axilla, Right	L Thumb, Right		K Nonautologous tissue substitute	
5 Axilla, Left	M Thumb, Left			
6 Upper Extremity, Right	N Index Finger, Right			
7 Upper Extremity, Left	P Index Finger, Left			
8 Upper Arm, Right	Q Middle Finger, Right			
9 Upper Arm, Left	R Middle Finger, Left			
B Elbow Region, Right	S Ring Finger, Right			
C Elbow Region, Left	T Ring Finger, Left			
D Lower Arm, Right	V Little Finger, Right			
F Lower Arm, Left	W Little Finger, Left			
G Wrist Region, Right				
H Wrist Region, Left				

DEVICE GROUP: Change, Insertion, Removal, Replacement, Revision, Supplement
Root Operations that always involve a device.

1ST - **0** Medical and Surgical

2ND - **X** Anatomical Regions, Upper Extremities

3RD - **W REVISION**

EXAMPLE: Reposition drain tube | CMS Ex: Adjustment pacemaker lead

REVISION: Correcting, to the extent possible, a portion of a malfunctioning device or the position of a displaced device.

EXPLANATION: May replace components of a device ...

Body Part – 4TH	Approach – 5TH	Device – 6TH	Qualifier – 7TH
6 Upper Extremity, Right	0 Open	0 Drainage device	Z No qualifier
7 Upper Extremity, Left	3 Percutaneous	3 Infusion device	
	4 Percutaneous endoscopic	7 Autologous tissue substitute	
	X External	J Synthetic substitute	
		K Nonautologous tissue substitute	
		Y Other device	

REGIONS UPPER EXT 0 X W

MOVE GROUP: Reattachment, (Reposition), Transfer, (Transplantation)
Root Operations that put in/put back or move some/all of a body part.

1ST - 0 Medical and Surgical	EXAMPLE: Transfer index finger to thumb	CMS Ex: Tendon transfer
2ND - X Anatomical Regions, Upper Extremities	TRANSFER: Moving, without taking out, all or a portion of a body part to another location to take over the function of all or a portion of a body part.	
3RD - X TRANSFER	EXPLANATION: The body part remains connected ...	

Body Part – 4TH	Approach – 5TH	Device – 6TH	Qualifier – 7TH
N Index Finger, Right	0 Open	Z No device	L Thumb, Right
P Index Finger, Left	0 Open	Z No device	M Thumb, Left

MOVE GROUP: Reattachment, (Reposition), (Transfer), Transplantation
Root Operations that put in/put back or move some/all of a body part.

1ST - 0 Medical and Surgical	EXAMPLE: Hand transplant	CMS Ex: Kidney transplant
2ND - X Anatomical Regions, Upper Extremities	TRANSPLANTATION: Putting in or on all or a portion of a living body part taken from another individual or animal to physically take the place and/or function of all or a portion of a similar body part.	
3RD - Y TRANSPLANTATION	EXPLANATION: May take over all or part of its function ...	

Body Part – 4TH	Approach – 5TH	Device – 6TH	Qualifier – 7TH
J Hand, Right K Hand, Left	0 Open	Z No device	0 Allogeneic 1 Syngeneic

Educational Annotations | Y – Anatomical Regions, Lower Extremities

Body System Specific Educational Annotations for the Anatomical Regions, Lower Extremities include:

- Anatomy and Physiology Review
- Anatomical Illustrations
- Definitions of Common Procedures
- AHA Coding Clinic® Reference Notations
- Body Part Key Listings
- Device Key Listings
- Device Aggregation Table Listings
- Coding Notes

Anatomy and Physiology Review of Anatomical Regions, Lower Extremities

BODY PART VALUES – Y - ANATOMICAL REGIONS, LOWER EXTREMITIES

Coding Guideline B2.1a - Body System, General Guideline – The procedure codes in the general anatomical regions body systems ~~should only~~ can be used when the procedure is performed on an anatomical region rather than a specific body part (e.g., root operations Control and Detachment, Drainage of a body cavity) or on the rare occasion when no information is available to support assignment of a code to a specific body part.
Examples: Control of postoperative hemorrhage is coded to the root operation Control found in the general anatomical regions body systems.
Chest tube drainage of the pleural cavity is coded to the root operation Drainage found in the general anatomical regions body systems. Suture repair of the abdominal wall is coded to the root operation Repair in the General Anatomical Regions body system.

1st Ray – The first digit of the foot and its associated first metatarsal bone.

2nd Ray – The second digit of the foot and its associated second metatarsal bone.

3rd Ray – The third digit of the foot and its associated third metatarsal bone.

4th Ray – The fourth digit of the foot and its associated fourth metatarsal bone.

5th Ray – The fifth digit of the foot and its associated fifth metatarsal bone.

1st Toe – The first digit of the foot.

2nd Toe – The second digit of the foot.

3rd Toe – The third digit of the foot.

4th Toe – The fourth digit of the foot.

5th Toe – The fifth digit of the foot.

Ankle Region – The multi-tissue-layered ankle joint area.

Buttock – The rounded lower portions of the posterior trunk including the gluteus muscles.

Femoral Region – The multi-tissue-layered area of the anterior upper inner portion of the thigh (also known as the femoral triangle). See also the body part "Upper Leg."

Foot – The portion of the lower extermity distal to the lower end of the tibia and fibula.

Hindquarter – The portion of the body including the lower extremity, buttock, and pelvis.

Inguinal Region – The multi-tissue-layered area between the lower abdomen, thigh, and pubic bone.

Knee Region – The multi-tissue-layered knee joint area.

Lower Extremity – The entire lower extremity (leg).

Lower Leg – The portion of the lower extermity distal to the knee.

Upper Leg – The portion of the lower extermity distal to the hip and proximal to the knee.

Educational Annotations | Y – Anatomical Regions, Lower Extremities

Anatomical Illustrations of Anatomical Regions, Lower Extremities

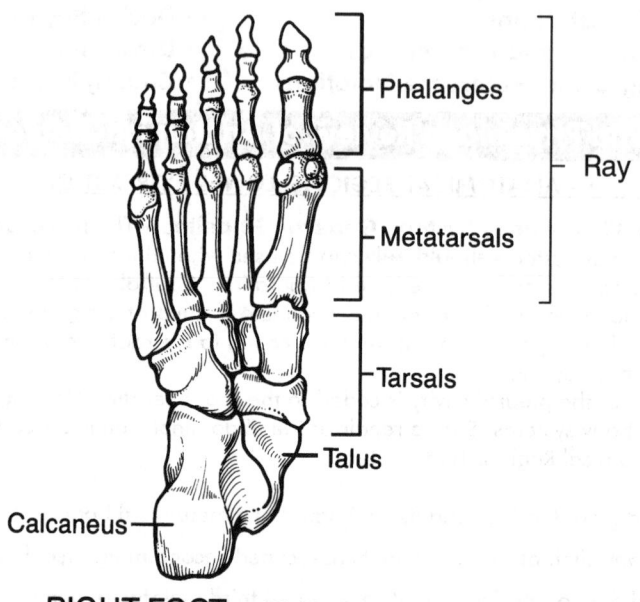

Phalanges

Ray

Metatarsals

Tarsals

Talus

Calcaneus

RIGHT FOOT — PLANTAR VIEW

Definitions of Common Procedures of Anatomical Regions, Lower Extremities

Buttock implants – The plastic surgical enhancement of the buttocks usually using solid silicone implants or by fat transfers.

Hindquarter amputation – The surgical detachment and removal of the entire leg including part or all of the buttock and pelvis.

Midfoot amputation – The surgical detachment and removal of the distal foot that is performed through the tarsal-metatarsal joints.

Educational Annotations | Y – Anatomical Regions, Lower Extremities

AHA Coding Clinic® Reference Notations of Anatomical Regions, Lower Extremities

ROOT OPERATION SPECIFIC - Y - ANATOMICAL REGIONS, LOWER EXTREMITIES

ALTERATION - 0

CHANGE - 2

CONTROL - 3

DETACHMENT - 6
Amputation of 1st toe at the interphalangeal joint ....AHA 15:2Q:p2
Midfoot amputation ....AHA 15:1Q:p28

DRAINAGE - 9
Incision and drainage of femoral region wound infection ....AHA 15:1Q:p22
Incision and drainage of inguinal region wound infection ....AHA 15:1Q:p22

EXCISION - B

INSERTION - H

INSPECTION - J

REATTACHMENT - M

REMOVAL - P

REPAIR - Q

SUPPLEMENT - U

REVISION - W

Body Part Key Listings of Anatomical Regions, Lower Extremities

See also Body Part Key in Appendix C

Hallux ....*use* 1st Toe, Left/Right

Inguinal canal ....*use* Inguinal Region, Bilateral/Left/Right

Inguinal triangle ....*use* Inguinal Region, Bilateral/Left/Right

Device Key Listings of Anatomical Regions, Lower Extremities

See also Device Key in Appendix D

Autograft ....*use* Autologous Tissue Substitute

Brachytherapy seeds ....*use* Radioactive Element

Cook Biodesign® Hernia Graft(s) ....*use* Nonautologous Tissue Substitute

Cook Biodesign® Layered Graft(s) ....*use* Nonautologous Tissue Substitute

Cook Zenapro™ Layered Graft(s) ....*use* Nonautologous Tissue Substitute

Tissue bank graft ....*use* Nonautologous Tissue Substitute

Device Aggregation Table Listings of Anatomical Regions, Lower Extremities

See also Device Aggregation Table in Appendix E

Specific Device	For Operation	In Body System	General Device
None Listed in Device Aggregation Table for this Body System			

Educational Annotations | Y – Anatomical Regions, Lower Extremities

Coding Notes of Anatomical Regions, Lower Extremities

Body System Relevant Coding Guidelines

General Guidelines
B2.1a

The procedure codes in the general anatomical regions body systems ~~should only~~ can be used when the procedure is performed on an anatomical region rather than a specific body part (e.g., root operations Control and Detachment, Drainage of a body cavity) or on the rare occasion when no information is available to support assignment of a code to a specific body part.

Examples: Control of postoperative hemorrhage is coded to the root operation Control found in the general anatomical regions body systems.

Chest tube drainage of the pleural cavity is coded to the root operation Drainage found in the general anatomical regions body systems. Suture repair of the abdominal wall is coded to the root operation Repair in the General Anatomical Regions body system.

Control vs. more definitive root operations
B3.7

The root operation Control is defined as, "Stopping, or attempting to stop, postprocedural or other acute bleeding." If an attempt to stop postprocedural or other acute bleeding is initially unsuccessful, and to stop the bleeding requires performing any of the definitive root operations Bypass, Detachment, Excision, Extraction, Reposition, Replacement, or Resection, then that root operation is coded instead of Control.

Example: Resection of spleen to stop ~~postprocedural~~ bleeding is coded to Resection instead of Control.

Body System Specific PCS Reference Manual Exercises

PCS CODE	Y – ANATOMICAL REGIONS, LOWER EXTREMITIES EXERCISES
0 Y 3 F 4 Z Z	Arthroscopy with drainage of hemarthrosis at previous operative site, right knee.
0 Y 6 2 0 Z Z	Right leg and hip amputation through ischium. (The "Hindquarter" body part includes amputation along any part of the hip bone.)
0 Y 6 C 0 Z 3	Right above-knee amputation, distal femur.
0 Y 6 H 0 Z 1	Right below-knee amputation, proximal tibia/fibula. (The qualifier "High" here means the portion of the tibia/fibula closest to the knee.)
0 Y 6 N 0 Z 9	Trans-metatarsal amputation of foot at left big toe. (A "Partial" amputation is through the shaft of the metatarsal bone.)
0 Y 6 W 0 Z 1	Left fourth toe amputation, mid-proximal phalanx. (The qualifier "High" here means anywhere along the proximal phalanx.)
0 Y U 6 4 J Z	Laparoscopic repair of left inguinal hernia with marlex plug.

OTHER OBJECTIVES GROUP: Alteration, (Creation), (Fusion)
Root Operations that define other objectives.

1ST - 0 Medical and Surgical **2ND - Y** Anatomical Regions, Lower Extremities **3RD - 0 ALTERATION**	EXAMPLE: Cosmetic buttock augmentation CMS Ex: Face lift
	ALTERATION: Modifying the anatomic structure of a body part without affecting the function of the body part.
	EXPLANATION: Principal purpose is to improve appearance

Body Part – 4TH		Approach – 5TH	Device – 6TH	Qualifier – 7TH
0 Buttock, Right 1 Buttock, Left 9 Lower Extremity, Right B Lower Extremity, Left C Upper Leg, Right D Upper Leg, Left	F Knee Region, Right G Knee Region, Left H Lower Leg, Right J Lower Leg, Left K Ankle Region, Right L Ankle Region, Left	0 Open 3 Percutaneous 4 Percutaneous endoscopic	7 Autologous tissue substitute J Synthetic substitute K Nonautologous tissue substitute Z No device	Z No qualifier

DEVICE GROUP: Change, Insertion, Removal, (Replacement), Revision, Supplement
Root Operations that always involve a device.

1ST - 0 Medical and Surgical **2ND - Y** Anatomical Regions, Lower Extremities **3RD - 2 CHANGE**	EXAMPLE: Exchange drain tube CMS Ex: Changing urinary catheter
	CHANGE: Taking out or off a device from a body part and putting back an identical or similar device in or on the same body part without cutting or puncturing the skin or a mucous membrane.
	EXPLANATION: ALL Changes use EXTERNAL approach only …

Body Part – 4TH	Approach – 5TH	Device – 6TH	Qualifier – 7TH
9 Lower Extremity, Right B Lower Extremity, Left	X External	0 Drainage device Y Other device	Z No qualifier

OTHER REPAIRS GROUP: Control, Repair
Root Operations that define other repairs.

1ST - 0 Medical and Surgical **2ND - Y** Anatomical Regions, Lower Extremities **3RD - 3 CONTROL**	EXAMPLE: Ligation post-op bleeder CMS Ex: Control post-op hemorrhage
	CONTROL: Stopping, or attempting to stop, postprocedural or other acute bleeding.
	EXPLANATION: Bleeding site coded to an anatomical region…

Body Part – 4TH		Approach – 5TH	Device – 6TH	Qualifier – 7TH
0 Buttock, Right 1 Buttock, Left 5 Inguinal Region, Right 6 Inguinal Region, Left 7 Femoral Region, Right 8 Femoral Region, Left 9 Lower Extremity, Right B Lower Extremity, Left C Upper Leg, Right D Upper Leg, Left	F Knee Region, Right G Knee Region, Left H Lower Leg, Right J Lower Leg, Left K Ankle Region, Right L Ankle Region, Left M Foot, Right N Foot, Left	0 Open 3 Percutaneous 4 Percutaneous endoscopic	Z No device	Z No qualifier

REGIONS LOWER EXT **0 Y 3**

EXCISION GROUP: Excision, (Resection), (Destruction), (Extraction), **Detachment**
Root Operations that take out some or all of a body part.

1ST - 0 Medical and Surgical
2ND - Y Anatomical Regions, Lower Extremities
3RD - 6 DETACHMENT

EXAMPLE: Below knee amputation | CMS Ex: Leg amputation

DETACHMENT: Cutting off all or portion of the upper or lower extremities.

EXPLANATION: Qualifier specifies amputation level ...

Body Part – 4TH		Approach – 5TH	Device – 6TH	Qualifier – 7TH
2 Hindquarter, Right 3 Hindquarter, Left 4 Hindquarter, Bilateral	7 Femoral Region, Right 8 Femoral Region, Left F Knee Region, Right G Knee Region, Left	0 Open	Z No device	Z No qualifier
C Upper Leg, Right D Upper Leg, Left H Lower Leg, Right J Lower Leg, Left		0 Open	Z No device	1 High 2 Mid 3 Low
M Foot, Right N Foot, Left		0 Open	Z No device	0 Complete 4 Complete 1st Ray 5 Complete 2nd Ray 6 Complete 3rd Ray 7 Complete 4th Ray 8 Complete 5th Ray 9 Partial 1st Ray B Partial 2nd Ray C Partial 3rd Ray D Partial 4th Ray F Partial 5th Ray
P 1st Toe, Right Q 1st Toe, Left R 2nd Toe, Right S 2nd Toe, Left T 3rd Toe, Right	U 3rd Toe, Left V 4th Toe, Right W 4th Toe, Left X 5th Toe, Right Y 5th Toe, Left	0 Open	Z No device	0 Complete 1 High 2 Mid 3 Low

DRAINAGE GROUP: Drainage, (Extirpation), (Fragmentation)				
Root Operations that take out solids/fluids/gases from a body part.				

1ST - 0 Medical and Surgical

2ND - Y Anatomical Regions, Lower Extremities

3RD - 9 DRAINAGE

EXAMPLE: I&D deep wound infection   CMS Ex: Thoracentesis

DRAINAGE: Taking or letting out fluids and/or gases from a body part.

EXPLANATION: Qualifier "X Diagnostic" indicates biopsy ...

Body Part – 4TH		Approach – 5TH	Device – 6TH	Qualifier – 7TH
0 Buttock, Right 1 Buttock, Left 5 Inguinal Region, Right 6 Inguinal Region, Left 7 Femoral Region, Right 8 Femoral Region, Left 9 Lower Extremity, Right B Lower Extremity, Left C Upper Leg, Right D Upper Leg, Left	F Knee Region, Right G Knee Region, Left H Lower Leg, Right J Lower Leg, Left K Ankle Region, Right L Ankle Region, Left M Foot, Right N Foot, Left	0 Open 3 Percutaneous 4 Percutaneous endoscopic	0 Drainage device	Z No qualifier
0 Buttock, Right 1 Buttock, Left 5 Inguinal Region, Right 6 Inguinal Region, Left 7 Femoral Region, Right 8 Femoral Region, Left 9 Lower Extremity, Right B Lower Extremity, Left C Upper Leg, Right D Upper Leg, Left	F Knee Region, Right G Knee Region, Left H Lower Leg, Right J Lower Leg, Left K Ankle Region, Right L Ankle Region, Left M Foot, Right N Foot, Left	0 Open 3 Percutaneous 4 Percutaneous endoscopic	Z No device	X Diagnostic Z No qualifier

EXCISION GROUP: Excision, (Resection), (Destruction), (Extraction), Detachment				
Root Operations that take out some or all of a body part.				

1ST - 0 Medical and Surgical

2ND - Y Anatomical Regions, Lower Extremities

3RD - B EXCISION

EXAMPLE: Excision tumor inguinal region   CMS Ex: Liver biopsy

EXCISION: Cutting out or off, without replacement, a portion of a body part.

EXPLANATION: Qualifier "X Diagnostic" indicates biopsy ...

Body Part – 4TH		Approach – 5TH	Device – 6TH	Qualifier – 7TH
0 Buttock, Right 1 Buttock, Left 5 Inguinal Region, Right 6 Inguinal Region, Left 7 Femoral Region, Right 8 Femoral Region, Left 9 Lower Extremity, Right B Lower Extremity, Left C Upper Leg, Right D Upper Leg, Left	F Knee Region, Right G Knee Region, Left H Lower Leg, Right J Lower Leg, Left K Ankle Region, Right L Ankle Region, Left M Foot, Right N Foot, Left	0 Open 3 Percutaneous 4 Percutaneous endoscopic	Z No device	X Diagnostic Z No qualifier

---

DEVICE GROUP: Change, Insertion, Removal, (Replacement), Revision, Supplement
Root Operations that always involve a device.

1ST – **0** Medical and Surgical

2ND – **Y** Anatomical Regions, Lower Extremities

3RD – **H** INSERTION

EXAMPLE: Implant infusion device | CMS Ex: Central venous catheter

INSERTION: Putting in a nonbiological appliance that monitors, assists, performs, or prevents a physiological function but does not physically take the place of a body part.

EXPLANATION: None

Body Part – 4TH		Approach – 5TH	Device – 6TH	Qualifier – 7TH
0 Buttock, Right	F Knee Region, Right	0 Open	1 Radioactive element	Z No qualifier
1 Buttock, Left	G Knee Region, Left	3 Percutaneous	3 Infusion device	
5 Inguinal Region, Right	H Lower Leg, Right	4 Percutaneous endoscopic	Y Other device	
6 Inguinal Region, Left	J Lower Leg, Left			
7 Femoral Region, Right	K Ankle Region, Right			
8 Femoral Region, Left	L Ankle Region, Left			
9 Lower Extremity, Right	M Foot, Right			
B Lower Extremity, Left	N Foot, Left			
C Upper Leg, Right				
D Upper Leg, Left				

EXAMINATION GROUP: Inspection, (Map)
Root Operations involving examination only.

1ST – **0** Medical and Surgical

2ND – **Y** Anatomical Regions, Lower Extremities

3RD – **J** INSPECTION

EXAMPLE: Exploration femoral region | CMS Ex: Colonoscopy

INSPECTION: Visually and/or manually exploring a body part.

EXPLANATION: Direct or instrumental visualization ...

Body Part – 4TH		Approach – 5TH	Device – 6TH	Qualifier – 7TH
0 Buttock, Right	E Femoral Region, Bilateral	0 Open	Z No device	Z No qualifier
1 Buttock, Left	F Knee Region, Right	3 Percutaneous		
5 Inguinal Region, Right	G Knee Region, Left	4 Percutaneous endoscopic		
6 Inguinal Region, Left	H Lower Leg, Right	X External		
7 Femoral Region, Right	J Lower Leg, Left			
8 Femoral Region, Left	K Ankle Region, Right			
9 Lower Extremity, Right	L Ankle Region, Left			
A Inguinal Region, Bilateral	M Foot, Right			
B Lower Extremity, Left	N Foot, Left			
C Upper Leg, Right				
D Upper Leg, Left				

MOVE GROUP: Reattachment, (Reposition), (Transfer), (Transplantation)
Root Operations that put in/put back or move some/all of a body part.

1ST - 0 Medical and Surgical	EXAMPLE: Reattachment severed 1st toe	CMS Ex: Reattachment hand
2ND - Y Anatomical Regions, Lower Extremities	REATTACHMENT: Putting back in or on all or a portion of a separated body part to its normal location or other suitable location.	
3RD - M REATTACHMENT	EXPLANATION: With/without reconnection of vessels/nerves…	

Body Part – 4TH		Approach – 5TH	Device – 6TH	Qualifier – 7TH
0 Buttock, Right	H Lower Leg, Right	0 Open	Z No device	Z No qualifier
1 Buttock, Left	J Lower Leg, Left			
2 Hindquarter, Right	K Ankle Region, Right			
3 Hindquarter, Left	L Ankle Region, Left			
4 Hindquarter, Bilateral	M Foot, Right			
5 Inguinal Region, Right	N Foot, Left			
6 Inguinal Region, Left	P 1st Toe, Right			
7 Femoral Region, Right	Q 1st Toe, Left			
8 Femoral Region, Left	R 2nd Toe, Right			
9 Lower Extremity, Right	S 2nd Toe, Left			
B Lower Extremity, Left	T 3rd Toe, Right			
C Upper Leg, Right	U 3rd Toe, Left			
D Upper Leg, Left	V 4th Toe, Right			
F Knee Region, Right	W 4th Toe, Left			
G Knee Region, Left	X 5th Toe, Right			
	Y 5th Toe, Left			

DEVICE GROUP: Change, Insertion, Removal, (Replacement), Revision, Supplement
Root Operations that always involve a device.

1ST - 0 Medical and Surgical	EXAMPLE: Removal drain tube	CMS Ex: Chest tube removal
2ND - Y Anatomical Regions, Lower Extremities	REMOVAL: Taking out or off a device from a body part.	
3RD - P REMOVAL	EXPLANATION: Removal device without reinsertion …	

Body Part – 4TH	Approach – 5TH	Device – 6TH	Qualifier – 7TH
9 Lower Extremity, Right	0 Open	0 Drainage device	Z No qualifier
B Lower Extremity, Left	3 Percutaneous	1 Radioactive element	
	4 Percutaneous endoscopic	3 Infusion device	
	X External	7 Autologous tissue substitute	
		J Synthetic substitute	
		K Nonautologous tissue substitute	
		Y Other device	

REGIONS LOWER EXT 0 Y P

OTHER REPAIRS GROUP: Control, Repair
Root Operations that define other repairs.

1ST – **0** Medical and Surgical	EXAMPLE: Repair upper leg	CMS Ex: Suture laceration
2ND – **Y** Anatomical Regions, Lower Extremities	**REPAIR:** Restoring, to the extent possible, a body part to its normal anatomic structure and function.	
3RD – **Q REPAIR**	EXPLANATION: Only when no other root operation applies ...	

Body Part – 4TH		Approach – 5TH	Device – 6TH	Qualifier – 7TH
0 Buttock, Right	K Ankle Region, Right	0 Open	Z No device	Z No qualifier
1 Buttock, Left	L Ankle Region, Left	3 Percutaneous		
5 Inguinal Region, Right	M Foot, Right	4 Percutaneous		
6 Inguinal Region, Left	N Foot, Left	endoscopic		
7 Femoral Region, Right	P 1st Toe, Right	X External		
8 Femoral Region, Left	Q 1st Toe, Left			
9 Lower Extremity, Right	R 2nd Toe, Right			
A Inguinal Region, Bilateral	S 2nd Toe, Left			
B Lower Extremity, Left	T 3rd Toe, Right			
C Upper Leg, Right	U 3rd Toe, Left			
D Upper Leg, Left	V 4th Toe, Right			
E Femoral Region, Bilateral	W 4th Toe, Left			
F Knee Region, Right	X 5th Toe, Right			
G Knee Region, Left	Y 5th Toe, Left			
H Lower Leg, Right				
J Lower Leg, Left				

DEVICE GROUP: Change, Insertion, Removal, (Replacement), Revision, Supplement
Root Operations that always involve a device.

1ST – **0** Medical and Surgical	EXAMPLE: Inguinal hernia repair with mesh	CMS Ex: Hernia with mesh
2ND – **Y** Anatomical Regions, Lower Extremities	**SUPPLEMENT:** Putting in or on biological or synthetic material that physically reinforces and/or augments the function of a portion of a body part.	
3RD – **U SUPPLEMENT**	EXPLANATION: Biological material from same individual ...	

Body Part – 4TH		Approach – 5TH	Device – 6TH	Qualifier – 7TH
0 Buttock, Right	K Ankle Region, Right	0 Open	7 Autologous tissue substitute	Z No qualifier
1 Buttock, Left	L Ankle Region, Left	4 Percutaneous endoscopic	J Synthetic substitute	
5 Inguinal Region, Right	M Foot, Right		K Nonautologous tissue substitute	
6 Inguinal Region, Left	N Foot, Left			
7 Femoral Region, Right	P 1st Toe, Right			
8 Femoral Region, Left	Q 1st Toe, Left			
9 Lower Extremity, Right	R 2nd Toe, Right			
A Inguinal Region, Bilateral	S 2nd Toe, Left			
B Lower Extremity, Left	T 3rd Toe, Right			
C Upper Leg, Right	U 3rd Toe, Left			
D Upper Leg, Left	V 4th Toe, Right			
E Femoral Region, Bilateral	W 4th Toe, Left			
F Knee Region, Right	X 5th Toe, Right			
G Knee Region, Left	Y 5th Toe, Left			
H Lower Leg, Right				
J Lower Leg, Left				

REGIONS LOWER EXT 0 Y Q

DEVICE GROUP: Change, Insertion, Removal, (Replacement), Revision, Supplement
Root Operations that always involve a device.

1ST - **0**   Medical and Surgical

2ND - **Y**   Anatomical Regions, Lower Extremities

3RD - **W REVISION**

EXAMPLE: Reposition drain tube   CMS Ex: Adjustment pacemaker lead

REVISION: Correcting, to the extent possible, a portion of a malfunctioning device or the position of a displaced device.

EXPLANATION: May replace components of a device ...

Body Part – 4TH	Approach – 5TH	Device – 6TH	Qualifier – 7TH
9 Lower Extremity, Right B Lower Extremity, Left	0 Open 3 Percutaneous 4 Percutaneous endoscopic X External	0 Drainage device 3 Infusion device 7 Autologous tissue substitute J Synthetic substitute K Nonautologous tissue substitute Y Other device	Z No qualifier

REGIONS LOWER EXT 0 Y W

<u>**NOTES**</u>

Educational Annotations | Section 1 – Obstetrics

Section Specific Educational Annotations for the Obstetrics Section include:

- Anatomy and Physiology Review
- Anatomical Illustrations
- Definitions of Common Procedures
- AHA Coding Clinic® Reference Notations
- Body Part Key Listings
- Device Key Listings
- Device Aggregation Table Listings
- Coding Notes

Anatomy and Physiology Review of Obstetrics

BODY PART VALUES – 0 - Obstetrics

Products of Conception – The fetus, placenta, and other tissue derived from a fertilized gestation.

Products of Conception, Ectopic – Products of conception that develop outside the uterus.

Products of Conception, Retained – Products of conception that remain in the uterus following delivery, termination of pregnancy, or miscarriage.

Anatomical Illustrations of Obstetrics

None for the Obstetrics Section

Definitions of Common Procedures of Obstetrics

Amniocentesis – The medical procedure of inserting a needle with ultrasound guidance through the abdominal wall and uterine wall, and then puncturing the amniotic sac to withdraw a small amount of amniotic fluid that is used for testing for fetal abnormalities, usually done early in the second trimester.

Amnioscopy – The instrumental visualization of the fetus and lower amniotic sac by using an amnioscope that is inserted into the vaginal canal and used in late pregnancy or during labor.

Cesarean section (C-section) – The surgical delivery of the fetus through an incision in the uterine wall. The classical c-section incision is a vertical incision in the abdomen and in the mid to upper portion of the uterus. The low cervical c-section incision is a transverse (horizontal) or vertical incision in the abdomen just above the pubis and in the lower portion of the uterus just above the cervix.

Forceps-assisted vaginal delivery – The use of special tools that are curved and shallow cup-shaped to assist delivering a fetus that is having difficulty passing through the birth canal. The descriptions of low, mid, or high forceps are based on the stage of fetal head engagement and station of progress entering and passing through the birth canal.

Removal of tubal pregnancy – The open or laparoscopic-approach surgical removal of an ectopic pregnancy (embryo attaches outside the uterus) that is attached in a fallopian tube. The fallopian tube may be incised (salpingostomy) or a segment may need to be excised (salpingectomy).

Vacuum-assisted vaginal delivery – The use of a special vacuum extractor with a soft plastic cup that attaches to the fetal head with suction to help deliver the fetus through the birth canal.

OBSTETRICS

1

Educational Annotations | Section 1 – Obstetrics

AHA Coding Clinic® Reference Notations of Obstetrics

ROOT OPERATION SPECIFIC - OBSTETRICS - Section 1

MISC
Induction of labor, IV oxytocin, peripheral vein ....AHA 14:4Q:p17
Induction of labor with Cervidil dinoprostone vaginal tampon...................AHA 14:2Q:p8
Pitocin to augment active labor ....AHA 14:2Q:p9

CHANGE - 2

DRAINAGE - 9
Artificial rupture of membranes ....AHA 14:2Q:p9
Laser microseptostomy for twin-twin transfusion syndrome ....AHA 14:3Q:p12

ABORTION - A

EXTRACTION - D
Cesarean section with vacuum assistance...AHA 14:4Q:p43
Vacuum assisted low forceps delivery ....AHA 16:1Q:p9
Vacuum D&C for blighted ovum ....AHA 14:4Q:p43

DELIVERY - E
Assisted vaginal delivery ....AHA 14:2Q:p9
Manually assisted vaginal delivery ....AHA 16:2Q:p34

INSERTION - H
Intrauterine pressure monitoring during labor ....AHA 13:2Q:p36

INSPECTION - J

REMOVAL - P

REPAIR - Q
Fetoscopic laser photocoagulation of vascular connections ....AHA 14:3Q:p12

REPOSITION - S

RESECTION - T
Excision/removal of fallopian tube ectopic pregnancy ....AHA 15:3Q:p31

TRANSPLANTATION - Y

Body Part Key Listings of Obstetrics

None for the Obstetrics Section

Device Key Listings of Obstetrics

None for the Obstetrics Section

Device Aggregation Table Listings of Obstetrics

None for the Obstetrics Section

OBSTETRICS

1

Educational Annotations | Section 1 – Obstetrics

Coding Notes of Obstetrics

Body System Relevant Coding Guidelines

C. Obstetrics Section

Products of conception

C1

Procedures performed on the products of conception are coded to the Obstetrics section. Procedures performed on the pregnant female other than the products of conception are coded to the appropriate root operation in the Medical and Surgical section.

Example: Amniocentesis is coded to the products of conception body part in the Obstetrics section. Repair of obstetric urethral laceration is coded to the urethra body part in the Medical and Surgical section.

Procedures following delivery or abortion

C2

Procedures performed following a delivery or abortion for curettage of the endometrium or evacuation of retained products of conception are all coded in the Obstetrics section, to the root operation Extraction and the body part Products of Conception, Retained. Diagnostic or therapeutic dilation and curettage performed during times other than the postpartum or post-abortion period are all coded in the Medical and Surgical section, to the root operation Extraction and the body part Endometrium.

Med/Surg Related Section Specific PCS Reference Manual Exercises

PCS CODE	1 – OBSTETRICS EXERCISES
1 0 9 0 3 Z A	Fetal spinal tap, percutaneous.
1 0 A 0 7 Z W	Abortion by dilation and evacuation following laminaria insertion.
1 0 A 0 7 Z X	Abortion by abortifacient insertion.
1 0 D 0 0 Z 2	Extraperitoneal c-section, low transverse incision.
1 0 E 0 X Z Z	Manually assisted spontaneous abortion. (Since the pregnancy was not artificially terminated, this is coded to Delivery, because it captures the procedure objective. The fact that it was an abortion will be identified in the diagnosis code.)
1 0 J 0 7 Z Z	Bimanual pregnancy examination.
1 0 P 0 7 3 Z	Transvaginal removal of fetal monitoring electrode.
1 0 Q 0 0 Z K	Open in utero repair of congenital diaphragmatic hernia. (Diaphragm is classified to the Respiratory body system in the Medical and Surgical section.)
1 0 T 2 4 Z Z	Laparoscopy with total excision of tubal pregnancy.
1 0 Y 0 4 Z S	Fetal kidney transplant, laparoscopic.

OBSTETRICS

1

Educational Annotations | Section 1 – Obstetrics

NOTES

OBSTETRICS SECTION:			
Change, Drainage, Abortion, Extraction, Delivery, Insertion, Inspection, Removal, Repair, Reposition, Resection, Transplanation			
Root Operations that are performed on the products of conception.			

1ST - **1** Obstetrics

2ND - **0** Pregnancy ♀

3RD - **2 CHANGE**

EXAMPLE: Exchanging intrauterine pressure monitor

CHANGE: Taking out or off a device from a body part and putting back an identical or similar device in or on the same body part without cutting or puncturing the skin or a mucous membrane.

EXPLANATION: None

Body Part – 4TH	Approach – 5TH	Device – 6TH	Qualifier – 7TH
0 Products of Conception	7 Via natural or artificial opening	3 Monitoring electrode Y Other device	Z No qualifier

OBSTETRICS SECTION:			
Change, Drainage, Abortion, Extraction, Delivery, Insertion, Inspection, Removal, Repair, Reposition, Resection, Transplanation			
Root Operations that are performed on the products of conception.			

1ST - **1** Obstetrics

2ND - **0** Pregnancy ♀

3RD - **9 DRAINAGE**

EXAMPLE: Amniocentesis, artificial rupture of membranes

DRAINAGE: Taking or letting out fluids and/or gases from a body part.

EXPLANATION: Qualifier identifies type of fluid

Body Part – 4TH	Approach – 5TH	Device – 6TH	Qualifier – 7TH
0 Products of Conception	0 Open 3 Percutaneous 4 Percutaneous endoscopic 7 Via natural or artificial opening 8 Via natural or artificial opening endoscopic	Z No device	9 Fetal blood A Fetal cerebrospinal fluid B Fetal fluid, other C Amniotic fluid, therapeutic D Fluid, other U Amniotic fluid, diagnostic

OBSTETRICS

109

OBSTETRICS SECTION:
Change, Drainage, Abortion, Extraction, Delivery, Insertion, Inspection, Removal, Repair, Reposition, Resection, Transplanation
Root Operations that are performed on the products of conception.

1ST - 1 Obstetrics	EXAMPLE: Therapeutic abortion
2ND - 0 Pregnancy ♀	**ABORTION:** Artificially terminating a pregnancy.
3RD - A ABORTION	EXPLANATION: None

Body Part – 4TH	Approach – 5TH	Device – 6TH	Qualifier – 7TH
0 Products of Conception	0 Open 3 Percutaneous 4 Percutaneous endoscopic 8 Via natural or artificial opening endoscopic	Z No device	Z No qualifier
0 Products of Conception	7 Via natural or artificial opening	Z No device	6 Vacuum W Laminaria X Abortifacient Z No qualifier

OBSTETRICS SECTION:
Change, Drainage, Abortion, Extraction, Delivery, Insertion, Inspection, Removal, Repair, Reposition, Resection, Transplanation
Root Operations that are performed on the products of conception.

1ST - 1 Obstetrics	EXAMPLE: Cesarean or forceps-assisted delivery
2ND - 0 Pregnancy ♀	**EXTRACTION:** Pulling or stripping out or off all or a portion of a body part by the use of force.
3RD - D EXTRACTION	EXPLANATION: Qualifier - type of instrumentation/assistance

Body Part – 4TH	Approach – 5TH	Device – 6TH	Qualifier – 7TH
0 Products of Conception	0 Open	Z No device	0 Classical 1 Low cervical 2 Extraperitoneal
0 Products of Conception	7 Via natural or artificial opening	Z No device	3 Low forceps 4 Mid forceps 5 High forceps 6 Vacuum 7 Internal version 8 Other
1 Products of Conception, Retained 2 Products of Conception, Ectopic	7 Via natural or artificial opening 8 Via natural or artificial opening endoscopic	Z No device	Z No qualifier

O B S T E T R I C S

1 0 A

OBSTETRICS SECTION:
Change, Drainage, Abortion, Extraction, Delivery, Insertion, Inspection, Removal, Repair, Reposition, Resection, Transplanation
Root Operations that are performed on the products of conception.

1ST – **1** Obstetrics

2ND – **0** Pregnancy ♀

3RD – **E DELIVERY**

EXAMPLE: Spontaneous vaginal delivery

DELIVERY: Assisting the passage of the products of conception from the genital canal.

EXPLANATION: Manually assisted delivery without instruments

Body Part – 4TH	Approach – 5TH	Device – 6TH	Qualifier – 7TH
0 Products of Conception	X External	Z No device	Z No qualifier

---

OBSTETRICS SECTION:
Change, Drainage, Abortion, Extraction, Delivery, Insertion, Inspection, Removal, Repair, Reposition, Resection, Transplanation
Root Operations that are performed on the products of conception.

1ST – **1** Obstetrics

2ND – **0** Pregnancy ♀

3RD – **H INSERTION**

EXAMPLE: Insertion intrauterine pressure monitor

INSERTION: Putting in a nonbiological appliance that monitors, assists, performs, or prevents a physiological function but does not physically take the place of a body part.

EXPLANATION: None

Body Part – 4TH	Approach – 5TH	Device – 6TH	Qualifier – 7TH
0 Products of Conception	0 Open 7 Via natural or artificial opening	3 Monitoring electrode Y Other device	Z No qualifier

OBSTETRICS SECTION:
Change, Drainage, Abortion, Extraction, Delivery, Insertion, Inspection, Removal, Repair, Reposition, Resection, Transplanation
Root Operations that are performed on the products of conception.

1ST - 1 Obstetrics

2ND - 0 Pregnancy ♀

3RD - J INSPECTION

EXAMPLE: Amnioscopy, bimanual pregnancy examination

INSPECTION: Visually and/or manually exploring a body part.

EXPLANATION: Direct or instrumental visualization ...

Body Part – 4TH	Approach – 5TH	Device – 6TH	Qualifier – 7TH
0 Products of Conception 1 Products of Conception, Retained 2 Products of Conception, Ectopic	0 Open 3 Percutaneous 4 Percutaneous endoscopic 7 Via natural or artificial opening 8 Via natural or artificial opening endoscopic X External	Z No device	Z No qualifier

OBSTETRICS SECTION:
Change, Drainage, Abortion, Extraction, Delivery, Insertion, Inspection, Removal, Repair, Reposition, Resection, Transplanation
Root Operations that are performed on the products of conception.

1ST - 1 Obstetrics

2ND - 0 Pregnancy ♀

3RD - P REMOVAL

EXAMPLE: Removal fetal monitoring electrode

REMOVAL: Taking out or off a device from a body part, region or orifice.

EXPLANATION: Removal device without reinsertion ...

Body Part – 4TH	Approach – 5TH	Device – 6TH	Qualifier – 7TH
0 Products of Conception	0 Open 7 Via natural or artificial opening	3 Monitoring electrode Y Other device	Z No qualifier

OBSTETRICS

1
0
J

OBSTETRICS SECTION:
Change, Drainage, Abortion, Extraction, Delivery, Insertion, Inspection, Removal, Repair, Reposition, Resection, Transplanation
Root Operations that are performed on the products of conception.

1ST - **1**   Obstetrics

2ND - **0**   Pregnancy ♀

3RD - **Q REPAIR**

EXAMPLE: In utero repair congenital diaphragmatic hernia

REPAIR: Restoring, to the extent possible, a body part to its normal anatomic structure and function.

EXPLANATION: Only when no other root operation applies ...

Body Part – 4TH	Approach – 5TH	Device – 6TH	Qualifier – 7TH
0 Products of Conception	0 Open 3 Percutaneous 4 Percutaneous endoscopic 7 Via natural or artificial opening 8 Via natural or artificial opening endoscopic	Y Other device Z No device	E Nervous System F Cardiovascular System G Lymphatics and Hemic H Eye J Ear, Nose and Sinus K Respiratory System L Mouth and Throat M Gastrointestinal System N Hepatobiliary and Pancreas P Endocrine System Q Skin R Musculoskeletal System S Urinary System T Female Reproductive System V Male Reproductive System Y Other Body System

---

OBSTETRICS SECTION:
Change, Drainage, Abortion, Extraction, Delivery, Insertion, Inspection, Removal, Repair, Reposition, Resection, Transplanation
Root Operations that are performed on the products of conception.

1ST - **1**   Obstetrics

2ND - **0**   Pregnancy ♀

3RD - **S REPOSITION**

EXAMPLE: Manual external version of fetus

REPOSITION: Moving to its normal location, or other suitable location, all or a portion of a body part.

EXPLANATION: May or may not be cut to be moved ...

Body Part – 4TH	Approach – 5TH	Device – 6TH	Qualifier – 7TH
0 Products of Conception	7 Via natural or artificial opening X External	Z No device	Z No qualifier
2 Products of Conception, Ectopic	0 Open 3 Percutaneous 4 Percutaneous endoscopic 7 Via natural or artificial opening 8 Via natural or artificial opening endoscopic	Z No device	Z No qualifier

OBSTETRICS

1 0 S

OBSTETRICS SECTION:

Change, Drainage, Abortion, Extraction, Delivery, Insertion, Inspection, Removal, Repair, Reposition, Resection, Transplanation

Root Operations that are performed on the products of conception.

1ST - 1 Obstetrics 2ND - 0 Pregnancy ♀ 3RD - T RESECTION	EXAMPLE: Surgical removal ectopic pregnancy
	RESECTION: Cutting out or off, without replacement, all of a body part.
	EXPLANATION: None

Body Part – 4TH	Approach – 5TH	Device – 6TH	Qualifier – 7TH
2 Products of Conception, Ectopic	0 Open 3 Percutaneous 4 Percutaneous endoscopic 7 Via natural or artificial opening 8 Via natural or artificial opening endoscopic	Z No device	Z No qualifier

OBSTETRICS SECTION:

Change, Drainage, Abortion, Extraction, Delivery, Insertion, Inspection, Removal, Repair, Reposition, Resection, Transplanation

Root Operations that are performed on the products of conception.

1ST - 1 Obstetrics 2ND - 0 Pregnancy ♀ 3RD - Y TRANSPLANTATION	EXAMPLE: Fetal kidney transplant
	TRANSPLANTATION: Putting in or on all or a portion of a living body part taken from another individual or animal to physically take the place and/or function of all or a portion of a similar body part.
	EXPLANATION: May take over all or part of its function …

Body Part – 4TH	Approach – 5TH	Device – 6TH	Qualifier – 7TH	
0 Products of Conception	3 Percutaneous 4 Percutaneous endoscopic 7 Via natural or artificial opening	Z No device	E Nervous System F Cardiovascular System G Lymphatics and Hemic H Eye J Ear, Nose and Sinus K Respiratory System L Mouth and Throat M Gastrointestinal System	N Hepatobiliary and Pancreas P Endocrine System Q Skin R Musculoskeletal System S Urinary System T Female Reproductive System V Male Reproductive System Y Other Body System

OBSTETRICS

10 T

Educational Annotations | Section 2 – Placement

Section Specific Educational Annotations for the Placement Section include:

- Anatomy and Physiology Review
- Anatomical Illustrations
- AHA Coding Clinic® Reference Notations
- Body Part Key Listings
- Device Key Listings
- Device Aggregation Table Listings
- Coding Notes

Anatomy and Physiology Review of Placement

BODY REGION VALUES – 2 - Placement

Abdominal Wall – The multi-tissue-layered covering of the abdominal and pelvic portions of the trunk.

Anorectal – The multi-tissue-layered area containing the anus and rectum.

Back – The multi-tissue-layered covering of the back portion of the trunk.

Chest Wall – The multi-tissue-layered covering of the thoracic portion of the trunk.

Ear – The organ of hearing comprised of the external ear (auricle or pinna), middle ear (malleus, incus, and stapes bones), and inner ear (cochlea).

Face – The multi-tissue-layered covering of the anterior portion of the head.

Female Genital Tract – The organs and structures of the reproductive systems.

Finger – A digit of the hand.

Foot – The portion of the lower extermity distal to the lower end of the tibia and fibula.

Hand – The portion of the upper extermity distal to the forearm.

Head – The portion of the human body above the neck.

Inguinal Region – The multi-tissue-layered area between the lower abdomen, thigh, and pubic bone.

Lower Arm – The portion of the upper extermity distal to the elbow.

Lower Extremity – The entire lower extremity (leg).

Lower Leg – The portion of the lower extermity distal to the knee.

Mouth and Pharynx – The portion of the head formed by the oral cavity and pharynx.

Nasal – The multi-tissue-layered area of the nose in the anterior portion of the head.

Neck – The portion of the human body above the trunk and below the head.

Thumb – The first digit of the hand.

Toe – A digit of the foot.

Upper Arm – The portion of the upper extermity distal to the shoulder and proximal to the elbow.

Upper Extremity – The entire upper extremity (arm).

Upper Leg – The portion of the lower extermity distal to the hip and proximal to the knee.

Urethra – The urethra is the musculomembranous tube which extends and carries urine from the bladder to the external urethral opening (meatus).

Anatomical Illustrations of Placement

None for the Placement Section

Educational Annotations | Section 2 – Placement

AHA Coding Clinic® Reference Notations of Placement

ROOT OPERATION SPECIFIC - PLACEMENT - Section 2
CHANGE - 0
COMPRESSION - 1
DRESSING - 2
IMMOBILIZATION - 3
PACKING - 4
REMOVAL - 5
TRACTION - 6
    Tongs used to stabilize cervical fracture ....AHA 13:2Q:p39

Body Part Key Listings of Placement

See also Body Part Key in Appendix C
Hallux ....*use* 1st Toe, Left/Right
Inguinal canal ....*use* Inguinal Region, Bilateral/Left/Right
Inguinal triangle ....*use* Inguinal Region, Bilateral/Left/Right

Device Key Listings of Placement

None for the Placement Section

Device Aggregation Table Listings of Placement

None for the Placement Section

Coding Notes of Placement

Med/Surg Related Section Specific PCS Reference Manual Exercises

PCS CODE	2 – PLACEMENT EXERCISES
2 W 0 P X 6 Z	Exchange of pressure dressing to left thigh.
2 W 1 8 X 7 Z	Placement of intermittent pneumatic compression device, covering entire right arm.
2 W 2 7 X 4 Z	Sterile dressing placement to left groin region.
2 W 3 2 X 3 Z	Placement of neck brace.
2 W 4 4 X 5 Z	Packing of wound, chest wall.
2 W 5 A X 1 Z	Removal of splint, right shoulder.
2 W 6 M X 0 Z	Mechanical traction of entire left leg.
2 Y 0 4 X 5 Z	Change of vaginal packing.
2 Y 4 2 X 5 Z	Placement of packing material, right ear.
2 Y 5 0 X 5 Z	Removal of packing material from pharynx.

PLACEMENT

2

PLACEMENT SECTION: Change, Compression, Dressing, Immobilization, Packing, Removal, Traction
Root Operations include only those that are performed without an incision or a puncture.

1ST - **2** Placement 2ND - **W** Anatomical Regions 3RD - **0 CHANGE**	EXAMPLE: Changing a cast
	CHANGE: Taking out or off a device from a body part and putting back an identical or similar device in or on the same body part without cutting or puncturing the skin or a mucous membrane.
	EXPLANATION: Performed without an incision or puncture ...

Body Region – 4TH		Approach – 5TH	Device – 6TH	Qualifier – 7TH
0 Head 2 Neck 3 Abdominal Wall 4 Chest Wall 5 Back 6 Inguinal Region, Right 7 Inguinal Region, Left 8 Upper Extremity, Right 9 Upper Extremity, Left A Upper Arm, Right B Upper Arm, Left C Lower Arm, Right D Lower Arm, Left E Hand, Right F Hand, Left	G Thumb, Right H Thumb, Left J Finger, Right K Finger, Left L Lower Extremity, Right M Lower Extremity, Left N Upper Leg, Right P Upper Leg, Left Q Lower Leg, Right R Lower Leg, Left S Foot, Right T Foot, Left U Toe, Right V Toe, Left	X External	0 Traction apparatus 1 Splint 2 Cast 3 Brace 4 Bandage 5 Packing material 6 Pressure dressing 7 Intermittent pressure device Y Other device	Z No qualifier
1 Face		X External	0 Traction apparatus 1 Splint 2 Cast 3 Brace 4 Bandage 5 Packing material 6 Pressure dressing 7 Intermittent pressure device 9 Wire Y Other device	Z No qualifier

P L A C E M E N T

2 W 0

PLACEMENT SECTION: Change, Compression, Dressing, Immobilization, Packing, Removal, Traction
Root Operations include only those that are performed without an incision or a puncture.

1ST – 2 Placement 2ND – W Anatomical Regions 3RD – 1 COMPRESSION	EXAMPLE: Application of pressure dressing
	COMPRESSION: Putting pressure on a body region.
	EXPLANATION: Performed without an incision or puncture …

Body Region – 4TH		Approach – 5TH	Device – 6TH	Qualifier – 7TH
0 Head 1 Face 2 Neck 3 Abdominal Wall 4 Chest Wall 5 Back 6 Inguinal Region, Right 7 Inguinal Region, Left 8 Upper Extremity, Right 9 Upper Extremity, Left A Upper Arm, Right B Upper Arm, Left C Lower Arm, Right D Lower Arm, Left E Hand, Right F Hand, Left	G Thumb, Right H Thumb, Left J Finger, Right K Finger, Left L Lower Extremity, Right M Lower Extremity, Left N Upper Leg, Right P Upper Leg, Left Q Lower Leg, Right R Lower Leg, Left S Foot, Right T Foot, Left U Toe, Right V Toe, Left	X External	6 Pressure dressing 7 Intermittent pressure device	Z No qualifier

PLACEMENT SECTION: Change, Compression, Dressing, Immobilization, Packing, Removal, Traction
Root Operations include only those that are performed without an incision or a puncture.

1ST – 2 Placement 2ND – W Anatomical Regions 3RD – 2 DRESSING	EXAMPLE: Bandage-type dressing
	DRESSING: Putting material on a body region for protection.
	EXPLANATION: Performed without an incision or puncture …

Body Region – 4TH		Approach – 5TH	Device – 6TH	Qualifier – 7TH
0 Head 1 Face 2 Neck 3 Abdominal Wall 4 Chest Wall 5 Back 6 Inguinal Region, Right 7 Inguinal Region, Left 8 Upper Extremity, Right 9 Upper Extremity, Left A Upper Arm, Right B Upper Arm, Left C Lower Arm, Right D Lower Arm, Left E Hand, Right F Hand, Left	G Thumb, Right H Thumb, Left J Finger, Right K Finger, Left L Lower Extremity, Right M Lower Extremity, Left N Upper Leg, Right P Upper Leg, Left Q Lower Leg, Right R Lower Leg, Left S Foot, Right T Foot, Left U Toe, Right V Toe, Left	X External	4 Bandage	Z No qualifier

PLACEMENT

2 W 1

PLACEMENT SECTION: Change, Compression, Dressing, Immobilization, Packing, Removal, Traction
Root Operations include only those that are performed without an incision or a puncture.

1ST – **2** Placement

2ND – **W** Anatomical Regions

3RD – **3 IMMOBILIZATION**

EXAMPLE: Application of brace or splint

IMMOBILIZATION: Limiting or preventing motion of a body region.

EXPLANATION: Performed without an incision or puncture …

Body Region – 4TH		Approach – 5TH	Device – 6TH	Qualifier – 7TH
0 Head	G Thumb, Right	X External	1 Splint	Z No qualifier
2 Neck	H Thumb, Left		2 Cast	
3 Abdominal Wall	J Finger, Right		3 Brace	
4 Chest Wall	K Finger, Left		Y Other device	
5 Back	L Lower Extremity, Right			
6 Inguinal Region, Right	M Lower Extremity, Left			
7 Inguinal Region, Left	N Upper Leg, Right			
8 Upper Extremity, Right	P Upper Leg, Left			
9 Upper Extremity, Left	Q Lower Leg, Right			
A Upper Arm, Right	R Lower Leg, Left			
B Upper Arm, Left	S Foot, Right			
C Lower Arm, Right	T Foot, Left			
D Lower Arm, Left	U Toe, Right			
E Hand, Right	V Toe, Left			
F Hand, Left				
1 Face		X External	1 Splint	Z No qualifier
			2 Cast	
			3 Brace	
			9 Wire	
			Y Other device	

PLACEMENT SECTION: Change, Compression, Dressing, Immobilization, Packing, Removal, Traction
Root Operations include only those that are performed without an incision or a puncture.

1ST – **2** Placement

2ND – **W** Anatomical Regions

3RD – **4 PACKING**

EXAMPLE: Open wound packing

PACKING: Putting material in a body region or orifice.

EXPLANATION: Performed without an incision or puncture …

Body Region – 4TH		Approach – 5TH	Device – 6TH	Qualifier – 7TH
0 Head	G Thumb, Right	X External	5 Packing material	Z No qualifier
1 Face	H Thumb, Left			
2 Neck	J Finger, Right			
3 Abdominal Wall	K Finger, Left			
4 Chest Wall	L Lower Extremity, Right			
5 Back	M Lower Extremity, Left			
6 Inguinal Region, Right	N Upper Leg, Right			
7 Inguinal Region, Left	P Upper Leg, Left			
8 Upper Extremity, Right	Q Lower Leg, Right			
9 Upper Extremity, Left	R Lower Leg, Left			
A Upper Arm, Right	S Foot, Right			
B Upper Arm, Left	T Foot, Left			
C Lower Arm, Right	U Toe, Right			
D Lower Arm, Left	V Toe, Left			
E Hand, Right				
F Hand, Left				

PLACEMENT SECTION: Change, Compression, Dressing, Immobilization, Packing, Removal, Traction
Root Operations include only those that are performed without an incision or a puncture.

1ST - 2 Placement	EXAMPLE: Cast removal
2ND - W Anatomical Regions	**REMOVAL:** Taking out or off a device from a body part.
3RD - 5 REMOVAL	EXPLANATION: Performed without an incision or puncture ...

Body Region – 4TH		Approach – 5TH	Device – 6TH	Qualifier – 7TH
0 Head	G Thumb, Right	X External	0 Traction apparatus	Z No qualifier
2 Neck	H Thumb, Left		1 Splint	
3 Abdominal Wall	J Finger, Right		2 Cast	
4 Chest Wall	K Finger, Left		3 Brace	
5 Back	L Lower Extremity, Right		4 Bandage	
6 Inguinal Region, Right	M Lower Extremity, Left		5 Packing material	
7 Inguinal Region, Left	N Upper Leg, Right		6 Pressure dressing	
8 Upper Extremity, Right	P Upper Leg, Left		7 Intermittent pressure device	
9 Upper Extremity, Left	Q Lower Leg, Right		Y Other device	
A Upper Arm, Right	R Lower Leg, Left			
B Upper Arm, Left	S Foot, Right			
C Lower Arm, Right	T Foot, Left			
D Lower Arm, Left	U Toe, Right			
E Hand, Right	V Toe, Left			
F Hand, Left				
1 Face		X External	0 Traction apparatus	Z No qualifier
			1 Splint	
			2 Cast	
			3 Brace	
			4 Bandage	
			5 Packing material	
			6 Pressure dressing	
			7 Intermittent pressure device	
			9 Wire	
			Y Other device	

PLACEMENT SECTION: Change, Compression, Dressing, Immobilization, Packing, Removal, Traction
Root Operations include only those that are performed without an incision or a puncture.

1ST - **2** Placement	EXAMPLE: Lumbar traction using traction table
2ND - **W** Anatomical Regions	**TRACTION:** Exerting a pulling force on a body region in a distal direction.
3RD - **6 TRACTION**	EXPLANATION: Performed without an incision or puncture ...

Body Region – 4TH		Approach – 5TH	Device – 6TH	Qualifier – 7TH
0 Head	G Thumb, Right	X External	0 Traction apparatus	Z No qualifier
1 Face	H Thumb, Left		Z No device	
2 Neck	J Finger, Right			
3 Abdominal Wall	K Finger, Left			
4 Chest Wall	L Lower Extremity, Right			
5 Back	M Lower Extremity, Left			
6 Inguinal Region, Right	N Upper Leg, Right			
7 Inguinal Region, Left	P Upper Leg, Left			
8 Upper Extremity, Right	Q Lower Leg, Right			
9 Upper Extremity, Left	R Lower Leg, Left			
A Upper Arm, Right	S Foot, Right			
B Upper Arm, Left	T Foot, Left			
C Lower Arm, Right	U Toe, Right			
D Lower Arm, Left	V Toe, Left			
E Hand, Right				
F Hand, Left				

PLACEMENT

2 W 6

PLACEMENT SECTION: Change, Compression, Dressing, Immobilization, Packing, Removal, Traction
Root Operations include only those that are performed without an incision or a puncture.

1ST - **2** Placement 2ND - **Y** Anatomical Orifices 3RD - **0** CHANGE	EXAMPLE: Replacing nasal packing **CHANGE:** Taking out or off a device from a body part and putting back an identical or similar device in or on the same body part without cutting or puncturing the skin or a mucous membrane. EXPLANATION: Performed without an incision or puncture ...

Body Region – 4TH	Approach – 5TH	Device – 6TH	Qualifier – 7TH
0 Mouth and Pharynx 1 Nasal 2 Ear 3 Anorectal 4 Female Genital Tract ♀ 5 Urethra	X External	5 Packing material	Z No qualifier

---

PLACEMENT SECTION: Change, Compression, Dressing, Immobilization, Packing, Removal, Traction
Root Operations include only those that are performed without an incision or a puncture.

1ST - **2** Placement 2ND - **Y** Anatomical Orifices 3RD - **4** PACKING	EXAMPLE: Insertion of nasal packing **PACKING:** Putting material in a body region or orifice. EXPLANATION: Performed without an incision or puncture ...

Body Region – 4TH	Approach – 5TH	Device – 6TH	Qualifier – 7TH
0 Mouth and Pharynx 1 Nasal 2 Ear 3 Anorectal 4 Female Genital Tract ♀ 5 Urethra	X External	5 Packing material	Z No qualifier

---

PLACEMENT SECTION: Change, Compression, Dressing, Immobilization, Packing, Removal, Traction
Root Operations include only those that are performed without an incision or a puncture.

1ST - **2** Placement 2ND - **Y** Anatomical Orifices 3RD - **5** REMOVAL	EXAMPLE: Removal of nasal packing **REMOVAL:** Taking out or off a device from a body part. EXPLANATION: Performed without an incision or puncture ...

Body Region – 4TH	Approach – 5TH	Device – 6TH	Qualifier – 7TH
0 Mouth and Pharynx 1 Nasal 2 Ear 3 Anorectal 4 Female Genital Tract ♀ 5 Urethra	X External	5 Packing material	Z No qualifier

Educational Annotations | Section 3 – Administration

Section Specific Educational Annotations for the Administration Section include:
- AHA Coding Clinic® Reference Notations
- Coding Notes

AHA Coding Clinic® Reference Notations of Administration

ROOT OPERATION SPECIFIC - ADMINISTRATION - Section 3
INTRODUCTION - 0

Chemoembolization of hepatic artery	AHA 15:1Q:p38
EGD with epinephrine injection	AHA 15:3Q:p24
Glucagon to flush bile duct stones	AHA 14:3Q:p11
Imaging report to identify the body part of an infusion device	AHA 14:3Q:p5
Immune globulin (Rh-D, anti-D), injection, intramuscular	AHA 14:4Q:p16
Induction of labor, IV oxytocin, peripheral vein	AHA 14:4Q:p17
Induction of labor with Cervidil dinoprostone vaginal tampon	AHA 14:2Q:p8
Infusion of thrombolytic therapy	AHA 14:4Q:p19
Injection of combination of drugs	AHA 14:4Q:p45
Injection of intrathecal chemotherapy	AHA 15:1Q:p31
Injection of Ovation® (extracellular matrix) into amputation wound	AHA 15:2Q:p27
Injection of sclerosing agent into an esophageal varix	AHA 13:1Q:p27
Injection of substances with vitrectomy	AHA 15:2Q:p24
Injection of talc in pleura for pleurodesis	AHA 15:2Q:p31
Instillation of saline and Seprafilm solution	AHA 14:4Q:p38
Intraoperative (open) placement of chemotherapy wafers	AHA 14:4Q:p34
Nasogastric (NG) tube used for both drainage and feeding	AHA 15:2Q:p29
Neulasta injection to prevent infection	AHA 14:2Q:p10
Seprafilm use during procedures	AHA 15:3Q:p29
tPA administration	AHA 13:4Q:p124

IRRIGATION - 1
TRANSFUSION - 2

Coding Notes of Administration

Med/Surg Related Section Specific PCS Reference Manual Exercises

PCS CODE	3 – ADMINISTRATION EXERCISES
3 0 2 4 3 G 0	Autologous bone marrow transplant via central venous line.
3 0 2 6 3 V 1	Transfusion of antihemophilic factor, (nonautologous) via arterial central line.
3 E 0 1 0 2 A	Implantation of anti-microbial envelope with cardiac defibrillator placement, open.
3 E 0 3 3 1 7	Systemic infusion of recombinant tissue plasminogen activator (r-tPA) via peripheral venous catheter.
3 E 0 4 3 6 Z	Infusion of total parenteral nutrition via central venous catheter.
3 E 0 G 8 G C	Esophagogastroscopy with botox injection into esophageal sphincter. (Botulinum toxin is a paralyzing agent with temporary effects; it does not sclerose or destroy the nerve.)
3 E 0 P 3 Q 1	Transabdominal in-vitro fertilization, implantation of donor ovum.
3 E 0 P 7 L Z	Transvaginal artificial insemination.
3 E 1 M 3 9 Z	Peritoneal dialysis via indwelling catheter.
3 E 1 U 3 8 Z	Percutaneous irrigation of knee joint.

ADMINISTRATION 3

Educational Annotations | Section 3 – Administration

NOTES

ADMINISTRATION SECTION: Introduction, Irrigation, Transfusion
Root Operations that define procedures where a diagnostic or therapeutic substance is given to the patient.

1ST - 3 Administration	EXAMPLE: Whole blood transfusion
2ND - 0 Circulatory	**TRANSFUSION:** Putting in blood or blood products.
3RD - 2 TRANSFUSION	EXPLANATION: Blood products, bone marrow, and stem cells

Body System Region – 4TH	Approach – 5TH	Substance – 6TH		Qualifier – 7TH
3 Peripheral Vein 4 Central Vein	0 Open 3 Percutaneous	A Stem cells, embryonic NC*		Z No qualifier
3 Peripheral Vein 4 Central Vein	0 Open 3 Percutaneous	G Bone marrow NC* X Stem cells, cord blood Y Stem cells, hematopoietic NC*		0 Autologous 2 Allogeneic, related 3 Allogeneic, unrelated 4 Allogeneic, unspecified
3 Peripheral Vein 4 Central Vein	0 Open 3 Percutaneous	H Whole blood J Serum albumin K Frozen plasma L Fresh plasma M Plasma cryoprecipitate N Red blood cells P Frozen red cells	Q White cells R Platelets S Globulin T Fibrinogen V Antihemophilic factors W Factor IX	0 Autologous 1 Nonautologous
5 Peripheral Artery 6 Central Artery	0 Open 3 Percutaneous	G Bone marrow NC* H Whole blood J Serum albumin K Frozen plasma L Fresh plasma M Plasma cryoprecipitate N Red blood cells P Frozen red cells	Q White cells R Platelets S Globulin T Fibrinogen V Antihemophilic factors W Factor IX X Stem cells, cord blood Y Stem cells, hematopoietic NC*	0 Autologous 1 Nonautologous
7 Products of Conception, Circulatory ♀	3 Percutaneous 7 Via natural or artificial opening	H Whole blood J Serum albumin K Frozen plasma L Fresh plasma M Plasma cryoprecipitate N Red blood cells P Frozen red cells	Q White cells R Platelets S Globulin T Fibrinogen V Antihemophilic factors W Factor IX	1 Nonautologous
8 Vein	0 Open 3 Percutaneous	B 4-Factor prothrombin complex concentrate		1 Nonautologous

NC* – Some procedures are considered non-covered by Medicare. See current Medicare Code Editor for details.

ADMINISTRATION SECTION: Introduction, Irrigation, Transfusion
Root Operations that define procedures where a diagnostic or therapeutic substance is given to the patient.

1ST - 3 Administration	EXAMPLE: Irrigation of catheter port
2ND - C Indwelling Device	**IRRIGATION:** Putting in or on a cleansing substance.
3RD - 1 IRRIGATION	EXPLANATION: Cleansing substance

Body System/Region – 4TH	Approach – 5TH	Substance – 6TH	Qualifier – 7TH
Z None	X External	8 Irrigating substance	Z No qualifier

ADMINISTRATION SECTION: Introduction, Irrigation, Transfusion

Root Operations that define procedures where a diagnostic or therapeutic substance is given to the patient.

1ST – **3** Administration

2ND – **E** Physiological Systems and Anatomical Regions

3RD – **0 INTRODUCTION**

EXAMPLE: Infusion of chemotherapy agent

INTRODUCTION: Putting in or on a therapeutic, diagnostic, nutritional, physiological, or prophylactic substance except blood or blood products.

EXPLANATION: Substances other than blood and cleansing ...

Body System/Region – 4TH	Approach – 5TH	Substance – 6TH	Qualifier – 7TH
0 Skin and Mucous Membranes	X External	0 Antineoplastic	5 Other antineoplastic M Monoclonal antibody
0 Skin and Mucous Membranes	X External	2 Anti-infective	8 Oxazolidinones 9 Other anti-infective
0 Skin and Mucous Membranes	X External	3 Anti-inflammatory 4 Serum, toxoid and vaccine B Local anesthetic K Other diagnostic substance M Pigment N Analgesics, hypnotics, sedatives T Destructive agent	Z No qualifier
0 Skin and Mucous Membranes	X External	G Other therapeutic substance	C Other substance
1 Subcutaneous Tissue	0 Open	2 Anti-infective	A Anti-infective envelope
1 Subcutaneous Tissue	3 Percutaneous	0 Antineoplastic	5 Other antineoplastic M Monoclonal antibody
1 Subcutaneous Tissue	3 Percutaneous	2 Anti-infective	8 Oxazolidinones 9 Other anti-infective A Anti-infective envelope
1 Subcutaneous Tissue	3 Percutaneous	3 Anti-inflammatory 4 Serum, toxoid and vaccine 6 Nutritional substance 7 Electrolytic and water balance substance B Local anesthetic H Radioactive substance K Other diagnostic substance N Analgesics, hypnotics, sedatives T Destructive agent	Z No qualifier
1 Subcutaneous Tissue	3 Percutaneous	G Other therapeutic substance	C Other substance
1 Subcutaneous Tissue	3 Percutaneous	V Hormone	G Insulin J Other hormone
2 Muscle	3 Percutaneous	0 Antineoplastic	5 Other antineoplastic M Monoclonal antibody
2 Muscle	3 Percutaneous	2 Anti-infective	8 Oxazolidinones 9 Other anti-infective

c o n t i n u e d ⇨

ADMINISTRATION 3 E 0

© 2016 Channel Publishing, Ltd.

3 E 0 INTRODUCTION – continued

Body System/Region – 4TH	Approach – 5TH	Substance – 6TH	Qualifier – 7TH
2 Muscle	3 Percutaneous	3 Anti-inflammatory 4 Serum, toxoid and vaccine 6 Nutritional substance 7 Electrolytic and water balance substance B Local anesthetic H Radioactive substance K Other diagnostic substance N Analgesics, hypnotics, sedatives T Destructive agent	Z No qualifier
2 Muscle	3 Percutaneous	G Other therapeutic substance	C Other substance
3 Peripheral Vein	0 Open	0 Antineoplastic	2 High-dose interleukin-2 3 Low-dose interleukin-2 5 Other antineoplastic M Monoclonal antibody P Clofarabine
3 Peripheral Vein	0 Open	1 Thrombolytic	6 Recombinant human-activated protein C 7 Other thrombolytic
3 Peripheral Vein	0 Open	2 Anti-infective	8 Oxazolidinones 9 Other anti-infective
3 Peripheral Vein	0 Open	3 Anti-inflammatory 4 Serum, toxoid and vaccine 6 Nutritional substance 7 Electrolytic and water balance substance F Intracirculatory anesthetic H Radioactive substance K Other diagnostic substance N Analgesics, hypnotics, sedatives P Platelet inhibitor R Antiarrhythmic T Destructive agent X Vasopressor	Z No qualifier
3 Peripheral Vein	0 Open	G Other therapeutic substance	C Other substance N Blood brain barrier disruption
3 Peripheral Vein	0 Open	U Pancreatic islet cells	0 Autologous 1 Nonautologous
3 Peripheral Vein	0 Open	V Hormone	G Insulin H Human B-type natriuretic peptide J Other hormone

ADMINISTRATION 3 E 0

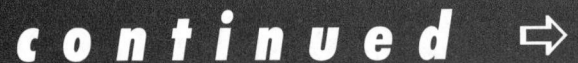

c o n t i n u e d ⇨

3 E 0 INTRODUCTION – continued

Body System/Region – 4TH	Approach – 5TH	Substance – 6TH	Qualifier – 7TH
3 Peripheral Vein	0 Open	W Immunotherapeutic	K Immunostimulator L Immunosuppressive
3 Peripheral Vein	3 Percutaneous	0 Antineoplastic	2 High-dose interleukin-2 3 Low-dose interleukin-2 5 Other antineoplastic M Monoclonal antibody P Clofarabine
3 Peripheral Vein	3 Percutaneous	1 Thrombolytic	6 Recombinant human-activated protein C 7 Other thrombolytic
3 Peripheral Vein	3 Percutaneous	2 Anti-infective	8 Oxazolidinones 9 Other anti-infective
3 Peripheral Vein	3 Percutaneous	3 Anti-inflammatory 4 Serum, toxoid and vaccine 6 Nutritional substance 7 Electrolytic and water balance substance F Intracirculatory anesthetic H Radioactive substance K Other diagnostic substance N Analgesics, hypnotics, sedatives P Platelet inhibitor R Antiarrhythmic T Destructive agent X Vasopressor	Z No qualifier
3 Peripheral Vein	3 Percutaneous	G Other therapeutic substance	C Other substance N Blood brain barrier disruption Q Glucarpidase
3 Peripheral Vein	3 Percutaneous	U Pancreatic islet cells	0 Autologous 1 Nonautologous
3 Peripheral Vein	3 Percutaneous	V Hormone	G Insulin H Human B-type natriuretic peptide J Other hormone
3 Peripheral Vein	3 Percutaneous	W Immunotherapeutic	K Immunostimulator L Immunosuppressive

continued ⇨

ADMINISTRATION 3 E 0

3   E   0   INTRODUCTION–*continued*

Body System/Region – 4TH	Approach – 5TH	Substance – 6TH	Qualifier – 7TH
4 Central Vein	0 Open	0 Antineoplastic	2 High-dose interleukin-2 3 Low-dose interleukin-2 5 Other antineoplastic M Monoclonal antibody P Clofarabine
4 Central Vein	0 Open	1 Thrombolytic	6 Recombinant human-activated protein C 7 Other thrombolytic
4 Central Vein	0 Open	2 Anti-infective	8 Oxazolidinones 9 Other anti-infective
4 Central Vein	0 Open	3 Anti-inflammatory 4 Serum, toxoid and vaccine 6 Nutritional substance 7 Electrolytic and water balance substance F Intracirculatory anesthetic H Radioactive substance K Other diagnostic substance N Analgesics, hypnotics, sedatives P Platelet inhibitor R Antiarrhythmic T Destructive agent X Vasopressor	Z No qualifier
4 Central Vein	0 Open	G Other therapeutic substance	C Other substance N Blood brain barrier disruption
4 Central Vein	0 Open	V Hormone	G Insulin H Human B-type natriuretic peptide J Other hormone
4 Central Vein	0 Open	W Immunotherapeutic	K Immunostimulator L Immunosuppressive

ADMINISTRATION 3 E 0

continued ⇨

3 E 0 INTRODUCTION—*continued*

Body System/Region – 4TH	Approach – 5TH	Substance – 6TH	Qualifier – 7TH
4 Central Vein	3 Percutaneous	0 Antineoplastic	2 High-dose interleukin-2 3 Low-dose interleukin-2 5 Other antineoplastic M Monoclonal antibody P Clofarabine
4 Central Vein	3 Percutaneous	1 Thrombolytic	6 Recombinant human-activated protein C 7 Other thrombolytic
4 Central Vein	3 Percutaneous	2 Anti-infective	8 Oxazolidinones 9 Other anti-infective
4 Central Vein	3 Percutaneous	3 Anti-inflammatory 4 Serum, toxoid and vaccine 6 Nutritional substance 7 Electrolytic and water balance substance F Intracirculatory anesthetic H Radioactive substance K Other diagnostic substance N Analgesics, hypnotics, sedatives P Platelet inhibitor R Antiarrhythmic T Destructive agent X Vasopressor	Z No qualifier
4 Central Vein	3 Percutaneous	G Other therapeutic substance	C Other substance N Blood brain barrier disruption Q Glucarpidase
4 Central Vein	3 Percutaneous	V Hormone	G Insulin H Human B-type natriuretic peptide J Other hormone
4 Central Vein	3 Percutaneous	W Immunotherapeutic	K Immunostimulator L Immunosuppressive

continued ⇨

3   E   0   INTRODUCTION – *continued*

Body System/Region – 4TH	Approach – 5TH	Substance – 6TH	Qualifier – 7TH
5 Peripheral Artery 6 Central Artery	0 Open 3 Percutaneous	0 Antineoplastic	2 High-dose interleukin-2 3 Low-dose interleukin-2 5 Other antineoplastic M Monoclonal antibody P Clofarabine
5 Peripheral Artery 6 Central Artery	0 Open 3 Percutaneous	1 Thrombolytic	6 Recombinant human-activated protein C 7 Other thrombolytic
5 Peripheral Artery 6 Central Artery	0 Open 3 Percutaneous	2 Anti-infective	8 Oxazolidinones 9 Other anti-infective
5 Peripheral Artery 6 Central Artery	0 Open 3 Percutaneous	3 Anti-inflammatory 4 Serum, toxoid and vaccine 6 Nutritional substance 7 Electrolytic and water balance substance F Intracirculatory anesthetic H Radioactive substance K Other diagnostic substance N Analgesics, hypnotics, sedatives P Platelet inhibitor R Antiarrhythmic T Destructive agent X Vasopressor	Z No qualifier
5 Peripheral Artery 6 Central Artery	0 Open 3 Percutaneous	G Other therapeutic substance	C Other substance N Blood brain barrier disruption
5 Peripheral Artery 6 Central Artery	0 Open 3 Percutaneous	V Hormone	G Insulin H Human B-type natriuretic peptide J Other hormone
5 Peripheral Artery 6 Central Artery	0 Open 3 Percutaneous	W Immunotherapeutic	K Immunostimulator L Immunosuppressive

ADMINISTRATION 3 E 0

continued ⇨

3   E   0   INTRODUCTION — *continued*

Body System/Region – 4TH	Approach – 5TH	Substance – 6TH	Qualifier – 7TH
7 Coronary Artery 8 Heart	0 Open 3 Percutaneous	1 Thrombolytic	6 Recombinant human-activated protein C 7 Other thrombolytic
7 Coronary Artery 8 Heart	0 Open 3 Percutaneous	G Other therapeutic substance	C Other substance
7 Coronary Artery 8 Heart	0 Open 3 Percutaneous	K Other diagnostic substance P Platelet inhibitor	Z No qualifier
9 Nose	3 Percutaneous 7 Via natural or artificial opening X External	0 Antineoplastic	5 Other antineoplastic M Monoclonal antibody
9 Nose	3 Percutaneous 7 Via natural or artificial opening X External	2 Anti-infective	8 Oxazolidinones 9 Other anti-infective
9 Nose	3 Percutaneous 7 Via natural or artificial opening X External	3 Anti-inflammatory 4 Serum, toxoid and vaccine B Local anesthetic H Radioactive substance K Other diagnostic substance N Analgesics, hypnotics, sedatives T Destructive agent	Z No qualifier
9 Nose	3 Percutaneous 7 Via natural or artificial opening X External	G Other therapeutic substance	C Other substance
A Bone Marrow	3 Percutaneous	0 Antineoplastic	5 Other antineoplastic M Monoclonal antibody
A Bone Marrow	3 Percutaneous	G Other therapeutic substance	C Other substance

continued ⇨

ADMINISTRATION 3 E 0

3   E   0   INTRODUCTION–*continued*

Body System/Region – 4TH	Approach – 5TH	Substance – 6TH	Qualifier – 7TH

B Ear	3 Percutaneous
	7 Via natural or
	   artificial opening
	X External
		0 Antineoplastic	4 Liquid brachytherapy
			   radioisotope
			5 Other antineoplastic
			M Monoclonal antibody

B Ear	3 Percutaneous 7 Via natural or artificial opening X External	2 Anti-infective	8 Oxazolidinones 9 Other anti-infective
B Ear	3 Percutaneous 7 Via natural or artificial opening X External	3 Anti-inflammatory B Local anesthetic H Radioactive substance K Other diagnostic substance N Analgesics, hypnotics, sedatives T Destructive agent	Z No qualifier
B Ear	3 Percutaneous 7 Via natural or artificial opening X External	G Other therapeutic substance	C Other substance

C Eye	3 Percutaneous
	7 Via natural or
	   artificial opening
	X External
		0 Antineoplastic	4 Liquid brachytherapy
			   radioisotope
			5 Other antineoplastic
			M Monoclonal antibody

C Eye	3 Percutaneous 7 Via natural or artificial opening X External	2 Anti-infective	8 Oxazolidinones 9 Other anti-infective
C Eye	3 Percutaneous 7 Via natural or artificial opening X External	3 Anti-inflammatory B Local anesthetic H Radioactive substance K Other diagnostic substance M Pigment N Analgesics, hypnotics, sedatives T Destructive agent	Z No qualifier
C Eye	3 Percutaneous 7 Via natural or artificial opening X External	G Other therapeutic substance	C Other substance
C Eye	3 Percutaneous 7 Via natural or artificial opening X External	S Gas	F Other gas

ADMINISTRATION 3 E 0

continued ⇨

3   E   0   INTRODUCTION – *continued*

Body System/Region – 4TH	Approach – 5TH	Substance – 6TH	Qualifier – 7TH
D Mouth and Pharynx	3 Percutaneous 7 Via natural or artificial opening X External	0 Antineoplastic	4 Liquid brachytherapy radioisotope 5 Other antineoplastic M Monoclonal antibody
D Mouth and Pharynx	3 Percutaneous 7 Via natural or artificial opening X External	2 Anti-infective	8 Oxazolidinones 9 Other anti-infective
D Mouth and Pharynx	3 Percutaneous 7 Via natural or artificial opening X External	3 Anti-inflammatory 4 Serum, toxoid and vaccine 6 Nutritional substance 7 Electrolytic and water balance substance B Local anesthetic H Radioactive substance K Other diagnostic substance N Analgesics, hypnotics, sedatives R Antiarrhythmic T Destructive agent	Z No qualifier
D Mouth and Pharynx	3 Percutaneous 7 Via natural or artificial opening X External	G Other therapeutic substance	C Other substance
E Products of Conception ♀ G Upper GI H Lower GI K Genitourinary Tract N Male Reproductive ♂	3 Percutaneous 7 Via natural or artificial opening 8 Via natural or artificial opening endoscopic	0 Antineoplastic	4 Liquid brachytherapy radioisotope 5 Other antineoplastic M Monoclonal antibody
E Products of Conception ♀ G Upper GI H Lower GI K Genitourinary Tract N Male Reproductive ♂	3 Percutaneous 7 Via natural or artificial opening 8 Via natural or artificial opening endoscopic	2 Anti-infective	8 Oxazolidinones 9 Other anti-infective
E Products of Conception ♀ G Upper GI H Lower GI K Genitourinary Tract N Male Reproductive ♂	3 Percutaneous 7 Via natural or artificial opening 8 Via natural or artificial opening endoscopic	3 Anti-inflammatory 6 Nutritional substance 7 Electrolytic and water balance substance B Local anesthetic H Radioactive substance K Other diagnostic substance N Analgesics, hypnotics, sedatives T Destructive agent	Z No qualifier

ADMINISTRATION 3 E 0

continued ⇨

3   E   0   INTRODUCTION – *continued*

Body System/Region – 4TH	Approach – 5TH	Substance – 6TH	Qualifier – 7TH
E Products of Conception ♀ G Upper GI H Lower GI K Genitourinary Tract N Male Reproductive ♂	3 Percutaneous 7 Via natural or artificial opening 8 Via natural or artificial opening endoscopic	G Other therapeutic substance	C Other substance
E Products of Conception ♀ G Upper GI H Lower GI K Genitourinary Tract N Male Reproductive ♂	3 Percutaneous 7 Via natural or artificial opening 8 Via natural or artificial opening endoscopic	S Gas	F Other gas
F Respiratory Tract	3 Percutaneous	0 Antineoplastic	4 Liquid brachytherapy radioisotope 5 Other antineoplastic M Monoclonal antibody
F Respiratory Tract	3 Percutaneous	2 Anti-infective	8 Oxazolidinones 9 Other anti-infective
F Respiratory Tract	3 Percutaneous	3 Anti-inflammatory 6 Nutritional substance 7 Electrolytic and water balance substance B Local anesthetic H Radioactive substance K Other diagnostic substance N Analgesics, hypnotics, sedatives T Destructive agent	Z No qualifier
F Respiratory Tract	3 Percutaneous	G Other therapeutic substance	C Other substance
F Respiratory Tract	3 Percutaneous	S Gas	D Nitric oxide F Other gas
F Respiratory Tract	7 Via natural or artificial opening 8 Via natural or artificial opening endoscopic	0 Antineoplastic	4 Liquid brachytherapy radioisotope 5 Other antineoplastic M Monoclonal antibody
F Respiratory Tract	7 Via natural or artificial opening 8 Via natural or artificial opening endoscopic	2 Anti-infective	8 Oxazolidinones 9 Other anti-infective

ADMINISTRATION 3 E 0

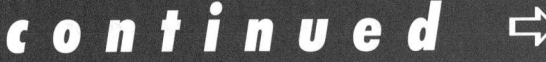
continued ⇨

3 E 0 INTRODUCTION – continued

ADMINISTRATION 3 E 0

Body System/Region – 4ᵀᴴ	Approach – 5ᵀᴴ	Substance – 6ᵀᴴ	Qualifier – 7ᵀᴴ
F Respiratory Tract	7 Via natural or artificial opening 8 Via natural or artificial opening endoscopic	3 Anti-inflammatory 6 Nutritional substance 7 Electrolytic and water balance substance B Local anesthetic D Inhalation anesthetic H Radioactive substance K Other diagnostic substance N Analgesics, hypnotics, sedatives T Destructive agent	Z No qualifier
F Respiratory Tract	7 Via natural or artificial opening 8 Via natural or artificial opening endoscopic	G Other therapeutic substance	C Other substance
F Respiratory Tract	7 Via natural or artificial opening 8 Via natural or artificial opening endoscopic	S Gas	D Nitric oxide F Other gas
J Biliary and Pancreatic Tract	3 Percutaneous 7 Via natural or artificial opening 8 Via natural or artificial opening endoscopic	0 Antineoplastic	4 Liquid brachytherapy radioisotope 5 Other antineoplastic M Monoclonal antibody
J Biliary and Pancreatic Tract	3 Percutaneous 7 Via natural or artificial opening 8 Via natural or artificial opening endoscopic	2 Anti-infective	8 Oxazolidinones 9 Other anti-infective
J Biliary and Pancreatic Tract	3 Percutaneous 7 Via natural or artificial opening 8 Via natural or artificial opening endoscopic	3 Anti-inflammatory 6 Nutritional substance 7 Electrolytic and water balance substance B Local anesthetic H Radioactive substance K Other diagnostic substance N Analgesics, hypnotics, sedatives T Destructive agent	Z No qualifier
J Biliary and Pancreatic Tract	3 Percutaneous 7 Via natural or artificial opening 8 Via natural or artificial opening endoscopic	G Other therapeutic substance	C Other substance

continued ⇨

3   E   0   INTRODUCTION – *continued*

Body System/Region – 4TH	Approach – 5TH	Substance – 6TH	Qualifier – 7TH
J Biliary and Pancreatic Tract	3 Percutaneous 7 Via natural or artificial opening 8 Via natural or artificial opening endoscopic	S Gas	F Other gas
J Biliary and Pancreatic Tract	3 Percutaneous 7 Via natural or artificial opening 8 Via natural or artificial opening endoscopic	U Pancreatic islet cells	0 Autologous 1 Nonautologous
L Pleural Cavity M Peritoneal Cavity	0 Open	5 Adhesion barrier	Z No qualifier
L Pleural Cavity M Peritoneal Cavity	3 Percutaneous	0 Antineoplastic	4 Liquid brachytherapy radioisotope 5 Other antineoplastic M Monoclonal antibody
L Pleural Cavity M Peritoneal Cavity	3 Percutaneous	2 Anti-infective	8 Oxazolidinones 9 Other anti-infective
L Pleural Cavity M Peritoneal Cavity	3 Percutaneous	3 Anti-inflammatory 6 Nutritional substance 7 Electrolytic and water balance substance B Local anesthetic H Radioactive substance K Other diagnostic substance N Analgesics, hypnotics, sedatives T Destructive agent	Z No qualifier
L Pleural Cavity M Peritoneal Cavity	3 Percutaneous	G Other therapeutic substance	C Other substance
L Pleural Cavity M Peritoneal Cavity	3 Percutaneous	S Gas	F Other gas
L Pleural Cavity M Peritoneal Cavity	7 Via natural or artificial opening	0 Antineoplastic	4 Liquid brachytherapy radioisotope 5 Other antineoplastic M Monoclonal antibody
L Pleural Cavity M Peritoneal Cavity	7 Via natural or artificial opening	S Gas	F Other gas

ADMINISTRATION 3 E 0

continued ⇨

3   E   0   INTRODUCTION – *continued*

Body System/Region – 4TH	Approach – 5TH	Substance – 6TH	Qualifier – 7TH
P Female Reproductive ♀	0 Open	5 Adhesion barrier	Z No qualifier
P Female Reproductive ♀	3 Percutaneous 7 Via natural or artificial opening	0 Antineoplastic	4 Liquid brachytherapy radioisotope 5 Other antineoplastic M Monoclonal antibody
P Female Reproductive ♀	3 Percutaneous 7 Via natural or artificial opening	2 Anti-infective	8 Oxazolidinones 9 Other anti-infective
P Female Reproductive ♀	3 Percutaneous 7 Via natural or artificial opening	3 Anti-inflammatory 6 Nutritional substance 7 Electrolytic and water balance substance B Local anesthetic H Radioactive substance K Other diagnostic substance L Sperm N Analgesics, hypnotics, sedatives T Destructive agent	Z No qualifier
P Female Reproductive ♀	3 Percutaneous 7 Via natural or artificial opening	G Other therapeutic substance	C Other substance
P Female Reproductive ♀	3 Percutaneous 7 Via natural or artificial opening	Q Fertilized ovum	0 Autologous 1 Nonautologous
P Female Reproductive ♀	3 Percutaneous 7 Via natural or artificial opening	S Gas	F Other gas
P Female Reproductive ♀	8 Via natural or artificial opening endoscopic	0 Antineoplastic	4 Liquid brachytherapy radioisotope 5 Other antineoplastic M Monoclonal antibody
P Female Reproductive ♀	8 Via natural or artificial opening endoscopic	2 Anti-infective	8 Oxazolidinones 9 Other anti-infective

ADMINISTRATION 3E0

continued ⇨

3   E   0   INTRODUCTION—*continued*

Body System/Region – 4TH	Approach – 5TH	Substance – 6TH	Qualifier – 7TH
P Female Reproductive ♀	8 Via natural or artificial opening endoscopic	3 Anti-inflammatory 6 Nutritional substance 7 Electrolytic and water balance substance B Local anesthetic H Radioactive substance K Other diagnostic substance N Analgesics, hypnotics, sedatives T Destructive agent	Z No qualifier
P Female Reproductive ♀	8 Via natural or artificial opening endoscopic	G Other therapeutic substance	C Other substance
P Female Reproductive ♀	8 Via natural or artificial opening endoscopic	S Gas	F Other gas
Q Cranial Cavity and Brain	0 Open 3 Percutaneous	0 Antineoplastic	4 Liquid brachytherapy radioisotope 5 Other antineoplastic M Monoclonal antibody
Q Cranial Cavity and Brain	0 Open 3 Percutaneous	2 Anti-infective	8 Oxazolidinones 9 Other anti-infective
Q Cranial Cavity and Brain	0 Open 3 Percutaneous	3 Anti-inflammatory 6 Nutritional substance 7 Electrolytic and water balance substance A Stem cells, embryonic B Local anesthetic H Radioactive substance K Other diagnostic substance N Analgesics, hypnotics, sedatives T Destructive agent	Z No qualifier
Q Cranial Cavity and Brain	0 Open 3 Percutaneous	E Stem cells, somatic	0 Autologous 1 Nonautologous
Q Cranial Cavity and Brain	0 Open 3 Percutaneous	G Other therapeutic substance	C Other substance
Q Cranial Cavity and Brain	0 Open 3 Percutaneous	S Gas	F Other gas

continued ⇨

ADMINISTRATION 3 E 0

3   E   0   INTRODUCTION – *continued*

Body System/Region – 4TH	Approach – 5TH	Substance – 6TH	Qualifier – 7TH
Q Cranial Cavity and Brain	7 Via natural or artificial opening	0 Antineoplastic	4 Liquid brachytherapy radioisotope 5 Other antineoplastic M Monoclonal antibody
Q Cranial Cavity and Brain	7 Via natural or artificial opening	S Gas	F Other gas
R Spinal Canal	0 Open	A Stem cells, embryonic	Z No qualifier
R Spinal Canal	0 Open	E Stem cells, somatic	0 Autologous 1 Nonautologous
R Spinal Canal	3 Percutaneous	0 Antineoplastic	2 High-dose Interleukin-2 3 Low-dose Interleukin-2 4 Liquid brachytherapy radioisotope 5 Other antineoplastic M Monoclonal antibody
R Spinal Canal	3 Percutaneous	2 Anti-infective	8 Oxazolidinones 9 Other anti-infective
R Spinal Canal	3 Percutaneous	3 Anti-inflammatory 6 Nutritional substance 7 Electrolytic and water balance substance A Stem cells, embryonic B Local anesthetic C Regional anesthetic H Radioactive substance K Other diagnostic substance N Analgesics, hypnotics, sedatives T Destructive agent	Z No qualifier
R Spinal Canal	3 Percutaneous	E Stem cells, somatic	0 Autologous 1 Nonautologous
R Spinal Canal	3 Percutaneous	G Other therapeutic substance	C Other substance
R Spinal Canal	3 Percutaneous	S Gas	F Other gas
R Spinal Canal	7 Via natural or artificial opening	S Gas	F Other gas

continued ⇨

A D M I N I S T R A T I O N 3 E 0

3　　E　　0　INTRODUCTION—*continued*

Body System/Region – 4TH	Approach – 5TH	Substance – 6TH	Qualifier – 7TH
S Epidural Space	3 Percutaneous	0 Antineoplastic	2 High-dose Interleukin-2 3 Low-dose Interleukin-2 4 Liquid brachytherapy radioisotope 5 Other antineoplastic M Monoclonal antibody
S Epidural Space	3 Percutaneous	2 Anti-infective	8 Oxazolidinones 9 Other anti-infective
S Epidural Space	3 Percutaneous	3 Anti-inflammatory 6 Nutritional substance 7 Electrolytic and water balance substance B Local anesthetic C Regional anesthetic H Radioactive substance K Other diagnostic substance N Analgesics, hypnotics, sedatives T Destructive agent	Z No qualifier
S Epidural Space	3 Percutaneous	G Other therapeutic substance	C Other substance
S Epidural Space	3 Percutaneous	S Gas	F Other gas
S Epidural Space	7 Via natural or artificial opening	S Gas	F Other gas
T Peripheral Nerves and Plexi X Cranial Nerves	3 Percutaneous	3 Anti-inflammatory B Local anesthetic C Regional anesthetic T Destructive agent	Z No qualifier
T Peripheral Nerves and Plexi X Cranial Nerves	3 Percutaneous	G Other therapeutic substance	C Other substance

continued ⇨

ADMINISTRATION 3 E 0

3   E   0   INTRODUCTION – *continued*

Body System/Region – 4TH	Approach – 5TH	Substance – 6TH	Qualifier – 7TH
U Joints	0 Open	2 Anti-infective	8 Oxazolidinones 9 Other anti-infective
U Joints	0 Open	G Other therapeutic substance	B Recombinant bone morphogenetic protein
U Joints	3 Percutaneous	0 Antineoplastic	4 Liquid brachytherapy radioisotope 5 Other antineoplastic M Monoclonal antibody
U Joints	3 Percutaneous	2 Anti-infective	8 Oxazolidinones 9 Other anti-infective
U Joints	3 Percutaneous	3 Anti-inflammatory 6 Nutritional substance 7 Electrolytic and water balance substance B Local anesthetic H Radioactive substance K Other diagnostic substance N Analgesics, hypnotics, sedatives T Destructive agent	Z No qualifier
U Joints	3 Percutaneous	G Other therapeutic substance	B Recombinant bone morphogenetic protein C Other substance
U Joints	3 Percutaneous	S Gas	F Other gas
V Bones	0 Open	G Other therapeutic substance	B Recombinant bone morphogenetic protein
V Bones	3 Percutaneous	0 Antineoplastic	5 Other antineoplastic M Monoclonal antibody
V Bones	3 Percutaneous	2 Anti-infective	8 Oxazolidinones 9 Other anti-infective
V Bones	3 Percutaneous	3 Anti-inflammatory 6 Nutritional substance 7 Electrolytic and water balance substance B Local anesthetic H Radioactive substance K Other diagnostic substance N Analgesics, hypnotics, sedatives T Destructive agent	Z No qualifier
V Bones	3 Percutaneous	G Other therapeutic substance	B Recombinant bone morphogenetic protein C Other substance

continued ⇨

3   E   0   INTRODUCTION – *continued*

Body System/Region – 4TH	Approach – 5TH	Substance – 6TH	Qualifier – 7TH
W Lymphatics	3 Percutaneous	0 Antineoplastic	5 Other antineoplastic M Monoclonal antibody
W Lymphatics	3 Percutaneous	2 Anti-infective	8 Oxazolidinones 9 Other anti-infective
W Lymphatics	3 Percutaneous	3 Anti-inflammatory 6 Nutritional substance 7 Electrolytic and water balance substance B Local anesthetic H Radioactive substance K Other diagnostic substance N Analgesics, hypnotics, sedatives T Destructive agent	Z No qualifier
W Lymphatics	3 Percutaneous	G Other therapeutic substance	C Other substance
Y Pericardial Cavity	3 Percutaneous	0 Antineoplastic	4 Liquid brachytherapy radioisotope 5 Other antineoplastic M Monoclonal antibody
Y Pericardial Cavity	3 Percutaneous	2 Anti-infective	8 Oxazolidinones 9 Other anti-infective
Y Pericardial Cavity	3 Percutaneous	3 Anti-inflammatory 6 Nutritional substance 7 Electrolytic and water balance substance B Local anesthetic H Radioactive substance K Other diagnostic substance N Analgesics, hypnotics, sedatives T Destructive agent	Z No qualifier
Y Pericardial Cavity	3 Percutaneous	G Other therapeutic substance	C Other substance
Y Pericardial Cavity	3 Percutaneous	S Gas	F Other gas
Y Pericardial Cavity	7 Via natural or artificial opening	0 Antineoplastic	4 Liquid brachytherapy radioisotope 5 Other antineoplastic M Monoclonal antibody
Y Pericardial Cavity	7 Via natural or artificial opening	S Gas	F Other gas

ADMINISTRATION 3 E 0

ADMINISTRATION SECTION: Introduction, Irrigation, Transfusion
Root Operations that define procedures where a diagnostic or therapeutic substance is given to the patient.

1ST – **3** Administration

2ND – **E** Physiological Systems and Anatomical Regions

3RD – **1** IRRIGATION

EXAMPLE: Flushing of eye

IRRIGATION: Putting in or on a cleansing substance.

EXPLANATION: Cleansing substance or dialysate

Body System/Region – 4TH	Approach – 5TH	Substance – 6TH	Qualifier – 7TH
0 Skin and Mucous Membranes C Eye	3 Percutaneous X External	8 Irrigating substance	X Diagnostic Z No qualifier
9 Nose B Ear F Respiratory Tract G Upper GI H Lower GI J Biliary and Pancreatic Tract K Genitourinary Tract N Male Reproductive ♂ P Female Reproductive ♀	3 Percutaneous 7 Via natural or artificial opening 8 Via natural or artificial opening endoscopic	8 Irrigating substance	X Diagnostic Z No qualifier
L Pleural Cavity Q Cranial Cavity and Brain R Spinal Canal S Epidural Space U Joints Y Pericardial Cavity	3 Percutaneous	8 Irrigating substance	X Diagnostic Z No qualifier
M Peritoneal Cavity	3 Percutaneous	8 Irrigating substance	X Diagnostic Z No qualifier
M Peritoneal Cavity	3 Percutaneous	9 Dialysate	Z No qualifier

Educational Annotations | Section 4 – Measurement and Monitoring

Section Specific Educational Annotations for the Measurement and Monitoring Section include:
- **AHA Coding Clinic® Reference Notations**
- **Coding Notes**

AHA Coding Clinic® Reference Notations of Measurement and Monitoring

ROOT OPERATION SPECIFIC - MEASUREMENT AND MONITORING - Section 4

MEASUREMENT - 0

Left heart cardiac catheterization .... AHA 13:3Q:p26

MONITORING - 1

Continuous arterial pressure monitoring... AHA 16:2Q:p33

EMG monitoring during surgery .... AHA 15:2Q:p14

Intraoperative neuromonitoring .... AHA 14:4Q:p28

.... AHA 15:1Q:p26

Coding Notes of Measurement and Monitoring

Med/Surg Related Section Specific PCS Reference Manual Exercises

PCS CODE	4 – MEASUREMENT AND MONITORING EXERCISES
4 A 0 2 3 N 8	Right and left heart cardiac catheterization with bilateral sampling and pressure measurements.
4 A 0 2 X M 4	Cardiac stress test, single measurement.
4 A 0 4 X J 1	Peripheral venous pulse, external, single measurement.
4 A 0 7 X 7 Z	Visual mobility test, single measurement.
4 A 0 8 X 0 Z	Olfactory acuity test, single measurement.
4 A 0 9 X C Z	Respiratory rate, external, single measurement.
4 A 0 C 8 5 Z	EGD with biliary flow measurement.
4 A 1 2 3 9 Z	Left ventricular cardiac output monitoring from pulmonary artery wedge (Swan-Ganz) catheter.
4 A 1 2 X 4 5	Holter monitoring.
4 A 1 H 7 C Z	Fetal heart rate monitoring, transvaginal.

MEASUREMENT

4

Educational Annotations | Section 4 – Measurement and Monitoring

<u>**NOTES**</u>

MEASUREMENT AND MONITORING SECTION: Measurment, Monitoring
Root Operations that define one procedure/level and a series of procedures/levels obtained at intervals.

1ST - **4** Measurement and Monitoring

2ND - **A** Physiological Systems

3RD - **0 MEASUREMENT**

EXAMPLE: EKG (single electrocardiogram)

MEASUREMENT: Determining the level of a physiological or physical function at a point in time.

EXPLANATION: Describes a single measurement

Body System – 4TH	Approach – 5TH	Function/Device – 6TH	Qualifier – 7TH
0 Central Nervous	0 Open	2 Conductivity 4 Electrical activity B Pressure	Z No qualifier
0 Central Nervous	3 Percutaneous	4 Electrical activity	Z No qualifier
0 Central Nervous	3 Percutaneous	B Pressure K Temperature R Saturation	D Intracranial
0 Central Nervous	7 Via natural or artificial opening	B Pressure K Temperature R Saturation	D Intracranial
0 Central Nervous	X External	2 Conductivity 4 Electrical activity	Z No qualifier
1 Peripheral Nervous	0 Open 3 Percutaneous X External	2 Conductivity	9 Sensory B Motor
1 Peripheral Nervous	0 Open 3 Percutaneous X External	4 Electrical activity	Z No qualifier
2 Cardiac	0 Open 3 Percutaneous	4 Electrical activity 9 Output C Rate F Rhythm H Sound P Action currents	Z No qualifier
2 Cardiac	0 Open 3 Percutaneous	N Sampling and pressure	6 Right heart 7 Left heart 8 Bilateral
2 Cardiac	X External	4 Electrical activity	A Guidance Z No qualifier
2 Cardiac	X External	9 Output C Rate F Rhythm H Sound P Action currents	Z No qualifier
2 Cardiac	X External	M Total activity	4 Stress

MEASUREMENT 4 A 0

continued ⇨

4 A 0 MEASUREMENT – *continued*

Body System – 4TH	Approach – 5TH	Function/Device – 6TH	Qualifier – 7TH
3 Arterial	0 Open 3 Percutaneous	5 Flow J Pulse	1 Peripheral 3 Pulmonary C Coronary
3 Arterial	0 Open 3 Percutaneous	B Pressure	1 Peripheral 3 Pulmonary C Coronary F Other Thoracic
3 Arterial	0 Open 3 Percutaneous	H Sound R Saturation	1 Peripheral
3 Arterial	X External	5 Flow B Pressure H Sound J Pulse R Saturation	1 Peripheral
4 Venous	0 Open 3 Percutaneous	5 Flow B Pressure J Pulse	0 Central 1 Peripheral 2 Portal 3 Pulmonary
4 Venous	0 Open 3 Percutaneous	R Saturation	1 Peripheral
4 Venous	X External	5 Flow B Pressure J Pulse R Saturation	1 Peripheral
5 Circulatory	X External	L Volume	Z No qualifier
6 Lymphatic	0 Open 3 Percutaneous	5 Flow B Pressure	Z No qualifier
7 Visual	X External	0 Acuity 7 Mobility B Pressure	Z No qualifier
8 Olfactory	X External	0 Acuity	Z No qualifier
9 Respiratory	7 Via natural or artificial opening 8 Via natural or artificial opening endoscopic X External	1 Capacity 5 Flow C Rate D Resistance L Volume M Total activity	Z No qualifier
B Gastrointestinal	7 Via natural or artificial opening 8 Via natural or artificial opening endoscopic	8 Motility B Pressure G Secretion	Z No qualifier

continued ⇨

4   A   0   MEASUREMENT – *continued*

Body System – 4TH	Approach – 5TH	Function/Device – 6TH	Qualifier – 7TH
C Biliary	3 Percutaneous 4 Percutaneous endoscopic 7 Via natural or artificial opening 8 Via natural or artificial opening endoscopic	5 Flow B Pressure	Z No qualifier
D Urinary	7 Via natural or artificial opening	3 Contractility 5 Flow B Pressure D Resistance L Volume	Z No qualifier
F Musculoskeletal	3 Percutaneous X External	3 Contractility	Z No qualifier
H Products of Conception, Cardiac ♀	7 Via natural or artificial opening 8 Via natural or artificial opening endoscopic X External	4 Electrical activity C Rate F Rhythm H Sound	Z No qualifier
J Products of Conception, Nervous ♀	7 Via natural or artificial opening 8 Via natural or artificial opening endoscopic X External	2 Conductivity 4 Electrical activity B Pressure	Z No qualifier
Z None	7 Via natural or artificial opening	6 Metabolism K Temperature	Z No qualifier
Z None	X External	6 Metabolism K Temperature Q Sleep	Z No qualifier

MEASUREMENT

4 A 0

MEASUREMENT AND MONITORING SECTION: Measurment, Monitoring
Root Operations that define one procedure/level and a series of procedures/levels obtained at intervals.

1ST – **4** Measurement and Monitoring

2ND – **A** Physiological Systems

3RD – **1 MONITORING**

EXAMPLE: Holter monitor

MONITORING: Determining the level of a physiological or physical function repetitively over a period of time.

EXPLANATION: Describes a series of measurements

Body System – 4TH	Approach – 5TH	Function/Device – 6TH	Qualifier – 7TH
0 Central Nervous	0 Open	2 Conductivity B Pressure	Z No qualifier
0 Central Nervous	0 Open	4 Electrical activity	G Intraoperative Z No qualifier
0 Central Nervous	3 Percutaneous	4 Electrical activity	G Intraoperative Z No qualifier
0 Central Nervous	3 Percutaneous	B Pressure K Temperature R Saturation	D Intracranial
0 Central Nervous	7 Via natural or artificial opening	B Pressure K Temperature R Saturation	D Intracranial
0 Central Nervous	X External	2 Conductivity	Z No qualifier
0 Central Nervous	X External	4 Electrical activity	G Intraoperative Z No qualifier
1 Peripheral Nervous	0 Open 3 Percutaneous X External	2 Conductivity	9 Sensory B Motor
1 Peripheral Nervous	0 Open 3 Percutaneous X External	4 Electrical activity	G Intraoperative Z No qualifier
2 Cardiac	0 Open 3 Percutaneous	4 Electrical activity 9 Output C Rate F Rhythm H Sound	Z No qualifier
2 Cardiac	X External	4 Electrical activity	5 Ambulatory Z No qualifier
2 Cardiac	X External	9 Output C Rate F Rhythm H Sound	Z No qualifier
2 Cardiac	X External	M Total activity	4 Stress
2 Cardiac	X External	S Vascular perfusion	H Indocyanine green dye
3 Arterial	0 Open 3 Percutaneous	5 Flow B Pressure J Pulse	1 Peripheral 3 Pulmonary C Coronary
3 Arterial	0 Open 3 Percutaneous	H Sound R Saturation	1 Peripheral

c o n t i n u e d ⇨

MEASUREMENT 4 A 1

4   A   1   MONITORING – continued

Body System – 4TH	Approach – 5TH	Function/Device – 6TH	Qualifier – 7TH
3 Arterial	X External	5 Flow B Pressure H Sound J Pulse R Saturation	1 Peripheral
4 Venous	0 Open 3 Percutaneous	5 Flow B Pressure J Pulse	0 Central 1 Peripheral 2 Portal 3 Pulmonary
4 Venous	0 Open 3 Percutaneous	R Saturation	0 Central 2 Portal 3 Pulmonary
4 Venous	X External	5 Flow B Pressure J Pulse	1 Peripheral
6 Lymphatic	0 Open 3 Percutaneous	5 Flow B Pressure	Z No qualifier
9 Respiratory	7 Via natural or artificial opening X External	1 Capacity 5 Flow C Rate D Resistance L Volume	Z No qualifier
B Gastrointestinal	7 Via natural or artificial opening 8 Via natural or artificial opening endoscopic	8 Motility B Pressure G Secretion	Z No qualifier
B Gastrointestinal	X External	S Vascular perfusion	H Indocyanine green dye
D Urinary	7 Via natural or artificial opening	3 Contractility 5 Flow B Pressure D Resistance L Volume	Z No qualifier
G Skin and Breast	X External	S Vascular perfusion	H Indocyanine green dye
H Products of Conception, Cardiac ♀	7 Via natural or artificial opening 8 Via natural or artificial opening endoscopic X External	4 Electrical activity C Rate F Rhythm H Sound	Z No qualifier
J Products of Conception, Nervous ♀	7 Via natural or artificial opening 8 Via natural or artificial opening endoscopic X External	2 Conductivity 4 Electrical activity B Pressure	Z No qualifier
Z None	7 Via natural or artificial opening	K Temperature	Z No qualifier
Z None	X External	K Temperature Q Sleep	Z No qualifier

MEASUREMENT

4 A 1

© 2016 Channel Publishing, Ltd.

MEASUREMENT AND MONITORING SECTION: Measurment, Monitoring
Root Operations that define one procedure/level and a series of procedures/levels obtained at intervals.

1ST – **4** Measurement and Monitoring

2ND – **B** Physiological Devices

3RD – **0 MEASUREMENT**

EXAMPLE: Pacemaker rate check

MEASUREMENT: Determining the level of a physiological or physical function at a point in time.

EXPLANATION: Describes a single measurement

Body System – 4TH	Approach – 5TH	Function/Device – 6TH	Qualifier – 7TH
0 Central Nervous 1 Peripheral Nervous F Musculoskeletal	X External	V Stimulator	Z No qualifier
2 Cardiac	X External	S Pacemaker T Defibrillator	Z No qualifier
9 Respiratory	X External	S Pacemaker	Z No qualifier

Educational Annotations | Section 5 – Extracorporeal Assistance and Performance

Section Specific Educational Annotations for the Extracorporeal Assistance and Performance Section include:
- AHA Coding Clinic® Reference Notations
- Coding Notes

AHA Coding Clinic® Reference Notations of Extracoporeal Assistance and Performance

ROOT OPERATION SPECIFIC - EXTRACORPOREAL ASSISTANCE AND PERFORMANCE - Section 5

ASSISTANCE - 0
BiPAP ventilatory support system	AHA 14:4Q:p9
Impella assistance/support	AHA 14:3Q:p19
Intra-aortic balloon pump	AHA 13:3Q:p18

PERFORMANCE - 1
Cardiopulmonary bypass	AHA 14:3Q:p17,20
	AHA 14:1Q:P10
	AHA 13:3Q:p18
Continuous cardiac pacing	AHA 13:3Q:p18
Extracoporeal liver assist device (ELAD) filtration	AHA 16:1Q:p28
Hemodialysis treatments, multiple	AHA 16:1Q:p29
Mechanical ventilation	AHA 14:4Q:p3
Mechanical ventilation, at night for sleep apnea	AHA 14:4Q:p11

RESTORATION - 2

Coding Notes of Extracoporeal Assistance and Performance

Med/Surg Related Section Specific PCS Reference Manual Exercises

PCS CODE	5 – EXTRACORPOREAL ASSISTANCE AND PERFORMANCE EXERCISES
5 A 0 2 1 1 5	Pulsatile compression boot with intermittent inflation. (This is coded to the function value Cardiac Output, because the purpose of such compression devices is to return blood to the heart faster.)
5 A 0 2 2 1 0	IABP (intra-aortic balloon pump) continuous.
5 A 0 9 3 5 8	IPPB (intermittent positive pressure breathing) for mobilization of secretions, 22 hours.
5 A 1 2 2 3 Z	Intra-operative cardiac pacing, continuous.
5 A 1 5 2 2 3	ECMO (extracorporeal membrane oxygenation), continuous.
5 A 1 9 3 5 Z	Intermittent mechanical ventilation, 16 hours.
5 A 1 9 4 5 Z	Controlled mechanical ventilation (CMV), 45 hours.
5 A 1 C 0 0 Z	Liver dialysis, single encounter.
5 A 1 D 6 0 Z	Renal dialysis, series of encounters.
5 A 2 2 0 4 Z	Cardiac countershock with successful conversion to sinus rhythm.

EXTRA ASSISTANCE 5

Educational Annotations | Section 5 – Extracorporeal Assistance and Performance

NOTES

EXTRACORPOREAL ASSISTANCE AND PERFORMANCE SECTION: Assistance, Performance, Restoration
Root Operations that use equipment to support a physiological function in some manner.

1ST - 5 Extracorporeal Assistance and Performance

2ND - A Physiological Systems

3RD - 0 ASSISTANCE

EXAMPLE: Intra-aortic balloon pump

ASSISTANCE: Taking over a portion of a physiological function by extracorporeal means.

EXPLANATION: Supports, but does not take over function …

Body System – 4TH	Duration – 5TH	Function – 6TH	Qualifier – 7TH
2 Cardiac	1 Intermittent 2 Continuous	1 Output	0 Balloon pump 5 Pulsatile compression 6 Other pump D Impeller pump
5 Circulatory	1 Intermittent 2 Continuous	2 Oxygenation	1 Hyperbaric C Supersaturated
9 Respiratory	3 Less than 24 consecutive hours 4 24-96 consecutive hours 5 Greater than 96 consecutive hours	5 Ventilation	7 Continuous positive airway pressure 8 Intermittent positive airway pressure 9 Continuous negative airway pressure B Intermittent negative airway pressure Z No qualifier

EXTRACORPOREAL ASSISTANCE AND PERFORMANCE SECTION: Assistance, Performance, Restoration
Root Operations that use equipment to support a physiological function in some manner.

1ST - 5 Extracorporeal Assistance and Performance

2ND - A Physiological Systems

3RD - 1 PEFORMANCE

EXAMPLE: Cardioplumonary bypass in CABG

PERFORMANCE: Completely taking over a physiological function by extracorporeal means.

EXPLANATION: Completely takes over function …

Body System – 4TH	Duration – 5TH	Function – 6TH	Qualifier – 7TH
2 Cardiac	0 Single	1 Output	2 Manual
2 Cardiac	1 Intermittent	3 Pacing	Z No qualifier
2 Cardiac	2 Continuous	1 Output 3 Pacing	Z No qualifier
5 Circulatory	2 Continuous	2 Oxygenation	3 Membrane
9 Respiratory	0 Single	5 Ventilation	4 Nonmechanical
9 Respiratory	3 Less than 24 consecutive hours 4 24-96 consecutive hours 5 Greater than 96 consecutive hours LOS*	5 Ventilation	Z No qualifier
C Biliary D Urinary	0 Single 6 Multiple	0 Filtration	Z No qualifier

LOS* – Procedure Inconsistent with LOS Edit – Code only when the respiratory ventilation is provided for greater than four consecutive days during the length of stay. See current Medicare Code Editor for details.

EXTRA ASSISTANCE 5 A 1

EXTRACORPOREAL ASSISTANCE AND PERFORMANCE SECTION: Assistance, Performance, Restoration
Root Operations that use equipment to support a physiological function in some manner.

1ST – **5** Extracorporeal Assistance and Performance	EXAMPLE: Cardiac defibrillation
2ND – **A** Physiological Systems	<u>RESTORATION:</u> Returning, or attempting to return, a physiological function to its original state by extracorporeal means.
3RD – **2 RESTORATION**	EXPLANATION: Defibrillation and cardioversion only …

Body System – 4TH	Duration – 5TH	Function – 6TH	Qualifier – 7TH
2 Cardiac	0 Single	4 Rhythm	Z No qualifier

Educational Annotations | Section 6 – Extracorporeal Therapies

Section Specific Educational Annotations for the Extracorporeal Therapies Section include:
- AHA Coding Clinic® Reference Notations
- Coding Notes

AHA Coding Clinic® Reference Notations of Extracorporeal Therapies

ROOT OPERATION SPECIFIC - EXTRACORPOREAL THERAPIES - Section 6
ATMOSPHERIC CONTROL - 0
DECOMPRESSION - 1
ELECTROMAGNETIC THERAPY - 2
HYPERTHERMIA - 3
HYPOTHERMIA - 4
PHERESIS - 5
PHOTOTHERAPY - 6
ULTRASOUND THERAPY - 7
    Ultrasound accelerated thrombolysis ....AHA 14:4Q:p19
ULTRVIOLET LIGHT THERAPY - 8
SHOCK WAVE THERAPY - 9

Coding Notes of Extracorporeal Therapies

Med/Surg Related Section Specific PCS Reference Manual Exercises

PCS CODE	6 – EXTRACORPOREAL THERAPIES EXERCISES
6 A 0 Z 1 Z Z	Antigen-free air conditioning, series treatment.
6 A 2 1 0 Z Z	Extracorporeal electromagnetic stimulation (EMS) for urinary incontinence, single treatment.
6 A 2 2 1 Z Z	TMS (transcranial magnetic stimulation), series treatment.
6 A 4 Z 0 Z Z	Whole body hypothermia, single treatment.
6 A 5 5 0 Z 2	Donor thrombocytapheresis, single encounter.
6 A 5 5 1 Z 3	Plasmapheresis, series treatment.
6 A 6 5 0 Z Z	Circulatory phototherapy, single encounter.
6 A 6 5 1 Z Z	Bili-lite phototherapy, series treatment.
6 A 7 5 0 Z Z	Therapeutic ultrasound of peripheral vessels, single treatment.
6 A 9 3 0 Z Z	Shock wave therapy of plantar fascia, single treatment.

Educational Annotations | Section 6 – Extracorporeal Therapies

<u>**NOTES**</u>

EXTRACORPOREAL THERAPIES SECTION: Atmospheric Control, Decompression, Electromagnetic Therapy, Hyperthermia, Hypothermia, Pheresis, Phototherapy, Ultrasound Therapy, Ultraviolet Light Therapy, Shock Wave Therapy, Perfusion
Root Operations that describe other extracorporeal procedures that are not defined by Assistance and Performance in Section 5.

1ST - **6** Extracorporeal Therapies

2ND - **A** Physiological Systems

3RD - **0** ATMOSPHERIC CONTROL

EXAMPLE: Antigen-free air conditioning

ATMOSPHERIC CONTROL:
Extracorporeal control of atmospheric pressure and composition.

EXPLANATION: Control of air composition and pressure ...

Body System – 4TH	Duration – 5TH	Qualifier – 6TH	Qualifier – 7TH
Z None	0 Single 1 Multiple	Z No qualifier	Z No qualifier

EXTRACORPOREAL THERAPIES SECTION: Atmospheric Control, Decompression, Electromagnetic Therapy, Hyperthermia, Hypothermia, Pheresis, Phototherapy, Ultrasound Therapy, Ultraviolet Light Therapy, Shock Wave Therapy, Perfusion
Root Operations that describe other extracorporeal procedures that are not defined by Assistance and Performance in Section 5.

1ST - **6** Extracorporeal Therapies

2ND - **A** Physiological Systems

3RD - **1** DECOMPRESSION

EXAMPLE: Decompression chamber treatment

DECOMPRESSION: Extracorporeal elimination of undissolved gas from body fluids.

EXPLANATION: Used only to treat the "bends" ...

Body System – 4TH	Duration – 5TH	Qualifier – 6TH	Qualifier – 7TH
5 Circulatory	0 Single 1 Multiple	Z No qualifier	Z No qualifier

---

EXTRACORPOREAL THERAPIES SECTION: Atmospheric Control, Decompression, Electromagnetic Therapy, Hyperthermia, Hypothermia, Pheresis, Phototherapy, Ultrasound Therapy, Ultraviolet Light Therapy, Shock Wave Therapy, Perfusion
Root Operations that describe other extracorporeal procedures that are not defined by Assistance and Performance in Section 5.

1ST - **6** Extracorporeal Therapies

2ND - **A** Physiological Systems

3RD - **2** ELECTROMAGNETIC THERAPY

EXAMPLE: Transcranial magnetic stimulation (TMS)

ELECTROMAGNETIC THERAPY:
Extracorporeal treatment by electromagnetic rays.

EXPLANATION: Electromagnetic energy to stimulate cells

Body System – 4TH	Duration – 5TH	Qualifier – 6TH	Qualifier – 7TH
1 Urinary 2 Central Nervous	0 Single 1 Multiple	Z No qualifier	Z No qualifier

---

EXTRACORPOREAL THERAPIES SECTION: Atmospheric Control, Decompression, Electromagnetic Therapy, Hyperthermia, Hypothermia, Pheresis, Phototherapy, Ultrasound Therapy, Ultraviolet Light Therapy, Shock Wave Therapy, Perfusion
Root Operations that describe other extracorporeal procedures that are not defined by Assistance and Performance in Section 5.

1ST - **6** Extracorporeal Therapies

2ND - **A** Physiological Systems

3RD - **3 HYPERTHERMIA**

EXAMPLE: Whole body hyperthermia

HYPERTHERMIA: Extracorporeal raising of body temperature.

EXPLANATION: Used to treat temperature imbalance …

Body System – 4TH	Duration – 5TH	Qualifier – 6TH	Qualifier – 7TH
Z None	0 Single 1 Multiple	Z No qualifier	Z No qualifier

EXTRACORPOREAL THERAPIES SECTION: Atmospheric Control, Decompression, Electromagnetic Therapy, Hyperthermia, Hypothermia, Pheresis, Phototherapy, Ultrasound Therapy, Ultraviolet Light Therapy, Shock Wave Therapy, Perfusion
Root Operations that describe other extracorporeal procedures that are not defined by Assistance and Performance in Section 5.

1ST - **6** Extracorporeal Therapies

2ND - **A** Physiological Systems

3RD - **4 HYPOTHERMIA**

EXAMPLE: Whole body hypothermia

HYPOTHERMIA: Extracorporeal lowering of body temperature.

EXPLANATION: Used to treat temperature imbalance …

Body System – 4TH	Duration – 5TH	Qualifier – 6TH	Qualifier – 7TH
Z None	0 Single 1 Multiple	Z No qualifier	Z No qualifier

EXTRACORPOREAL THERAPIES SECTION: Atmospheric Control, Decompression, Electromagnetic Therapy, Hyperthermia, Hypothermia, Pheresis, Phototherapy, Ultrasound Therapy, Ultraviolet Light Therapy, Shock Wave Therapy, Perfusion
Root Operations that describe other extracorporeal procedures that are not defined by Assistance and Performance in Section 5.

1ST - **6** Extracorporeal Therapies

2ND - **A** Physiological Systems

3RD - **5 PHERESIS**

EXAMPLE: Therapeutic leukapheresis

PHERESIS: Extracorporeal separation of blood products.

EXPLANATION: Used to separate and remove blood products

Body System – 4TH	Duration – 5TH	Qualifier – 6TH	Qualifier – 7TH
5 Circulatory	0 Single 1 Multiple	Z No qualifier	0 Erythrocytes 1 Leukocytes 2 Platelets 3 Plasma T Stem cells, cord blood V Stem cells, hematopoietic

E X T R A T H E R A P I E S 6 A 3

EXTRACORPOREAL THERAPIES SECTION: Atmospheric Control, Decompression, Electromagnetic Therapy, Hyperthermia, Hypothermia, Pheresis, Phototherapy, Ultrasound Therapy, Ultraviolet Light Therapy, Shock Wave Therapy, Perfusion
Root Operations that describe other extracorporeal procedures that are not defined by Assistance and Performance in Section 5.

1ST – **6** Extracorporeal Therapies

2ND – **A** Physiological Systems

3RD – **6 PHOTOTHERAPY**

EXAMPLE: Phototherapy of circulatory system

PHOTOTHERAPY: Extracorporeal treatment by light rays.

EXPLANATION: Uses light rays for treatment ...

Body System – 4TH	Duration – 5TH	Qualifier – 6TH	Qualifier – 7TH
0 Skin	0 Single	Z No qualifier	Z No qualifier
5 Circulatory	1 Multiple		

EXTRACORPOREAL THERAPIES SECTION: Atmospheric Control, Decompression, Electromagnetic Therapy, Hyperthermia, Hypothermia, Pheresis, Phototherapy, Ultrasound Therapy, Ultraviolet Light Therapy, Shock Wave Therapy, Perfusion
Root Operations that describe other extracorporeal procedures that are not defined by Assistance and Performance in Section 5.

1ST – **6** Extracorporeal Therapies

2ND – **A** Physiological Systems

3RD – **7 ULTRASOUND THERAPY**

EXAMPLE: Therapeutic ultrasound of vessels

ULTRASOUND THERAPY: Extracorporeal treatment by ultrasound.

EXPLANATION: Therapeutic use of ultrasound waves

Body System – 4TH	Duration – 5TH	Qualifier – 6TH	Qualifier – 7TH
5 Circulatory	0 Single	Z No qualifier	4 Head and Neck Vessels
	1 Multiple		5 Heart
			6 Peripheral Vessels
			7 Other Vessels
			Z No qualifier

EXTRACORPOREAL THERAPIES SECTION: Atmospheric Control, Decompression, Electromagnetic Therapy, Hyperthermia, Hypothermia, Pheresis, Phototherapy, Ultrasound Therapy, Ultraviolet Light Therapy, Shock Wave Therapy, Perfusion
Root Operations that describe other extracorporeal procedures that are not defined by Assistance and Performance in Section 5.

1ST – **6** Extracorporeal Therapies

2ND – **A** Physiological Systems

3RD – **8** ULTRAVIOLET LIGHT THERAPY

EXAMPLE: Ultraviolet light therapy of newborns

ULTRAVIOLET LIGHT THERAPY: Extracorporeal treatment by ultraviolet light.

EXPLANATION: Uses ultraviolet light for treatment

Body System – 4TH	Duration – 5TH	Qualifier – 6TH	Qualifier – 7TH
0 Skin	0 Single	Z No qualifier	Z No qualifier
	1 Multiple		

EXTRA THERAPIES 6 A 8

EXTRACORPOREAL THERAPIES SECTION: Atmospheric Control, Decompression, Electromagnetic Therapy, Hyperthermia, Hypothermia, Pheresis, Phototherapy, Ultrasound Therapy, Ultraviolet Light Therapy, Shock Wave Therapy, Perfusion
Root Operations that describe other extracorporeal procedures that are not defined by Assistance and Performance in Section 5.

1ST – **6** Extracorporeal Therapies

2ND – **A** Physiological Systems

3RD – **9 SHOCK WAVE THERAPY**

EXAMPLE: Shock wave treatment of fascia

SHOCK WAVE THERAPY: Extracorporeal treatment by shock waves.

EXPLANATION: Uses pulses of sound waves for treatment

Body System – 4TH	Duration – 5TH	Qualifier – 6TH	Qualifier – 7TH
3 Musculoskeletal	0 Single 1 Multiple	Z No qualifier	Z No qualifier

---

EXTRACORPOREAL THERAPIES SECTION: Atmospheric Control, Decompression, Electromagnetic Therapy, Hyperthermia, Hypothermia, Pheresis, Phototherapy, Ultrasound Therapy, Ultraviolet Light Therapy, Shock Wave Therapy, Perfusion
Root Operations that describe other extracorporeal procedures that are not defined by Assistance and Performance in Section 5.

1ST – **6** Extracorporeal Therapies

2ND – **A** Physiological Systems

3RD – **B PERFUSION**

EXAMPLE: Perfusion of donor organ

PERFUSION: Extracorporeal treatment by diffusion of therapeutic fluid.

EXPLANATION: Perfusion of donor organ

Body System – 4TH	Duration – 5TH	Qualifier – 6TH	Qualifier – 7TH
5 Circulatory B Respiratory System F Hepatobiliary System and Pancreas T Urinary System	0 Single	B Donor organ	Z No qualifier

Educational Annotations | Section 7 – Osteopathic

Section Specific Educational Annotations for the Osteopathic Section include:

- AHA Coding Clinic® Reference Notations
- Coding Notes

AHA Coding Clinic® Reference Notations of Osteopathic

ROOT OPERATION SPECIFIC - OSTEOPATHIC - Section 7
TREATMENT - 0

Coding Notes of Osteopathic

Med/Surg Related Section Specific PCS Reference Manual Exercises

PCS CODE	7 – OSTEOPATHIC EXERCISES
7 W 0 0 X 5 Z	Low velocity-high amplitude osteopathic treatment of head.
7 W 0 1 X 0 Z	Articulatory osteopathic treatment of cervical region.
7 W 0 4 X 4 Z	Indirect osteopathic treatment of sacrum.
7 W 0 6 X 8 Z	Isotonic muscle energy treatment of right leg.
7 W 0 7 X 6 Z	Lymphatic pump osteopathic treatment of left axilla.

OSTEOPATHIC

7

Educational Annotations | Section 7 – Osteopathic

<u>**NOTES**</u>

OSTEOPATHIC SECTION: Treatment	
Root Operation that defines osteopathic treatment.	

1ST - 7 Osteopathic

2ND - W Anatomical Regions

3RD - 0 TREATMENT

EXAMPLE: Articulopathy osteopathic treatment

TREATMENT: Manual treatment to eliminate or alleviate somatic dysfunction and related disorders.

EXPLANATION: Uses only osteopathic methods and treatments

Body Region – 4TH	Approach – 5TH	Method – 6TH	Qualifier – 7TH
0 Head	X External	0 Articulatory-raising	Z None
1 Cervical		1 Fascial release	
2 Thoracic		2 General mobilization	
3 Lumbar		3 High velocity-low amplitude	
4 Sacrum		4 Indirect	
5 Pelvis		5 Low velocity-high amplitude	
6 Lower Extremities		6 Lymphatic pump	
7 Upper Extremities		7 Muscle energy-isometric	
8 Rib Cage		8 Muscle energy-isotonic	
9 Abdomen		9 Other method	

OSTEOPATHIC 7 W 0

NOTES

Educational Annotations | Section 8 – Other Procedures

Section Specific Educational Annotations for the Other Procedures Section include:
- AHA Coding Clinic® Reference Notations
- Coding Notes

AHA Coding Clinic® Reference Notations of Other Procedures

ROOT OPERATION SPECIFIC - OTHER PROCEDURES - Section 8
COLLECTION - 6
NEAR INFRARED SPECTROSCOPY - D
COMPUTER ASSISTED PROCEDURE - B
ROBOTIC ASSISTED PROCEDURE - C
    Radical prostatectomy, robotic-assisted, with bilateral resection of
        vas deferens and seminal vesicles ....AHA 14:4Q:p33
    Robotic assisted procedure ....AHA 15:1Q:p33
ACUPUNCTURE - 0
THERAPEUTIC MASSAGE - 1
OTHER METHOD - Y

Coding Notes of Other Procedures

Med/Surg Related Section Specific PCS Reference Manual Exercises

PCS CODE	8 – OTHER PROCEDURES EXERCISES
8E023DZ	Near infrared spectroscopy of leg vessels.
8E09XBG	CT computer assisted sinus surgery. (The primary procedure is coded separately.)
8E0W0CZ	Robotic assisted open prostatectomy. (The primary procedure is coded separately.)
8E0WXY8	Suture removal, abdominal wall.
8E0ZXY6	Isolation after infectious disease exposure.

OTHER PROCEDURES 8

Educational Annotations | Section 8 – Other Procedures

NOTES

OTHER PROCEDURES SECTION: Other Procedures
Root Operation that defines procedures not included in the Medical and Medical/Surgical related sections.

1ST - **8** Other Procedures

2ND - **C** Indwelling Device

3RD - **0** OTHER PROCEDURES

EXAMPLE: None

OTHER PROCEDURES: Methodologies which attempt to remediate or cure a disorder or disease.

EXPLANATION: Procedures not included elsewhere

Body Region – 4TH	Approach – 5TH	Method – 6TH	Qualifier – 7TH
1 Nervous System	X External	6 Collection	J Cerebrospinal fluid L Other fluid
2 Circulatory System	X External	6 Collection	K Blood L Other fluid

OTHER PROCEDURES SECTION: Other Procedures
Root Operation that defines procedures not included in the Medical and Medical/Surgical related sections.

1ST - **8** Other Procedures

2ND - **E** Physiological Systems and Anatomical Regions

3RD - **0** OTHER PROCEDURES

EXAMPLE: Suture removal

OTHER PROCEDURES: Methodologies which attempt to remediate or cure a disorder or disease.

EXPLANATION: Procedures not included elsewhere

Body Region – 4TH	Approach – 5TH	Method – 6TH	Qualifier – 7TH
1 Nervous System U Female Reproductive System ♀	X External	Y Other method	7 Examination
2 Circulatory System	3 Percutaneous	D Near infrared spectroscopy	Z No qualifier
9 Head and Neck Region W Trunk Region	0 Open 3 Percutaneous 4 Percutaneous endoscopic 7 Via natural or artificial opening 8 Via natural or artificial opening endoscopic	C Robotic assisted procedure	Z No qualifier
9 Head and Neck Region W Trunk Region	X External	B Computer assisted procedure	F With fluoroscopy G With computerized tomography H With magnetic resonance imaging Z No qualifier
9 Head and Neck Region W Trunk Region	X External	C Robotic assisted procedure	Z No qualifier
9 Head and Neck Region W Trunk Region	X External	Y Other method	8 Suture removal

OTHER PROCEDURES 8 E 0

continued ⇨

| 8 | E | 0 | OTHER PROCEDURES —*continued* |

Body Region – 4TH	Approach – 5TH	Method – 6TH	Qualifier – 7TH
H Integumentary System and Breast	3 Percutaneous	0 Acupuncture	0 Anesthesia Z No qualifier
H Integumentary System and Breast ♀	X External	6 Collection	2 Breast milk
H Integumentary System and Breast	X External	Y Other method	9 Piercing
K Musculoskeletal System	X External	1 Therapeutic massage	Z No qualifier
K Musculoskeletal System	X External	Y Other method	7 Examination
V Male Reproductive System	X External	1 Therapeutic massage	C Prostate ♂ D Rectum
V Male Reproductive System ♂	X External	6 Collection	3 Sperm
X Upper Extremity Y Lower Extremity	0 Open 3 Percutaneous 4 Percutaneous endoscopic	C Robotic assisted procedure	Z No qualifier
X Upper Extremity Y Lower Extremity	X External	B Computer assisted procedure	F With fluoroscopy G With computerized tomography H With magnetic resonance imaging Z No qualifier
X Upper Extremity Y Lower Extremity	X External	C Robotic assisted procedure	Z No qualifier
X Upper Extremity Y Lower Extremity	X External	Y Other method	8 Suture removal
Z None	X External	Y Other method	1 In vitro fertilization 4 Yoga therapy 5 Meditation 6 Isolation

Educational Annotations | Section 9 – Chiropractic

Section Specific Educational Annotations for the Chiropractic Section include:
- AHA Coding Clinic® Reference Notations
- Coding Notes

AHA Coding Clinic® Reference Notations of Chiropractic

ROOT OPERATION SPECIFIC - CHIROPRACTIC - Section 9
MANIPULATION - B

Coding Notes of Chiropractic

Med/Surg Related Section Specific PCS Reference Manual Exercises

PCS CODE	9 – CHIROPRACTIC EXERCISES
9 W B 0 X K Z	Mechanically-assisted chiropractic manipulation of head.
9 W B 3 X G Z	Chiropractic treatment of lumbar region using long lever specific contact.
9 W B 4 X J Z	Chiropractic treatment of sacrum using long and short lever specific contact.
9 W B 6 X D Z	Chiropractic extra-articular treatment of hip region.
9 W B 9 X C Z	Chiropractic manipulation of abdominal region, indirect visceral.

CHIROPRACTIC 9

Educational Annotations | Section 9 – Chiropractic

<u>NOTES</u>

CHIROPRACTIC SECTION: Manipulation
Root Operation that defines chiropractic procedures.

1ST - **9** Chiropractic

2ND - **W** Anatomical Regions

3RD - **B MANIPULATION**

EXAMPLE: Chiropractic manipulation of spine

MANIPULATION: Manual procedure that involves a directed thrust to move a joint past the physiological range of motion, without exceeding the anatomical limit.

EXPLANATION: None

Body Region – 4TH	Approach – 5TH	Method – 6TH	Qualifier – 7TH
0 Head	X External	B Non-manual	Z None
1 Cervical		C Indirect visceral	
2 Thoracic		D Extra-articular	
3 Lumbar		F Direct visceral	
4 Sacrum		G Long lever specific contact	
5 Pelvis		H Short lever specific contact	
6 Lower Extremities		J Long and short lever specific contact	
7 Upper Extremities		K Mechanically assisted	
8 Rib Cage		L Other method	
9 Abdomen			

C
H
I
R
O
P
R
A
C
T
I
C

9

W

B

NOTES

Educational Annotations | Section B – Imaging

Section Specific Educational Annotations for the Imaging Section include:
- AHA Coding Clinic® Reference Notations
- Coding Notes

AHA Coding Clinic® Reference Notations of Imaging

<u>ROOT TYPE SPECIFIC - IMAGING - Section B</u>
PLAIN RADIOGRAPHY - 0
FLUOROSCOPY - 1
　　Fluoroscopic guidance of central venous catheter ....AHA 15:4Q:p30
COMPUTERIZED TOMOGRAPHY (CT SCAN) - 2
MAGNETIC RESONANCE IMAGING (MRI) - 3
ULTRASONOGRAPHY - 4
　　Ultrasonic guidance during ERCP ....AHA 14:3Q:p15

Coding Notes of Imaging

<u>Ancillary Section Specific PCS Reference Manual Exercises</u>

PCS CODE	B – IMAGING EXERCISES
B 2 1 5 1 Z Z	Left ventriculography using low osmolar contrast.
B 3 4 2 Z Z 3	Intravascular ultrasound, left subclavian artery.
B 4 1 G 1 Z Z	Fluoroscopic guidance for percutaneous transluminal angioplasty (PTA) of left common femoral artery, low osmolar contrast.
B 5 1 8 1 Z A	Fluoroscopic guidance for insertion of central venous catheter in SVC, low osmolar contrast.
B B 2 4 0 Z Z	CT scan of bilateral lungs, high osmolar contrast with densitometry.
B D 1 1 Y Z Z	Esophageal videofluoroscopy study with oral barium contrast.
B F 4 3 Z Z Z	Endoluminal ultrasound of gallbladder and bile ducts.
B P 0 J Z Z Z	Portable X-ray study of right radius/ulna shaft, standard series.
B W 2 1 Z Z Z	Non-contrast CT of abdomen and pelvis.
B Y 4 D Z Z Z	Routine fetal ultrasound, second trimester twin gestation.

IMAGING

B

Educational Annotations | Section B – Imaging

NOTES

1ST – B Imaging	EXAMPLE: Chest X-ray
2ND – 0 Central Nervous System	**PLAIN RADIOGRAPHY:** Planar display of an image developed from the capture of external ionizing radiation on photographic or photoconductive plate.
3RD – 0 **PLAIN RADIOGRAPHY**	

Body Part – 4TH	Contrast – 5TH	Qualifier – 6TH	Qualifier – 7TH
B Spinal Cord	0 High osmolar 1 Low osmolar Y Other contrast Z None	Z None	Z None

1ST – B Imaging	EXAMPLE: Fluoroscopic guidance
2ND – 0 Central Nervous System	**FLUOROSCOPY:** Single plane or bi-plane real time display of an image developed from the capture of external ionizing radiation on a fluorescent screen. The image may also be stored by either digital or analog means.
3RD – 1 **FLUOROSCOPY**	

Body Part – 4TH	Contrast – 5TH	Qualifier – 6TH	Qualifier – 7TH
B Spinal Cord	0 High osmolar 1 Low osmolar Y Other contrast Z None	Z None	Z None

1ST – B Imaging	EXAMPLE: CT Scan of head
2ND – 0 Central Nervous System	**COMPUTERIZED TOMOGRAPHY (CT Scan):** Computer reformatted digital display of multiplanar images developed from the capture of multiple exposures of external ionizing radiation.
3RD – 2 **COMPUTERIZED TOMOGRAPHY** (CT Scan)	

Body Part – 4TH	Contrast – 5TH	Qualifier – 6TH	Qualifier – 7TH
0 Brain 7 Cisterna 8 Cerebral Ventricle(s) 9 Sella Turcica/Pituitary Gland B Spinal Cord	0 High osmolar 1 Low osmolar Y Other contrast	0 Unenhanced and enhanced Z None	Z None
0 Brain 7 Cisterna 8 Cerebral Ventricle(s) 9 Sella Turcica/Pituitary Gland B Spinal Cord	Z None	Z None	Z None

IMAGING

B02

MAGNETIC RESONANCE IMAGING (MRI)

1ST – B Imaging
2ND – 0 Central Nervous System
3RD – 3 MAGNETIC RESONANCE IMAGING (MRI)

EXAMPLE: MRI of knee

MAGNETIC RESONANCE IMAGING (MRI): Computer reformatted digital display of multiplanar images developed from the capture of radiofrequency signals emitted by nuclei in a body site excited within a magnetic field.

Body Part – 4TH	Contrast – 5TH	Qualifier – 6TH	Qualifier – 7TH
0 Brain 9 Sella Turcica/Pituitary Gland B Spinal Cord C Acoustic Nerves	Y Other contrast	0 Unenhanced and enhanced Z None	Z None
0 Brain 9 Sella Turcica/Pituitary Gland B Spinal Cord C Acoustic Nerves	Z None	Z None	Z None

ULTRASONOGRAPHY

1ST – B Imaging
2ND – 0 Central Nervous System
3RD – 4 ULTRASONOGRAPHY

EXAMPLE: Abdominal ultrasound

ULTRASONOGRAPHY: Real time display of images of anatomy or flow information developed from the capture of reflected and attenuated high frequency sound waves.

Body Part – 4TH	Contrast – 5TH	Qualifier – 6TH	Qualifier – 7TH
0 Brain B Spinal Cord	Z None	Z None	Z None

PLAIN RADIOGRAPHY

1ST – B Imaging
2ND – 2 Heart
3RD – 0 PLAIN RADIOGRAPHY

EXAMPLE: Chest X-ray

PLAIN RADIOGRAPHY: Planar display of an image developed from the capture of external ionizing radiation on photographic or photoconductive plate.

Body Part – 4TH	Contrast – 5TH	Qualifier – 6TH	Qualifier – 7TH
0 Coronary Artery, Single 1 Coronary Arteries, Multiple 2 Coronary Artery Bypass Graft, Single 3 Coronary Artery Bypass Grafts, Multiple 4 Heart, Right 5 Heart, Left 6 Heart, Right and Left 7 Internal Mammary Bypass Graft, Right 8 Internal Mammary Bypass Graft, Left F Bypass Graft, Other	0 High osmolar 1 Low osmolar Y Other contrast	Z None	Z None

1ST - B Imaging	EXAMPLE: Fluoroscopic guidance
2ND - 2 Heart	**FLUOROSCOPY:** Single plane or bi-plane real time display of an image developed from the capture of external ionizing radiation on a fluorescent screen. The image may also be stored by either digital or analog means.
3RD - 1 FLUOROSCOPY	

Body Part – 4TH	Contrast – 5TH	Qualifier – 6TH	Qualifier – 7TH
0 Coronary Artery, Single 1 Coronary Arteries, Multiple 2 Coronary Artery Bypass Graft, Single 3 Coronary Artery Bypass Grafts, Multiple	0 High osmolar 1 Low osmolar Y Other contrast	1 Laser	0 Intraoperative
0 Coronary Artery, Single 1 Coronary Arteries, Multiple 2 Coronary Artery Bypass Graft, Single 3 Coronary Artery Bypass Grafts, Multiple	0 High osmolar 1 Low osmolar Y Other contrast	Z None	Z None
4 Heart, Right 5 Heart, Left 6 Heart, Right and Left 7 Internal Mammary Bypass Graft, Right 8 Internal Mammary Bypass Graft, Left F Bypass Graft, Other	0 High osmolar 1 Low osmolar Y Other contrast	Z None	Z None

1ST - B Imaging	EXAMPLE: CT Scan of head
2ND - 2 Heart	**COMPUTERIZED TOMOGRAPHY (CT Scan):** Computer reformatted digital display of multiplanar images developed from the capture of multiple exposures of external ionizing radiation.
3RD - 2 COMPUTERIZED TOMOGRAPHY (CT Scan)	

Body Part – 4TH	Contrast – 5TH	Qualifier – 6TH	Qualifier – 7TH
1 Coronary Arteries, Multiple 3 Coronary Artery Bypass Grafts, Multiple 6 Heart, Right and Left	0 High osmolar 1 Low osmolar Y Other contrast	0 Unenhanced and enhanced Z None	Z None
1 Coronary Arteries, Multiple 3 Coronary Artery Bypass Grafts, Multiple 6 Heart, Right and Left	Z None	2 Intravascular optical coherence Z None	Z None

1ST - B Imaging	EXAMPLE: MRI of knee
2ND - 2 Heart	**MAGNETIC RESONANCE IMAGING (MRI):** Computer reformatted digital display of multiplanar images developed from the capture of radiofrequency signals emitted by nuclei in a body site excited within a magnetic field.
3RD - 3 MAGNETIC RESONANCE IMAGING (MRI)	

Body Part – 4TH	Contrast – 5TH	Qualifier – 6TH	Qualifier – 7TH
1 Coronary Arteries, Multiple 3 Coronary Artery Bypass Grafts, Multiple 6 Heart, Right and Left	Y Other contrast	0 Unenhanced and enhanced Z None	Z None
1 Coronary Arteries, Multiple 3 Coronary Artery Bypass Grafts, Multiple 6 Heart, Right and Left	Z None	Z None	Z None

IMAGING

B 2 3

1ST - B Imaging	EXAMPLE: Abdominal ultrasound
2ND - 2 Heart	ULTRASONOGRAPHY: Real time display of images of anatomy or flow information developed from the capture of reflected and attenuated high frequency sound waves.
3RD - 4 ULTRASONOGRAPHY	

Body Part – 4TH	Contrast – 5TH	Qualifier – 6TH	Qualifier – 7TH
0　Coronary Artery, Single 1　Coronary Arteries, Multiple 4　Heart, Right 5　Heart, Left 6　Heart, Right and Left B　Heart with Aorta C　Pericardium D　Pediatric Heart	Y　Other contrast	Z　None	Z　None
0　Coronary Artery, Single 1　Coronary Arteries, Multiple 4　Heart, Right 5　Heart, Left 6　Heart, Right and Left B　Heart with Aorta C　Pericardium D　Pediatric Heart	Z　None	Z　None	3　Intravascular 4　Trans esophageal Z　None

1ST - B Imaging	EXAMPLE: Chest X-ray
2ND - 3 Upper Arteries	PLAIN RADIOGRAPHY: Planar display of an image developed from the capture of external ionizing radiation on photographic or photoconductive plate.
3RD - 0 PLAIN RADIOGRAPHY	

Body Part – 4TH	Contrast – 5TH	Qualifier – 6TH	Qualifier – 7TH
0　Thoracic Aorta 1　Brachiocephalic-Subclavian Artery, Right 2　Subclavian Artery, Left 3　Common Carotid Artery, Right 4　Common Carotid Artery, Left 5　Common Carotid Arteries, Bilateral 6　Internal Carotid Artery, Right 7　Internal Carotid Artery, Left 8　Internal Carotid Arteries, Bilateral 9　External Carotid Artery, Right B　External Carotid Artery, Left C　External Carotid Arteries, Bilateral D　Vertebral Artery, Right F　Vertebral Artery, Left G　Vertebral Arteries, Bilateral H　Upper Extremity Arteries, Right J　Upper Extremity Arteries, Left K　Upper Extremity Arteries, Bilateral L　Intercostal and Bronchial Arteries M　Spinal Arteries N　Upper Arteries, Other P　Thoraco-Abdominal Aorta Q　Cervico-Cerebral Arch R　Intracranial Arteries S　Pulmonary Artery, Right T　Pulmonary Artery, Left	0　High osmolar 1　Low osmolar Y　Other contrast Z　None	Z　None	Z　None

I M A G I N G

B 2 4

1ST - B Imaging	EXAMPLE: Fluoroscopic guidance
2ND - 3 Upper Arteries	**FLUOROSCOPY:** Single plane or bi-plane real time display of an image developed from the capture of external ionizing radiation on a fluorescent screen. The image may also be stored by either digital or analog means.
3RD - 1 FLUOROSCOPY	

Body Part – 4TH		Contrast – 5TH	Qualifier – 6TH	Qualifier – 7TH
0 Thoracic Aorta		0 High osmolar	1 Laser	0 Intraoperative
1 Brachiocephalic-Subclavian Artery, Right		1 Low osmolar		
2 Subclavian Artery, Left		Y Other contrast		
3 Common Carotid Artery, Right				
4 Common Carotid Artery, Left				
5 Common Carotid Arteries, Bilateral				
6 Internal Carotid Artery, Right				
7 Internal Carotid Artery, Left				
8 Internal Carotid Arteries, Bilateral				
9 External Carotid Artery, Right				
B External Carotid Artery, Left				
C External Carotid Arteries, Bilateral				
D Vertebral Artery, Right				
F Vertebral Artery, Left				
G Vertebral Arteries, Bilateral				
H Upper Extremity Arteries, Right				
J Upper Extremity Arteries, Left				
K Upper Extremity Arteries, Bilateral				
L Intercostal and Bronchial Arteries				
M Spinal Arteries				
N Upper Arteries, Other	R Intracranial Arteries			
P Thoraco-Abdominal Aorta	S Pulmonary Artery, Right			
Q Cervico-Cerebral Arch	T Pulmonary Artery, Left			
0 Thoracic Aorta		0 High osmolar	Z None	Z None
1 Brachiocephalic-Subclavian Artery, Right		1 Low osmolar		
2 Subclavian Artery, Left		Y Other contrast		
3 Common Carotid Artery, Right				
4 Common Carotid Artery, Left				
5 Common Carotid Arteries, Bilateral				
6 Internal Carotid Artery, Right				
7 Internal Carotid Artery, Left				
8 Internal Carotid Arteries, Bilateral				
9 External Carotid Artery, Right				
B External Carotid Artery, Left				
C External Carotid Arteries, Bilateral				
D Vertebral Artery, Right				
F Vertebral Artery, Left				
G Vertebral Arteries, Bilateral				
H Upper Extremity Arteries, Right				
J Upper Extremity Arteries, Left				
K Upper Extremity Arteries, Bilateral				
L Intercostal and Bronchial Arteries				
M Spinal Arteries				
N Upper Arteries, Other	R Intracranial Arteries			
P Thoraco-Abdominal Aorta	S Pulmonary Artery, Right			
Q Cervico-Cerebral Arch	T Pulmonary Artery, Left			

IMAGING

B 3 1

continued ⇨

B 3 1 — FLUOROSCOPY — continued

Body Part – 4TH	Contrast – 5TH	Qualifier – 6TH	Qualifier – 7TH
0 Thoracic Aorta 1 Brachiocephalic-Subclavian Artery, Right 2 Subclavian Artery, Left 3 Common Carotid Artery, Right 4 Common Carotid Artery, Left 5 Common Carotid Arteries, Bilateral 6 Internal Carotid Artery, Right 7 Internal Carotid Artery, Left 8 Internal Carotid Arteries, Bilateral 9 External Carotid Artery, Right B External Carotid Artery, Left C External Carotid Arteries, Bilateral D Vertebral Artery, Right F Vertebral Artery, Left G Vertebral Arteries, Bilateral H Upper Extremity Arteries, Right J Upper Extremity Arteries, Left K Upper Extremity Arteries, Bilateral L Intercostal and Bronchial Arteries M Spinal Arteries N Upper Arteries, Other R Intracranial Arteries P Thoraco-Abdominal Aorta S Pulmonary Artery, Right Q Cervico-Cerebral Arch T Pulmonary Artery, Left	Z None	Z None	Z None

1ST – B Imaging
2ND – 3 Upper Arteries
3RD – 2 COMPUTERIZED TOMOGRAPHY (CT Scan)

EXAMPLE: CT Scan of head

COMPUTERIZED TOMOGRAPHY (CT Scan): Computer reformatted digital display of multiplanar images developed from the capture of multiple exposures of external ionizing radiation.

Body Part – 4TH	Contrast – 5TH	Qualifier – 6TH	Qualifier – 7TH
0 Thoracic Aorta 5 Common Carotid Arteries, Bilateral 8 Internal Carotid Arteries, Bilateral G Vertebral Arteries, Bilateral R Intracranial Arteries S Pulmonary Artery, Right T Pulmonary Artery, Left	0 High osmolar 1 Low osmolar Y Other contrast	Z None	Z None
0 Thoracic Aorta 5 Common Carotid Arteries, Bilateral 8 Internal Carotid Arteries, Bilateral G Vertebral Arteries, Bilateral R Intracranial Arteries S Pulmonary Artery, Right T Pulmonary Artery, Left	Z None	2 Intravascular optical coherence Z None	Z None

IMAGING

B 3 1

1ST - **B** Imaging 2ND - **3** Upper Arteries 3RD - **3** MAGNETIC RESONANCE IMAGING (MRI)		EXAMPLE: MRI of knee
		MAGNETIC RESONANCE IMAGING (MRI): Computer reformatted digital display of multiplanar images developed from the capture of radiofrequency signals emitted by nuclei in a body site excited within a magnetic field.

Body Part – 4TH	Contrast – 5TH	Qualifier – 6TH	Qualifier – 7TH
0 Thoracic Aorta 5 Common Carotid Arteries, Bilateral 8 Internal Carotid Arteries, Bilateral G Vertebral Arteries, Bilateral H Upper Extremity Arteries, Right J Upper Extremity Arteries, Left K Upper Extremity Arteries, Bilateral M Spinal Arteries Q Cervico-Cerebral Arch R Intracranial Arteries	Y Other contrast	0 Unenhanced and enhanced Z None	Z None
0 Thoracic Aorta 5 Common Carotid Arteries, Bilateral 8 Internal Carotid Arteries, Bilateral G Vertebral Arteries, Bilateral H Upper Extremity Arteries, Right J Upper Extremity Arteries, Left K Upper Extremity Arteries, Bilateral M Spinal Arteries Q Cervico-Cerebral Arch R Intracranial Arteries	Z None	Z None	Z None

1ST - **B** Imaging 2ND - **3** Upper Arteries 3RD - **4** ULTRASONOGRAPHY		EXAMPLE: Abdominal ultrasound
		ULTRASONOGRAPHY: Real time display of images of anatomy or flow information developed from the capture of reflected and attenuated high frequency sound waves.

Body Part – 4TH	Contrast – 5TH	Qualifier – 6TH	Qualifier – 7TH
0 Thoracic Aorta 1 Brachiocephalic-Subclavian Artery, Right 2 Subclavian Artery, Left 3 Common Carotid Artery, Right 4 Common Carotid Artery, Left 5 Common Carotid Arteries, Bilateral 6 Internal Carotid Artery, Right 7 Internal Carotid Artery, Left 8 Internal Carotid Arteries, Bilateral H Upper Extremity Arteries, Right J Upper Extremity Arteries, Left K Upper Extremity Arteries, Bilateral R Intracranial Arteries S Pulmonary Artery, Right T Pulmonary Artery, Left V Ophthalmic Arteries	Z None	Z None	3 Intravascular Z None

1ST - **B** Imaging

2ND - **4** Lower Arteries

3RD - **0** PLAIN RADIOGRAPHY

EXAMPLE: Chest X-ray

PLAIN RADIOGRAPHY: Planar display of an image developed from the capture of external ionizing radiation on photographic or photoconductive plate.

Body Part – 4TH	Contrast – 5TH	Qualifier – 6TH	Qualifier – 7TH
0 Abdominal Aorta	0 High osmolar	Z None	Z None
2 Hepatic Artery	1 Low osmolar		
3 Splenic Arteries	Y Other contrast		
4 Superior Mesenteric Artery			
5 Inferior Mesenteric Artery			
6 Renal Artery, Right			
7 Renal Artery, Left			
8 Renal Arteries, Bilateral			
9 Lumbar Arteries			
B Intra-Abdominal Arteries, Other			
C Pelvic Arteries			
D Aorta and Bilateral Lower Extremity Arteries			
F Lower Extremity Arteries, Right			
G Lower Extremity Arteries, Left			
J Lower Arteries, Other			
M Renal Artery Transplant			

1ST - **B** Imaging 2ND - **4** Lower Arteries 3RD - **1 FLUOROSCOPY**	EXAMPLE: Fluoroscopic guidance **FLUOROSCOPY:** Single plane or bi-plane real time display of an image developed from the capture of external ionizing radiation on a fluorescent screen. The image may also be stored by either digital or analog means.

Body Part – 4TH	Contrast – 5TH	Qualifier – 6TH	Qualifier – 7TH
0 Abdominal Aorta 2 Hepatic Artery 3 Splenic Arteries 4 Superior Mesenteric Artery 5 Inferior Mesenteric Artery 6 Renal Artery, Right 7 Renal Artery, Left 8 Renal Arteries, Bilateral 9 Lumbar Arteries B Intra-Abdominal Arteries, Other C Pelvic Arteries D Aorta and Bilateral Lower Extremity Arteries F Lower Extremity Arteries, Right G Lower Extremity Arteries, Left J Lower Arteries, Other	0 High osmolar 1 Low osmolar Y Other contrast	1 Laser	0 Intraoperative
0 Abdominal Aorta 2 Hepatic Artery 3 Splenic Arteries 4 Superior Mesenteric Artery 5 Inferior Mesenteric Artery 6 Renal Artery, Right 7 Renal Artery, Left 8 Renal Arteries, Bilateral 9 Lumbar Arteries B Intra-Abdominal Arteries, Other C Pelvic Arteries D Aorta and Bilateral Lower Extremity Arteries F Lower Extremity Arteries, Right G Lower Extremity Arteries, Left J Lower Arteries, Other	0 High osmolar 1 Low osmolar Y Other contrast	Z None	Z None
0 Abdominal Aorta 2 Hepatic Artery 3 Splenic Arteries 4 Superior Mesenteric Artery 5 Inferior Mesenteric Artery 6 Renal Artery, Right 7 Renal Artery, Left 8 Renal Arteries, Bilateral 9 Lumbar Arteries B Intra-Abdominal Arteries, Other C Pelvic Arteries D Aorta and Bilateral Lower Extremity Arteries F Lower Extremity Arteries, Right G Lower Extremity Arteries, Left J Lower Arteries, Other	Z None	Z None	Z None

IMAGING

B 4 1

1ST – **B** Imaging 2ND – **4** Lower Arteries 3RD – **2 COMPUTERIZED TOMOGRAPHY** (CT Scan)	EXAMPLE: CT Scan of head **COMPUTERIZED TOMOGRAPHY (CT Scan):** Computer reformatted digital display of multiplanar images developed from the capture of multiple exposures of external ionizing radiation.		
Body Part – 4TH	**Contrast – 5TH**	**Qualifier – 6TH**	**Qualifier – 7TH**
0 Abdominal Aorta 1 Celiac Artery 4 Superior Mesenteric Artery 8 Renal Arteries, Bilateral C Pelvic Arteries F Lower Extremity Arteries, Right G Lower Extremity Arteries, Left H Lower Extremity Arteries, Bilateral M Renal Artery Transplant	0 High osmolar 1 Low osmolar Y Other contrast	Z None	Z None
0 Abdominal Aorta 1 Celiac Artery 4 Superior Mesenteric Artery 8 Renal Arteries, Bilateral C Pelvic Arteries F Lower Extremity Arteries, Right G Lower Extremity Arteries, Left H Lower Extremity Arteries, Bilateral M Renal Artery Transplant	Z None	2 Intravascular optical coherence Z None	Z None

1ST – **B** Imaging 2ND – **4** Lower Arteries 3RD – **3 MAGNETIC RESONANCE IMAGING (MRI)**	EXAMPLE: MRI of knee **MAGNETIC RESONANCE IMAGING (MRI):** Computer reformatted digital display of multiplanar images developed from the capture of radiofrequency signals emitted by nuclei in a body site excited within a magnetic field.		
Body Part – 4TH	**Contrast – 5TH**	**Qualifier – 6TH**	**Qualifier – 7TH**
0 Abdominal Aorta 1 Celiac Artery 4 Superior Mesenteric Artery 8 Renal Arteries, Bilateral C Pelvic Arteries F Lower Extremity Arteries, Right G Lower Extremity Arteries, Left H Lower Extremity Arteries, Bilateral	Y Other contrast	0 Unenhanced and enhanced Z None	Z None
0 Abdominal Aorta 1 Celiac Artery 4 Superior Mesenteric Artery 8 Renal Arteries, Bilateral C Pelvic Arteries F Lower Extremity Arteries, Right G Lower Extremity Arteries, Left H Lower Extremity Arteries, Bilateral	Z None	Z None	Z None

IMAGING

B 4 2

1ST - B Imaging	EXAMPLE: Abdominal ultrasound
2ND - 4 Lower Arteries	**ULTRASONOGRAPHY:** Real time display of images of anatomy or flow information developed from the capture of reflected and attenuated high frequency sound waves.
3RD - 4 ULTRASONOGRAPHY	

Body Part – 4TH	Contrast – 5TH	Qualifier – 6TH	Qualifier – 7TH
0 Abdominal Aorta 4 Superior Mesenteric Artery 5 Inferior Mesenteric Artery 6 Renal Artery, Right 7 Renal Artery, Left 8 Renal Arteries, Bilateral B Intra-Abdominal Arteries, Other F Lower Extremity Arteries, Right G Lower Extremity Arteries, Left H Lower Extremity Arteries, Bilateral K Celiac and Mesenteric Arteries L Femoral Artery N Penile Arteries	Z None	Z None	3 Intravascular Z None

1ST - B Imaging	EXAMPLE: Chest X-ray
2ND - 5 Veins	**PLAIN RADIOGRAPHY:** Planar display of an image developed from the capture of external ionizing radiation on photographic or photoconductive plate.
3RD - 0 PLAIN RADIOGRAPHY	

Body Part – 4TH		Contrast – 5TH	Qualifier – 6TH	Qualifier – 7TH
0 Epidural Veins 1 Cerebral and Cerebellar Veins 2 Intracranial Sinuses 3 Jugular Veins, Right 4 Jugular Veins, Left 5 Jugular Veins, Bilateral 6 Subclavian Vein, Right 7 Subclavian Vein, Left 8 Superior Vena Cava 9 Inferior Vena Cava B Lower Extremity Veins, Right C Lower Extremity Veins, Left D Lower Extremity Veins, Bilateral F Pelvic (Iliac) Veins, Right	G Pelvic (Iliac) Veins, Left H Pelvic (Iliac) Veins, Bilateral J Renal Vein, Right K Renal Vein, Left L Renal Veins, Bilateral M Upper Extremity Veins, Right N Upper Extremity Veins, Left P Upper Extremity Veins, Bilateral Q Pulmonary Vein, Right R Pulmonary Vein, Left S Pulmonary Veins, Bilateral T Portal and Splanchnic Veins V Veins, Other W Dialysis Shunt/Fistula	0 High osmolar 1 Low osmolar Y Other contrast	Z None	Z None

IMAGING

B 50

1ST - B Imaging	EXAMPLE: Fluoroscopic guidance
2ND - 5 Veins	**FLUOROSCOPY:** Single plane or bi-plane real time display of an image developed from the capture of external ionizing radiation on a fluorescent screen. The image may also be stored by either digital or analog means.
3RD - 1 FLUOROSCOPY	

Body Part – 4TH		Contrast – 5TH	Qualifier – 6TH	Qualifier – 7TH
0 Epidural Veins 1 Cerebral and Cerebellar Veins 2 Intracranial Sinuses 3 Jugular Veins, Right 4 Jugular Veins, Left 5 Jugular Veins, Bilateral 6 Subclavian Vein, Right 7 Subclavian Vein, Left 8 Superior Vena Cava 9 Inferior Vena Cava B Lower Extremity Veins, Right C Lower Extremity Veins, Left D Lower Extremity Veins, Bilateral F Pelvic (Iliac) Veins, Right	G Pelvic (Iliac) Veins, Left H Pelvic (Iliac) Veins, Bilateral J Renal Vein, Right K Renal Vein, Left L Renal Veins, Bilateral M Upper Extremity Veins, Right N Upper Extremity Veins, Left P Upper Extremity Veins, Bilateral Q Pulmonary Vein, Right R Pulmonary Vein, Left S Pulmonary Veins, Bilateral T Portal and Splanchnic Veins V Veins, Other W Dialysis Shunt/Fistula	0 High osmolar 1 Low osmolar Y Other contrast Z None	Z None	A Guidance Z None

1ST - B Imaging	EXAMPLE: CT Scan of head
2ND - 5 Veins	**COMPUTERIZED TOMOGRAPHY (CT Scan):** Computer reformatted digital display of multiplanar images developed from the capture of multiple exposures of external ionizing radiation.
3RD - 2 COMPUTERIZED TOMOGRAPHY (CT Scan)	

Body Part – 4TH		Contrast – 5TH	Qualifier – 6TH	Qualifier – 7TH
2 Intracranial Sinuses 8 Superior Vena Cava 9 Inferior Vena Cava F Pelvic (Iliac) Veins, Right G Pelvic (Iliac) Veins, Left H Pelvic (Iliac) Veins, Bilateral	J Renal Vein, Right K Renal Vein, Left L Renal Veins, Bilateral Q Pulmonary Vein, Right R Pulmonary Vein, Left S Pulmonary Veins, Bilateral T Portal and Splanchnic Veins	0 High osmolar 1 Low osmolar Y Other contrast	0 Unenhanced and enhanced Z None	Z None
2 Intracranial Sinuses 8 Superior Vena Cava 9 Inferior Vena Cava F Pelvic (Iliac) Veins, Right G Pelvic (Iliac) Veins, Left H Pelvic (Iliac) Veins, Bilateral	J Renal Vein, Right K Renal Vein, Left L Renal Veins, Bilateral Q Pulmonary Vein, Right R Pulmonary Vein, Left S Pulmonary Veins, Bilateral T Portal and Splanchnic Veins	Z None	2 Intravascular optical coherence Z None	Z None

1ST - **B** Imaging 2ND - **5** Veins 3RD - **3** MAGNETIC RESONANCE IMAGING (MRI)		EXAMPLE: MRI of knee **MAGNETIC RESONANCE IMAGING (MRI):** Computer reformatted digital display of multiplanar images developed from the capture of radiofrequency signals emitted by nuclei in a body site excited within a magnetic field.			
Body Part – 4TH		**Contrast – 5TH**	**Qualifier – 6TH**	**Qualifier – 7TH**	
1 Cerebral and Cerebellar Veins 2 Intracranial Sinuses 5 Jugular Veins, Bilateral 8 Superior Vena Cava 9 Inferior Vena Cava B Lower Extremity Veins, Right C Lower Extremity Veins, Left D Lower Extremity Veins, Bilateral	H Pelvic (Iliac) Veins, Bilateral L Renal Veins, Bilateral M Upper Extremity Veins, Right N Upper Extremity Veins, Left P Upper Extremity Veins, Bilateral S Pulmonary Veins, Bilateral T Portal and Splanchnic Veins V Veins, Other	Y Other contrast	0 Unenhanced and enhanced Z None	Z None	
1 Cerebral and Cerebellar Veins 2 Intracranial Sinuses 5 Jugular Veins, Bilateral 8 Superior Vena Cava 9 Inferior Vena Cava B Lower Extremity Veins, Right C Lower Extremity Veins, Left D Lower Extremity Veins, Bilateral	H Pelvic (Iliac) Veins, Bilateral L Renal Veins, Bilateral M Upper Extremity Veins, Right N Upper Extremity Veins, Left P Upper Extremity Veins, Bilateral S Pulmonary Veins, Bilateral T Portal and Splanchnic Veins V Veins, Other	Z None	Z None	Z None	

1ST - **B** Imaging 2ND - **5** Veins 3RD - **4** ULTRASONOGRAPHY		EXAMPLE: Abdominal ultrasound **ULTRASONOGRAPHY:** Real time display of images of anatomy or flow information developed from the capture of reflected and attenuated high frequency sound waves.			
Body Part – 4TH		**Contrast – 5TH**	**Qualifier – 6TH**	**Qualifier – 7TH**	
3 Jugular Veins, Right 4 Jugular Veins, Left 6 Subclavian Vein, Right 7 Subclavian Vein, Left 8 Superior Vena Cava 9 Inferior Vena Cava B Lower Extremity Veins, Right C Lower Extremity Veins, Left	D Lower Extremity Veins, Bilateral J Renal Vein, Right K Renal Vein, Left L Renal Veins, Bilateral M Upper Extremity Veins, Right N Upper Extremity Veins, Left P Upper Extremity Veins, Bilateral T Portal and Splanchnic Veins	Z None	Z None	3 Intravascular A Guidance Z None	

IMAGING

B 5 4

Table 1

1ST – B Imaging 2ND – 7 Lymphatic System 3RD – 0 PLAIN RADIOGRAPHY	EXAMPLE: Chest X-ray PLAIN RADIOGRAPHY: Planar display of an image developed from the capture of external ionizing radiation on photographic or photoconductive plate.		
Body Part – 4TH	**Contrast – 5TH**	**Qualifier – 6TH**	**Qualifier – 7TH**
0 Abdominal/Retroperitoneal Lymphatics, Unilateral 1 Abdominal/Retroperitoneal Lymphatics, Bilateral 4 Lymphatics, Head and Neck 5 Upper Extremity Lymphatics, Right 6 Upper Extremity Lymphatics, Left 7 Upper Extremity Lymphatics, Bilateral 8 Lower Extremity Lymphatics, Right 9 Lower Extremity Lymphatics, Left B Lower Extremity Lymphatics, Bilateral C Lymphatics, Pelvic	0 High osmolar 1 Low osmolar Y Other contrast	Z None	Z None

Table 2

1ST – B Imaging 2ND – 8 Eye 3RD – 0 PLAIN RADIOGRAPHY	EXAMPLE: Chest X-ray PLAIN RADIOGRAPHY: Planar display of an image developed from the capture of external ionizing radiation on photographic or photoconductive plate.		
Body Part – 4TH	**Contrast – 5TH**	**Qualifier – 6TH**	**Qualifier – 7TH**
0 Lacrimal Duct, Right 1 Lacrimal Duct, Left 2 Lacrimal Ducts, Bilateral	0 High osmolar 1 Low osmolar Y Other contrast	Z None	Z None
3 Optic Foramina, Right 4 Optic Foramina, Left 5 Eye, Right 6 Eye, Left 7 Eyes, Bilateral	Z None	Z None	Z None

Table 3

1ST – B Imaging 2ND – 8 Eye 3RD – 2 COMPUTERIZED TOMOGRAPHY (CT Scan)	EXAMPLE: CT Scan of head COMPUTERIZED TOMOGRAPHY (CT Scan): Computer reformatted digital display of multiplanar images developed from the capture of multiple exposures of external ionizing radiation.		
Body Part – 4TH	**Contrast – 5TH**	**Qualifier – 6TH**	**Qualifier – 7TH**
5 Eye, Right 6 Eye, Left 7 Eyes, Bilateral	0 High osmolar 1 Low osmolar Y Other contrast	0 Unenhanced and enhanced Z None	Z None
5 Eye, Right 6 Eye, Left 7 Eyes, Bilateral	Z None	Z None	Z None

1ST - B Imaging 2ND - 8 Eye 3RD - 3 MAGNETIC RESONANCE IMAGING (MRI)	EXAMPLE: MRI of knee **MAGNETIC RESONANCE IMAGING (MRI):** Computer reformatted digital display of multiplanar images developed from the capture of radiofrequency signals emitted by nuclei in a body site excited within a magnetic field.		
Body Part – 4TH	**Contrast – 5TH**	**Qualifier – 6TH**	**Qualifier – 7TH**
5　Eye, Right 6　Eye, Left 7　Eyes, Bilateral	Y　Other contrast	0　Unenhanced and enhanced Z　None	Z　None
5　Eye, Right 6　Eye, Left 7　Eyes, Bilateral	Z　None	Z　None	Z　None

1ST - B Imaging 2ND - 8 Eye 3RD - 4 ULTRASONOGRAPHY	EXAMPLE: Abdominal ultrasound **ULTRASONOGRAPHY:** Real time display of images of anatomy or flow information developed from the capture of reflected and attenuated high frequency sound waves.		
Body Part – 4TH	**Contrast – 5TH**	**Qualifier – 6TH**	**Qualifier – 7TH**
5　Eye, Right 6　Eye, Left 7　Eyes, Bilateral	Z　None	Z　None	Z　None

1ST - B Imaging 2ND - 9 Ear, Nose, Mouth and Throat 3RD - 0 PLAIN RADIOGRAPHY	EXAMPLE: Chest X-ray **PLAIN RADIOGRAPHY:** Planar display of an image developed from the capture of external ionizing radiation on photographic or photoconductive plate.		
Body Part – 4TH	**Contrast – 5TH**	**Qualifier – 6TH**	**Qualifier – 7TH**
2　Paranasal Sinuses F　Nasopharynx/Oropharynx H　Mastoids	Z　None	Z　None	Z　None
4　Parotid Gland, Right 5　Parotid Gland, Left 6　Parotid Glands, Bilateral 7　Submandibular Gland, Right 8　Submandibular Gland, Left 9　Submandibular Glands, Bilateral B　Salivary Gland, Right C　Salivary Gland, Left D　Salivary Glands, Bilateral	0　High osmolar 1　Low osmolar Y　Other contrast	Z　None	Z　None

IMAGING

B90

1ST - B Imaging 2ND - 9 Ear, Nose, Mouth and Throat 3RD - 1 FLUOROSCOPY	EXAMPLE: Fluoroscopic guidance **FLUOROSCOPY:** Single plane or bi-plane real time display of an image developed from the capture of external ionizing radiation on a fluorescent screen. The image may also be stored by either digital or analog means.		
Body Part – 4TH	**Contrast – 5TH**	**Qualifier – 6TH**	**Qualifier – 7TH**
G Pharynx and Epiglottis J Larynx	Y Other contrast Z None	Z None	Z None

1ST - B Imaging 2ND - 9 Ear, Nose, Mouth and Throat 3RD - 2 COMPUTERIZED TOMOGRAPHY (CT Scan)	EXAMPLE: CT Scan of head **COMPUTERIZED TOMOGRAPHY (CT Scan):** Computer reformatted digital display of multiplanar images developed from the capture of multiple exposures of external ionizing radiation.		
Body Part – 4TH	**Contrast – 5TH**	**Qualifier – 6TH**	**Qualifier – 7TH**
0 Ear D Salivary Glands, Bilateral 2 Paranasal Sinuses F Nasopharynx/ 6 Parotid Glands, Bilateral Oropharynx 9 Submandibular Glands, J Larynx Bilateral	0 High osmolar 1 Low osmolar Y Other contrast	0 Unenhanced and enhanced Z None	Z None
0 Ear D Salivary Glands, Bilateral 2 Paranasal Sinuses F Nasopharynx/ 6 Parotid Glands, Bilateral Oropharynx 9 Submandibular Glands, J Larynx Bilateral	Z None	Z None	Z None

1ST - B Imaging 2ND - 9 Ear, Nose, Mouth and Throat 3RD - 3 MAGNETIC RESONANCE IMAGING (MRI)	EXAMPLE: MRI of knee **MAGNETIC RESONANCE IMAGING (MRI):** Computer reformatted digital display of multiplanar images developed from the capture of radiofrequency signals emitted by nuclei in a body site excited within a magnetic field.		
Body Part – 4TH	**Contrast – 5TH**	**Qualifier – 6TH**	**Qualifier – 7TH**
0 Ear D Salivary Glands, Bilateral 2 Paranasal Sinuses F Nasopharynx/ 6 Parotid Glands, Bilateral Oropharynx 9 Submandibular Glands, J Larynx Bilateral	Y Other contrast	0 Unenhanced and enhanced Z None	Z None
0 Ear D Salivary Glands, Bilateral 2 Paranasal Sinuses F Nasopharynx/ 6 Parotid Glands, Bilateral Oropharynx 9 Submandibular Glands, J Larynx Bilateral	Z None	Z None	Z None

I
M
A
G
I
N
G

B
9
1

1ST - **B** Imaging	EXAMPLE: Chest X-ray
2ND - **B** Respiratory System	**PLAIN RADIOGRAPHY:** Planar display of an image developed from the capture of external ionizing radiation on photographic or photoconductive plate.
3RD - **0 PLAIN RADIOGRAPHY**	

Body Part – 4TH	Contrast – 5TH	Qualifier – 6TH	Qualifier – 7TH
7 Tracheobronchial Tree, Right 8 Tracheobronchial Tree, Left 9 Tracheobronchial Trees, Bilateral	Y Other contrast	Z None	Z None
D Upper Airways	Z None	Z None	Z None

1ST - **B** Imaging	EXAMPLE: Fluoroscopic guidance
2ND - **B** Respiratory System	**FLUOROSCOPY:** Single plane or bi-plane real time display of an image developed from the capture of external ionizing radiation on a fluorescent screen. The image may also be stored by either digital or analog means.
3RD - **1 FLUOROSCOPY**	

Body Part – 4TH	Contrast – 5TH	Qualifier – 6TH	Qualifier – 7TH
2 Lung, Right 3 Lung, Left 4 Lungs, Bilateral 6 Diaphragm C Mediastinum D Upper Airways	Z None	Z None	Z None
7 Tracheobronchial Tree, Right 8 Tracheobronchial Tree, Left 9 Tracheobronchial Trees, Bilateral	Y Other contrast	Z None	Z None

1ST - **B** Imaging	EXAMPLE: CT Scan of head
2ND - **B** Respiratory System	**COMPUTERIZED TOMOGRAPHY (CT Scan):** Computer reformatted digital display of multiplanar images developed from the capture of multiple exposures of external ionizing radiation.
3RD - **2 COMPUTERIZED TOMOGRAPHY** (CT Scan)	

Body Part – 4TH	Contrast – 5TH	Qualifier – 6TH	Qualifier – 7TH
4 Lungs, Bilateral 7 Tracheobronchial Tree, Right 8 Tracheobronchial Tree, Left 9 Tracheobronchial Trees, Bilateral F Trachea/Airways	0 High osmolar 1 Low osmolar Y Other contrast	0 Unenhanced and enhanced Z None	Z None
4 Lungs, Bilateral 7 Tracheobronchial Tree, Right 8 Tracheobronchial Tree, Left 9 Tracheobronchial Trees, Bilateral F Trachea/Airways	Z None	Z None	Z None

IMAGING

B B 2

MAGNETIC RESONANCE IMAGING (MRI)

1ST – B	Imaging
2ND – B	Respiratory System
3RD – 3	MAGNETIC RESONANCE IMAGING (MRI)

EXAMPLE: MRI of knee

MAGNETIC RESONANCE IMAGING (MRI): Computer reformatted digital display of multiplanar images developed from the capture of radiofrequency signals emitted by nuclei in a body site excited within a magnetic field.

Body Part – 4TH	Contrast – 5TH	Qualifier – 6TH	Qualifier – 7TH
G Lung Apices	Y Other contrast	0 Unenhanced and enhanced Z None	Z None
G Lung Apices	Z None	Z None	Z None

1ST – B	Imaging
2ND – B	Respiratory System
3RD – 4	ULTRASONOGRAPHY

EXAMPLE: Abdominal ultrasound

ULTRASONOGRAPHY: Real time display of images of anatomy or flow information developed from the capture of reflected and attenuated high frequency sound waves.

Body Part – 4TH	Contrast – 5TH	Qualifier – 6TH	Qualifier – 7TH
B Pleura C Mediastinum	Z None	Z None	Z None

1ST – B	Imaging
2ND – D	Gastrointestinal System
3RD – 1	FLUOROSCOPY

EXAMPLE: Fluoroscopic guidance

FLUOROSCOPY: Single plane or bi-plane real time display of an image developed from the capture of external ionizing radiation on a fluorescent screen. The image may also be stored by either digital or analog means.

Body Part – 4TH		Contrast – 5TH	Qualifier – 6TH	Qualifier – 7TH
1 Esophagus	5 Upper GI	Y Other contrast	Z None	Z None
2 Stomach	6 Upper GI and Small Bowel	Z None		
3 Small Bowel	9 Duodenum			
4 Colon	B Mouth/Oropharynx			

IMAGING BB3

1ST - **B** Imaging 2ND - **D** Gastrointestinal System 3RD - **2 COMPUTERIZED TOMOGRAPHY** (CT Scan)	EXAMPLE: CT Scan of head **COMPUTERIZED TOMOGRAPHY (CT Scan):** Computer reformatted digital display of multiplanar images developed from the capture of multiple exposures of external ionizing radiation.

Body Part – 4TH	Contrast – 5TH	Qualifier – 6TH	Qualifier – 7TH
4 Colon	0 High osmolar 1 Low osmolar Y Other contrast	0 Unenhanced and enhanced Z None	Z None
4 Colon	Z None	Z None	Z None

1ST - **B** Imaging 2ND - **D** Gastrointestinal System 3RD - **4 ULTRASONOGRAPHY**	EXAMPLE: Abdominal ultrasound **ULTRASONOGRAPHY:** Real time display of images of anatomy or flow information developed from the capture of reflected and attenuated high frequency sound waves.

Body Part – 4TH	Contrast – 5TH	Qualifier – 6TH	Qualifier – 7TH
1 Esophagus 8 Appendix 2 Stomach 9 Duodenum 7 Gastrointestinal Tract C Rectum	Z None	Z None	Z None

1ST - **B** Imaging 2ND - **F** Hepatobiliary System and Pancreas 3RD - **0 PLAIN RADIOGRAPHY**	EXAMPLE: Chest X-ray **PLAIN RADIOGRAPHY:** Planar display of an image developed from the capture of external ionizing radiation on photographic or photoconductive plate.

Body Part – 4TH	Contrast – 5TH	Qualifier – 6TH	Qualifier – 7TH
0 Bile Ducts 3 Gallbladder and Bile Ducts C Hepatobiliary System, All	0 High osmolar 1 Low osmolar Y Other contrast	Z None	Z None

IMAGING

B F 0

1ˢᵀ – B Imaging
2ᴺᴰ – F Hepatobiliary System and Pancreas
3ᴿᴰ – 1 FLUOROSCOPY

EXAMPLE: Fluoroscopic guidance

FLUOROSCOPY: Single plane or bi-plane real time display of an image developed from the capture of external ionizing radiation on a fluorescent screen. The image may also be stored by either digital or analog means.

Body Part – 4ᵀᴴ	Contrast – 5ᵀᴴ	Qualifier – 6ᵀᴴ	Qualifier – 7ᵀᴴ
0 Bile Ducts 1 Biliary and Pancreatic Ducts 2 Gallbladder 3 Gallbladder and Bile Ducts 4 Gallbladder, Bile Ducts and Pancreatic Ducts 8 Pancreatic Ducts	0 High osmolar 1 Low osmolar Y Other contrast	Z None	Z None

1ˢᵀ – B Imaging
2ᴺᴰ – F Hepatobiliary System and Pancreas
3ᴿᴰ – 2 COMPUTERIZED TOMOGRAPHY (CT Scan)

EXAMPLE: CT Scan of head

COMPUTERIZED TOMOGRAPHY (CT Scan): Computer reformatted digital display of multiplanar images developed from the capture of multiple exposures of external ionizing radiation.

Body Part – 4ᵀᴴ	Contrast – 5ᵀᴴ	Qualifier – 6ᵀᴴ	Qualifier – 7ᵀᴴ
5 Liver 6 Liver and Spleen 7 Pancreas C Hepatobiliary System, All	0 High osmolar 1 Low osmolar Y Other contrast	0 Unenhanced and enhanced Z None	Z None
5 Liver 6 Liver and Spleen 7 Pancreas C Hepatobiliary System, All	Z None	Z None	Z None

1ˢᵀ – B Imaging
2ᴺᴰ – F Hepatobiliary System and Pancreas
3ᴿᴰ – 3 MAGNETIC RESONANCE IMAGING (MRI)

EXAMPLE: MRI of knee

MAGNETIC RESONANCE IMAGING (MRI): Computer reformatted digital display of multiplanar images developed from the capture of radiofrequency signals emitted by nuclei in a body site excited within a magnetic field.

Body Part – 4ᵀᴴ	Contrast – 5ᵀᴴ	Qualifier – 6ᵀᴴ	Qualifier – 7ᵀᴴ
5 Liver 6 Liver and Spleen 7 Pancreas	Y Other contrast	0 Unenhanced and enhanced Z None	Z None
5 Liver 6 Liver and Spleen 7 Pancreas	Z None	Z None	Z None

© 2016 Channel Publishing, Ltd.

1ST - B Imaging 2ND - F Hepatobiliary System and Pancreas 3RD - 4 ULTRASONOGRAPHY	EXAMPLE: Abdominal ultrasound ULTRASONOGRAPHY: Real time display of images of anatomy or flow information developed from the capture of reflected and attenuated high frequency sound waves.		
Body Part – 4TH	**Contrast – 5TH**	**Qualifier – 6TH**	**Qualifier – 7TH**
0 Bile Ducts 2 Gallbladder 3 Gallbladder and Bile Ducts 5 Liver 6 Liver and Spleen 7 Pancreas C Hepatobiliary System, All	Z None	Z None	Z None

1ST - B Imaging 2ND - G Endocrine System 3RD - 2 COMPUTERIZED TOMOGRAPHY (CT Scan)	EXAMPLE: CT Scan of head COMPUTERIZED TOMOGRAPHY (CT Scan): Computer reformatted digital display of multiplanar images developed from the capture of multiple exposures of external ionizing radiation.		
Body Part – 4TH	**Contrast – 5TH**	**Qualifier – 6TH**	**Qualifier – 7TH**
2 Adrenal Glands, Bilateral 3 Parathyroid Glands 4 Thyroid Gland	0 High osmolar 1 Low osmolar Y Other contrast	0 Unenhanced and enhanced Z None	Z None
2 Adrenal Glands, Bilateral 3 Parathyroid Glands 4 Thyroid Gland	Z None	Z None	Z None

1ST - B Imaging 2ND - G Endocrine System 3RD - 3 MAGNETIC RESONANCE IMAGING (MRI)	EXAMPLE: MRI of knee MAGNETIC RESONANCE IMAGING (MRI): Computer reformatted digital display of multiplanar images developed from the capture of radiofrequency signals emitted by nuclei in a body site excited within a magnetic field.		
Body Part – 4TH	**Contrast – 5TH**	**Qualifier – 6TH**	**Qualifier – 7TH**
2 Adrenal Glands, Bilateral 3 Parathyroid Glands 4 Thyroid Gland	Y Other contrast	0 Unenhanced and enhanced Z None	Z None
2 Adrenal Glands, Bilateral 3 Parathyroid Glands 4 Thyroid Gland	Z None	Z None	Z None

IMAGING

B G 3

1ST – B Imaging 2ND – G Endocrine System 3RD – 4 ULTRASONOGRAPHY	EXAMPLE: Abdominal ultrasound ULTRASONOGRAPHY: Real time display of images of anatomy or flow information developed from the capture of reflected and attenuated high frequency sound waves.		
Body Part – 4TH	**Contrast – 5TH**	**Qualifier – 6TH**	**Qualifier – 7TH**
0 Adrenal Gland, Right 1 Adrenal Gland, Left 2 Adrenal Glands, Bilateral 3 Parathyroid Glands 4 Thyroid Gland	Z None	Z None	Z None

1ST – B Imaging 2ND – H Skin, Subcutaneous Tissue and Breast 3RD – 0 PLAIN RADIOGRAPHY	EXAMPLE: Chest X-ray PLAIN RADIOGRAPHY: Planar display of an image developed from the capture of external ionizing radiation on photographic or photoconductive plate.		
Body Part – 4TH	**Contrast – 5TH**	**Qualifier – 6TH**	**Qualifier – 7TH**
0 Breast, Right 1 Breast, Left 2 Breasts, Bilateral	Z None	Z None	Z None
3 Single Mammary Duct, Right 4 Single Mammary Duct, Left 5 Multiple Mammary Ducts, Right 6 Multiple Mammary Ducts, Left	0 High osmolar 1 Low osmolar Y Other contrast Z None	Z None	Z None

IMAGING

BG4

1ST - **B** Imaging 2ND - **H** Skin, Subcutaneous Tissue and Breast 3RD - **3** MAGNETIC RESONANCE IMAGING (MRI)	EXAMPLE: MRI of knee
	MAGNETIC RESONANCE IMAGING (MRI): Computer reformatted digital display of multiplanar images developed from the capture of radiofrequency signals emitted by nuclei in a body site excited within a magnetic field.

Body Part – 4TH	Contrast – 5TH	Qualifier – 6TH	Qualifier – 7TH
0 Breast, Right 1 Breast, Left 2 Breasts, Bilateral D Subcutaneous Tissue, Head/Neck F Subcutaneous Tissue, Upper Extremity G Subcutaneous Tissue, Thorax H Subcutaneous Tissue, Abdomen and Pelvis J Subcutaneous Tissue, Lower Extremity	Y Other contrast	0 Unenhanced and enhanced Z None	Z None
0 Breast, Right 1 Breast, Left 2 Breasts, Bilateral D Subcutaneous Tissue, Head/Neck F Subcutaneous Tissue, Upper Extremity G Subcutaneous Tissue, Thorax H Subcutaneous Tissue, Abdomen and Pelvis J Subcutaneous Tissue, Lower Extremity	Z None	Z None	Z None

1ST - **B** Imaging 2ND - **H** Skin, Subcutaneous Tissue and Breast 3RD - **4** ULTRASONOGRAPHY	EXAMPLE: Abdominal ultrasound
	ULTRASONOGRAPHY: Real time display of images of anatomy or flow information developed from the capture of reflected and attenuated high frequency sound waves.

Body Part – 4TH		Contrast – 5TH	Qualifier – 6TH	Qualifier – 7TH
0 Breast, Right 1 Breast, Left 2 Breasts, Bilateral 7 Extremity, Upper	8 Extremity, Lower 9 Abdominal Wall B Chest Wall C Head and Neck	Z None	Z None	Z None

1ST – B Imaging
2ND – L Connective Tissue
3RD – 3 MAGNETIC RESONANCE IMAGING (MRI)

EXAMPLE: MRI of knee

MAGNETIC RESONANCE IMAGING (MRI):
Computer reformatted digital display of multiplanar images developed from the capture of radiofrequency signals emitted by nuclei in a body site excited within a magnetic field.

Body Part – 4TH	Contrast – 5TH	Qualifier – 6TH	Qualifier – 7TH
0 Connective Tissue, Upper Extremity 1 Connective Tissue, Lower Extremity 2 Tendons, Upper Extremity 3 Tendons, Lower Extremity	Y Other contrast	0 Unenhanced and enhanced Z None	Z None
0 Connective Tissue, Upper Extremity 1 Connective Tissue, Lower Extremity 2 Tendons, Upper Extremity 3 Tendons, Lower Extremity	Z None	Z None	Z None

1ST – B Imaging
2ND – L Connective Tissue
3RD – 4 ULTRASONOGRAPHY

EXAMPLE: Abdominal ultrasound

ULTRASONOGRAPHY: Real time display
of images of anatomy or flow information developed from the capture of reflected and attenuated high frequency sound waves.

Body Part – 4TH	Contrast – 5TH	Qualifier – 6TH	Qualifier – 7TH
0 Connective Tissue, Upper Extremity 1 Connective Tissue, Lower Extremity 2 Tendons, Upper Extremity 3 Tendons, Lower Extremity	Z None	Z None	Z None

1ST – B Imaging
2ND – N Skull and Facial Bones
3RD – 0 PLAIN RADIOGRAPHY

EXAMPLE: Chest X-ray

PLAIN RADIOGRAPHY: Planar display of an
image developed from the capture of external ionizing radiation on photographic or photoconductive plate.

Body Part – 4TH		Contrast – 5TH	Qualifier – 6TH	Qualifier – 7TH
0 Skull 1 Orbit, Right 2 Orbit, Left 3 Orbits, Bilateral 4 Nasal Bones 5 Facial Bones 6 Mandible	B Zygomatic Arch, Right C Zygomatic Arch, Left D Zygomatic Arches, Bilateral G Tooth, Single H Teeth, Multiple J Teeth, All	Z None	Z None	Z None
7 Temporomandibular Joint, Right 8 Temporomandibular Joint, Left 9 Temporomandibular Joints, Bilateral		0 High osmolar 1 Low osmolar Y Other contrast Z None	Z None	Z None

IMAGING

BL3

1ST - **B** Imaging 2ND - **N** Skull and Facial Bones 3RD - **1** FLUOROSCOPY	EXAMPLE: Fluoroscopic guidance
	FLUOROSCOPY: Single plane or bi-plane real time display of an image developed from the capture of external ionizing radiation on a fluorescent screen. The image may also be stored by either digital or analog means.

Body Part – 4TH	Contrast – 5TH	Qualifier – 6TH	Qualifier – 7TH
7 Temporomandibular Joint, Right 8 Temporomandibular Joint, Left 9 Temporomandibular Joints, Bilateral	0 High osmolar 1 Low osmolar Y Other contrast Z None	Z None	Z None

1ST - **B** Imaging 2ND - **N** Skull and Facial Bones 3RD - **2** COMPUTERIZED TOMOGRAPHY (CT Scan)	EXAMPLE: CT Scan of head
	COMPUTERIZED TOMOGRAPHY (CT Scan): Computer reformatted digital display of multiplanar images developed from the capture of multiple exposures of external ionizing radiation.

Body Part – 4TH	Contrast – 5TH	Qualifier – 6TH	Qualifier – 7TH
0 Skull 6 Mandible 3 Orbits, Bilateral 9 Temporomandibular Joints, 5 Facial Bones Bilateral F Temporal Bones	0 High osmolar 1 Low osmolar Y Other contrast Z None	Z None	Z None

1ST - **B** Imaging 2ND - **N** Skull and Facial Bones 3RD - **3** MAGNETIC RESONANCE IMAGING (MRI)	EXAMPLE: MRI of knee
	MAGNETIC RESONANCE IMAGING (MRI): Computer reformatted digital display of multiplanar images developed from the capture of radiofrequency signals emitted by nuclei in a body site excited within a magnetic field.

Body Part – 4TH	Contrast – 5TH	Qualifier – 6TH	Qualifier – 7TH
9 Temporomandibular Joints, Bilateral	Y Other contrast Z None	Z None	Z None

IMAGING

B N 3

1ST - B Imaging
2ND - P Non-Axial Upper Bones
3RD - 0 PLAIN RADIOGRAPHY

EXAMPLE: Chest X-ray

PLAIN RADIOGRAPHY: Planar display of an image developed from the capture of external ionizing radiation on photographic or photoconductive plate.

Body Part – 4TH		Contrast – 5TH	Qualifier – 6TH	Qualifier – 7TH
0 Sternoclavicular Joint, Right	A Humerus, Right	Z None	Z None	Z None
1 Sternoclavicular Joint, Left	B Humerus, Left			
2 Sternoclavicular Joints, Bilateral	E Upper Arm, Right			
3 Acromioclavicular Joints, Bilateral	F Upper Arm, Left			
4 Clavicle, Right	J Forearm, Right			
5 Clavicle, Left	K Forearm, Left			
6 Scapula, Right	N Hand, Right			
7 Scapula, Left	P Hand, Left			
	R Finger(s), Right			
	S Finger(s), Left			
	X Ribs, Right			
	Y Ribs, Left			
8 Shoulder, Right	G Elbow, Right	0 High osmolar	Z None	Z None
9 Shoulder, Left	H Elbow, Left	1 Low osmolar		
C Hand/Finger Joint, Right	L Wrist, Right	Y Other contrast		
D Hand/Finger Joint, Left	M Wrist, Left	Z None		

1ST - B Imaging
2ND - P Non-Axial Upper Bones
3RD - 1 FLUOROSCOPY

EXAMPLE: Fluoroscopic guidance

FLUOROSCOPY: Single plane or bi-plane real time display of an image developed from the capture of external ionizing radiation on a fluorescent screen. The image may also be stored by either digital or analog means.

Body Part – 4TH		Contrast – 5TH	Qualifier – 6TH	Qualifier – 7TH
0 Sternoclavicular Joint, Right	A Humerus, Right	Z None	Z None	Z None
1 Sternoclavicular Joint, Left	B Humerus, Left			
2 Sternoclavicular Joints, Bilateral	E Upper Arm, Right			
3 Acromioclavicular Joints, Bilateral	F Upper Arm, Left			
4 Clavicle, Right	J Forearm, Right			
5 Clavicle, Left	K Forearm, Left			
6 Scapula, Right	N Hand, Right			
7 Scapula, Left	P Hand, Left			
	R Finger(s), Right			
	S Finger(s), Left			
	X Ribs, Right			
	Y Ribs, Left			
8 Shoulder, Right		0 High osmolar	Z None	Z None
9 Shoulder, Left		1 Low osmolar		
L Wrist, Right		Y Other contrast		
M Wrist, Left		Z None		
C Hand/Finger Joint, Right		0 High osmolar	Z None	Z None
D Hand/Finger Joint, Left		1 Low osmolar		
G Elbow, Right		Y Other contrast		
H Elbow, Left				

IMAGING

BP0

1ST - **B** Imaging 2ND - **P** Non-Axial Upper Bones 3RD - **2 COMPUTERIZED TOMOGRAPHY** (CT Scan)	EXAMPLE: CT Scan of head **COMPUTERIZED TOMOGRAPHY (CT Scan):** Computer reformatted digital display of multiplanar images developed from the capture of multiple exposures of external ionizing radiation.

Body Part – 4TH		Contrast – 5TH	Qualifier – 6TH	Qualifier – 7TH
0 Sternoclavicular Joint, Right 1 Sternoclavicular Joint, Left W Thorax		0 High osmolar 1 Low osmolar Y Other contrast	Z None	Z None
2 Sternoclavicular Joints, Bilateral 3 Acromioclavicular Joints, Bilateral 4 Clavicle, Right 5 Clavicle, Left 6 Scapula, Right 7 Scapula, Left 8 Shoulder, Right 9 Shoulder, Left A Humerus, Right B Humerus, Left E Upper Arm, Right F Upper Arm, Left G Elbow, Right	H Elbow, Left J Forearm, Right K Forearm, Left L Wrist, Right M Wrist, Left N Hand, Right P Hand, Left Q Hands and Wrists, Bilateral R Finger(s), Right S Finger(s), Left T Upper Extremity, Right U Upper Extremity, Left V Upper Extremities, Bilateral X Ribs, Right Y Ribs, Left	0 High osmolar 1 Low osmolar Y Other contrast Z None	Z None	Z None
C Hand/Finger Joint, Right D Hand/Finger Joint, Left		Z None	Z None	Z None

1ST - **B** Imaging 2ND - **P** Non-Axial Upper Bones 3RD - **3 MAGNETIC RESONANCE IMAGING (MRI)**	EXAMPLE: MRI of knee **MAGNETIC RESONANCE IMAGING (MRI):** Computer reformatted digital display of multiplanar images developed from the capture of radiofrequency signals emitted by nuclei in a body site excited within a magnetic field.

Body Part – 4TH		Contrast – 5TH	Qualifier – 6TH	Qualifier – 7TH
8 Shoulder, Right 9 Shoulder, Left C Hand/Finger Joint, Right D Hand/Finger Joint, Left E Upper Arm, Right F Upper Arm, Left	G Elbow, Right H Elbow, Left J Forearm, Right K Forearm, Left L Wrist, Right M Wrist, Left	Y Other contrast	0 Unenhanced and enhanced Z None	Z None
8 Shoulder, Right 9 Shoulder, Left C Hand/Finger Joint, Right D Hand/Finger Joint, Left E Upper Arm, Right F Upper Arm, Left	G Elbow, Right H Elbow, Left J Forearm, Right K Forearm, Left L Wrist, Right M Wrist, Left	Z None	Z None	Z None

IMAGING

B P 3

1ST - **B** Imaging

2ND - **P** Non-Axial Upper Bones

3RD - **4 ULTRASONOGRAPHY**

EXAMPLE: Abdominal ultrasound

ULTRASONOGRAPHY: Real time display of images of anatomy or flow information developed from the capture of reflected and attenuated high frequency sound waves.

Body Part – 4TH		Contrast – 5TH	Qualifier – 6TH	Qualifier – 7TH
8 Shoulder, Right	L Wrist, Right	Z None	Z None	1 Densitometry
9 Shoulder, Left	M Wrist, Left			Z None
G Elbow, Right	N Hand, Right			
H Elbow, Left	P Hand, Left			

1ST - **B** Imaging

2ND - **Q** Non-Axial Lower Bones

3RD - **0 PLAIN RADIOGRAPHY**

EXAMPLE: Chest X-ray

PLAIN RADIOGRAPHY: Planar display of an image developed from the capture of external ionizing radiation on photographic or photoconductive plate.

Body Part – 4TH		Contrast – 5TH	Qualifier – 6TH	Qualifier – 7TH
0 Hip, Right		0 High osmolar	Z None	Z None
1 Hip, Left		1 Low osmolar		
		Y Other contrast		
0 Hip, Right		Z None	Z None	1 Densitometry
1 Hip, Left				Z None
3 Femur, Right		Z None	Z None	1 Densitometry
4 Femur, Left				Z None
7 Knee, Right		0 High osmolar	Z None	Z None
8 Knee, Left		1 Low osmolar		
G Ankle, Right		Y Other contrast		
H Ankle, Left		Z None		
D Lower Leg, Right	M Foot, Left	Z None	Z None	Z None
F Lower Leg, Left	P Toe(s), Right			
J Calcaneus, Right	Q Toe(s), Left			
K Calcaneus, Left	V Patella, Right			
L Foot, Right	W Patella, Left			
X Foot/Toe Joint, Right		0 High osmolar	Z None	Z None
Y Foot/Toe Joint, Left		1 Low osmolar		
		Y Other contrast		

IMAGING

BP4

1ST - **B** Imaging		EXAMPLE: Fluoroscopic guidance

2ND - **Q** Non-Axial Lower Bones

3RD - **1** FLUOROSCOPY

FLUOROSCOPY: Single plane or bi-plane real time display of an image developed from the capture of external ionizing radiation on a fluorescent screen. The image may also be stored by either digital or analog means.

Body Part – 4TH		Contrast – 5TH	Qualifier – 6TH	Qualifier – 7TH
0 Hip, Right 1 Hip, Left 7 Knee, Right 8 Knee, Left	G Ankle, Right H Ankle, Left X Foot/Toe Joint, Right Y Foot/Toe Joint, Left	0 High osmolar 1 Low osmolar Y Other contrast Z None	Z None	Z None
3 Femur, Right 4 Femur, Left D Lower Leg, Right F Lower Leg, Left J Calcaneus, Right K Calcaneus, Left	L Foot, Right M Foot, Left P Toe(s), Right Q Toe(s), Left V Patella, Right W Patella, Left	Z None	Z None	Z None

1ST - **B** Imaging		EXAMPLE: CT Scan of head

2ND - **Q** Non-Axial Lower Bones

3RD - **2** COMPUTERIZED TOMOGRAPHY (CT Scan)

COMPUTERIZED TOMOGRAPHY (CT Scan): Computer reformatted digital display of multiplanar images developed from the capture of multiple exposures of external ionizing radiation.

Body Part – 4TH		Contrast – 5TH	Qualifier – 6TH	Qualifier – 7TH
0 Hip, Right 1 Hip, Left 3 Femur, Right 4 Femur, Left 7 Knee, Right 8 Knee, Left D Lower Leg, Right F Lower Leg, Left G Ankle, Right H Ankle, Left J Calcaneus, Right	K Calcaneus, Left L Foot, Right M Foot, Left P Toe(s), Right Q Toe(s), Left R Lower Extremity, Right S Lower Extremity, Left V Patella, Right W Patella, Left X Foot/Toe Joint, Right Y Foot/Toe Joint, Left	0 High osmolar 1 Low osmolar Y Other contrast Z None	Z None	Z None
B Tibia/Fibula, Right C Tibia/Fibula, Left		0 High osmolar 1 Low osmolar Y Other contrast	Z None	Z None

IMAGING

B Q 2

1ST – B Imaging 2ND – Q Non-Axial Lower Bones 3RD – 3 MAGNETIC RESONANCE IMAGING (MRI)	EXAMPLE: MRI of knee **MAGNETIC RESONANCE IMAGING (MRI):** Computer reformatted digital display of multiplanar images developed from the capture of radiofrequency signals emitted by nuclei in a body site excited within a magnetic field.		
Body Part – 4TH	**Contrast – 5TH**	**Qualifier – 6TH**	**Qualifier – 7TH**
0 Hip, Right H Ankle, Left 1 Hip, Left J Calcaneus, Right 3 Femur, Right K Calcaneus, Left 4 Femur, Left L Foot, Right 7 Knee, Right M Foot, Left 8 Knee, Left P Toe(s), Right D Lower Leg, Right Q Toe(s), Left F Lower Leg, Left V Patella, Right G Ankle, Right W Patella, Left	Y Other contrast	0 Unenhanced and enhanced Z None	Z None
0 Hip, Right H Ankle, Left 1 Hip, Left J Calcaneus, Right 3 Femur, Right K Calcaneus, Left 4 Femur, Left L Foot, Right 7 Knee, Right M Foot, Left 8 Knee, Left P Toe(s), Right D Lower Leg, Right Q Toe(s), Left F Lower Leg, Left V Patella, Right G Ankle, Right W Patella, Left	Z None	Z None	Z None

1ST – B Imaging 2ND – Q Non-Axial Lower Bones 3RD – 4 ULTRASONOGRAPHY	EXAMPLE: Abdominal ultrasound **ULTRASONOGRAPHY:** Real time display of images of anatomy or flow information developed from the capture of reflected and attenuated high frequency sound waves.		
Body Part – 4TH	**Contrast – 5TH**	**Qualifier – 6TH**	**Qualifier – 7TH**
0 Hip, Right 7 Knee, Right 1 Hip, Left 8 Knee, Left 2 Hips, Bilateral 9 Knees, Bilateral	Z None	Z None	Z None

IMAGING

BQ3

1ST - B Imaging		EXAMPLE: Chest X-ray
2ND - R Axial Skeleton, Except Skull and Facial Bones		**PLAIN RADIOGRAPHY:** Planar display of an image developed from the capture of external ionizing radiation on photographic or photoconductive plate.
3RD - 0 PLAIN RADIOGRAPHY		

Body Part – 4TH		Contrast – 5TH	Qualifier – 6TH	Qualifier – 7TH
0 Cervical Spine 7 Thoracic Spine	9 Lumbar Spine G Whole Spine	Z None	Z None	1 Densitometry Z None
1 Cervical Disc(s) 2 Thoracic Disc(s) 3 Lumbar Disc(s)	4 Cervical Facet Joint(s) 5 Thoracic Facet Joint(s) 6 Lumbar Facet Joint(s) D Sacroiliac Joints	0 High osmolar 1 Low osmolar Y Other contrast Z None	Z None	Z None
8 Thoracolumbar Joint B Lumbosacral Joint	C Pelvis F Sacrum and Coccyx H Sternum	Z None	Z None	Z None

1ST - B Imaging		EXAMPLE: Fluoroscopic guidance
2ND - R Axial Skeleton, Except Skull and Facial Bones		**FLUOROSCOPY:** Single plane or bi-plane real time display of an image developed from the capture of external ionizing radiation on a fluorescent screen. The image may also be stored by either digital or analog means.
3RD - 1 FLUOROSCOPY		

Body Part – 4TH		Contrast – 5TH	Qualifier – 6TH	Qualifier – 7TH
0 Cervical Spine 1 Cervical Disc(s) 2 Thoracic Disc(s) 3 Lumbar Disc(s) 4 Cervical Facet Joint(s) 5 Thoracic Facet Joint(s) 6 Lumbar Facet Joint(s) 7 Thoracic Spine	8 Thoracolumbar Joint 9 Lumbar Spine B Lumbosacral Joint C Pelvis D Sacroiliac Joints F Sacrum and Coccyx G Whole Spine H Sternum	0 High osmolar 1 Low osmolar Y Other contrast Z None	Z None	Z None

IMAGING

BR1

1ST – **B** Imaging 2ND – **R** Axial Skeleton, Except Skull and Facial Bones 3RD – **2 COMPUTERIZED TOMOGRAPHY** (CT Scan)	EXAMPLE: CT Scan of head **COMPUTERIZED TOMOGRAPHY (CT Scan):** Computer reformatted digital display of multiplanar images developed from the capture of multiple exposures of external ionizing radiation.		
Body Part – 4TH	**Contrast – 5TH**	**Qualifier – 6TH**	**Qualifier – 7TH**
0　Cervical Spine　　C　Pelvis 7　Thoracic Spine　　D　Sacroiliac Joints 9　Lumbar Spine　　　F　Sacrum and Coccyx	0　High osmolar 1　Low osmolar Y　Other contrast Z　None	Z　None	Z　None

1ST – **B** Imaging 2ND – **R** Axial Skeleton, Except Skull and Facial Bones 3RD – **3 MAGNETIC RESONANCE IMAGING (MRI)**	EXAMPLE: MRI of knee **MAGNETIC RESONANCE IMAGING (MRI):** Computer reformatted digital display of multiplanar images developed from the capture of radiofrequency signals emitted by nuclei in a body site excited within a magnetic field.		
Body Part – 4TH	**Contrast – 5TH**	**Qualifier – 6TH**	**Qualifier – 7TH**
0　Cervical Spine　　　7　Thoracic Spine 1　Cervical Disc(s)　　9　Lumbar Spine 2　Thoracic Disc(s)　　C　Pelvis 3　Lumbar Disc(s)　　F　Sacrum and Coccyx	Y　Other contrast	0　Unenhanced and enhanced Z　None	Z　None
0　Cervical Spine　　　7　Thoracic Spine 1　Cervical Disc(s)　　9　Lumbar Spine 2　Thoracic Disc(s)　　C　Pelvis 3　Lumbar Disc(s)　　F　Sacrum and Coccyx	Z　None	Z　None	Z　None

1ST – **B** Imaging 2ND – **R** Axial Skeleton, Except Skull and Facial Bones 3RD – **4 ULTRASONOGRAPHY**	EXAMPLE: Abdominal ultrasound **ULTRASONOGRAPHY:** Real time display of images of anatomy or flow information developed from the capture of reflected and attenuated high frequency sound waves.		
Body Part – 4TH	**Contrast – 5TH**	**Qualifier – 6TH**	**Qualifier – 7TH**
0　Cervical Spine 7　Thoracic Spine 9　Lumbar Spine F　Sacrum and Coccyx	Z　None	Z　None	Z　None

IMAGING

BR2

1ST – B Imaging
2ND – T Urinary System
3RD – 0 PLAIN RADIOGRAPHY

EXAMPLE: Chest X-ray

PLAIN RADIOGRAPHY: Planar display of an image developed from the capture of external ionizing radiation on photographic or photoconductive plate.

Body Part – 4TH		Contrast – 5TH	Qualifier – 6TH	Qualifier – 7TH
0 Bladder	5 Urethra	0 High osmolar	Z None	Z None
1 Kidney, Right	6 Ureter, Right	1 Low osmolar		
2 Kidney, Left	7 Ureter, Left	Y Other contrast		
3 Kidneys, Bilateral	8 Ureters, Bilateral	Z None		
4 Kidneys, Ureters and Bladder	B Bladder and Urethra			
	C Ileal Diversion Loop			

1ST – B Imaging
2ND – T Urinary System
3RD – 1 FLUOROSCOPY

EXAMPLE: Fluoroscopic guidance

FLUOROSCOPY: Single plane or bi-plane real time display of an image developed from the capture of external ionizing radiation on a fluorescent screen. The image may also be stored by either digital or analog means.

Body Part – 4TH		Contrast – 5TH	Qualifier – 6TH	Qualifier – 7TH
0 Bladder	B Bladder and Urethra	0 High osmolar	Z None	Z None
1 Kidney, Right	C Ileal Diversion Loop	1 Low osmolar		
2 Kidney, Left	D Kidney, Ureter and Bladder, Right	Y Other contrast		
3 Kidneys, Bilateral		Z None		
4 Kidneys, Ureters and Bladder	F Kidney, Ureter and Bladder, Left			
5 Urethra	G Ileal Loop, Ureters and Kidneys			
6 Ureter, Right				
7 Ureter, Left				

1ST – B Imaging
2ND – T Urinary System
3RD – 2 COMPUTERIZED TOMOGRAPHY (CT Scan)

EXAMPLE: CT Scan of head

COMPUTERIZED TOMOGRAPHY (CT Scan): Computer reformatted digital display of multiplanar images developed from the capture of multiple exposures of external ionizing radiation.

Body Part – 4TH		Contrast – 5TH	Qualifier – 6TH	Qualifier – 7TH
0 Bladder	3 Kidneys, Bilateral	0 High osmolar	0 Unenhanced and enhanced	Z None
1 Kidney, Right	9 Kidney Transplant	1 Low osmolar		
2 Kidney, Left		Y Other contrast	Z None	
0 Bladder	3 Kidneys, Bilateral	Z None	Z None	Z None
1 Kidney, Right	9 Kidney Transplant			
2 Kidney, Left				

MAGNETIC RESONANCE IMAGING (MRI)

1ST – **B** Imaging
2ND – **T** Urinary System
3RD – **3** MAGNETIC RESONANCE IMAGING (MRI)

EXAMPLE: MRI of knee

MAGNETIC RESONANCE IMAGING (MRI): Computer reformatted digital display of multiplanar images developed from the capture of radiofrequency signals emitted by nuclei in a body site excited within a magnetic field.

Body Part – 4TH		Contrast – 5TH	Qualifier – 6TH	Qualifier – 7TH
0 Bladder	3 Kidneys, Bilateral	Y Other contrast	0 Unenhanced and enhanced	Z None
1 Kidney, Right	9 Kidney Transplant		Z None	
2 Kidney, Left				
0 Bladder	3 Kidneys, Bilateral	Z None	Z None	Z None
1 Kidney, Right	9 Kidney Transplant			
2 Kidney, Left				

ULTRASONOGRAPHY

1ST – **B** Imaging
2ND – **T** Urinary System
3RD – **4** ULTRASONOGRAPHY

EXAMPLE: Abdominal ultrasound

ULTRASONOGRAPHY: Real time display of images of anatomy or flow information developed from the capture of reflected and attenuated high frequency sound waves.

Body Part – 4TH		Contrast – 5TH	Qualifier – 6TH	Qualifier – 7TH
0 Bladder	6 Ureter, Right	Z None	Z None	Z None
1 Kidney, Right	7 Ureter, Left			
2 Kidney, Left	8 Ureters, Bilateral			
3 Kidneys, Bilateral	9 Kidney Transplant			
5 Urethra	J Kidneys and Bladder			

PLAIN RADIOGRAPHY

1ST – **B** Imaging
2ND – **U** Female Reproductive System ♀
3RD – **0** PLAIN RADIOGRAPHY

EXAMPLE: Chest X-ray

PLAIN RADIOGRAPHY: Planar display of an image developed from the capture of external ionizing radiation on photographic or photoconductive plate.

Body Part – 4TH		Contrast – 5TH	Qualifier – 6TH	Qualifier – 7TH
0 Fallopian Tube, Right	6 Uterus	0 High osmolar	Z None	Z None
1 Fallopian Tube, Left	8 Uterus and Fallopian	1 Low osmolar		
2 Fallopian Tubes, Bilateral	Tubes	Y Other contrast		
	9 Vagina			

IMAGING

B T 3

1st - B Imaging
2nd - U Female Reproductive System ♀
3rd - 1 FLUOROSCOPY

EXAMPLE: Fluoroscopic guidance

FLUOROSCOPY: Single plane or bi-plane real time display of an image developed from the capture of external ionizing radiation on a fluorescent screen. The image may also be stored by either digital or analog means.

Body Part – 4TH		Contrast – 5TH	Qualifier – 6TH	Qualifier – 7TH
0 Fallopian Tube, Right	6 Uterus	0 High osmolar	Z None	Z None
1 Fallopian Tube, Left	8 Uterus and Fallopian	1 Low osmolar		
2 Fallopian Tubes, Bilateral	Tubes	Y Other contrast		
	9 Vagina	Z None		

1st - B Imaging
2nd - U Female Reproductive System ♀
3rd - 3 MAGNETIC RESONANCE IMAGING (MRI)

EXAMPLE: MRI of knee

MAGNETIC RESONANCE IMAGING (MRI): Computer reformatted digital display of multiplanar images developed from the capture of radiofrequency signals emitted by nuclei in a body site excited within a magnetic field.

Body Part – 4TH		Contrast – 5TH	Qualifier – 6TH	Qualifier – 7TH
3 Ovary, Right	9 Vagina	Y Other contrast	0 Unenhanced and enhanced	Z None
4 Ovary, Left	B Pregnant Uterus		Z None	
5 Ovaries, Bilateral	C Uterus and Ovaries			
6 Uterus				
3 Ovary, Right	9 Vagina	Z None	Z None	Z None
4 Ovary, Left	B Pregnant Uterus			
5 Ovaries, Bilateral	C Uterus and Ovaries			
6 Uterus				

1st - B Imaging
2nd - U Female Reproductive System ♀
3rd - 4 ULTRASONOGRAPHY

EXAMPLE: Abdominal ultrasound

ULTRASONOGRAPHY: Real time display of images of anatomy or flow information developed from the capture of reflected and attenuated high frequency sound waves.

Body Part – 4TH		Contrast – 5TH	Qualifier – 6TH	Qualifier – 7TH
0 Fallopian Tube, Right	4 Ovary, Left	Y Other contrast	Z None	Z None
1 Fallopian Tube, Left	5 Ovaries, Bilateral	Z None		
2 Fallopian Tubes, Bilateral	6 Uterus			
3 Ovary, Right	C Uterus and Ovaries			

IMAGING

B U 4

1ST – **B** Imaging

2ND – **V** Male Reproductive System ♂

3RD – **0** PLAIN RADIOGRAPHY

EXAMPLE: Chest X-ray

PLAIN RADIOGRAPHY: Planar display of an image developed from the capture of external ionizing radiation on photographic or photoconductive plate.

Body Part – 4TH		Contrast – 5TH	Qualifier – 6TH	Qualifier – 7TH
0 Corpora Cavernosa	5 Testicle, Right	0 High osmolar	Z None	Z None
1 Epididymis, Right	6 Testicle, Left	1 Low osmolar		
2 Epididymis, Left	8 Vasa Vasorum	Y Other contrast		
3 Prostate				

1ST – **B** Imaging

2ND – **V** Male Reproductive System ♂

3RD – **1** FLUOROSCOPY

EXAMPLE: Fluoroscopic guidance

FLUOROSCOPY: Single plane or bi-plane real time display of an image developed from the capture of external ionizing radiation on a fluorescent screen. The image may also be stored by either digital or analog means.

Body Part – 4TH	Contrast – 5TH	Qualifier – 6TH	Qualifier – 7TH
0 Corpora Cavernosa	0 High osmolar	Z None	Z None
8 Vasa Vasorum	1 Low osmolar		
	Y Other contrast		
	Z None		

1ST – **B** Imaging

2ND – **V** Male Reproductive System ♂

3RD – **2** COMPUTERIZED TOMOGRAPHY (CT Scan)

EXAMPLE: CT Scan of head

COMPUTERIZED TOMOGRAPHY (CT Scan): Computer reformatted digital display of multiplanar images developed from the capture of multiple exposures of external ionizing radiation.

Body Part – 4TH	Contrast – 5TH	Qualifier – 6TH	Qualifier – 7TH
3 Prostate	0 High osmolar	0 Unenhanced	Z None
	1 Low osmolar	and enhanced	
	Y Other contrast	Z None	
3 Prostate	Z None	Z None	Z None

I M A G I N G

B V 0

MRI — Male Reproductive System

1ST - B Imaging 2ND - V Male Reproductive System ♂ 3RD - 3 MAGNETIC RESONANCE IMAGING (MRI)	EXAMPLE: MRI of knee **MAGNETIC RESONANCE IMAGING (MRI):** Computer reformatted digital display of multiplanar images developed from the capture of radiofrequency signals emitted by nuclei in a body site excited within a magnetic field.

Body Part – 4TH		Contrast – 5TH	Qualifier – 6TH	Qualifier – 7TH
0 Corpora Cavernosa 3 Prostate 4 Scrotum	5 Testicle, Right 6 Testicle, Left 7 Testicles, Bilateral	Y Other contrast	0 Unenhanced and enhanced Z None	Z None
0 Corpora Cavernosa 3 Prostate 4 Scrotum	5 Testicle, Right 6 Testicle, Left 7 Testicles, Bilateral	Z None	Z None	Z None

Ultrasonography — Male Reproductive System

1ST - B Imaging 2ND - V Male Reproductive System ♂ 3RD - 4 ULTRASONOGRAPHY	EXAMPLE: Abdominal ultrasound **ULTRASONOGRAPHY:** Real time display of images of anatomy or flow information developed from the capture of reflected and attenuated high frequency sound waves.

Body Part – 4TH	Contrast – 5TH	Qualifier – 6TH	Qualifier – 7TH
4 Scrotum 9 Prostate and Seminal Vesicles B Penis	Z None	Z None	Z None

Plain Radiography — Anatomical Regions

1ST - B Imaging 2ND - W Anatomical regions 3RD - 0 PLAIN RADIOGRAPHY	EXAMPLE: Chest X-ray **PLAIN RADIOGRAPHY:** Planar display of an image developed from the capture of external ionizing radiation on photographic or photoconductive plate.

Body Part – 4TH		Contrast – 5TH	Qualifier – 6TH	Qualifier – 7TH
0 Abdomen 1 Abdomen and Pelvis 3 Chest B Long Bones, All	C Lower Extremity J Upper Extremity K Whole Body L Whole Skeleton M Whole Body, Infant	Z None	Z None	Z None

IMAGING

B W 0

1ST - B	Imaging	EXAMPLE: Fluoroscopic guidance
2ND - W	Anatomical Regions	**FLUOROSCOPY:** Single plane or bi-plane real time display of an image developed from the capture of external ionizing radiation on a fluorescent screen. The image may also be stored by either digital or analog means.
3RD - 1	**FLUOROSCOPY**	

Body Part – 4TH		Contrast – 5TH	Qualifier – 6TH	Qualifier – 7TH
1 Abdomen and Pelvis 9 Head and Neck C Lower Extremity J Upper Extremity		0 High osmolar 1 Low osmolar Y Other contrast Z None	Z None	Z None

1ST - B	Imaging	EXAMPLE: CT Scan of head
2ND - W	Anatomical Regions	**COMPUTERIZED TOMOGRAPHY (CT Scan):** Computer reformatted digital display of multiplanar images developed from the capture of multiple exposures of external ionizing radiation.
3RD - 2	**COMPUTERIZED TOMOGRAPHY** (CT Scan)	

Body Part – 4TH		Contrast – 5TH	Qualifier – 6TH	Qualifier – 7TH
0 Abdomen 1 Abdomen and Pelvis 4 Chest and Abdomen 5 Chest, Abdomen and Pelvis	8 Head 9 Head and Neck F Neck G Pelvic Region	0 High osmolar 1 Low osmolar Y Other contrast	0 Unenhanced and enhanced Z None	Z None
0 Abdomen 1 Abdomen and Pelvis 4 Chest and Abdomen 5 Chest, Abdomen and Pelvis	8 Head 9 Head and Neck F Neck G Pelvic Region	Z None	Z None	Z None

1ST - B	Imaging	EXAMPLE: MRI of knee
2ND - W	Anatomical Regions	**MAGNETIC RESONANCE IMAGING (MRI):** Computer reformatted digital display of multiplanar images developed from the capture of radiofrequency signals emitted by nuclei in a body site excited within a magnetic field.
3RD - 3	**MAGNETIC RESONANCE IMAGING (MRI)**	

Body Part – 4TH		Contrast – 5TH	Qualifier – 6TH	Qualifier – 7TH
0 Abdomen 8 Head F Neck	G Pelvic Region H Retroperitoneum P Brachial Plexus	Y Other contrast	0 Unenhanced and enhanced Z None	Z None
0 Abdomen 8 Head F Neck	G Pelvic Region H Retroperitoneum P Brachial Plexus	Z None	Z None	Z None
3 Chest		Y Other contrast	0 Unenhanced and enhanced Z None	Z None

IMAGING

BW1

Table 1

1ST – B Imaging 2ND – W Anatomical Regions 3RD – 4 ULTRASONOGRAPHY	EXAMPLE: Abdominal ultrasound **ULTRASONOGRAPHY:** Real time display of images of anatomy or flow information developed from the capture of reflected and attenuated high frequency sound waves.		
Body Part – 4TH	**Contrast – 5TH**	**Qualifier – 6TH**	**Qualifier – 7TH**
0 Abdomen 1 Abdomen and Pelvis F Neck G Pelvic Region	Z None	Z None	Z None

Table 2

1ST – B Imaging 2ND – Y Fetus and Obstetrical ♀ 3RD – 3 MAGNETIC RESONANCE IMAGING (MRI)	EXAMPLE: MRI of knee **MAGNETIC RESONANCE IMAGING (MRI):** Computer reformatted digital display of multiplanar images developed from the capture of radiofrequency signals emitted by nuclei in a body site excited within a magnetic field.		
Body Part – 4TH	**Contrast – 5TH**	**Qualifier – 6TH**	**Qualifier – 7TH**
0 Fetal Head 4 Fetal Spine 1 Fetal Heart 5 Fetal Extremities 2 Fetal Thorax 6 Whole Fetus 3 Fetal Abdomen	Y Other contrast	0 Unenhanced and enhanced Z None	Z None
0 Fetal Head 4 Fetal Spine 1 Fetal Heart 5 Fetal Extremities 2 Fetal Thorax 6 Whole Fetus 3 Fetal Abdomen	Z None	Z None	Z None

Table 3

1ST – B Imaging 2ND – Y Fetus and Obstetrical ♀ 3RD – 4 ULTRASONOGRAPHY	EXAMPLE: Abdominal ultrasound **ULTRASONOGRAPHY:** Real time display of images of anatomy or flow information developed from the capture of reflected and attenuated high frequency sound waves.		
Body Part – 4TH	**Contrast – 5TH**	**Qualifier – 6TH**	**Qualifier – 7TH**
7 Fetal Umbilical Cord 8 Placenta 9 First Trimester, Single Fetus B First Trimester, Multiple Gestation C Second Trimester, Single Fetus D Second Trimester, Multiple Gestation F Third Trimester, Single Fetus G Third Trimester, Multiple Gestation	Z None	Z None	Z None

IMAGING

B Y 4

<u>**NOTES**</u>

IMAGING

B
Y

Educational Annotations | Section C – Nuclear Medicine

Section Specific Educational Annotations for the Nuclear Medicine Section include:
- AHA Coding Clinic® Reference Notations
- Coding Notes

AHA Coding Clinic® Reference Notations of Nuclear Medicine

ROOT TYPE SPECIFIC - NUCLEAR MEDICINE - Section C
PLANAR NUCLEAR MEDICINE IMAGING - 1
TOMOGRAPHIC (TOMO) NUCLEAR MEDICINE IMAGING - 2
POSITRON EMMISION TOMOGRAPHY (PET) - 3
NONIMAGING NUCLEAR MEDICINE UPTAKE - 4
NONIMAGING NUCLEAR MEDICINE PROBE - 5
NONIMAGING NUCLEAR MEDICINE ASSAY - 6
SYSTEMIC NUCLEAR MEDICINE THERAPY - 7

Coding Notes of Nuclear Medicine

Ancillary Section Specific PCS Reference Manual Exercises

PCS CODE	C – NUCLEAR MEDICINE EXERCISES
C 0 3 0 B Z Z	Carbon 11 PET scan of brain with quantification.
C 0 5 0 V Z Z	Xenon gas nonimaging probe of brain.
C 2 2 6 Y Z Z	Tomo scan of right and left heart, unspecified radiopharmaceutical, qualitative gated rest.
C 2 3 G Q Z Z	PET scan of myocardium using rubidium.
C 7 6 3 H Z Z	Iodinated albumin nuclear medicine assay, blood plasma volume study.
C D 1 5 Y Z Z	Upper GI scan, radiopharmaceutical unspecified, for gastric emptying.
C H 2 2 S Z Z	Thallous chloride tomographic scan of bilateral breasts.
C P 1 5 1 Z Z	Uniplanar scan of spine using technetium oxidronate, with first pass study.
C T 6 3 1 Z Z	Technetium pentetate assay of kidneys, ureters, and bladder.
C W 1 B L Z Z	Gallium citrate scan of head and neck, single plane imaging.

NUCLEAR MEDICINE C

Educational Annotations | Section C – Nuclear Medicine

NOTES

| 1ST - C Nuclear Medicine |
| 2ND - 0 Central Nervous System |
| 3RD - 1 PLANAR NUCLEAR MEDICINE IMAGING |

EXAMPLE: Gallium scan, single plane image

PLANAR NUCLEAR MEDICINE IMAGING: Introduction of radioactive materials into the body for single plane display of images developed from the capture of radioactive emissions.

Body Part – 4TH	Radionuclide – 5TH	Qualifier – 6TH	Qualifier – 7TH
0　Brain	1　Technetium 99m (Tc-99m) Y　Other radionuclide	Z　None	Z　None
5　Cerebrospinal Fluid	D　Indium 111 (In-111) Y　Other radionuclide	Z　None	Z　None
Y　Central Nervous System	Y　Other radionuclide	Z　None	Z　None

| 1ST - C Nuclear Medicine |
| 2ND - 0 Central Nervous System |
| 3RD - 2 TOMOGRAPHIC (TOMO) NUCLEAR MEDICINE IMAGING |

EXAMPLE: Tomo scan of breast

TOMOGRAPHIC (TOMO) NUCLEAR MEDICINE IMAGING: Introduction of radioactive materials into the body for three dimensional display of images developed from the capture of radioactive emissions.

Body Part – 4TH	Radionuclide – 5TH	Qualifier – 6TH	Qualifier – 7TH
0　Brain	1　Technetium 99m (Tc-99m) F　Iodine 123 (I-123) S　Thallium 201 (Tl-201) Y　Other radionuclide	Z　None	Z　None
5　Cerebrospinal Fluid	D　Indium 111 (In-111) Y　Other radionuclide	Z　None	Z　None
Y　Central Nervous System	Y　Other radionuclide	Z　None	Z　None

| 1ST - C Nuclear Medicine |
| 2ND - 0 Central Nervous System |
| 3RD - 3 POSITRON EMISSION (PET) TOMOGRAPHIC IMAGING |

EXAMPLE: PET scan of brain

POSITRON EMISSION TOMOGRAPHIC (PET) IMAGING: Introduction of radioactive materials into the body for three dimensional display of images developed from the simultaneous capture, 180 degrees apart, of radioactive emissions.

Body Part – 4TH	Radionuclide – 5TH	Qualifier – 6TH	Qualifier – 7TH
0　Brain	B　Carbon 11 (C-11) K　Fluorine 18 (F-18) M　Oxygen 15 (O-15) Y　Other radionuclide	Z　None	Z　None
Y　Central Nervous System	Y　Other radionuclide	Z　None	Z　None

NUCLEAR MEDICINE C 03

1ST – **C** Nuclear Medicine

2ND – **0** Central Nervous System

3RD – **5** NONIMAGING NUCLEAR MEDICINE PROBE

EXAMPLE: Xenon gas nonimaging probe of brain

NONIMAGING NUCLEAR MEDICINE PROBE: Introduction of radioactive materials into the body for the study of distribution and fate of certain substances by the detection of radioactive emissions; or, alternatively, measurement of absorption of radioactive emissions from an external source.

Body Part – 4TH	Radionuclide – 5TH	Qualifier – 6TH	Qualifier – 7TH
0 Brain	V Xenon 133 (Xe-133) Y Other radionuclide	Z None	Z None
Y Central Nervous System	Y Other radionuclide	Z None	Z None

1ST – **C** Nuclear Medicine

2ND – **2** Heart

3RD – **1** PLANAR NUCLEAR MEDICINE IMAGING

EXAMPLE: Gallium scan, single plane image

PLANAR NUCLEAR MEDICINE IMAGING: Introduction of radioactive materials into the body for single plane display of images developed from the capture of radioactive emissions.

Body Part – 4TH	Radionuclide – 5TH	Qualifier – 6TH	Qualifier – 7TH
6 Heart, Right and Left	1 Technetium 99m (Tc-99m) Y Other radionuclide	Z None	Z None
G Myocardium	1 Technetium 99m (Tc-99m) D Indium 111 (In-111) S Thallium 201 (Tl-201) Y Other radionuclide Z None	Z None	Z None
Y Heart	Y Other radionuclide	Z None	Z None

1ST – **C** Nuclear Medicine

2ND – **2** Heart

3RD – **2** TOMOGRAPHIC (TOMO) NUCLEAR MEDICINE IMAGING

EXAMPLE: Tomo scan of breast

TOMOGRAPHIC (TOMO) NUCLEAR MEDICINE IMAGING: Introduction of radioactive materials into the body for three dimensional display of images developed from the capture of radioactive emissions.

Body Part – 4TH	Radionuclide – 5TH	Qualifier – 6TH	Qualifier – 7TH
6 Heart, Right and Left	1 Technetium 99m (Tc-99m) Y Other radionuclide	Z None	Z None
G Myocardium	1 Technetium 99m (Tc-99m) D Indium 111 (In-111) K Fluorine 18 (F-18) S Thallium 201 (Tl-201) Y Other radionuclide Z None	Z None	Z None
Y Heart	Y Other radionuclide	Z None	Z None

NUCLEAR MEDICINE C 0 5

1ST - C Nuclear Medicine 2ND - 2 Heart 3RD - 3 POSITRON EMISSION (PET) TOMOGRAPHIC IMAGING	EXAMPLE: PET scan of brain **POSITRON EMISSION TOMOGRAPHIC (PET) IMAGING:** Introduction of radioactive materials into the body for three dimensional display of images developed from the simultaneous capture, 180 degrees apart, of radioactive emissions.

Body Part – 4TH	Radionuclide – 5TH	Qualifier – 6TH	Qualifier – 7TH
G Myocardium	K Fluorine 18 (F-18) M Oxygen 15 (O-15) Q Rubidium 82 (Rb-82) R Nitrogen 13 (N-13) Y Other radionuclide	Z None	Z None
Y Heart	Y Other radionuclide	Z None	Z None

1ST - C Nuclear Medicine 2ND - 2 Heart 3RD - 5 NONIMAGING NUCLEAR MEDICINE PROBE	EXAMPLE: Xenon gas nonimaging probe of brain **NONIMAGING NUCLEAR MEDICINE PROBE:** Introduction of radioactive materials into the body for the study of distribution and fate of certain substances by the detection of radioactive emissions; or, alternatively, measurement of absorption of radioactive emissions from an external source.

Body Part – 4TH	Radionuclide – 5TH	Qualifier – 6TH	Qualifier – 7TH
6 Heart, Right and Left	1 Technetium 99m (Tc-99m) Y Other radionuclide	Z None	Z None
Y Heart	Y Other radionuclide	Z None	Z None

1ST - C Nuclear Medicine 2ND - 5 Veins 3RD - 1 PLANAR NUCLEAR MEDICINE IMAGING	EXAMPLE: Gallium scan, single plane image **PLANAR NUCLEAR MEDICINE IMAGING:** Introduction of radioactive materials into the body for single plane display of images developed from the capture of radioactive emissions.

Body Part – 4TH	Radionuclide – 5TH	Qualifier – 6TH	Qualifier – 7TH
B Lower Extremity Veins, Right C Lower Extremity Veins, Left D Lower Extremity Veins, Bilateral N Upper Extremity Veins, Right P Upper Extremity Veins, Left Q Upper Extremity Veins, Bilateral R Central Veins	1 Technetium 99m (Tc-99m) Y Other radionuclide	Z None	Z None
Y Veins	Y Other radionuclide	Z None	Z None

NUCLEAR MEDICINE C 5 1

1ST – **C** Nuclear Medicine 2ND – **7** Lymphatic and Hematologic System 3RD – **1** PLANAR NUCLEAR MEDICINE IMAGING	EXAMPLE: Gallium scan, single plane image **PLANAR NUCLEAR MEDICINE IMAGING:** Introduction of radioactive materials into the body for single plane display of images developed from the capture of radioactive emissions.

Body Part – 4TH	Radionuclide – 5TH	Qualifier – 6TH	Qualifier – 7TH
0 Bone Marrow	1 Technetium 99m (Tc-99m) D Indium 111 (In-111) Y Other radionuclide	Z None	Z None
2 Spleen 5 Lymphatics, Head and Neck D Lymphatics, Pelvic J Lymphatics, Head K Lymphatics, Neck L Lymphatics, Upper Chest M Lymphatics, Trunk N Lymphatics, Upper Extremity P Lymphatics, Lower Extremity	1 Technetium 99m (Tc-99m) Y Other radionuclide	Z None	Z None
3 Blood	D Indium 111 (In-111) Y Other radionuclide	Z None	Z None
Y Lymphatic and Hematologic System	Y Other radionuclide	Z None	Z None

---

1ST – **C** Nuclear Medicine 2ND – **7** Lymphatic and Hematologic System 3RD – **2** TOMOGRAPHIC (TOMO) NUCLEAR MEDICINE IMAGING	EXAMPLE: Tomo scan of breast **TOMOGRAPHIC (TOMO) NUCLEAR MEDICINE IMAGING:** Introduction of radioactive materials into the body for three dimensional display of images developed from the capture of radioactive emissions.

Body Part – 4TH	Radionuclide – 5TH	Qualifier – 6TH	Qualifier – 7TH
2 Spleen	1 Technetium 99m (Tc-99m) Y Other radionuclide	Z None	Z None
Y Lymphatic and Hematologic System	Y Other radionuclide	Z None	Z None

---

1ST – **C** Nuclear Medicine 2ND – **7** Lymphatic and Hematologic System 3RD – **5** NONIMAGING NUCLEAR MEDICINE PROBE	EXAMPLE: Xenon gas nonimaging probe of brain **NONIMAGING NUCLEAR MEDICINE PROBE:** Introduction of radioactive materials into the body for the study of distribution and fate of certain substances by the detection of radioactive emissions; or, alternatively, measurement of absorption of radioactive emissions from an external source.

Body Part – 4TH	Radionuclide – 5TH	Qualifier – 6TH	Qualifier – 7TH
5 Lymphatics, Head and Neck D Lymphatics, Pelvic J Lymphatics, Head K Lymphatics, Neck L Lymphatics, Upper Chest M Lymphatics, Trunk N Lymphatics, Upper Extremity P Lymphatics, Lower Extremity	1 Technetium 99m (Tc-99m) Y Other radionuclide	Z None	Z None
Y Lymphatic and Hematologic System	Y Other radionuclide	Z None	Z None

NUCLEAR MEDICINE C 7 1

1ST - C Nuclear Medicine	EXAMPLE: Technetium assay of kidneys
2ND - 7 Lymphatic and Hematologic System	**NONIMAGING NUCLEAR MEDICINE ASSAY:** Introduction of radioactive materials into the body for the study of body fluids and blood elements, by the detection of radioactive emissions.
3RD - 6 NONIMAGING NUCLEAR MEDICINE ASSAY	

Body Part – 4TH	Radionuclide – 5TH	Qualifier – 6TH	Qualifier – 7TH
3　Blood	1　Technetium 99m (Tc-99m) 7　Cobalt 58 (Co-58) C　Cobalt 57 (Co-57) D　Indium 111 (In-111) H　Iodine 125 (I-125) W　Chromium (Cr-51) Y　Other radionuclide	Z　None	Z　None
Y　Lymphatic and Hematologic System	Y　Other radionuclide	Z　None	Z　None

1ST - C Nuclear Medicine	EXAMPLE: Gallium scan, single plane image
2ND - 8 Eye	**PLANAR NUCLEAR MEDICINE IMAGING:** Introduction of radioactive materials into the body for single plane display of images developed from the capture of radioactive emissions.
3RD - 1 PLANAR NUCLEAR MEDICINE IMAGING	

Body Part – 4TH	Radionuclide – 5TH	Qualifier – 6TH	Qualifier – 7TH
9　Lacrimal Ducts, Bilateral	1　Technetium 99m (Tc-99m) Y　Other radionuclide	Z　None	Z　None
Y　Eye	Y　Other radionuclide	Z　None	Z　None

1ST - C Nuclear Medicine	EXAMPLE: Gallium scan, single plane image
2ND - 9 Ear, Nose, Mouth and Throat	**PLANAR NUCLEAR MEDICINE IMAGING:** Introduction of radioactive materials into the body for single plane display of images developed from the capture of radioactive emissions.
3RD - 1 PLANAR NUCLEAR MEDICINE IMAGING	

Body Part – 4TH	Radionuclide – 5TH	Qualifier – 6TH	Qualifier – 7TH
B　Salivary Glands, Bilateral	1　Technetium 99m (Tc-99m) Y　Other radionuclide	Z　None	Z　None
Y　Ear, Nose, Mouth and Throat	Y　Other radionuclide	Z　None	Z　None

NUCLEAR MEDICINE C 91

1ST - **C** Nuclear Medicine

2ND - **B** Respiratory System

3RD - **1** PLANAR NUCLEAR MEDICINE IMAGING

EXAMPLE: Gallium scan, single plane image

PLANAR NUCLEAR MEDICINE IMAGING: Introduction of radioactive materials into the body for single plane display of images developed from the capture of radioactive emissions.

Body Part – 4TH	Radionuclide – 5TH	Qualifier – 6TH	Qualifier – 7TH
2 Lungs and Bronchi	1 Technetium 99m (Tc-99m) 9 Krypton (Kr-81m) T Xenon 127 (Xe-127) V Xenon 133 (Xe-133) Y Other radionuclide	Z None	Z None
Y Respiratory System	Y Other radionuclide	Z None	Z None

1ST - **C** Nuclear Medicine

2ND - **B** Respiratory System

3RD - **2** TOMOGRAPHIC (TOMO) NUCLEAR MEDICINE IMAGING

EXAMPLE: Tomo scan of breast

TOMOGRAPHIC (TOMO) NUCLEAR MEDICINE IMAGING: Introduction of radioactive materials into the body for three dimensional display of images developed from the capture of radioactive emissions.

Body Part – 4TH	Radionuclide – 5TH	Qualifier – 6TH	Qualifier – 7TH
2 Lungs and Bronchi	1 Technetium 99m (Tc-99m) 9 Krypton (Kr-81m) Y Other radionuclide	Z None	Z None
Y Respiratory System	Y Other radionuclide	Z None	Z None

1ST - **C** Nuclear Medicine

2ND - **B** Respiratory System

3RD - **3** POSITRON EMISSION (PET) TOMOGRAPHIC IMAGING

EXAMPLE: PET scan of brain

POSITRON EMISSION TOMOGRAPHIC (PET) IMAGING: Introduction of radioactive materials into the body for three dimensional display of images developed from the simultaneous capture, 180 degrees apart, of radioactive emissions.

Body Part – 4TH	Radionuclide – 5TH	Qualifier – 6TH	Qualifier – 7TH
2 Lungs and Bronchi	K Fluorine 18 (F-18) Y Other radionuclide	Z None	Z None
Y Respiratory System	Y Other radionuclide	Z None	Z None

1ST - C Nuclear Medicine
2ND - D Gastrointestinal System
3RD - 1 PLANAR NUCLEAR MEDICINE IMAGING

EXAMPLE: Gallium scan, single plane image

PLANAR NUCLEAR MEDICINE IMAGING: Introduction of radioactive materials into the body for single plane display of images developed from the capture of radioactive emissions.

Body Part – 4TH	Radionuclide – 5TH	Qualifier – 6TH	Qualifier – 7TH
5 Upper Gastrointestinal Tract 7 Gastrointestinal Tract	1 Technetium 99m (Tc-99m) D Indium 111 (In-111) Y Other radionuclide	Z None	Z None
Y Digestive System	Y Other radionuclide	Z None	Z None

1ST - C Nuclear Medicine
2ND - D Gastrointestinal System
3RD - 2 TOMOGRAPHIC (TOMO) NUCLEAR MEDICINE IMAGING

EXAMPLE: Tomo scan of breast

TOMOGRAPHIC (TOMO) NUCLEAR MEDICINE IMAGING: Introduction of radioactive materials into the body for three dimensional display of images developed from the capture of radioactive emissions.

Body Part – 4TH	Radionuclide – 5TH	Qualifier – 6TH	Qualifier – 7TH
7 Gastrointestinal Tract	1 Technetium 99m (Tc-99m) D Indium 111 (In-111) Y Other radionuclide	Z None	Z None
Y Digestive System	Y Other radionuclide	Z None	Z None

1ST - C Nuclear Medicine
2ND - F Hepatobiliary System and Pancreas
3RD - 1 PLANAR NUCLEAR MEDICINE IMAGING

EXAMPLE: Gallium scan, single plane image

PLANAR NUCLEAR MEDICINE IMAGING: Introduction of radioactive materials into the body for single plane display of images developed from the capture of radioactive emissions.

Body Part – 4TH	Radionuclide – 5TH	Qualifier – 6TH	Qualifier – 7TH
4 Gallbladder 5 Liver 6 Liver and Spleen C Hepatobiliary System, All	1 Technetium 99m (Tc-99m) Y Other radionuclide	Z None	Z None
Y Hepatobiliary System and Pancreas	Y Other radionuclide	Z None	Z None

NUCLEAR MEDICINE C F 1

1ST - **C** Nuclear Medicine 2ND - **F** Hepatobiliary System and Pancreas 3RD - **2** TOMOGRAPHIC (TOMO) NUCLEAR MEDICINE IMAGING	EXAMPLE: Tomo scan of breast **TOMOGRAPHIC (TOMO) NUCLEAR MEDICINE IMAGING:** Introduction of radioactive materials into the body for three dimensional display of images developed from the capture of radioactive emissions.

Body Part – 4TH	Radionuclide – 5TH	Qualifier – 6TH	Qualifier – 7TH
4 Gallbladder 5 Liver 6 Liver and Spleen	1 Technetium 99m (Tc-99m) Y Other radionuclide	Z None	Z None
Y Hepatobiliary System and Pancreas	Y Other radionuclide	Z None	Z None

1ST - **C** Nuclear Medicine 2ND - **G** Endocrine System 3RD - **1** PLANAR NUCLEAR MEDICINE IMAGING	EXAMPLE: Gallium scan, single plane image **PLANAR NUCLEAR MEDICINE IMAGING:** Introduction of radioactive materials into the body for single plane display of images developed from the capture of radioactive emissions.

Body Part – 4TH	Radionuclide – 5TH	Qualifier – 6TH	Qualifier – 7TH
1 Parathyroid Glands	1 Technetium 99m (Tc-99m) S Thallium 201 (Tl-201) Y Other radionuclide	Z None	Z None
2 Thyroid Gland	1 Technetium 99m (Tc-99m) F Iodine 123 (I-123) G Iodine 131 (I-131) Y Other radionuclide	Z None	Z None
4 Adrenal Glands, Bilateral	G Iodine 131 (I-131) Y Other radionuclide	Z None	Z None
Y Endocrine System	Y Other radionuclide	Z None	Z None

1ST - **C** Nuclear Medicine 2ND - **G** Endocrine System 3RD - **2** TOMOGRAPHIC (TOMO) NUCLEAR MEDICINE IMAGING	EXAMPLE: Tomo scan of breast **TOMOGRAPHIC (TOMO) NUCLEAR MEDICINE IMAGING:** Introduction of radioactive materials into the body for three dimensional display of images developed from the capture of radioactive emissions.

Body Part – 4TH	Radionuclide – 5TH	Qualifier – 6TH	Qualifier – 7TH
1 Parathyroid Glands	1 Technetium 99m (Tc-99m) S Thallium 201 (Tl-201) Y Other radionuclide	Z None	Z None
Y Endocrine System	Y Other radionuclide	Z None	Z None

1ST - C Nuclear Medicine 2ND - G Endocrine System 3RD - 4 NONIMAGING NUCLEAR MEDICINE UPTAKE	EXAMPLE: Iodine uptake test of thyroid **NONIMAGING NUCLEAR MEDICINE UPTAKE:** Introduction of radioactive materials into the body for measurements of organ function, from the detection of radioactive emissions.

Body Part – 4TH	Radionuclide – 5TH	Qualifier – 6TH	Qualifier – 7TH
2　Thyroid Gland	1　Technetium 99m (Tc-99m) F　Iodine 123 (I-123) G　Iodine 131 (I-131) Y　Other radionuclide	Z　None	Z　None
Y　Endocrine System	Y　Other radionuclide	Z　None	Z　None

1ST - C Nuclear Medicine 2ND - H Skin, Subcutaneous Tissue and Breast 3RD - 1 PLANAR NUCLEAR MEDICINE IMAGING	EXAMPLE: Gallium scan, single plane image **PLANAR NUCLEAR MEDICINE IMAGING:** Introduction of radioactive materials into the body for single plane display of images developed from the capture of radioactive emissions.

Body Part – 4TH	Radionuclide – 5TH	Qualifier – 6TH	Qualifier – 7TH
0　Breast, Right 1　Breast, Left 2　Breasts, Bilateral	1　Technetium 99m (Tc-99m) S　Thallium 201 (Tl-201) Y　Other radionuclide	Z　None	Z　None
Y　Skin, Subcutaneous Tissue and Breast	Y　Other radionuclide	Z　None	Z　None

1ST - C Nuclear Medicine 2ND - H Skin, Subcutaneous Tissue and Breast 3RD - 2 TOMOGRAPHIC (TOMO) NUCLEAR MEDICINE IMAGING	EXAMPLE: Tomo scan of breast **TOMOGRAPHIC (TOMO) NUCLEAR MEDICINE IMAGING:** Introduction of radioactive materials into the body for three dimensional display of images developed from the capture of radioactive emissions.

Body Part – 4TH	Radionuclide – 5TH	Qualifier – 6TH	Qualifier – 7TH
0　Breast, Right 1　Breast, Left 2　Breasts, Bilateral	1　Technetium 99m (Tc-99m) S　Thallium 201 (Tl-201) Y　Other radionuclide	Z　None	Z　None
Y　Skin, Subcutaneous Tissue and Breast	Y　Other radionuclide	Z　None	Z　None

NUCLEAR MEDICINE C H 2

1ST – **C** Nuclear Medicine

2ND – **P** Musculoskeletal System

3RD – **1** PLANAR NUCLEAR MEDICINE IMAGING

EXAMPLE: Gallium scan, single plane image

PLANAR NUCLEAR MEDICINE IMAGING: Introduction of radioactive materials into the body for single plane display of images developed from the capture of radioactive emissions.

Body Part – 4TH	Radionuclide – 5TH	Qualifier – 6TH	Qualifier – 7TH
1 Skull 4 Thorax 5 Spine 6 Pelvis 7 Spine and Pelvis 8 Upper Extremity, Right 9 Upper Extremity, Left B Upper Extremities, Bilateral C Lower Extremity, Right D Lower Extremity, Left F Lower Extremities, Bilateral Z Musculoskeletal System, All	1 Technetium 99m (Tc-99m) Y Other radionuclide	Z None	Z None
Y Musculoskeletal System, Other	Y Other radionuclide	Z None	Z None

1ST – **C** Nuclear Medicine

2ND – **P** Musculoskeletal System

3RD – **2** TOMOGRAPHIC (TOMO) NUCLEAR MEDICINE IMAGING

EXAMPLE: Tomo scan of breast

TOMOGRAPHIC (TOMO) NUCLEAR MEDICINE IMAGING: Introduction of radioactive materials into the body for three dimensional display of images developed from the capture of radioactive emissions.

Body Part – 4TH	Radionuclide – 5TH	Qualifier – 6TH	Qualifier – 7TH
1 Skull 2 Cervical Spine 3 Skull and Cervical Spine 4 Thorax 6 Pelvis 7 Spine and Pelvis 8 Upper Extremity, Right 9 Upper Extremity, Left B Upper Extremities, Bilateral C Lower Extremity, Right D Lower Extremity, Left F Lower Extremities, Bilateral G Thoracic Spine H Lumbar Spine J Thoracolumbar Spine	1 Technetium 99m (Tc-99m) Y Other radionuclide	Z None	Z None
Y Musculoskeletal System, Other	Y Other radionuclide	Z None	Z None

1ST - **C** Nuclear Medicine	EXAMPLE: Xenon gas nonimaging probe of brain
2ND - **P** Musculoskeletal System	**NONIMAGING NUCLEAR MEDICINE PROBE:** Introduction of radioactive materials into the body for the study of distribution and fate of certain substances by the detection of radioactive emissions; or, alternatively, measurement of absorption of radioactive emissions from an external source.
3RD - **5** NONIMAGING NUCLEAR MEDICINE PROBE	

Body Part – 4TH	Radionuclide – 5TH	Qualifier – 6TH	Qualifier – 7TH
5 Spine N Upper Extremities P Lower Extremities	Z None	Z None	Z None
Y Musculoskeletal System, Other	Y Other radionuclide	Z None	Z None

1ST - **C** Nuclear Medicine	EXAMPLE: Gallium scan, single plane image
2ND - **T** Urinary System	**PLANAR NUCLEAR MEDICINE IMAGING:** Introduction of radioactive materials into the body for single plane display of images developed from the capture of radioactive emissions.
3RD - **1** PLANAR NUCLEAR MEDICINE IMAGING	

Body Part – 4TH	Radionuclide – 5TH	Qualifier – 6TH	Qualifier – 7TH
3 Kidneys, Ureters and Bladder	1 Technetium 99m (Tc-99m) F Iodine 123 (I-123) G Iodine 131 (I-131) Y Other radionuclide	Z None	Z None
H Bladder and Ureters	1 Technetium 99m (Tc-99m) Y Other radionuclide	Z None	Z None
Y Urinary System	Y Other radionuclide	Z None	Z None

1ST - **C** Nuclear Medicine	EXAMPLE: Tomo scan of breast
2ND - **T** Urinary System	**TOMOGRAPHIC (TOMO) NUCLEAR MEDICINE IMAGING:** Introduction of radioactive materials into the body for three dimensional display of images developed from the capture of radioactive emissions.
3RD - **2** TOMOGRAPHIC (TOMO) NUCLEAR MEDICINE IMAGING	

Body Part – 4TH	Radionuclide – 5TH	Qualifier – 6TH	Qualifier – 7TH
3 Kidneys, Ureters and Bladder	1 Technetium 99m (Tc-99m) Y Other radionuclide	Z None	Z None
Y Urinary System	Y Other radionuclide	Z None	Z None

NUCLEAR MEDICINE C T 2

1ST – C	Nuclear Medicine
2ND – T	Urinary System
3RD – 6	NONIMAGING NUCLEAR MEDICINE ASSAY

EXAMPLE: Technetium assay of kidneys

NONIMAGING NUCLEAR MEDICINE ASSAY: Introduction of radioactive materials into the body for the study of body fluids and blood elements, by the detection of radioactive emissions.

Body Part – 4TH	Radionuclide – 5TH	Qualifier – 6TH	Qualifier – 7TH
3 Kidneys, Ureters and Bladder	1 Technetium 99m (Tc-99m) F Iodine 123 (I-123) G Iodine 131 (I-131) H Iodine 125 (I-125) Y Other radionuclide	Z None	Z None
Y Urinary System	Y Other radionuclide	Z None	Z None

1ST – C	Nuclear Medicine
2ND – V	Male Reproductive System
3RD – 1	PLANAR NUCLEAR MEDICINE IMAGING

EXAMPLE: Gallium scan, single plane image

PLANAR NUCLEAR MEDICINE IMAGING: Introduction of radioactive materials into the body for single plane display of images developed from the capture of radioactive emissions.

Body Part – 4TH	Radionuclide – 5TH	Qualifier – 6TH	Qualifier – 7TH
9 Testicles, Bilateral ♂	1 Technetium 99m (Tc-99m) Y Other radionuclide	Z None	Z None
Y Male Reproductive System ♂	Y Other radionuclide	Z None	Z None

1ST - C Nuclear Medicine	EXAMPLE: Gallium scan, single plane image
2ND - W Anatomical Regions	**PLANAR NUCLEAR MEDICINE IMAGING:**
3RD - 1 PLANAR NUCLEAR MEDICINE IMAGING	Introduction of radioactive materials into the body for single plane display of images developed from the capture of radioactive emissions.

Body Part – 4TH	Radionuclide – 5TH	Qualifier – 6TH	Qualifier – 7TH
0 Abdomen 1 Abdomen and Pelvis 4 Chest and Abdomen 6 Chest and Neck B Head and Neck D Lower Extremity J Pelvic Region M Upper Extremity N Whole Body	1 Technetium 99m (Tc-99m) D Indium 111 (In-111) F Iodine 123 (I-123) G Iodine 131 (I-131) L Gallium 67 (Ga-67) S Thallium 201 (Tl-201) Y Other radionuclide	Z None	Z None
3 Chest	1 Technetium 99m (Tc-99m) D Indium 111 (In-111) F Iodine 123 (I-123) G Iodine 131 (I-131) K Fluorine 18 (F-18) L Gallium 67 (Ga-67) S Thallium 201 (Tl-201) Y Other radionuclide	Z None	Z None
Y Anatomical Regions, Multiple	Y Other radionuclide	Z None	Z None
Z Anatomical Region, Other	Z None	Z None	Z None

1ST - C Nuclear Medicine	EXAMPLE: Tomo scan of breast
2ND - W Anatomical Regions	**TOMOGRAPHIC (TOMO) NUCLEAR MEDICINE IMAGING:** Introduction of
3RD - 2 TOMOGRAPHIC (TOMO) NUCLEAR MEDICINE IMAGING	radioactive materials into the body for three dimensional display of images developed from the capture of radioactive emissions.

Body Part – 4TH	Radionuclide – 5TH	Qualifier – 6TH	Qualifier – 7TH
0 Abdomen 1 Abdomen and Pelvis 3 Chest 4 Chest and Abdomen 6 Chest and Neck B Head and Neck D Lower Extremity J Pelvic Region M Upper Extremity	1 Technetium 99m (Tc-99m) D Indium 111 (In-111) F Iodine 123 (I-123) G Iodine 131 (I-131) K Fluorine 18 (F-18) L Gallium 67 (Ga-67) S Thallium 201 (Tl-201) Y Other radionuclide	Z None	Z None
Y Anatomical Regions, Multiple	Y Other radionuclide	Z None	Z None

NUCLEAR MEDICINE C W 2

Table CW3 (PET) — Positron Emission Tomographic Imaging

1ST – C	Nuclear Medicine
2ND – W	Anatomical Regions
3RD – 3	POSITRON EMISSION (PET) TOMOGRAPHIC IMAGING

EXAMPLE: PET scan of brain

POSITRON EMISSION TOMOGRAPHIC (PET) IMAGING: Introduction of radioactive materials into the body for three dimensional display of images developed from the simultaneous capture, 180 degrees apart, of radioactive emissions.

Body Part – 4TH	Radionuclide – 5TH	Qualifier – 6TH	Qualifier – 7TH
N Whole Body	Y Other radionuclide	Z None	Z None

Table CW5 — Nonimaging Nuclear Medicine Probe

1ST – C	Nuclear Medicine
2ND – W	Anatomical Regions
3RD – 5	NONIMAGING NUCLEAR MEDICINE PROBE

EXAMPLE: Xenon gas nonimaging probe of brain

NONIMAGING NUCLEAR MEDICINE PROBE: Introduction of radioactive materials into the body for the study of distribution and fate of certain substances by the detection of radioactive emissions; or, alternatively, measurement of absorption of radioactive emissions from an external source.

Body Part – 4TH	Radionuclide – 5TH	Qualifier – 6TH	Qualifier – 7TH
0 Abdomen 1 Abdomen and Pelvis 3 Chest 4 Chest and Abdomen 6 Chest and Neck B Head and Neck D Lower Extremity J Pelvic Region M Upper Extremity	1 Technetium 99m (Tc-99m) D Indium 111 (In-111) Y Other radionuclide	Z None	Z None

Table CW7 — Systemic Nuclear Medicine Therapy

1ST – C	Nuclear Medicine
2ND – W	Anatomical Regions
3RD – 7	SYSTEMIC NUCLEAR MEDICINE THERAPY

EXAMPLE: None

SYSTEMIC NUCLEAR MEDICINE THERAPY: Introduction of unsealed radioactive materials into the body for treatment.

Body Part – 4TH	Radionuclide – 5TH	Qualifier – 6TH	Qualifier – 7TH
0 Abdomen 3 Chest	N Phosphorus 32 (P-32) Y Other radionuclide	Z None	Z None
G Thyroid	G Iodine 131 (I-131) Y Other radionuclide	Z None	Z None
N Whole Body	8 Samarium 153 (Sm-153) G Iodine 131 (I-131) N Phosphorus 32 (P-32) P Strontium 89 (Sr-89) Y Other radionuclide	Z None	Z None
Y Anatomical Regions, Multiple	Y Other radionuclide	Z None	Z None

Educational Annotations | Section D – Radiation Therapy

Section Specific Educational Annotations for the Radiation Therapy Section include:
- AHA Coding Clinic® Reference Notations
- Coding Notes

AHA Coding Clinic® Reference Notations of Radiation Therapy

ROOT TYPE SPECIFIC - RADIATION THERAPY - Section D
BEAM RADIATION - 0
BRACHYTHERAPY - 1
STEREOTACTIC RADIOSURGERY - 3
OTHER RADIATION - Y

Coding Notes of Radiation Therapy

Ancillary Section Specific PCS Reference Manual Exercises

PCS CODE	D – RADIATION THERAPY EXERCISES
D 0 0 1 1 Z Z	8 MeV photon beam radiation to brain.
D 0 1 6 B 9 Z	LDR brachytherapy to spinal cord using iodine.
D 8 Y 0 F Z Z	Plaque radiation of left eye, single port.
D 9 Y 5 7 Z Z	Contact radiation of tongue.
D D Y 5 C Z Z	IORT of colon, 3 ports.
D F 0 3 4 Z Z	Heavy particle radiation treatment of pancreas, four risk sites.
D M 0 1 3 Z Z	Electron radiation treatment of right breast, custom device.
D V 1 0 9 B Z	HDR Brachytherapy of prostate using Palladium 103.
D W Y 5 G F Z	Whole body Phosphorus 32 administration with risk to hematopoetic system.
D W Y 6 8 Z Z	Hyperthermia oncology treatment of pelvic region.

RADIATION THERAPY D

Educational Annotations | Section D – Radiation Therapy

NOTES

1ST - D Radiation Therapy

2ND - 0 Central and Peripheral Nervous System

3RD - 0 BEAM RADIATION

EXAMPLE: External beam radiation

MODALITY: BEAM RADIATION

Treatment Site – 4TH	Modality Qualifier – 5TH	Isotope – 6TH	Qualifier – 7TH
0 Brain 1 Brain Stem 6 Spinal Cord 7 Peripheral Nerve	0 Photons <1 MeV 1 Photons 1 - 10 MeV 2 Photons >10 MeV 4 Heavy particles (protons, ions) 5 Neutrons 6 Neutron capture	Z None	Z None
0 Brain 1 Brain Stem 6 Spinal Cord 7 Peripheral Nerve	3 Electrons	Z None	0 Intraoperative Z None

---

1ST - D Radiation Therapy

2ND - 0 Central and Peripheral Nervous System

3RD - 1 BRACHYTHERAPY

EXAMPLE: Insertion of radioactive material

MODALITY: BRACHYTHERAPY

Treatment Site – 4TH	Modality Qualifier – 5TH	Isotope – 6TH	Qualifier – 7TH
0 Brain 1 Brain Stem 6 Spinal Cord 7 Peripheral Nerve	9 High dose rate (HDR) B Low dose rate (LDR)	7 Cesium 137 (Cs-137) 8 Iridium 192 (Ir-192) 9 Iodine 125 (I-125) B Palladium 103 (Pd-103) C Californium 252 (Cf-252) Y Other isotope	Z None

---

1ST - D Radiation Therapy

2ND - 0 Central and Peripheral Nervous System

3RD - 2 STEREOTACTIC RADIOSURGERY

EXAMPLE: Particulate stereotactic radiosurgery

MODALITY: STEREOTACTIC RADIOSURGERY

Treatment Site – 4TH	Modality Qualifier – 5TH	Isotope – 6TH	Qualifier – 7TH
0 Brain 1 Brain Stem 6 Spinal Cord 7 Peripheral Nerve	D Stereotactic other photon radiosurgery H Stereotactic particulate radiosurgery J Stereotactic gamma beam radiosurgery	Z None	Z None

1ST – D Radiation Therapy
2ND – 0 Central and Peripheral Nervous System
3RD – Y OTHER RADIATION

EXAMPLE: Laser interstitial thermal therapy

MODALITY: OTHER RADIATION

Treatment Site – 4TH	Modality Qualifier – 5TH	Isotope – 6TH	Qualifier – 7TH
0 Brain	7 Contact radiation	Z None	Z None
1 Brain Stem	8 Hyperthermia		
6 Spinal Cord	F Plaque radiation		
7 Peripheral Nerve	K Laser interstitial thermal therapy		

1ST – D Radiation Therapy
2ND – 7 Lymphatic and Hematologic System
3RD – 0 BEAM RADIATION

EXAMPLE: External beam radiation

MODALITY: BEAM RADIATION

Treatment Site – 4TH	Modality Qualifier – 5TH	Isotope – 6TH	Qualifier – 7TH
0 Bone Marrow	0 Photons <1 MeV	Z None	Z None
1 Thymus	1 Photons 1 - 10 MeV		
2 Spleen	2 Photons >10 MeV		
3 Lymphatics, Neck	4 Heavy particles (protons, ions)		
4 Lymphatics, Axillary	5 Neutrons		
5 Lymphatics, Thorax	6 Neutron capture		
6 Lymphatics, Abdomen			
7 Lymphatics, Pelvis			
8 Lymphatics, Inguinal			
0 Bone Marrow	3 Electrons	Z None	0 Intraoperative
1 Thymus			Z None
2 Spleen			
3 Lymphatics, Neck			
4 Lymphatics, Axillary			
5 Lymphatics, Thorax			
6 Lymphatics, Abdomen			
7 Lymphatics, Pelvis			
8 Lymphatics, Inguinal			

RADIATION THERAPY D 0 Y

| 1ST - D Radiation Therapy 2ND - 7 Lymphatic and Hematologic System 3RD - 1 BRACHYTHERAPY | EXAMPLE: Insertion of radioactive material MODALITY: BRACHYTHERAPY |

Treatment Site – 4TH	Modality Qualifier – 5TH	Isotope – 6TH	Qualifier – 7TH
0 Bone Marrow 1 Thymus 2 Spleen 3 Lymphatics, Neck 4 Lymphatics, Axillary 5 Lymphatics, Thorax 6 Lymphatics, Abdomen 7 Lymphatics, Pelvis 8 Lymphatics, Inguinal	9 High dose rate (HDR) B Low dose rate (LDR)	7 Cesium 137 (Cs-137) 8 Iridium 192 (Ir-192) 9 Iodine 125 (I-125) B Palladium 103 (Pd-103) C Californium 252 (Cf-252) Y Other isotope	Z None

| 1ST - D Radiation Therapy 2ND - 7 Lymphatic and Hematologic System 3RD - 2 STEREOTACTIC RADIOSURGERY | EXAMPLE: Particulate stereotactic radiosurgery MODALITY: STEREOTACTIC RADIOSURGERY |

Treatment Site – 4TH	Modality Qualifier – 5TH	Isotope – 6TH	Qualifier – 7TH
0 Bone Marrow 1 Thymus 2 Spleen 3 Lymphatics, Neck 4 Lymphatics, Axillary 5 Lymphatics, Thorax 6 Lymphatics, Abdomen 7 Lymphatics, Pelvis 8 Lymphatics, Inguinal	D Stereotactic other photon radiosurgery H Stereotactic particulate radiosurgery J Stereotactic gamma beam radiosurgery	Z None	Z None

| 1ST - D Radiation Therapy 2ND - 7 Lymphatic and Hematologic System 3RD - Y OTHER RADIATION | EXAMPLE: Laser interstitial thermal therapy MODALITY: OTHER RADIATION |

Treatment Site – 4TH	Modality Qualifier – 5TH	Isotope – 6TH	Qualifier – 7TH
0 Bone Marrow 1 Thymus 2 Spleen 3 Lymphatics, Neck 4 Lymphatics, Axillary 5 Lymphatics, Thorax 6 Lymphatics, Abdomen 7 Lymphatics, Pelvis 8 Lymphatics, Inguinal	8 Hyperthermia F Plaque radiation	Z None	Z None

RADIATION THERAPY D 7 Y

1ST - D Radiation Therapy	EXAMPLE: External beam radiation
2ND - 8 Eye	MODALITY: BEAM RADIATION
3RD - 0 BEAM RADIATION	

Treatment Site – 4TH	Modality Qualifier – 5TH	Isotope – 6TH	Qualifier – 7TH
0 Eye	0 Photons <1 MeV 1 Photons 1 - 10 MeV 2 Photons >10 MeV 4 Heavy particles (protons, ions) 5 Neutrons 6 Neutron capture	Z None	Z None
0 Eye	3 Electrons	Z None	0 Intraoperative Z None

1ST - D Radiation Therapy	EXAMPLE: Insertion of radioactive material
2ND - 8 Eye	MODALITY: BRACHYTHERAPY
3RD - 1 BRACHYTHERAPY	

Treatment Site – 4TH	Modality Qualifier – 5TH	Isotope – 6TH	Qualifier – 7TH
0 Eye	9 High dose rate (HDR) B Low dose rate (LDR)	7 Cesium 137 (Cs-137) 8 Iridium 192 (Ir-192) 9 Iodine 125 (I-125) B Palladium 103 (Pd-103) C Californium 252 (Cf-252) Y Other isotope	Z None

1ST - D Radiation Therapy	EXAMPLE: Particulate stereotactic radiosurgery
2ND - 8 Eye	MODALITY: STEREOTACTIC RADIOSURGERY
3RD - 2 STEREOTACTIC RADIOSURGERY	

Treatment Site – 4TH	Modality Qualifier – 5TH	Isotope – 6TH	Qualifier – 7TH
0 Eye	D Stereotactic other photon radiosurgery H Stereotactic particulate radiosurgery J Stereotactic gamma beam radiosurgery	Z None	Z None

---

1ST – **D** Radiation Therapy

2ND – **8** Eye

3RD – **Y** OTHER RADIATION

EXAMPLE: Laser interstitial thermal therapy

MODALITY: OTHER RADIATION

Treatment Site – 4TH	Modality Qualifier – 5TH	Isotope – 6TH	Qualifier – 7TH
0 Eye	7 Contact radiation 8 Hyperthermia F Plaque radiation	Z None	Z None

---

1ST – **D** Radiation Therapy

2ND – **9** Ear, Nose, Mouth and Throat

3RD – **0** BEAM RADIATION

EXAMPLE: External beam radiation

MODALITY: BEAM RADIATION

Treatment Site – 4TH	Modality Qualifier – 5TH	Isotope – 6TH	Qualifier – 7TH
0 Ear 7 Sinuses 1 Nose 8 Hard Palate 3 Hypopharynx 9 Soft Palate 4 Mouth B Larynx 5 Tongue D Nasopharynx 6 Salivary Glands F Oropharynx	0 Photons <1 MeV 1 Photons 1 - 10 MeV 2 Photons >10 MeV 4 Heavy particles (protons, ions) 5 Neutrons 6 Neutron capture	Z None	Z None
0 Ear 7 Sinuses 1 Nose 8 Hard Palate 3 Hypopharynx 9 Soft Palate 4 Mouth B Larynx 5 Tongue D Nasopharynx 6 Salivary Glands F Oropharynx	3 Electrons	Z None	0 Intraoperative Z None

---

1ST – **D** Radiation Therapy

2ND – **9** Ear, Nose, Mouth and Throat

3RD – **1** BRACHYTHERAPY

EXAMPLE: Insertion of radioactive material

MODALITY: BRACHYTHERAPY

Treatment Site – 4TH	Modality Qualifier – 5TH	Isotope – 6TH	Qualifier – 7TH

0 Ear   7 Sinuses
1 Nose   8 Hard Palate
3 Hypopharynx   9 Soft Palate
4 Mouth   B Larynx
5 Tongue   D Nasopharynx
6 Salivary Glands F Oropharynx
	9 High dose rate (HDR)
	B Low dose rate (LDR)
		7 Cesium 137
		    (Cs-137)
		8 Iridium 192
		    (Ir-192)
		9 Iodine 125
		    (I-125)
		B Palladium 103
		    (Pd-103)
		C Californium
		    252 (Cf-252)
		Y Other isotope
			Z None

RADIATION THERAPY D 9 1

1ST – **D** Radiation Therapy

2ND – **9** Ear, Nose, Mouth and Throat

3RD – **2** STEREOTACTIC RADIOSURGERY

EXAMPLE: Particulate stereotactic radiosurgery

MODALITY: STEREOTACTIC RADIOSURGERY

Treatment Site – 4TH		Modality Qualifier – 5TH	Isotope – 6TH	Qualifier – 7TH
0 Ear	8 Hard Palate	D Stereotactic other photon radiosurgery	Z None	Z None
1 Nose	9 Soft Palate	H Stereotactic particulate radiosurgery		
4 Mouth	B Larynx	J Stereotactic gamma beam		
5 Tongue	C Pharynx	radiosurgery		
6 Salivary Glands	D Nasopharynx			
7 Sinuses				

1ST – **D** Radiation Therapy

2ND – **9** Ear, Nose, Mouth and Throat

3RD – **Y** OTHER RADIATION

EXAMPLE: Laser interstitial thermal therapy

MODALITY: OTHER RADIATION

Treatment Site – 4TH		Modality Qualifier – 5TH	Isotope – 6TH	Qualifier – 7TH
0 Ear	7 Sinuses	7 Contact radiation	Z None	Z None
1 Nose	8 Hard Palate	8 Hyperthermia		
5 Tongue	9 Soft Palate	F Plaque radiation		
6 Salivary Glands				
3 Hypopharynx		7 Contact radiation	Z None	Z None
F Oropharynx		8 Hyperthermia		
4 Mouth		7 Contact radiation	Z None	Z None
B Larynx		8 Hyperthermia		
D Nasopharynx		C Intraoperative radiation therapy (IORT)		
		F Plaque radiation		
C Pharynx		C Intraoperative radiation therapy (IORT)	Z None	Z None
		F Plaque radiation		

1ST – **D** Radiation Therapy

2ND – **B** Respiratory System

3RD – **0** BEAM RADIATION

EXAMPLE: External beam radiation

MODALITY: BEAM RADIATION

Treatment Site – 4TH		Modality Qualifier – 5TH	Isotope – 6TH	Qualifier – 7TH
0 Trachea	6 Mediastinum	0 Photons <1 MeV	Z None	Z None
1 Bronchus	7 Chest Wall	1 Photons 1 - 10 MeV		
2 Lung	8 Diaphragm	2 Photons >10 MeV		
5 Pleura		4 Heavy particles (protons, ions)		
		5 Neutrons		
		6 Neutron capture		
0 Trachea	6 Mediastinum	3 Electrons	Z None	0 Intraoperative
1 Bronchus	7 Chest Wall			Z None
2 Lung	8 Diaphragm			
5 Pleura				

1ST - D Radiation Therapy
2ND - B Respiratory System
3RD - 1 BRACHYTHERAPY

EXAMPLE: Insertion of radioactive material

MODALITY: BRACHYTHERAPY

Treatment Site – 4TH		Modality Qualifier – 5TH	Isotope – 6TH	Qualifier – 7TH

0 Trachea
1 Bronchus
2 Lung
5 Pleura
	6 Mediastinum
	7 Chest Wall
	8 Diaphragm
		9 High dose rate (HDR)
		B Low dose rate (LDR)
			7 Cesium 137
			  (Cs-137)
			8 Iridium 192
			  (Ir-192)
			9 Iodine 125
			  (I-125)
			B Palladium 103
			  (Pd-103)
			C Californium
			  252 (Cf-252)
			Y Other isotope
				Z None

1ST - D Radiation Therapy
2ND - B Respiratory System
3RD - 2 STEREOTACTIC RADIOSURGERY

EXAMPLE: Particulate stereotactic radiosurgery

MODALITY: STEREOTACTIC RADIOSURGERY

Treatment Site – 4TH		Modality Qualifier – 5TH	Isotope – 6TH	Qualifier – 7TH
0 Trachea 1 Bronchus 2 Lung 5 Pleura	6 Mediastinum 7 Chest Wall 8 Diaphragm	D Stereotactic other photon radiosurgery H Stereotactic particulate radiosurgery J Stereotactic gamma beam radiosurgery	Z None	Z None

1ST - D Radiation Therapy
2ND - B Respiratory System
3RD - Y OTHER RADIATION

EXAMPLE: Laser interstitial thermal therapy

MODALITY: OTHER RADIATION

Treatment Site – 4TH		Modality Qualifier – 5TH	Isotope – 6TH	Qualifier – 7TH
0 Trachea 1 Bronchus 2 Lung 5 Pleura	6 Mediastinum 7 Chest Wall 8 Diaphragm	7 Contact radiation 8 Hyperthermia F Plaque radiation K Laser interstitial thermal therapy	Z None	Z None

R A D I A T I O N T H E R A P Y D B Y

1ST - D Radiation Therapy
2ND - D Gastrointestinal System
3RD - 0 BEAM RADIATION

EXAMPLE: External beam radiation

MODALITY: BEAM RADIATION

Treatment Site – 4TH				Modality Qualifier – 5TH		Isotope – 6TH		Qualifier – 7TH	
0	Esophagus	4	Ileum	0	Photons <1 MeV	Z	None	Z	None
1	Stomach	5	Colon	1	Photons 1 - 10 MeV				
2	Duodenum	7	Rectum	2	Photons >10 MeV				
3	Jejunum			4	Heavy particles (protons, ions)				
				5	Neutrons				
				6	Neutron capture				
0	Esophagus	4	Ileum	3	Electrons	Z	None	0	Intraoperative
1	Stomach	5	Colon					Z	None
2	Duodenum	7	Rectum						
3	Jejunum								

1ST - D Radiation Therapy
2ND - D Gastrointestinal System
3RD - 1 BRACHYTHERAPY

EXAMPLE: Insertion of radioactive material

MODALITY: BRACHYTHERAPY

Treatment Site – 4TH				Modality Qualifier – 5TH		Isotope – 6TH		Qualifier – 7TH	
0	Esophagus	4	Ileum	9	High dose rate (HDR)	7	Cesium 137 (Cs-137)	Z	None
1	Stomach	5	Colon	B	Low dose rate (LDR)	8	Iridium 192 (Ir-192)		
2	Duodenum	7	Rectum			9	Iodine 125 (I-125)		
3	Jejunum					B	Palladium 103 (Pd-103)		
						C	Californium 252 (Cf-252)		
						Y	Other isotope		

1ST - D Radiation Therapy
2ND - D Gastrointestinal System
3RD - 2 STEREOTACTIC RADIOSURGERY

EXAMPLE: Particulate stereotactic radiosurgery

MODALITY: STEREOTACTIC RADIOSURGERY

Treatment Site – 4TH				Modality Qualifier – 5TH		Isotope – 6TH		Qualifier – 7TH	
0	Esophagus	4	Ileum	D	Stereotactic other photon radiosurgery	Z	None	Z	None
1	Stomach	5	Colon	H	Stereotactic particulate radiosurgery				
2	Duodenum	7	Rectum	J	Stereotactic gamma beam radiosurgery				
3	Jejunum								

1ST – **D** Radiation Therapy
2ND – **D** Gastrointestinal System
3RD – **Y** OTHER RADIATION

EXAMPLE: Laser interstitial thermal therapy

MODALITY: OTHER RADIATION

Treatment Site – 4TH	Modality Qualifier – 5TH	Isotope – 6TH	Qualifier – 7TH
0 Esophagus	7 Contact radiation 8 Hyperthermia F Plaque radiation K Laser interstitial thermal therapy	Z None	Z None
1 Stomach 2 Duodenum 3 Jejunum 4 Ileum 5 Colon 7 Rectum	7 Contact radiation 8 Hyperthermia C Intraoperative radiation therapy (IORT) F Plaque radiation K Laser interstitial thermal therapy	Z None	Z None
8 Anus	C Intraoperative radiation therapy (IORT) F Plaque radiation K Laser interstitial thermal therapy	Z None	Z None

1ST – **D** Radiation Therapy
2ND – **F** Hepatobiliary System and Pancreas
3RD – **0** BEAM RADIATION

EXAMPLE: External beam radiation

MODALITY: BEAM RADIATION

Treatment Site – 4TH	Modality Qualifier – 5TH	Isotope – 6TH	Qualifier – 7TH
0 Liver 1 Gallbladder 2 Bile Ducts 3 Pancreas	0 Photons <1 MeV 1 Photons 1 - 10 MeV 2 Photons >10 MeV 4 Heavy particles (protons, ions) 5 Neutrons 6 Neutron capture	Z None	Z None
0 Liver 1 Gallbladder 2 Bile Ducts 3 Pancreas	3 Electrons	Z None	0 Intraoperative Z None

RADIATION THERAPY D F 0

1ST - D Radiation Therapy 2ND - F Hepatobiliary System and Pancreas 3RD - 1 BRACHYTHERAPY	EXAMPLE: Insertion of radioactive material MODALITY: BRACHYTHERAPY

Treatment Site – 4TH	Modality Qualifier – 5TH	Isotope – 6TH	Qualifier – 7TH

0 Liver
1 Gallbladder
2 Bile Ducts
3 Pancreas
	9 High dose rate (HDR)
	B Low dose rate (LDR)
		7 Cesium 137
		  (Cs-137)
		8 Iridium 192
		  (Ir-192)
		9 Iodine 125
		  (I-125)
		B Palladium 103
		  (Pd-103)
		C Californium
		  252 (Cf-252)
		Y Other isotope
			Z None

1ST - D Radiation Therapy 2ND - F Hepatobiliary System and Pancreas 3RD - 2 STEREOTACTIC RADIOSURGERY	EXAMPLE: Particulate stereotactic radiosurgery MODALITY: STEREOTACTIC RADIOSURGERY

Treatment Site – 4TH	Modality Qualifier – 5TH	Isotope – 6TH	Qualifier – 7TH
0 Liver 1 Gallbladder 2 Bile Ducts 3 Pancreas	D Stereotactic other photon radiosurgery H Stereotactic particulate radiosurgery J Stereotactic gamma beam radiosurgery	Z None	Z None

1ST - D Radiation Therapy 2ND - F Hepatobiliary System and Pancreas 3RD - Y OTHER RADIATION	EXAMPLE: Laser interstitial thermal therapy MODALITY: OTHER RADIATION

Treatment Site – 4TH	Modality Qualifier – 5TH	Isotope – 6TH	Qualifier – 7TH
0 Liver 1 Gallbladder 2 Bile Ducts 3 Pancreas	7 Contact radiation 8 Hyperthermia C Intraoperative radiation therapy (IORT) F Plaque radiation K Laser interstitial thermal therapy	Z None	Z None

RADIATION THERAPY D F 1

1ST - D Radiation Therapy
2ND - G Endocrine System
3RD - 0 BEAM RADIATION

EXAMPLE: External beam radiation

MODALITY: BEAM RADIATION

Treatment Site – 4TH	Modality Qualifier – 5TH	Isotope – 6TH	Qualifier – 7TH
0 Pituitary Gland 1 Pineal Body 2 Adrenal Glands 4 Parathyroid Glands 5 Thyroid	0 Photons <1 MeV 1 Photons 1 - 10 MeV 2 Photons >10 MeV 5 Neutrons 6 Neutron capture	Z None	Z None
0 Pituitary Gland 1 Pineal Body 2 Adrenal Glands 4 Parathyroid Glands 5 Thyroid	3 Electrons	Z None	0 Intraoperative Z None

1ST - D Radiation Therapy
2ND - G Endocrine System
3RD - 1 BRACHYTHERAPY

EXAMPLE: Insertion of radioactive material

MODALITY: BRACHYTHERAPY

Treatment Site – 4TH	Modality Qualifier – 5TH	Isotope – 6TH	Qualifier – 7TH
0 Pituitary Gland 1 Pineal Body 2 Adrenal Glands 4 Parathyroid Glands 5 Thyroid	9 High dose rate (HDR) B Low dose rate (LDR)	7 Cesium 137 (Cs-137) 8 Iridium 192 (Ir-192) 9 Iodine 125 (I-125) B Palladium 103 (Pd-103) C Californium 252 (Cf-252) Y Other isotope	Z None

1ST - D Radiation Therapy
2ND - G Endocrine System
3RD - 2 STEREOTACTIC RADIOSURGERY

EXAMPLE: Particulate stereotactic radiosurgery

MODALITY: STEREOTACTIC RADIOSURGERY

Treatment Site – 4TH	Modality Qualifier – 5TH	Isotope – 6TH	Qualifier – 7TH
0 Pituitary Gland 1 Pineal Body 2 Adrenal Glands 4 Parathyroid Glands 5 Thyroid	D Stereotactic other photon radiosurgery H Stereotactic particulate radiosurgery J Stereotactic gamma beam radiosurgery	Z None	Z None

RADIATION THERAPY D G 2

1ST - **D** Radiation Therapy
2ND - **G** Endocrine System
3RD - **Y** OTHER RADIATION

EXAMPLE: Laser interstitial thermal therapy

MODALITY: OTHER RADIATION

Treatment Site – 4TH	Modality Qualifier – 5TH	Isotope – 6TH	Qualifier – 7TH
0 Pituitary Gland 1 Pineal Body 2 Adrenal Glands 4 Parathyroid Glands 5 Thyroid	7 Contact radiation 8 Hyperthermia F Plaque radiation K Laser interstitial thermal therapy	Z None	Z None

1ST - **D** Radiation Therapy
2ND - **H** Skin
3RD - **0** BEAM RADIATION

EXAMPLE: External beam radiation

MODALITY: BEAM RADIATION

Treatment Site – 4TH		Modality Qualifier – 5TH	Isotope – 6TH	Qualifier – 7TH
2 Skin, Face 3 Skin, Neck 4 Skin, Arm 6 Skin, Chest	7 Skin, Back 8 Skin, Abdomen 9 Skin, Buttock B Skin, Leg	0 Photons <1 MeV 1 Photons 1 - 10 MeV 2 Photons >10 MeV 4 Heavy particles (protons, ions) 5 Neutrons 6 Neutron capture	Z None	Z None
2 Skin, Face 3 Skin, Neck 4 Skin, Arm 6 Skin, Chest	7 Skin, Back 8 Skin, Abdomen 9 Skin, Buttock B Skin, Leg	3 Electrons	Z None	0 Intraoperative Z None

1ST - **D** Radiation Therapy
2ND - **H** Skin
3RD - **Y** OTHER RADIATION

EXAMPLE: Laser interstitial thermal therapy

MODALITY: OTHER RADIATION

Treatment Site – 4TH		Modality Qualifier – 5TH	Isotope – 6TH	Qualifier – 7TH
2 Skin, Face 3 Skin, Neck 4 Skin, Arm 6 Skin, Chest	7 Skin, Back 8 Skin, Abdomen 9 Skin, Buttock B Skin, Leg	7 Contact radiation 8 Hyperthermia F Plaque radiation	Z None	Z None
5 Skin, Hand C Skin, Foot		F Plaque radiation	Z None	Z None

1ST - D Radiation Therapy
2ND - M Breast
3RD - 0 BEAM RADIATION

EXAMPLE: External beam radiation

MODALITY: BEAM RADIATION

Treatment Site – 4TH	Modality Qualifier – 5TH	Isotope – 6TH	Qualifier – 7TH
0 Breast, Left 1 Breast, Right	0 Photons <1 MeV 1 Photons 1 - 10 MeV 2 Photons >10 MeV 4 Heavy particles (protons, ions) 5 Neutrons 6 Neutron capture	Z None	Z None
0 Breast, Left 1 Breast, Right	3 Electrons	Z None	0 Intraoperative Z None

1ST - D Radiation Therapy
2ND - M Breast
3RD - 1 BRACHYTHERAPY

EXAMPLE: Insertion of radioactive material

MODALITY: BRACHYTHERAPY

Treatment Site – 4TH	Modality Qualifier – 5TH	Isotope – 6TH	Qualifier – 7TH
0 Breast, Left 1 Breast, Right	9 High dose rate (HDR) B Low dose rate (LDR)	7 Cesium 137 (Cs-137) 8 Iridium 192 (Ir-192) 9 Iodine 125 (I-125) B Palladium 103 (Pd-103) C Californium 252 (Cf-252) Y Other isotope	Z None

1ST - D Radiation Therapy
2ND - M Breast
3RD - 2 STEREOTACTIC RADIOSURGERY

EXAMPLE: Particulate stereotactic radiosurgery

MODALITY: STEREOTACTIC RADIOSURGERY

Treatment Site – 4TH	Modality Qualifier – 5TH	Isotope – 6TH	Qualifier – 7TH
0 Breast, Left 1 Breast, Right	D Stereotactic other photon radiosurgery H Stereotactic particulate radiosurgery J Stereotactic gamma beam radiosurgery	Z None	Z None

RADIATION THERAPY D M 2

1ST – D Radiation Therapy
2ND – M Breast
3RD – Y OTHER RADIATION

EXAMPLE: Laser interstitial thermal therapy

MODALITY: OTHER RADIATION

Treatment Site – 4TH	Modality Qualifier – 5TH	Isotope – 6TH	Qualifier – 7TH
0 Breast, Left 1 Breast, Right	7 Contact radiation 8 Hyperthermia F Plaque radiation K Laser interstitial thermal therapy	Z None	Z None

1ST – D Radiation Therapy
2ND – P Musculoskeletal System
3RD – 0 BEAM RADIATION

EXAMPLE: External beam radiation

MODALITY: BEAM RADIATION

Treatment Site – 4TH		Modality Qualifier – 5TH	Isotope – 6TH	Qualifier – 7TH
0 Skull 2 Maxilla 3 Mandible 4 Sternum 5 Rib(s) 6 Humerus	7 Radius/Ulna 8 Pelvic Bones 9 Femur B Tibia/Fibula C Other Bone	0 Photons <1 MeV 1 Photons 1 - 10 MeV 2 Photons >10 MeV 4 Heavy particles (protons, ions) 5 Neutrons 6 Neutron capture	Z None	Z None
0 Skull 2 Maxilla 3 Mandible 4 Sternum 5 Rib(s) 6 Humerus	7 Radius/Ulna 8 Pelvic Bones 9 Femur B Tibia/Fibula C Other Bone	3 Electrons	Z None	0 Intraoperative Z None

1ST – D Radiation Therapy
2ND – P Musculoskeletal System
3RD – Y OTHER RADIATION

EXAMPLE: Laser interstitial thermal therapy

MODALITY: OTHER RADIATION

Treatment Site – 4TH		Modality Qualifier – 5TH	Isotope – 6TH	Qualifier – 7TH
0 Skull 2 Maxilla 3 Mandible 4 Sternum 5 Rib(s) 6 Humerus	7 Radius/Ulna 8 Pelvic Bones 9 Femur B Tibia/Fibula C Other Bone	7 Contact radiation 8 Hyperthermia F Plaque radiation	Z None	Z None

RADIATION THERAPY D M Y

1ST - D Radiation Therapy
2ND - T Urinary System
3RD - 0 BEAM RADIATION

EXAMPLE: External beam radiation

MODALITY: BEAM RADIATION

Treatment Site – 4TH	Modality Qualifier – 5TH	Isotope – 6TH	Qualifier – 7TH
0 Kidney 1 Ureter 2 Bladder 3 Urethra	0 Photons <1 MeV 1 Photons 1 - 10 MeV 2 Photons >10 MeV 4 Heavy particles (protons, ions) 5 Neutrons 6 Neutron capture	Z None	Z None
0 Kidney 1 Ureter 2 Bladder 3 Urethra	3 Electrons	Z None	0 Intraoperative Z None

1ST - D Radiation Therapy
2ND - T Urinary System
3RD - 1 BRACHYTHERAPY

EXAMPLE: Insertion of radioactive material

MODALITY: BRACHYTHERAPY

Treatment Site – 4TH	Modality Qualifier – 5TH	Isotope – 6TH	Qualifier – 7TH
0 Kidney 1 Ureter 2 Bladder 3 Urethra	9 High dose rate (HDR) B Low dose rate (LDR)	7 Cesium 137 (Cs-137) 8 Iridium 192 (Ir-192) 9 Iodine 125 (I-125) B Palladium 103 (Pd-103) C Californium 252 (Cf-252) Y Other isotope	Z None

1ST - D Radiation Therapy
2ND - T Urinary System
3RD - 2 STEREOTACTIC RADIOSURGERY

EXAMPLE: Particulate stereotactic radiosurgery

MODALITY: STEREOTACTIC RADIOSURGERY

Treatment Site – 4TH	Modality Qualifier – 5TH	Isotope – 6TH	Qualifier – 7TH
0 Kidney 1 Ureter 2 Bladder 3 Urethra	D Stereotactic other photon radiosurgery H Stereotactic particulate radiosurgery J Stereotactic gamma beam radiosurgery	Z None	Z None

RADIATION THERAPY D T 2

1ST – D Radiation Therapy
2ND – T Urinary System
3RD – Y OTHER RADIATION

EXAMPLE: Laser interstitial thermal therapy

MODALITY: OTHER RADIATION

Treatment Site – 4TH	Modality Qualifier – 5TH	Isotope – 6TH	Qualifier – 7TH
0 Kidney 1 Ureter 2 Bladder 3 Urethra	7 Contact radiation 8 Hyperthermia C Intraoperative radiation therapy (IORT) F Plaque radiation	Z None	Z None

1ST – D Radiation Therapy
2ND – U Female Reproductive System ♀
3RD – 0 BEAM RADIATION

EXAMPLE: External beam radiation

MODALITY: BEAM RADIATION

Treatment Site – 4TH	Modality Qualifier – 5TH	Isotope – 6TH	Qualifier – 7TH
0 Ovary 1 Cervix 2 Uterus	0 Photons <1 MeV 1 Photons 1 - 10 MeV 2 Photons >10 MeV 4 Heavy particles (protons, ions) 5 Neutrons 6 Neutron capture	Z None	Z None
0 Ovary 1 Cervix 2 Uterus	3 Electrons	Z None	0 Intraoperative Z None

1ST – D Radiation Therapy
2ND – U Female Reproductive System ♀
3RD – 1 BRACHYTHERAPY

EXAMPLE: Insertion of radioactive material

MODALITY: BRACHYTHERAPY

Treatment Site – 4TH	Modality Qualifier – 5TH	Isotope – 6TH	Qualifier – 7TH
0 Ovary 1 Cervix 2 Uterus	9 High dose rate (HDR) B Low dose rate (LDR)	7 Cesium 137 (Cs-137) 8 Iridium 192 (Ir-192) 9 Iodine 125 (I-125) B Palladium 103 (Pd-103) C Californium 252 (Cf-252) Y Other isotope	Z None

RADIATION THERAPY DTY

Block 1

1ST – **D** Radiation Therapy
2ND – **U** Female Reproductive System ♀
3RD – **2** STEREOTACTIC RADIOSURGERY

EXAMPLE: Particulate stereotactic radiosurgery

MODALITY: STEREOTACTIC RADIOSURGERY

Treatment Site – 4TH	Modality Qualifier – 5TH	Isotope – 6TH	Qualifier – 7TH
0 Ovary 1 Cervix 2 Uterus	D Stereotactic other photon radiosurgery H Stereotactic particulate radiosurgery J Stereotactic gamma beam radiosurgery	Z None	Z None

Block 2

1ST – **D** Radiation Therapy
2ND – **U** Female Reproductive System ♀
3RD – **Y** OTHER RADIATION

EXAMPLE: Laser interstitial thermal therapy

MODALITY: OTHER RADIATION

Treatment Site – 4TH	Modality Qualifier – 5TH	Isotope – 6TH	Qualifier – 7TH
0 Ovary 1 Cervix 2 Uterus	7 Contact radiation 8 Hyperthermia C Intraoperative radiation therapy (IORT) F Plaque radiation	Z None	Z None

Block 3

1ST – **D** Radiation Therapy
2ND – **V** Male Reproductive System ♂
3RD – **0** BEAM RADIATION

EXAMPLE: External beam radiation

MODALITY: BEAM RADIATION

Treatment Site – 4TH	Modality Qualifier – 5TH	Isotope – 6TH	Qualifier – 7TH
0 Prostate 1 Testis	0 Photons <1 MeV 1 Photons 1 - 10 MeV 2 Photons >10 MeV 4 Heavy particles (protons, ions) 5 Neutrons 6 Neutron capture	Z None	Z None
0 Prostate 1 Testis	3 Electrons	Z None	0 Intraoperative Z None

RADIATION THERAPY **D V 0**

Table 1

1ST – **D** Radiation Therapy
2ND – **V** Male Reproductive System ♂
3RD – **1** BRACHYTHERAPY

EXAMPLE: Insertion of radioactive material

MODALITY: BRACHYTHERAPY

Treatment Site – 4TH	Modality Qualifier – 5TH	Isotope – 6TH	Qualifier – 7TH
0 Prostate 1 Testis	9 High dose rate (HDR) B Low dose rate (LDR)	7 Cesium 137 (Cs-137) 8 Iridium 192 (Ir-192) 9 Iodine 125 (I-125) B Palladium 103 (Pd-103) C Californium 252 (Cf-252) Y Other isotope	Z None

Table 2

1ST – **D** Radiation Therapy
2ND – **V** Male Reproductive System ♂
3RD – **2** STEREOTACTIC RADIOSURGERY

EXAMPLE: Particulate stereotactic radiosurgery

MODALITY: STEREOTACTIC RADIOSURGERY

Treatment Site – 4TH	Modality Qualifier – 5TH	Isotope – 6TH	Qualifier – 7TH
0 Prostate 1 Testis	D Stereotactic other photon radiosurgery H Stereotactic particulate radiosurgery J Stereotactic gamma beam radiosurgery	Z None	Z None

Table 3

1ST – **D** Radiation Therapy
2ND – **V** Male Reproductive System ♂
3RD – **Y** OTHER RADIATION

EXAMPLE: Laser interstitial thermal therapy

MODALITY: OTHER RADIATION

Treatment Site – 4TH	Modality Qualifier – 5TH	Isotope – 6TH	Qualifier – 7TH
0 Prostate	7 Contact radiation 8 Hyperthermia C Intraoperative radiation therapy (IORT) F Plaque radiation K Laser interstitial thermal therapy	Z None	Z None
1 Testis	7 Contact radiation 8 Hyperthermia F Plaque radiation	Z None	Z None

RADIATION THERAPY **D V 1**

1ST - D Radiation Therapy
2ND - W Anatomical Regions
3RD - 0 BEAM RADIATION

EXAMPLE: External beam radiation

MODALITY: BEAM RADIATION

Treatment Site – 4TH	Modality Qualifier – 5TH	Isotope – 6TH	Qualifier – 7TH
1 Head and Neck 2 Chest 3 Abdomen 4 Hemibody 5 Whole Body 6 Pelvic Region	0 Photons <1 MeV 1 Photons 1 - 10 MeV 2 Photons >10 MeV 4 Heavy particles (protons, ions) 5 Neutrons 6 Neutron capture	Z None	Z None
1 Head and Neck 2 Chest 3 Abdomen 4 Hemibody 5 Whole Body 6 Pelvic Region	3 Electrons	Z None	0 Intraoperative Z None

1ST - D Radiation Therapy
2ND - W Anatomical Regions
3RD - 1 BRACHYTHERAPY

EXAMPLE: Insertion of radioactive material

MODALITY: BRACHYTHERAPY

Treatment Site – 4TH	Modality Qualifier – 5TH	Isotope – 6TH	Qualifier – 7TH
1 Head and Neck 2 Chest 3 Abdomen 6 Pelvic Region	9 High dose rate (HDR) B Low dose rate (LDR)	7 Cesium 137 (Cs-137) 8 Iridium 192 (Ir-192) 9 Iodine 125 (I-125) B Palladium 103 (Pd-103) C Californium 252 (Cf-252) Y Other isotope	Z None

1ST - D Radiation Therapy
2ND - W Anatomical Regions
3RD - 2 STEREOTACTIC RADIOSURGERY

EXAMPLE: Particulate stereotactic radiosurgery

MODALITY: STEREOTACTIC RADIOSURGERY

Treatment Site – 4TH	Modality Qualifier – 5TH	Isotope – 6TH	Qualifier – 7TH
1 Head and Neck 2 Chest 3 Abdomen 6 Pelvic Region	D Stereotactic other photon radiosurgery H Stereotactic particulate radiosurgery J Stereotactic gamma beam radiosurgery	Z None	Z None

RADIATION THERAPY D W 2

1ST – **D** Radiation Therapy
2ND – **W** Anatomical Regions
3RD – **Y** OTHER RADIATION

EXAMPLE: Laser interstitial thermal therapy

MODALITY: OTHER RADIATION

Treatment Site – 4TH	Modality Qualifier – 5TH	Isotope – 6TH	Qualifier – 7TH
1 Head and Neck 2 Chest 3 Abdomen 4 Hemibody 6 Pelvic Region	7 Contact radiation 8 Hyperthermia F Plaque radiation	Z None	Z None
5 Whole Body	7 Contact radiation 8 Hyperthermia F Plaque radiation	Z None	Z None
5 Whole Body	G Isotope administration	D Iodine 131 (I-131) F Phosphorus 32 (P-32) G Strontium 89 (Sr-89) H Strontium 90 (Sr-90) Y Other isotope	Z None

RADIATION THERAPY D W Y

© 2016 Channel Publishing, Ltd.

Educational Annotations | Section F – Physical Rehabilitation and Diagnostic Audiology

Section Specific Educational Annotations for the Physical Rehabilitation and Diagnostic Audiology Section include:
- AHA Coding Clinic® Reference Notations
- Coding Notes

AHA Coding Clinic® Reference Notations of Physical Rehabilitation and Diagnostic Audiology

ROOT TYPE SPECIFIC - PHYSICAL REHABILITATION AND DIAGNOSTIC AUDIOLOGY - Section F
SPEECH ASSESSMENT - 0
MOTOR AND/OR NERVE FUNCTION ASSESSMENT - 1
ACTIVITIES OF DAILY LIVING ASSESSMENT - 2
HEARING ASSESSMENT - 3
HEARING AID ASSESSMENT - 4
VESTIBULAR ASSESSMENT - 5
SPEECH TREATMENT - 6
MOTOR TREATMENT - 7
ACTIVITIES OF DAILY LIVING TREATMENT - 8
HEARING TREATMENT - 9
COCHLEAR IMPLANT TREATMENT - B
VESTIBULAR TREATMENT - C
DEVICE FITTING - D
CAREGIVER TRAINING - F

Coding Notes of Physical Rehabilitation and Diagnostic Audiology

Ancillary Section Specific PCS Reference Manual Exercises

PCS CODE	F – PHYSICAL REHABILITATION AND DIAGNOSTIC AUDIOLOGY EXERCISES
F 0 0 Z H Y Z	Bedside swallow assessment using assessment kit.
F 0 2 Z F Z Z	Verbal assessment of patient's pain level.
F 0 7 L 0 Z Z	Physical therapy for range of motion and mobility, patient right hip, no special equipment.
F 0 7 M 6 Z Z	Group musculoskeletal balance training exercises, whole body, no special equipment. (Balance training is included in the Motor Treatment reference table under Therapeutic Exercise.)
F 0 9 Z 2 K Z	Individual therapy for auditory processing using tape recorder. (Tape recorder is listed in the equipment reference table under Audiovisual Equipment.)
F 0 D Z 7 E Z	Application of short arm cast in rehabilitation setting. (Inhibitory cast is listed in the equipment reference table under E, Orthosis.)
F 0 D Z 8 U Z	Individual fitting of left eye prosthesis.
F 0 F Z 8 Z Z	Caregiver training in airway clearance techniques.
F 0 F Z J M Z	Caregiver training in communication skills using manual communication board. (Manual communication board is listed in the equipment reference table under M, Augmentative/ Alternative Communication.)
F 1 3 Z 3 1 Z	Bekesy assessment using audiometer.

Educational Annotations

Section F – Physical Rehabilitation and Diagnostic Audiology

NOTES

1ST - **F**   Physical Rehabilitation and Diagnostic Audiology
2ND - **0**   Rehabilitation
3RD - **0**   SPEECH ASSESSMENT

SPEECH ASSESSMENT:

Measurement of speech and related functions.

Body System/Region – 4TH	Type Qualifier – 5TH	Equipment – 6TH	Qualifier 7TH
3 Neurological System - Whole Body	G Communicative/cognitive integration skills	K Audiovisual M Augmentative/alternative communication P Computer Y Other equipment Z None	Z None
Z None	0 Filtered speech 3 Staggered spondaic word Q Performance intensity phonetically balanced speech discrimination R Brief tone stimuli S Distorted speech T Dichotic stimuli V Temporal ordering of stimuli W Masking patterns	1 Audiometer 2 Sound field/booth K Audiovisual Z None	Z None
Z None	1 Speech threshold 2 Speech/word recognition	1 Audiometer 2 Sound field/booth 9 Cochlear implant K Audiovisual Z None	Z None
Z None	4 Sensorineural acuity level	1 Audiometer 2 Sound field/booth Z None	Z None
Z None	5 Synthetic sentence identification	1 Audiometer 2 Sound field/booth 9 Cochlear implant K Audiovisual	Z None
Z None	6 Speech and/or language screening 7 Nonspoken language 8 Receptive/expressive language C Aphasia G Communicative/cognitive integration skills L Augmentative/alternative communication system	K Audiovisual M Augmentative/alternative communication P Computer Y Other equipment Z None	Z None
Z None	9 Articulation/phonology	K Audiovisual P Computer Q Speech analysis Y Other equipment Z None	Z None

continued ⇨

REHAB & AUDIOLOGY **F 0 0**

F 0 0 SPEECH ASSESSMENT —continued

Body System/Region – 4TH	Type Qualifier – 5TH	Equipment – 6TH	Qualifier 7TH
Z None	B Motor speech	K Audiovisual N Biosensory feedback P Computer Q Speech analysis T Aerodynamic function Y Other equipment Z None	Z None
Z None	D Fluency	K Audiovisual N Biosensory feedback P Computer Q Speech analysis S Voice analysis T Aerodynamic function Y Other equipment Z None	Z None
Z None	F Voice	K Audiovisual N Biosensory feedback P Computer S Voice analysis T Aerodynamic function Y Other equipment Z None	Z None
Z None	H Bedside swallowing and oral function P Oral peripheral mechanism	Y Other equipment Z None	Z None
Z None	J Instrumental swallowing and oral function	T Aerodynamic function W Swallowing Y Other equipment	Z None
Z None	K Orofacial myofunctional	K Audiovisual P Computer Y Other equipment Z None	Z None
Z None	M Voice prosthetic	K Audiovisual P Computer S Voice analysis V Speech prosthesis Y Other equipment Z None	Z None
Z None	N Non-invasive instrumental status	N Biosensory feedback P Computer Q Speech analysis S Voice analysis T Aerodynamic function Y Other equipment	Z None
Z None	X Other specified central auditory processing	Z None	Z None

1ST - **F** Physical Rehabilitation and Diagnostic Audiology
2ND - **0** Rehabilitation
3RD - **1 MOTOR AND/OR NERVE FUNCTION ASSESSMENT**

MOTOR AND/OR NERVE FUNCTION ASSESSMENT: Measurement of motor, nerve, and related functions.

Body System/Region — 4TH	Type Qualifier — 5TH	Equipment — 6TH	Qualifier 7TH
0 Neurological System - Head and Neck 1 Neurological System - Upper Back / Upper Extremity 2 Neurological System - Lower Back / Lower Extremity 3 Neurological System - Whole Body	0 Muscle performance	E Orthosis F Assistive, adaptive, supportive or protective U Prosthesis Y Other equipment Z None	Z None
0 Neurological System - Head and Neck 1 Neurological System - Upper Back / Upper Extremity 2 Neurological System - Lower Back / Lower Extremity 3 Neurological System - Whole Body	1 Integumentary integrity 3 Coordination/dexterity 4 Motor function G Reflex integrity	Z None	Z None
0 Neurological System - Head and Neck 1 Neurological System - Upper Back / Upper Extremity 2 Neurological System - Lower Back / Lower Extremity 3 Neurological System - Whole Body	5 Range of motion and joint integrity 6 Sensory awareness/processing/ integrity	Y Other equipment Z None	Z None

continued ⇨

REHAB & AUDIOLOGY F 0 1

F 0 1 MOTOR ASSESSMENT –*continued*

Body System/Region – 4TH	Type Qualifier – 5TH	Equipment – 6TH	Qualifier 7TH
D Integumentary System - Head and Neck F Integumentary System - Upper Back/Upper Extremity G Integumentary System - Lower Back/Lower Extremity H Integumentary System - Whole Body J Musculoskeletal System - Head and Neck K Musculoskeletal System - Upper Back/Upper Extremity L Musculoskeletal System - Lower Back/Lower Extremity M Musculoskeletal System - Whole Body	0 Muscle performance	E Orthosis F Assistive, adaptive, supportive or protective U Prosthesis Y Other equipment Z None	Z None
D Integumentary System - Head and Neck F Integumentary System - Upper Back/Upper Extremity G Integumentary System - Lower Back/Lower Extremity H Integumentary System - Whole Body J Musculoskeletal System - Head and Neck K Musculoskeletal System - Upper Back/Upper Extremity L Musculoskeletal System - Lower Back/Lower Extremity M Musculoskeletal System - Whole Body	1 Integumentary integrity	Z None	Z None

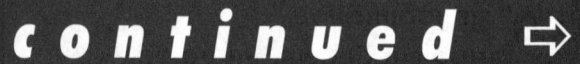
continued ⇨

REHAB & AUDIOLOGY F 0 1

F 0 1 MOTOR ASSESSMENT – *continued*

Body System/Region – 4TH	Type Qualifier – 5TH	Equipment – 6TH	Qualifier 7TH
D Integumentary System - Head and Neck F Integumentary System - Upper Back/Upper Extremity G Integumentary System - Lower Back/Lower Extremity H Integumentary System - Whole Body J Musculoskeletal System - Head and Neck K Musculoskeletal System - Upper Back/Upper Extremity L Musculoskeletal System - Lower Back/Lower Extremity M Musculoskeletal System - Whole Body	5 Range of motion and joint integrity 6 Sensory awareness/processing/ integrity	Y Other equipment Z None	Z None
N Genitourinary System	0 Muscle performance	E Orthosis F Assistive, adaptive, supportive or protective U Prosthesis Y Other equipment Z None	Z None
Z None	2 Visual motor integration	K Audiovisual M Augmentative/alternative communication N Biosensory feedback P Computer Q Speech analysis S Voice analysis Y Other equipment Z None	Z None
Z None	7 Facial nerve function	7 Electrophysiologic	Z None
Z None	9 Somatosensory evoked potentials	J Somatosensory	Z None
Z None	B Bed Mobility C Transfer F Wheelchair mobility	E Orthosis F Assistive, adaptive, supportive or protective U Prosthesis Z None	Z None
Z None	D Gait and/or balance	E Orthosis F Assistive, adaptive, supportive or protective U Prosthesis Y Other equipment Z None	Z None

REHAB & AUDIOLOGY F 0 1

1ST - **F** Physical Rehabilitation and Diagnostic Audiology
2ND - **0** Rehabilitation
3RD - **2** ACTIVITIES OF DAILY LIVING ASSESSMENT

ACTIVITIES OF DAILY LIVING ASSESSMENT: Measurement of functional level for activities of daily living.

Body System/Region – 4TH	Type Qualifier – 5TH	Equipment – 6TH	Qualifier 7TH
0 Neurological System - Head and Neck	9 Cranial nerve integrity D Neuromotor development	Y Other equipment Z None	Z None
1 Neurological System - Upper Back/Upper Extremity 2 Neurological System - Lower Back/Lower Extremity 3 Neurological System - Whole Body	D Neuromotor development	Y Other equipment Z None	Z None
4 Circulatory System - Head and Neck 5 Circulatory System - Upper Back/Upper Extremity 6 Circulatory System - Lower Back/Lower Extremity 8 Respiratory System - Head and Neck 9 Respiratory System - Upper Back/Upper Extremity B Respiratory System - Lower Back/Lower Extremity	G Ventilation, respiration and circulation	C Mechanical G Aerobic endurance and conditioning Y Other equipment Z None	Z None
7 Circulatory System - Whole Body C Respiratory System - Whole Body	7 Aerobic capacity and endurance	E Orthosis G Aerobic endurance and conditioning U Prosthesis Y Other equipment Z None	Z None
7 Circulatory System - Whole Body C Respiratory System - Whole Body	G Ventilation, respiration and circulation	C Mechanical G Aerobic endurance and conditioning Y Other equipment Z None	Z None
Z None	0 Bathing/showering 1 Dressing 3 Grooming/personal hygiene 4 Home management	E Orthosis F Assistive, adaptive, supportive or protective U Prosthesis Z None	Z None
Z None	2 Feeding/eating 8 Anthropometric characteristics F Pain	Y Other equipment Z None	Z None

REHAB & AUDIOLOGY F02

© 2016 Channel Publishing, Ltd.

continued ⇨

F 0 2 ACTVITIES ASSESSMENT —continued

Body System/Region – 4TH	Type Qualifier – 5TH	Equipment – 6TH	Qualifier 7TH
Z None	5 Perceptual processing	K Audiovisual M Augmentative/alternative communication N Biosensory feedback P Computer Q Speech analysis S Voice analysis Y Other equipment Z None	Z None
Z None	6 Psychosocial skills	Z None	Z None
Z None	B Environmental, home and work barriers C Ergonomics and body mechanics	E Orthosis F Assistive, adaptive, supportive or protective U Prosthesis Y Other equipment Z None	Z None
Z None	H Vocational activities and functional community or work reintegration skills	E Orthosis F Assistive, adaptive, supportive or protective G Aerobic endurance and conditioning U Prosthesis Y Other equipment Z None	Z None

1ST – F	Physical Rehabilitation and Diagnostic Audiology
2ND – 0	Rehabilitation
3RD – 6	**SPEECH TREATMENT**

SPEECH TREATMENT: Application of techniques to improve, augment, or compensate for speech and related functional impairment.

Body System/Region – 4TH	Type Qualifier – 5TH	Equipment – 6TH	Qualifier 7TH
3 Neurological System - Whole Body	6 Communicative/cognitive integration skills	K Audiovisual M Augmentative/alternative communication P Computer Y Other equipment Z None	Z None
Z None	0 Nonspoken language 3 Aphasia 6 Communicative/cognitive integration skills	K Audiovisual M Augmentative/alternative communication P Computer Y Other equipment Z None	Z None
Z None	1 Speech-language pathology and related disorders counseling 2 Speech-language pathology and related disorders prevention	K Audiovisual Z None	Z None
Z None	4 Articulation/phonology	K Audiovisual P Computer Q Speech analysis T Aerodynamic function Y Other equipment Z None	Z None
Z None	5 Aural rehabilitation	K Audiovisual L Assistive listening M Augmentative/alternative communication N Biosensory feedback P Computer Q Speech analysis S Voice analysis Y Other equipment Z None	Z None
Z None	7 Fluency	4 Electroacoustic immitance/acoustic reflex K Audiovisual N Biosensory feedback Q Speech analysis S Voice analysis T Aerodynamic function Y Other equipment Z None	Z None

REHAB & AUDIOLOGY F 0 6

continued ⇨

F 0 6 SPEECH TREATMENT —*continued*

Body System/Region – 4TH	Type Qualifier – 5TH	Equipment – 6TH	Qualifier 7TH
Z None	8 Motor speech	K Audiovisual N Biosensory feedback P Computer Q Speech analysis S Voice analysis T Aerodynamic function Y Other equipment Z None	Z None
Z None	9 Orofacial myofunctional	K Audiovisual P Computer Y Other equipment Z None	Z None
Z None	B Receptive/expressive language	K Audiovisual L Assistive listening M Augmentative/alternative communication P Computer Y Other equipment Z None	Z None
Z None	C Voice	K Audiovisual N Biosensory feedback P Computer S Voice analysis T Aerodynamic function V Speech prosthesis Y Other equipment Z None	Z None
Z None	D Swallowing dysfunction	M Augmentative/alternative communication T Aerodynamic function V Speech prosthesis Y Other equipment Z None	Z None

REHAB & AUDIOLOGY **F 0 6**

1ST - **F**	Physical Rehabilitation and Diagnostic Audiology	**MOTOR TREATMENT:** Exercise or activities to increase or facilitate motor function.
2ND - **0**	Rehabilitation	
3RD - **7**	**MOTOR TREATMENT**	

Body System/Region – 4TH	Type Qualifier – 5TH	Equipment – 6TH	Qualifier 7TH
0 Neurological System - Head and Neck	0 Range of motion and joint mobility	E Orthosis	Z None
1 Neurological System - Upper Back/Upper Extremity	1 Muscle performance	F Assistive, adaptive, supportive or protective	
2 Neurological System - Lower Back/Lower Extremity	2 Coordination/dexterity	U Prosthesis	
3 Neurological System - Whole Body	3 Motor function	Y Other equipment	
D Integumentary System - Head and Neck		Z None	
F Integumentary System - Upper Back/Upper Extremity			
G Integumentary System - Lower Back/Lower Extremity			
H Integumentary System - Whole Body			
J Musculoskeletal System - Head and Neck			
K Musculoskeletal System - Upper Back/Upper Extremity			
L Musculoskeletal System - Lower Back/Lower Extremity			
M Musculoskeletal System - Whole Body			

continued ⇨

F 0 7 MOTOR TREATMENT —*continued*

Body System/Region – 4TH	Type Qualifier – 5TH	Equipment – 6TH	Qualifier 7TH
0 Neurological System - Head and Neck 1 Neurological System - Upper Back/Upper Extremity 2 Neurological System - Lower Back/Lower Extremity 3 Neurological System - Whole Body D Integumentary System - Head and Neck F Integumentary System - Upper Back/Upper Extremity G Integumentary System - Lower Back/Lower Extremity H Integumentary System - Whole Body J Musculoskeletal System - Head and Neck K Musculoskeletal System - Upper Back/Upper Extremity L Musculoskeletal System - Lower Back/Lower Extremity M Musculoskeletal System - Whole Body	6 Therapeutic exercise	B Physical Agents C Mechanical D Electrotherapeutic E Orthosis F Assistive, adaptive, supportive or protective G Aerobic endurance and conditioning H Mechanical or electromechanical U Prosthesis Y Other equipment Z None	Z None

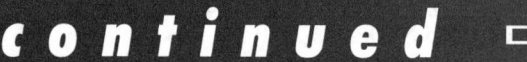

continued ⇨

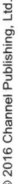

REHAB & AUDIOLOGY F 0 7

© 2016 Channel Publishing, Ltd.

F 0 7 MOTOR TREATMENT – *continued*

Body System/Region – 4TH	Type Qualifier – 5TH	Equipment – 6TH	Qualifier 7TH
0 Neurological System - Head and Neck 1 Neurological System - Upper Back/Upper Extremity 2 Neurological System - Lower Back/Lower Extremity 3 Neurological System - Whole Body D Integumentary System - Head and Neck F Integumentary System - Upper Back/Upper Extremity G Integumentary System - Lower Back/Lower Extremity H Integumentary System - Whole Body J Musculoskeletal System - Head and Neck K Musculoskeletal System - Upper Back/Upper Extremity L Musculoskeletal System - Lower Back/Lower Extremity M Musculoskeletal System - Whole Body	7 Manual therapy techniques	Z None	Z None
4 Circulatory System - Head and Neck 5 Circulatory System - Upper Back/Upper Extremity 6 Circulatory System - Lower Back/Lower Extremity 7 Circulatory System - Whole Body 8 Respiratory System - Head and Neck 9 Respiratory System - Upper Back/Upper Extremity B Respiratory System - Lower Back/Lower Extremity C Respiratory System - Whole Body	6 Therapeutic exercise	B Physical Agents C Mechanical D Electrotherapeutic E Orthosis F Assistive, adaptive, supportive or protective G Aerobic endurance and conditioning H Mechanical or electromechanical U Prosthesis Y Other equipment Z None	Z None

continued

F 0 7 MOTOR TREATMENT — *continued*

Body System/Region – 4TH	Type Qualifier – 5TH	Equipment – 6TH	Qualifier 7TH
N Genitourinary System	1 Muscle performance	E Orthosis F Assistive, adaptive, supportive or protective U Prosthesis Y Other equipment Z None	Z None
N Genitourinary System	6 Therapeutic exercise	B Physical Agents C Mechanical D Electrotherapeutic E Orthosis F Assistive, adaptive, supportive or protective G Aerobic endurance and conditioning H Mechanical or electromechanical U Prosthesis Y Other equipment Z None	Z None
Z None	4 Wheelchair mobility	D Electrotherapeutic E Orthosis F Assistive, adaptive, supportive or protective U Prosthesis Y Other equipment Z None	Z None
Z None	5 Bed mobility	C Mechanical E Orthosis F Assistive, adaptive, supportive or protective U Prosthesis Y Other equipment Z None	Z None
Z None	8 Transfer training	C Mechanical D Electrotherapeutic E Orthosis F Assistive, adaptive, supportive or protective U Prosthesis Y Other equipment Z None	Z None
Z None	9 Gait training/functional ambulation	C Mechanical D Electrotherapeutic E Orthosis F Assistive, adaptive, supportive or protective U Prosthesis Y Other equipment Z None	Z None

REHAB & AUDIOLOGY F 0 7

1ST – F	Physical Rehabilitation and Diagnostic Audiology
2ND – 0	Rehabilitation
3RD – 8	**ACTIVITIES OF DAILY LIVING TREATMENT**

ACTIVITIES OF DAILY LIVING TREATMENT: Exercise or activities to facilitate functional competence for activities of daily living.

Body System/Region – 4TH	Type Qualifier – 5TH	Equipment – 6TH	Qualifier 7TH
D Integumentary System - Head and Neck F Integumentary System - Upper Back/Upper Extremity G Integumentary System - Lower Back/Lower Extremity H Integumentary System - Whole Body J Musculoskeletal System - Head and Neck K Musculoskeletal System - Upper Back/Upper Extremity L Musculoskeletal System - Lower Back/Lower Extremity M Musculoskeletal System - Whole Body	5 Wound Management	B Physical Agents C Mechanical D Electrotherapeutic E Orthosis F Assistive, adaptive, supportive or protective U Prosthesis Y Other equipment Z None	Z None
Z None	0 Bathing/showering techniques 1 Dressing techniques 2 Grooming/personal hygiene	E Orthosis F Assistive, adaptive, supportive or protective U Prosthesis Y Other equipment Z None	Z None
Z None	3 Feeding/eating	C Mechanical D Electrotherapeutic E Orthosis F Assistive, adaptive, supportive or protective U Prosthesis Y Other equipment Z None	Z None
Z None	4 Home management	D Electrotherapeutic E Orthosis F Assistive, adaptive, supportive or protective U Prosthesis Y Other equipment Z None	Z None
Z None	6 Psychosocial skills	Z None	Z None
Z None	7 Vocational activities and functional community or work reintegration skills	B Physical Agents C Mechanical D Electrotherapeutic E Orthosis F Assistive, adaptive, supportive or protective G Aerobic endurance and conditioning U Prosthesis Y Other equipment Z None	Z None

1ST - F Physical Rehabilitation and Diagnostic Audiology
2ND - 0 Rehabilitation
3RD - 9 HEARING TREATMENT

HEARING TREATMENT: Application of techniques to improve, augment, or compensate for hearing and related functional impairment.

Body System/Region – 4TH	Type Qualifier – 5TH	Equipment – 6TH	Qualifier 7TH
Z None	0 Hearing and related disorders counseling 1 Hearing and related disorders prevention	K Audiovisual Z None	Z None
Z None	2 Auditory processing	K Audiovisual L Assistive listening P Computer Y Other equipment Z None	Z None
Z None	3 Cerumen management	X Cerumen management Z None	Z None

1ST - F Physical Rehabilitation and Diagnostic Audiology
2ND - 0 Rehabilitation
3RD - B COCHLEAR IMPLANT TREATMENT

COCHLEAR IMPLANT TREATMENT: Application of techniques to improve the communication abilities of individuals with cochlear implant.

Body System/Region – 4TH	Type Qualifier – 5TH	Equipment – 6TH	Qualifier 7TH
Z None	0 Cochlear implant rehabilitation	1 Audiometer 2 Sound field/booth 9 Cochlear implant K Audiovisual P Computer Y Other equipment	Z None

REHAB & AUDIOLOGY F 0 B

1ST - F Physical Rehabilitation and Diagnostic Audiology
2ND - 0 Rehabilitation
3RD - C VESTIBULAR TREATMENT

VESTIBULAR TREATMENT: Application of techniques to improve, augment, or compensate for vestibular and related functional impairment.

Body System/Region – 4TH	Type Qualifier – 5TH	Equipment – 6TH	Qualifier 7TH
3 Neurological System - Whole Body H Integumentary System - Whole Body M Musculoskeletal System - Whole Body	3 Postural control	E Orthosis F Assistive, adaptive, supportive or protective U Prosthesis Y Other equipment Z None	Z None
Z None	0 Vestibular	8 Vestibular/balance Z None	Z None
Z None	1 Perceptual processing 2 Visual motor integration	K Audiovisual L Assistive listening N Biosensory feedback P Computer Q Speech analysis S Voice analysis T Aerodynamic function Y Other equipment Z None	Z None

1ST - F Physical Rehabilitation and Diagnostic Audiology
2ND - 0 Rehabilitation
3RD - D DEVICE FITTING

DEVICE FITTING: Fitting of a device designed to facilitate or support achievement of a higher level of function.

Body System/Region – 4TH	Type Qualifier – 5TH	Equipment – 6TH	Qualifier 7TH
Z None	0 Tinnitus masker	5 Hearing aid selection/fitting/test Z None	Z None
Z None	1 Monaural hearing aid 2 Binaural hearing aid 5 Assistive listening device	1 Audiometer 2 Sound field/booth 5 Hearing aid selection/fitting/test K Audiovisual L Assistive listening Z None	Z None
Z None	3 Augmentative/alternative communication system	M Augmentative/alternative communication	Z None
Z None	4 Voice prosthetic	S Voice analysis V Speech prosthesis	Z None
Z None	6 Dynamic orthosis 7 Static orthosis 8 Prosthesis 9 Assistive, adaptive, supportive or protective devices	E Orthosis F Assistive, adaptive, supportive or protective U Prosthesis Z None	Z None

REHAB & AUDIOLOGY F 0 C

1ST - F Physical Rehabilitation and Diagnostic Audiology
2ND - 0 Rehabilitation
3RD - F CAREGIVER TRAINING

CAREGIVER TRAINING: Training in activities to support patient's optimal level of function.

Body System/Region – 4TH	Type Qualifier – 5TH	Equipment – 6TH	Qualifier 7TH
Z None	0 Bathing/showering technique 1 Dressing 2 Feeding and eating 3 Grooming/personal hygiene 4 Bed mobility 5 Transfer 6 Wheelchair mobility 7 Therapeutic exercise 8 Airway clearance techniques 9 Wound management B Vocational activities and functional community or work reintegration skills C Gait training/functional ambulation D Application, proper use and care of devices F Application, proper use and care of orthoses G Application, proper use and care of prosthesis H Home management	E Orthosis F Assistive, adaptive, supportive or protective U Prosthesis Z None	Z None
Z None	J Communication skills	K Audiovisual L Assistive Listening M Augmentative/alternative communication P Computer Z None	Z None

REHAB & AUDIOLOGY

F 0 F

1ST - F	Physical Rehabilitation and Diagnostic Audiology	**HEARING ASSESSMENT:** Measurement of hearing and related functions.
2ND - 1	Diagnostic Audiology	
3RD - 3	HEARING ASSESSMENT	

Body System/Region – 4TH	Type Qualifier – 5TH	Equipment – 6TH	Qualifier 7TH
Z None	0 Hearing screening	0 Occupational hearing 1 Audiometer 2 Sound field/booth 3 Tympanometer 8 Vestibular/balance 9 Cochlear implant Z None	Z None
Z None	1 Pure tone audiometry, air 2 Pure tone audiometry, air and bone	0 Occupational hearing 1 Audiometer 2 Sound field/booth Z None	Z None
Z None	3 Bekesy audiometry 6 Visual reinforcement audiometry 9 Short increment sensitivity index B Stenger C Pure tone stenger	1 Audiometer 2 Sound field/booth Z None	Z None
Z None	4 Conditioned play audiometry 5 Select picture audiometry	1 Audiometer 2 Sound field/booth K Audiovisual Z None	Z None
Z None	7 Alternate binaural or monaural loudness balance	1 Audiometer K Audiovisual Z None	Z None
Z None	8 Tone decay D Tympanometry F Eustachian tube function G Acoustic reflex patterns H Acoustic reflex threshold J Acoustic reflex decay	3 Tympanometer 4 Electroacoustic immitance/acoustic reflex Z None	Z None
Z None	K Electrocochleography L Auditory evoked potentials	7 Electrophysiologic Z None	Z None
Z None	M Evoked otoacoustic emissions, screening N Evoked otoacoustic emissions, diagnostic	6 Otoacoustic emission (OAE) Z None	Z None
Z None	P Aural rehabilitation status	1 Audiometer 2 Sound field/booth 4 Electroacoustic immitance/acoustic reflex 9 Cochlear implant K Audiovisual L Assistive listening P Computer Z None	Z None
Z None	Q Auditory processing	K Audiovisual P Computer Y Other equipment Z None	Z None

REHAB & AUDIOLOGY F13

1ST - F	Physical Rehabilitation and Diagnostic Audiology
2ND - 1	Diagnostic Audiology
3RD - 4	HEARING AID ASSESSMENT

HEARING AID ASSESSMENT:
Measurement of the appropriateness and/or effectiveness of a hearing device.

Body System/Region – 4TH	Type Qualifier – 5TH	Equipment – 6TH	Qualifier 7TH
Z None	0 Cochlear implant	1 Audiometer 2 Sound field/booth 3 Tympanometer 4 Electroacoustic immitance/acoustic reflex 5 Hearing Aid Selection/fitting/test 7 Electrophysiologic 9 Cochlear implant K Audiovisual L Assistive listening P Computer Y Other equipment Z None	Z None
Z None	1 Ear canal probe microphone 6 Binaural electroacoustic hearing aid check 8 Monaural electroacoustic hearing aid check	5 Hearing Aid Selection/fitting/test Z None	Z None
Z None	2 Monaural hearing aid 3 Binaural hearing aid	1 Audiometer 2 Sound field/booth 3 Tympanometer 4 Electroacoustic immitance/acoustic reflex 5 Hearing Aid Selection/fitting/test K Audiovisual L Assistive listening P Computer Z None	Z None
Z None	4 Assistive listening system/device selection	1 Audiometer 2 Sound field/booth 3 Tympanometer 4 Electroacoustic immitance/acoustic reflex K Audiovisual L Assistive listening Z None	Z None
Z None	5 Sensory aids	1 Audiometer 2 Sound field/booth 3 Tympanometer 4 Electroacoustic immitance/acoustic reflex 5 Hearing Aid Selection/fitting/test K Audiovisual L Assistive listening Z None	Z None
Z None	7 Ear protector attentuation	0 Occupational hearing Z None	Z None

REHAB & AUDIOLOGY F14

1ST - **F** Physical Rehabilitation and Diagnostic Audiology 2ND - **1** Diagnostic Audiology 3RD - **5** VESTIBULAR ASSESSMENT	**VESTIBULAR ASSESSMENT:** Measurement of the vestibular system and related functions.

Body System/Region — 4TH	Type Qualifier — 5TH	Equipment — 6TH	Qualifier 7TH
Z None	0 Bithermal, binaural caloric irrigation 1 Bithermal, monaural caloric irrigation 2 Unithermal binaural screen 3 Oscillating tracking 4 Sinusoidal vertical axis rotational 5 Dix-Hallpike dynamic 6 Computerized dynamic posturography	8 Vestibular/balance Z None	Z None
Z None	7 Tinnitus masker	5 Hearing aid selection/fitting/test Z None	Z None

Educational Annotations | Section G – Mental Health

Section Specific Educational Annotations for the Mental Health Section include:
- AHA Coding Clinic® Reference Notations
- Coding Notes

AHA Coding Clinic® Reference Notations of Mental Health

ROOT TYPE SPECIFIC - MENTAL HEALTH - Section G
PSYCHOLOGICAL TESTS - 1
CRISIS INTERVENTION - 2
INDIVIDUAL PSYCHOTHERAPY - 5
COUNSELING - 6
FAMILY PSYCHOTHERAPY - 7
ELECTROCONVULSIVE THERAPY - B
BIOFEEDBACK - C
HYPNOSIS - F
NARCOSYNTHESIS - G
GROUP THERAPY - H
LIGHT THERAPY - J

Coding Notes of Mental Health

Ancillary Section Specific PCS Reference Manual Exercises

PCS CODE	G – MENTAL HEALTH EXERCISES
G Z 1 0 Z Z Z	Developmental testing.
G Z 1 3 Z Z Z	Neuropsychological testing.
G Z 2 Z Z Z Z	Crisis intervention.
G Z 5 8 Z Z Z	Cognitive-behavioral psychotherapy, individual.
G Z 6 1 Z Z Z	Vocational counseling.
G Z 7 2 Z Z Z	Family psychotherapy.
G Z B 1 Z Z Z	ECT (Electroconvulsive therapy), unilateral, multiple seizure.
G Z F Z Z Z Z	Hypnosis.
G Z G Z Z Z Z	Narcosynthesis.
G Z J Z Z Z Z	Light therapy.

MENTAL HEALTH G

Educational Annotations | Section G – Mental Health

<u>**NOTES**</u>

MENTAL HEALTH G

1ST - G Mental Health 2ND - Z None 3RD - 1 PSYCHOLOGICAL TESTS	PSYCHOLOGICAL TESTS: The administration and interpretation of standardized psychological tests and measurement instruments for the assessment of psychological function.		
Qualifier – 4TH	**Qualifier – 5TH**	**Qualifier – 6TH**	**Qualifier – 7TH**
0 Developmental 1 Personality and behavioral 2 Intellectual and psychoeducational 3 Neuropsychological 4 Neurobehavioral and cognitive status	Z None	Z None	Z None

1ST - G Mental Health 2ND - Z None 3RD - 2 CRISIS INTERVENTION	CRISIS INTERVENTION: Treatment of a traumatized, acutely disturbed or distressed individual for the purpose of short-term stabilization.		
Qualifier – 4TH	**Qualifier – 5TH**	**Qualifier – 6TH**	**Qualifier – 7TH**
Z None	Z None	Z None	Z None

1ST - G Mental Health 2ND - Z None 3RD - 3 MEDICATION MANAGEMENT	MEDICATION MANAGEMENT: Monitoring and adjusting the use of medications for the treatment of a mental health disorder.		
Qualifier – 4TH	**Qualifier – 5TH**	**Qualifier – 6TH**	**Qualifier – 7TH**
Z None	Z None	Z None	Z None

MENTAL HEALTH

GZ3

1ST – G Mental Health 2ND – Z None 3RD – 5 INDIVIDUAL PSYCHOTHERAPY	**INDIVIDUAL PSYCHOTHERAPY:** Treatment of an individual with a mental health disorder by behavioral, cognitive, psychoanalytic, psychodynamic or psychophysiological means to improve functioning or well-being.		
Qualifier – 4TH	**Qualifier – 5TH**	**Qualifier – 6TH**	**Qualifier – 7TH**
0 Interactive 1 Behavioral 2 Cognitive 3 Interpersonal 4 Psychoanalysis 5 Psychodynamic 6 Supportive 8 Cognitive-Behavioral 9 Psychophysiological	Z None	Z None	Z None

1ST – G Mental Health 2ND – Z None 3RD – 6 COUNSELING	**COUNSELING:** The application of psychological methods to treat an individual with normal developmental issues and psychological problems in order to increase function, improve well-being, alleviate distress, maladjustment or resolve crises.		
Qualifier – 4TH	**Qualifier – 5TH**	**Qualifier – 6TH**	**Qualifier – 7TH**
0 Educational 1 Vocational 3 Other counseling	Z None	Z None	Z None

1ST – G Mental Health 2ND – Z None 3RD – 7 FAMILY PSYCHOTHERAPY	**FAMILY PSYCHOTHERAPY:** Treatment that includes one or more family members of an individual with a mental health disorder by behavioral, cognitive, psychoanalytic, psychodynamic or psychophysiological means to improve functioning or well-being.		
Qualifier – 4TH	**Qualifier – 5TH**	**Qualifier – 6TH**	**Qualifier – 7TH**
2 Other family psychotherapy	Z None	Z None	Z None

MENTAL HEALTH G Z 5

1ST - G Mental Health	**ELECTROCONVULSIVE THERAPY:** The application of controlled electrical voltages to treat a mental health disorder.		
2ND - Z None			
3RD - B ELECTROCONVULSIVE THERAPY			

Qualifier – 4TH	Qualifier – 5TH	Qualifier – 6TH	Qualifier – 7TH
0 Unilateral-single seizure 1 Unilateral-multiple seizure 2 Bilateral-single seizure 3 Bilateral-multiple seizure 4 Other electroconvulsive therapy	Z None	Z None	Z None

1ST - G Mental Health	**BIOFEEDBACK:** Provision of information from the monitoring and regulating of physiological processes in conjunction with cognitive-behavioral techniques to improve patient functioning or ell-being.		
2ND - Z None			
3RD - C BIOFEEDBACK			

Qualifier – 4TH	Qualifier – 5TH	Qualifier – 6TH	Qualifier – 7TH
9 Other biofeedback	Z None	Z None	Z None

1ST - G Mental Health	**HYPNOSIS:** Induction of a state of heightened suggestibility by auditory, visual and tactile techniques to elicit an emotional or behavioral response.		
2ND - Z None			
3RD - F HYPNOSIS			

Qualifier – 4TH	Qualifier – 5TH	Qualifier – 6TH	Qualifier – 7TH
Z None	Z None	Z None	Z None

1ST - **G** Mental Health

2ND - **Z** None

3RD - **G** NARCOSYNTHESIS

NARCOSYNTHESIS: Administration of intravenous barbiturates in order to release suppressed or repressed thoughts.

Qualifier – 4TH	Qualifier — 5TH	Qualifier — 6TH	Qualifier — 7TH
Z None	Z None	Z None	Z None

1ST - **G** Mental Health

2ND - **Z** None

3RD - **H** GROUP PSYCHOTHERAPY

GROUP PSYCHOTHERAPY: Treatment of two or more individuals with a mental health disorder by behavioral, cognitive, psychoanalytic, psychodynamic or psychophysiological means to improve functioning or well-being.

Qualifier – 4TH	Qualifier — 5TH	Qualifier — 6TH	Qualifier — 7TH
Z None	Z None	Z None	Z None

1ST - **G** Mental Health

2ND - **Z** None

3RD - **J** LIGHT THERAPY

LIGHT THERAPY: Application of specialized light treatments to improve functioning or well-being.

Qualifier – 4TH	Qualifier — 5TH	Qualifier — 6TH	Qualifier — 7TH
Z None	Z None	Z None	Z None

MENTAL HEALTH

GZG

Educational Annotations | Section H – Substance Abuse

Section Specific Educational Annotations for the Substance Abuse Section include:
- AHA Coding Clinic® Reference Notations
- Coding Notes

AHA Coding Clinic® Reference Notations of Substance Abuse

ROOT TYPE SPECIFIC - SUBSTANCE ABUSE TREATMENT - Section H
DETOXIFICATION SERVICES - 2
INDIVIDUAL COUNSELING - 3
GROUP COUNSELING - 4
INDIVIDUAL PSYCHOTHERAPY - 5
FAMILY COUNSELING - 6
MEDICATION MANAGEMENT - 8
PHARMACOTHERAPY - 9

Coding Notes of Substance Abuse

Ancillary Section Specific PCS Reference Manual Exercises

PCS CODE	H – SUBSTANCE ABUSE EXERCISES
H Z 2 Z Z Z Z	Patient in for alcohol detoxification treatment.
H Z 3 C Z Z Z	Post-test infectious disease counseling for IV drug abuser.
H Z 4 2 Z Z Z	Group cognitive-behavioral counseling for substance abuse.
H Z 4 7 Z Z Z	Group motivational counseling.
H Z 5 3 Z Z Z	Individual 12-step psychotherapy for substance abuse.
H Z 5 4 Z Z Z	Individual interpersonal psychotherapy for drug abuse.
H Z 5 C Z Z Z	Psychodynamic psychotherapy for drug dependent patient.
H Z 6 3 Z Z Z	Substance abuse treatment family counseling.
H Z 8 1 Z Z Z	Medication monitoring of patient on methadone maintenance.
H Z 9 4 Z Z Z	Naltrexone treatment for drug dependency.

SUBSTANCE ABUSE H

Educational Annotations | Section H – Substance Abuse

NOTES

1ST - **H** Substance Abuse Treatment 2ND - **Z** None 3RD - **2** DETOXIFICATION SERVICES	DETOXIFICATION SERVICES: Detoxification from alcohol and/or drugs.		
Qualifier – 4TH	**Qualifier – 5TH**	**Qualifier – 6TH**	**Qualifier – 7TH**
Z None	Z None	Z None	Z None

1ST - **H** Substance Abuse Treatment 2ND - **Z** None 3RD - **3** INDIVIDUAL COUNSELING	INDIVIDUAL COUNSELING: The application of psychological methods to treat an individual with addictive behavior.		
Qualifier – 4TH	**Qualifier – 5TH**	**Qualifier – 6TH**	**Qualifier – 7TH**
0 Cognitive 1 Behavioral 2 Cognitive-behavioral 3 12-Step 4 Interpersonal 5 Vocational 6 Psychoeducation 7 Motivational enhancement 8 Confrontational 9 Continuing care B Spiritual C Pre/post-test infectious disease	Z None	Z None	Z None

1ST - **H** Substance Abuse Treatment 2ND - **Z** None 3RD - **4** GROUP COUNSELING	GROUP COUNSELING: The application of psychological methods to treat two or more individuals with addictive behavior.		
Qualifier – 4TH	**Qualifier – 5TH**	**Qualifier – 6TH**	**Qualifier – 7TH**
0 Cognitive 1 Behavioral 2 Cognitive-behavioral 3 12-Step 4 Interpersonal 5 Vocational 6 Psychoeducation 7 Motivational enhancement 8 Confrontational 9 Continuing care B Spiritual C Pre/post-test infectious disease	Z None	Z None	Z None

SUBSTANCE ABUSE **H Z 4**

1ST - **H** Substance Abuse Treatment

2ND - **Z** None

3RD - **5 INDIVIDUAL PSYCHOTHERAPY**

INDIVIDUAL PSYCHOTHERAPY:
Treatment of an individual with addictive behavior by behavioral, cognitive, psychoanalytic, psychodynamic or psychophysiological means.

Qualifier – 4TH	Qualifier – 5TH	Qualifier – 6TH	Qualifier – 7TH
0 Cognitive	Z None	Z None	Z None
1 Behavioral			
2 Cognitive-behavioral			
3 12-Step			
4 Interpersonal			
5 Interactive			
6 Psychoeducation			
7 Motivational enhancement			
8 Confrontational			
9 Supportive			
B Psychoanalysis			
C Psychodynamic			
D Psychophysiological			

1ST - **H** Substance Abuse Treatment

2ND - **Z** None

3RD - **6 FAMILY COUNSELING**

FAMILY COUNSELING: The application of psychological methods that includes one or more family members to treat an individual with addictive behavior.

Qualifier – 4TH	Qualifier – 5TH	Qualifier – 6TH	Qualifier – 7TH
3 Other family counseling	Z None	Z None	Z None

1ST - **H** Substance Abuse Treatment

2ND - **Z** None

3RD - **8 MEDICATION MANAGEMENT**

MEDICATION MANAGEMENT:
Monitoring and adjusting the use of replacement medications for the treatment of addiction.

Qualifier – 4TH	Qualifier – 5TH	Qualifier – 6TH	Qualifier – 7TH
0 Nicotine replacement	Z None	Z None	Z None
1 Methadone maintenance			
2 Levo-alpha-acetyl-methadol (LAAM)			
3 Antabuse			
4 Naltrexone			
5 Naloxone			
6 Clonidine			
7 Bupropion			
8 Psychiatric medication			
9 Other replacement medication			

SUBSTANCE ABUSE HZ5

1ST - H Substance Abuse Treatment

2ND - Z None

3RD - 9 PHARMACOTHERAPY

PHARMACOTHERAPY: The use of replacement medications for the treatment of addiction.

Qualifier – 4TH	Qualifier – 5TH	Qualifier – 6TH	Qualifier – 7TH
0 Nicotine replacement	Z None	Z None	Z None
1 Methadone maintenance			
2 Levo-alpha-acetyl-methadol (LAAM)			
3 Antabuse			
4 Naltrexone			
5 Naloxone			
6 Clonidine			
7 Bupropion			
8 Psychiatric medication			
9 Other replacement medication			

SUBSTANCE ABUSE

HZ9

NOTES

© 2016 Channel Publishing, Ltd.

Educational Annotations | Section X – New Technology

Section Specific Educational Annotations for the New Technology Section include:
- AHA Coding Clinic® Reference Notations
- Coding Notes

NEW TECHNOLOGY – SECTION X
Section X New Technology is the section in ICD-10-PCS for codes that uniquely identify procedures requested via the New Technology Application Process, and for codes that capture new technologies not currently classified in ICD-10-PCS.

This section may include codes for medical and surgical procedures, medical and surgical-related procedures, or ancillary procedures designated as new technology.

In section X, the seven characters are defined as follows:
- First character: section (X)
- Second character: body system
- Third character: operation
- Fourth character: body part
- Fifth character: approach
- Sixth character: device/substance/technology
- Seventh character: new technology group

The New Technology section includes infusions of new technology drugs, and can potentially include a wide range of other new technology medical, surgical, and ancillary procedures. The example below is for infusion of a new technology drug.

Coding Note: Seventh Character New Technology Group
In ICD-10-PCS, the type of information specified in the seventh character is called the qualifier, and the information specified depends on the section. In this section, the seventh character is used exclusively to indicate the new technology group.

The New Technology Group is a number or letter that changes each year that new technology codes are added to the system. For example, Section X codes added for the first year have the seventh character value 1, New Technology Group 1, and the next year that Section X codes are added have the seventh character value 2 New Technology Group 2, and so on.

Changing the seventh character New Technology Group to a unique value every year that there are new codes in this section allows the ICD-10-PCS to "recycle" the values in the third, fourth, and sixth characters as needed. This avoids the creation of duplicate codes, because the root operation, body part, and device/substance/technology values can specify a different meaning with every new technology group, if needed. Having a unique value for the New Technology Group maximizes the flexibility and capacity of section X over its lifespan, and allows it to evolve as medical technology evolves.

Body System Values
Second character body systems in this section do not change from year to year. They are a fixed set of values that combine the uses of body system, body region, and physiological system as specified in other sections in ICD-10-PCS. As a result, the second character body system values are broader values. This allows body part values to be as general or specific as they need to be to efficiently represent the body part applicable to a new technology.

Root Operations
Third character root operations in this section use the same root operation values as their counterparts in other sections of ICD-10-PCS. The example above uses the root operation value Introduction. This root operation has the same definition as its counterpart in section 3 of ICD-10-PCS, as given below.

- 0 – Introduction: Putting in or on a therapeutic, diagnostic, nutritional, physiological, or prophylactic substance except blood or blood products

Continued on next page

Educational Annotations | Section X – New Technology

Continued from previous page

Body Part Values
Fourth character body part values in this section use the same body part values as their closest counterparts in other sections of ICD-10-PCS. The example above uses the body part value 4 Central Vein. This is its closest counterpart in section 3 of ICD-10-PCS.

Device/Substance/Technology Values
In this section, the sixth character contains a general description of the key feature of the new technology. The example above uses the device/substance/technology value 2 Ceftazidime-Avibactam Anti-infective.

AHA Coding Clinic® Reference Notations of New Technology

<u>ROOT OPERATION SPECIFIC - NEW TECHNOLOGY - Section X</u>
EXTIRPATION - C
    Orbital atherectomy and drug-eluting balloon angioplasty of
       coronary artery ....AHA 15:4Q:p13
INTRODUCTION - 0
    Blincyto infusion (blinatumomab) ....AHA 15:4Q:p14
    Introduction of idarucizumab prior to surgery ....AHA 15:4Q:p13
MISC

Device Key Listings of New Technology

See also Device Key in Appendix D
EDWARDS INTUITY Elite valve system ....*use* Zooplastic Tisssue, Rapid Deployment Technique
INTUITY Elite valve system, EDWARDS ....*use* Zooplastic Tisssue, Rapid Deployment Technique
MAGEC® Spinal Bracing and Distraction System ....*use* Magnetically Controlled Growth Rod(s)
MICRODERM™ Biologic Wound Matrix ....*use* Skin Substitute, Porcine Liver Derived
nanoLOCK™ interbody fusion device ....*use* Interbody Fusion Device, Nanotextured Surface
Perceval sutureless valve ....*use* Zooplastic Tisssue, Rapid Deployment Technique
Spiral growth rod(s), magnetically controlled..........*use* Magnetically Controlled Growth Rod(s)
Sutureless valve, Perceval ....*use* Zooplastic Tisssue, Rapid Deployment Technique

Coding Notes of New Technology

Ancillary Section Specific PCS Reference Manual Exercises

PCS CODE	X – NEW TECHNOLOGY EXERCISES
X W 0 3 3 2 1	Infusion of ceftazidime via peripheral venous catheter.

Body System Relevant Coding Guidelines

D. New Technology Section – Section X

General guidelines

D1
    Section X codes are standalone codes. They are not supplemental codes. Section X codes fully represent the specific procedure described in the code title, and do not require any additional codes from other sections of ICD-10-PCS. When section X contains a code title which describes a specific new technology procedure, only that X code is reported for the procedure. There is no need to report a broader, non-specific code in another section of ICD-10-PCS.
    Example: XW04321 Introduction of Ceftazidime-Avibactam Anti-infective into Central Vein, Percutaneous Approach, New Technology Group 1, can be coded to indicate that Ceftazidime-Avibactam Anti-infective was administered via a central vein. A separate code from table 3E0 in the Administration section of ICD-10-PCS is not coded in addition to this code.

1ST - **X** New Technology 2ND - **2** Cardiovascular System 3RD - **A ASSISTANCE**	EXAMPLE: Cerebral embolic filtration
	ASSISTANCE: Taking over a portion of a physiological function by extracorporeal means.
	EXPLANATION: Supports, but does not take over function …

Body Part – 4TH	Approach – 5TH	Device/Substance/Technology – 6TH	Qualifier – 7TH
5 Innominate Artery and Left Common Carotid Artery	3 Percutaneous	1 Cerebral embolic filtration, dual filter	2 New Technology Group 2

1ST - **X** New Technology 2ND - **2** Cardiovascular System 3RD - **C EXTIRPATION**	EXAMPLE: Removal coronary artery plaque
	EXTIRPATION: Taking or cutting out solid matter from a body part.
	EXPLANATION: Abnormal byproduct or foreign body …

Body Part – 4TH	Approach – 5TH	Device/Substance/Technology – 6TH	Qualifier – 7TH
0 Coronary Artery, One Artery 1 Coronary Artery, Two Arteries 2 Coronary Artery, Three Arteries 3 Coronary Artery, Four or More Arteries	3 Percutaneous	6 Orbital atherectomy technology	1 New Technology Group 1

1ST - **X** New Technology 2ND - **2** Cardiovascular System 3RD - **R REPLACEMENT**	EXAMPLE: Rapid deployment technique aortic valve replacement
	REPLACEMENT: Putting in or on biological or synthetic material that physically takes the place and/or function of all or a portion of a body part.
	EXPLANATION: Includes taking out body part, or eradication …

Body Part – 4TH	Approach – 5TH	Device/Substance/Technology – 6TH	Qualifier – 7TH
F Aortic Valve	0 Open 3 Percutaneous 4 Percutaneous endoscopic	3 Zooplastic tissue, rapid deployment technique	2 New Technology Group 2

1ST - **X** New Technology 2ND - **H** Skin, Subcutaneous Tissue, Fascia and Breast 3RD - **R REPLACEMENT**	EXAMPLE: Porcine liver derived skin substitute
	REPLACEMENT: Putting in or on biological or synthetic material that physically takes the place and/or function of all or a portion of a body part.
	EXPLANATION: Includes taking out body part, or eradication …

Body Part – 4TH	Approach – 5TH	Device/Substance/Technology – 6TH	Qualifier – 7TH
P Skin	X External	L Skin substitute, porcine liver derived	2 New Technology Group 2

1ST - X New Technology 2ND - N Bones 3RD - S REPOSITION	EXAMPLE: Adjusting magnetically controlled growth rod(s)
	REPOSITION: Moving to its normal location, or other suitable location, all or a portion of a body part.
	EXPLANATION: The body part is moved to a new location ...

Body Part – 4TH	Approach – 5TH	Device/Substance/Technology – 6TH	Qualifier – 7TH
0 Lumbar Vertebra 3 Cervical Vertebra 4 Thoracic Vertebra	0 Open 4 Percutaneous endoscopic	3 Magnetically controlled growth rod(s)	2 New Technology Group 2

1ST - X New Technology 2ND - R Joints 3RD - 2 MONITORING	EXAMPLE: Holter monitor
	MONITORING: Determining the level of a physiological or physical function repetitively over a period of time.
	EXPLANATION: Describes a series of measurements

Body Part – 4TH	Approach – 5TH	Device/Substance/Technology – 6TH	Qualifier – 7TH
G Knee Joint, Right H Knee Joint, Left	0 Open	2 Intraoperative knee replacement sensor	1 New Technology Group 1

1ST - X New Technology 2ND - R Joints 3RD - G FUSION	EXAMPLE: Nanotextured surface interbody fusion device
	FUSION: Joining together portions of an articular body part rendering the articular body part immobile.
	EXPLANATION: Use of fixation device, graft, or other means ...

Body Part – 4TH	Approach – 5TH	Device/Substance/Technology – 6TH	Qualifier – 7TH
0 Occipital-cervical Joint 1 Cervical Vertebral Joint 2 Cervical Vertebral Joints, 2 or more 4 Cervicothoracic Vertebral Joint 6 Thoracic Vertebral Joint 7 Thoracic Vertebral Joints, 2 to 7 8 Thoracic Vertebral Joints, 8 or more A Thoracolumbar Vertebral Joint B Lumbar Vertebral Joint C Lumbar Vertebral Joints, 2 or more D Lumbosacral Joint	0 Open	9 Interbody fusion device, nanotextured surface	2 New Technology Group 2

N E W T E C H N O L O G Y X N S

1ST – **X** New Technology

2ND – **W** Anatomical Regions

3RD – **0 INTRODUCTION**

EXAMPLE: Infusion of substance

INTRODUCTION: Putting in or on a therapeutic, diagnostic, nutritional, physiological, or prophylactic substance except blood or blood products.

EXPLANATION: Substances other than blood ...

Body Part – 4TH	Approach – 5TH	Device/Substance/Technology – 6TH	Qualifier – 7TH
3 Peripheral Vein	3 Percutaneous	2 Ceftazidime-avibactam anti-infective 3 Idarucizumab, Dabigatran reversal agent 4 Isavuconazole anti-infective 5 Blinatumomab antineoplastic immunotherapy	1 New Technology Group 1
3 Peripheral Vein	3 Percutaneous	7 Andexanet alfa, Factor Xa inhibitor reversal agent 9 Defibrotide sodium anticoagulant	2 New Technology Group 2
4 Central Vein	3 Percutaneous	2 Ceftazidime-avibactam anti-infective 3 Idarucizumab, Dabigatran reversal agent 4 Isavuconazole anti-infective 5 Blinatumomab antineoplastic immunotherapy	1 New Technology Group 1
4 Central Vein	3 Percutaneous	7 Andexanet alfa, Factor Xa inhibitor reversal agent 9 Defibrotide sodium anticoagulant	2 New Technology Group 2
D Mouth and Pharynx	X External	8 Uridine triacetate	2 New Technology Group 2

NEW TECHNOLOGY X W 0

NOTES

APPENDIX A
ROOT OPERATIONS OF THE MEDICAL AND SURGICAL SECTION

APPENDIX A contains the following parts:
PART 1: Groups of Similar Root Operations (Medical and Surgical Section)
PART 2: Alphabetic Listing of Root Operations (Medical and Surgical Section)

PART 1: Groups of Similar Root Operations (Medical and Surgical Section)

The Root Operations of the Medical and Surgical section are divided into logical groups that share similar attributes. Each root operation chart group includes: root operation name, objective of the procedure, site of the procedure, and an example of that root operation. These root operation chart groups are:
- Root operations that take out some or all of a body part
- Root operations that take out solids/fluids/gases from a body part
- Root operations involving cutting or separation only
- Root operations that put in/put back or move some/all of a body part
- Root operations that alter the diameter/route of a tubular body part
- Root operations that always involve a device
- Root operations involving examination only
- Root operations that define other repairs
- Root operations that define other objectives

Bold word(s) within each chart identify the concept that help differentiate it from other root operations within that chart.

Root operations that take out some or all of a body part

Root Operation	Objective of Procedure	Site of Procedure	Example
Excision	Cutting out/off without replacement	**Some** of a body part	Breast lumpectomy
Resection	Cutting out/off without replacement	**All** of a body part	Total mastectomy
Detachment	Cutting out/off without replacement	**Extremity only**, any level	Amputation above elbow
Destruction	**Eradicating** without replacement	Some/all of a body part	Fulguration of endometrium
Extraction	**Pulling out** or off without replacement	Some/all of a body part	Suction D&C

Root operations that take out solids/fluids/gases from a body part

Root Operation	Objective of Procedure	Site of Procedure	Example
Drainage	Taking/letting out **fluids/gases**	Within a body part	Incision and drainage
Extirpation	Taking/cutting out **solid matter**	Within a body part	Thrombectomy
Fragmentation	**Breaking** solid matter into pieces	Within a body part	Lithotripsy

Root operations involving cutting or separation only

Root Operation	Objective of Procedure	Site of Procedure	Example
Division	Cutting into/**separating** a body part	Within a body part	Neurotomy
Release	**Freeing** a body part from constraint	Around a body part	Adhesiolysis

APPENDIX A

Root operations that put in/put back or move some/all of a body part

Root Operation	Objective of Procedure	Site of Procedure	Example
Transplantation	**Putting in** a living body part from a person/animal	Some/all of a body part	Kidney transplant
Reattachment	**Putting back** a detached body part	Some/all of a body part	Reattach finger
Transfer	**Moving** a body part to **function for** a similar body part	Some/all of a body part	Skin transfer flap
Reposition	**Moving** a body part to **normal** or other suitable location	Some/all of a body part	Move undescended testicle

Root operations that alter the diameter/route of a tubular body part

Root Operation	Objective of Procedure	Site of Procedure	Example
Restriction	**Partially** closing orifice/lumen	Tubular body part	Gastroesophageal fundoplication
Occlusion	**Completely** closing orifice/lumen	Tubular body part	Fallopian tube ligation
Dilation	**Expanding** orifice/lumen	Tubular body part	Percutaneous transluminal coronary angioplasty (PTCA)
Bypass	**Altering route** of passage	Tubular body part	Coronary artery bypass graft (CABG)

Root operations that always involve a device

Root Operation	Objective of Procedure	Site of Procedure	Example
Insertion	Putting in **non-biological** device	In/on a body part	Central line insertion
Replacement	Putting in device that **replaces** a body part	Some/all of a body part	Total hip replacement
Supplement	Putting in device that **reinforces** or augments a body part	In/on a body part	Abdominal wall herniorrhaphy using mesh
Change	**Exchanging** device without cutting/puncturing	In/on a body part	Drainage tube change
Removal	**Taking out** device	In/on a body part	Central line removal
Revision	**Correcting** a malfunctioning/displaced device	In/on a body part	Revision of pacemaker insertion

Root operations involving examination only

Root Operation	Objective of Procedure	Site of Procedure	Example
Inspection	Visual/manual **exploration**	Some/all of a body part	Diagnostic cystoscopy
Map	**Locating** electrical impulses/functional areas	Brain/cardiac conduction mechanism	Cardiac mapping

Root operations that define other repairs

Root Operation	Objective of Procedure	Site of Procedure	Example
Control	Stopping/attempting to stop **postprocedural bleeding**	Anatomical region	Post-prostatectomy bleeding control
Repair	**Restoring** body part to its normal structure	Some/all of a body part	Suture laceration

Root operations that define other objectives

Root Operation	Objective of Procedure	Site of Procedure	Example
Fusion	Rendering joint **immobile**	Joint	Spinal fusion
Alteration	**Modifying** body part for cosmetic purposes without affecting function	Some/all of a body part	Face lift
Creation	**Forming** a new body part to replicate the function of an absent body part	Some/all of a body part	Artificial vagina/penis

PART 2: Alphabetic Listing of Root Operations (Medical and Surgical Section)

The Root Operations of the Medical and Surgical section are listed below in alphabetic order and include information detailing each root operation. Each root operation chart includes:

- Root Operation value and title
- Definition
- Explanation
- Examples

0 ALTERATION	DEFINITION: Modifying the anatomic structure of a body part without affecting the function of the body part
EXPLANATION:	Principal purpose is to improve appearance
EXAMPLES:	Face lift, breast augmentation

1 BYPASS	DEFINITION: Altering the route of passage of the contents of a tubular body part
EXPLANATION:	Rerouting contents of a body part to a downstream area of the normal route, to a similar route and body part, or to an abnormal route and dissimilar body part. Includes one or more anastomoses, with or without the use of a device
EXAMPLES:	Coronary artery bypass, colostomy formation

2 CHANGE	DEFINITION: Taking out or off a device from a body part and putting back an identical or similar device in or on the same body part without cutting or puncturing the skin or a mucous membrane
EXPLANATION:	All CHANGE procedures are coded using the approach EXTERNAL
EXAMPLES:	Urinary catheter change, gastrostomy tube change

3 CONTROL	DEFINITION: Stopping, or attempting to stop, postprocedural bleeding or other acute bleeding
EXPLANATION:	The site of the bleeding is coded as an anatomical region and not to a specific body part
EXAMPLES:	Control of post-prostatectomy hemorrhage, control of intracranial subdural hemorrhage, control of bleeding duodenal ulcer, control of retroperitoneal hemorrhage

4 CREATION	DEFINITION: Putting in or on biological or synthetic material to form a new body part that to the extent possible replicates the anatomic structure or function of an absent body part
EXPLANATION:	Used for gender reassignment surgery and corrective procedures in individuals with congenital anomalies
EXAMPLES:	Creation of vagina in a male, creation of right and left atrioventricular valve from common atrioventricualr valve

5 DESTRUCTION

DEFINITION: Physical eradication of all or a portion of a body part by the direct use of energy, force, or a destructive agent

EXPLANATION: None of the body part is physically taken out

EXAMPLES: Fulguration of rectal polyp, cautery of skin lesion

6 DETACHMENT

DEFINITION: Cutting off all or portion of the upper or lower extremities

EXPLANATION: The body part value is the site of the detachment, with a qualifier if applicable to further specify the level where the extremity was detached

EXAMPLES: Below knee amputation, disarticulation of shoulder

7 DILATION

DEFINITION: Expanding an orifice or the lumen of a tubular body part

EXPLANATION: The orifice can be a natural orifice or an artificially created orifice. Accomplished by stretching a tubular body part using intraluminal pressure or by cutting part of the orifice or wall of the tubular body part.

EXAMPLES: Percutaneous transluminal angioplasty, pyloromyotomy

8 DIVISION

DEFINITION: Cutting into a body part, without draining fluids and/or gases from the body part, in order to separate or transect a body part

EXPLANATION: All or a portion of the body part is separated into two or more portions

EXAMPLES: Spinal cordotomy, osteotomy

9 DRAINAGE

DEFINITION: Taking or letting out fluids and/or gases from a body part

EXPLANATION: The qualifier DIAGNOSTIC is used to identify drainage procedures that are biopsies

EXAMPLES: Thoracentesis, incision and drainage

B EXCISION

DEFINITION: Cutting out or off, without replacement, a portion of a body part

EXPLANATION: The qualifier DIAGNOSTIC is used to identify excision procedures that are biopsies

EXAMPLES: Partial nephrectomy, liver biopsy

C EXTIRPATION

DEFINITION: Taking or cutting out solid matter from a body part

EXPLANATION: The solid matter may be an abnormal byproduct of a biological function or a foreign body; it may be imbedded in a body part or in the lumen of a tubular body part. The solid matter may or may not have been previously broken into pieces.

EXAMPLES: Thrombectomy, choledocholithotomy

D EXTRACTION

DEFINITION: Pulling or stripping out or off all or a portion of a body part by the use of force

EXPLANATION: The qualifier DIAGNOSTIC is used to identify extraction procedures that are biopsies

EXAMPLES: Dilation and curettage, vein stripping

F FRAGMENTATION

DEFINITION: Breaking solid matter in a body part into pieces

EXPLANATION: Physical force (e.g., manual, ultrasonic) applied directly or indirectly is used to break the solid matter into pieces. The solid matter may be an abnormal byproduct of a biological function or a foreign body. The pieces of solid matter are not taken out.

EXAMPLES: Extracorporeal shockwave lithotripsy, transurethral lithotripsy

G FUSION

DEFINITION: Joining together portions of an articular body part rendering the articular body part immobile

EXPLANATION: The body part is joined together by fixation device, bone graft, or other means

EXAMPLES: Spinal fusion, ankle arthrodesis

H INSERTION

DEFINITION: Putting in a nonbiological appliance that monitors, assists, performs or prevents a physiological function but does not physically take the place of a body part

EXPLANATION: None

EXAMPLES: Insertion of radioactive implant, insertion of central venous catheter

J INSPECTION

DEFINITION: Visually and/or manually exploring a body part

EXPLANATION: Visual exploration may be performed with or without optical instrumentation. Manual exploration may be performed directly or through intervening body layers

EXAMPLES: Diagnostic arthroscopy, exploratory laparotomy

K MAP

DEFINITION: Locating the route of passage of electrical impulses and/or locating functional areas in a body part

EXPLANATION: Applicable only to the cardiac conduction mechanism and the central nervous system

EXAMPLES: Cardiac mapping, cortical mapping

L OCCLUSION

DEFINITION: Completely closing an orifice or the lumen of a tubular body part

EXPLANATION: The orifice can be a natural orifice or an artificially created orifice

EXAMPLES: Fallopian tube ligation, ligation of inferior vena cava

M REATTACHMENT

DEFINITION: Putting back in or on all or a portion of a separated body part to its normal location or other suitable location

EXPLANATION: Vascular circulation and nervous pathways may or may not be reestablished

EXAMPLES: Reattachment of hand, reattachment of avulsed kidney

N RELEASE

DEFINITION: Freeing a body part from an abnormal physical constraint by cutting or by the use of force

EXPLANATION: Some of the restraining tissue may be taken out but none of the body part is taken out

EXAMPLES: Adhesiolysis, carpal tunnel release

P REMOVAL

DEFINITION: Taking out or off a device from a body part

EXPLANATION: If a device is taken out and a similar device put in without cutting or puncturing the skin or mucous membrane, the procedure is coded to the root operation CHANGE. Otherwise, the procedure for taking out a device is coded to the root operation REMOVAL.

EXAMPLES: Drainage tube removal, cardiac pacemaker removal

Q REPAIR

DEFINITION: Restoring, to the extent possible, a body part to its normal anatomic structure and function

EXPLANATION: Used only when the method to accomplish the repair is not one of the other root operations

EXAMPLES: Colostomy takedown, suture of laceration

R REPLACEMENT

DEFINITION: Putting in or on biological or synthetic material that physically takes the place and/or function of all or a portion of a body part

EXPLANATION: The body part may have been taken out or replaced, or may be taken out, physically eradicated, or rendered non-functional during the REPLACEMENT procedure. A REMOVAL procedure is coded for taking out the device used in a previous replacement procedure.

EXAMPLES: Total hip replacement, bone graft, free skin graft

S REPOSITION

DEFINITION: Moving to its normal location, or other suitable location, all or a portion of a body part

EXPLANATION: The body part is moved to a new location from an abnormal location, or from a normal location where it is not functioning correctly. The body part may or may not be cut out or off to be moved to the new location.

EXAMPLES: Reposition of undescended testicle, fracture reduction

T RESECTION

DEFINITION: Cutting out or off, without replacement, all of a body part

EXPLANATION: None

EXAMPLES: Total nephrectomy, total lobectomy of lung

V RESTRICTION	DEFINITION: Partially closing an orifice or the lumen of a tubular body part
EXPLANATION:	The orifice can be a natural orifice or an artificially created orifice
EXAMPLES:	Esophagogastric fundoplication, cervical cerclage

W REVISION	DEFINITION: Correcting, to the extent possible, a portion of a malfunctioning device or the position of a displaced device
EXPLANATION:	Revision can include correcting a malfunctioning or displaced device by taking out or putting in components of the device such as a screw or pin
EXAMPLES:	Adjustment of position of pacemaker lead, recementing of hip prosthesis

U SUPPLEMENT	DEFINITION: Putting in or on biologic or synthetic material that physically reinforces and/or augments the function of a portion of a body part
EXPLANATION:	The biological material is non-living, or is living and from the same individual. The body part may have been previously replaced, and the Supplement procedure is performed to physically reinforce and/or augment the function of the replaced body part.
EXAMPLES:	Herniorrhaphy using mesh, free nerve graft, mitral valve ring annuloplasty, put a new acetabular liner in a previous hip replacement

X TRANSFER	DEFINITION: Moving, without taking out, all or a portion of a body part to another location to take over the function of all or a portion of a body part
EXPLANATION:	The body part transferred remains connected to its vascular and nervous supply
EXAMPLES:	Tendon transfer, skin pedicle flap transfer

Y TRANSPLANTATION	DEFINITION: Putting in or on all or a portion of a living body part taken from another individual or animal to physically take the place and/or function of all or a portion of a similar body part
EXPLANATION:	The native body part may or may not be taken out, and the transplanted body part may take over all or a portion of its function
EXAMPLES:	Kidney transplant, heart transplant

Root operation/type definitions, explanations, and examples of the Medical- and Surgical-Related Section and the Ancillary Section are found at the specific code tables in their respective sections.

APPENDIX B
APPROACH DEFINITIONS OF THE MEDICAL AND SURGICAL SECTION

0 OPEN	DEFINITION: Cutting through the skin or mucous membrane and any other body layers necessary to expose the site of the procedure
EXPLANATION:	Includes "laparoscopic-assisted" open approach procedures
EXAMPLES:	Kidney tranplant, laparoscopic-assisted sigmoidectomy

3 PERCUTANEOUS	DEFINITION: Entry, by puncture or minor incision, of instrumentation through the skin or mucous membrane and any other body layers necessary to reach the site of the procedure
EXPLANATION:	Includes procedures performed percutaneously via device placed for the procedure
EXAMPLES:	Needle biopsy of liver, fragmentation of kidney stone performed via percutaneous nephrostomy

4 PERCUTANEOUS ENDOSCOPIC	DEFINITION: Entry, by puncture or minor incision, of instrumentation through the skin or mucous membrane and any other body layers necessary to reach and visualize the site of the procedure
EXPLANATION:	Percutaneous procedures using visualization
EXAMPLES:	Laparoscopic cholecystectomy, arthroscopy

7 VIA NATURAL OR ARTIFICIAL OPENING	DEFINITION: Entry of instrumentation through a natural or artificial external opening to reach the site of the procedure
EXPLANATION:	Access entry through natural or artificial external opening WITHOUT visualization
EXAMPLES:	Insertion of urinary catheter, insertion of endotracheal tube

8 VIA NATURAL OR ARTIFICIAL OPENING ENDOSCOPIC	DEFINITION: Entry of instrumentation through a natural or artificial external opening to reach and visualize the site of the procedure
EXPLANATION:	Access entry through natural or artificial external opening using visualization
EXAMPLES:	Bronchoscopy, colonoscopy with biopsy

F VIA NATURAL OR ARTIFICIAL OPENING WITH PERCUTANEOUS ENDOSCOPIC ASSISTANCE	DEFINITION: Entry of instrumentation through a natural or artificial external opening and entry, by puncture or minor incision, of instrumentation through the skin or mucous membrane and any other body layers necessary to aid in the performance of the procedure
EXPLANATION:	Access entry through natural or artificial external opening AND using a separate percutaneous visualization
EXAMPLES:	Laparoscopic-assisted vaginal hysterectomy

X EXTERNAL	DEFINITION: Procedures performed directly on the skin or mucous membrane and procedures performed indirectly by the application of external force through the skin or mucous membrane
EXPLANATION:	Includes procedures performed within an orifice on structures that are visible without the aid of any instrumentation
EXAMPLES:	Closed reduction of fracture, suture of laceration, tonsillectomy

NOTES

BODY PART	USE:
Abdominal aortic plexus	use Abdominal Sympathetic Nerve
Abdominal esophagus	use Esophagus, Lower
Abductor hallucis muscle	use Foot Muscle, Left/Right
Accessory cephalic vein	use Cephalic Vein, Left/Right
Accessory obturator nerve	use Lumbar Plexus
Accessory phrenic nerve	use Phrenic Nerve
Accessory spleen	use Spleen
Acetabulofemoral joint	use Hip Joint, Left/Right
Achilles tendon	use Lower Leg Tendon, Left/Right
Acromioclavicular ligament	use Shoulder Bursa and Ligament, Left/Right
Acromion (process)	use Scapula, Left/Right
Adductor brevis muscle	use Upper Leg Muscle, Left/Right
Adductor hallucis muscle	use Foot Muscle, Left/Right
Adductor longus muscle	use Upper Leg Muscle, Left/Right
Adductor magnus muscle	
Adenohypophysis	use Pituitary Gland
Alar ligament of axis	use Head and Neck Bursa and Ligament
Alveolar process of mandible	use Mandible, Left/Right
Alveolar process of maxilla	use Maxilla, Left/Right
Anal orifice	use Anus
Anatomical snuffbox	use Lower Arm and Wrist Muscle, Left/Right
Angular artery	use Face Artery
Angular vein	use Face Vein, Left/Right
Annular ligament	use Elbow Bursa and Ligament, Left/Right
Anorectal junction	use Rectum
Ansa cervicalis	use Cervical Plexus
Antebrachial fascia	use Subcutaneous Tissue and Fascia, Lower Arm, Left/Right
Anterior cerebral artery	use Intracranial Artery
Anterior cerebral vein	use Intracranial Vein
Anterior choroidal artery	use Intracranial Artery
Anterior circumflex humeral artery	use Axillary Artery, Left/Right
Anterior communicating artery	use Intracranial Artery
Anterior cruciate ligament (ACL)	use Knee Bursa and Ligament, Left/Right
Anterior crural nerve	use Femoral Nerve
Anterior facial vein	use Face Vein, Left/Right
Anterior intercostal artery	use Internal Mammary Artery, Left/Right
Anterior interosseous nerve	use Median Nerve
Anterior lateral malleolar artery	use Anterior Tibial Artery, Left/Right
Anterior lingual gland	use Minor Salivary Gland
Anterior medial malleolar artery	use Anterior Tibial Artery, Left/Right
Anterior (pectoral) lymph node	use Lymphatic, Axillary, Left/Right
Anterior spinal artery	use Vertebral Artery, Left/Right

BODY PART	USE:
Anterior tibial recurrent artery	use Anterior Tibial Artery, Left/Right
Anterior ulnar recurrent artery	use Ulnar Artery, Left/Right
Anterior vagal trunk	use Vagus Nerve
Anterior vertebral muscle	use Neck Muscle, Left/Right
Antihelix	use External Ear, Bilateral/Left/Right
Antitragus	
Antrum of Highmore	use Maxillary Sinus, Left/Right
Aortic annulus	use Aortic Valve
Aortic arch	use Thoracic Aorta, Ascending/Arch
Aortic intercostal artery	use Upper Artery
Apical (subclavicular) lymph node	use Lymphatic, Axillary, Left/Right
Apneustic center	use Pons
Aqueduct of Sylvius	use Cerebral Ventricle
Aqueous humour	use Anterior Chamber, Left/Right
Arachnoid mater, intracranial	use Cerebral Meninges
Arachnoid mater, spinal	use Spinal Meninges
Arcuate artery	use Foot Artery, Left/Right
Areola	use Nipple, Left/Right
Arterial canal (duct)	use Pulmonary Artery, Left
Aryepiglottic fold	use Larynx
Arytenoid cartilage	
Arytenoid muscle	use Neck Muscle, Left/Right
Ascending aorta	use Thoracic Aorta, Ascending/Arch
Ascending palatine artery	use Face Artery
Ascending pharyngeal artery	use External Carotid Artery, Left/Right
Atlantoaxial joint	use Cervical Vertebral Joint
Atrioventricular node	use Conduction Mechanism
Atrium dextrum cordis	use Atrium, Right
Atrium pulmonale	use Atrium, Left
Auditory tube	use Eustachian Tube, Left/Right
Auerbach's (myenteric) plexus	use Abdominal Sympathetic Nerve
Auricle	use External Ear, Bilateral/Left/Right
Auricularis muscle	use Head Muscle
Axillary fascia	use Subcutaneous Tissue and Fascia, Upper Arm, Left/Right
Axillary nerve	use Brachial Plexus
Bartholin's (greater vestibular) gland	use Vestibular Gland
Basal (internal) cerebral vein	use Intracranial Vein
Basal nuclei	use Basal Ganglia
Base of tongue	use Pharynx
Basilar artery	use Intracranial Artery
Basis pontis	use Pons
Biceps brachii muscle	use Upper Arm Muscle, Left/Right
Biceps femoris muscle	use Upper Leg Muscle, Left/Right
Bicipital aponeurosis	use Subcutaneous Tissue and Fascia, Lower Arm, Left/Right
Bicuspid valve	use Mitral Valve
Body of femur	use Femoral Shaft, Left/Right
Body of fibula	use Fibula, Left/Right

BODY PART	USE:
Bony labyrinth	*use* Inner Ear, Left/Right
Bony orbit	*use* Orbit, Left/Right
Bony vestibule	*use* Inner Ear, Left/Right
Botallo's duct	*use* Pulmonary Artery, Left
Brachial (lateral) lymph node	*use* Lymphatic, Axillary, Left/Right
Brachialis muscle	*use* Upper Arm Muscle, Left/Right
Brachiocephalic artery Brachiocephalic trunk	*use* Innominate Artery
Brachiocephalic vein	*use* Innominate Vein, Left/Right
Brachioradialis muscle	*use* Lower Arm and Wrist Muscle, Left/Right
Broad ligament	*use* Uterine Supporting Structure
Bronchial artery	*use* Upper Artery
Bronchus intermedius	*use* Main Bronchus, Right
Buccal gland	*use* Buccal Mucosa
Buccinator lymph node	*use* Lymphatic, Head
Buccinator muscle	*use* Facial Muscle
Bulbospongiosus muscle	*use* Perineum Muscle
Bulbourethral (Cowper's) gland	*use* Urethra
Bundle of His Bundle of Kent	*use* Conduction Mechanism
Calcaneocuboid joint	*use* Tarsal Joint, Left/Right
Calcaneocuboid ligament	*use* Foot Bursa and Ligament, Left/Right
Calcaneofibular ligament	*use* Ankle Bursa and Ligament, Left/Right
Calcaneus	*use* Tarsal, Left/Right
Capitate bone	*use* Carpal, Left/Right
Cardia	*use* Esophagogastric Junction
Cardiac plexus	*use* Thoracic Sympathetic Nerve
Cardioesophageal junction	*use* Esophagogastric Junction
Caroticotympanic artery	*use* Internal Carotid Artery, Left/Right
Carotid glomus	*use* Carotid Body, Bilateral/Left/Right
Carotid sinus	*use* Internal Carotid Artery, Left/Right
Carotid sinus nerve	*use* Glossopharyngeal Nerve
Carpometacarpal (CMC) joint	*use* Metacarpocarpal Joint, Left/Right
Carpometacarpal ligament	*use* Hand Bursa and Ligament, Left/Right
Cauda equina	*use* Lumbar Spinal Cord
Cavernous plexus	*use* Head and Neck Sympathetic Nerve
Celiac (solar) plexus Celiac ganglion	*use* Abdominal Sympathetic Nerve
Celiac lymph node	*use* Lymphatic, Aortic
Celiac trunk	*use* Celiac Artery
Central axillary lymph node	*use* Lymphatic, Axillary, Left/Right
Cerebral aqueduct (Sylvius)	*use* Cerebral Ventricle
Cerebrum	*use* Brain
Cervical esophagus	*use* Esophagus, Upper
Cervical facet joint	*use* Cervical Vertebral Joint(s)

BODY PART	USE:
Cervical ganglion	*use* Head and Neck Sympathetic Nerve
Cervical interspinous ligament Cervical intertransverse ligament Cervical ligamentum flavum	*use* Head and Neck Bursa and Ligament
Cervical lymph node	*use* Lymphatic, Neck, Left/Right
Cervicothoracic facet joint	*use* Cervicothoracic Vertebral Joint
Choana	*use* Nasopharynx
Chondroglossus muscle	*use* Tongue, Palate, Pharynx Muscle
Chorda tympani	*use* Facial Nerve
Choroid plexus	*use* Cerebral Ventricle
Ciliary body	*use* Eye, Left/Right
Ciliary ganglion	*use* Head and Neck Sympathetic Nerve
Circle of Willis	*use* Intracranial Artery
Circumflex iliac artery	*use* Femoral Artery, Left/Right
Claustrum	*use* Basal Ganglia
Coccygeal body	*use* Coccygeal Glomus
Coccygeus muscle	*use* Trunk Muscle, Left/Right
Cochlea	*use* Inner Ear, Left/Right
Cochlear nerve	*use* Acoustic Nerve
Columella	*use* Nose
Common digital vein	*use* Foot Vein, Left/Right
Common facial vein	*use* Face Vein, Left/Right
Common fibular nerve	*use* Peroneal Nerve
Common hepatic artery	*use* Hepatic Artery
Common iliac (subaortic) lymph node	*use* Lymphatic, Pelvis
Common interosseous artery	*use* Ulnar Artery, Left/Right
Common peroneal nerve	*use* Peroneal Nerve
Condyloid process	*use* Mandible, Left/Right
Conus arteriosus	*use* Ventricle, Right
Conus medullaris	*use* Lumbar Spinal Cord
Coracoacromial ligament	*use* Shoulder Bursa and Ligament, Left/Right
Coracobrachialis muscle	*use* Upper Arm Muscle, Left/Right
Coracoclavicular ligament Coracohumeral ligament	*use* Shoulder Bursa and Ligament, Left/Right
Coracoid process	*use* Scapula, Left/Right
Corniculate cartilage	*use* Larynx
Corpus callosum	*use* Brain
Corpus cavernosum Corpus spongiosum	*use* Penis
Corpus striatum	*use* Basal Ganglia
Corrugator supercilii muscle	*use* Facial Muscle
Costocervical trunk	*use* Subclavian Artery, Left/Right
Costoclavicular ligament	*use* Shoulder Bursa and Ligament, Left/Right
Costotransverse joint	*use* Thoracic Vertebral Joint
Costotransverse ligament	*use* Thorax Bursa and Ligament, Left/Right
Costovertebral joint	*use* Thoracic Vertebral Joint

BODY PART	USE:
Costoxiphoid ligament	use Thorax Bursa and Ligament, Left/Right
Cowper's (bulbourethral) gland	use Urethra
Cremaster muscle	use Perineum Muscle
Cribriform plate	use Ethmoid Bone, Left/Right
Cricoid cartilage	use Trachea
Cricothyroid artery	use Thyroid Artery, Left/Right
Cricothyroid muscle	use Neck Muscle, Left/Right
Crural fascia	use Subcutaneous Tissue and Fascia, Upper Leg, Left/Right
Cubital lymph node	use Lymphatic, Upper Extremity, Left/Right
Cubital nerve	use Ulnar Nerve
Cuboid bone	use Tarsal, Left/Right
Cuboideonavicular joint	use Tarsal Joint, Left/Right
Culmen	use Cerebellum
Cuneiform cartilage	use Larynx
Cuneonavicular joint	use Tarsal Joint, Left/Right
Cuneonavicular ligament	use Foot Bursa and Ligament, Left/Right
Cutaneous (transverse) cervical nerve	use Cervical Plexus
Deep cervical fascia	use Subcutaneous Tissue and Fascia, Anterior Neck
Deep cervical vein	use Vertebral Vein, Left/Right
Deep circumflex iliac artery	use External Iliac Artery, Left/Right
Deep facial vein	use Face Vein, Left/Right
Deep femoral artery	use Femoral Artery, Left/Right
Deep femoral (profunda femoris) vein	use Femoral Vein, Left/Right
Deep palmar arch	use Hand Artery, Left/Right
Deep transverse perineal muscle	use Perineum Muscle
Deferential artery	use Internal Iliac Artery, Left/Right
Deltoid fascia	use Subcutaneous Tissue and Fascia, Upper Arm, Left/Right
Deltoid ligament	use Ankle Bursa and Ligament, Left/Right
Deltoid muscle	use Shoulder Muscle, Left/Right
Deltopectoral (infraclavicular) lymph node	use Lymphatic, Upper Extremity, Left/Right
Denticulate (dentate) ligament	use Spinal Meninges
Depressor anguli oris muscle	use Facial Muscle
Depressor labii inferioris muscle	
Depressor septi nasi muscle	
Depressor supercilii muscle	
Dermis	use Skin
Descending genicular artery	use Femoral Artery, Left/Right
Diaphragma sellae	use Dura Mater
Distal humerus	use Humeral Shaft, Left/Right

BODY PART	USE:
Distal humerus, involving joint	use Elbow Joint, Left/Right
Distal radioulnar joint	use Wrist Joint, Left/Right
Dorsal digital nerve	use Radial Nerve
Dorsal metacarpal vein	use Hand Vein, Left/Right
Dorsal metatarsal artery	use Foot Artery, Left/Right
Dorsal metatarsal vein	use Foot Vein, Left/Right
Dorsal scapular artery	use Subclavian Artery, Left/Right
Dorsal scapular nerve	use Brachial Plexus
Dorsal venous arch	use Foot Vein, Left/Right
Dorsalis pedis artery	use Anterior Tibial Artery, Left/Right
Duct of Santorini	use Pancreatic Duct, Accessory
Duct of Wirsung	use Pancreatic Duct
Ductus deferens	use Vas Deferens, Bilateral/Left/Right
Duodenal ampulla	use Ampulla of Vater
Duodenojejunal flexure	use Jejunum
Dura mater, intracranial	use Dura Mater
Dura mater, spinal	use Spinal Meninges
Dural venous sinus	use Intracranial Vein
Earlobe	use External Ear, Bilateral/Left/Right
Eighth cranial nerve	use Acoustic Nerve
Ejaculatory duct	use Vas Deferens, Bilateral/Left/Right
Eleventh cranial nerve	use Accessory Nerve
Encephalon	use Brain
Ependyma	use Cerebral Ventricle
Epidermis	use Skin
Epidural space intracranial	use Epidural Space
Epidural space, spinal	use Spinal Canal
Epiploic foramen	use Peritoneum
Epithalamus	use Thalamus
Epitrochlear lymph node	use Lymphatic, Upper Extremity, Left/Right
Erector spinae muscle	use Trunk Muscle, Left/Right
Esophageal artery	use Upper Artery
Esophageal plexus	use Thoracic Sympathetic Nerve
Ethmoidal air cell	use Ethmoid Sinus, Left/Right
Extensor carpi radialis muscle	use Lower Arm and Wrist Muscle, Left/Right
Extensor carpi ulnaris muscle	
Extensor digitorum brevis muscle	use Foot Muscle, Left/Right
Extensor digitorum longus muscle	use Lower Leg Muscle, Left/Right
Extensor hallucis brevis muscle	use Foot Muscle, Left/Right
Extensor hallucis longus muscle	use Lower Leg Muscle, Left/Right
External anal sphincter	use Anal Sphincter
External auditory meatus	use External Auditory Canal, Left/Right
External maxillary artery	use Face Artery
External naris	use Nose
External oblique aponeurosis	use Subcutaneous Tissue and Fascia, Trunk
External oblique muscle	use Abdomen Muscle, Left/Right

BODY PART	USE:
External popliteal nerve	use Peroneal Nerve
External pudendal artery	use Femoral Artery, Left/Right
External pudendal vein	use Greater Saphenous Vein, Left/Right
External urethral sphincter	use Urethra
Extradural space, intracranial	use Epidural Space
Extradural space, spinal	use Spinal Canal
Facial artery	use Face Artery
False vocal cord	use Larynx
Falx cerebri	use Dura Mater
Fascia lata	use Subcutaneous Tissue and Fascia, Upper Leg, Left/Right
Femoral head	use Upper Femur, Left/Right
Femoral lymph node	use Lymphatic, Lower Extremity, Left/Right
Femoropatellar joint	use Knee Joint, Left/Right / use Knee Joint, Femoral Surface, Left/Right
Femorotibial joint	use Knee Joint, Left/Right / use Knee Joint, Tibial Surface, Left/Right
Fibular artery	use Peroneal Artery, Left/Right
Fibularis brevis muscle / Fibularis longus muscle	use Lower Leg Muscle, Left/Right
Fifth cranial nerve	use Trigeminal Nerve
Filum terminale	use Spinal Meninges
First cranial nerve	use Olfactory Nerve
First intercostal nerve	use Brachial Plexus
Flexor carpi radialis muscle / Flexor carpi ulnaris muscle	use Lower Arm and Wrist Muscle, Left/Right
Flexor digitorum brevis muscle	use Foot Muscle, Left/Right
Flexor digitorum longus muscle	use Lower Leg Muscle, Left/Right
Flexor hallucis brevis muscle	use Foot Muscle, Left/Right
Flexor hallucis longus muscle	use Lower Leg Muscle, Left/Right
Flexor pollicis longus muscle	use Lower Arm and Wrist Muscle, Left/Right
Foramen magnum	use Occipital Bone, Left/Right
Foramen of Monro (intraventricular)	use Cerebral Ventricle
Foreskin	use Prepuce
Fossa of Rosenmuller	use Nasopharynx
Fourth cranial nerve	use Trochlear Nerve
Fourth ventricle	use Cerebral Ventricle
Fovea	use Retina, Left/Right
Frenulum labii inferioris	use Lower Lip
Frenulum labii superioris	use Upper Lip
Frenulum linguae	use Tongue
Frontal lobe	use Cerebral Hemisphere
Frontal vein	use Face Vein, Left/Right
Fundus uteri	use Uterus

BODY PART	USE:
Galea aponeurotica	use Subcutaneous Tissue and Fascia, Scalp
Ganglion impar (ganglion of Walther)	use Sacral Sympathetic Nerve
Gasserian ganglion	use Trigeminal Nerve
Gastric lymph node	use Lymphatic, Aortic
Gastric plexus	use Abdominal Sympathetic Nerve
Gastrocnemius muscle	use Lower Leg Muscle, Left/Right
Gastrocolic ligament / Gastrocolic omentum	use Greater Omentum
Gastroduodenal artery	use Hepatic Artery
Gastroesophageal (GE) junction	use Esophagogastric Junction
Gastrohepatic omentum	use Lesser Omentum
Gastrophrenic ligament / Gastrosplenic ligament	use Greater Omentum
Gemellus muscle	use Hip Muscle, Left/Right
Geniculate ganglion	use Facial Nerve
Geniculate nucleus	use Thalamus
Genioglossus muscle	use Tongue, Palate, Pharynx Muscle
Genitofemoral nerve	use Lumbar Plexus
Glans penis	use Prepuce
Glenohumeral joint	use Shoulder Joint, Left/Right
Glenohumeral ligament	use Shoulder Bursa and Ligament, Left/Right
Glenoid fossa (of scapula)	use Glenoid Cavity, Left/Right
Glenoid ligament (labrum)	use Shoulder Joint, Left/Right
Globus pallidus	use Basal Ganglia
Glossoepiglottic fold	use Epiglottis
Glottis	use Larynx
Gluteal lymph node	use Lymphatic, Pelvis
Gluteal vein	use Hypogastric Vein, Left/Right
Gluteus maximus muscle / Gluteus medius muscle / Gluteus minimus muscle	use Hip Muscle, Left/Right
Gracilis muscle	use Upper Leg Muscle, Left/Right
Great auricular nerve	use Cervical Plexus
Great cerebral vein	use Intracranial Vein
Great saphenous vein	use Greater Saphenous Vein, Left/Right
Greater alar cartilage	use Nose
Greater occipital nerve	use Cervical Nerve
Greater splanchnic nerve	use Thoracic Sympathetic Nerve
Greater superficial petrosal nerve	use Facial Nerve
Greater trochanter	use Upper Femur, Left/Right
Greater tuberosity	use Humeral Head, Left/Right
Greater vestibular (Bartholin's) gland	use Vestibular Gland
Greater wing	use Sphenoid Bone, Left/Right
Hallux	use 1st Toe, Left/Right
Hamate bone	use Carpal, Left/Right
Head of fibula	use Fibula, Left/Right
Helix	use External Ear, Bilateral/Left/Right
Hepatic artery proper	use Hepatic Artery
Hepatic flexure	use Ascending Colon
Hepatic lymph node	use Lymphatic, Aortic

BODY PART	USE:
Hepatic plexus	use Abdominal Sympathetic Nerve
Hepatic portal vein	use Portal Vein
Hepatogastric ligament	use Lesser Omentum
Hepatopancreatic ampulla	use Ampulla of Vater
Humeroradial joint	use Elbow Joint, Left/Right
Humeroulnar joint	
Humerus, distal	use Humeral Shaft, Left/Right
Hyoglossus muscle	use Tongue, Palate, Pharynx Muscle
Hyoid artery	use Thyroid Artery, Left/Right
Hypogastric artery	use Internal Iliac Artery, Left/Right
Hypopharynx	use Pharynx
Hypophysis	use Pituitary Gland
Hypothenar muscle	use Hand Muscle, Left/Right
Ileal artery	use Superior Mesenteric Artery
Ileocolic artery	
Ileocolic vein	use Colic Vein
Iliac crest	use Pelvic Bone, Left/Right
Iliac fascia	use Subcutaneous Tissue and Fascia, Upper Leg, Left/Right
Iliac lymph node	use Lymphatic, Pelvis
Iliacus muscle	use Hip Muscle, Left/Right
Iliofemoral ligament	use Hip Bursa and Ligament, Left/Right
Iliohypogastric nerve	use Lumbar Plexus
Ilioinguinal nerve	
Iliolumbar artery	use Internal Iliac Artery, Left/Right
Iliolumbar ligament	use Trunk Bursa and Ligament, Left/Right
Iliotibial tract (band)	use Subcutaneous Tissue and Fascia, Upper Leg, Left/Right
Ilium	use Pelvic Bone, Left/Right
Incus	use Auditory Ossicle, Left/Right
Inferior cardiac nerve	use Thoracic Sympathetic Nerve
Inferior cerebellar vein	use Intracranial Vein
Inferior cerebral vein	
Inferior epigastric artery	use External Iliac Artery, Left/Right
Inferior epigastric lymph node	use Lymphatic, Pelvis
Inferior genicular artery	use Popliteal Artery, Left/Right
Inferior gluteal artery	use Internal Iliac Artery, Left/Right
Inferior gluteal nerve	use Sacral Plexus
Inferior hypogastric plexus	use Abdominal Sympathetic Nerve
Inferior labial artery	use Face Artery
Inferior longitudinal muscle	use Tongue, Palate, Pharynx Muscle
Inferior mesenteric ganglion	use Abdominal Sympathetic Nerve
Inferior mesenteric lymph node	use Lymphatic, Mesenteric
Inferior mesenteric plexus	use Abdominal Sympathetic Nerve
Inferior oblique muscle	use Extraocular Muscle, Left/Right
Inferior pancreatico-duodenal artery	use Superior Mesenteric Artery
Inferior phrenic artery	use Abdominal Aorta
Inferior rectus muscle	use Extraocular Muscle, Left/Right
Inferior suprarenal artery	use Renal Artery, Left/Right
Inferior tarsal plate	use Lower Eyelid, Left/Right

BODY PART	USE:
Inferior thyroid vein	use Innominate Vein, Left/Right
Inferior tibiofibular joint	use Ankle Joint, Left/Right
Inferior turbinate	use Nasal Turbinate
Inferior ulnar collateral artery	use Brachial Artery, Left/Right
Inferior vesical artery	use Internal Iliac Artery, Left/Right
Infraauricular lymph node	use Lymphatic, Head
Infraclavicular (delto-pectoral) lymph node	use Lymphatic, Upper Extremity, Left/Right
Infrahyoid muscle	use Neck Muscle, Left/Right
Infraparotid lymph node	use Lymphatic, Head
Infraspinatus fascia	use Subcutaneous Tissue and Fascia, Upper Arm, Left/Right
Infraspinatus muscle	use Shoulder Muscle, Left/Right
Infundibulopelvic ligament	use Uterine Supporting Structure
Inguinal canal	use Inguinal Region, Bilateral/Left/Right
Inguinal triangle	
Interatrial septum	use Atrial Septum
Intercarpal joint	use Carpal Joint, Left/Right
Intercarpal ligament	use Hand Bursa and Ligament, Left/Right
Interclavicular ligament	use Shoulder Bursa and Ligament, Left/Right
Intercostal lymph node	use Lymphatic, Thorax
Intercostal muscle	use Thorax Muscle, Left/Right
Intercostal nerve	use Thoracic Nerve
Intercostobrachial nerve	
Intercuneiform joint	use Tarsal Joint, Left/Right
Intercuneiform ligament	use Foot Bursa and Ligament, Left/Right
Intermediate bronchus	use Main Bronchus, Right
Intermediate cuneiform bone	use Tarsal, Left/Right
Internal (basal) cerebral vein	use Intracranial Vein
Internal anal sphincter	use Anal Sphincter
Internal carotid artery, intracranial portion	use Intracranial Artery
Internal carotid plexus	use Head and Neck Sympathetic Nerve
Internal iliac vein	use Hypogastric Vein, Left/Right
Internal maxillary artery	use External Carotid Artery, Left/Right
Internal naris	use Nose
Internal oblique muscle	use Abdomen Muscle, Left/Right
Internal pudendal artery	use Internal Iliac Artery, Left/Right
Internal pudendal vein	use Hypogastric Vein, Left/Right
Internal thoracic artery	use Internal Mammary Artery, Left/Right Subclavian Artery, Left/Right
Internal urethral sphincter	use Urethra
Interphalangeal (IP) joint	use Finger Phalangeal Joint, Left/Right Toe Phalangeal Joint, Left/Right
Interphalangeal ligament	use Hand Bursa and Ligament, Left/Right Foot Bursa and Ligament, Left/Right

BODY PART	USE:
Interspinalis muscle	*use* Trunk Muscle, Left/Right
Interspinous ligament	*use* Head and Neck Bursa and Ligament
	use Trunk Bursa and Ligament, Left/Right
Intertransversarius muscle	*use* Trunk Muscle, Left/Right
Intertransverse ligament	*use* Trunk Bursa and Ligament, Left/Right
Interventricular foramen (Monro)	*use* Cerebral Ventricle
Interventricular septum	*use* Ventricular Septum
Intestinal lymphatic trunk	*use* Cisterna Chyli
Ischiatic nerve	*use* Sciatic Nerve
Ischiocavernosus muscle	*use* Perineum Muscle
Ischiofemoral ligament	*use* Hip Bursa and Ligament, Left/Right
Ischium	*use* Pelvic Bone, Left/Right
Jejunal artery	*use* Superior Mesenteric Artery
Jugular body	*use* Glomus Jugulare
Jugular lymph node	*use* Lymphatic, Neck, Left/Right
Labia majora Labia minora	*use* Vulva
Labial gland	*use* Upper Lip, Lower Lip
Lacrimal canaliculus	*use* Lacrimal Duct, Left/Right
Lacrimal punctum Lacrimal sac	
Laryngopharynx	*use* Pharynx
Lateral (brachial) lymph node	*use* Lymphatic, Axillary, Left/Right
Lateral canthus	*use* Upper Eyelid, Left/Right
Lateral collateral ligament (LCL)	*use* Knee Bursa and Ligament, Left/Right
Lateral condyle of femur	*use* Lower Femur, Left/Right
Lateral condyle of tibia	*use* Tibia, Left/Right
Lateral cuneiform bone	*use* Tarsal, Left/Right
Lateral epicondyle of femur	*use* Lower Femur, Left/Right
Lateral epicondyle of humerus	*use* Humeral Shaft, Left/Right
Lateral femoral cutaneous nerve	*use* Lumbar Plexus
Lateral malleolus	*use* Fibula, Left/Right
Lateral meniscus	*use* Knee Joint, Left/Right
Lateral nasal cartilage	*use* Nose
Lateral plantar artery	*use* Foot Artery, Left/Right
Lateral plantar nerve	*use* Tibial Nerve
Lateral rectus muscle	*use* Extraocular Muscle, Left/Right
Lateral sacral artery	*use* Internal Iliac Artery, Left/Right
Lateral sacral vein	*use* Hypogastric Vein, Left/Right
Lateral sural cutaneous nerve	*use* Peroneal Nerve
Lateral tarsal artery	*use* Foot Artery, Left/Right
Lateral temporo-mandibular ligament	*use* Head and Neck Bursa and Ligament
Lateral thoracic artery	*use* Axillary Artery, Left/Right
Latissimus dorsi muscle	*use* Trunk Muscle, Left/Right
Least splanchnic nerve	*use* Thoracic Sympathetic Nerve

BODY PART	USE:
Left ascending lumbar vein	*use* Hemiazygos Vein
Left atrioventricular valve	*use* Mitral Valve
Left auricular appendix	*use* Atrium, Left
Left colic vein	*use* Colic Vein
Left coronary sulcus	*use* Heart, Left
Left gastric artery	*use* Gastric Artery
Left gastroepiploic artery	*use* Splenic Artery
Left gastroepiploic vein	*use* Splenic Vein
Left inferior phrenic vein	*use* Renal Vein, Left
Left inferior pulmonary vein	*use* Pulmonary Vein, Left
Left jugular trunk	*use* Thoracic Duct
Left lateral ventricle	*use* Cerebral Ventricle
Left ovarian vein Left second lumbar vein	*use* Renal Vein, Left
Left subclavian trunk	*use* Thoracic Duct
Left subcostal vein	*use* Hemiazygos Vein
Left superior pulmonary vein	*use* Pulmonary Vein, Left
Left suprarenal vein Left testicular vein	*use* Renal Vein, Left
Leptomeninges, intracranial	*use* Cerebral Meninges
Leptomeninges, spinal	*use* Spinal Meninges
Lesser alar cartilage	*use* Nose
Lesser occipital nerve	*use* Cervical Plexus
Lesser splanchnic nerve	*use* Thoracic Sympathetic Nerve
Lesser trochanter	*use* Upper Femur, Left/Right
Lesser tuberosity	*use* Humeral Head, Left/Right
Lesser wing	*use* Sphenoid Bone, Left/Right
Levator anguli oris muscle	*use* Facial Muscle
Levator ani muscle	*use* Perineum Muscle
Levator labii superioris alaeque nasi muscle Levator labii superioris muscle	*use* Facial Muscle
Levator palpebrae superioris muscle	*use* Upper Eyelid, Left/Right
Levator scapulae muscle	*use* Neck Muscle, Left/Right
Levator veli palatini muscle	*use* Tongue, Palate, Pharynx Muscle
Levatores costarum muscle	*use* Thorax Muscle, Left/Right
Ligament of head of fibula	*use* Knee Bursa and Ligament, Left/Right
Ligament of the lateral malleolus	*use* Ankle Bursa and Ligament, Left/Right
Ligamentum flavum	*use* Trunk Bursa and Ligament, Left/Right
Lingual artery	*use* External Carotid Artery, Left/Right
Lingual tonsil	*use* Tongue
Locus ceruleus	*use* Pons
Long thoracic nerve	*use* Brachial Plexus
Lumbar artery	*use* Abdominal Aorta
Lumbar facet joint	*use* Lumbar Vertebral Joint
Lumbar ganglion	*use* Lumbar Sympathetic Nerve

BODY PART	USE:
Lumbar lymph node	use Lymphatic, Aortic
Lumbar lymphatic trunk	use Cisterna Chyli
Lumbar splanchnic nerve	use Lumbar Sympathetic Nerve
Lumbosacral facet joint	use Lumbosacral Joint
Lumbosacral trunk	use Lumbar Nerve
Lunate bone	use Carpal, Left/Right
Lunotriquetral ligament	use Hand Bursa and Ligament, Left/Right
Macula	use Retina, Left/Right
Malleus	use Auditory Ossicle, Left/Right
Mammary duct Mammary gland	use Breast, Bilateral/Left/Right
Mammillary body	use Hypothalamus
Mandibular nerve	use Trigeminal Nerve
Mandibular notch	use Mandible, Left/Right
Manubrium	use Sternum
Masseter muscle	use Head Muscle
Masseteric fascia	use Subcutaneous Tissue and Fascia, Face
Mastoid air cells	use Mastoid Sinus, Left/Right
Mastoid (postauricular) lymph node	use Lymphatic, Neck, Left/Right
Mastoid process	use Temporal Bone, Left/Right
Maxillary artery	use External Carotid Artery, Left/Right
Maxillary nerve	use Trigeminal Nerve
Medial canthus	use Lower Eyelid, Left/Right
Medial collateral ligament (MCL)	use Knee Bursa and Ligament, Left/Right
Medial condyle of femur	use Lower Femur, Left/Right
Medial condyle of tibia	use Tibia, Left/Right
Medial cuneiform bone	use Tarsal, Left/Right
Medial epicondyle of femur	use Lower Femur, Left/Right
Medial epicondyle of humerus	use Humeral Shaft, Left/Right
Medial malleolus	use Tibia, Left/Right
Medial meniscus	use Knee Joint, Left/Right
Medial plantar artery	use Foot Artery, Left/Right
Medial plantar nerve Medial popliteal nerve	use Tibial Nerve
Medial rectus muscle	use Extraocular Muscle, Left/Right
Medial sural cutaneous nerve	use Tibial Nerve
Median antebrachial vein Median cubital vein	use Basilic Vein, Left/Right
Median sacral artery	use Abdominal Aorta
Mediastinal lymph node	use Lymphatic, Thorax
Meissner's (submucous) plexus	use Abdominal Sympathetic Nerve
Membranous urethra	use Urethra
Mental foramen	use Mandible, Left/Right
Mentalis muscle	use Facial Muscle
Mesoappendix Mesocolon	use Mesentery
Metacarpal ligament Metacarpophalangeal ligament	use Hand Bursa and Ligament, Left/Right

BODY PART	USE:
Metatarsal ligament	use Foot Bursa and Ligament, Left/Right
Metatarsophalangeal (MTP) joint	use Metatarsal-Phalangeal Joint, Left/Right
Metatarsophalangeal ligament	use Foot Bursa and Ligament, Left/Right
Metathalamus	use Thalamus
Midcarpal joint	use Carpal Joint, Left/Right
Middle cardiac nerve	use Thoracic Sympathetic Nerve
Middle cerebral artery	use Intracranial Artery
Middle cerebral vein	use Intracranial Vein
Middle colic vein	use Colic Vein
Middle genicular artery	use Popliteal Artery, Left/Right
Middle hemorrhoidal vein	use Hypogastric Vein, Left/Right
Middle rectal artery	use Internal Iliac Artery, Left/Right
Middle suprarenal artery	use Abdominal Aorta
Middle temporal artery	use Temporal Artery, Left/Right
Middle turbinate	use Nasal Turbinate
Mitral annulus	use Mitral Valve
Molar gland	use Buccal Mucosa
Musculocutaneous nerve	use Brachial Plexus
Musculophrenic artery	use Internal Mammary Artery, Left/Right
Musculospiral nerve	use Radial Nerve
Myelencephalon	use Medulla Oblongata
Myenteric (Auerbach's) plexus	use Abdominal Sympathetic Nerve
Myometrium	use Uterus
Nail bed, Nail plate	use Finger Nail, Toe Nail
Nasal cavity	use Nose
Nasal concha	use Nasal Turbinate
Nasalis muscle	use Facial Muscle
Nasolacrimal duct	use Lacrimal Duct, Left/Right
Navicular bone	use Tarsal, Left/Right
Neck of femur	use Upper Femur, Left/Right
Neck of humerus (anatomical) (surgical)	use Humeral Head, Left/Right
Nerve to the stapedius	use Facial Nerve
Neurohypophysis	use Pituitary Gland
Ninth cranial nerve	use Glossopharyngeal Nerve
Nostril	use Nose
Obturator artery	use Internal Iliac Artery, Left/Right
Obturator lymph node	use Lymphatic, Pelvis
Obturator muscle	use Hip Muscle, Left/Right
Obturator nerve	use Lumbar Plexus
Obturator vein	use Hypogastric Vein, Left/Right
Obtuse margin	use Heart, Left
Occipital artery	use External Carotid Artery, Left/Right
Occipital lobe	use Cerebral Hemisphere
Occipital lymph node	use Lymphatic, Neck, Left/Right
Occipitofrontalis muscle	use Facial Muscle
Olecranon bursa	use Elbow Bursa and Ligament, Left/Right
Olecranon process	use Ulna, Left/Right
Olfactory bulb	use Olfactory Nerve
Ophthalmic artery	use Intracranial Artery
Ophthalmic nerve	use Trigeminal Nerve
Ophthalmic vein	use Intracranial Vein

BODY PART	USE:
Optic chiasma	*use* Optic Nerve
Optic disc	*use* Retina, Left/Right
Optic foramen	*use* Sphenoid Bone, Left/Right
Orbicularis oculi muscle	*use* Upper Eyelid, Left/Right
Orbicularis oris muscle	*use* Facial Muscle
Orbital fascia	*use* Subcutaneous Tissue and Fascia, Face
Orbital portion of: ethmoid bone, frontal bone, lacrimal bone, maxilla, palatine bone, sphenoid bone, zygomatic bone	*use* Orbit, Left/Right
Oropharynx	*use* Pharynx
Otic ganglion	*use* Head and Neck Sympathetic Nerve
Oval window	*use* Middle Ear, Left/Right
Ovarian artery	*use* Abdominal Aorta
Ovarian ligament	*use* Uterine Supporting Structure
Oviduct	*use* Fallopian Tube, Left/Right
Palatine gland	*use* Buccal Mucosa
Palatine tonsil	*use* Tonsils
Palatine uvula	*use* Uvula
Palatoglossal muscle Palatopharyngeal muscle	*use* Tongue, Palate, Pharynx Muscle
Palmar cutaneous nerve	*use* Median Nerve, Radial Nerve
Palmar fascia (aponeurosis)	*use* Subcutaneous Tissue and Fascia, Hand, Left/Right
Palmar interosseous muscle	*use* Hand Muscle, Left/Right
Palmar ulnocarpal ligament	*use* Wrist Bursa and Ligament, Left/Right
Palmar (volar) digital vein Palmar (volar) metacarpal vein	*use* Hand Vein, Left/Right
Palmaris longus muscle	*use* Lower Arm and Wrist Muscle, Left/Right
Pancreatic artery	*use* Splenic Artery
Pancreatic plexus	*use* Abdominal Sympathetic Nerve
Pancreatic vein	*use* Splenic Vein
Pancreaticosplenic lymph node Paraaortic lymph node	*use* Lymphatic, Aortic
Pararectal lymph node	*use* Lymphatic, Mesenteric
Parasternal lymph node Paratracheal lymph node	*use* Lymphatic, Thorax
Paraurethral (Skene's) gland	*use* Vestibular Gland
Parietal lobe	*use* Cerebral Hemisphere
Parotid lymph node	*use* Lymphatic, Head
Parotid plexus	*use* Facial Nerve
Pars flaccida	*use* Tympanic Membrane, Left/Right
Patellar ligament	*use* Knee Bursa and Ligament, Left/Right
Patellar tendon	*use* Knee Tendon, Left/Right
Patellofemoral joint	*use* Knee Joint, Left/Right *use* Knee Joint, Femoral Surface, Left/Right

BODY PART	USE:
Pectineus muscle	*use* Upper Leg Muscle, Left/Right
Pectoral (anterior) lymph node	*use* Lymphatic, Axillary, Left/Right
Pectoral fascia	*use* Subcutaneous Tissue and Fascia, Chest
Pectoralis major muscle Pectoralis minor muscle	*use* Thorax Muscle, Left/Right
Pelvic splanchnic nerve	*use* Abdominal Sympathetic Nerve Sacral Sympathetic Nerve
Penile urethra	*use* Urethra
Pericardiophrenic artery	*use* Internal Mammary Artery, Left/Right
Perimetrium	*use* Uterus
Peroneus brevis muscle Peroneus longus muscle	*use* Lower Leg Muscle, Left/Right
Petrous part of temporal bone	*use* Temporal Bone, Left/Right
Pharyngeal constrictor muscle	*use* Tongue, Palate, Pharynx Muscle
Pharyngeal plexus	*use* Vagus Nerve
Pharyngeal recess	*use* Nasopharynx
Pharyngeal tonsil	*use* Adenoids
Pharyngotympanic tube	*use* Eustachian Tube, Left/Right
Pia mater, intracranial	*use* Cerebral Meninges
Pia mater, spinal	*use* Spinal Meninges
Pinna	*use* External Ear, Bilateral/Left/Right
Piriform recess (sinus)	*use* Pharynx
Piriformis muscle	*use* Hip Muscle, Left/Right
Pisiform bone	*use* Carpal, Left/Right
Pisohamate ligament Pisometacarpal ligament	*use* Hand Bursa and Ligament, Left/Right
Plantar digital vein	*use* Foot Vein, Left/Right
Plantar fascia (aponeurosis)	*use* Subcutaneous Tissue and Fascia, Foot, Left/Right
Plantar metatarsal vein Plantar venous arch	*use* Foot Vein, Left/Right
Platysma muscle	*use* Neck Muscle, Left/Right
Plica semilunaris	*use* Conjunctiva, Left/Right
Pneumogastric nerve	*use* Vagus Nerve
Pneumotaxic center Pontine tegmentum	*use* Pons
Popliteal ligament	*use* Knee Bursa and Ligament, Left/Right
Popliteal lymph node	*use* Lymphatic, Lower Extremity, Left/Right
Popliteal vein	*use* Femoral Vein, Left/Right
Popliteus muscle	*use* Lower Leg Muscle, Left/Right
Postauricular (mastoid) lymph node	*use* Lymphatic, Neck, Left/Right
Postcava	*use* Inferior Vena Cava
Posterior (subscapular) lymph node	*use* Lymphatic, Axillary, Left/Right
Posterior auricular artery	*use* External Carotid Artery, Left/Right
Posterior auricular nerve	*use* Facial Nerve
Posterior auricular vein	*use* External Jugular Vein, Left/Right
Posterior cerebral artery	*use* Intracranial Artery

BODY PART	USE:
Posterior chamber	use Eye, Left/Right
Posterior circumflex humeral artery	use Axillary Artery, Left/Right
Posterior communicating artery	use Intracranial Artery
Posterior cruciate ligament (PCL)	use Knee Bursa and Ligament, Left/Right
Posterior facial (retro-mandibular) vein	use Face Vein, Left/Right
Posterior femoral cutaneous nerve	use Sacral Plexus
Posterior inferior cerebellar artery (PICA)	use Intracranial Artery
Posterior interosseous nerve	use Radial Nerve
Posterior labial nerve Posterior scrotal nerve	use Pudendal Nerve
Posterior spinal artery	use Vertebral Artery, Left/Right
Posterior tibial recurrent artery	use Anterior Tibial Artery, Left/Right
Posterior ulnar recurrent artery	use Ulnar Artery, Left/Right
Posterior vagal trunk	use Vagus Nerve
Preauricular lymph node	use Lymphatic, Head
Precava	use Superior Vena Cava
Prepatellar bursa	use Knee Bursa and Ligament, Left/Right
Pretracheal fascia	use Subcutaneous Tissue and Fascia, Anterior Neck
Prevertebral fascia	use Subcutaneous Tissue and Fascia, Posterior Neck
Princeps pollicis artery	use Hand Artery, Left/Right
Procerus muscle	use Facial Muscle
Profunda brachii	use Brachial Artery, Left/Right
Profunda femoris (deep femoral) vein	use Femoral Vein, Left/Right
Pronator quadratus muscle Pronator teres muscle	use Lower Arm and Wrist Muscle, Left/Right
Prostatic urethra	use Urethra
Proximal radioulnar joint	use Elbow Joint, Left/Right
Psoas muscle	use Hip Muscle, Left/Right
Pterygoid muscle	use Head Muscle
Pterygoid process	use Sphenoid Bone, Left/Right
Pterygopalatine (spheno-palatine) ganglion	use Head and Neck Sympathetic Nerve
Pubic ligament	use Trunk Bursa and Ligament, Left/Right
Pubis	use Pelvic Bone, Left/Right
Pubofemoral ligament	use Hip Bursa and Ligament, Left/Right
Pudendal nerve	use Sacral Plexus
Pulmoaortic canal	use Pulmonary Artery, Left
Pulmonary annulus	use Pulmonary Valve
Pulmonary plexus	use Vagus Nerve/Thoracic Sympathetic Nerve

BODY PART	USE:
Pulmonic valve	use Pulmonary Valve
Pulvinar	use Thalamus
Pyloric antrum Pyloric canal Pyloric sphincter	use Stomach, Pylorus
Pyramidalis muscle	use Abdomen Muscle, Left/Right
Quadrangular cartilage	use Nasal Septum
Quadrate lobe	use Liver
Quadratus femoris muscle	use Hip Muscle, Left/Right
Quadratus lumborum muscle	use Trunk Muscle, Left/Right
Quadratus plantae muscle	use Foot Muscle, Left/Right
Quadriceps (femoris)	use Upper Leg Muscle, Left/Right
Radial collateral carpal ligament	use Wrist Bursa and Ligament, Left/Right
Radial collateral ligament	use Elbow Bursa and Ligament, Left/Right
Radial notch	use Ulna, Left/Right
Radial recurrent artery	use Radial Artery, Left/Right
Radial vein	use Brachial Vein, Left/Right
Radialis indicis	use Hand Artery, Left/Right
Radiocarpal joint	use Wrist Joint, Left/Right
Radiocarpal ligament Radioulnar ligament	use Wrist Bursa and Ligament, Left/Right
Rectosigmoid junction	use Sigmoid Colon
Rectus abdominis muscle	use Abdomen Muscle, Left/Right
Rectus femoris muscle	use Upper Leg Muscle, Left/Right
Recurrent laryngeal nerve	use Vagus Nerve
Renal calyx Renal capsule Renal cortex	use Kidney, Bilateral/Left/Right
Renal plexus	use Abdominal Sympathetic Nerve
Renal segment	use Kidney, Bilateral/Left/Right
Renal segmental artery	use Renal Artery, Left/Right
Retroperitoneal lymph node	use Lymphatic, Aortic
Retroperitoneal space	use Retroperitoneum
Retropharyngeal lymph node	use Lymphatic, Neck, Left/Right
Retropubic space	use Pelvic Cavity
Rhinopharynx	use Nasopharynx
Rhomboid major muscle Rhomboid minor muscle	use Trunk Muscle, Left/Right
Right ascending lumbar vein	use Azygos Vein
Right atrioventricular valve	use Tricuspid Valve
Right auricular appendix	use Atrium, Right
Right colic vein	use Colic Vein
Right coronary sulcus	use Heart, Right
Right gastric artery	use Gastric Artery
Right gastroepiploic vein	use Superior Mesenteric Vein
Right inferior phrenic vein	use Inferior Vena Cava
Right inferior pulmonary vein	use Pulmonary Vein, Right
Right jugular trunk	use Lymphatic, Right Neck
Right lateral ventricle	use Cerebral Ventricle

BODY PART	USE:
Right lymphatic duct	use Lymphatic, Right Neck
Right ovarian vein	use Inferior Vena Cava
Right second lumbar vein	
Right subclavian trunk	use Lymphatic, Right Neck
Right subcostal vein	use Azygos Vein
Right superior pulmonary vein	use Pulmonary Vein, Right
Right suprarenal vein	use Inferior Vena Cava
Right testicular vein	
Rima glottidis	use Larynx
Risorius muscle	use Facial Muscle
Round ligament of uterus	use Uterine Supporting Structure
Round window	use Inner Ear, Left/Right
Sacral ganglion	use Sacral Sympathetic Nerve
Sacral lymph node	use Lymphatic, Pelvis
Sacral splanchnic nerve	use Sacral Sympathetic Nerve
Sacrococcygeal ligament	use Trunk Bursa and Ligament, Left/Right
Sacrococcygeal symphysis	use Sacrococcygeal Joint
Sacroiliac ligament	use Trunk Bursa and Ligament,
Sacrospinous ligament	Left/Right
Sacrotuberous ligament	
Salpingopharyngeus muscle	use Tongue, Palate, Pharynx Muscle
Salpinx	use Fallopian Tube, Left/Right
Saphenous nerve	use Femoral Nerve
Sartorius muscle	use Upper Leg Muscle, Left/Right
Scalene muscle	use Neck Muscle, Left/Right
Scaphoid bone	use Carpal, Left/Right
Scapholunate ligament	use Hand Bursa and Ligament,
Scaphotrapezium ligament	Left/Right
Scarpa's (vestibular) ganglion	use Acoustic Nerve
Sebaceous gland	use Skin
Second cranial nerve	use Optic Nerve
Sella turcica	use Sphenoid Bone, Left/Right
Semicircular canal	use Inner Ear, Left/Right
Semimembranosus muscle	use Upper Leg Muscle, Left/Right
Semitendinosus muscle	
Septal cartilage	use Nasal Septum
Serratus anterior muscle	use Thorax Muscle, Left/Right
Serratus posterior muscle	use Trunk Muscle, Left/Right
Seventh cranial nerve	use Facial Nerve
Short gastric artery	use Splenic Artery
Sigmoid artery	use Inferior Mesenteric Artery
Sigmoid flexure	use Sigmoid Colon
Sigmoid vein	use Inferior Mesenteric Vein
Sinoatrial node	use Conduction Mechanism
Sinus venosus	use Atrium, Right
Sixth cranial nerve	use Abducens Nerve
Skene's (paraurethral) gland	use Vestibular Gland
Small saphenous vein	use Lesser Saphenous Vein, Left/Right
Solar (celiac) plexus	use Abdominal Sympathetic Nerve
Soleus muscle	use Lower Leg Muscle, Left/Right

BODY PART	USE:
Sphenomandibular ligament	use Head and Neck Bursa and Ligament
Sphenopalatine (pterygo-palatine) ganglion	use Head and Neck Sympathetic Nerve
Spinal nerve, cervical	use Cervical Nerve
Spinal nerve, lumbar	use Lumbar Nerve
Spinal nerve, sacral	use Sacral Nerve
Spinal nerve, thoracic	use Thoracic Nerve
Spinous process	use Cervical, Thoracic, Lumbar Vertebra
Spiral ganglion	use Acoustic Nerve
Splenic flexure	use Transverse Colon
Splenic plexus	use Abdominal Sympathetic Nerve
Splenius capitis muscle	use Head Muscle
Splenius cervicis muscle	use Neck Muscle, Left/Right
Stapes	use Auditory Ossicle, Left/Right
Stellate ganglion	use Head and Neck Sympathetic Nerve
Stensen's duct	use Parotid Duct, Left/Right
Sternoclavicular ligament	use Shoulder Bursa and Ligament, Left/Right
Sternocleidomastoid artery	use Thyroid Artery, Left/Right
Sternocleidomastoid muscle	use Neck Muscle, Left/Right
Sternocostal ligament	use Thorax Bursa and Ligament, Left/Right
Styloglossus muscle	use Tongue, Palate, Pharynx Muscle
Stylomandibular ligament	use Head and Neck Bursa and Ligament
Stylopharyngeus muscle	use Tongue, Palate, Pharynx Muscle
Subacromial bursa	use Shoulder Bursa and Ligament, Left/Right
Subaortic (common iliac) lymph node	use Lymphatic, Pelvis
Subarachnoid space, intracranial	use Subarachnoid Space
Subarachnoid space, spinal	use Spinal Canal
Subclavicular (apical) lymph node	use Lymphatic, Axillary, Left/Right
Subclavius muscle	use Thorax Muscle, Left/Right
Subclavius nerve	use Brachial Plexus
Subcostal artery	use Upper Artery
Subcostal muscle	use Thorax Muscle, Left/Right
Subcostal nerve	use Thoracic Nerve
Subdural space, intracranial	use Subdural Space
Subdural space, spinal	use Spinal Canal
Submandibular ganglion	use Facial Nerve Head and Neck Sympathetic Nerve
Submandibular gland	use Submaxillary Gland, Left/Right
Submandibular lymph node	use Lymphatic, Head
Submaxillary ganglion	use Head and Neck Sympathetic Nerve

BODY PART	USE:
Submaxillary lymph node	use Lymphatic, Head
Submental artery	use Face Artery
Submental lymph node	use Lymphatic, Head
Submucous (Meissner's) plexus	use Abdominal Sympathetic Nerve
Suboccipital nerve	use Cervical Nerve
Suboccipital venous plexus	use Vertebral Vein, Left/Right
Subparotid lymph node	use Lymphatic, Head
Subscapular aponeurosis	use Subcutaneous Tissue and Fascia, Upper Arm, Left/Right
Subscapular artery	use Axillary Artery, Left/Right
Subscapular (posterior) lymph node	use Lymphatic, Axillary, Left/Right
Subscapularis muscle	use Shoulder Muscle, Left/Right
Substantia nigra	use Basal Ganglia
Subtalar (talocalcaneal) joint	use Tarsal Joint, Left/Right
Subtalar ligament	use Foot Bursa and Ligament, Left/Right
Subthalamic nucleus	use Basal Ganglia
Superficial circumflex iliac vein	use Greater Saphenous Vein, Left/Right
Superficial epigastric artery	use Femoral Artery, Left/Right
Superficial epigastric vein	use Greater Saphenous Vein, Left/Right
Superficial palmar arch	use Hand Artery, Left/Right
Superficial palmar venous arch	use Hand Vein, Left/Right
Superficial temporal artery	use Temporal Artery, Left/Right
Superficial transverse perineal muscle	use Perineum Muscle
Superior cardiac nerve	use Thoracic Sympathetic Nerve
Superior cerebellar vein	use Intracranial Vein
Superior cerebral vein	
Superior clunic (cluneal) nerve	use Lumbar Nerve
Superior epigastric artery	use Internal Mammary Artery, Left/Right
Superior genicular artery	use Popliteal Artery, Left/Right
Superior gluteal artery	use Internal Iliac Artery, Left/Right
Superior gluteal nerve	use Lumbar Plexus
Superior hypogastric plexus	use Abdominal Sympathetic Nerve
Superior labial artery	use Face Artery
Superior laryngeal artery	use Thyroid Artery, Left/Right
Superior laryngeal nerve	use Vagus Nerve
Superior longitudinal muscle	use Tongue, Palate, Pharynx Muscle
Superior mesenteric ganglion	use Abdominal Sympathetic Nerve
Superior mesenteric lymph node	use Lymphatic, Mesenteric
Superior mesenteric plexus	use Abdominal Sympathetic Nerve

BODY PART	USE:
Superior oblique muscle	use Extraocular Muscle, Left/Right
Superior olivary nucleus	use Pons
Superior rectal artery	use Inferior Mesenteric Artery
Superior rectal vein	use Inferior Mesenteric Vein
Superior rectus muscle	use Extraocular Muscle, Left/Right
Superior tarsal plate	use Upper Eyelid, Left/Right
Superior thoracic artery	use Axillary Artery, Left/Right
Superior thyroid artery	use External Carotid Artery, Left/Right Thyroid Artery, Left/Right
Superior turbinate	use Nasal Turbinate
Superior ulnar collateral artery	use Brachial Artery, Left/Right
Supraclavicular (Virchow's) lymph node	use Lymphatic, Neck, Left/Right
Supraclavicular nerve	use Cervical Plexus
Suprahyoid lymph node	use Lymphatic, Head
Suprahyoid muscle	use Neck Muscle, Left/Right
Suprainguinal lymph node	use Lymphatic, Pelvis
Supraorbital vein	use Face Vein, Left/Right
Suprarenal gland	use Adrenal Gland, Bilateral/Left/Right
Suprarenal plexus	use Abdominal Sympathetic Nerve
Suprascapular nerve	use Brachial Plexus
Supraspinatus fascia	use Subcutaneous Tissue and Fascia, Upper Arm, Left/Right
Supraspinatus muscle	use Shoulder Muscle, Left/Right
Supraspinous ligament	use Trunk Bursa and Ligament, Left/Right
Suprasternal notch	use Sternum
Supratrochlear lymph node	use Lymphatic, Upper Extremity, Left/Right
Sural artery	use Popliteal Artery, Left/Right
Sweat gland	use Skin
Talocalcaneal (subtalar) joint	use Tarsal Joint, Left/Right
Talocalcaneal ligament	use Foot Bursa and Ligament, Left/Right
Talocalcaneonavicular joint	use Tarsal Joint, Left/Right
Talocalcaneonavicular ligament	use Foot Bursa and Ligament, Left/Right
Talocrural joint	use Ankle Joint, Left/Right
Talofibular ligament	use Ankle Bursa and Ligament, Left/Right
Talus bone	use Tarsal, Left/Right
Tarsometatarsal joint	use Metatarsal-Tarsal Joint, Left/Right
Tarsometatarsal ligament	use Foot Bursa and Ligament, Left/Right
Temporal lobe	use Cerebral Hemisphere
Temporalis muscle	use Head Muscle
Temporoparietalis muscle	
Tensor fasciae latae muscle	use Hip Muscle, Left/Right
Tensor veli palatini muscle	use Tongue, Palate, Pharynx Muscle
Tenth cranial nerve	use Vagus Nerve

BODY PART	USE:
Tentorium cerebelli	use Dura Mater
Teres major muscle	use Shoulder Muscle, Left/Right
Teres minor muscle	
Testicular artery	use Abdominal Aorta
Thenar muscle	use Hand Muscle, Left/Right
Third cranial nerve	use Oculomotor Nerve
Third occipital nerve	use Cervical Nerve
Third ventricle	use Cerebral Ventricle
Thoracic aortic plexus	use Thoracic Sympathetic Nerve
Thoracic esophagus	use Esophagus, Middle
Thoracic facet joint	use Thoracic Vertebral Joint
Thoracic ganglion	use Thoracic Sympathetic Nerve
Thoracoacromial artery	use Axillary Artery, Left/Right
Thoracolumbar facet joint	use Thoracolumbar Vertebral Joint
Thymus gland	use Thymus
Thyroarytenoid muscle	use Neck Muscle, Left/Right
Thyrocervical trunk	use Thyroid Artery, Left/Right
Thyroid cartilage	use Larynx
Tibialis anterior muscle	use Lower Leg Muscle, Left/Right
Tibialis posterior muscle	
Tibiofemoral joint	use Knee Joint, Left/Right
	use Knee Joint, Tibial Surface, Left/Right
Tongue, base of	use Pharynx
Tracheobronchial lymph node	use Lymphatic, Thorax
Tragus	use External Ear, Bilateral/Left/Right
Transversalis fascia	use Subcutaneous Tissue and Fascia, Trunk
Transverse (cutaneous) cervical nerve	use Cervical Plexus
Transverse acetabular ligament	use Hip Bursa and Ligament, Left/Right
Transverse facial artery	use Temporal Artery, Left/Right
Transverse humeral ligament	use Shoulder Bursa and Ligament, Left/Right
Transverse ligament of atlas	use Head and Neck Bursa and Ligament
Transverse scapular ligament	use Shoulder Bursa and Ligament, Left/Right
Transverse thoracis muscle	use Thorax Muscle, Left/Right
Transversospinalis muscle	use Trunk Muscle, Left/Right
Transversus abdominis muscle	use Abdomen Muscle, Left/Right
Trapezium bone	use Carpal, Left/Right
Trapezius muscle	use Trunk Muscle, Left/Right
Trapezoid bone	use Carpal, Left/Right
Triceps brachii muscle	use Upper Arm Muscle, Left/Right
Tricuspid annulus	use Tricuspid Valve
Trifacial nerve	use Trigeminal Nerve
Trigone of bladder	use Bladder
Triquetral bone	use Carpal, Left/Right
Trochanteric bursa	use Hip Bursa and Ligament, Left/Right
Twelfth cranial nerve	use Hypoglossal Nerve

BODY PART	USE:
Tympanic cavity	use Middle Ear, Left/Right
Tympanic nerve	use Glossopharyngeal Nerve
Tympanic part of temporal bone	use Temporal Bone, Left/Right
Ulnar collateral carpal ligament	use Wrist Bursa and Ligament, Left/Right
Ulnar collateral ligament	use Elbow Bursa and Ligament, Left/Right
Ulnar notch	use Radius, Left/Right
Ulnar vein	use Brachial Vein, Left/Right
Umbilical artery	use Internal Iliac Artery, Left/Right
Ureteral orifice	use Ureter, Bilateral/Left/Right
Ureteropelvic junction (UPJ)	use Kidney Pelvis, Left/Right
Ureterovesical orifice	use Ureter, Bilateral/Left/Right
Uterine artery	use Internal Iliac Artery, Left/Right
Uterine cornu	use Uterus
Uterine tube	use Fallopian Tube, Left/Right
Uterine vein	use Hypogastric Vein, Left/Right
Vaginal artery	use Internal Iliac Artery, Left/Right
Vaginal vein	use Hypogastric Vein, Left/Right
Vastus intermedius muscle	use Upper Leg Muscle, Left/Right
Vastus lateralis muscle	
Vastus medialis muscle	
Ventricular fold	use Larynx
Vermiform appendix	use Appendix
Vermilion border	use Upper Lip, Lower Lip
Vertebral arch	use Cervical, Thoracic, Lumbar Vertebra
Vertebral canal	use Spinal Canal
Vertebral foramen	use Cervical, Thoracic, Lumbar Vertebra
Vertebral lamina	
Vertebral pedicle	
Vesical vein	use Hypogastric Vein, Left/Right
Vestibular nerve	use Acoustic Nerve
Vestibular (Scarpa's) ganglion	
Vestibulocochlear nerve	
Virchow's (supraclavicular) lymph node	use Lymphatic, Neck, Left/Right
Vitreous body	use Vitreous, Left/Right
Vocal fold	use Vocal Cord, Left/Right
Volar (palmar) digital vein	use Hand Vein, Left/Right
Volar (palmar) metacarpal vein	
Vomer bone	use Nasal Septum
Vomer of nasal septum	use Nasal Bone
Xiphoid process	use Sternum
Zonule of Zinn	use Lens, Left/Right
Zygomatic process of frontal bone	use Frontal Bone, Left/Right
Zygomatic process of temporal bone	use Temporal Bone, Left/Right
Zygomaticus muscle	use Facial Muscle

APPENDIX C

DEVICE	USE:
3f (Aortic) Bioprosthesis valve	*use* Zooplastic Tissue in Heart and Great Vessels
AbioCor® Total Replacement Heart	*use* Synthetic Substitute
Absolute Pro Vascular (OTW) Self-Expanding Stent System	*use* Intraluminal Device
Acculink (RX) Carotid Stent System	*use* Intraluminal Device
Acellular Hydrated Dermis	*use* Nonautologous Tissue Substitute
Acetabular cup	*use* Liner in Lower Joints
Activa PC neurostimulator	*use* Stimulator Generator, Multiple Array for Insertion in Subcutaneous Tissue and Fascia
Activa RC neurostimulator	*use* Stimulator Generator, Multiple Array Rechargeable for Insertion in Subcutaneous Tissue and Fascia
Activa SC neurostimulator	*use* Stimulator Generator, Single Array for Insertion in Subcutaneous Tissue and Fascia
ACUITY™ Steerable Lead	*use* Cardiac Lead, Pacemaker for Insertion in Heart and Great Vessels Cardiac Lead, Defibrillator for Insertion in Heart and Great Vessels
Advisa (MRI)	*use* Pacemaker, Dual Chamber for Insertion in Subcutaneous Tissue and Fascia
AFX® Endovascular AAA System	*use* Intraluminal Device
AMPLATZER® Muscular VSD Occluder	*use* Synthetic Substitute
AMS 800® Urinary Control System	*use* Artificial Sphincter in Urinary System
AneuRx® AAA Advantage®	*use* Intraluminal Device
Annuloplasty ring	*use* Synthetic Substitute
Artificial anal sphincter (AAS)	*use* Artificial Sphincter in Gastrointestinal System
Artificial bowel sphincter (neosphincter)	*use* Artificial Sphincter in Gastrointestinal System
Artificial urinary sphincter (AUS)	*use* Artificial Sphincter in Urinary System
Ascenda Intrathecal Catheter	*use* Infusion Device
Assurant (Cobalt) stent	*use* Intraluminal Device
Attain Ability® lead	*use* Cardiac Lead, Pacemaker for Insertion in Heart and Great Vessels Cardiac Lead, Defibrillator for Insertion in Heart and Great Vessels
Attain StarFix® (OTW) lead	*use* Cardiac Lead, Pacemaker for Insertion in Heart and Great Vessels Cardiac Lead, Defibrillator for Insertion in Heart and Great Vessels
Autograft	*use* Autologous Tissue Substitute
Autologous artery graft	*use* Autologous Arterial Tissue in Heart and Great Vessels Autologous Arterial Tissue in Upper Arteries, Lower Arteries Autologous Arterial Tissue in Upper Veins, Lower Veins
Autologous vein graft	*use* Autologous Venous Tissue in Heart and Great Vessels Autologous Venous Tissue in Upper Arteries, Lower Arteries Autologous Venous Tissue in Upper Veins, Lower Veins
Axial Lumbar Interbody Fusion System	*use* Interbody Fusion Device in Lower Joints
AxiaLIF® System	*use* Interbody Fusion Device in Lower Joints
BAK/C® Interbody Cervical Fusion System	*use* Interbody Fusion Device in Upper Joints
Bard® Composix® (E/X)(LP) mesh	*use* Synthetic Substitute
Bard® Composix® Kugel® patch	*use* Synthetic Substitute
Bard® Dulex™ mesh	*use* Synthetic Substitute
Bard® Ventralex™ hernia patch	*use* Synthetic Substitute
Baroreflex Activation Therapy® (BAT®)	*use* Stimulator Lead in Upper Arteries Stimulator Generator in Subcutaneous Tissue and Fascia
Berlin Heart Ventricular Assist Device	*use* Implantable Heart Assist System in Heart and Great Vessels
Bioactive embolization coil(s)	*use* Intraluminal Device, Bioactive in Upper Arteries
Biventricular external heart assist system	*use* External Heart Assist System in Heart and Great Vessels
Blood glucose monitoring system	*use* Monitoring Device
Bone anchored hearing device	*use* Hearing Device, Bone Conduction for Insertion in Ear, Nose, Sinus Hearing Device in Head and Facial Bones
Bone bank bone graft	*use* Nonautologous Tissue Substitute
Bone screw (interlocking) (lag) (pedicle) (recessed)	*use* Internal Fixation Device in Head and Facial Bones, Upper Bones, Lower Bones
Bovine pericardial valve	*use* Zooplastic Tissue in Heart and Great Vessels
Bovine pericardium graft	*use* Zooplastic Tissue in Heart and Great Vessels
Brachytherapy seeds	*use* Radioactive Element
BRYAN® Cervical Disc System	*use* Synthetic Substitute

DEVICE	USE:
BVS 5000 Ventricular Assist Device	use External Heart Assist System in Heart and Great Vessels
Cardiac contractility modulation lead	use Cardiac Lead in Heart and Great Vessels
Cardiac event recorder	use Monitoring Device
Cardiac resynchronization therapy (CRT) lead	use Cardiac Lead, Pacemaker for Insertion in Heart and Great Vessels Cardiac Lead, Defibrillator for Insertion in Heart and Great Vessels
CardioMEMS® pressure sensor	use Monitoring Device, Pressure Sensor for Insertion in Heart and Great Vessels
Carotid (artery) sinus (baroreceptor) lead	use Stimulator Lead in Upper Arteries
Carotid WALLSTENT® Monorail® Endoprosthesis	use Intraluminal Device
Centrimag® Blood Pump	use External Heart Assist System in Heart and Great Vessels
Ceramic on ceramic bearing surface	use Synthetic Substitute, Ceramic for Replacement in Lower Joints
Clamp and rod internal fixation system (CRIF)	use Internal Fixation Device in Upper Bones, Lower Bones
CoAxia NeuroFlo catheter	use Intraluminal Device
Cobalt/chromium head and polyethylene socket	use Synthetic Substitute, Metal on Polyethylene for Replacement in Lower Joints
Cobalt/chromium head and socket	use Synthetic Substitute, Metal for Replacement in Lower Joints
Cochlear implant (CI), multiple channel (electrode)	use Hearing Device, Multiple Channel Cochlear Prosthesis for Insertion in Ear, Nose, Sinus
Cochlear implant (CI), single channel (electrode)	use Hearing Device, Single Channel Cochlear Prosthesis for Insertion in Ear, Nose, Sinus
COGNIS® CRT-D	use Cardiac Resynchronization Defibrillator Pulse Generator for Insertion in Subcutaneous Tissue and Fascia
Colonic Z-Stent®	use Intraluminal Device
Complete (SE) stent	use Intraluminal Device
Concerto II CRT-D	use Cardiac Resynchronization Defibrillator Pulse Generator for Insertion in Subcutaneous Tissue and Fascia
CONSERVE® PLUS Total Resurfacing Hip System	use Resurfacing Device in Lower Joints
Consulta CRT-D	use Cardiac Resynchronization Defibrillator Pulse Generator for Insertion in Subcutaneous Tissue and Fascia
Consulta CRT-P	use Cardiac Resynchronization Pacemaker Pulse Generator for Insertion in Subcutaneous Tissue and Fascia
CONTAK RENEWAL® 3 RF (HE) CRT-D	use Cardiac Resynchronization Defibrillator Pulse Generator for Insertion in Subcutaneous Tissue and Fascia
Contegra Pulmonary Valved Conduit	use Zooplastic Tissue in Heart and Great Vessels
Continuous Glucose Monitoring (CGM) device	use Monitoring Device
Cook Biodesign® Fistula Plug(s)	use Nonautologous Tissue Substitute
Cook Biodesign® Hernia Graft(s)	use Nonautologous Tissue Substitute
Cook Biodesign® Layered Graft(s)	use Nonautologous Tissue Substitute
Cook Zenapro™ Layered Graft(s)	use Nonautologous Tissue Substitute
Cook Zenith AAA Endovascular Graft	use Intraluminal Device, Branched or Fenestrated, One or Two Arteries for Restriction in Lower Arteries use Intraluminal Device, Branched or Fenestrated, Three or More Arteries for Restriction in Lower Arteries use Intraluminal Device
CoreValve transcatheter aortic valve	use Zooplastic Tissue in Heart and Great Vessels
Cormet Hip Resurfacing System	use Resurfacing Device in Lower Joints
CoRoent® XL	use Interbody Fusion Device in Lower Joints
Corox OTW (Bipolar) Lead	use Cardiac Lead, Pacemaker for Insertion in Heart and Great Vessels Cardiac Lead, Defibrillator for Insertion in Heart and Great Vessels
Cortical strip neurostimulator lead	use Neurostimulator Lead in Central Nervous System
Cultured epidermal cell autograft	use Autologous Tissue Substitute
CYPHER® Stent	use Intraluminal Device, Drug-eluting in Heart and Great Vessels
Cystostomy tube	use Drainage Device
DBS lead	use Neurostimulator Lead in Central Nervous System
DeBakey Left Ventricular Assist Device	use Implantable Heart Assist System in Heart and Great Vessels
Deep brain neurostimulator lead	use Neurostimulator Lead in Central Nervous System
Delta frame external fixator	use External Fixation Device, Hybrid for Insertion in Upper Bones, Lower Bones External Fixation Device, Hybrid for Reposition in Upper Bones, Lower Bones
Delta III Reverse shoulder prosthesis	use Synthetic Substitute, Reverse Ball and Socket for Replacement in Upper Joints
Diaphragmatic pacemaker generator	use Stimulator Generator in Subcutaneous Tissue and Fascia
Direct Lateral Interbody Fusion (DLIF) device	use Interbody Fusion Device in Lower Joints

DEVICE	USE:
Driver stent (RX) (OTW)	*use* Intraluminal Device
DuraHeart Left Ventricular Assist System	*use* Implantable Heart Assist System in Heart and Great Vessels
Durata® Defibrillation Lead	*use* Cardiac Lead, Defibrillator for Insertion in Heart and Great Vessels
Dynesys® Dynamic Stabilization System	*use* Spinal Stabilization Device, Pedicle-Based for Insertion in Upper Joints, Lower Joints
E-Luminexx™ (Biliary) (Vascular) Stent	*use* Intraluminal Device
EDWARDS INTUITY Elite valve system	*use* Zooplastic Tissue, Rapid Deployment Technique in New Technology
Electrical bone growth stimulator (EBGS)	*use* Bone Growth Stimulator in Head and Facial Bones, Upper Bones, Lower Bones
Electrical muscle stimulation (EMS) lead	*use* Stimulator Lead in Muscles
Electronic muscle stimulator lead	*use* Stimulator Lead in Muscles
Embolization coil(s)	*use* Intraluminal Device
Endeavor® (III) (IV) (Sprint) Zotarolimus-eluting Coronary Stent System	*use* Intraluminal Device, Drug-eluting in Heart and Great Vessels
Endologix AFX® Endovascular AAA System	*use* Intraluminal Device
EndoSure® sensor	*use* Monitoring Device, Pressure Sensor for Insertion in Heart and Great Vessels
ENDOTAK RELIANCE® (G) Defibrillation Lead	*use* Cardiac Lead, Defibrillator for Insertion in Heart and Great Vessels
Endotracheal tube (cuffed) (double-lumen)	*use* Intraluminal Device, Endotracheal Airway in Respiratory System
Endurant® Endovascular Stent Graft	*use* Intraluminal Device
Endurant® II AAA stent graft system	*use* Intraluminal Device
EnRhythm	*use* Pacemaker, Dual Chamber for Insertion in Subcutaneous Tissue and Fascia
Enterra gastric neurostimulator	*use* Stimulator Generator, Multiple Array for Insertion in Subcutaneous Tissue and Fascia
Epic™ Stented Tissue Valve (aortic)	*use* Zooplastic Tissue in Heart and Great Vessels
Epicel® cultured epidermal autograft	*use* Autologous Tissue Substitute
Esophageal obturator airway (EOA)	*use* Intraluminal Device, Airway in Gastrointestinal System
Esteem® implantable hearing system	*use* Hearing Device in Ear, Nose, Sinus
Evera (XT) (S) (DR/VR)	*use* Defibrillator Generator for Insertion in Subcutaneous Tissue and Fascia
Everolimus-eluting coronary stent	*use* Intraluminal Device, Drug-eluting in Heart and Great Vessels
Ex-PRESS™ mini glaucoma shunt	*use* Synthetic Substitute
EXCLUDER® AAA Endoprothesis	*use* Intraluminal Device, Branched or Fenestrated, One or Two Arteries for Restriction in Lower Arteries *use* Intraluminal Device, Branched or Fenestrated, Three or More Arteries for Restriction in Lower Arteries *use* Intraluminal Device
EXCLUDER® IBE Endoprothesis	*use* Intraluminal Device, Branched or Fenestrated, One or Two Arteries for Restriction in Lower Arteries
Express® (LD) Premounted Stent System	*use* Intraluminal Device
Express® Biliary SD Monorail® Premounted Stent System	*use* Intraluminal Device
Express® SD Renal Monorail® Premounted Stent System	*use* Intraluminal Device
External fixator	*use* External Fixation Device in Head and Facial Bones, Upper Bones, Lower Bones, Upper Joints, Lower Joints
EXtreme Lateral Interbody Fusion (XLIF) device	*use* Interbody Fusion Device in Lower Joints
Facet replacement spinal stabilization device	*use* Spinal Stabilization Device, Facet Replacement for Insertion in Upper Joints, Lower Joints
FLAIR® Endovascular Stent Graft	*use* Intraluminal Device
Flexible Composite Mesh	*use* Synthetic Substitute
Foley catheter	*use* Drainage Device
Formula™ Balloon-Expandable Renal Stent System	*use* Intraluminal Device
Freestyle (Stentless) Aortic Root Bioprosthesis	*use* Zooplastic Tissue in Heart and Great Vessels
Fusion screw (compression) (lag) (locking)	*use* Internal Fixation Device in Upper Joints, Lower Joints
Gastric electrical stimulation (GES) lead	*use* Stimulator Lead in Gastrointestinal System
Gastric pacemaker lead	*use* Stimulator Lead in Gastrointestinal System
GORE® DUALMESH®	*use* Synthetic Substitute
GORE EXCLUDER® AAA Endoprothesis	*use* Intraluminal Device, Branched or Fenestrated, One or Two Arteries for Restriction in Lower Arteries *use* Intraluminal Device, Branched or Fenestrated, Three or More Arteries for Restriction in Lower Arteries *use* Intraluminal Device

DEVICE	USE:
GORE EXCLUDER® IBE Endoprothesis	*use* Intraluminal Device, Branched or Fenestrated, One or Two Arteries for Restriction in Lower Arteries
GORE TAG® Thoracic Endoprothesis	*use* Intraluminal Device
Guedel airway	*use* Intraluminal Device, Airway in Mouth and Throat
Hancock Bioprosthesis (aortic) (mitral) valve	*use* Zooplastic Tissue in Heart and Great Vessels
Hancock Bioprosthetic Valved Conduit	*use* Zooplastic Tissue in Heart and Great Vessels
HeartMate II® Left Ventricular Assist Device (LVAD)	*use* Implantable Heart Assist System in Heart and Great Vessels
HeartMate XVE® Left Ventricular Assist Device (LVAD)	*use* Implantable Heart Assist System in Heart and Great Vessels
Herculink (RX) Elite Renal Stent System	*use* Intraluminal Device
Hip (joint) liner	*use* Liner in Lower Joints
Holter valve ventricular shunt	*use* Synthetic Substitute
Ilizarov external fixator	*use* External Fixation Device, Ring for Insertion in Upper Bones, Lower Bones External Fixation Device, Ring for Reposition in Upper Bones, Lower Bones
Ilizarov-Vecklich device	*use* External Fixation Device, Limb Lengthening for Insertion in Upper Bones, Lower Bones
Implantable cardioverter-defibrillator (ICD)	*use* Defibrillator Generator for Insertion in Subcutaneous Tissue and Fascia
Implantable drug infusion pump (anti-spasmodic) (chemotherapy) (pain)	*use* Infusion Device, Pump in Subcutaneous Tissue and Fascia
Implantable glucose monitoring device	*use* Monitoring Device
Implantable hemodynamic monitor (IHM)	*use* Monitoring Device, Hemodynamic for Insertion in Subcutaneous Tissue and Fascia
Implantable hemodynamic monitoring system (IHMS)	*use* Monitoring Device, Hemodynamic for Insertion in Subcutaneous Tissue and Fascia
Implantable Miniature Telescope™ (IMT)	*use* Synthetic Substitute, Intraocular Telescope for Replacement in Eye
Implanted (venous) (access) port	*use* Vascular Access Device, Reservoir in Subcutaneous Tissue and Fascia
InDura, intrathecal catheter (1P) (spinal)	*use* Infusion Device
Injection reservoir, port	*use* Vascular Access Device, Reservoir in Subcutaneous Tissue and Fascia
Injection reservoir, pump	*use* Infusion Device, Pump in Subcutaneous Tissue and Fascia
Interbody fusion (spine) cage	*use* Interbody Fusion Device in Upper Joints, Lower Joints
Interspinous process spinal stabilization device	*use* Spinal Stabilization Device, Interspinous Process for Insertion in Upper Joints, Lower Joints
InterStim® Therapy lead	*use* Neurostimulator Lead in Peripheral Nervous System
InterStim® Therapy neurostimulator	*use* Stimulator Generator, Single Array for Insertion in Subcutaneous Tissue and Fascia
Intramedullary (IM) rod (nail)	*use* Internal Fixation Device, Intramedullary in Upper Bones, Lower Bones
Intramedullary skeletal kinetic distractor (ISKD)	*use* Internal Fixation Device, Intramedullary in Upper Bones, Lower Bones
Intrauterine device (IUD)	*use* Contraceptive Device in Female Reproductive System
INTUITY Elite valve system, EDWARDS	*use* Zooplastic Tissue, Rapid Deployment Technique in New Technology
Itrel (3) (4) neurostimulator	*use* Stimulator Generator, Single Array for Insertion in Subcutaneous Tissue and Fascia
Joint fixation plate	*use* Internal Fixation Device in Upper Joints, Lower Joints
Joint liner (insert)	*use* Liner in Lower Joints
Joint spacer (antibiotic)	*use* Spacer in Upper Joints, Lower Joints
Kappa	*use* Pacemaker, Dual Chamber for Insertion in Subcutaneous Tissue and Fascia
Kirschner wire (K-wire)	*use* Internal Fixation Device in Head and Facial Bones, Upper Bones, Lower Bones, Upper Joints, Lower Joints
Knee (implant) insert	*use* Liner in Lower Joints
Kuntscher nail	*use* Internal Fixation Device, Intramedullary in Upper Bones, Lower Bones
LAP-BAND® adjustable gastric banding system	*use* Extraluminal Device
LifeStent® (Flexstar) (XL) Vascular Stent System	*use* Intraluminal Device
LIVIAN™ CRT-D	*use* Cardiac Resynchronization Defibrillator Pulse Generator for Insertion in Subcutaneous Tissue and Fascia
Loop recorder, implantable	*use* Monitoring Device
MAGEC® Spinal Bracing and Distraction System	*use* Magnetically Controlled Growth Rod(s) in New Technology
Mark IV Breathing Pacemaker System	*use* Stimulator Generator in Subcutaneous Tissue and Fascia
Maximo II DR (VR)	*use* Defibrillator Generator for Insertion in Subcutaneous Tissue and Fascia
Maximo II DR CRT-D	*use* Cardiac Resynchronization Defibrillator Pulse Generator for Insertion in Subcutaneous Tissue and Fascia
Medtronic Endurant® II AAA stent graft system	*use* Intraluminal Device
Melody® transcatheter pulmonary valve	*use* Zooplastic Tissue in Heart and Great Vessels
Metal on metal bearing surface	*use* Synthetic Substitute, Metal for Replacement in Lower Joints

DEVICE	USE:
Micro-Driver stent (RX) (OTW)	*use* Intraluminal Device
MicroMed HeartAssist	*use* Implantable Heart Assist System in Heart and Great Vessels
Micrus CERECYTE microcoil	*use* Intraluminal Device, Bioactive in Upper Arteries
MIRODERM™ Biologic Wound Matrix	*use* Skin Substitute, Porcine Liver Derived in New Technology
MitraClip valve repair system	*use* Synthetic Substitute
Mitroflow® Aortic Pericardial Heart Valve	*use* Zooplastic Tissue in Heart and Great Vessels
Mosaic Bioprosthesis (aortic) (mitral) valve	*use* Zooplastic Tissue in Heart and Great Vessels
MULTI-LINK (VISION) (MINI-VISION) (ULTRA) Coronary Stent System	*use* Intraluminal Device
nanoLOCK™ interbody fusion device	*use* Interbody Fusion Device, Nanotextured Surface in New Technology
Nasopharyngeal airway (NPA)	*use* Intraluminal Device, Airway in Ear, Nose, Sinus
Neuromuscular electrical stimulation (NEMS) lead	*use* Stimulator Lead in Muscles
Neurostimulator generator, multiple channel	*use* Stimulator Generator, Multiple Array for Insertion in Subcutaneous Tissue and Fascia
Neurostimulator generator, multiple channel rechargeable	*use* Stimulator Generator, Multiple Array Rechargeable for Insertion in Subcutaneous Tissue and Fascia
Neurostimulator generator, single channel	*use* Stimulator Generator, Single Array for Insertion in Subcutaneous Tissue and Fascia
Neurostimulator generator, single channel rechargeable	*use* Stimulator Generator, Single Array Rechargeable for Insertion in Subcutaneous Tissue and Fascia
Neutralization plate	*use* Internal Fixation Device in Head and Facial Bones, Upper Bones, Lower Bones
Nitinol framed polymer mesh	*use* Synthetic Substitute
Non-tunneled central venous catheter	*use* Infusion Device
Novacor Left Ventricular Assist Device	*use* Implantable Heart Assist System in Heart and Great Vessels
Novation® Ceramic AHS® (Articulation Hip System)	*use* Synthetic Substitute, Ceramic for Replacement in Lower Joints
Omnilink Elite Vascular Balloon Expandable Stent System	*use* Intraluminal Device
Open Pivot Aortic Valve Graft (AVG)	*use* Synthetic Substitute
Open Pivot (mechanical) valve	*use* Synthetic Substitute
Optimizer™ III implantable pulse generator	*use* Contractility Modulation Device for Insertion in Subcutaneous Tissue and Fascia
Oropharyngeal airway (OPA)	*use* Intraluminal Device, Airway in Mouth and Throat
Ovatio™ CRT-D	*use* Cardiac Resynchronization Defibrillator Pulse Generator for Insertion in Subcutaneous Tissue and Fascia
Oxidized zirconium ceramic hip bearing surface	*use* Synthetic Substitute, Ceramic on Polyethylene for Replacement in Lower Joints
Paclitaxel-eluting coronary stent	*use* Intraluminal Device, Drug-eluting in Heart and Great Vessels
Paclitaxel-eluting peripheral stent	*use* Intraluminal Device, Drug-eluting in Upper Arteries, Lower Arteries
Partially absorbable mesh	*use* Synthetic Substitute
Pedicle-based dynamic stabilization device	*use* Spinal Stabilization Device, Pedicle-Based for Insertion in Upper Joints, Lower Joints
Perceval sutureless valve	*use* Zooplastic Tissue, Rapid Deployment Technique in New Technology
Percutaneous endoscopic gastrojejunostomy (PEG/J) tube	*use* Feeding Device in Gastrointestinal System
Percutaneous endoscopic gastrostomy (PEG) tube	*use* Feeding Device in Gastrointestinal System
Percutaneous nephrostomy catheter	*use* Drainage Device
Peripherally inserted central catheter (PICC)	*use* Infusion Device
Pessary ring	*use* Intraluminal Device, Pessary in Female Reproductive System
Phrenic nerve stimulator generator	*use* Stimulator Generator in Subcutaneous Tissue and Fascia
Phrenic nerve stimulator lead	*use* Diaphragmatic Pacemaker Lead in Respiratory System
PHYSIOMESH™ Flexible Composite Mesh	*use* Synthetic Substitute
Pipeline™ Embolization device (PED)	*use* Intraluminal Device
Polyethylene socket	*use* Synthetic Substitute, Polyethylene for Replacement in Lower Joints
Polymethylmethacrylate (PMMA)	*use* Synthetic Substitute
Polypropylene mesh	*use* Synthetic Substitute
Porcine (bioprosthetic) valve	*use* Zooplastic Tissue in Heart and Great Vessels
PRESTIGE® Cervical Disc	*use* Synthetic Substitute
PrimeAdvanced neurostimulator (SureScan) (MRI Safe)	*use* Stimulator Generator, Multiple Array for Insertion in Subcutaneous Tissue and Fascia
PROCEED™ Ventral Patch	*use* Synthetic Substitute
Prodisc-C	*use* Synthetic Substitute
Prodisc-L	*use* Synthetic Substitute

DEVICE	USE:
PROLENE Polypropylene Hernia System (PHS)	*use* Synthetic Substitute
Protecta XT CRT-D	*use* Cardiac Resynchronization Defibrillator Pulse Generator for Insertion in Subcutaneous Tissue and Fascia
Protecta XT DR (XT VR)	*use* Defibrillator Generator for Insertion in Subcutaneous Tissue and Fascia
Protégé® RX Carotid Stent System	*use* Intraluminal Device
Pump reservoir	*use* Infusion Device, Pump in Subcutaneous Tissue and Fascia
REALIZE® Adjustable Gastric Band	*use* Extraluminal Device
Rebound HRD® (Hernia Repair Device)	*use* Synthetic Substitute
RestoreAdvanced neurostimulator (SureScan) (MRI Safe)	*use* Stimulator Generator, Multiple Array Rechargeable for Insertion in Subcutaneous Tissue and Fascia
RestoreSensor neurostimulator (SureScan) (MRI Safe)	*use* Stimulator Generator, Multiple Array Rechargeable for Insertion in Subcutaneous Tissue and Fascia
RestoreUltra neurostimulator (SureScan) (MRI Safe)	*use* Stimulator Generator, Multiple Array Rechargeable for Insertion in Subcutaneous Tissue and Fascia
Reveal (DX) (XT)	*use* Monitoring Device
Reverse® Shoulder Prosthesis	*use* Synthetic Substitute, Reverse Ball and Socket for Replacement in Upper Joints
Revo MRI™ SureScan® pacemaker	*use* Pacemaker, Dual Chamber for Insertion in Subcutaneous Tissue and Fascia
Rheos® System device	*use* Stimulator Generator in Subcutaneous Tissue and Fascia
Rheos® System lead	*use* Stimulator Lead in Upper Arteries
RNS System lead	*use* Neurostimulator Lead in Central Nervous System
RNS system neurostimulator generator	*use* Neurostimulator Generator in Head and Facial Bones
Sacral nerve modulation (SNM) lead	*use* Stimulator Lead in Urinary System
Sacral neuromodulation lead	*use* Stimulator Lead in Urinary System
SAPIEN transcatheter aortic valve	*use* Zooplastic Tissue in Heart and Great Vessels
Secura (DR) (VR)	*use* Defibrillator Generator for Insertion in Subcutaneous Tissue and Fascia
Sheffield hybrid external fixator	*use* External Fixation Device, Hybrid for Insertion in Upper Bones, Lower Bones External Fixation Device, Hybrid for Reposition in Upper Bones, Lower Bones
Sheffield ring external fixator	*use* External Fixation Device, Ring for Insertion in Upper Bones, Lower Bones External Fixation Device, Ring for Reposition in Upper Bones, Lower Bones
Single lead pacemaker (atrium) (ventricle)	*use* Pacemaker, Single Chamber for Insertion in Subcutaneous Tissue and Fascia
Single lead rate responsive pacemaker (atrium) (ventricle)	*use* Pacemaker, Single Chamber Rate Responsive for Insertion in Subcutaneous Tissue and Fascia
Sirolimus-eluting coronary stent	*use* Intraluminal Device, Drug-eluting in Heart and Great Vessels
SJM Biocor® Stented Valve System	*use* Zooplastic Tissue in Heart and Great Vessels
Spinal cord neurostimulator lead	*use* Neurostimulator Lead in Central Nervous System
Spinal growth rod(s), magnetically controlled	*use* Magnetically Controlled Growth Rod(s) in New Technology
Spiration IBV™ Valve System	*use* Intraluminal Device, Endobronchial Valve in Respiratory System
Stent, intraluminal (cardiovascular) (gastrointestinal) (hepatobiliary) (urinary)	*use* Intraluminal Device
Stented tissue valve	*use* Zooplastic Tissue in Heart and Great Vessels
Stratos LV	*use* Cardiac Resynchronization Pacemaker Pulse Generator for Insertion in Subcutaneous Tissue and Fascia
Subcutaneous injection reservoir, port	*use* Vascular Access Device, Reservoir in Subcutaneous Tissue and Fascia
Subcutaneous injection reservoir, pump	*use* Infusion Device, Pump in Subcutaneous Tissue and Fascia
Subdermal progesterone implant	*use* Contraceptive Device in Subcutaneous Tissue and Fascia
Sutureless valve, Perceval	*use* Zooplastic Tissue, Rapid Deployment Technique in New Technology
SynCardia Total Artificial Heart	*use* Synthetic Substitute
Synchra CRT-P	*use* Cardiac Resynchronization Pacemaker Pulse Generator for Insertion in Subcutaneous Tissue and Fascia
SynchroMed pump	*use* Infusion Device, Pump in Subcutaneous Tissue and Fascia
Talent® Converter	*use* Intraluminal Device
Talent® Occluder	*use* Intraluminal Device
Talent® Stent Graft (abdominal) (thoracic)	*use* Intraluminal Device
TandemHeart® System	*use* External Heart Assist System in Heart and Great Vessels
TAXUS® Liberté® Paclitaxel-eluting Coronary Stent System	*use* Intraluminal Device, Drug-eluting in Heart and Great Vessels
Therapeutic occlusion coil(s)	*use* Intraluminal Device

DEVICE	USE:
Thoracostomy tube	*use* Drainage Device
Thoratec IVAD (Implantable Ventricular Assist Device)	*use* Implantable Heart Assist System in Heart and Great Vessels
Thoratec Paracorporeal Ventricular Assist Device	*use* External Heart Assist System in Heart and Great Vessels
Tibial insert	*use* Liner in Lower Joints
TigerPaw® system for closure of left atrial appendage	*use* Extraluminal Device
Tissue bank graft	*use* Nonautologous Tissue Substitute
Tissue expander (inflatable) (injectable)	*use* Tissue Expander in Skin and Breast Tissue Expander in Subcutaneous Tissue and Fascia
Titanium Sternal Fixation System (TSFS)	*use* Internal Fixation Device, Rigid Plate for Insertion in Upper Bones Internal Fixation Device, Rigid Plate for Reposition in Upper Bones
Total artificial (replacement) heart	*use* Synthetic Substitute
Tracheostomy tube	*use* Tracheostomy Device in Respiratory System
Trifecta™ Valve (aortic)	*use* Zooplastic Tissue in Heart and Great Vessels
Tunneled central venous catheter	*use* Vascular Access Device in Subcutaneous Tissue and Fascia
Tunneled spinal (intrathecal) catheter	*use* Infusion Device
Two lead pacemaker	*use* Pacemaker, Dual Chamber for Insertion in Subcutaneous Tissue and Fascia
Ultraflex™ Precision Colonic Stent System	*use* Intraluminal Device
ULTRAPRO Hernia System (UHS)	*use* Synthetic Substitute
ULTRAPRO Partially Absorbable Lightweight Mesh	*use* Synthetic Substitute
ULTRAPRO Plug	*use* Synthetic Substitute
Ultrasonic osteogenic stimulator	*use* Bone Growth Stimulator in Head and Facial Bones, Upper Bones, Lower Bones
Ultrasound bone healing system	*use* Bone Growth Stimulator in Head and Facial Bones, Upper Bones, Lower Bones
Uniplanar external fixator	*use* External Fixation Device, Monoplanar for Insertion in Upper Bones, Lower Bones External Fixation Device, Monoplanar for Reposition in Upper Bones, Lower Bones
Urinary incontinence stimulator lead	*use* Stimulator Lead in Urinary System
Vaginal pessary	*use* Intraluminal Device, Pessary in Female Reproductive System
Valiant Thoracic Stent Graft	*use* Intraluminal Device
Vectra® Vascular Access Graft	*use* Vascular Access Device in Subcutaneous Tissue and Fascia
Ventrio™ Hernia Patch	*use* Synthetic Substitute
Versa	*use* Pacemaker, Dual Chamber for Insertion in Subcutaneous Tissue and Fascia
Virtuoso (II) (DR) (VR)	*use* Defibrillator Generator for Insertion in Subcutaneous Tissue and Fascia
Viva (XT) (S)	*use* Cardiac Resynchronization Defibrillator Pulse Generator for Insertion in Subcutaneous Tissue and Fascia
WALLSTENT® Endoprosthesis	*use* Intraluminal Device
X-STOP® Spacer	*use* Spinal Stabilization Device, Interspinous Process for Insertion in Upper Joints, Lower Joints
Xact Carotid Stent System	*use* Intraluminal Device
Xenograft	*use* Zooplastic Tissue in Heart and Great Vessels
XIENCE Everolimus Eluting Coronary Stent System	*use* Intraluminal Device, Drug-eluting in Heart and Great Vessels
XLIF® System	*use* Interbody Fusion Device in Lower Joints
Zenith AAA Endovascular Graft	*use* Intraluminal Device, Branched or Fenestrated, One or Two Arteries for Restriction in Lower Arteries *use* Intraluminal Device, Branched or Fenestrated, Three or More Arteries for Restriction in Lower Arteries *use* Intraluminal Device
Zenith Flex® AAA Endovascular Graft	*use* Intraluminal Device
Zenith TX2® TAA Endovascular Graft	*use* Intraluminal Device
Zenith® Renu™ AAA Ancillary Graft	*use* Intraluminal Device
Zilver® PTX® (paclitaxel) Drug-Eluting Peripheral Stent	*use* Intraluminal Device, Drug-eluting in Upper Arteries, Lower Arteries
Zimmer® NexGen® LPS Mobile Bearing Knee	*use* Synthetic Substitute
Zimmer® NexGen® LPS-Flex Mobile Knee	*use* Synthetic Substitute
Zotarolimus-eluting coronary stent	*use* Intraluminal Device, Drug-eluting in Heart and Great Vessels

NOTES

Specific Device	Operation	In Body System	General Device
Autologous Arterial Tissue	All applicable	Heart and Great Vessels Lower Arteries, Lower Veins Upper Arteries, Upper Veins	7 Autologous Tissue Substitute
Autologous Venous Tissue	All applicable	Heart and Great Vessels Lower Arteries, Lower Veins Upper Arteries, Upper Veins	7 Autologous Tissue Substitute
Cardiac Lead, Defibrillator	Insertion	Heart and Great Vessels	M Cardiac Lead
Cardiac Lead, Pacemaker	Insertion	Heart and Great Vessels	M Cardiac Lead
Cardiac Resynchronization Defibrillator Pulse Generator	Insertion	Subcutaneous Tissue and Fascia	P Cardiac Rhythm Related Device
Cardiac Resynchronization Pacemaker Pulse Generator	Insertion	Subcutaneous Tissue and Fascia	P Cardiac Rhythm Related Device
Contractility Modulation Device	Insertion	Subcutaneous Tissue and Fascia	P Cardiac Rhythm Related Device
Defibrillator Generator	Insertion	Subcutaneous Tissue and Fascia	P Cardiac Rhythm Related Device
Epiretinal Visual Prosthesis	All applicable	Eye	J Synthetic Substitute
External Fixation Device, Hybrid	Insertion	Lower Bones, Upper Bones	5 External Fixation Device
External Fixation Device, Hybrid	Reposition	Lower Bones, Upper Bones	5 External Fixation Device
External Fixation Device, Limb Lengthening	Insertion	Lower Bones, Upper Bones	5 External Fixation Device
External Fixation Device, Monoplanar	Insertion	Lower Bones, Upper Bones	5 External Fixation Device
External Fixation Device, Monoplanar	Reposition	Lower Bones, Upper Bones	5 External Fixation Device
External Fixation Device, Ring	Insertion	Lower Bones, Upper Bones	5 External Fixation Device
External Fixation Device, Ring	Reposition	Lower Bones, Upper Bones	5 External Fixation Device
Hearing Device, Bone Conduction	Insertion	Ear, Nose, Sinus	S Hearing Device
Hearing Device, Multiple Channel Cochlear Prosthesis	Insertion	Ear, Nose, Sinus	S Hearing Device
Hearing Device, Single Channel Cochlear Prosthesis	Insertion	Ear, Nose, Sinus	S Hearing Device
Internal Fixation Device, Intramedullary	All applicable	Lower Bones, Upper Bones	4 Internal Fixation Device
Internal Fixation Device, Rigid Plate	Insertion	Upper Bones	4 Internal Fixation Device
Internal Fixation Device, Rigid Plate	Reposition	Upper Bones	4 Internal Fixation Device
Intraluminal Device, Airway	All applicable	Ear, Nose, Sinus Gastrointestinal System Mouth and Throat	D Intraluminal Device
Intraluminal Device, Bioactive	All applicable	Upper Arteries	D Intraluminal Device
Intraluminal Device, Branched or Fenestrated, One or Two Arteries	Restriction	Heart and Great Vessels Lower Arteries	D Intraluminal Device
Intraluminal Device, Branched or Fenestrated, Three or More Arteries	Restriction	Heart and Great Vessels Lower Arteries	D Intraluminal Device
Intraluminal Device, Drug-eluting	All applicable	Heart and Great Vessels Lower Arteries, Upper Arteries	D Intraluminal Device
Intraluminal Device, Drug-eluting, Four or More	All applicable	Heart and Great Vessels Lower Arteries, Upper Arteries	D Intraluminal Device
Intraluminal Device, Drug-eluting, Three	All applicable	Heart and Great Vessels Lower Arteries, Upper Arteries	D Intraluminal Device
Intraluminal Device, Drug-eluting, Two	All applicable	Heart and Great Vessels Lower Arteries, Upper Arteries	D Intraluminal Device
Intraluminal Device, Endobronchial Valve	All applicable	Respiratory System	D Intraluminal Device
Intraluminal Device, Endotracheal Airway	All applicable	Respiratory System	D Intraluminal Device
Intraluminal Device, Four or More	All applicable	Heart and Great Vessels Lower Arteries, Upper Arteries	D Intraluminal Device
Intraluminal Device, Pessary	All applicable	Female Reproductive System	D Intraluminal Device
Intraluminal Device, Radioactive	All applicable	Heart and Great Vessels	D Intraluminal Device
Intraluminal Device, Three	All applicable	Heart and Great Vessels Lower Arteries, Upper Arteries	D Intraluminal Device
Intraluminal Device, Two	All applicable	Heart and Great Vessels Lower Arteries, Upper Arteries	D Intraluminal Device
Monitoring Device, Hemodynamic	Insertion	Subcutaneous Tissue and Fascia	2 Monitoring Device
Monitoring Device, Pressure Sensor	Insertion	Heart and Great Vessels	2 Monitoring Device
Pacemaker, Dual Chamber	Insertion	Subcutaneous Tissue and Fascia	P Cardiac Rhythm Related Device
Pacemaker, Single Chamber	Insertion	Subcutaneous Tissue and Fascia	P Cardiac Rhythm Related Device
Pacemaker, Single Chamber Rate Responsive	Insertion	Subcutaneous Tissue and Fascia	P Cardiac Rhythm Related Device

Specific Device	Operation	In Body System	General Device
Spinal Stabilization Device, Facet Replacement	Insertion	Lower Joints, Upper Joints	4 Internal Fixation Device
Spinal Stabilization Device, Interspinous Process	Insertion	Lower Joints, Upper Joints	4 Internal Fixation Device
Spinal Stabilization Device, Pedicle-Based	Insertion	Lower Joints, Upper Joints	4 Internal Fixation Device
Stimulator Generator, Multiple Array	Insertion	Subcutaneous Tissue and Fascia	M Stimulator Generator
Stimulator Generator, Multiple Array Rechargeable	Insertion	Subcutaneous Tissue and Fascia	M Stimulator Generator
Stimulator Generator, Single Array	Insertion	Subcutaneous Tissue and Fascia	M Stimulator Generator
Stimulator Generator, Single Array Rechargeable	Insertion	Subcutaneous Tissue and Fascia	M Stimulator Generator
Synthetic Substitute, Ceramic	Replacement	Lower Joints	J Synthetic Substitute
Synthetic Substitute, Ceramic on Polyethylene	Replacement	Lower Joints	J Synthetic Substitute
Synthetic Substitute, Intraocular Telescope	Replacement	Eye	J Synthetic Substitute
Synthetic Substitute, Metal	Replacement	Lower Joints	J Synthetic Substitute
Synthetic Substitute, Metal on Polyethylene	Replacement	Lower Joints	J Synthetic Substitute
Synthetic Substitute, Polyethylene	Replacement	Lower Joints	J Synthetic Substitute
Synthetic Substitute, Reverse Ball and Socket	Replacement	Upper Joints	J Synthetic Substitute
Synthetic Substitute, Unicondylar	Replacement	Lower Joints	J Synthetic Substitute

APPENDIX F – QUALIFIER KEY
PHYSICAL REHABILITATION AND DIAGNOSTIC AUDIOLOGY

Acoustic Reflex Decay	Definition: Measures reduction in size/strength of acoustic reflex over time Includes/Examples: Includes site of lesion test
Acoustic Reflex Patterns	Definition: Defines site of lesion based upon presence/absence of acoustic reflexes with ipsilateral vs. contralateral stimulation
Acoustic Reflex Threshold	Definition: Determines minimal intensity that acoustic reflex occurs with ipsilateral and/or contralateral stimulation
Aerobic Capacity and Endurance	Definition: Measures autonomic responses to positional changes; perceived exertion, dyspnea or angina during activity; performance during exercise protocols; standard vital signs; and blood gas analysis or oxygen consumption
Alternate Binaural or Monaural Loudness Balance	Definition: Determines auditory stimulus parameter that yields the same objective sensation Includes/Examples: Sound intensities that yield same loudness perception
Anthropometric Characteristics	Definition: Measures edema, body fat composition, height, weight, length and girth
Aphasia (Assessment)	Definition: Measures expressive and receptive speech and language function including reading and writing
Aphasia (Treatment)	Definition: Applying techniques to improve, augment, or compensate for receptive/expressive language impairments
Articulation/Phonology (Assessment)	Definition: Measures speech production
Articulation/Phonology (Treatment)	Definition: Applying techniques to correct, improve, or compensate for speech productive impairment
Assistive Listening Device	Definition: Assists in use of effective and appropriate assistive listening device/system
Assistive Listening System/Device Selection	Definition: Measures the effectiveness and appropriateness of assistive listening systems/devices
Assistive, Adaptive, Supportive or Protective Devices	Explanation: Devices to facilitate or support achievement of a higher level of function in wheelchair mobility; bed mobility; transfer or ambulation ability; bath and showering ability; dressing; grooming; personal hygiene; play or leisure
Auditory Evoked Potentials	Definition: Measures electric responses produced by the VIIIth cranial nerve and brainstem following auditory stimulation
Auditory Processing (Assessment)	Definition: Evaluates ability to receive and process auditory information and comprehension of spoken language
Auditory Processing (Treatment)	Definition: Applying techniques to improve the receiving and processing of auditory information and comprehension of spoken language
Augmentative/Alternative Communication System (Assessment)	Definition: Determines the appropriateness of aids, techniques, symbols, and/or strategies to augment or replace speech and enhance communication Includes/Examples: Includes the use of telephones, writing equipment, emergency equipment, and TDD
Augmentative/Alternative Communication System (Treatment)	Includes/Examples: Includes augmentative communication devices and aids
Aural Rehabilitation	Definition: Applying techniques to improve the communication abilities associated with hearing loss
Aural Rehabilitation Status	Definition: Measures impact of a hearing loss including evaluation of receptive and expressive communication skills
Bathing/Showering	Includes/Examples: Includes obtaining and using supplies; soaping, rinsing, and drying body parts; maintaining bathing position; and transferring to and from bathing positions
Bathing/Showering Techniques	Definition: Activities to facilitate obtaining and using supplies, soaping, rinsing and drying body parts, maintaining bathing position, and transferring to and from bathing positions
Bed Mobility (Assessment)	Definition: Transitional movement within bed
Bed Mobility (Treatment)	Definition: Exercise or activities to facilitate transitional movements within bed
Bedside Swallowing and Oral Function	Includes/Examples: Bedside swallowing includes assessment of sucking, masticating, coughing, and swallowing. Oral function includes assessment of musculature for controlled movements, structures and functions to determine coordination and phonation

Bekesy Audiometry	Definition: Uses an instrument that provides a choice of discrete or continuously varying pure tones; choice of pulsed or continuous signal
Binaural Electroacoustic Hearing Aid Check	Definition: Determines mechanical and electroacoustic function of bilateral hearing aids using hearing aid test box
Binaural Hearing Aid (Assessment)	Definition: Measures the candidacy, effectiveness, and appropriateness of hearing aids Explanation: Measures bilateral fit
Binaural Hearing Aid (Treatment)	Explanation: Assists in achieving maximum understanding and performance
Bithermal, Binaural Caloric Irrigation	Definition: Measures the rhythmic eye movements stimulated by changing the temperature of the vestibular system
Bithermal, Monaural Caloric Irrigation	Definition: Measures the rhythmic eye movements stimulated by changing the temperature of the vestibular system in one ear
Brief Tone Stimuli	Definition: Measures specific central auditory process
Cerumen Management	Definition: Includes examination of external auditory canal and tympanic membrane and removal of cerumen from external ear canal
Cochlear Implant	Definition: Measures candidacy for cochlear implant
Cochlear Implant Rehabilitation	Definition: Applying techniques to improve the communication abilities of individuals with cochlear implant; includes programming the device, providing patients/families with information
Communicative/Cognitive Integration Skills (Assessment)	Definition: Measures ability to use higher cortical functions Includes/Examples: Includes orientation, recognition, attention span, initiation and termination of activity, memory, sequencing, categorizing, concept formation, spatial operations, judgment, problem solving, generalization and pragmatic communication
Communicative/Cognitive Integration Skills (Treatment)	Definition: Activities to facilitate the use of higher cortical functions Includes/Examples: Includes level of arousal, orientation, recognition, attention span, initiation and termination of activity, memory sequencing, judgment and problem solving, learning and generalization, and pragmatic communication
Computerized Dynamic Posturography	Definition: Measures the status of the peripheral and central vestibular system and the sensory/motor component of balance; evaluates the efficacy of vestibular rehabilitation
Conditioned Play Audiometry	Definition: Behavioral measures using nonspeech and speech stimuli to obtain frequency-specific and ear-specific information on auditory status from the patient Explanation: Obtains speech reception threshold by having patient point to pictures of spondaic words
Coordination/Dexterity (Assessment)	Definition: Measures large and small muscle groups for controlled goal-directed movements Explanation: Dexterity includes object manipulation
Coordination/Dexterity (Treatment)	Definition: Exercise or activities to facilitate gross coordination and fine coordination
Cranial Nerve Integrity	Definition: Measures cranial nerve sensory and motor functions, including tastes, smell and facial expression
Dichotic Stimuli	Definition: Measures specific central auditory process
Distorted Speech	Definition: Measures specific central auditory process
Dix-Hallpike Dynamic	Definition: Measures nystagmus following Dix-Hallpike maneuver
Dressing	Includes/Examples: Includes selecting clothing and accessories, obtaining clothing from storage, dressing and, fastening and adjusting clothing and shoes, and applying and removing personal devices, prosthesis or orthosis
Dressing Techniques	Definition: Activities to facilitate selecting clothing and accessories, dressing and undressing, adjusting clothing and shoes, applying and removing devices, prostheses or orthoses
Dynamic Orthosis	Includes/Examples: Includes customized and prefabricated splints, inhibitory casts, spinal and other braces, and protective devices; allows motion through transfer of movement from other body parts or by use of outside forces
Ear Canal Probe Microphone	Definition: Real ear measures
Ear Protector Attentuation	Definition: Measures ear protector fit and effectiveness
Electrocochleography	Definition: Measures the VIIIth cranial nerve action potential
Environmental, Home and Work Barriers	Definition: Measures current and potential barriers to optimal function, including safety hazards, access problems and home or office design

© 2016 Channel Publishing, Ltd.

A P P E N D I X   F

Ergonomics and Body Mechanics	Definition: Ergonomic measurement of job tasks, work hardening or work conditioning needs; functional capacity; and body mechanics
Eustachian Tube Function	Definition: Measures eustachian tube function and patency of eustachian tube
Evoked Otoacoustic Emissions, Diagnostic	Definition: Measures auditory evoked potentials in a diagnostic format
Evoked Otoacoustic Emissions, Screening	Definition: Measures auditory evoked potentials in a screening format
Facial Nerve Function	Definition: Measures electrical activity of the VIIth cranial nerve (facial nerve)
Feeding/Eating (Assessment)	Includes/Examples: Includes setting up food, selecting and using utensils and tableware, bringing food or drink to mouth, cleaning face, hands, and clothing, and management of alternative methods of nourishment
Feeding/Eating (Treatment)	Definition: Exercise or activities to facilitate setting up food, selecting and using utensils and tableware, bringing food or drink to mouth, cleaning face, hands, and clothing, and management of alternative methods of nourishment
Filtered Speech	Definition: Uses high or low pass filtered speech stimuli to assess central auditory processing disorders, site of lesion testing
Fluency (Assessment)	Definition: Measures speech fluency or stuttering
Fluency (Treatment)	Definition: Applying techniques to improve and augment fluent speech
Gait and/or Balance	Definition: Measures biomechanical, arthrokinematic and other spatial and temporal characteristics of gait and balance
Gait Training/Functional Ambulation	Definition: Exercise or activities to facilitate ambulation on a variety of surfaces and in a variety of environments
Grooming/Personal Hygiene (Assessment)	Includes/Examples: Includes ability to obtain and use supplies in a sequential fashion, general grooming, oral hygiene, toilet hygiene, personal care devices, including care for artificial airways
Grooming/Personal Hygiene (Treatment)	Definition: Activities to facilitate obtaining and using supplies in a sequential fashion: general grooming, oral hygiene, toilet hygiene, cleaning body, and personal care devices, including artificial airways
Hearing and Related Disorders Counseling	Definition: Provides patients/families/caregivers with information, support, referrals to facilitate recovery from a communication disorder Includes/Examples: Includes strategies for psychosocial adjustment to hearing loss for clients and families/caregivers
Hearing and Related Disorders Prevention	Definition: Provides patients/families/caregivers with information and support to prevent communication disorders
Hearing Screening	Definition: Pass/refer measures designed to identify need for further audiologic assessment
Home Management (Assessment)	Definition: Obtaining and maintaining personal and household possessions and environment Includes/Examples: Includes clothing care, cleaning, meal preparation and cleanup, shopping, money management, household maintenance, safety procedures, and childcare/parenting
Home Management (Treatment)	Definition: Activities to facilitate obtaining and maintaining personal household possessions and environment Includes/Examples: Includes clothing care, cleaning, meal preparation and clean-up, shopping, money management, household maintenance, safety procedures, childcare/parenting
Instrumental Swallowing and Oral Function	Definition: Measures swallowing function using instrumental diagnostic procedures Explanation: Methods include videofluoroscopy, ultrasound, manometry, endoscopy
Integumentary Integrity	Includes/Examples: Includes burns, skin conditions, ecchymosis, bleeding, blisters, scar tissue, wounds and other traumas, tissue mobility, turgor and texture
Manual Therapy Techniques	Definition: Techniques in which the therapist uses his/her hands to administer skilled movements Includes/Examples: Includes connective tissue massage, joint mobilization and manipulation, manual lymph drainage, manual traction, soft tissue mobilization and manipulation
Masking Patterns	Definition: Measures central auditory processing status
Monaural Electroacoustic Hearing Aid Check	Definition: Determines mechanical and electroacoustic function of one hearing aid using hearing aid test box

APPENDIX F

Monaural Hearing Aid (Assessment)	Definition: Measures the candidacy, effectiveness, and appropriateness of a hearing aid Explanation: Measures unilateral fit
Monaural Hearing Aid (Treatment)	Explanation: Assists in achieving maximum understanding and performance
Motor Function (Assessment)	Definition: Measures the body's functional and versatile movement patterns Includes/Examples: Includes motor assessment scales, analysis of head, trunk and limb movement, and assessment of motor learning
Motor Function (Treatment)	Definition: Exercise or activities to facilitate crossing midline, laterality, bilateral integration, praxis, neuromuscular relaxation, inhibition, facilitation, motor function and motor learning
Motor Speech (Assessment)	Definition: Measures neurological motor aspects of speech production
Motor Speech (Treatment)	Definition: Applying techniques to improve and augment the impaired neurological motor aspects of speech production
Muscle Performance (Assessment)	Definition: Measures muscle strength, power and endurance using manual testing, dynamometry or computer-assisted electromechanical muscle test; functional muscle strength, power and endurance; muscle pain, tone, or soreness; or pelvic-floor musculature Explanation: Muscle endurance refers to the ability to contract a muscle repeatedly over time
Muscle Performance (Treatment)	Definition: Exercise or activities to increase the capacity of a muscle to do work in terms of strength, power, and/or endurance Explanation: Muscle strength is the force exerted to overcome resistance in one maximal effort. Muscle power is work produced per unit of time, or the product of strength and speed. Muscle endurance is the ability to contract a muscle repeatedly over time
Neuromotor Development	Definition: Measures motor development, righting and equilibrium reactions, and reflex and equilibrium reactions
Neurophysiologic Intraoperative	Definition: Monitors neural status during surgery
Non-invasive Instrumental Status	Definition: Instrumental measures of oral, nasal, vocal, and velopharyngeal functions as they pertain to speech production
Nonspoken Language (Assessment)	Definition: Measures nonspoken language (print, sign, symbols) for communication
Nonspoken Language (Treatment)	Definition: Applying techniques that improve, augment, or compensate spoken communication
Oral Peripheral Mechanism	Definition: Structural measures of face, jaw, lips, tongue, teeth, hard and soft palate, pharynx as related to speech production
Orofacial Myofunctional (Assessment)	Definition: Measures orofacial myofunctional patterns for speech and related functions
Orofacial Myofunctional (Treatment)	Definition: Applying techniques to improve, alter, or augment impaired orofacial myofunctional patterns and related speech production errors
Oscillating Tracking	Definition: Measures ability to visually track
Pain	Definition: Measures muscle soreness, pain and soreness with joint movement, and pain perception Includes/Examples: Includes questionnaires, graphs, symptom magnification scales or visual analog scales
Perceptual Processing (Assessment)	Definition: Measures stereognosis, kinesthesia, body schema, right-left discrimination, form constancy, position in space, visual closure, figure-ground, depth perception, spatial relations and topographical orientation
Perceptual Processing (Treatment)	Definition: Exercise and activities to facilitate perceptual processing Explanation: Includes stereognosis, kinesthesia, body schema, right-left discrimination, form constancy, position in space, visual closure, figure-ground, depth perception, spatial relations, and topographical orientation Includes/Examples: Includes stereognosis, kinesthesia, body schema, right-left discrimination, form constancy, position in space, visual closure, figure-ground, depth perception, spatial relations, and topographical orientation
Performance Intensity Phonetically Balanced Speech Discrimination	Definition: Measures word recognition over varying intensity levels
Postural Control	Definition: Exercise or activities to increase postural alignment and control
Prosthesis	Explanation: Artificial substitutes for missing body parts that augment performance or function

Psychosocial Skills (Assessment)	Definition: The ability to interact in society and to process emotions Includes/Examples: Includes psychological (values, interests, self-concept); social (role performance, social conduct, interpersonal skills, self expression); self-management (coping skills, time management, self-control)
Psychosocial Skills (Treatment)	Definition: The ability to interact in society and to process emotions Includes/Examples: Includes psychological (values, interests, self-concept); social (role performance, social conduct, interpersonal skills, self expression); self-management (coping skills, time management, self-control)
Pure Tone Audiometry, Air	Definition: Air-conduction pure tone threshold measures with appropriate masking
Pure Tone Audiometry, Air and Bone	Definition: Air-conduction and bone-conduction pure tone threshold measures with appropriate masking
Pure Tone Stenger	Definition: Measures unilateral nonorganic hearing loss based on simultaneous presentation of pure tones of differing volume
Range of Motion and Joint Integrity	Definition: Measures quantity, quality, grade, and classification of joint movement and/or mobility Explanation: Range of Motion is the space, distance or angle through which movement occurs at a joint or series of joints. Joint integrity is the conformance of joints to expected anatomic, biomechanical and kinematic norms
Range of Motion and Joint Mobility	Definition: Exercise or activities to increase muscle length and joint mobility
Receptive/Expressive Language (Assessment)	Definition: Measures receptive and expressive language
Receptive/Expressive Language (Treatment)	Definition: Applying techniques to improve and augment receptive/expressive language
Reflex Integrity	Definition: Measures the presence, absence, or exaggeration of developmentally appropriate, pathologic or normal reflexes
Select Picture Audiometry	Definition: Establishes hearing threshold levels for speech using pictures
Sensorineural Acuity Level	Definition: Measures sensorineural acuity masking presented via bone conduction
Sensory Aids	Definition: Determines the appropriateness of a sensory prosthetic device, other than a hearing aid or assistive listening system/device
Sensory Awareness/Processing/Integrity	Includes/Examples: Includes light touch, pressure, temperature, pain, sharp/dull, proprioception, vestibular, visual, auditory, gustatory, and olfactory
Short Increment Sensitivity Index	Definition: Measures the ear's ability to detect small intensity changes; site of lesion test requiring a behavioral response
Sinusoidal Vertical Axis Rotational	Definition: Measures nystagmus following rotation
Somatosensory Evoked Potentials	Definition: Measures neural activity from sites throughout the body
Speech and/or Language Screening	Definition: Identifies need for further speech and/or language evaluation
Speech Threshold	Definition: Measures minimal intensity needed to repeat spondaic words
Speech-Language Pathology and Related Disorders Counseling	Definition: Provides patients/families with information, support, referrals to facilitate recovery from a communication disorder
Speech-Language Pathology and Related Disorders Prevention	Definition: Applying techniques to avoid or minimize onset and/or development of a communication disorder
Speech/Word Recognition	Definition: Measures ability to repeat/identify single syllable words; scores given as a percentage; includes word recognition/speech discrimination
Staggered Spondaic Word	Definition: Measures central auditory processing site of lesion based upon dichotic presentation of spondaic words
Static Orthosis	Includes/Examples: Includes customized and prefabricated splints, inhibitory casts, spinal and other braces, and protective devices; has no moving parts, maintains joint(s) in desired position
Stenger	Definition: Measures unilateral nonorganic hearing loss based on simultaneous presentation of signals of differing volume
Swallowing Dysfunction	Definition: Activities to improve swallowing function in coordination with respiratory function Includes/Examples: Includes function and coordination of sucking, mastication, coughing, swallowing
Synthetic Sentence Identification	Definition: Measures central auditory dysfunction using identification of third order approximations of sentences and competing messages

APPENDIX F

Temporal Ordering of Stimuli	Definition: Measures specific central auditory process
Therapeutic Exercise	Definition: Exercise or activities to facilitate sensory awareness, sensory processing, sensory integration, balance training, conditioning, reconditioning Includes/Examples: Includes developmental activities, breathing exercises, aerobic endurance activities, aquatic exercises, stretching and ventilatory muscle training
Tinnitus Masker (Assessment)	Definition: Determines candidacy for tinnitus masker
Tinnitus Masker (Treatment)	Explanation: Used to verify physical fit, acoustic appropriateness, and benefit; assists in achieving maximum benefit
Tone Decay	Definition: Measures decrease in hearing sensitivity to a tone; site of lesion test requiring a behavioral response
Transfer	Definition: Transitional movement from one surface to another
Transfer Training	Definition: Exercise or activities to facilitate movement from one surface to another
Tympanometry	Definition: Measures the integrity of the middle ear; measures ease at which sound flows through the tympanic membrane while air pressure against the membrane is varied
Unithermal Binaural Screen	Definition: Measures the rhythmic eye movements stimulated by changing the temperature of the vestibular system in both ears using warm water, screening format
Ventilation, Respiration and Circulation	Definition: Measures ventilatory muscle strength, power and endurance, pulmonary function and ventilatory mechanics Includes/Examples: Includes ability to clear airway, activities that aggravate or relieve edema, pain, dyspnea or other symptoms, chest wall mobility, cardiopulmonary response to performance of ADL and IAD, cough and sputum, standard vital signs
Vestibular	Definition: Applying techniques to compensate for balance disorders; includes habituation, exercise therapy, and balance retraining
Visual Motor Integration (Assessment)	Definition: Coordinating the interaction of information from the eyes with body movement during activity
Visual Motor Integration (Treatment)	Definition: Exercise or activities to facilitate coordinating the interaction of information from eyes with body movement during activity
Visual Reinforcement Audiometry	Definition: Behavioral measures using nonspeech and speech stimuli to obtain frequency/ear-specific information on auditory status Includes/Examples: Includes a conditioned response of looking toward a visual reinforcer (e.g., lights, animated toy) every time auditory stimuli are heard
Vocational Activities and Functional Community or Work Reintegration Skills (Assessment)	Definition: Measures environmental, home, work (job/school/play) barriers that keep patients from functioning optimally in their environment Includes/Examples: Includes assessment of vocational skill and interests, environment of work (job/school/play), injury potential and injury prevention or reduction, ergonomic stressors, transportation skills, and ability to access and use community resources
Vocational Activities and Functional Community or Work Reintegration Skills (Treatment)	Definition: Activities to facilitate vocational exploration, body mechanics training, job acquisition, and environmental or work (job/school/play) task adaptation Includes/Examples: Includes injury prevention and reduction, ergonomic stressor reduction, job coaching and simulation, work hardening and conditioning, driving training, transportation skills, and use of community resources
Voice (Assessment)	Definition: Measures vocal structure, function and production
Voice (Treatment)	Definition: Applying techniques to improve voice and vocal function
Voice Prosthetic (Assessment)	Definition: Determines the appropriateness of voice prosthetic/adaptive device to enhance or facilitate communication
Voice Prosthetic (Treatment)	Includes/Examples: Includes electrolarynx, and other assistive, adaptive, supportive devices
Wheelchair Mobility (Assessment)	Definition: Measures fit and functional abilities within wheelchair in a variety of environments
Wheelchair Mobility (Treatment)	Definition: Management, maintenance and controlled operation of a wheelchair, scooter or other device, in and on a variety of surfaces and environments
Wound Management	Includes/Examples: Includes non-selective and selective debridement (enzymes, autolysis, sharp debridement), dressings (wound coverings, hydrogel, vacuum-assisted closure), topical agents, etc.

APPENDIX G – QUALIFIER KEY FOR MENTAL HEALTH

Behavioral	Definition: Primarily to modify behavior Includes/Examples: Includes modeling and role playing, positive reinforcement of target behaviors, response cost, and training of self-management skills
Cognitive	Definition: Primarily to correct cognitive distortions and errors
Cognitive-Behavioral	Definition: Combining cognitive and behavioral treatment strategies to improve functioning Explanation: Maladaptive responses are examined to determine how cognitions relate to behavior patterns in response to an event. Uses learning principles and information-processing models
Developmental	Definition: Age-normed developmental status of cognitive, social and adaptive behavior skills
Intellectual and Psychoeducational	Definition: Intellectual abilities, academic achievement and learning capabilities (including behaviors and emotional factors affecting learning)
Interactive	Definition: Uses primarily physical aids and other forms of non-oral interaction with a patient who is physically, psychologically or developmentally unable to use ordinary language for communication Includes/Examples: Includes. the use of toys in symbolic play
Interpersonal	Definition: Helps an individual make changes in interpersonal behaviors to reduce psychological dysfunction Includes/Examples: Includes exploratory techniques, encouragement of affective expression, clarification of patient statements, analysis of communication patterns, use of therapy relationship and behavior change techniques
Neurobehavioral and Cognitive Status	Definition: Includes neurobehavioral status exam, interview(s), and observation for the clinical assessment of thinking, reasoning and judgment, acquired knowledge, attention, memory, visual spatial abilities, language functions, and planning
Neuropsychological	Definition: Thinking, reasoning and judgment, acquired knowledge, attention, memory, visual spatial abilities, language functions, planning
Personality and Behavioral	Definition: Mood, emotion, behavior, social functioning, psychopathological conditions, personality traits and characteristics
Psychoanalysis	Definition: Methods of obtaining a detailed account of past and present mental and emotional experiences to determine the source and eliminate or diminish the undesirable effects of unconscious conflicts Explanation: Accomplished by making the individual aware of their existence, origin, and inappropriate expression in emotions and behavior
Psychodynamic	Definition: Exploration of past and present emotional experiences to understand motives and drives using insight-oriented techniques to reduce the undesirable effects of internal conflicts on emotions and behavior Explanation: Techniques include empathetic listening, clarifying self-defeating behavior patterns, and exploring adaptive alternatives
Psychophysiological	Definition: Monitoring and alteration of physiological processes to help the individual associate physiological reactions combined with cognitive and behavioral strategies to gain improved control of these processes to help the individual cope more effectively
Supportive	Definition: Formation of therapeutic relationship primarily for providing emotional support to prevent further deterioration in functioning during periods of particular stress Explanation: Often used in conjunction with other therapeutic approaches
Vocational	Definition: Exploration of vocational interests, aptitudes and required adaptive behavior skills to develop and carry out a plan for achieving a successful vocational placement Includes/Examples: Includes enhancing work related adjustment and/or pursuing viable options in training education or preparation

NOTES

© 2016 Channel Publishing, Ltd.

NOTES

SUBSTANCE	USE:
AIGISRx Antibacterial Envelope Antimicrobial envelope	*use* Anti-Infective Envelope
Bone morphogenetic protein 2 (BMP 2)	*use* Recombinant Bone Morphogenetic Protein
Clolar	*use* Clofarabine
Defitelio	*use* Defibrotide Sodium Anticoagulant
Factor Xa Inhibitor Reversal Agent, Andexanet Alfa	*use* Andexanet Alfa, Factor Xa Inhibitor Reversal Agent
Kcentra	*use* 4-Factor Prothrombin Complex Concentrate
Nesiritide	*use* Human B-type Natriuretic Peptide
rhBMP-2	*use* Recombinant Bone Morphogenetic Protein
Seprafilm	*use* Adhesion Barrier
Tissue Plasminogen Activator (tPA) (r-tPA)	*use* Other Thrombolytic
Vistogard®	*use* Uridine Triacetate
Voraxaze	*use* Glucarpidase
Zyvox	*use* Oxazolidinones

A
P
P
E
N
D
I
X

H

DEVICE	USE:
EDWARDS INTUITY Elite valve system	*use* Zooplastic Tissue, Rapid Deployment Technique in New Technology
INTUITY Elite valve system, EDWARDS	*use* Zooplastic Tissue, Rapid Deployment Technique in New Technology
MAGEC® Spinal Bracing and Distraction System	*use* Magnetically Controlled Growth Rod(s) in New Technology
MIRODERM™ Biologic Wound Matrix	*use* Skin Substitute, Porcine Liver Derived in New Technology
nanoLOCK™ interbody fusion device	*use* Interbody Fusion Device, Nanotextured Surface in New Technology
Perceval sutureless valve	*use* Zooplastic Tissue, Rapid Deployment Technique in New Technology
Spinal growth rod(s), magnetically controlled	*use* Magnetically Controlled Growth Rod(s) in New Technology
Sutureless valve, Perceval	*use* Zooplastic Tissue, Rapid Deployment Technique in New Technology